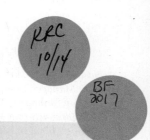

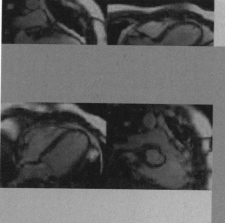

Noninvasive Cardiovascular Imaging:

A Multimodality Approach

EDITOR

MARIO J. GARCIA, MD

Director, Cardiac Imaging
Mount Sinai Heart
Professor of Medicine & Radiology
Mount Sinai School of Medicine
New York, New York

 Wolters Kluwer | Lippincott Williams & Wilkins
Health
Philadelphia · Baltimore · New York · London
Buenos Aires · Hong Kong · Sydney · Tokyo

Acquisitions Editor: Frances R. Destefano
Product Manager: Leanne McMillan
Production Manager: Alicia Jackson
Senior Manufacturing Manager: Ben Rivera
Marketing Manager: Kimberly Schonberger
Design Coordinator: Stephen Druding
Production Service: SPi Technologies India Pvt. Ltd.

Library of Congress Cataloging-in-Publication Data

Noninvasive cardiovascular imaging : a multimodality approach / editor, Mario J. Garcia.
      p. ; cm.
  Includes bibliographical references and index.
  ISBN 978-0-7817-9535-7 (alk. paper)
  1. Cardiovascular system–Imaging. I. Garcia, Mario J.
  [DNLM: 1. Cardiovascular Diseases–diagnosis. 2. Diagnostic Imaging–methods.
WG 141 N8137 2009]
  RC683.5.I42N65 2009
  616.1'0754–dc22
                                                          2009024850

Care has been taken to confirm the accuracy of the information presented and to describe generally accepted practices. However, the authors, editors, and publisher are not responsible for errors or omissions or for any consequences from application of the information in this book and make no warranty, expressed or implied, with respect to the currency, completeness, or accuracy of the contents of the publication. Application of the information in a particular situation remains the professional responsibility of the practitioner.

The authors, editors, and publisher have exerted every effort to ensure that drug selection and dosage set forth in this text are in accordance with current recommendations and practice at the time of publication. However, in view of ongoing research, changes in government regulations, and the constant flow of information relating to drug therapy and drug reactions, the reader is urged to check the package insert for each drug for any change in indications and dosage and for added warnings and precautions. This is particularly important when the recommended agent is a new or infrequently employed drug.

Some drugs and medical devices presented in the publication have Food and Drug Administration (FDA) clearance for limited use in restricted research settings. It is the responsibility of the health care provider to ascertain the FDA status of each drug or device planned for use in their clinical practice.

To purchase additional copies of this book, call our customer service department at (800) 638-3030 or fax orders to (301) 223-2320. International customers should call (301) 223-2300.

Visit Lippincott Williams & Wilkins on the Internet: at LWW.com. Lippincott Williams & Wilkins customer service representatives are available from 8:30 am to 6 pm, EST.

10 9 8 7 6 5 4 3 2 1

In my life experience, as a practicing cardiovascular specialist, I have witnessed the great improvement in life expectancy and quality of life of patients with cardiovascular disease. Most of our success has been attributed to the development of novel therapeutic strategies, which undeniably have been remarkable. Yet, the impact that our enhanced diagnostic abilities have made in recognizing the disease at earlier stages and in guiding the selection and evaluating the effect of treatment cannot be ignored. Most of the advancement in cardiovascular diagnosis has taken place based on the field of cardiovascular imaging, both due to technological breakthroughs and through the development of expertise.

The role of the cardiovascular diagnostician has been evolving, and to the critical role of the stethoscope, sophisticated imaging techniques have been added, including ultrasound, magnetic resonance, computed tomography, and nuclear scintigraphic imaging. One may look at this evolution with nostalgia and be critical of the "lost clinical skills" of the younger generation, or take a more pragmatic approach and recognize the value brought by the adoption of new technology. It is critical, however, that we continue to measure the value, cost, and benefits provided by technology as we evolve, and that we evaluate each technology for its ability to answer a clinical question in comparison to other competing technologies. Within the context the concept of the multimodality imaging approach is emerging, with the cardiovascular specialist who, rather than promoting a specific imaging test, continues to serve the role of an expert diagnostician, presently choosing the most effective single or combined imaging modalities to solve an enigma.

This textbook represents a remarkable accomplishment in the cardiovascular literature. The editor, Dr. Mario J. Garcia, an outstanding clinician, also recognized as an expert leader in multiple imaging fields, provides a new framework where the diagnosis to cardiovascular disease is approached from a multimodality perspective. The different background and expertise of the contributing authors provides a perfect balance to accomplish the objectives of this book, which will be equally appealing to the clinical as well as to the noninvasive imaging expert.

I recommend on the highest terms the textbook "Noninvasive Cardiovascular Imaging: A Multimodality Approach" as a "must" to read and/or to have access to all cardiovascular and noninvasive imaging specialists, as well as by students and health care providers interested in such contemporary and important diagnostic field.

Valentin Fuster, MD, PhD
Director, Mount Sinai Heart
Richard Gorlin/Heart Research Foundation
Professor of Cardiology
Mount Sinai School of Medicine
New York, New York

Preface

Soon after I developed a passion for the field of cardiovascular medicine, I realized that I had to choose a career path, and like most of my colleagues and fellows, I wondered about how to make such a difficult decision. I also once liked the thrill of holding a sharp object in my hand and I felt quite comfortable wearing lead. In fact, during the first year of my cardiology training, not been adequately exposed yet, I did not have an appreciation for the value of noninvasive imaging.

Quite often, the positive influence of a mentor steers you. I was very fortunate during my second year when I chose to take an elective in echocardiography with a great teacher. Ira Cohen was a skilled echocardiographer but I did not see him as such. I saw a remarkable clinical cardiologist with a superb ability to solve a clinical dilemma by applying the extrasensorial ability provided by an ultrasound machine. I knew at that time that from then on the only places where I would play with sharps would be my kitchen and my woodworking shop. Then is when I started my career in cardiovascular imaging. I spent one year at the Massachusetts General Hospital learning nuclear cardiology followed by another year at Cleveland Clinic learning echocardiography.

In the late 1990s, I was fortunate to start a collaboration with a group of engineers and physicists at Picker Medical in Highlight Heights, OH, a company that was ready to release a 4-slice multidetector CT scanner. Working with this group, I learned that technical development can be steered in the right direction to meet a clinical need or be derailed in a pathway that ends without finding a clinical application. We knew back then that there was one clinical need that was not met by noninvasive imaging, the evaluation of the coronary anatomy. I was lucky to be in the right place and time and contribute to the birth of CT coronary angiography.

In the last few years, I completed the circle through learning cardiac MRI, without doubt the most challenging and complex among all the cardiovascular imaging modalities. Although I may seem like a perpetual student on a constant search for new thrills, I always kept my hands on clinical practice and applied imaging modalities as tools to solve clinical questions. I cannot overemphasize the value of practicing medicine as part of the learning process. Only through clinical practice we learn the value and limitations of technology, we discover unmet clinical needs, and we find new applications. Also, through clinical practice I learned that quite often we have different methods to conduct an investigation and that the best choice is not always clear. Moreover, that one of the risks of approaching a clinical question from a diagnostic modality perspective is to develop a bias against other possibly more valuable and cost-effective alternatives. In an era where the escalating costs of medical imaging are been scrutinized, more than ever it is paramount for the practitioner to understand the relative value, limitations, and complementary roles of different diagnostic imaging strategies in clinical decision making.

With this in mind, I designed this textbook of cardiovascular imaging to serve as a guide for both the imaging specialist and the clinical cardiologist to help select and maximize the value of noninvasive imaging tests to answer specific clinical questions. The textbook contains fifty-one chapters divided into nine sections. The first section covers the basic physical principles, instrumentation, and protocols for each noninvasive cardiovascular imaging modality. The second section covers the application of imaging tests for the evaluation of common cardiovascular symptoms and syndromes. Sections III through VIII address specific cardiovascular disease entities. Finally, section IX includes a guide for the systematic review of incidental extracardiac findings, a very important task that is becoming more relevant for cardiologists embarking in the interpretation of tomographic chest studies.

Each disease-entity chapter has been structured in a similar format to cover principles of epidemiology, clinical presentation, pathophysiology, diagnostic imaging, and treatment and includes an online question and answer section to test the reader's knowledge. Ample number of figures and movies complement each chapter to illustrate the key learning points.

I cannot praise enough the remarkable job done by each chapter's authors. They demonstrated a level of expertise and put forth an effort far beyond my expectations. I have been blessed with their contribution to make this project a reality and I will be forever grateful to all of them.

Mario J. Garcia, MD

Contributors

Nikolaos Alexopoulos, MD
Division of Cardiology
Department of Medicine
Emory University
Atlanta, Georgia

Craig R. Asher, MD
Cardiology Fellowship Director
Department of Cardiovascular Medicine
Cleveland Clinic Foundation
Weston, Florida

Juan J. Badimon, PhD, FAHA, FACC
Atherothrombosis Research Unit
Cardiovascular Institute
Mount Sinai School of Medicine
New York, New York

Anthony A. Bavry, MD, MPH
Associate Professor of Medicine
Division of Cardiovascular Medicine
Gainesville, Florida

Susan M. Begelman, MD
Genentech, Inc.
South San Francisco, California

Robert O. Bonow, MD
Division of Cardiology
Northwestern University Feinberg School of Medicine
Bluhm Cardiovascular Institute
Northwestern Memorial Hospital
Chicago, Illinois

Andrew D. Boyd, MD
Research Assistant Professor
Department of Biomedical and Health Information Sciences
University of Illinois at Chicago
Chicago, Illinois

Carlos Capuñay, MD
Invited Professor
Favaloro University School of Medicine
Sub-Head, Department of Computed Tornography
Sub-Head, Department of Research Affairs
Diagnostico, MAIPU
Av. Maipu
Buenos Aires, CABA, Argentina

Patricia Carrascosa, MD, PhD
Associate Professor of Radiology
Buenos Aires University School of Medicine
Head, Department of Computed Tornography
Head, Department of Research Affairs
Diagnostico, MAIPU
Av. Maipu
Buenos Aires, CABA, Argentina

Ramon Castello, MD, FACC, FASE
Director of Echocardiography
Apex Cardiovascular Group
St Lukes Hospital
Jacksonville, Florida

George P. Chatzimavroudis, PhD
Associate Professor
Department of Chemical and Biomedical
   Engineering
Cleveland State University
Cleveland, Ohio

Hina Chaudhry, MD
Senior Faculty
Department of Medicine
Division of Cardiology
Mount Sinai School of Medicine
New York, New York

Ji Chen, PhD
Assistant Professor of Radiology
Department of Radiology
Emory University School of Medicine
Atlanta, Georgia

Emil I. Cohen, MD
Assistant Professor
Department of Radiology
Georgetown University Hospital
Washington, DC

Lori B. Croft, MD
Mount Sinai Hospital
New York, New York

Hug Cuéllar, MD
Medical Doctor
Servei de Radiologia
Institut Diagnostic per l'Imatge
Hospital Vall d' Hebron
Barcelona, Spain

Ronan J. Curtin
Department of Cardiovascular Medicine
Heart and Vascular Institute
Cleveland Clinic
Cleveland, Ohio

Manisha Das, MD
Gill Heart Institute and Division
   of Cardiology
University of Kentucky
Lexington, Kentucky

Sabe De, MD
Clinical Scholar
Department of Cardiovascular Medicine
Cleveland Clinic Foundation
Cleveland, Ohio

Jose Alberto de Augustin, MD
Associate Professor
Department of Cardiology
Complutense University
Medical Doctor
Department of Cardiology
Clinic Hospital San Carlos
Madrid, Spain

Antonio De Miguel, MD
Atherothrombosis Research Unit
Cardiovascular Institute
Mount Sinai School of Medicine
New York, New York
Cardiology Department
Hospital de León
León, Spain

Milind Y. Desai, MD
Staff Cardiologist
Section of Cardiac Imaging
Division of Cardiovascular Medicine
Cleveland Clinic
Assistant Professor of Medicine & Radiology
Joint appointment in Cardiology and Radiology
Lerner College of Medicine
Case Western Reserve University
Cleveland, Ohio

Jennifer A. Dickerson, MD
Assistant Professor
Internal Medicine
Division of Cardiovascular Medicine
Davis Heart Lung Research Institute
The Ohio State University
Columbus, Ohio

Ennis J. Duffis, MD
University of Massachusetts Medical School
Worcester, Massachusetts

W. Lane Duvall, MD
Assistant Professor
Department of Medicine
Mount Sinai School of Medicine
Assistant Director of the Cardiac Care unit
Department of Medicine
Mount Sinai Medical Center
New York, New York

Arturo Evangelista, MD, FESC
Director of Imaging
Department of Cardiology
Servei de Cardiología
Area del Cor
Hospital Universitari Vall d'Hebron
Barcelona, Spain

Tracy L. Faber, PhD
Assistant Professor of Radiology
Department of Radiology
Emory University School of Medicine
Atlanta, Georgia

Zahi A. Fayad
Mount Sinai School of Medicine
Translational and Molecular Imaging Institute

Avi Fischer, MD
Assistant Professor
Department of Medicine/Cardiology
Mount Sinai School of Medicine
Director, Pacemaker and Defibrillator Therapy
Department of Cardiology
Mount Sinai Medical Center
New York, New York

Brian Fonseca, MD
Assistant Professor
Department of Pediatric Cardiology
University of Colorado Denver
Assistant Professor
Department of Pediatric Cardiology
The Children's Hospital
Aurora, Colorado

Fetnat Fouad-Tarazi, MD
Heart and Vascular Institute
Division of Cardiovascular Medicine
Cleveland Clinic
E.P Section
Syncope Clinic
Cleveland, Ohio

Ruvin S. Gabriel BHB, MBCGB, FRACP
Advanced Cardiovascular Imaging Fellow
Department of Heart and Vascular Institute
Cleveland Clinic
Cleveland, Ohio

James R. Galt, PhD
Assistant Professor of Radiology
Department of Radiology
Emory University School of Medicine
Atlanta, Georgia

Ernest V. Garcia, PhD
Professor of Radiology
Department of Radiology
Emory University Hospital
Emory University School of Medicine
Atlanta, Georgia

Mario J. Garcia, MD
Director, Cardiac Imaging
Professor of Medicine & Radiology
Mount Sinai School of Medicine
Mount Sinai Heart
New York, New York

Juan Gaztanaga, MD
Cardiovascular Institute
Mount Sinai Hospital
New York, New York

Martin E. Goldman, MD
The Zena and Michael A. Wiener Cardiovascular Institute and
The Marie-Josee and Henry R. Kravis Cardiovascular
    Health Center
The Mount Sinai School of Medicine
New York, New York

Neil Greenberg, PhD
Project Staff
Heart and Vascular Institute
Cleveland Clinic
Cleveland, Ohio

Brian Griffin, MD, FACC
Section of Cardiovascular Imaging
Department of Cardiovascular Medicine
Cleveland Clinic
Cleveland, Ohio

Richard A. Grimm, DO
Section of Cardiovascular Imaging
Heart and Vascular Institute
Cleveland Clinic
Cleveland, Ohio

Rebecca T. Hahn, MD
Assistant Professor of Clinical Medicine
Division of Cardiology
Columbia University College of Physicians & Surgeons
New York, New York

Sandra S. Halliburton, PhD
Cardiac Imaging Scientist
Cardiovascular Imaging Laboratory
Imaging Institute
Cleveland Clinic
Cleveland, Ohio

Milena J. Henzlova, MD, PhD
Professor of Medicine
Director, Nuclear Cardiology
Department of Cardiology
Mount Sinai Medical Center
New York, New York

Dawn-Alita Hernandez, MD, MSPH, FCCP
Assistant Professor of Medicine
Division of Pulmonary/Critical Care and Sleep Medicine
Health Science Campus
University of Toledo
Toledo, Ohio

Carolyn Y. Ho, MD
Medical Director
Cardiovascular Genetics Center
Division of Cardiovascular Medicine
Brigham and Women's Hospital
Boston, Massachusetts

Randolph Hutter, MD
Zena and Michael A. Weiner
Cardiovascular Institute
Mount Sinai School of Medicine
Mount Sinai Medical Center
New York, New York

Borja Ibanez, MD
Atherothrombosis Research Unit
Cardiovascular Institute
Mount Sinai School of Medicine
New York, New York
Interventional Cardiology Laboratory
Cardiology Department
Fundación Jiménez
Díaz-Capio, Madrid, Spain

Wael A. Jaber, MD
Division of Cardiovascular Medicine
Heart and Vascular Institute
Cleveland Clinic
Cleveland, Ohio

Luis J. Jimenez-Borreguero, MD
Department of Cardiology
University Hospital Dela Princessa
Madrid, Spain

Samir R. Kapadia, MD
Division of Cardiovascular Medicine
Cleveland Clinic
Cleveland, Ohio

Samer J. Khouri, MD, FACC, FASE
Associate Professor of Medicine
Division of Cardiovascular Medicine
Health Science Campus
University of Toledo
Toledo, Ohio

Jacobo Kirsch, MD
Associate Staff
Department of Radiology
Cleveland Clinic Florida
Weston, Florida

Allan L. Klein, MD, FRCP(C), FACC, FAHA, FASE
Professor of Medicine
Lerner College of Medicine of Case Western University
Director
Cardiovascular Imaging Research
Department of Cardiovascular Medicine
Cleveland Clinic
Cleveland, Ohio

Pranay Krishnan, MD
Department of Radiology
Mount Sinai Medical Center
New York, New York

Deborah Kwon, MD
Section of Cardiovascular Imaging
Department of Cardiovascular Medicine
Cleveland Clinic
Cleveland, Ohio

Wyman W. Lai, MD, MPH
Associate Professor of Pediatrics and Radiology
Division of Pediatric Radiology
Mount Sinai Medical Center
New York, New York

Neal Lakdawala, MD
Fellow of Cardiovascular Medicine
Division of Cardiovascular Medicine
Brigham and Women's Hospital
Post Doctoral Research Fellow
Harvard Medical School
Boston, Massachusetts

Bruce F. Landeck, II, MD, MS
Assistant Professor
Department of Pediatric Cardiology
University of Colorado Denver
Assistant Professor
Department of Pediatric Cardiology
The Children's Hospital
Aurora, Colorado

Roberto M. Lang, MD
The University of Chicago
Chicago, Illinois

Stamatios Lerakis, MD
Associate Professor
Division of Cardiology
Department of Medicine
Emory University
Atlanta, Georgia

Robert A. Lookstein, MD
Department of Radiology
Mount Sinai Medical Center
New York, New York

Kameswari Maganti, MD
Division of Cardiology
Northwestern University Feinberg School of Medicine
Bluhm Cardiovascular Institute
Northwestern Memorial Hospital
Chicago, Ilinois

Venkatesh Mani, PhD
Instructor
Department of Radiology
Mount Sinai School of Medicine
Translational and Molecular Imaging Institute
New York, New York

Kenneth Mayuga, MD
Clinical Fellow
Division of Cardiovascular Medicine
University of California Davis Medical Center
Sacramento, California

Dalton McLean, MD
Division of Cardiology
Department of Medicine
Emory University
Atlanta, Georgia

Jose L. Merino, MD, FESC
Arrhtyhmia Research Unit
University Hospital La Paz
Madrid, Spain

Marc A. Miller, MD
The Zena and Michael A. Wiener Cardiovascular
    Institute and
The Marie-Josee and Henry R. Kravis Cardiovascular
    Health Center
Mount Sinai School of Medicine
New York, New York

Majaz Moonis, MD
University of Massachusetts Medical School
Worcester, Massachusetts

Victor Mor-Avi, PhD
University of Chicago Medical Center
Section of Cardiology
The University of Chicago
Chicago, Illinois

Debabrata Mukherjee, MD
Director of Cardiac Catheterization Laboratories
Division of Cardiovascular Medicine
Gill Heart Institute
Gill Foundation Professor of Interventional Cardiology
University of Kentucky
Lexington, Kentucky

Gian M. Novaro, MD
Director, Echocardiography
Department of Cardiology
Cleveland Clinic Florida
Staff
Department of Cardiology
Cleveland Clinic Florida Hospital
Weston, Florida

Jeffrey W. Olin, DO
Professor of Medicine
Director, Vascular Medicine
Zena and Michael A. Wiener Cardiovascular
    Institute and
Marie-Josée and Henry R. Kravis Center for
    Cardiovascular Health
Mount Sinai School of Medicine
New York, New York

Utpal Pandya, MD
Assistant Professor of Medicine
Division of Cardiovascular Medicine
Health Science Campus
University of Toledo
Toledo, Ohio

Victor Pineda, MD
Medical Doctor (Staff)
Servei de Radiologia
Institut Diagnostic per l'Imatge
Hospital Vall d' Hebron
Barcelona, Spain

Susanna Prat-Gonzalez, MD
Post Doctoral Fellow
Cardiovascular Institute
Mount Sinai Hospital
New York, New York

Paolo Raggi, MD
Professor Medicine and Radiology
Director Emory Cardiac Imaging Center
Emory University School of Medicine
Atlanta, Georgia

Subha V. Raman, MD, MSEE, FACC
Associate Professor of Internal Medicine
The Ohio State University
Medical Director
Cardiac CT/MR
Ohio State University Health System
Columbus, Ohio

John P. Reilly, MD, FACC, FSCAI
Director of Cardiovascular CT
Department of Cardiology
Ochsner Health System
New Orleans, Louisiana

Vera H. Rigolin, MD
Division of Cardiology
Northwestern University Feinberg School of Medicine
Bluhm Cardiovascular Institute, Northwestern Memorial Hospital
Chicago, Illinois

Leonardo Rodriguez
Cardiovascular Imaging
Heart and Vascular Institute
Cleveland Clinic
Cleveland, Ohio

James H.F. Rudd
HEFCE Senior Lecturer
Division of Cardiovascular Medicine
University of Cambridge
Honorary Consultant Cardiologist
Addenbrooke's Hospital
Cambridge, United Kingdom

Deepa Sangani, MD
Section of Cardiac Imaging
Cleveland Clinic Florida
Weston, Florida

Javier Sanz, MD
Assistant Professor of Medicine (Cardiology)
Cardiovascular Institute
Mount Sinai Hospital
New York, New York

Randolph M. Setser, DSc
Cardiovascular Imaging Laboratory
Imaging Institute
Cleveland Clinic
Cleveland, Ohio

Michael Shapiro, MD
Cardiovascular Division
Oregon Health and Science University
Portland, Oregon

Raj Shekar, PhD
Associate Professor
Department of Diagnostic Radiology
and Nuclear Medicine
University of Maryland School of Medicine
Baltimore, Maryland

Michael Shen, MD, MS, FACC, FASNC
Section of Cardiac Imaging
Cleveland Clinic Florida
Weston, Florida

Takahiro Shiota, MD
Professor of Medicine
Division of Cardiovascular Medicine
Cleveland Clinic
Cleveland, Ohio

Jeffrey S. Soble, MD
Associate Professor of Medicine
Director of Clinical Cardiology
Rush Medical Center
Director of Noninvasive Cardiology
Director of Cardiology Information Systems
Rush Medical College
Chicago, Illinois

Lissa Sugeng, MD
The University of Chicago
Chicago, Illinois

James D. Thomas, MD
Department of Cardiovascular Medicine
Cleveland Clinic Foundation
Cleveland, Ohio

Dennis A. Tighe, MD
University of Massachusetts Medical School
Worcester, Massachusetts

Richard W. Troughton, MD, MB, CHB, Ph.D, FRACP
Associate Professor in Medicine
University of Otago, Christchurch
Christchurch, New Zealand

David Verhaert, MD
Department of Cardiovascular Medicine
Cleveland Clinic
Cleveland, Ohio

Huijan Wang, MD

Kevin Wei, MD
Assistant Professor of Medicine
Oregon Health and Science University
Portland, Oregon

Raymond Wong, MD
Heart and Vascular Institute
Cleveland Clinic
Cleveland, Ohio

Adel Younoszai, MD
Associate Professor
Director
Cardiac and Fetal Imaging
Department of Pediatric Cardiology
University of Colorado Denver
Director
Cardiac and Fetal Imaging
Department of Pediatric Cardiology
The Children's Hospital
Aurora, Colorado

José Luis Zamorano, MD
Professor of Medicine
Director of Cardiovascular Imaging Unit
Hospital Clinico San Carlos
Plaza de Cristo Rey
Madrid, Spain

Contents

Physical Principles of Echocardiography

1

David Verhaert
James D. Thomas

1. INTRODUCTION

The field of cardiac ultrasound has rapidly evolved during the last two decades. Continuous improvements in equipment and technology have led to a widespread acceptance and use of echocardiography as a first-line diagnostic test before alternative cardiac imaging modalities are even considered. In spite of these advances, it is still essential for practitioners to have a good understanding of the basic physical principles underlying cardiac ultrasound. First, a good insight in the fundamental concepts of ultrasound physics and a notion of the limitations and potential pitfalls of this technique are necessary for correct interpretation and proper clinical decision making. Second, knowing how to apply the technology in different clinical settings is crucial for the acquisition of optimal quality data, even with current advances in echocardiography instrumentation. The basic principles of sound wave mechanics, image acquisition, and Doppler echocardiography will, therefore, be reviewed in this chapter.

2. KEY CONCEPTS OF ULTRASOUND

Sound waves are mechanical waves, implying a physical interaction between the wave and a medium that results in regions where the density and pressure of the medium are higher (compression) alternating with regions with lower pressure and density (rarefaction). Mechanical waves can travel through a medium by two different means: as longitudinal waves (causing particles to vibrate in the same direction as the line of propagation) or as transverse waves (causing vibrations perpendicular to the wave propagation direction). Sound waves are typically longitudinal waves and can be represented graphically as sine waves (Fig. 1.1). Note that this graph can be considered in two ways, either a moment in time showing pressure variations along the propagation path of the ultrasonic wave or as the temporal evolution of pressure at a single point. Like all waves, sound can be specified by four fundamental characteristics:

- Frequency (f), described as cycles per second or hertz
- Propagation velocity (c)
- Wavelength (λ)
- Amplitude (A), described in an absolute sense by units of pressure or in a relative sense by decibels

2.1. Frequency

The frequency of a sound wave describes the number of compression–rarefaction episodes occurring per second. While the human auditory spectrum involves frequencies between 20 Hz and 20 kHz, diagnostic medical ultrasound typically uses frequencies between 1 and 20 million cycles per second (1 to 20 MHz). The reciprocal of frequency is the time needed for one cycle, defined as the period (P). Thus, a frequency of 5 MHz can be converted to a period of 0.2 μs.

2.2. Propagation velocity

The velocity of sound waves depends on the stiffness and density of the medium, specifically the square root of the elastic modulus K divided by the density ρ : $c = (K/\rho)^{1/2}$. For example, the speed of sound through air is approximately 340 m/s, depending on the temperature and pressure of the air, while the propagation velocity in water is about 1,500 m/s. Since water is over 800 times denser than air, this seems counterintuitive, until we realize that water is approximately 20,000 times stiffer than air, which more than makes up the difference. In human tissue, ultrasound is assumed to travel at a constant speed of 1,540 m/s, although in reality it is a few percent slower in fat than muscle.

2.3. Wavelength

The wavelength is a measure of distance. Because the propagation velocity of ultrasound within the heart is constant, the wavelength for any transducer frequency can be calculated as $\lambda = c/f$. As a consequence, typical wavelengths in ultrasound range from about 770 (at a frequency of 2 MHz) to 77 μm (at 20 MHz). Wavelength is a very important parameter as it will determine the axial resolution (the ability to differentiate two different structures in depth), which is no greater than one to two wavelengths. Higher frequencies or shorter wavelengths will obviously result in better resolution, although at the cost of a decreased penetration depth.

2.4. Amplitude

The amplitude is a term to describe the intensity or loudness of sound. The amplitude of ultrasound waves is given by the pressure of particle compression and rarefaction and depends on the voltage that drives the transducer. Amplitude is important for two reasons. First, larger amplitude signals penetrate more deeply into the patient and will yield stronger returning echoes. Second, high intensity sound waves have the potential for causing tissue damage, termed in general bioeffects.

By definition, the amplitude is peak negative (or rarefaction) pressure, typically expressed in megapascals (MPa), where 1 mm Hg = 133.3 Pa. Diagnostic ultrasound can have pressures of several megapascals, representing pressures as high as 50 atmospheres.

To better describe the biological impact of ultrasound, the *mechanical index* (MI) has been devised, given by the pressure (in MPa) divided by the square root of the imaging frequency (in MHz) ultrasound (Fig. 1.1) and can be described in decibels (dB).

1

A Amplitude (dB)

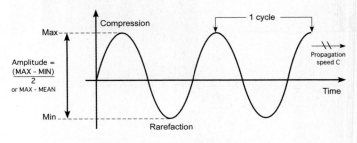

- Duration of 1 cycle = 1 period (P)
- Frequency = number of cycles / sec (Mz) = 1/P

B Amplitude

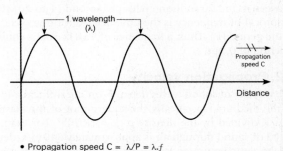

- Propagation speed C = $\lambda/P = \lambda \cdot f$

Figure 1.1 Schematic diagram of an ultrasound wave traveling in time (**A**) and in space (**B**).

Decibels are units based on a logarithmic power ratio between a measured value V to a reference value R of acoustic pressure, as given by the equation **dB = 20 log (V/R)**. As such, increasing the driving voltage by a factor of 100 will increase the transmit power with $20 \times \log(100/1) = 40$ dB. Conversely, decreasing the transmit voltage by a factor of two implies a $20 \times \log(0.5) = 20 \times (-3) = -6$ dB decrease.

The logarithmic compression of signal amplitude into a decibel scale provides a very effective tool to deal with the large dynamic range of returning echoes and allows very weak signals to be displayed alongside signals of much higher amplitude, as will be discussed later.

3. INTERACTION OF ULTRASOUND WITH TISSUE

3.1. Reflection

When an ultrasonic beam travels through a homogeneous medium, it follows a straight path. Tissue within a patient, however, is never homogeneous, and as the beam hits a boundary between two different media, part of the acoustic energy is reflected and part will continue its path into the second medium. Ultrasound is based on reflection, and the amount of reflection that will occur depends on the acoustic impedance mismatch at the interface (Fig. 1.2).

The acoustic impedance Z depends on the tissue density (ρ) and on the propagation velocity (c) and can be defined by the expression: $Z = \rho \times c$, with ρ in kg/m^3 and c in m/s, and Z has units of kg/s $\cdot$ m^2, termed the Rayl.

Reflection occurs by transitioning from a structure with higher impedance to one with lower impedance, or vice versa. The larger the mismatch, the larger is the reflection. The percentage of energy reflected at an interface is determined by the equation: $(Z_2 - Z_1/Z_2 + Z_1)^2$

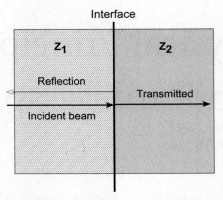

Figure 1.2 Acoustic impedance mismatch and reflection of ultrasound. Z_1 and Z_2 represent the acoustic impedance in media 1 and 2, respectively.

Imagine using a transducer with a high impedance crystal (e.g., 35 MRayls) in direct contact with a patient (the impedance of tissue being approximately 2 MRayls). As can be predicted from the above equation, the percentage reflection will be $[(35 - 2)/(35 + 2)]^2 = (33/37)^2 = 80\%$. In other words, only 20% of the energy will effectively be transmitted into the patient. And of course, the same low transmission rate will occur once more when the signal that is reflected back from the patient encounters the same large acoustic impedance mismatch again, implying that eventually only a very weak signal will be received by the transducer. This is why matching layers with intermediate impedance are used to minimize the large acoustic impedance mismatch between the crystal and tissue, thereby increasing both transmit and receive efficiencies.

The opposite problem occurs at most biological interfaces. For example, the 6% difference in Z between blood and myocardium translates into <0.1% reflection in ultrasound, illustrating the challenge of detecting endocardial borders.

Depending on the geometry of the reflecting surface, there are basically three different types of reflection (Fig. 1.3):

1. Specular reflection occurs when the reflecting surface is large and smooth with respect to the wavelength; the angle of reflection will equal the angle of incidence in the same plane. This type of reflection is similar to light being reflected from a mirror. Good examples of specular reflectors in echocardiography are pacemaker wires, valves, calcifications, etc.
2. Scattering occurs when the sound wave encounters structures that are smaller than a wavelength, causing the sound energy to be radiated in all directions. Only a small amount of the scattered signal will return to the receiving transducer. As such, the amplitude of a scattered signal will be much lower than the amplitude of the signal returning from a specular reflector. A typical scatterer in cardiac ultrasound is a moving red blood cell (7 to 10 µm), which is important for the generation of Doppler-shifted echoes.
3. When a sound wave strikes a rather large but irregular surface, it will cause a specular reflection in addition to a scattered field.

While the strength of the reflected echo is greater for specular reflection, the amount of ultrasound received at the transducer by specular reflection is highly angle-dependent. With the transducer perpendicular to the reflecting surface, most of the returning energy will reach the transducer (Fig. 1.4A). With increasing angle, however, more energy will be directed away from the

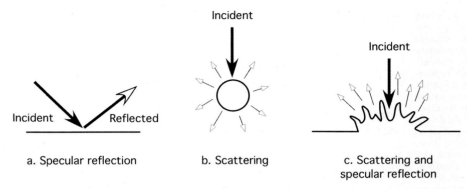

Figure 1.3 Specular, scattering, and mixed reflectors (see text for details).

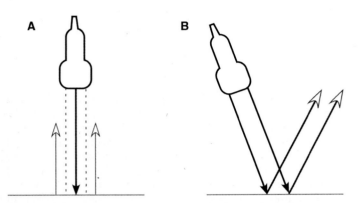

Figure 1.4 **A**: Transducer held perpendicular to the reflecting surface. **B**: Angulation of the transducer results in specular reflection being directed away from the transducer face.

transducer (Fig. 1.4B) and in the worst case (structure parallel to the ultrasound beam) only a minimal portion of the reflected energy will strike the transducer face. This accounts for the echo "dropout" of endocardium sometimes seen when scanning the left ventricle from an apical window. Most tissues have rough or uneven surfaces, resulting in scattering. Scattered energy may not have the same amount of energy as the energy returning from a specular reflector, but it will propagate in all directions and is therefore less angle-dependent.

3.2. Refraction

When an ultrasound beam strikes an interface between two media, a portion of the energy will be reflected (depending on

the acoustic mismatch), but the remainder will continue its path into the second medium. The path of the transmitted beam is not necessarily a straight line, but may be bent due to a change in the speed of sound in the two media, a phenomenon seen when a spoon placed in a glass of water appears bent due to the reduced speed of light in water.

Refraction is dictated by Snell's law: $c_i \times \sin \theta_i = c_t \times \sin \theta_t$. Figure 1.5A–C illustrates how a change in propagation velocity may lead to refraction when an ultrasound beam reaches an interface. Note that when the speed of sound in the transmitted medium exceeds that of the incident medium, there is an angle given by $\sin^{-1}(c_i/c_t)$ beyond which transmission cannot occur (since the sine can never be greater than one), producing 100% reflection at the interface. This phenomenon, familiar to those who swim underwater, is fortunately rarely important in echocardiography, due to the similarity of the speed of sound in all biological media.

Refraction may be better understood by the concept of a horizontal wavefront approaching an interface. When the wavefront is parallel to the interface (wavefront direction perpendicular to the interface, Fig. 1.6A), no refraction will occur, whatever the difference in propagation velocity between two media. When the wavefront approaches the interface at an angle as depicted in Figure 1.6B, the left edge of the wavefront will accelerate earlier than the right edge (as the propagation velocity of sound is higher in the second medium than in the first medium). As a consequence, the left edge will have traveled further in distance than the right edge by the time the right edge reaches the interface. The resultant wavefront will, therefore, be distorted and its course will be altered.

As ultrasound travels through a biologic medium, its signal strength will gradually decrease. This reduction in energy is not only due to reflection and scattering, but also due to absorption

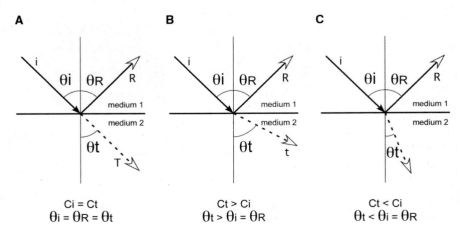

Figure 1.5 **A**: A sound beam strikes an interface between two media of different acoustic impedance; the propagation velocity in both media is equal, however, and no refraction occurs. **B**: The propagation velocity is higher in the second medium and the transmitted beam will be deflected to the right with an angle that is greater than the angle of incidence. **C**: The speed of sound is slower in the second medium; consequently, the beam will be deflected to the left at an angle of transmission that is less than the angle of incidence. i, incident beam; r, reflected beam; t, transmitted beam; θ_i, angle of incident beam; θ_r, angle of reflected beam; θ_t, angle of transmitted beam; C_i, propagation velocity of the incident beam; C_t, propagation velocity of the transmitted beam.

Figure 1.6 Refraction. **A**: when the wavefront is parallel to the interface, no refraction occurs. **B**: When the wavefront approaches the interface at an angle, the left edge of the wavefront will accelerate earlier than the right edge (as the propagation velocity of sound is higher in the second medium than in the first medium). As a consequence, the left edge will have traveled further in distance than the right edge by the time the right edge reaches the interface. The resultant wavefront will, therefore, be distorted and its course will be altered.

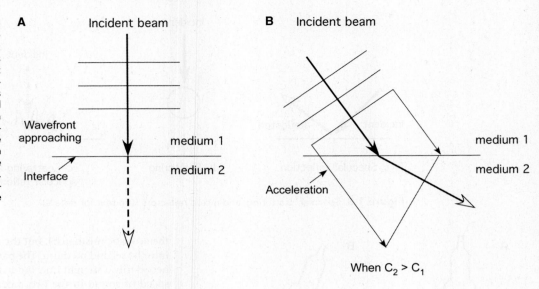

of ultrasound energy by conversion to heat, a process called attenuation. As mentioned earlier, attenuation is frequency (and thus wavelength) dependent and results in an exponential decay in signal strength. Although many factors influence this, the useful depth of penetration is typically limited to 200 wavelengths, corresponding to a penetration depth of 12 cm for a 2.5 MHz transducer and 6 cm for a 5 MHz transducer (remember: $\lambda = c/f$). Attenuation will thus guide the need for a specific transducer frequency in particular clinical situations, and as such there is always a trade-off to be made between penetration and resolution. As a general rule, the highest frequency should be used that still allows visualization of important distal structures like the posterior wall of the left ventricle. A good illustration is the use of higher frequency probes (3.5 to 5 MHz) in pediatric patients, whereas thick-chested subjects or patients with chronic obstructive pulmonary disease will usually require the use of lower frequency transducers (2.5 MHz or lower).

A high acoustic impedance mismatch causes substantial attenuation of signal strength. A good example is the presence of air between the transducer and cardiac tissue (emphysematous lungs, subcutaneous emphysema, or pneumomediastinum), resulting in poor image quality. To optimize image quality in transthoracic echocardiography, water-soluble gels are generally used to create an airless contact between the transducer and the patient's skin.

4. TRANSDUCERS

The ultrasound transducer is a device that works bidirectionally by both transmitting acoustic energy and receiving signals reflected back from tissues. This dual function of transducers is based on a crystal or ceramic material that exhibits the piezoelectric effect, a property that allows transformation of energy from mechanical to electrical, and vice versa. When an alternating electrical field is applied across a piezoelectric crystal, the polarized molecules (dipoles) will align with the induced electrical field. The alternating electrical current causes the molecules within the crystal to vibrate and will alternately compress and expand the crystal, thereby generating an ultrasound wave. A higher voltage will lead to a proportionally larger mechanical deformation, thus generating a higher amplitude signal. Conversely, when a mechanical stress is applied on a crystal (an ultrasound wave striking the piezoelectric element!), it will

lead to a minuscule movement of the individual dipoles and induce an electric field that can be detected by electrodes (Fig. 1.7). As such, the transducer also serves as a receiver because these small electrical signals can be amplified, processed, and consequently displayed by an ultrasound machine. While some naturally occurring crystals (such as quartz or lithium sulfate) exhibit piezoelectric properties, all transducers nowadays use exotic composite materials with increased efficiency in terms of sensitivity and bandwidth.

Figure 1.8 gives an illustration of the elementary components of a single disk-shaped ultrasound transducer.

4.1. The ultrasound beam

The sound energy produced by a transducer will be transmitted in the form of a beam. The beam configuration will vary predictably with distance from the transducer and can be represented as in Figure 1.9. In the immediate vicinity of the transducer, the beam will start out well columnated with the same dimension as the crystal diameter. With increasing depth, the beam will eventually start to diverge. The initial portion of the beam close to the transducer is called the near-field or Fresnel zone. The diverging portion is referred to as the far-field or the Fraunhofer zone, and the junction between near and far fields is the transition zone.

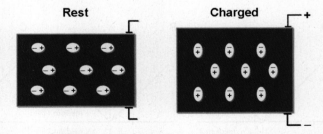

• **On transmit, electricity vibrates the crystal, emitting ultrasound**

• **On receive, ultrasound vibrations generate an electric signal**

Figure 1.7 Piezoelectric effect. Dipoles within the crystal will line up when an electric charge is placed across the crystal. This leads to physical vibration of these molecules, thereby producing an ultrasonic wave. Conversely, when the crystal is hit by an ultrasound wave, the vibrating molecules will generate an electric current.

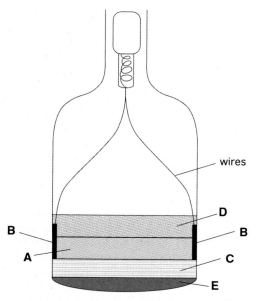

Figure 1.8 Transducer components. **A:** The piezoelectric crystal converts electrical energy into an ultrasound wave that is transmitted into the patient. At the same time, it serves as a receiver by transforming the returning echo into a voltage that is further processed by the system. The characteristic frequency of a transducer is determined by the thickness of the crystal. Larger structures vibrate more slowly, so there is an inverse relationship between the crystal thickness and the operating frequency of the transducer. **B:** Electrodes transmit an electrical current to the crystal and also record the voltage that is created by the reflected echoes. **C:** Impedance matching layer(s): To minimize reflective losses due to the acoustic impedance mismatch at the skin surface. The matching layer will typically be one-quarter wavelength thick. As such, a sound wave traveling through the matching layer will have undergone a 90° phase shift. The reflection from the surface of the matching layer will undergo another 90° phase shift, resulting in a 180° shift which is consistent with the distance of one half wavelength. Two waves, 180° out of phase will lead to destructive interference and thus cancel out reflections from the surface. **D:** A damping or backing material is used to decrease the number of cycles in the pulse sequence. As will be discussed later, the axial resolution of an ultrasonic system depends not only on wavelength but also on the pulse duration. Long pulses (composed of many cycles) result in poor range resolution. By placing a backing material behind the piezoelectric element, the "ringdown" (the length of time the crystal rings in response to excitation) can be decreased. Besides improving axial resolution, backing material will also increase the bandwidth (the range of frequencies over which the transducer can respond). **E:** An acoustic lens may be used to focus the beam.

The near-field length can be calculated from the formula $NFL = D^2/4\lambda$, where D is the diameter of the transducer face and λ is the wavelength of the transmitted pulse. This equation indicates that small increases in the crystal diameter will result in a much greater length of the near zone; higher frequencies (thus smaller wavelengths) will also result in a longer NFL. The angle of divergence θ beyond the transition zone can be derived from the formula $\sin \theta = 1.22\lambda/D$. An increase in frequency and transducer size will thus not only result in a longer NFL but also decrease the spread of sound energy by producing a narrower, more intense beam. Narrower beams result in better lateral resolution and are more intense, generating stronger echoes. Images from structures in the far field on the other hand are poor in quality because of the wider beam width (leading to a decreased lateral resolution) as well as higher attenuation. Although one might conclude that for optimal ultrasound imaging a large-diameter transducer with a high operating fre-

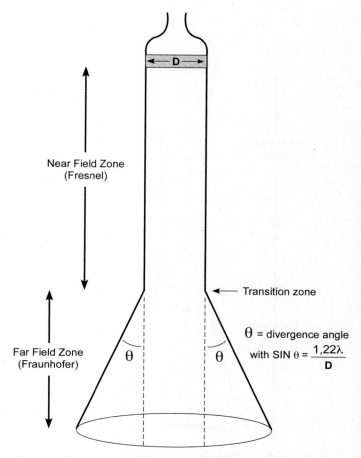

Figure 1.9 Beam configuration for a simple, disk-shaped crystal.

quency is needed, both the size of the intercostal spaces and the greater attenuation of high frequencies prevent this approach from being practical.

In addition to modifying the transducer size and frequency, the shape of the beam can also be altered by focusing (Fig. 1.10). Focusing is a process that will bring the narrowest portion of the beam closer to the transducer face. If attenuation is ignored, the beam intensity will be maximal at the focal zone, implying a maximal intensity for the echoes from all structures within the focal zone. Beyond the focal zone, the beam will diverge rapidly, and it should be noted that the angle of divergence in the far field will always be greater for a focused beam than for an unfocused beam. A beam that converges and diverges very quickly is said to have a shallow depth of field. Focusing can be achieved by making the surface of the piezoelectric crystal concave, by adding an acoustic lens to the front of the piezoelectric element as shown in Figure 1.8, or by electronic activation sequencing, a process called phasing. Modern transducers allow manipulation of the focal zone during the examination and can even focus at more than one depth at a time.

Phased array transducers are comprised of multiple elements. The individual elements lie in close apposition of each other, but function independently, and therefore, require separate insulating layers and electrical connections similar to the single disk-shaped transducer as described above. As each element is very narrow, the divergence of the beam will be very wide and the individual elements can be considered to emit a spherical wavefront. By precisely timing the discharge of multiple crystals, it is possible to

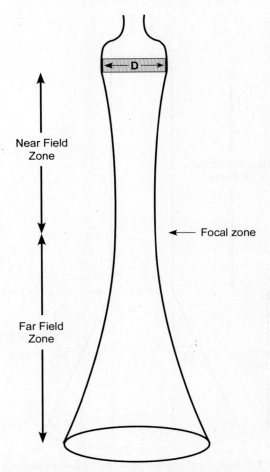

Figure 1.10 A focused beam. While the focal zone can be adjusted, the beam width will still depend on depth and on the transducer diameter.

direct a wavefront in an arbitrary direction, which allows steering and varying the focus without moving parts as in mechanical sector scanning. Electronic beam steering is achieved using the principle of summation of time-sequenced wavelets, a concept that was first described by Huygens. The method of beam steering is depicted in Figures 1.11 and 1.12.

Phased array transducers not only work in the transmit mode but also in the receive mode. As the beam will have a certain width, echoes returning from a specific reflector at the center of the sound beam will arrive at the individual transducer elements in the array at different times. Dynamic receive focusing is accomplished by introducing a specific phase delay of the electrical signals transferred by the individual elements; the computer will thus align and summate the signals returning from a specific target in the focal region. Conversely, the same phase delay will not result in the summation of signals coming from reflectors at the same depth but outside the focal zone (outside the area of interest). Echoes from reflectors outside the focal region will, therefore, be out of phase and can be partially canceled out with appropriate filtering.

The newest generation of transducers are two-dimensional array transducers with a matrix of transducer elements. Multiple elements in both the lateral and elevation planes allow steering and focusing in both the lateral and elevational dimension, which is essential for three-dimensional imaging (Fig. 1.13). The piezoelectric crystal is, therefore, cut into multiple (3,000 to 6,000) equal-sized minute square elements with laser technology, each individually addressed electronically. The matrix array transducer will then produce a pyramidal scan.

It should be noted that in addition to the main ultrasound beam, dispersion of ultrasound energy laterally from a simple disk-shaped transducer will lead to concentrations of energy in regions outside the central beam. Side lobes will thus arise at an angle θ from the central beam as given by the equation $\sin \theta = n\lambda/D$, where n indicates the sequential side lobes and

Figure 1.11 Time delays between the excitation pulses produce a series of wavelets propagating slightly behind each other. By connecting the tangential surface of each of the individual spherical waves, a new wavefront is created that will propagate at an angle to the transducer face. The steering angle will be proportional to the time delay between activation of the individual elements.

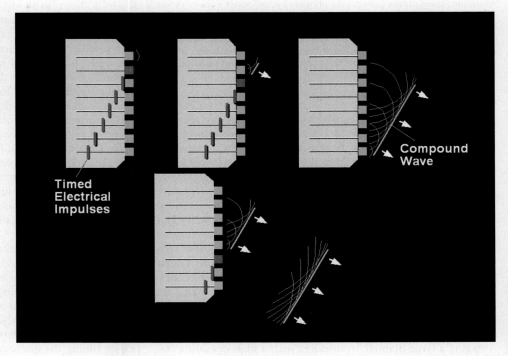

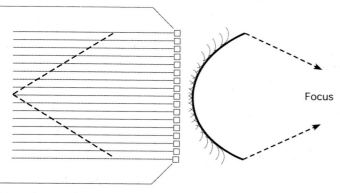

Figure 1.12 By activating the elements at the margin of the array slightly before those of the center, an activation sequence will be created that will result in the transmission of a focused beam. A single transmit focus will improve the resolution in the focal region; outside this region, dispersion of the beam will cause significant degradation of image resolution.

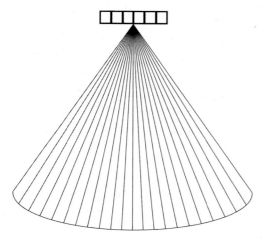

Figure 1.13 Steering also allows the creation of a sector image with a narrow apex and a broad far field. The application of a specific phase delay will result in a particular angle by which the ultrasound beams fans out.

D represents the transducer diameter (Fig. 1.14A). Side lobes will arise at points where the distance traversed by the ultrasound pulse starting from opposite edges of the crystal differs by exactly one wavelength: as such the sound waves of opposing edges will be in phase and the energy will summate in a region of high intensity. In between these side lobes, sound waves will arrive out of phase and phase cancellation will occur, resulting in a lower intensity sound field. The intensity of side lobes will decrease more radially away from the main beam. Side lobes are a potential source of artifacts, because echoes arising from strong reflectors in the path of side lobes may be displayed as though originating from the central beam.

In phased array transducers, constructive interference will occur at points where the distance traveled by the wavefronts arising from different crystal elements differs exactly by one wavelength (Fig. 1.14B). This will then lead to the formation of the so-called grating lobes. The angular location of grating lobes relative to the main beam is given by the same expression $\sin \theta = n\lambda/D$, where D is the center-to-center spacing of the array elements. For an array transducer with an operating frequency of 3.5 MHz ($\lambda = 0.44$ mm) and a 2 mm center-to-

center spacing of the elements, the values are $\sin \theta = 0.44/2 = 0.22$; θ can then be calculated as $\sin^{-1}(0.22) = 13°$, implying a first-order grating lobe at a 13° angle from the main beam axis and a second-order grating lobe at 26°. The problem of grating lobes, leading to artifacts and images cluttered with meaningless echoes can be minimized by using lower frequency transducers and decreasing the center-to-center spacing of elements. As such, once $\lambda/D > 1$, θ will be >90°, and grating lobe artifacts should be absent unless the main beam is deflected away from the center.

4.2. Resolution

Three different types of spatial resolution can be determined according to the dimensions of a beam: axial resolution (also referred to as depth, longitudinal, or range), lateral resolution, and elevational resolution.

Axial resolution implies the ability to resolve two different structures separated in depth. It depends on transducer frequency, bandwidth, and pulse length. The smallest resolvable distance between two reflectors is one wavelength; consequently shorter wavelengths (using higher frequency transducers) result in better axial resolution. If the spatial pulse length (defined as wavelength multiplied by the number of cycles) becomes too long (longer than twice the actual separation distance), returning echoes from two adjacent structures may connect, resulting in poor axial resolution. Shorter pulses, therefore, result in both improved axial resolution and increased bandwidth.

Lateral resolution is the ability to resolve two side-by-side structures as separate (producing two different echoes) and depends on beam width. A narrower beam results in better lateral resolution; lateral resolution will, therefore, be best at the focus but decreases rapidly in the far field. The same principle holds true for **elevational resolution** which equals the elevation beam width. Elevational resolution determines the actual thickness of the slab of tissue that is displayed in a two-dimensional slice.

Temporal resolution on the other hand pertains to the ability to distinguish closely timed events (rapidly moving structures, flow patterns) and display them as separate events in time. If an image was created by transmitting one, very wide beam, lateral resolution would obviously be very poor. As a consequence, an image (or frame) is produced by transmitting multiple acoustic lines (pulses or beams) repeatedly in varying directions. The number of scan lines in each frame will determine the scan-line density of the image. The disadvantage of scanned modalities (two-dimensional imaging and color Doppler), however, is that it takes much more time to complete such a full frame (frame time being determined as the number of lines in the image multiplied by the time required to produce each single line). The finite speed of sound in tissue obviously limits the maximum number of acoustic lines or pulses that can be transmitted in 1 s. As a general rule, the more lines transmitted per frame (higher line density) and the more time needed to process one display line (greater image depth), the longer the frame time and the worse the temporal resolution. Temporal resolution is defined by the frame rate, which is the reciprocal of the frame time. The pulse repetition period is the time needed for a pulse to travel from the transducer to the tissue and back and can be calculated as PRP = $2d/c$ (d being imaging depth which is doubled because of the round trip effect; c is the speed of sound in tissue which is 1,540 m/s). The pulse repetition frequency (PRF) (the reciprocal of the pulse repetition period, $c/2d$) will thus determine the number of scan lines per

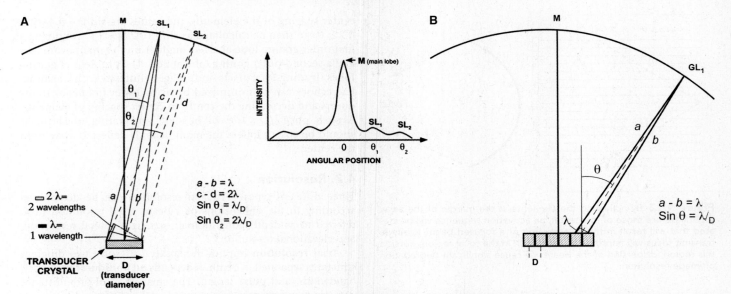

Figure 1.14 A: Although the main ultrasound beam is centrally directed, energy will also radiate in a diverging manner. Side lobes will occur at points where the distance traversed by the pulse from opposite edges of the crystal differs by exactly one or multiple wavelengths, which leads to constructive interference. Side lobe 1 (SL$_1$) will arise at an angle θ_1 because the path length for a pulse starting from the left edge of the crystal (distance a) is exactly one wavelength greater than the path length for a pulse starting from the right edge of the crystal (distance b). A second-order side lobe (SL$_2$) will then occur at an angle θ_2 when the difference in distance between opposite edges (c and d) is exactly two wavelengths. As shown, the energy in these extraneous beams is much weaker and decreases rapidly more radially away from the main beam. (Adapted from Geiser EA. In: Skorton DJ, Schelbert AR, Wolf GL, Brundage BH, eds. *Marcus Cardiac Imaging*. 2nd Ed. Philadelphia, Pa: WB Saunders; 1996:P280, Chapter 25.). **B:** Grating lobes exist because of constructive interference at points where the path length for an ultrasound pulse between two crystal elements differs by exactly one (or multiple) wavelength. The location of grating lobes can be predicted by the formula sin $\theta = n\lambda/D$, where D is the center-to-center spacing of the crystal elements.

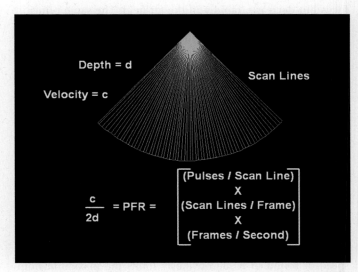

Figure 1.15 Temporal and spatial trade-offs determined by the PRF.

frame multiplied by the number of frames per second (Fig. 1.15). Given the known speed of sound, this can be simplified to give PRF (kHz) = 77/d, where d is imaging depth in centimeter. Dividing this by the number of lines/frame, will yield the frame rate: FR (Hz) = 77,000/[d (cm) × N (number of scan lines)]. Consequently, there is always a trade-off to be made between spatial and temporal resolutions. An increase in line density will enhance spatial resolution, but will reduce the frame rate. In the past 15 years, parallel processing has made it possible to process multiple scan lines simultaneously, resulting in a dramatic increase in color Doppler and two-dimensional frame rate. Parallel processing has also been an essential breakthrough for real-time three-dimensional scanning with parallelism up to 16:1 or beyond (Fig. 1.16).

4.3. Harmonic imaging

Tissue harmonic imaging is based on transmitting at a fundamental frequency and receiving the returning signal at twice the frequency (the second harmonic). The generation of this harmonic signal can be explained by the nonlinear propagation of sound through tissue. The stiffness of the medium increases slightly during compression and decreases during rarefaction, thereby altering the propagation speed. This means that the wave peaks will travel slightly faster than the wave troughs, causing a gradual change in the shape of the ultrasound wave to a more saw-tooth shaped signal composed of frequencies at multiples of the fundamental frequency (tissue harmonics, Fig. 1.17). Harmonic generation grows linearly with propagation depth and is related to the square of the signal amplitude. This means that there is very little harmonic signal related to near-field artifacts (ribs, lung interface, etc.) or from weak side-lobe and grating-lobe artifacts. By filtering out all but the harmonic signal, these troublesome artifacts are significantly reduced. Since harmonic energy at most is about 20 dB below the fundamental signal, harmonic imaging requires exceptionally low-noise amplifiers. It further must have a very sharp receive filter, so as to exclude the much stronger fundamental signal. Finally, the transmitted pulse train must be longer to more narrowly define the output spectrum. If the pulse is too brief, the spectrum will be so broad that the fundamental and harmonic spectra will overlap. This latter point is a potential downside of harmonic imaging, as the longer pulse trains mean thin objects (e.g., valves) may appear thicker. The formation of an

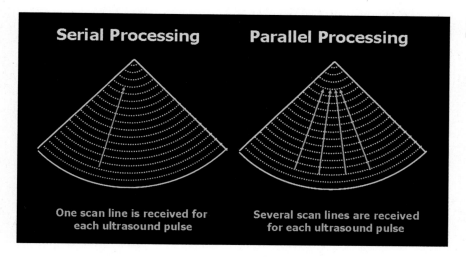

Figure 1.16 Parallel processing to improve frame rate.

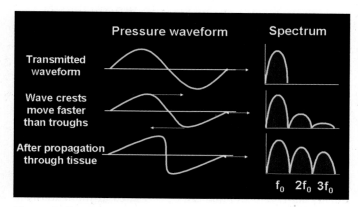

Figure 1.17 Harmonic generation. The propagation of sound through tissue is nonlinear, leading to a gradual change in the shape of the ultrasound wave as it propagates through the body (saw-tooth shape). Harmonic energy (at multiples of the fundamental frequency) appears in the waves as they propagate deeper into the chest.

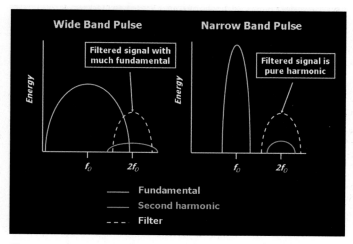

Figure 1.18 By filtering out the fundamental frequency on reception of the ultrasound signal, only the harmonics will be displayed, resulting in a significant improvement of transthoracic image quality. Contamination of the harmonic image by fundamental signal will degrade the quality of the harmonic image and is avoided by limiting the overlap between the fundamental (transmit) and harmonic (receive) bandwidths, a process called narrowbanding.

image by using only the second-harmonic energy in the returning echoes has, therefore, resulted in a marked increase in image quality of transthoracic echocardiography, particularly in technically difficult patients (Fig. 1.18).

5. DOPPLER ECHOCARDIOGRAPHY

The Doppler Effect is based on the change in frequency of a sound wave compared to the emitted frequency when the sound wave is reflected by a moving target (e.g., backscattered signal from a red blood cell). When the moving object is moving toward the observer (the transducer), there will be a positive shift to a higher frequency than the emitted wave. When the target moves away from the transducer, a negative Doppler shift produces a lower frequency. The Doppler Effect is observed regularly in daily life, for example, the change in the pitch of a car siren or a train whistle as it approaches or moves away from the observer (Fig. 1.19).

The Doppler shift (F_d) can be defined as the difference in frequency between the received frequency (F_r) and the transmitted frequency (F_t): $F_d = F_r - F_t$. Although higher velocities will obviously result in greater Doppler shifts, the degree of the shift will also depend on the transmitted frequency, the cosine of the insonification angle, and the sound velocity.

The Doppler shift is expressed in the equation: $F_d = 2F_t \times v \times \cos(\theta)/c$, where c is the propagation speed of sound in blood (1,540 m/s), θ is the insonification angle, and v is the velocity of the target. The Doppler Effect will thus critically depend on the relative position between the transducer and the direction of the moving object. As the angle varies from 0° (i.e., blood moving directly toward the transducer) through 90° (across the ultrasound beam) to 180° (away from the transducer), the cosine will change from 1 through 0 to –1, respectively. As such, no Doppler shift will be recorded if the ultrasound beam is perpendicular to blood flow. Therefore, the sonographer should always try to align the ultrasound beam as parallel as possible with the blood flow direction. While small deviations from a parallel intercept angle (<20°) are acceptable (cos 20° = 0.94), a misalignment of 60° will lead to a 50% underestimation of blood flow velocity (cos 60° = 0.5).

The small difference between the transmitted and received signals is extracted in the ultrasound front end by a process termed quadrature demodulation. The frequency content of this Doppler spectrum is then analyzed by a mathematical process called the Fourier Transform, which converts a signal that varies in time in

Figure 1.19 Illustration of the Doppler principle. As an ambulance with wailing siren moves toward an observer, it will cause a higher pitch due to compression of the wavelength in the direction of the observer. The opposite will occur as it moves away. The shift in frequency is proportional to the speed of the ambulance.

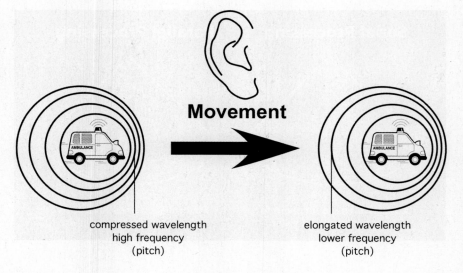

compressed wavelength
high frequency
(pitch)

Movement

elongated wavelength
lower frequency
(pitch)

the component frequencies within that signal. The derived frequency shifts can then be converted by the Doppler equation into a range of velocities to be presented on a spectral display in which the horizontal axis corresponds to time, and the vertical axis corresponds to the derived velocity. By convention, signals above the baseline represent positive frequency shifts (flow toward the transducer) and conversely for signals below the baseline. The amplitude of the signal is displayed by variations in brightness level (grayscale). Each pixel on a Doppler display will thus include information on blood flow velocity, blood flow direction, and signal amplitude at a particular point in time.

Three principal modalities are used in Doppler echocardiography: continuous-wave Doppler, pulsed Doppler, and color Doppler flow mapping. Each modality is processed differently, and each has distinct strengths and weaknesses.

5.1. Continuous-Wave Doppler

Transmitting and receiving continuously is the hallmark of continuous-wave Doppler. As it is difficult to transmit and receive continuously (thus simultaneously) on the same crystal, continuous-wave Doppler requires at least two crystals. An important advantage of this modality is that it allows detection of very high velocity flows. This is illustrated in Figure 1.20 where a typical display of aortic stenosis velocity is shown. The disadvantage of continuous-wave Doppler is that as it records all frequency shifts along the entire ultrasound beam, no information is given as to where along the scan line the velocity arises, referred to as range ambiguity. Since high velocity flow typically occurs in only a few locations in the heart, this usually is not a major problem, and pulsed and color Doppler can help localize the flow by identifying regions of aliasing (see below). Also, since the maximal velocity can only be measured if the insonification angle is parallel to the direction of flow, it is important to interrogate stenotic valves (particularly the aortic valve) from a variety of windows.

5.2. Pulsed Doppler

Pulsed Doppler allows the sonographer to interrogate (sample) the blood flow velocity at a particular depth rather than across the entire scanning line as in continuous-wave Doppler. The frequency shift that occurs at this sample volume is then translated into a particular velocity. To do this, the transducer sends out a burst of ultrasound and then turns off. The reflected waves

will return to the transducer after an interval determined by the depth of interrogation; at exactly that moment the transducer turns into the receiver mode. The duration of the receive phase is determined by the sample volume. For an interrogation depth D, the entire distance traveled by the ultrasound pulse is $2 \times D$. As the speed of sound in tissue is constant, a complete cycle of transmitting–waiting–receiving will obviously take longer for increasing depths. As explained above, the *pulse repetition period* (the time between two transmit events) is determined by the finite speed of sound, and this will set a limit to the number of pulses that can be transmitted per second, defined as the PRF. The deeper the interrogation depth, the lower the PRF. This is important because the lower the PRF, the lower the maximal frequency shift (velocity) that can be measured unambiguously as illustrated in Figure 1.21. To accurately determine the frequency of a waveform, one should sample at least twice during each cycle. A frequency greater than half the sampling rate will lead to aliasing, causing the Doppler signal to wrap around the spectral display, making it impossible to determine the peak velocity

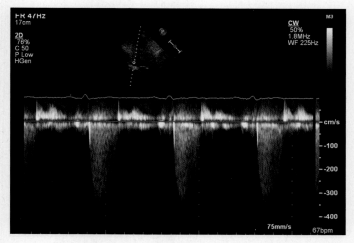

Figure 1.20 Spectral display of high velocity flow through a stenotic aortic valve. The signal is smooth in contour and clearly defines the onset and end of flow. It is easy to determine the direction of flow (away from the transducer) as well as the maximal flow velocity (3.5 m/s). The velocity curve is filled in because all blood flow velocities along the entire scan line (also the lower velocities) are recorded and represented.

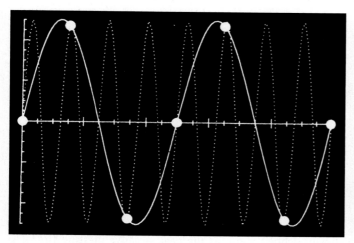

Figure 1.21 To fully resolve a waveform, it must be sampled at least twice per cycle. While the solid white waveform is completely determined by the white dots, it is obvious that these same white dots are too sparsely spaced to determine the underlying dotted signal. As such, this higher frequency signal can be mistaken for a much lower frequency signal, a phenomenon referred to as aliasing. Conversely, continuous-wave Doppler will never show aliasing (virtually no limit with respect to the maximum detectable Doppler shift), since the receiving is continuous and not the isolated sampling times of pulsed Doppler.

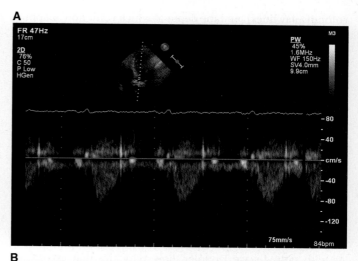

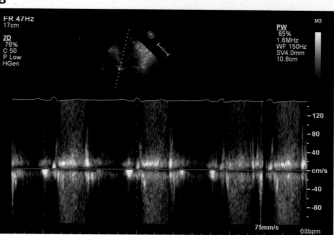

Figure 1.22 Pulsed-wave Doppler in a patient with aortic stenosis. (**A**) With the sample volume positioned in the LVOT, it is possible to accurately determine the blood flow velocity before acceleration occurs through the stenotic aortic valve. (**B**) When the sample volume is positioned somewhat higher (closer to the aortic valve), flow velocity exceeds the Nyquist limit and aliasing (velocity "wraparound") occurs.

(Fig. 1.22B). The greatest Doppler shift detectable (the Nyquist limit) is thus half the PRF: F_d (max) = PRF/2. To avoid aliasing from a pulsed Doppler interrogation, one could use continuous-wave Doppler (at the price of range ambiguity), make use of a transducer with a lower operating frequency or decrease the depth of interrogation by changing the view. If the velocity of interest exceeds the Nyquist limit by less than twofold, it is possible to restore the wrapped-around signal into the right position by shifting the baseline on the display. Finally, in high PRF mode, multiple pulses are transmitted at intervals equal to, say, one fourth the pulse repetition period (the time needed for a pulse to travel down and return from the interrogation depth). These additional wavefronts will add (return in the same phase), which allows the machine to sample at higher rates and potentially eliminates aliasing. However, there is no way to make out which of the four pulses is responsible for a particular echo; as four different sample volumes appear along the scan line, some degree of range ambiguity is introduced again. This range ambiguity is obvious in high PRF mode, as shallower sample volumes are displayed on the guiding image. What is often overlooked is that standard pulsed Doppler will always include the possibility of signals coming from depths that are two, three, or four times the interrogated depth.

The size of the sample volume is also used as a variable by adjusting the length of the pulse train sent out. Longer trains have greater sensitivity for weak signals, but at the expense of sampling over a larger volume, thus increasing the risk of contamination from adjacent flow.

5.3. Color Doppler

Color Doppler is based on the pulsed Doppler principle in that brief pulses of ultrasound are sent. However, instead of one sample volume (gate) on the receiving end, multiple sample volumes are evaluated along each individual sampling line. When a burst of ultrasound is transmitted, the returning signals

are received from each gate along that scan line. Since the color Doppler field contains many scan lines, the detailed spectral analysis of Fourier transformation (in which up to 128 samples are stored before analysis) is impractical. Instead, a packet of only six or eight pulses is used to produce one color Doppler display line. Instead of Fourier processing, a technique called autocorrelation is used where successive returning pulses are compared for changes in phase, a positive phase shift representing forward flow, and conversely for a negative shift. By averaging the phase shift (velocity) and amplitude of multiple color Doppler pulses together, it is possible to obtain a fairly precise estimate of mean velocity along the scan line, though not nearly with the velocity resolution of pulsed Doppler. Larger packet sizes will result in better color resolution but at the price of worse temporal resolution as the process of averaging more scan lines needs to be repeated for each display line across the image plane. The speed with which the image can be updated (the frame rate achieved) will thus depend on the packet size (number of acoustic lines needed to generate one color display line), the color sector size (which determines the number of color display lines), and the depth at which color flow mapping is performed (as this will affect the PRF just as for conventional pulsed Doppler). Finally, since the color-coded velocity patterns are superimposed on a two-dimensional reference image, it is obvious that the single acoustic lines needed to build up the two-dimensional image will also reduce the total frame time. Hence, frame rate for color Doppler imaging is only a fraction of B-mode imaging.

The frequency shifts (velocities) are encoded using a color scale displaying flow toward the transducer in red and away in blue. Different shades are applied for velocities relative to the Nyquist limit. A great variability between individual velocity estimates in the packet indicates turbulence and can be represented by an additional color (typically green or yellow). The color bar, always shown with color Doppler imaging, is the key to color interpretation. In addition to flow direction, the color bar reveals the mean velocity at which aliasing will occur. As with pulsed-wave Doppler, flow velocities that exceed the Nyquist limit (implying a sampling rate less than twice per cycle for that particular velocity/frequency) will cause aliasing of the color signal. This is visualized as a sudden "wraparound" from bright blue to bright red (or vice versa) of the velocity signal and should not be mistaken for blood traveling in a direction opposite to what would be expected (Fig. 1.23).

Changing the PRF or the color scale will not only affect the maximal velocity at which aliasing occurs, but also the minimal velocity displayed (since the color display has a set number of red or blue display hues evenly spread out between 0 cm/s and the aliasing velocity). It may also change the Doppler wall filters (high-pass filters designed to minimize low velocity "clutter" in the image) and may thus be helpful in the detection of low velocity flow (for instance a small left-to-right shunt through a patent foramen ovale). On the other hand, low scale settings will exaggerate the size of a regurgitant jet by encoding stagnant blood entrained by the jet, an issue that must be considered when assessing the severity of a regurgitant lesion.

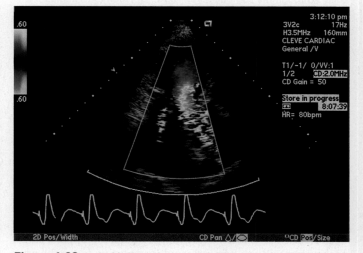

Figure 1.23 Apical long-axis view. Normal LV outflow is shown with aliasing from blue to yellow-red as the blood flow velocity exceeds the Nyquist limit of 60 cm/s (indicated by the value at the lower end of the color bar). Interpretation of the color bar helps the reader to asses flow direction and velocity. Both values at the upper and the lower ends of the color bar indicate the scale settings. The black band in the middle of the color bar (around the baseline) indicates the range of velocities that are not visualized (the cutoff frequency of the color wall filters).

6. INSTRUMENT SETTINGS

In order to derive the maximum diagnostic benefit from the ultrasound technology, every sonographer and echocardiographer should have sufficient training and knowledge to operate the echo machine effectively. Standard imaging control systems available on most platforms allow manipulation of:

Power output, or transmit power, governs the excitation voltage that is applied to the transducer crystal in order to generate an ultrasound signal. An increase in the amplitude of the voltage supply will cause a parallel increase in the amplitude of the acoustic pressure wave that is emitted, causing a higher intensity signal. Power output is often specified in two ways: first in decibels, where 0 dB represents maximal power output and values below 0 are reduced on the logarithmic decibel scale; second, to reflect the level of energy delivered into the body, the MI is shown, defined above as the peak negative pressure (in MPa) divided by the square root of the imaging frequency (in MHz). In general, the lowest transmit power should be used that allows proper diagnosis. If an excessive increase in transmit power is necessary to see far into the image, one might consider choosing a transducer at a lower frequency instead.

Gain is essentially a receiver function. Gain refers to the amplification of the returning signal. As such, it does not affect the risk of bioeffects. Increasing the gain will enhance the brightness of the whole image and is sometimes necessary to amplify small signals into a range that allows them to be displayed and perceived by the human eye. However, changing the gain will not necessarily improve image quality as it does not affect the overall signal-to-noise ratio. Using a higher receiver gain will increase the noise to a similar degree as the signal.

Dynamic range or compression refers to a technique that converts the enormous range in amplitude of signals returning from the patient (say, a 10,000-fold difference in acoustic strength between the faintest and strongest signals, mainly due to the exponential decay of ultrasound signal with increasing depth.) into a much narrower and manageable range. This is made possible by logarithmical compression of all signals into approximately 100 different shades of brightness (gray-scale values) visible to the human eye and suitable for display on the viewing monitor. The amount of compression (referring to the number of gray-scale levels present in the image) can be adjusted, with a broader dynamic range setting indicating more shades of gray ("softening" the image) and a smaller dynamic range resulting in a more prominent contrast between lighter and darker areas. In effect, logarithmic compression converts the exponential decay in signal strength with depth into a linear one.

Time-gain compensation: Even after logarithmic compression, there remains a linear decrease in signal strength with imaging depth. This is compensated for by time-gain compensation, which is designed to show structures of the same acoustic strength as echoes of equal amplitude, whatever their depth. Most echo machines have a column of approximately ten time-gain compensation slides, each slide representing a specific depth zone within the image, starting from the transducer face at the top. Although most machines offer time-gain compensation based on a preset built into the system (allowing the control slides to be left in a vertical line), some situations will require careful adjustment of the slides in order to optimize the image.

Focal depth: Refers to the depth at which the ultrasound beam is narrowest just before fanning out into the far field. This will be the region where the lateral resolution is maximal and so the focus should always be positioned at or just behind the region of interest. Some machines can focus at two depths simultaneously by sending out double pulses for each scan line, focusing each independently.

Image depth: As mentioned above, the depth that is displayed on the monitor will affect the PRF and thereby frame rate and may be important in terms of temporal resolution and aliasing in Doppler studies. Magnification ("zoom" or "regional expansion selection") modes will produce a magnified image in a selected area of interest with increased frame rate and spatial resolution.

Finally, additional manipulation of the signal before and after it is digitized (preprocessing and postprocessing, respectively) by algorithms specific for a particular instrument will further optimize image quality before it is displayed on the monitor.

7. IMAGING ARTIFACTS

Ultrasound artifacts are commonly encountered during echocardiographic evaluation of a patient and may lead the interpreter into making an inaccurate diagnosis. Artifacts include the appearance of structures that do not correspond with an anatomic tissue structure (at least not at that location) or the creation of an image with clearly different characteristics than its corresponding anatomic structure (different size and shape). It also includes failure to visualize structures (missing images). Many artifacts are based on the physical properties of ultrasound itself and thus require a basic understanding of some concepts described above. We will briefly review the most common artifacts and discuss how these pitfalls can be recognized and potentially avoided.

7.1. Degraded images

The most "common" artifact is *suboptimal image quality*, often referred to as "technically difficult study" by sonographers. Poor image quality results from poor penetration of ultrasound and is caused by interposition of tissues with inconsistent impedance between the transducer and the heart (e.g., air due to subcutaneous emphysema, adipose tissue in the obese or bone in patients with narrow intercostal spaces). A low signal-to-noise ratio will obviously compromise proper diagnosis and often precludes quantitative analysis. As mentioned above, overall image quality can be improved by the use of harmonic imaging, by choosing a lower operating frequency or by scanning from a different acoustic window.

Reverberation is the result of ultrasound bouncing back and forth between a highly reflective structure and another strong specular reflector. Reverberations appear as multiple parallel, irregular dense lines extending away from the transducer into the far field (Fig. 1.24A). These reverberations may limit evaluation of structures in the far field. In addition, as the ultrasound pulses will make repeated journeys before arriving at the transducer face, reverberation may result in the replication of the reverberating structures and the structures in between them at multiple distances from the primary target (Fig. 1.24B).

Noise is another cause of image degradation. It can be caused by excessive gain settings, but also by electrical interference with other devices (for instance electrocautery in the operating room, Fig. 1.25).

Beam width artifacts arise from the fact that the lateral resolution will decrease with increasing depth. As the ultrasound beam fans out in the far field, it becomes more difficult to discern two adjacent structures as distinct entities. Once two structures lie closer to each other than the lateral resolution, they will appear as one single image (superimposed).

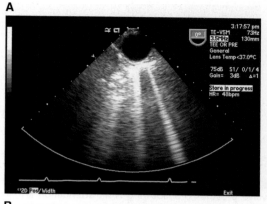

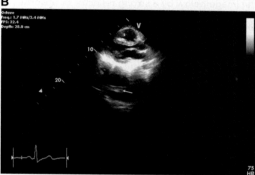

Figure 1.24 A: The descending aorta, evaluated by transesophageal echocardiography. The hyper-reflective aortic wall commonly results in linear reverberations directed away from the transducer (*arrows*). This is also referred to as "comet tail" effect. **B:** Reverberation often creates a double image, caused by ultrasound bouncing back and forth between hyper-reflective structures (in this case the hyper-reflective posterior pericardium, leading to the replication of the interventricular septum (*arrow*) and RV and LV cavities at a greater depth).

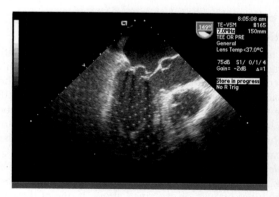

Figure 1.25 Noise caused by electrical interference during intraoperative echocardiography.

7.2. Missing structures

Acoustic shadowing: Highly reflective structures (specular reflectors) block the transmission of ultrasound more distally, resulting in poor or even no visualization of these far-field structures. A good example is the presence of a mechanical mitral valve prosthesis which prevents good visualization of the left atrium from an apical window (Fig. 1.26). Choosing another window (subcostal) or transesophageal imaging offers a solution.

Enhancement artifacts are actually the opposite of attenuation artifacts. When ultrasound passes through tissue or a

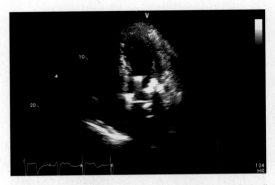

Figure 1.26 Acoustic shadowing (*) in a patient with a ball-in-cage mitral valve prosthesis. Shadowing is an attenuation artifact that is cast on the image below by a strong reflector or absorber. Reflection or absorption of ultrasound decreases the beam intensity dramatically, causing attenuation of underlying structures.

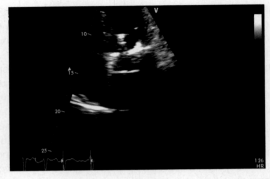

Figure 1.27 Same patient as in Figure 1.26. The ball appears larger and distorted due to the slowed transmission of ultrasound through the silastic rubber of the ball.

structure that is less absorbing than normal (e.g., a cyst), it will experience less attenuation, leading to enhancement of the amplitude of the echoes below the weak reflector. This can be adjusted by decreasing the time-gain compensation in the vertical plane.

Echo Dropout is often the reason why the endocardial border of the lateral wall is not well visualized in the apical view. Ultrasound imaging is based on specular reflection. Reflection will be maximal when the beam strikes the interface in a perpendicular fashion. Conversely, when the incident angle is parallel to the heart wall (as occurs with scanning from an apical window), there will be little specular reflection and thus not much echo returning from the ventricular walls to the transducer face. This can have important consequences (e.g., when interpreting stress echocardiography). Evaluation from another view (parasternal view) or the use of contrast agents helps the reader to overcome these problems.

7.3. Falsely perceived objects, misregistered locations, and speed error artifacts

Refraction artifacts occur when a sound beam is deflected from its original pathway as it passes through a medium with different acoustic impedance, as predicted by Snell's law. When the bent acoustic line strikes a reflector, it will create an artifactual image that is laterally displaced from the true structure because the transducer can only assume that that the beam followed a straight course. Refraction artifacts may disappear by changing the scanning angle.

Side Lobe and grating lobe artifacts. In addition to the central beam, transducers will produce lower intensity side lobes and grating lobes off-axis, as explained above. If one of these peripheral beams hits a strong reflector, the returning echo signal may erroneously be assumed to come from the main beam and thus subsequently displayed centrally (in a laterally displaced position) on the screen. This is a major source of cavity clutter signals which sometimes can be misinterpreted as thrombus or mass. The use of harmonic imaging (producing much lower intensity side lobes) resulted in a significant reduction in this type of artifacts. Altering the scanning angle can also be helpful.

Speed error artifact. Echocardiography is based on the assumption that the speed of sound in tissue is 1,540 m/s and constant. Accordingly, the ultrasound system will base its calculations of depth and distance on the time interval between transmitting a pulse and receiving an echo. Obviously, errors will arise whenever ultrasound travels through a medium with a different prop-

agation velocity. A good illustration is the distorted echo image of a ball and cage valve: as the propagation speed of ultrasound decreases by about half when passing through the silastic rubber of the ball, echoes will arrive later in time and produce an image that is much deeper (an elongated ball) than in reality (Fig. 1.27).

8. PRINCIPLES OF FLOW DYNAMICS

Within the circulatory system, blood flow is governed by the principles of conservation of mass, energy, and momentum. These three principles are central concepts in echocardiography and are applied on a daily basis to determine the severity of cardiac flow abnormalities.

a. **The principle of *conservation of mass*** states that in a closed system of flow, whatever volume of flow that comes in must also go out. In other words, flow must be continuous when going from one point to another, and this forms the basis of the continuity equation. Volumetric flow (Q) through a rigid tube can then be calculated as the product of V (mean spatial velocity) and the cross-sectional flow area:

$$Q = V \times \text{area} \qquad \text{(Eq. 1.1)}$$

For a constant flow rate, it can be predicted that a sudden change in cross-sectional area (e.g., flow through a stenotic aortic valve) will result in a parallel change (increase) in flow velocity. The continuity equation will thus allow us to evaluate the extent of a sudden change in caliber of a flow conduit because the Doppler principle enables us to measure flow velocities at different points along the flow trajectory (Fig. 1.28).

In the case of aortic stenosis, it is possible to calculate the valve area by measuring:

1. Left ventricular outflow tract (LVOT) flow from the product of LVOT area (calculated as $\pi D^2/4$, where D is the diameter of the LVOT) and the velocity in the LVOT (measured with pulsed Doppler by placing the sample volume in the LVOT at the same level that D was measured).
2. The velocity across the stenotic orifice derived by continuous-wave Doppler.
3. Rather than using one particular velocity value, most equations will use the time velocity integral (TVI, expressed in units of length) which represents the changing velocity profile during the cardiac cycle.

b. The **principle of *conservation of momentum*** states that the momentum across a jet remains constant throughout the

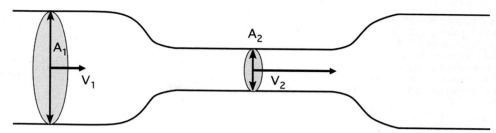

Figure 1.28 Illustration of the continuity equation: A_1 represents a cross-sectional area which usually is known and A_2 the unknown cross-sectional area of the restricted orifice. V_1 and V_2 are the average flow velocities at A_1 and A_2, respectively. The law of conservation of mass dictates that $Q_1 = Q_2$, thus $A_1 \times V_1 = A_2 \times V_2$. This equation can now be rewritten as $A_2 = A_1 \times \frac{V_1}{V_2}$. Hence, the continuity equation allows us to assess the severity of a stenotic lesion.

extent of the jet. Momentum equals mass multiplied by velocity and can be calculated for fluids as

$$M = \rho \times Q \times V \qquad \text{(Eq. 1.2)}$$

where ρ, density, V, velocity, and Q, flow rate. Knowing that $Q = V \times$ area (A), the equation becomes $M = \rho \times A \times V^2$.

Jet momentum is important as it is one of the best predictors of jet appearance by color flow mapping when evaluating the severity of a regurgitant lesion. Since jet momentum is proportional to jet area and the square of jet velocity, and knowing that momentum remains unchanged through the length of the jet, it becomes clear that as the regurgitant area distal to the regurgitant orifice increases, velocity will equally decrease downstream of the jet. Theoretically, this concept could be used to quantify the regurgitant orifice area by measuring the flow momentum in the receiving chamber (left atrium for mitral regurgitation) and obtaining the maximal jet velocity though the regurgitant orifice with continuous-wave Doppler. However, because the velocity profile downstream of the regurgitant jet is not uniform (decreasing when moving radially away from the centerline), an integral equation must be applied to account for this axisymmetric flow pattern, and the velocities in these jets typically exceed the Nyquist velocity and so cannot be directly measured. In addition, this equation would only be applicable for free jets; eccentric jets undergo jet constraint and distortion by adjacent walls. These eccentrically directed jets will typically flatten out along the wall and invariably appear smaller than similar sized central jets, when imaged by color Doppler (the Coanda effect). This, in turn, may lead to an underestimation of the severity of the regurgitation. While conservation of momentum may not be practical for regurgitation assessment, it provides a theoretical basis for the fact that high pressure (velocity) jets appear larger than low pressure jets, even if the actual flow rates are identical. Thus, the same regurgitant flow will appear larger across a mitral valve than across a tricuspid valve, provided the left ventricular (LV) and right ventricular (RV) systolic pressures are in normal range.

c. **The principle of _conservation of energy_** states that within a closed system, the total amount of energy must remain constant. Although energy can neither be created nor destroyed, it can change states. When blood is forced through a stenotic valve, the velocity (_kinetic energy_) will increase as demonstrated above. However, an increase in kinetic energy implies a proportional decrease in _potential energy_ (a loss of pressure or force exerted by the fluid on the vessel wall). In a pulsatile system, acceleration and deceleration of flow will lead to some additional energy losses caused by inertial forces. Viscous friction will finally also lead to a small additional loss of energy in the form of heat.

This relationship is contained in the complete **Bernoulli equation** which includes terms for pressure, kinetic energy, inertial forces, and heat losses (heat being related to blood viscosity and velocity) and is expressed as

$$\Delta P = \frac{1}{2}\rho\left[(v_2^2) - (v_2^1)\right] + M\left(\frac{dv}{dt}\right) + R(v) \qquad \text{(Eq. 1.3)}$$

where

- ΔP is the pressure difference across the stenosis (pressure gradient);
- $\frac{1}{2}\rho\left[(v_2^2) - (v_2^1)\right]$ corresponds to the change in kinetic energy as blood is accelerated through a stenosis. Kinetic energy is thus directly proportional to the velocity of blood squared as well as to the blood density;
- $M\left(\frac{dv}{dt}\right)$ represents the energy needed to accelerate a mass M of blood; M is a somewhat vague concept related to the effective volume of blood being accelerated through the smallest structure in the region of interest and is on the same order of magnitude as a sphere contained within the diameter of this structure;
- $R(v)$ accounts for energy losses associated with viscous and friction effects (leading to heat generation) and is most important for flow in tubes, such as the vascular tree.

Fortunately, for flow through a restrictive orifice (e.g., narrowed valves), these last two terms can be neglected and eliminated from the Bernoulli equation and the equation becomes

$$\Delta P = \frac{1}{2}\rho\left[(v_2^2 - v_1^2)\right] \qquad \text{(Eq. 1.4)}$$

When the normal density for blood is now inserted into the equation, by using units of millimeters of mercury for pressure, the equation can be written as

$$\Delta P = 4(v_2^2 - v_1^2) \qquad \text{(Eq. 1.5)}$$

Finally, if the distal velocity v_2 is much greater than the proximal velocity v_1 ($v_1 < 1$ m/s), the kinetic energy proximally will be small compared to the distal kinetic energy. In that case, v_1 can be eliminated without introducing a great error and this finally leads to the modified or simplified Bernoulli equation: $\Delta P = 4v_2^2$. Computationally, this may be easier to calculate in one's head as $2v_2^2$.

Once the proximal velocity exceeds 1 m/s, this proximal term can no longer be ignored and the Bernoulli equation in its "more complete" form $\Delta P = 4(v_2^2 - v_1^2)$ should be applied.

The simplified Bernoulli equation has been repeatedly validated against invasive measures of pressure decay and has become pivotal in the noninvasive assessment of intracardiac pressures in patients with valvular lesions or shunts.

Figure 1.29 A,B: Conservation of energy and the phenomenon of pressure recovery. 1) E_p represents potential energy, 2) E_k represents kinetic energy. Note that the potential energy will never return to its original state downstream of a stenosis due to energy losses related to the effects of turbulence. 3) pressure recovery observed distal of the stenosis.

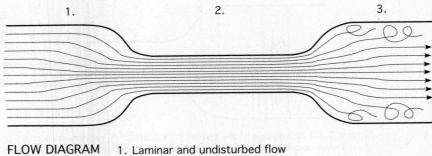

FLOW DIAGRAM

1. Laminar and undisturbed flow

2. Flow going through a narrow region, resulting in flow acceleration

3. Flow deceleration distal to the stenosis. Exit effect resulting in turbulence (whirling vortices on the edges of the jet)

This same principle can also be applied to account for the phenomenon of pressure recovery (Fig. 1.29). When blood flows in parallel streamlines toward a stenotic lesion, blood flow velocity will gradually increase until it reaches a maximum within (or actually just distal to) the stenosis, at the vena contracta. This change in velocity leads to a rise in kinetic energy (and a parallel fall in potential energy) as explained above. Once the streamlines arrive again at a region with a larger diameter, kinetic energy (velocity) will decrease again and (as predicted by the law of conservation of energy) there is a possible return to potential energy. This phenomenon is referred to as "pressure recovery" and is one of the reasons why Doppler-derived gradients tend to be higher than catheter-derived gradients. Because catheters are necessarily positioned downstream of the stenotic valve (beyond the vena contracta), some degree of pressure recovery may have occurred which translates into a smaller pressure gradient compared to the pressure gradient measured with Doppler (which is based on the velocity at the vena contracta). Fortunately, for the diagnostic accuracy of the Bernoulli equation, pressure recovery is a relatively minor issue for native stenotic and regurgitant lesions, as the reduction in kinetic energy is "wasted" into other forms of energy, like sound (from a murmur) or heat (from turbulent friction), rather than an increase in pressure. One circumstance where significant pressure recover does occur is with bileaflet mechanical valve prosthesis. The slight flair between the leaflets allows blood flow to slow down without turbulence, leading to 20% to 30% pressure recovery.

9. FUTURE DIRECTIONS

Although ultrasound imaging will always be limited by the physical constraints described in this chapter, it will likely remain as the primary diagnostic modality in cardiovascular medicine for the foreseeable future. The key advantages of ultrasound are its biological safety, portability, and low cost. Throughout the last decade, the introduction of parallel processing, miniaturized electronic transducer components, and the implementation of harmonic imaging and ultrasound contrast agents have dramatically reduced the number of nondiagnostic studies. The next few decades will likely bring a transition from two- and three-dimensional ultrasound, together with simpler and more robust quantification methods for evaluating global and regional myocardial mechanics and flow quantification. Meanwhile, having a full understanding of the physical principles and instrumentation will allow the cardiac sonographer and imaging physician to attain optimal image quality and thus reach maximal diagnostic certainty.

SUGGESTED READINGS

1. Weyman A. Physical principles of ultrasound. In: Weyman A, ed. *Principles and Practice of Echocardiography*. 2nd Ed. Philadelphia, Pa: Lea & Febiger; 1994.
2. Otto C. Principles of echocardiographic image acquisition and Doppler analysis. In: Otto C, ed. *Textbook of Clinical Echocardiography*. 3rd Ed. Philadelphia, Pa: WB Saunders; 2004.
3. Feigenbaum H. Physics and instrumentation. In: Feigenbaum H, Armstrong WF, Ryan T, eds. *Echocardiography*. 6th Ed. Philadelphia, Pa: Lippincott Williams & Wilkins; 2004.
4. Zagebski J. *Essentials of Ultrasound Physics*. St Louis, Mo: Mosby; 1996.
5. Hatle L, Angelsen B. *Doppler Ultrasound in Cardiology: Physical Principles and Clinical Application*. Philadelphia, Pa: Lea & Febiger; 1982.
6. Miele FR. *Essentials of Ultrasound Physics: The Board Review Book*. Forney, Tex: Pegasus Lectures, Inc; 2008.
7. Thomas JD, Rubin DN. Tissue harmonic imaging: Why does it work? *J Am Soc Echocardiogr*. 1998;11:803–808.
8. Kremkau FW. *Diagnostic Ultrasound: Principles and Instruments*. 6th Ed. Philadelphia, Pa: WB Saunders; 2002.
9. Thomas JD. Principles of imaging. In: Fozzard HA, Haber E, Jenning RB, Katz AM, eds. *The Heart and Cardiovascular System*. 2nd Ed. New York: Raven Press; 1996.

The Echocardiographic Examination

2

Juan Gaztanaga
Ramon Castello

1. INTRODUCTION

1.1. Historical perspective

The beginning of ultrasound has its roots in Vienna in 1761, where a physician named Leopold Auenbrugger used reflected sound from the human body to study a variety of diseases. It was not until two centuries later that Drs Inge Edler and Helmuth Hertz conducted the initial experiments using reflected sound waves to examine the cardiac structures, in 1954.[1] Through their experiments they were able to record oscillations from the heart onto paper. This was the initiation of M-mode echocardiography. Hertz later went on to detect myxomas and atrial thrombi using this method.[2]

Doppler technology first made its introduction into cardiology when Dr Satomura studied the velocity of cardiac tissues and blood[3] using the principles described by Christian Doppler in 1842. Doppler eventually made its way into regular clinical use when the first duplex scanner was introduced in 1974.[4]

In 1968, the first phased array scanner was created by Dr Somer.[5] In 1973, Bom et al.[6] described real-time imaging of the heart using a prototype multiple element echocardiographic instrument with a linear transducer. Through these advances clinical echocardiography has developed into the noninvasive workhorse we know today. It is the most versatile and used noninvasive imaging modality in cardiology.

1.2. Overview

In order to perform a complete optimal echocardiographic examination in a timely manner, the sonographer must be familiar with the ultrasound system. He or she must know where to find the different knob settings and screen displays as well as how to adjust them to obtain the best images (Fig. 2.1). To begin, the echocardiogram (ECG) signal must be clearly seen on the display screen. When the first image is acquired, gain setting, depth and plane of the examination must be adjusted to display the optimal image. These settings have to be adjusted constantly as one progresses through the examination. In addition to these, several other settings like focus, zoom/high resolution display (RES), freeze, pulsed wave (PW) Doppler, continuous wave (CW) Doppler, color Doppler, M-mode, tissue Doppler imaging (TDI) are commonly utilized during an exam. In most hospitals the echocardiography exam is performed by trained technicians who spend the workday performing up to 8 to 12 studies. In otter settings the exams may be performed by a physician. Although most exams are interpreted by cardiovascular specialists, many internists, emergency room physicians, intensivists, and anesthesiologists have undergone appropriate training and gained the expertise to perform limited echocardiographic examinations relevant to their field of practice. There are three levels of training in echocardiography.[7] Table 2.1 shows the requirements needed for each. Level 1 training is defined as the minimal introductory training that must be achieved by all specialists in adult cardiovascular medicine. This level includes a basic understanding of ultrasound physics, anatomy, physiology as well as technical aspects of performing the exam. This level of training is not sufficient for a physician to perform and interpret ECGs independently. Level 2 training is the minimum recommended training for a physician to perform and interpret ECGs independently. Level 3 training is the highest level attainable and allows a physician to be the director of an echocardiography laboratory. As the director, he or she is responsible for quality control as well as the training of physicians and sonographers in the lab.

2. TRANSTHORACIC EXAMINATION

2.1. Patient preparation

Transthoracic echocardiography is the most widely used imaging tool in the cardiology practice. It has revolutionized patient care over the years and has become the backbone for cardiovascular diagnosis. It has several different roles in the hospital setting in addition to the outpatient setting. Typically there are three different types of patients for which echocardiography is used in hospital inpatient care. The first type and most common is the patient who is not critically ill and is able to be transported to the echocardiography lab for a full and thorough examination. In these patients there are typically no external constraints which may hinder the exam. The patient is able to lie supine on the examination table, change positions, and follow breathing instructions from the sonographer during the exam to obtain the best possible images in the different imaging planes. Three electrocardiographic leads are placed upon the patient in order to obtain simultaneous ECG display. These exams can typically take between 20 and 30 min to complete for an experienced sonographer.

The remaining two inpatient scenarios are more challenging for the sonographer. The echocardiographic examination for the patient in the intensive care unit setting has several obstacles. Typically these patients are intubated and have mechanical ventilation which limits echocardiographic windows. These patients are critically ill and are more likely to have multisystem disease including airway disease which further affects the ability to acquire adequate imaging windows. In general patients are not able to be positioned or follow breathing instructions in order to acquire optimal images in the different echocardiographic plains. These exams are much more time consuming because of the complicated patient as well as the travel and setup time for the sonographer to move from patient room to patient room.

The last clinical inpatient scenario is the emergency setting that can occur anywhere in the hospital with the potential for impending patient mortality. These can be patients who arrive

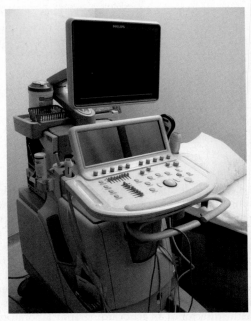

Figure 2.1 Display screen and control panel of a Philips ie33 ultrasound machine.

TABLE 2.1
PHYSICIAN TRAINING REQUIREMENTS FOR THE PERFORMANCE AND INTERPRETATION OF ADULT TRANSTHORACIC ECG

Training level	Duration of training (months)	Minimum total number of exams performed	Minimum total number of exams interpreted
Level 1	3	75	150
Level 2	6	150	300
Level 3	12	300	750

Figure 2.2 Different transducer positions used in a transthoracic ECG examination.

to the emergency department with hemodynamic instability or patients who are on the hospital floors and are deteriorating quickly. In these situations the patient is unable to comply with instructions and the exam must be quick and focused on answering the critical question of the physician team caring for the patient. One of the reasons why echocardiography can never be replaced is because of its versatility and mobility in these critical clinical situations, when compared to other noninvasive imaging modalities.

The outpatient setting is the most optimal situation for an echocardiographic exam. Patients are usually healthy and are able to cooperate with the sonographer to obtain best quality images.

2.2. Two-dimensional imaging planes and M-mode

The echocardiographic examination is based on obtaining optimal images for evaluation of the heart. The American Society of Echocardiography developed nomenclature and standards for performing an ECG.[8] The initial step in beginning an ECG is using the correct position to place the transducer. There are various locations that can be used to place the transducer and each will give a different image plane.[9] The first of the possible positions to place the transducer (from cranial to caudal) is the suprasternal view, which is when the transducer is placed at the suprasternal notch. The next position is left parasternal, which is at the third and fourth intercostal spaces in between the sternum and midclavicular line. The following position is the apical window, where the transducer is positioned over the maximal apical impulse. Finally, the subcostal window is when the transducer is placed midline below the sternum after the last ribs (Fig. 2.2).

The imaging planes are divided into three categories, short axis, long axis, and four chambers. The long-axis imaging plane is equivalent to the long axis of the left ventricle (LV) and is perpendicular to the dorsal/ventral plane of the body. Short-axis imaging planes transect the LV perpendicular to the long axis, creating a circular LV. The four-chamber imaging plane is both parallel to the long axis of the ventricle and also parallel to the dorsal/ventral plane of the body (Fig. 2.3). In order to name the images, the American Society of Echocardiography has recommended combining the transducer location with the imaging plane. For

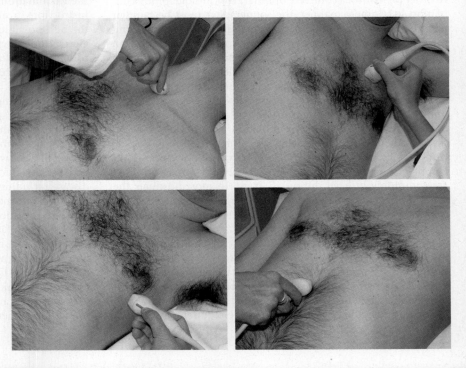

aorta, the pointer of the transducer must be rotated 90° clockwise until it is directed toward the dorsal surface. This view also allows visualization of the right pulmonary artery in its long axis.

The parasternal short axis of the LV is acquired by positioning the transducer pointer directed toward the right midclavicle. This will produce short-axis circular images of the LV (Fig. 2.5). One must make fine minimal positional adjustments in order to obtain the smallest circular ventricle, which correctly represents the actual short axis of the LV. At times moving from one intercostal space above or below may also improve the window. Rotating the pointer of the transducer clockwise 90°, the long axis of the LV is obtained. As seen in Figure 2.6 this plane allows visualization of the left ventricular outflow tract (LVOT), aortic and mitral valves, anteroseptal, apical and posterior segments of the LV as well as the left atrium (LA). In addition the right ventricle (RV) is sitting above the LV in this plane. When the long axis is not acquired completely perpendicular to the short axis, the image is said to be foreshortened and appears smaller than actual size. In this imaging plane the sonographer must make fine adjustments of the transducer to acquire the largest size of the LV, in order to avoid foreshortening.

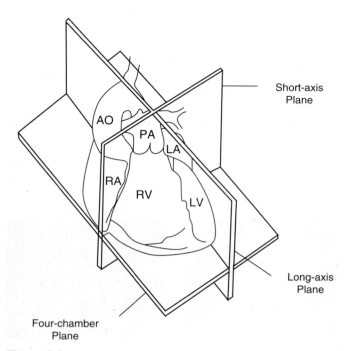

Figure 2.3 Three imaging planes of the heart used in echocardiography: short axis, long axis, and four chamber.

example, obtaining short-axis imaging planes by positioning the transducer at the left parasternal region would produce a type of image called parasternal short axis.

In order to acquire these optimal imaging planes the position of the patient's body must also be maneuvered in order to maximize the imaging windows. For both the suprasternal and subcostal views, the patient must be lying supine. For the apical views, the image quality is improved if the patient lies in a left lateral decubitus position, while left parasternal window is best visualized when the patient is able to lie in between supine and left lateral decubitus positions.

The suprasternal window allows one to assess the long axis of the ascending aorta, left aortic arch, and descending aorta when the transducer pointer is directed toward the right supraclavicular region (Fig. 2.4). In order to obtain the short-axis image of the

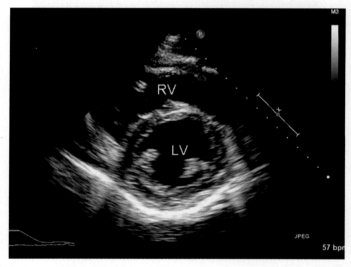

Figure 2.5 Parasternal short-axis window. LV, left ventricle; RV, right ventricle.

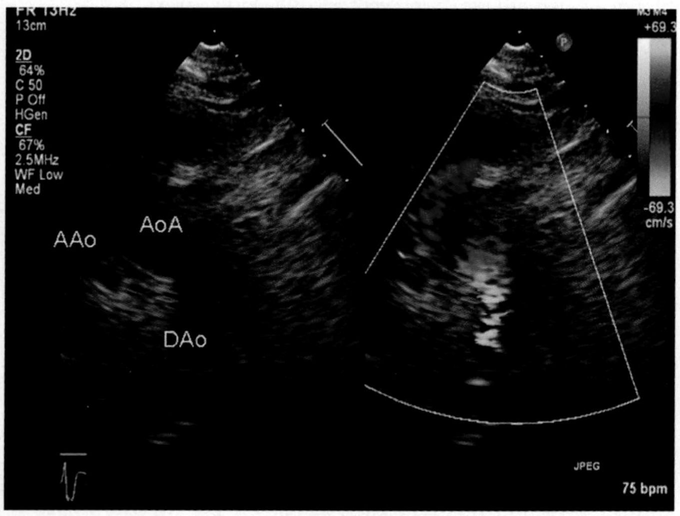

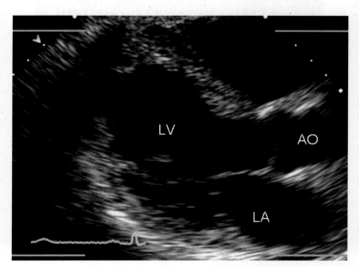

Figure 2.4 Suprasternal window showing the ascending aorta (AAo), left aortic arch (AoA), and descending aorta (DAo). Corresponding color Doppler image shown on the right panel.

Figure 2.6 Parasternal long-axis window. LA, Left atrium; LV, left ventricle; Ao, aorta.

In order to obtain the long axis of the RV and right atrium (RA), the probe must be tilted inferiorly and medially from the original position used to acquire the left parasternal long axis (Fig. 2.7). This view is used to evaluate the tricuspid valve structure as well as tricuspid valve regurgitation and RV pressure.

From the apical transducer position, one can acquire the long-axis four, five-, two-, and three-chamber views. The four-chamber image is obtained by placing the transducer at the maximal impulse and directing the transducer pointer down toward the floor while tilting the top of the probe inferolaterally. This will result in a four-chamber image with the LV and LA on the right side of the image. The LV in the four-chamber is comprised of the septal, apical, and lateral wall segments. Again the sonographer must make fine movements of the transducer to "open" up the LV and avoid foreshortening, which will underestimate the size and function (Figs. 2.8 and 2.9). By rotating the transducer slightly clockwise the LVOT and aortic valve will come into the image; this represents the five-chamber view (Fig. 2.10). Rotating the transducer counterclockwise 70 to 90° from the four-chamber view will produce the two-chamber view (Fig. 2.11). This allows

for evaluation of the anterior, apical, and inferior wall segments of the LV. Rotation of the transducer further in the counterclockwise direction will "open" the LVOT and produce the apical three-chamber view (Fig. 2.12).

The subcostal window can be very useful when a patient has lung disease and the chest windows are inadequate. The subcostal views are obtained by positioning the transducer in the midline below the last ribs. Directing the pointer of the transducer down toward the exam table and bringing down the end of the probe toward the patient reveal the hepatic veins and inferior vena cava (IVC). To further examine the IVC, the transducer can be rotated to the right flank of the patient, which will allow to show a true

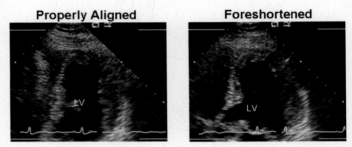

Figure 2.9 Example of foreshortened and properly aligned apical four-chamber images.

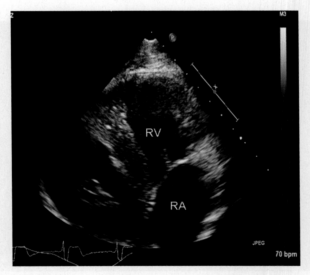

Figure 2.7 Parasternal long axis of RV and RA. RV, right ventricle; RA, right atrium.

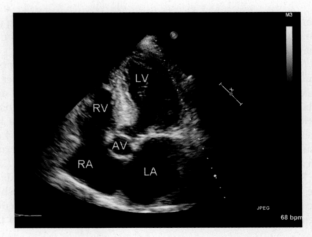

Figure 2.10 Apical five-chamber image. RV, right ventricle; RA, right atrium; LA, left atrium; LV, left ventricle, AV, aortic valve.

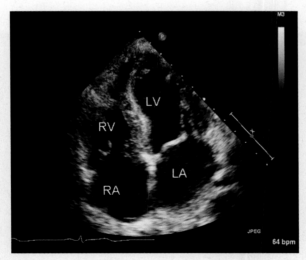

Figure 2.8 Apical four-chamber image. RV, right ventricle; RA, right atrium; LA, left atrium; LV, left ventricle.

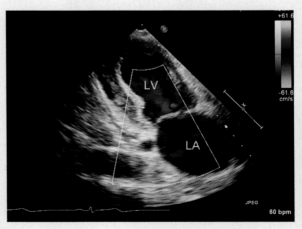

Figure 2.11 Apical two-chamber image. LA, left atrium; LV, left ventricle.

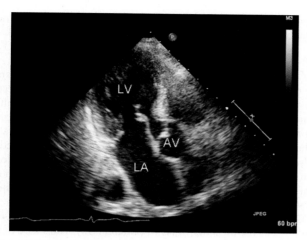

Figure 2.12 Apical three-chamber image. LV, left ventricle; LA, left atrium; AV, aortic valve.

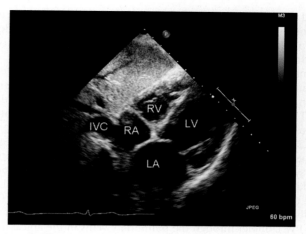

Figure 2.13 Subcostal four-chamber image. RV, right ventricle; RA, right atrium; LA, left atrium; LV, left ventricle; IVC, inferior vena cava.

long axis of this vessel. The subcostal four-chamber can also be viewed by tilting the transducer superiorly to the left midclavicle. This produces an image that is similar to the apical four-chamber but rotated 90° clockwise (Fig. 2.13). This is an optimal view for evaluating the interatrial septum as well as pericardial effusions.

M-mode echocardiography still continues to play an important role in the diagnostic exam, although at a substantially limited function. M-mode has the ability to delineate cardiac structures and allows another point of view to evaluate cardiac function. The best M-mode images are acquired by first obtaining a two-dimensional echocardiographic image and then placing the cursor through the region of interest (Fig. 2.14). M-mode is complimentary to the two-dimensional and Doppler examination. M-mode is used to help assess left ventricular function, cardiomyopathies, valvular disease as well as pericardial disease. An M-mode through the LV in the parasternal long axis two-dimension imaging plane allows for function evaluation. Functional measurements of the LV including end-diastolic volume and left ventricular end-

systolic volume can be obtained from M-mode images, but these estimated measurements are unreliable in patients with regional wall motion abnormalities or distorted ventricular geometries. M-mode evaluation of systolic anterior motion (SAM) of the mitral valve in hypertrophic cardiomyopathy (HCM), premature closure of the mitral valve in aortic regurgitation, and right ventricular diastolic compression in tamponade are paramount in the diagnosis of these pathologies.

2.3. Pulsed Doppler examination

Doppler echocardiography is used for the evaluation of pressure gradients, valvular stenosis, and regurgitation by measuring blood flow velocities in the different chambers of the heart. The three modalities of Doppler that are used are PW, CW, and color.

PW Doppler uses one crystal that intermittently emits a short ultrasound wave and pauses to receive the reflected signal prior to emitting the next ultrasound wave. This has several clinical applications including evaluating diastolic function, LVOT velocities,

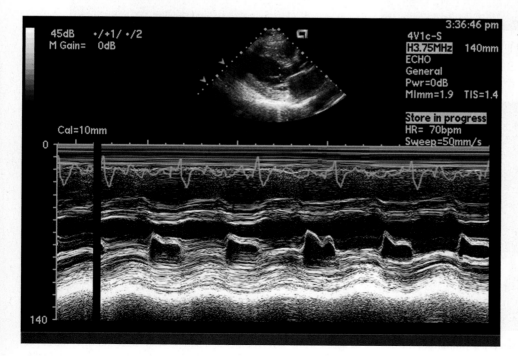

Figure 2.14 M-mode image obtained from the parasternal long-axis view at the level of the mitral leaflet tips.

and mitral inflow velocities. Specific measurements and calculations will be reviewed later in this chapter. Measurement is done by placing the sample volume in the region of interest.

Interrogation of the LV inflow is performed by placing the sample volume at the tips of the mitral valve in the apical four-chamber view. This gives the early LV filling (E) and atrial contraction (A) velocities as well as the mitral valve deceleration time (DT) (Fig. 2.15). These constitute the basic criteria for the evaluation of diastolic function (Chapter 16).

The mitral annular or myocardial longitudinal velocities may be examined by PW Doppler, and these are useful for evaluation of systolic and diastolic function. The sample volume is placed either at the medial or lateral annulus of the mitral valve. There are normally three velocity waves that are observed: systolic (S'), early diastolic (E'), and late diastolic (A') (Fig. 2.16).

PW Doppler through the pulmonary veins in the apical four-chamber view is also useful for the evaluation of diastolic function. The normal pulmonary venous flow pattern has typically three phases and three to four waves. The antegrade systolic flow can contain one or two waves (S1 and S2), the diastolic antegrade flow correspondent to ventricular diastole (D), and the retrograde atrial flow correspondent to atrial contraction (AR, Fig. 2.17).

2.4. Continuous wave Doppler examination

CW Doppler uses two crystals in the transducer, one which emits the ultrasound wave and the other which receives the reflected wave. The transducer is constantly emitting and receiving ultrasound waves. It also has numerous clinical applications. By placing the sample volume through the aortic valve or mitral valve, either regurgitation or stenosis can be determined. Compared to pulsed Doppler, CW Doppler cannot be obtained at specific location and provides the maximal velocity across a pathway. On the other hand, it allows detecting high velocity ranges, such as those present across stenotic valves.

CW Doppler is also used for the evaluation of dynamic LVOT gradients in the presence of HCM (Chapter 35). The shape of the curve seen in HCM patients is typically "dagger" like (Fig. 2.18).

The use of echocardiography for the evaluation of pulmonary hypertension is very common and easy. This is accomplished by using CW Doppler through the tricuspid valve. This measures the velocity of the tricuspid regurgitation which in turn can be used for the calculation of right ventricular systolic pressure (RVSP) using the simplified Bernouilli equation: $\Delta P = 4V^2$.

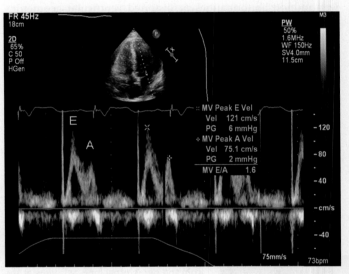

Figure 2.15 PW Doppler of mitral valve inflow. E, early LV filling; A, atrial contraction.

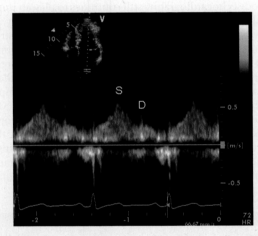

Figure 2.17 PW Doppler recording of the right pulmonary venous flow.

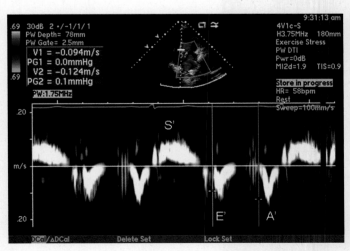

Figure 2.16 PW Doppler obtained at the basal septum from the apical four-chamber view.

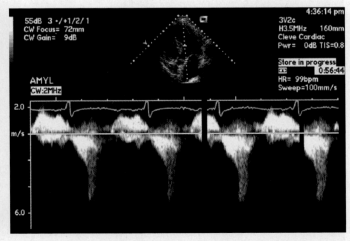

Figure 2.18 CW Doppler of a patient with HCM and dynamic LV outflow tract obstruction, showing the typical "dagger" like appearance.

2.5. Color Doppler examination

Color Doppler is the most common form of Doppler used in cardiac evaluation. It is used mostly for the assessment of valvular regurgitation. The velocity and direction of blood is assessed from a two-dimensional map of color-encoded velocities. If there is blood flowing toward the transducer the color will appear red, and if the flow of blood is away from the transducer the color will appear blue, as long as these do not exceed the Nyquist limit determined by the pulsed repetition frequency (Chapter 1).

Visual assessment of regurgitation using color Doppler is common practice in determining its severity (Fig. 2.19). It can also be used to evaluate the direction of the regurgitant jet in the case of mitral valve regurgitation, which can aid the surgeon in determining whether or not the valve can be repaired or if it has to be replaced. Color Doppler is also used for the evaluation of patent foramen ovale, atrial or ventricular septal defects, which are assessed using the subcostal four-chamber view.

Color M-Mode Doppler echocardiography has several uses including evaluation of diastolic function[10] as well as regurgitation and intracavitary obstruction. Color M-mode of the left ventricular inflow (Fig. 2.20) and PW Doppler of the mitral inflow, pulmonary veins, and mitral anulus make up the Doppler criteria for diastolic dysfunction (Chapter 16).

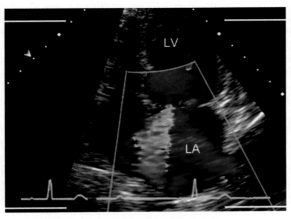

Figure 2.19 Color Doppler obtained in a patient with moderate MR. LA, left atrium; LV, left ventricle.

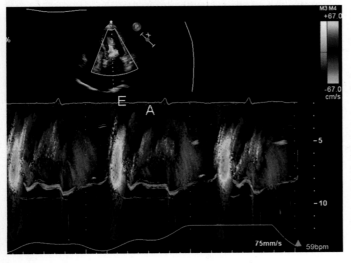

Figure 2.20 Color M-mode Doppler of the LV inflow.

3. TRANSESOPHAGEAL EXAMINATION

3.1. Patient preparation

Transesophageal echocardiography has become a very valuable diagnostic tool for multiple indications and has opened a new window to the heart that was not available before its existence. Unlike conventional transthoracic echocardiography, transesophageal echocardiography is a semi-invasive procedure that should be performed only by a properly trained physician who understands the contraindications and the potential complications of the procedure. In addition to being performed by highly skilled physician with advanced level II or level III training, the transesophageal study should be performed in a properly equipped room. The room should have an oxygen outlet and suction facilities. Oximetry should be available to be used in all patients who receive sedation, especially those with lung disease. The policies on procedure of different laboratories vary significantly and all of them should reflect the attention to detail that should be placed when performing a potentially harmful procedure. The patient should receive instruction via conversation or pamphlets prior to having the procedure. Different guidelines exist as to the fasting time the patient should be on, which is typically 4-8 h of fasting for a full meal, so most patients in whom these studies are performed in the morning are kept Nil Per Os (NPO) after midnight.

The majority of patients receive moderate sedation and Joint Commission on Accreditation of Healthcare Organizations (JCAHO) mandates that an assessment for moderate sedation be performed prior to the procedure. In addition, a "time out" or verification of the patient's identity, the procedure to be performed, and two forms of identity need to be verified by the team involved in the procedure prior to starting. Following informed consent, moderate conscious sedation as well as topical anesthesia of the hypopharynx is attempted. A 20-gauge intravenous cannula is inserted for administration of medications as well as for injection of agitated saline for contrast studies. Lidocaine hydrochloride is routinely used for topical anesthesia, which should cover the posterior pharynx and the tongue. Particular care should be taken to ask the patient to advance the tongue forward to reach areas of the hypopharynx, otherwise the patient will not be properly anesthetized. For moderate sedation, most laboratories utilize midazolam or diprivan and fentanyl with the assistance of anesthesiology for deeper sedation. It is greatly important that reversing agents are also available at the time of the study.

Conscious sedation is utilized in approximately 85% of the patients in the United States. The goal of the sedation is to make the procedure comfortable to the patient; however, it is important to maintain a low level of sedation not only for safety reasons, but also because the patients will be often asked to perform certain actions during the test. This is particularly important when evaluating patients for the presence of patent foramen ovale and maneuvers such as Valsalva or cough will be required from those patients in order to obtain an adequate study.

The practice of utilization of anticholinergic agents is abandoned in most laboratories. Salivation is handled by suction. In addition, antibiotic prophylaxis is not used routinely even in the patient with prosthetic heart valves.

3.2. Two-dimensional imaging plates

With the advances of transesophageal echocardiography transducers and particularly with the use of multiplane steering probes, the number of potential planes and views is virtually infinite. For that reason, it is important to follow a clear and precise protocol that can be consistent throughout. Although the main objective of the transesophageal echocardiogram is to answer the clinical questions, accreditation of laboratory depends on that the sequence as well as all anatomical structures will be investigated in every study.

There are several imaging views or sides as well as different imaging planes within the view. Those imaging views can be grouped as basal, four-chamber, transgastric, and aortic views. The basal views are obtained with a transesophageal probe located in the mid esophagus. By flexing and making appropriate contact with the esophagus, a short-axis view of the aortic valve, LA, superior vena cava, pulmonary artery, RV, and RA can typically be seen (Fig. 2.21).

The aortic valve is best visualized at an angle of 45° to 50°. In that same view, the left main is normally visualized as well as a small portion of the right coronary artery. The three leaflets of the aortic valve should be clearly seen in this view. By withdrawing the probe slightly, excellent views of the left atrial appendage (LAA) can be obtained. The LAA has a comma shape with the apex pointing anteriorly (Fig. 2.22). The gut pectinate muscles can be easily identified and need to be differentiated from small thrombi. An adequate scanning of the LA implies different imaging views from 0° all the way to 130°. In the same plane, located more anteriorly, the pulmonary artery and pulmonary valve can be seen. The actual bifurcation of the main pulmonary artery is often obtained and also up to 6 or 7 cm of the right pulmonary artery. This view can be particularly useful for the detection of pulmonary embolism.

The RA, interatrial septum, and LA are also visualized from the basal views. The four-chamber views are obtained at different levels of the esophagus with the transducer being more parallel to the main axis of the esophagus. Although these pose the risk of losing contact with the esophagus, it is actually the best way to obtain views of the LV and RV (Fig. 2.23). The entire LV can be visualized by moving the transducer from 0° to 180°. The images obtained are equivalent to four-chamber, two-chamber, and apical long-axis views. Typically, the apex is in the far field and is not visualized well, thus transesophageal echocardiography (TEE) should not be considered the test of choice to evaluate for an apical thrombus.

The mitral valve is seen very well from the midesophageal position. Normally the depth will be reduced or mechanisms to increase the resolution will be implemented. Once again, a continuous sweep from 0° to 180° would allow one to identify the individual scallops of the anterior and posterior mitral leaflets. Appropriate knowledge of the anatomy of the scallops is extremely useful to help guide mitral valve repair both preoperatively and intraoperatively.

At 120° to 150°, an optimal view of the LVOT could be obtained and is easily able to identify the ascending aorta and the aortic valve for evaluation of aortic regurgitation.

Transgastric views are obtained after careful advancement of the transesophageal probe into the stomach and using some degree of flexion. Short axis of the LV and RV can be obtained (Fig. 2.24). These are very useful views to monitor ischemia during noncardiac surgery. From the transgastric views, both LV and RV can be visualized in both short-axis and long-axis views. The mitral valve can also be assessed from the transgastric views and the relation of the leaflets and the commissures is probably best accomplished from this view.

One of the main uses of the transesophageal echocardiography is to visualize the thoracic aorta. The ascending aorta is very well visualized by TEE; approximately up to 4 to 5 cm above the aortic annulus can be seen on almost every study from the midesophageal views at 120° to 150°. By rotating the probe, it is easy to obtain short-axis sections of the descending aorta. Particular care needs to be given to examine and withdraw the probe very slowly to scan the entire thoracic aorta both horizontally and longitudinally by moving the transesophageal steering plane.

The aortic arch can also be well visualized and it is typically seen when the circular shape of the descending aorta turns into

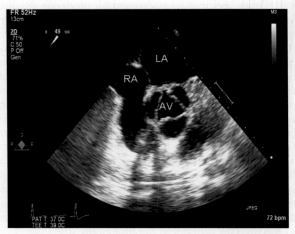

Figure 2.21 Transesophageal echocardiographic short-axis view of the aortic valve. RA, right atrium; LA, left atrium; AV, aortic valve.

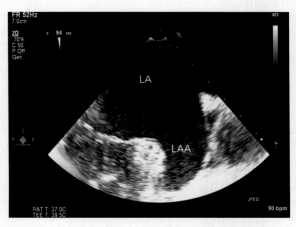

Figure 2.22 Transesophageal echocardiographic view of the LAA. LA, left atrium; LAA, left atrial appendage.

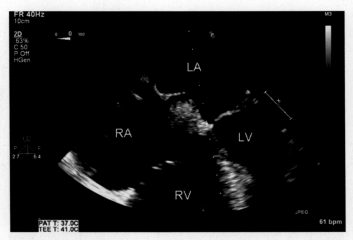

Figure 2.23 Transesophageal echocardiographic four-chamber view. RV, right ventricle; RA, right atrium; LA, left atrium; LV, left ventricle.

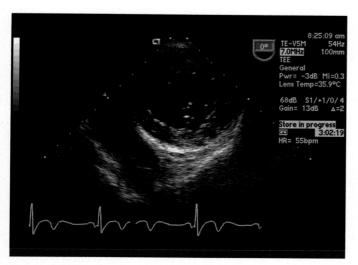

Figure 2.24 Transgastric echocardiographic short-axis view of the LV.

a more oval shape image. Also, important landmarks are the innominate and the left subclavian artery.

A blind zone between the ascending aorta and the aortic arch is always present during transesophageal examinations due to the interposition of the trachea. This may be an obstacle to visualize very localized type II aortic dissections; however, this is rather exceptional.

3.3. Pulsed Doppler examination

PW Doppler is utilized during transesophageal echocardiography as much as it is in transthoracic echocardiography. Certain structures that are visualized primarily with transesophageal echo are more the subject of Doppler interrogation. Specifically, PW Doppler is utilized to interrogate the pulmonary veins. Two to four pulmonary veins may be interrogated in each study. Color flow Doppler can be very useful to guide the placement of the PW Doppler sample at the point of maximal velocity or highest color hue. Careful examination of the pulmonary venous flow pattern can be utilized to evaluate diastolic parameters of both the LA and the LV.

In addition, one of the main uses of pulmonary venous flow analysis is the estimation or semiquantitation of mitral regurgitation (MR). Systolic reversal of the antegrade component is a very specific sign of severe MR. It is very important to be able to evaluate the flow in the four pulmonary veins or at the minimum two pulmonary veins, one in either side when evaluating eccentric mitral regurgitant jets. The determinants of the different components of the pulmonary vein flows have been extensively studied and these components are influenced by several factors including rhythm, left ventricular systolic function, cardiac output, diastolic properties of the LV, and left atrial pressures.

Another structure that is uniquely evaluated with PW Doppler during transesophageal examinations is the LAA. Until the advent of transesophageal echocardiography, the LAA could be hardly visualized and certainly could not be examined. Transesophageal echocardiography provides excellent visualization of this small, but important structure.[11,12] The LAA contains 90% of the thrombi that are formed in patients with atrial fibrillation; therefore, its examination is essential for risk stratification. In addition, PW Doppler can be very useful to evaluate also the mechanical function of the LAA. Several studies have shown that the magnitude of the LAA velocities is in direct relation to

the contractile properties of this structure.[13-15] In addition, it is possible to evaluate the fibrillatory waves and count the number of contractions per minute in patients with atrial arrhythmias such as atrial fibrillation or flutter. Studies have also shown that when there is a stagnant flow in the LAA, the velocities tend to be significantly decreased. Low atrial appendage velocities have been considered a marker for blood stagnation and therefore thrombus formation in patients with atrial fibrillation or atrial dysfunction. Because of the careful evaluation of LAA flow, it has been possible to demonstrate the stagnant or stunning status of the LAA following cardioversion. Following cardioversion, the electrical activity may be resumed but the mechanical activity of the LAA may take weeks to resume. That has been associated with a vulnerable period for thromboembolism and has explained the need for anticoagulation in the postcardioversion period. Typically, the LAA velocities as well as the more organized A wave of the mitral inflow may be decreased immediately following cardioversion and those velocities would increase as the mechanical activity recovers.

Limited visualization of the coronary arteries may be obtained from a transesophageal echocardiogram. The left main coronary artery can be visualized in over 95% of the individuals. The bifurcation between left anterior descending (LAD) and circumflex is also readily visualized. Because of the course of the left anterior descending artery parallel to the Doppler beam, it is quite often possible to measure coronary artery flow. Typical coronary artery flow has two components, systolic and diastolic with a diastolic predominance. Several studies have utilized this technique to calculate and evaluate coronary flow reserve.[16] This is a rather simple technique by which after obtaining baseline coronary artery flow, a vasodilator can be intravenously injected and the ratio of postvasodilator and prevasodilator velocities is a surrogate of a coronary flow reserve. Dipyridamole and adenosine have been utilized for that purpose.

Mitral inflow can certainly be obtained from the four-chamber view by placing the sample volume either at the annulus or at the tips of the mitral leaflets. Depending on different protocols, some laboratories prefer to invert the spectral display to make them similar to images obtained by transthoracic echocardiography. The parameters that are typically utilized are similar to those in transthoracic including E and A wave DT and E velocity variation. The use of an AccuMeter can be very helpful to visualize variations that occurred during the respiratory cycle. However, in the absence of the respirometer, a low sweep recording speed (25 to 30 m/s) can be utilized to look for those with significant variations. Such variations become important in cases of suspected constrictive pericarditis.

As it was mentioned previously, diastolic function evaluation can be obtained by combining mitral inflow velocities with pulmonary venous flow velocities. Several earlier studies showed that the combination can be very helpful although some of these parameters have become obsolete following the clinical inauguration of Doppler tissue imaging, which is typically not available in most transesophageal probes.

3.4. Continuous wave Doppler examination

CW Doppler has multiple applications during transesophageal echocardiography.

The most common utilization probably is the estimation of the RVSP or pulmonary artery pressure based on the tricuspid regurgitation velocity. Although tricuspid regurgitation is probably best visualized in the four-chamber view, the best way to align the CW Doppler beam with most of tricuspid regurgitant jets is by looking at the tricuspid valve from a 90° angle. Obviously, the operator needs to take into account the Doppler angle between the main direction of the regurgitation and the Doppler beam, not to underestimate the true velocity of the tricuspid regurgitation. Again, different protocols determine whether the spectral Doppler is inverted or not for the measurement of tricuspid regurgitation.

Another very common use for the CW Doppler during transesophageal echocardiography is the calculation of the severity of MR. CW Doppler of the mitral regurgitant jet is an intrinsical part to calculate the regurgitant volume (RV) by the proximal isovelocity surface area (PISA) method. Therefore, again, particular care should be taken to align the mitral regurgitant jet with a CW Doppler beam to obtain an adequate Doppler envelope that can be traced for PISA calculations.

CW Doppler of the MR can also be utilized to semiquantitate the severity of MR. The intensity and duration of the signal (not the velocity) are proportional to the amount of regurgitant flow. It also can be very helpful to quantitate the mitral regurgitant jet. Typically, mitral valve prolapse jets tend to be late systolic and can be clearly seen in CW Doppler displays. By looking at the intensity of the jet, CW Doppler can be helpful in discerning whether the regurgitant jet area represents a significant regurgitant jet or not. Finally, the spectral display obtained with CW Doppler of the MR can be utilized to calculate the DP/Dt, which is an index of left ventricular contractility.

Doppler can also be utilized to calculate the aortic valve gradient in aortic stenosis. Transesophageal echocardiography is not always suitable for this assessment since it is often difficult to be parallel to the main direction of the aortic stenosis jet. Color flow Doppler can be very useful on such evaluation. The most successful imaging planes are transgastric views with extreme retroflection at 0° or mild anteflexion at a 90° angle. Color flow Doppler can be useful to align the CW Doppler beam with area of maximal color disturbance.

3.5. Color Doppler examination

Color Doppler is by far the most common form of Doppler utilized in transesophageal echocardiography. It is virtually utilized in every single case to estimate the severity of valvular regurgitation or intracardiac shunts. Quantitative methods to assess MR are multiple including the maximal regurgitant area, the vena contracta, and the PISA method. Color flow Doppler is also particularly important to visualize the direction of a particular regurgitant jet, which could also give important clues to the mechanism of the regurgitation.

Flail leaflets tend to create very eccentric jets that loose their momentum when in contact with the atrial walls, an effect known as the Coanda effect. Depending on the imaging plane, some of these eccentric and flattened jets can look very small thus underestimating the severity of regurgitation.

Color flow Doppler can be virtually utilized for the evaluation of regurgitation of any of the four valves. For tricuspid regurgitation, the midesophageal view with a 0° (four-chamber) or 90° angle is probably the most effective. For the evaluation of aortic regurgitation, a short-axis view of the aortic valve at 50° is utilized to measure the area of the regurgitant jet. At 180°, the ratio of the LVOT to the aortic regurgitation jet width is the preferred view for such estimation. Pulmonary regurgitation can be seen both in a short-axis view at 0° or a longitudinal view at 90°.

For the evaluation of the mitral valve, color flow Doppler is essential not only to quantitate the severity of the jet, but also to evaluate the mechanism of MR. This is of particular importance when evaluating prior to mitral valve repair. Obtaining short-axis views of the mitral valve with superimposed color Doppler provides excellent visualization of the scallops involved in the MR mechanism.

4. STRESS ECHOCARDIOGRAPHY

Stress echocardiography is one of the most challenging modalities in the practice of echocardiography. The difficulties are multiple including the need to acquire and interpret appropriately regional wall motion abnormalities, the need to acquire transient events such as ischemia in a very short period of time, and finally the ability to acquire and display the images in a way where baseline and peak stress images are easily comparable side by side. In clinical practice, there are two main modalities of stress echocardiography: exercise echocardiography performed either on a treadmill[17] or bicycle[18] and pharmacologic stress testing performed primarily by dobutamine,[19] although alternatively dipyridamole[20] echocardiography can also be used. For exercise stress echocardiography there are several protocols available. The most common treadmill protocols are Bruce and modified Bruce. Most echocardiography laboratories would require patients to be fasting for at least 2 to 3 h prior to the procedure.

For dobutamine echocardiography, there are multiple protocols depending on the objective of the stress test. The objectives can be separated in two main groups, those studies aimed to evaluate myocardial ischemia and those studies aimed to evaluate myocardial viability. Like with exercise echocardiography, most echocardiography laboratories require patients to be fasting 2 to 3 h prior to the performance of a dobutamine echocardiography exam.

4.1. Preparation of the patient

Because of the intrinsic risk of stress studies, stress echocardiograms need to be performed in specifically equipped rooms with the necessary space to comfortably accommodate a treadmill or a bicycle as well as an ultrasound machine and access to oxygen and resuscitation equipment. Studies also need to be performed under the supervision of qualified, trained personnel.

For an exercise treadmill stress echocardiographic exam the patient is prepared in the usual way: Most protocols call for discontinuation of anti-ischemic therapy for diagnostic studies, but not for prognostic studies. Standard positioning of the ECG electrodes is employed with slight modification of the apical electrodes to allow for the placement of the ultrasound probe. The exercise protocol should be selected in accordance with the exercise capacity of the patient. Exercise testing is always preferable to pharmacologic as long as the patient is able to exercise and patients should undergo maximal symptom-related stress whenever possible.

Echocardiographic images are obtained prior to the exercise and immediately after. The critical element of the success of the test is the ability to capture the poststress images as quickly as possible. That requires the room to be arranged in such a way that the bed can be close to the treadmill so that the patient can return to the bed and be scanned as quickly as possible after finishing the exercise portion. Optimally, all images should be obtained within 45 s of completion of the stress test.

Bicycle stress testing may be performed in either an upright or supine position. The preparation for the patient is similar or identical to that for a treadmill test. The main advantage of bicycle protocols is that they allow obtaining images through peak exercise, with the avoidance of "cool down" phenomenon. This has resulted in a slightly higher sensitivity noted in some comparative studies. However in the United States, bicycle protocols are less utilized due to the difficulty of patients to exercise on a bike versus walking on a treadmill.

The most common form of pharmacologic echocardiography in the United States is dobutamine stress. Dobutamine is usually administered incrementally starting at a dose of 5 mcg/kg/min and increasing up to 40 mcg in 3-min stages. Occasionally, the peak dose can be increased up to 50 mcg/kg/min. In diagnostic studies where induction of ischemia is the goal of the study, atropine is commonly utilized in order to obtain an adequate heart rate blood pressure product.

Multiple protocols exist as to how to administer atropine, but the most successful ones include equal increments of atropine in early stages of the stress in order to create a rather smooth increase in heart rate. In patients, in whom, diagnosis of coronary artery disease is the reason for the study it is particularly important to discontinue β-blockade prior to the examination. In prognostic studies such as preoperative validation of treatments, etc., maintenance of β-blockers is widely accepted acknowledging that the studies may be negative at the heart rate blood pressure product obtained. This approach is particularly helpful when assessing patients preoperatively so that an adequate margin of ischemia-free heart rate range is to be known.

Dobutamine carries some side effects that reflect consequences of sympathomimetic stimulation. The most common side effects include hypotension, headache, anxiety, and arrhythmias. The most common arrhythmias are ventricular extrasystoles and non-sustained atrial arrhythmias. Ventricular fibrillation and death have been reported. Since dobutamine is a β-mimetic and therefore a vasodilator, it is not uncommon to develop no change in blood pressure or hypotension at the end of the peak dose. In patients that have been fasting and are relatively hypovolemic, dobutamine can induce dynamic LVOT obstruction. Unlike in exercise stress testing where the development of hypotension has a very ominous prognosis, in dobutamine stress testing it is a rather benign phenomenon.

4.2. Two-dimensional examination

The display of stress echocardiography is rather different from routine transthoracic echocardiography. The advent of digital echocardiography has revolutionized the use of stress echocardiography. Typically, images of the LV from different views are obtained in such a way that the 17 segments of the LV can be adequately displayed. The cornerstone of the interpretation of a stress echocardiography is the side-by-side comparison of the resting images to the peak images. In the case of exercise echocardiography, baseline images are compared to peak exercise images. In the case of dobutamine echocardiography, echocardiographic images are obtained and compared at the different dose stages of dobutamine. Different institutions have been using different protocols. There is more uniformity in the display of the exercise ECG.

By convention, the most commonly used views to evaluate the LV are the parasternal long-axis and short-axis views and an apical four-chamber and two-chamber view. More recently, some laboratories have been using only apical views to display all left ventricular segments. In those protocols, the apical long-axis view is added to the apical four-chamber and two-chamber views and parasternal views are not obtained at all. The rationale behind utilizing apical views only is that it allows one to obtain all peak images from one view which results in a shorter acquisition of the poststress images and avoids cool down. Regardless of the protocols employed, the digital displays include one or multiple cycles that are displayed side by side with corresponding views, that way

regional wall motion abnormalities at rest or peak exercise can be easily compared.

The American Society of Echocardiography has developed a wall motion score attributing a score to different regional wall motion abnormalities. That way quantitative measurement of the wall motion abnormalities per view can be compared and also serially followed. Many current reporting systems allow one to not only determine qualitative measurements of range (of the patient's regional wall motion abnormalities), but also the overall wall motion scoring of the different images obtained. With dobutamine echocardiography, the display is typically different and done in a wide screen format. Each screen represents four views corresponding to a particular stage of the test. Again, there is significant variation on the protocols and the times at which images are captured and also stored. The initial dobutamine protocols typically included baseline, low dose, peak dose, and recovery. Recently, many laboratories have switched to a display that includes baseline, intermediate stages and peak dobutamine dose. In order to easily compare wall motion abnormalities at different stages the final images are shuffled so that the same particular view is seen at the stages that have been predetermined per protocol, i.e., baseline, low dose, etc.

The interpretation of stress echocardiography relies primarily on the semiquantitative or quantitative interpretation of wall motion abnormalities. The presence or absence of wall motion abnormalities has to be analyzed at rest and at peak exercise when performing an exercise stress test. The LV is divided into 17 segments according to the new classification of the American Society of Echocardiography.[21,22] Different scoring systems have been utilized, but the most accepted is

1. Score of 1 for normal regions
2. Score of 2 for hypokinesis
3. Score of 3 for akinesis
4. Score of 4 for dyskinesis
5. Score of 5 for aneurysm

A score index per view or per ventricle can be developed by averaging the individual scores divided by the number of segments evaluated. In that way, serial studies are easily performed.

The normal response to exercise is an increase in global and segmental contractility. Some protocols call that hyperdynamic response. Depending on the threshold to increase sensitivity, a normal study would require all segments to become hyperdynamic. Some authors have considered a test abnormal if the contractility of a particular segment at peak exercise remains normal and not hyperdynamic. By using this criterion, sensitivity increases, but the specificity of the test significantly decreases.

Most commonly, ischemia is defined as the occurrence of new regional wall motion abnormalities. This is considered when a normal segment becomes hypokinetic, akinetic, or dyskinetic. Ischemia is also considered when there is a worsening of existing wall motion abnormalities. Obviously, the interpretation of worsening wall motion abnormalities is more difficult, requires more expertise, and certainly is subjected to a more widespread variability.

When using dobutamine echocardiography, other situations are commonly encountered. Some segments have wall motion abnormalities at rest but demonstrate continuous improvement during the infusion of dobutamine. Those segments are then considered viable, but nonischemic. Another response to dobutamine is what is known as the biphasic response, whereas a hypokinetic segment improves its contractility at low dose and worsens at peak dose. Those segments are then considered viable and ischemic and are the ones that respond best to revascularization. Finally, a segment that is abnormal at rest and does not change at low or peak dose dobutamine is considered infracted and nonviable. In patients who have an uncomplicated myocardial infarction and globally decreased left ventricular function, viability shown by stress echocardiography is associated with improved survival.[23]

4.3. Pulsed Doppler examination

Conventional Doppler, i.e., continuous or PW Doppler, is seldom used in routine stress echocardiography. However, it can be very useful in some specific indications and also in new emergent techniques. PW Doppler of the mitral inflow allows one to evaluate diastolic function along with a systolic function evaluation done based on wall motion analysis. Several studies have shown that ischemia may occur in the absence of systolic dysfunction. Ischemia may induce diastolic dysfunction post exercise compared to resting patterns. Some laboratories, therefore, routinely evaluate the mitral inflow pattern at rest and peak exercise and at rest and peak dobutamine. A more thorough analysis of diastolic function during stress testing can be done by obtaining not only mitral inflow patterns but also Doppler tissue analysis to estimate the left ventricular end-diastolic pressure. While these approaches are attractive from a physiologic standpoint, they are hard to apply in clinical practice, particularly in the case of exercise echocardiography where time is of the essence. However, with dobutamine echocardiography when the peak stage can be extended as necessary, those extra variables can be easily obtained and can add to the diagnostic armamentarium provided by stress echocardiography.

4.4. Continuous wave Doppler examination

Another common utilization of Doppler in stress echocardiography is CW Doppler for the evaluation of patients with aortic stenosis. Many patients with left ventricular dysfunction may have what is known as low-gradient aortic stenosis. Dobutamine studies can be utilized to risk-stratify and correctly classify those patients, so that the patients with primary cardiomyopathy versus those with cardiomyopathy secondary to aortic stenosis can be identified.

Some laboratories are very keen on routinely calculating pulmonary artery pressures during the performance of exercise echocardiography. Obviously, this is of great interest in patients with dyspnea on exertion and in those in whom pulmonary hypertension is of clinical significance.

For those calculations, CW Doppler of the tricuspid regurgitation, typically guided by color flow Doppler, is obtained at rest and the resting pulmonary artery pressure is then calculated. At peak exercise, the maximal tricuspid regurgitant jet velocity is again obtained and the peak exercise pulmonary artery pressure can be obtained.

CW Doppler is also very useful in the stress evaluation of patients with other valvulopathies. In addition to patients with aortic stenosis, those with mitral stenosis are occasionally stressed. Classic indications are discrepancies between symptoms and resting gradient in mitral valve areas (MVAs). Exercise echocardiography can be very useful in that particular setting and both the mean exercise mitral gradient as well as the peak pulmonary artery pressure can be obtained. Although these cases are uncommon given the scarcity of mitral stenosis and rheumatic heart disease in the United States, stress echocardiography is a valuable tool in the clinical management of those patients.[24]

4.5. Color Doppler examination

Color flow Doppler can also be utilized in conjunction with conventional two-dimensional stress echocardiography. The most common use of color Doppler is the evaluation of MR. Several studies have shown that ischemia may induce MR. In fact, some studies show that worsening MR is associated with the incidence of pulmonary edema,[25] as well as a higher sensitivity for ischemia. Only a few studies have shown this and color flow Doppler is not routinely utilized in most stress laboratories. One limitation that must be recognized is that the frame rate limitation of ultrasound systems during color Doppler imaging may difficult the visualization and quantification of regurgitant lesions at higher rates.

5. CONTRAST ECHOCARDIOGRAPHY

5.1. Contrast microbubbles: physical, chemical, and biological properties

Ultrasound contrast agents have a defined role in clinical echocardiography, patient management, and research. The currently approved echocardiographic agents share the common indication of left ventricular opacification and enhancement of left ventricular endocardial borders in patients with fairly difficult ECGs under resting conditions. Ultrasound contrast agents are made of microbubbles that possess thin and permeable shells and are filled with high molecular weight gas, i.e., perfluorocarbon with slow diffusion and dissolution within the blood stream. The two approved contrast agents on the market today are Definity and Optison. They both contain perfluten (octafluoropropane) as the gas in the core but they differ in their outer shells. Optison has an outer shell which consists of albumin, while Definity has an outer shell consisting of phospholipids. The size of both contrast agents is equal to that of a red blood cell measuring mostly <10 μm. Following an intravenous injection the microbubbles transit rapidly and reach the left-sided cardiac chambers and myocardium, which highlight left ventricular function or similar anatomies.

Both Definity and Optison have different protocols for injection. Definity is intended to be used only after it has been activated. Once it has warmed to room temperature the vial must be placed in a Vialmix, which is made to be used only for Definity. It has a 45 s mixing cycle, which is necessary for appropriate contrast activation. Once completed, Definity is given by bolus or by diluting 1.5 mL of activated contrast with 8.5 mL of preservative-free saline in a 10-mL syringe. The initial injection is up to 3 mL administered slowly over 10 s with a subsequent injection of 1 to 2 mL. The total dose of Definity should not exceed 1.6 mL.[26] Optison has a different preparation than that of Definity. Optison must also be refrigerated, allowed to warm, and comes in vials of 3 mL. The vial must be gently rotated in order to resuspend the contrast, which like Definity also becomes a milky white color. Optison is injected in doses of 0.5 mL at a time through either a 20-gauge or a larger intravenous catheter at a rate of ≤1 mL/s. Injection is followed by a saline flush. Doses can be given in increments of 0.5 mL for optimal images but cannot exceed more than 5 mL in any 10-min interval. The total dose should not exceed 8.7 mL in any given study.[27] Contrast agents should not be given to hemodynamically unstable patients or those with known cardiac shunts because of the theoretical risk of stroke.

The successful use of contrast agents requires a very adequate combined use of the appropriate ultrasound techniques along with the appropriate agents. In that regard advancements in both different contrast agents and ultrasound techniques have resulted in excellent results when combined appropriately. The interaction between microbubbles and ultrasound results in the oscillation of the microbubbles. That oscillation creates nonlinear components or harmonic imaging. Different specific contrast images can be obtained depending on the acoustic intensity or mechanical index of the ultrasound beam.

It is important to note that in addition to resonanance when ultrasound is applied, high intensity ultrasound will disrupt and eliminate most microbubble contrast agents. In fact, continuous imaging at high mechanical index results in the destruction of microbubbles. When this is utilized for left ventricular opacification, it may result in "swirling artifact." This effect is utilized when doing myocardial perfusion to obtain an area of destruction and replenishment by new bubbles.

5.2. Endocardial border enhancement

Real-time imaging of wall motion and left ventricular opacification can only be achieved with methods, such as low-mechanical index imaging, that protect bubbles without destroying them. A mechanical index of 0.7 and higher will likely destroy microbubbles and they cannot be used for ventricular border enhancement. Different techniques are accepted to modify the stream of echos and process from the linear scatters to nonlinear scatters. Techniques such as pulse inversion or amplitude modulations are utilized; therefore, bubbles can be detected in real time.

Clinical applications on several studies have demonstrated that the use of contrast echocardiography improves the readability, accuracy, and reproducibility of echocardiography for both qualitative and quantitative assessments of left ventricular structure and function (Fig. 2.25).[28] Contrast also facilitates the identification of intracardiac masses such as tumors and thrombi,[29] improved visualization of the RV, and can also be used to enhance Doppler signals utilized to evaluate above disease.

Initial studies with contrast agents employed fundamental ultrasound frequencies with relatively poor success. The combination of harmonic imaging revolutionized the use of contrast and made it effective in over 90% of clinically challenging studies. The use of contrast echocardiographic agents is particularly helpful in those patients in whom, due to body habitus such as obesity or lung disease or due to the special circumstances such as ventilators or critically ill patients, their images are presumably difficult.

For this reason contrast agents have also been shown to be particularly helpful with stress echocardiography. They are implemented in both exercise and dobutamine echocardiography

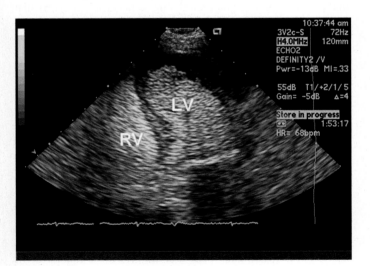

Figure 2.25 Image of contrast enhanced four-chamber view of the LV. RV, right ventricle; LV, left ventricle.

where defining wall motion abnormalities accurately is of critical importance.[30] Several studies have recently shown that contrast echocardiography significantly improves the correlation of left ventricular ejection fraction obtained by echocardiography compared to that with accepted "gold standards."[31] Contrast enhanced two-dimension echocardiography has excellent correlation with radionuclide, magnetic resonance, and CT measurements of left ventricular volumes and ejection fraction. Contrast echocardiography also significantly improves the interobserver variability as well as the confidence of the interpreting physician. Multiple studies have shown that the interobserver variability is related to the quality of the images. Therefore, contrast echocardiography decreases the interobserver variability by providing better quality images of the left ventricular or endocardial borders. The ability of contrast enhanced echocardiography to "rescue" any clinically difficult studies cannot be predicted from the baseline images. However, studies have shown that in several different groups of patients contrast echocardiography results in >90% success to evaluate both regional and global left ventricular function. This is of particular importance in those groups of patients in whom it traditionally is assumed that good images cannot be obtained. Particular interest is the group of the patients with significant or morbid obesity. Those patients are known to have a great percentage of cardiovascular abnormalities, but also at times cannot be properly assessed due to limitations posed by their own weight. In that regard ultrasound and contrast enhanced echocardiography appears particularly suitable, since there are no limitations based on weight, as there would be when they are subjected to techniques such as radionuclide imaging or left ventricular angiography.

5.3. Myocardial perfusion imaging

Because the compressed microbubbles can enter the myocardial vasculature, in theory they can be used to evaluate myocardial perfusion for detection of ischemia.[32] In addition they also have the ability to detect perfusion defects in patients with acute coronary syndromes.[33] If these contrast agents are able to detect myocardial infarctions by perfusion defects, it is reasonable to think that they also have the ability to detect viability. This has been shown in patients who have had myocardial infarctions and have hypokinetic myocardial segments with normal perfusion by contrast echocardiography. Contrast echocardiography can detect viability as well or better than dobutamine echocardiography and thallium scinigraphy.[34,35] However, clinical studies that have attempted to validate contrast ultrasound for these applications have yielded mixed results. Currently none of the commercially available agents are approved for these particular indications.

Two new agents are being evaluated in phase III research studies for evaluation of myocardial perfusion and diagnosis of coronary artery disease. Those are CARDIOsphere manufactured by POINT Biomedical Inc., San Carlos, California, and Imagify manufactured by Acusphere Inc, Watertown, Massachusetts. Their particular capsule structure that is relatively stiff makes those agents more suitable for intermittent harmonic power Doppler at higher levels of mechanical index.

The requirements of myocardial perfusion by echocardiography are different from those of left ventricular opacification. Myocardial perfusion requires the ability to deplete myocardial region of microspheres by a pulse of ultrasound, which destroys the microbubbles, and then assess the rapidity of replenishment as a surrogate for myocardial blood flow. Normally contrast can take up to five to seven cardiac cycles for myocardial replenishment, if it necessitates any longer it is pathologic. In another technique to obtain myocardial perfusion the bubbles are managed by a low mechanical index and they are not destroyed until a backward flow of contrast remains within the microvasculature bed.

Finally, another area where contrast echocardiography is being studied is in heart failure. Patients who present to the hospital with their first episode of decompensated heart failure and have no prior cardiac history have either an ischemic or nonischemic mechanism. Contrast echocardiography has shown to be able to correctly diagnose significant coronary atherosclerosis in this population with high sensitivity and specificity.[36]

6. ANALYSIS, CALCULATIONS, AND INTERPRETATION

6.1. Cardiac and vessel dimensions

Quantification in echocardiography is one of the most essential components of an adequately interpreted echocardiogram. One of the biggest criticisms of echocardiography over the years is that it is felt to be a very subjective operator dependent technique. Although there is a certain component of subjectivity in the way studies are performed, interpretation by ability can be substantially reduced by introducing quantitative parameters as often as possible. Quality of echocardiography reporting is very much linked to the amount of "thoughtful" quantifications. Because of the proliferation of mathematical algorithms and the ability of producing multiple numbers from certain ultrasound devices, many echocardiographic reports are cluttered with numbers of data that may or may not be meaningful to the clinician requesting the ECG.

Balancing clinical information and adequate quantification is extremely important in order to produce a quality echocardiographic report. This does not imply producing as many numbers as possible but rather utilizing meaningful numbers that will result in helping physicians using the echo services. In addition, quantification is a very important component of reproducibility and serial assessment of certain diseases. One of the most common parameters, i.e., left ventricular ejection fraction, is to be followed serially in many clinical circumstances. For an adequate quantification, it is essential that strict protocols are followed clinically. It is also essential that measurements are obtained according to strict guidelines. One of the most difficult areas in echocardiography is the performance of good, clean serial measurements to provide a longitudinal follow-up in patients' clinical conditions.

Different professional echocardiographic societies have provided their guidelines regarding common measurements and structures that should be routinely measured and therefore quantitative. Some of them have been implemented for many years and non-echocardiographer physicians are familiar with those. Examples of these are ejection fraction or left atrial size by diameter. Others have been introduced relatively recently and due to a variety of reasons including complexity of the parameter or difficulty in obtaining it accurately or simply lack of immediate clinical benefit result in less widespread understanding of these variables. Examples of these include regurgitant orifice area for aortic regurgitation, mitral valvuloplasty score, or dimensionless index for aortic valve stenosis. In order to present some of the most common clinically relevant quantitative parameters and formulas in echocardiography, we will go over those divided by two-dimensional and M-mode and Doppler and exercise stress quantifications.

The single most sought after echocardiographic parameter is the calculation of ejection fraction. This should be routinely calculated on every echocardiographic report as recommended by the American Society of Echocardiography. Reports indicating normal systolic function are probably not enough in a quality echocardiographic report. Over the years, multiple formulas have been devised to estimate left ventricular ejection fraction accurately. Some of the methods are based on M-mode parameters and some are based on two-dimensional parameters. Because the accuracy of the calculation of ejection fraction is related to the presence or absence of regional wall motion abnormalities, it is generally agreed that two-dimensional based methods are the most accurate and thus are recommended by the American Society of Echocardiography.

However, there are some single dimension based formulas that can be accurate in the absence of regional wall motion abnormalities or even in the presence of not very extensive regional wall motion abnormalities. An example of this is the ejection fraction calculated by the modified Quinones equation. This formula is based on the measurements of the end-diastolic diameter and the end-systolic diameter squared. In addition, the formula introduces a correction factor for apical contraction that goes from +15% given to a normal apical contraction to −10% given to a frankly dyskinetic apex. This particular formula is used routinely at the Mayo Clinic echocardiographic laboratory and has proved to be very accurate even in the presence of regional wall motion abnormalities. The formula is

$$\% \text{increment } D^2 = (\text{LVED } D^2 - \text{LVES } D^2)/(\text{LVED } D^2) \quad \text{(Eq. 2.1)}$$
$$\text{LVEF} = (\%\Delta D^2) + [(1 - \%\Delta D^2)(\%\Delta L)]$$

Simplified Quinones equation is as follows:

$$\text{LVEF} = (\text{LVED } D^2 - \text{LVES } D^2)/(\text{LVED } D^2 \times 100\% + K). \quad \text{(Eq. 2.2)}$$

LVEDD is the left ventricular end-diastole dimension; LVESD is left ventricular end-systolic dimension; and K is correction for apical contraction (10% normal apex, 5% hypokinetic apex, 0% akinetic apex, −5% dyskinetic apex, and −10% apical aneurysm).

These diastolic and systolic diameters can be obtained by M-mode, which is preferable to obtaining them by using calipers on two-dimensional images, so that the diameters obtained are perpendicular to the main axis of the longitudinal axis of the LV.

Another quantitative set of parameters relate to left ventricular geometry. These include the calculation of left ventricular mass and left ventricular mass index as well as an index of concentricity. In order to calculate all these parameters, one must classify them into four categories of left ventricular geometry, i.e., normal geometry, concentric remodeling, concentric left ventricular hypertrophy, and eccentric left ventricular hypertrophy.

The left ventricular mass can be calculated based on single dimension parameters and is also based on two-dimensional parameters. The American Society of Echocardiography's formula is as follows:

$$\begin{aligned}\text{Left ventricular mass (gram)} = {} & 0.8[1.04\,(\text{LVEDD} + \text{IVSD} + \text{PWD})3 \\ & - (\text{LVEDD})3] + 0.6 \end{aligned} \quad \text{(Eq. 2.3)}$$

where LVEDD is the left ventricular end-diastole diameter; IVSD is the thickness of the intraventricular septum in diastole; and PWD is the posterior wall thickness in diastole. The index of concentricity is calculated as:

$$\text{RWT} = 2 \times \text{PWD}/\text{LVEDD} \quad \text{(Eq. 2.4)}$$

where RWT stands for relative wall thickness. A relative wall thickness >0.42 classifies LV mass increase as concentric. The quantification of left ventricular mass and left ventricular mass index is of particular importance because the definition of left ventricular hypertrophy, which unfortunately is done by the majority of laboratories in an "eyeball fashion," should be based on the measurement of the left ventricular mass. Left ventricular hypertrophy is defined as increased left ventricular mass index. Unfortunately, in many laboratories that eyeball this parameter, the majority of hearts classified as left ventricular hypertrophy are really hearts with concentric left ventricular remodeling.

The third parameter that is becoming more and more important is the left atrial volume. Over the years, it is becoming clear that the traditional measurement of the left atrial diameter is inaccurate for the evaluation of the true left atrial size. Left atrial diameter assumes that the enlargement of the LA is uniform. However, multiple studies have shown that enlargement of the LA is certainly not uniform in all directions but rather follows a certain axis more than others. For that reason, evaluations of the left atrial volume are probably the most accurate and therefore constitute the goal standard for left atrial size. Surrogates of three-dimensional left atrial enlargement can be obtained by calculating the left atrial volume based on the biplane method. It is calculated by tracing the area of the LA in the four-chamber and in the two-chamber view. The left atrial volume formula is as follows:

$$LA\ volume = (0.85) \times A_1 \times A_2/L$$
$$\text{The left atrial volume index (LAVI)} = LA\ volume/BSA \tag{Eq. 2.5}$$

where A_1 is the maximal planimeter left atrial area in the apical four-chamber view and A_2 is the maximal planimeter left atrial area in the apical two-chamber view. L is the length measured from back wall to line across mitral valve hinge points. The apical four-chamber view and two-chamber view should be used in the equation.

6.2. Transvalvular flows and gradients

Transvalvular flows and gradients are based on Doppler echocardiographic imaging. Blood flow velocities across a valve can be measured by CW Doppler. It measures all velocities in its ultrasound path. Most measurements are acquired in the apical window where the three-, four-, and five-chamber views can be visualized. CW Doppler has the ability to measure blood flow velocities throughout the cardiac cycle, which includes reverse flow as well as forward flow. This allows one to examine both valvular stenosis and regurgitation. In addition to these measurements, these velocities can be used to determine pressure gradients across the valves to evaluate for stenosis[37] and therefore different intracardiac pressures as well.

In order to acquire the pressure gradient across a valve using the velocity obtained by CW Doppler, the modified Bernoulli equation is used:

$$\Delta P = 4(v_2 - v_1)^2. \tag{Eq. 2.6}$$

where v_2 is the peak velocity across at the valve orifice at that instant in time and $v1$ is the velocity proximal to the orifice, as determined by pulsed Doppler. In most clinical situations, $v1$ is negligible and the simplified Bernouilli equation is then used:

$$\Delta P = 4v_2^2. \tag{Eq. 2.7}$$

The velocity acquired is the maximal or peak velocity, which in turn correlates with the peak pressure gradient. Typically for the evaluation of valvular stenoses, the mean pressure gradient is the accepted measurement for examination and diagnosis. The mean gradient across a valve is the average pressure gradient throughout the entire cardiac cycle. This value is acquired by tracing the velocity outline on the CW Doppler image, which is then calculated and displayed by the built-in software on the echocardiography machine.

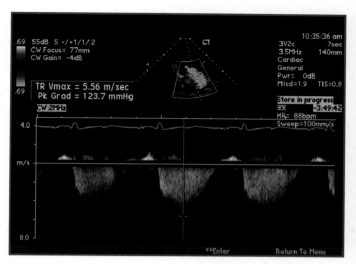

Figure 2.26 PW Doppler image through the tricuspid valve in a patient with severe pulmonary hypertension.

Transvalvular gradients are also used to determine intracardiac pressures. This noninvasive method has been validated by invasive catherization.[38,39] The most common and requested intracardiac pressure on an echocardiography exam is the RVSP, which is

$$RVSP = 4v^2 + RA\ pressure. \tag{Eq. 2.8}$$

This is obtained by placing the CW Doppler through the tricuspid valve to measure the velocity of regurgitation (Fig. 2.26). Again the velocity is plugged into the simplified Bernoulli equation above and then must be added to the RA pressure. The value of the RA pressure is dependent upon the IVC, which is imaged in the subcostal view. If the IVC is not dilated (<2 cm) and compresses, it is given a value between 5 and 10 mm Hg. If the IVC is either dilated or plethoric then the RA is given a value of 15 mm Hg. If finally the IVC is both dilated and plethoric, then a pressure of 20 mm Hg is used for the RA. In addition to the RVSP, several other intracardiac pressures can be evaluated by Doppler.

6.3. Valve area determination

One of the most important values which are acquired in an echocardiography examination is the valve area. The most common valve area which is evaluated is that of the aortic valve, since calcified aortic stenosis of the elderly is not uncommon. Mitral valve stenosis in the United States has become scarce secondary to the dramatic fall of rheumatic heart disease in the last half century. However, it is still occasionally seen in immigrants from second and third world countries. The aortic valve area (AVA) is calculated by using the continuity equation which is

$$A_1 \times V_1 = A_2 \times V_2 \tag{Eq. 2.9}$$

where A_1 is the known area proximal to the valve, which is taken at the LVOT; V_1 is the velocity measured proximal to the valve (LVOT); and V_2 is the maximal measured velocity of the aortic stenosis jet. Velocities are obtained using either CW or PW Doppler. With these known variables the AVA equation becomes

$$AVA = A_1 \times (V_1/V_2). \tag{Eq. 2.10}$$

MVA is evaluated by a different method, which is known as pressure half-time (PHT). This is the time it takes for the peak pressure gradient to reach half its original value.[40] This was originally evaluated by catheterization but has also been validated in echocardiography.[41] The MVA is related to PHT by the following equation:

$$MVA = 220/PHT. \tag{Eq. 2.11}$$

The simplest way of calculating the PHT is by using the DT obtained by CW Doppler of the mitral valve and using the following equation:

$$PHT = 0.29 \times DT. \tag{Eq. 2.12}$$

Using the PHT for the MVA and the continuity equation for the AVA in combination with the velocities and pressure gradients across the valves allows one to properly assess these valves for stenosis. PHT is also used to evaluate aortic regurgitation. If the PHT of the aortic regurgitation Doppler velocity is <250 ms, the degree of regurgitation is considered severe.[42,43]

6.4. Regurgitant flow and orifice calculations

One of the most frequent reasons for requesting an echocardiogram is the assessment of a murmur which was auscultated on a physical exam. Generally the amount of regurgitation found is trivial to mild but significant regurgitation is not too uncommon either. Severity of regurgitation is usually assessed by color Doppler in an "eyeball" fashion and is usually adequate; however, calculated regurgitant orifice areas and volumes are a necessity for a correct diagnosis. The most widely accepted and used method for evaluating valvular regurgitant orifice area is PISA.[44–46] This method is based on two concepts, the continuity principle and flow convergence. For example in MR, when blood is forced from the large ventricle through a small orifice, the blood accelerates until it reaches its maximal velocity at the narrowest portion of the orifice. The acceleration occurs at different levels of "hemispheres" where the center of the sphere is the orifice (Fig. 2.27). There are an infinite number of hemispheres of varying velocities as the blood converges upon the orifice. Following the continuity principle, the volume of blood moving through a conduit per unit time is called the flow rate, which is equal to the cross-sectional area multiplied by the velocity of the blood. Therefore, flow rate is equal at any particular hemisphere. Hence, we use the same equation which was used for defining the AVA:

$$A_1 \times V_1 = A_2 \times V_2 \tag{Eq. 2.13}$$

The continuity principle holds true for backward flow (regurgitation) as well as forward flow.

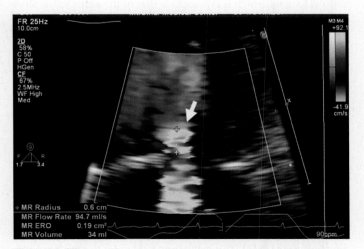

Figure 2.27 Color flow Doppler image obtained from a patient with severe MR demonstrating the hemispheric region of proximal flow convergence used for the calculation of regurgitant volume and orifice by the PISA method.

The initial step is to acquire the regurgitant jet by color Doppler. If we follow the example of MR, we will image the valve in the apical four-chamber view. Since the flow from the ventricle to the mitral valve is moving away from the probe, the color of the regurgitant blood will be blue until the blood reaches the aliasing velocity at which point the color turns orange-yellow. By adjusting the Nyquist limit, one can move the color transition point closer or farther away from the orifice. The Nyquist limit is defined as the velocity at which the color flow changes from blue to red or red to blue. If one measures the distance (radius) from the transition point to the center of the orifice, this gives the area for that particular hemisphere and thus allows one to calculate the area of the regurgitant orifice by the following equation:

$$A_{Hemisphere} = 2\pi r^2 \tag{Eq. 2.14}$$

It is important to measure the radius from the outer edge of blue to the center of the regurgitant orifice. The following step is to measure the maximal velocity of the MR jet at the regurgitant orifice by CW Doppler. Finally we can calculate the effective regurgitant orifice area (EROA) by using the continuity equation and modifying it with the values acquired as follows:

$$EROA \times V_{max\ at\ orifice} = 2\pi r^2 \times Nyquist\ limit_{velocity}$$
$$EROA = 2\pi r^2 \times Nyquist\ limit_{velocity} / V_{max\ at\ orifice} \tag{Eq. 2.15}$$

Once the EROA is calculated, the RV and regurgitant fraction (RF) are easily obtained. Since volume = area × velocity–time integral (VTI), one can trace the VTI of the MR jet on the CW image and then calculate the RV using the following equation:

$$RV = EROA \times VTI. \tag{Eq. 2.16}$$

Once this is known, then the mitral RF is calculated by the ratio of RV over total systemic stroke volume (Q_s). Systemic stroke volume equals LVOT area × LVOT VTI. Using these values, one can determine the severity of valvular regurgitation. Many of these calculations can be performed by the built-in software of the echocardiography machines. Along these lines, one can also calculate the significance of an intracardiac shunt by measuring the ratio of the pulmonic stroke volume to the systemic stroke volume with the following equation:

$$Q_p / Q_s = RVOT_{area} \times RVOT_{VTI} / LVOT_{area} \times LVOT_{VTI} \tag{Eq. 2.17}$$

If the ratio is >1.5, then the shunt is significant and closure is indicated.

7. FUTURE DIRECTIONS

As was reviewed in the introduction the roots of echocardiography are very old compared to the newer imaging technologies available, but this field continues to evolve and grow exponentially. Recently, three-dimensional echocardiography has begun to make its appearances in the clinical world. Left ventricular volumes assessed with contrast enhanced three-dimensional echocardiography were found to be similar to those values obtained with cardiac magnetic resonance imaging.[47] In addition, it can be utilized for the evaluation of valve areas,[48,49] as well as several other clinical indications. The utility of three-dimensional echocardiography has not reached the general cardiology world as yet. It remains mostly an investigative tool at most academic centers, while it is not being utilized at all in most community hospitals. Improvements in software, advantages over two-dimensional echocardiography, and increased knowledge in the community will aid in its acceptance and general use in the clinical setting. Another area of echocardiography which has a bright future and can revolutionize clinical care will be contrast perfusion imaging. With the advent of new contrast agents designed specifically for perfusion on the verge of gaining FDA approval in the near future, it opens a new realm of utility for echocardiography. As was mentioned previously, contrast echocardiography has shown the ability to detect ischemia[32] as well as perfusion defects in patients with acute coronary syndromes.[33] This could be another potential tool used in the emergency department setting for the rapid risk stratification of patients arriving with chest pain. These are evaluations that can be done at the bedside and offer a great advantage over more modern and expensive imaging modalities.

REFERENCES

1. Edler I, Lindstrom K. The history of echocardiography. *Ultrasound Med Biol.* 2004;30:1565–1644.
2. Effert S, Domanig E. Diagnosis of intra-auricular tumors & large thrombi with the aid of ultrasonic echography. *Dtsch Med Wochenschr.* 1959;84:6–8.
3. Satomura S. A study on examining the heart with ultrasonics. I Principles; II Instrument. *Jpn Circ J.* 1956;20:227–228.
4. Barber FE, Baker DW, Nation AW, et al. Ultrasonic duplex echo-Doppler scanner. *IEEE Trans Biomed Eng.* 1974;21:109–113.
5. Somer JC. Electronic sector scanning for ultrasonic diagnosis. *Ultrasonics.* 1968;6:153–159.
6. Bom N, Lancee CT, van Zwieten G, et al. Multiscan echocardiography. I. Technical description. *Circulation.* 1973;48:1066–1074.
7. Quinones MA, Douglas PS, Foster E, et al. American College of Cardiology/American Heart Association clinical competence statement on echocardiography: A report of the American College of Cardiology/American Heart Association/American College of Physicians–American Society of Internal Medicine Task Force on Clinical Competence. *Circulation.* 2003;107:1068–1089.
8. Henry WL, DeMaria A, Gramiak R, et al. Report of the American Society of Echocardiography Committee on Nomenclature and Standards in Two-dimensional Echocardiography. *Circulation.* 1980;62:212–217.
9. Tajik AJ, Seward JB, Hagler DJ, et al. Two-dimensional real-time ultrasonic imaging of the heart and great vessels. Technique, image orientation, structure identification, and validation. *Mayo Clin Proc.* 1978;53:271–303.
10. Garcia MJ, Smedira NG, Greenberg NL, et al. Color M-mode Doppler flow propagation velocity is a preload insensitive index of left ventricular relaxation: Animal and human validation. *J Am Coll Cardiol.* 2000;35:201–208.
11. Klein AL, Grimm RA, Murray RD, et al. Use of transesophageal echocardiography to guide cardioversion in patients with atrial fibrillation. *N Engl J Med.* 2001;344:1411–1420.
12. Klein AL, Grimm RA, Black IW, et al. Cardioversion guided by transesophageal echocardiography: The ACUTE Pilot Study. A randomized, controlled trial. assessment of cardioversion using transesophageal echocardiography. *Ann Intern Med.* 1997;126:200–209.
13. Garcia-Fernandez MA, Torrecilla EG, San Roman D, et al. Left atrial appendage Doppler flow patterns: Implications on thrombus formation. *Am Heart J.* 1992;124:955–961.
14. Li YH, Lai LP, Shyu KG, et al. Clinical implications of left atrial appendage flow patterns in nonrheumatic atrial fibrillation. *Chest.* 1994;105:748–752.
15. Heppell RM, Berkin KE, McLenachan JM, et al. Haemostatic and haemodynamic abnormalities associated with left atrial thrombosis in non-rheumatic atrial fibrillation. *Heart.* 1997;77:407–411.
16. Redberg RF, Sobol Y, Chou TM, et al. Adenosine-induced coronary vasodilation during transesophageal Doppler echocardiography. Rapid and safe measurement of coronary flow reserve ratio can predict significant left anterior descending coronary stenosis. *Circulation.* 1995;92:190–196.
17. Roger VL, Pellikka PA, Oh JK, et al. Stress echocardiography. Part I. Exercise echocardiography: Techniques, implementation, clinical applications, and correlations. *Mayo Clin Proc.* 1995;70:5–15.
18. Badruddin SM, Ahmad A, Mickelson J, et al. Supine bicycle versus post-treadmill exercise echocardiography in the detection of myocardial ischemia: A randomized single-blind crossover trial. *J Am Coll Cardiol.* 1999;33:1485–1490.
19. Ho FM, Huang PJ, Liau CS, et al. Dobutamine stress echocardiography compared with dipyridamole thallium-201 single-photon emission computed tomography in detecting coronary artery disease. *Eur Heart J.* 1995;16:570–575.
20. Fragasso G, Lu C, Dabrowski P, et al. Comparison of stress/rest myocardial perfusion tomography, dipyridamole and dobutamine stress echocardiography for the detection of coronary disease in hypertensive patients with chest pain and positive exercise test. *J Am Coll Cardiol.* 1999;34:441–447.
21. Lang RM, Bierig M, Devereux RB, et al. Recommendations for chamber quantification: A report from the American Society of Echocardiography's Guidelines and Standards Committee and the Chamber Quantification Writing Group, developed in conjunction with the European Association of Echocardiography, a branch of the European Society of Cardiology. *J Am Soc Echocardiogr.* 2005;18:1440–1463.
22. Cerqueira MD, Weissman NJ, Dilsizian V, et al. Standardized myocardial segmentation and nomenclature for tomographic imaging of the heart: A statement for healthcare professionals from the Cardiac Imaging Committee of the Council on Clinical Cardiology of the American Heart Association. *Circulation.* 2002;105:539–542.
23. Picano E, Sicari R, Landi P, et al. Prognostic value of myocardial viability in medically treated patients with global left ventricular dysfunction early after an acute uncomplicated myocardial infarction: A dobutamine stress echocardiographic study. *Circulation.* 1998;98:1078–1084.
24. Tunick PA, Freedberg RS, Gargiulo A, et al. Exercise Doppler echocardiography as an aid to clinical decision making in mitral valve disease. *J Am Soc Echocardiogr.* 1992;5:225–230.
25. Pierard LA, Lancellotti P. The role of ischemic mitral regurgitation in the pathogenesis of acute pulmonary edema. *N Engl J Med.* 2004;351:1627–1634.
26. Lantheus Medical Imaging I. Definity Package Insert. In; 2008.
27. GE Healthcare I. Optison Package Insert. In; 2008.
28. Thomson HL, Basmadjian AJ, Rainbird AJ, et al. Contrast echocardiography improves the accuracy and reproducibility of left ventricular remodeling measurements: a prospective, randomly assigned, blinded study. *J Am Coll Cardiol.* 2001;38:867–875.
29. Kirkpatrick JN, Wong T, Bednarz JE, et al. Differential diagnosis of cardiac masses using contrast echocardiographic perfusion imaging. *J Am Coll Cardiol.* 2004;43:1412–1419.
30. Rainbird AJ, Mulvagh SL, Oh JK, et al. Contrast dobutamine stress echocardiography: clinical practice assessment in 300 consecutive patients. *J Am Soc Echocardiogr.* 2001;14:378–385.
31. Hundley WG, Kizilbash AM, Afridi I, et al. Administration of an intravenous perfluorocarbon contrast agent improves echocardiographic determination of left ventricular volumes and ejection fraction: Comparison with cine magnetic resonance imaging. *J Am Coll Cardiol.* 1998;32:1426–1432.
32. Kaul S, Senior R, Dittrich H, et al. Detection of coronary artery disease with myocardial contrast echocardiography: Comparison with 99mTc-sestamibi single-photon emission computed tomography. *Circulation.* 1997;96:785–792.
33. Kang DH, Kang SJ, Song JM, et al. Efficacy of myocardial contrast echocardiography in the diagnosis and risk stratification of acute coronary syndrome. *Am J Cardiol.* 2005;96:1498–1502.
34. Shimoni S, Frangogiannis NG, Aggeli CJ, et al. Identification of hibernating myocardium with quantitative intravenous myocardial contrast echocardiography: Comparison with dobutamine echocardiography and thallium-201 scintigraphy. *Circulation.* 2003;107:538–544.
35. Nagueh SF, Vaduganathan P, Ali N, et al. Identification of hibernating myocardium: comparative accuracy of myocardial contrast echocardiography, rest-redistribution thallium-201 tomography and dobutamine echocardiography. *J Am Coll Cardiol.* 1997;29:985–993.
36. Senior R, Janardhanan R, Jeetley P, et al. Myocardial contrast echocardiography for distinguishing ischemic from nonischemic first-onset acute heart failure: Insights into the mechanism of acute heart failure. *Circulation.* 2005;112:1587–1593.
37. Currie PJ, Seward JB, Reeder GS, et al. Continuous-wave Doppler echocardiographic assessment of severity of calcific aortic stenosis: A simultaneous Doppler-catheter correlative study in 100 adult patients. *Circulation.* 1985;71:1162–1169.
38. Currie PJ, Seward JB, Chan KL, et al. Continuous wave Doppler determination of right ventricular pressure: A simultaneous Doppler-catheterization study in 127 patients. *J Am Coll Cardiol.* 1985;6:750–756.
39. Currie PJ, Hagler DJ, Seward JB, et al. Instantaneous pressure gradient: a simultaneous Doppler and dual catheter correlative study. *J Am Coll Cardiol.* 1986;7:800–806.
40. Libanoff AJ, Rodbard S. Atrioventricular pressure half-time. Measure of mitral valve orifice area. *Circulation.* 1968;38:144–150.
41. Hatle L, Angelsen B, Tromsdal A. Noninvasive assessment of atrioventricular pressure half-time by Doppler ultrasound. *Circulation.* 1979;60:1096–1104.
42. Labovitz AJ, Ferrara RP, Kern MJ, et al. Quantitative evaluation of aortic insufficiency by continuous wave Doppler echocardiography. *J Am Coll Cardiol.* 1986;8:1341–1347.
43. Samstad SO, Hegrenaes L, Skjaerpe T, et al. Half time of the diastolic aortoventricular pressure difference by continuous wave Doppler ultrasound: A measure of the severity of aortic regurgitation? *Br Heart J.* 1989;61:336–343.
44. Dujardin KS, Enriquez-Sarano M, Bailey KR, et al. Grading of mitral regurgitation by quantitative Doppler echocardiography: Calibration by left ventricular angiography in routine clinical practice. *Circulation.* 1997;96:3409–3415.
45. Tribouilloy CM, Enriquez-Sarano M, Fett SL, et al. Application of the proximal flow convergence method to calculate the effective regurgitant orifice area in aortic regurgitation. *J Am Coll Cardiol.* 1998;32:1032–1039.
46. Rivera JM, Vandervoort PM, Mele D, et al. Quantification of tricuspid regurgitation by means of the proximal flow convergence method: A clinical study. *Am Heart J.* 1994;127:1354–1362.
47. Jenkins C, Moir S, Chan J, et al. Left ventricular volume measurement with echocardiography: A comparison of left ventricular opacification, three-dimensional echocardiography, or both with magnetic resonance imaging. *Eur Heart J.* 2009 Jan; 30(1): 98–106.
48. Blot-Souletie N, Hebrard A, Acar P, et al. Comparison of accuracy of aortic valve area assessment in aortic stenosis by real time three-dimensional echocardiography in biplane mode versus two-dimensional transthoracic and transesophageal echocardiography. *Echocardiography.* 2007;24:1065–1072.
49. Zamorano J, Cordeiro P, Sugeng L, et al. Real-time three-dimensional echocardiography for rheumatic mitral valve stenosis evaluation: An accurate and novel approach. *J Am Coll Cardiol.* 2004;43:2091–2096.

3

The Vascular Ultrasound Examination

Susan M. Begelman

1. INTRODUCTION

1.1. Historical perspectives

Modern day use of Duplex ultrasound for the noninvasive diagnosis of vascular disease began in the 1950s and early 1960s with the advent and subsequent application of continuous wave (CW) Doppler to evaluate arteries.[1] The potential for noninvasive imaging would not be realized until the 1970s when advancements in technology allowed characterization of flow directionality and determination of vessel location within tissues.[2,3] Advances in signal processing allowing simultaneous display of Doppler information and B-mode (gray scale) images and development of a method to display blood flow in real-time using color occurred in the late 1970s and early 1980s.[4,5] Initially developed to assess the carotid circulation, application of duplex ultrasound, expanded to other vascular beds with later improvements in this technology. Today, duplex ultrasound is an essential tool for the noninvasive diagnosis of vascular disease.

1.2. General ultrasound principles

Duplex ultrasound combines gray scale imaging (B-mode, or brightness mode) and pulsed Doppler to enable vessel visualization and quantitative hemodynamic assessment. Waveform analysis includes evaluation of phase, shape and spectrum, and velocity (measurement of the latter is critical to interpret the degree of arterial stenosis). Normal peripheral arteries have triphasic appearance (Fig. 3.1). Each cardiac contraction results in forward flow, followed by flow reversal during early diastole and a second forward component (due to elastic recoil of the vessel) during late diastole. The flow within a normal vessel is laminar; blood cells travel within a limited range of speed resulting in a narrow Doppler waveform and a clear spectral window. However, at vessel bifurcations, curves, and within areas of stenosis, the range of speed with which blood cells travel increases, resulting in spectral broadening (Fig. 3.2). The Doppler waveform morphology also reflects the resistance to flow by the tissues supplied by that artery. High resistive signals are seen in arteries that have a low metabolic demand in the resting state (e.g., peripheral arteries when limb muscles are not being used, mesenteric arteries when an individual has been fasting); whereas arteries supplying the brain, liver, and kidney have low resistive signals (Figs. 3.3 and 3.4). A high resistive waveform is triphasic. A low resistive waveform will not exhibit a flow reversal component and will have continuous flow during diastole. Venous signals are more complex since they reflect body positioning, arterial flow, venous capacitance, muscle activity (specifically in the calf), and respiration. With proper patient positioning, the Doppler signal is phasic, due to respiration and cardiac pulsation (Fig. 3.5).

Color Doppler is a qualitative tool that can provide additional information for vessel identification (e.g., the presence of flow, differentiation of an artery from a vein from soft tissue) and detection of disease (e.g., color bruit due to vessel vibration, aliasing) (Fig. 3.2). Assignment of color is arbitrary and requires that the operator understands vessel orientation relative to the ultrasound beam. By convention, many laboratories choose to orient the transducer so that flow appears red within arteries and blue within veins.

Power Doppler, a method of color-flow imaging, displays signal intensity or power. While power Doppler cannot be used to determine flow direction, it is more sensitive in detecting presence or absence of any flow. It is less dependent on the Doppler beam angle of incidence and is not affected by aliasing. As a result, this modality is often used to assess a vessel for a high-grade stenosis versus complete occlusion and to detect the presence of collateral vessels.

1.3. General equipment and patient requirements

The Intersocietal Commission for the Accreditation of Vascular Laboratories published standards outlining required instrument characteristics for noninvasive vascular ultrasound testing (Table 3.1).[6] As the transducer frequency increases, detail resolution improves, but penetration decreases. Therefore, lower frequency transducers (e.g., 3 MHz) are required to study the aorta, mesenteric, and renal vessels, whereas higher frequency transducers (e.g., 5 to 10 MHz) are used to image the carotid and peripheral arteries. The degree of arterial stenosis is determined by measuring flow velocity calculated by the machine using the simplified Bernouilli equation (Table 3.2). The accuracy flow velocity and hence degree of stenosis depend on the magnitude of the Doppler angle of incidence, which is the angle between the long axis orientation of the vessel and the insonation beam of the transducer. A 90° angle is used during B-mode imaging. However, a 60° angle for vascular imaging with pulsed Doppler is optimal (Fig. 3.4). While measurement error is less significant with smaller angles, substantial measurement errors occur once the 60° angle is exceeded, since as the angle varies from 0° to 90°, the cosine decreases from 1 to 0 (see Chapter 1).

Once a vascular ultrasound is ordered, the patient is provided with information about test preparation and performance.[7] Each study will take 15 to 60 min to perform. The patient may feel some discomfort associated with the applied pressure of the transducer but there are no known associated risks with the performance of vascular ultrasound. It is recommended to inform the patient ahead of time that the results will not be immediately available upon test completion.

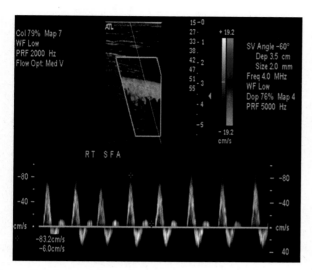

Figure 3.1 Image of a normal femoral artery obtained while the patient was resting comfortably. The triphasic waveform is characterized by reversal of flow in early diastole but absence of flow during late diastole. This is a high resistance signal.

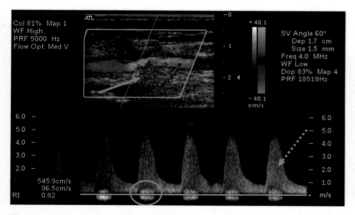

Figure 3.2 Image of an abnormal peripheral artery obtained while the patient was resting comfortably. Note the elevation in the PSV (545.9 cm/s), color bruit artifact (*solid arrow*), spectral broadening (*dotted arrow*), and Doppler bruit (*circle*). These findings are consistent with a 50% to 99% stenosis (the proximal arterial segment had a normal PSV).

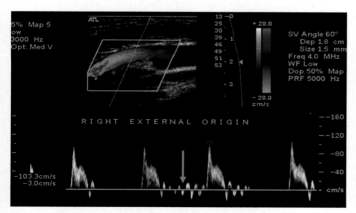

Figure 3.3 Normal waveform tracing of the ECA, which has a high resistive signal. The oscillations in the waveform (*arrow*) are due to the performance of a temporal tap.

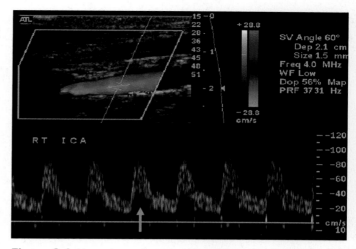

Figure 3.4 Normal waveform tracing of the ICA, which has a low resistive signal, obtained with an angle of insonation at 60°. Note the continuous flow throughout diastole. There is a clear spectral window and the velocity is below 100 cm/s, consistent with <50% ICA stenosis.

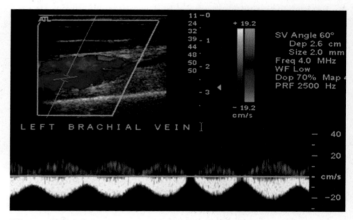

Figure 3.5 Normal spontaneous, phasic venous flow in the brachial vein **(bright signal)**. The faint signal is an artifact.

TABLE 3.1
REQUIRED INSTRUMENT CHARACTERISTICS

1. A range of imaging frequencies appropriate for the vessels and structures evaluated must be available
2. Doppler frequencies appropriate for the vessels evaluated must be available
3. Range-gated Doppler must be provided with the ability to adjust the position of the range gate within the area of interest
4. The Doppler angle must be measurable and adjustable
5. The instrument must provide a visual display and an audible output, as well as a permanent recording of the Doppler waveform and image

TABLE 3.2
THE DOPPLER EQUATION

$$f_D = \frac{2f_0 v \cos\theta}{c}$$

f_D is the Doppler frequency or shift (measured by the system);
f_0 is the transmit frequency;
v is the flow velocity;
θ is the Doppler angle;
c is the speed of sound (1,540 m/s in soft tissue);
2 reflects the roundtrip transmission of the sound beam.

2. CAROTID ARTERY EXAMINATION

2.1. Patient preparation

Access to the neck is required. Most often it is preferred that the patient changes into a gown. The patient should lie supine on the examination table with a small towel placed beneath the head so that the neck is slightly hyperextended, unless contraindicated or the patient is unable to do so (e.g., cervical arthritis). The patient should turn his head to the side contralateral to the one that will be scanned. Most carotid ultrasound studies will be performed using a high-frequency transducer (e.g., 7.5 MHz). Imaging may be limited in patients who have had recent neck surgery, have a dressing, sutures, or staples in the area to be examined, a history of neck radiation, and in those who are unable to lie flat, still, or extend their necks, and have thick and/or muscular necks. Sometimes visualization may improve by having the patient reach for his or her hips, which lowers the shoulders.

2.2. B-mode imaging

The study begins with a survey of the cervical vessels using transverse and longitudinal views to identify vessel anatomy and disease. Scanning begins at the base of the neck and proceeds up to the jaw to view the common carotid artery (CCA), internal carotid artery (ICA), external carotid artery (ECA), internal jugular vein (IJV), and vertebral artery. The right CCA originates from the innominate artery and its origin can be visualized in many patients. The origin of the left CCA, which comes off the aortic arch, is rarely observed. Using B-mode imaging, one can identify the IJV by its compressibility with light pressure. The CCA is more pulsatile, uniform in size, and has thicker walls.

The CCA typically bifurcates into the ICA and ECA at the level of C3–C4. The ECA lies in an anteromedial plane and is typically smaller than the ICA, which can be found in a posterolateral plane. The vertebral artery lies low in the neck and is seen in segments. The CCA may be used as a landmark to identify the vertebral artery by tipping the transducer head inferolaterally.

Once the vessels are identified, atherosclerotic plaque is documented if present, including its extent, location, contour, texture, and appearance. Echogenicity increases with increasing calcification; plaque with a large lipid component is less echogenic. Significant plaque calcification may produce acoustic shadowing, prohibiting visualization of the arterial lumen (Fig. 3.6). Homogeneous plaque has a uniform acoustic texture, whereas heterogeneous plaque has a complex acoustic appearance. While in most cases one is able to describe plaque surface as smooth or irregular, ulceration may not be accurately identified. Despite their reflective nature on ultrasound, stents can be visualized and their presence, location, and any architectural abnormalities, such as a stent fracture, should be noted.

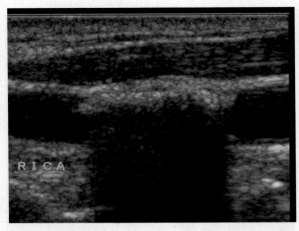

Figure 3.6 Calcified plaque in the ICA causes acoustic shadowing, prohibiting visualization of the vessel lumen.

2.3. Color Doppler examination

Color Doppler examination assists with vessel differentiation. Flow direction of the carotid artery and the IJV is represented by different colors. Cervical artery branches of the ECA help identify this artery since the ICA will not have branches in the neck. Color Doppler is used also to detect areas of flow disturbance when plaque or a dissection is present. A general imaging survey should be performed using this imaging modality. Flow separation, or boundary layer separation, is a normal flow disturbance within the carotid bulb in which flow reversal occurs at the posterolateral wall (Fig. 3.7). Low velocity flow through a narrow channel often occurs when high-grade stenosis is present. If color Doppler does not detect flow, power Doppler may be useful.

2.4. Pulsed Doppler examination

A complete examination of the CCA, ICA, ECA, and vertebral artery is required to record both peak systolic velocity (PSV) and end-diastolic velocity (EDV). Imaging the subclavian arteries bilaterally and the innominate artery is recommended since the information obtained is useful to interpret abnormal carotid waveforms. Using a 60°

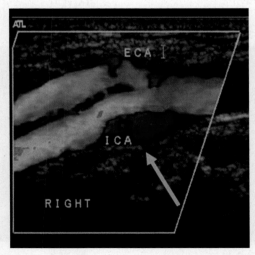

Figure 3.7 Color Doppler image from the carotid artery at the bifurcation. Flow separation, or boundary layer separation, within the carotid bulb results in flow reversal demonstrated in blue.

angle, small sample volume, and longitudinal view, the transducer is advanced along the arterial tree with a continuous sweeping motion. This approach decreases the likelihood that a short, focal stenosis will be missed. A smaller Doppler angle may be required if an artery is tortuous or to image the distal ICA since it often dives deep into the neck. Any change in the angle used should be documented for comparison of flow velocity at subsequent examinations.

The approach to imaging the cervical arteries using pulsed Doppler is similar to that described in Section 2.2. The normal CCA Doppler waveform morphology will appear to be a combination of both the low resistive ICA and the high resistive ECA. The CCA signal may change when a distal high-grade stenosis or occlusion is present. For example, the CCA may have a high resistive signal when the ICA is occluded due to shunting of blood to the ECA (Fig. 3.8). When this occurs, the contralateral CCA may demonstrate a compensatory rise in its EDV. Proximal disease also alters waveform morphology and comparison with the contralateral CCA assists in the proper diagnosis of the underlying pathology. For example, if the CCA has a stenosis at its origin, the detected waveform typically has an overall lower flow velocity with a longer time to peak (lower waveform slope or longer acceleration time [AT]) compared with the contralateral CCA waveform. Similar findings occur with right innominate artery stenosis. Additionally, waveform morphology reflects cardiac function. While tachycardia, bradycardia, and arrhythmias are easily identifiable, dampened waveforms may be due to low cardiac output (e.g., congestive heart failure, significant aortic stenosis) and aortic regurgitation can result in reflection of the waveform during diastole (Fig. 3.9). Changes due to cardiac disease should be detected in both carotid arteries.

Aside from waveform morphology there is a technique, which is useful to differentiate the ECA from the ICA. During the pulsed Doppler examination the sonographer places the index and middle fingers over the superficial temporal artery and with light pressure, repetitively compresses the vessel. Oscillations from this "temporal tap" will be reflected in the waveform if one is imaging the ECA, not ICA (Fig. 3.3).

ICA stenosis due to atherosclerosis most often occurs at the artery's origin and causes a velocity shift. The maximal velocity at the stenosis should be documented, as well as the prestenotic vessel segment length (waveform may be dampened), and the poststenotic vessel segment length (site of great turbulence and spectral broadening) (Fig. 3.10). An increase in compensatory

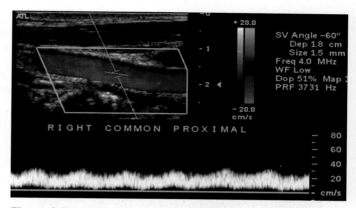

Figure 3.9 Low flow velocity with a long AT and a monophasic waveform, despite normal color flow and an artery that appears patent, is present when there is proximal disease as with innominate artery stenosis or cardiac disease (e.g., severe aortic stenosis, poor cardiac output).

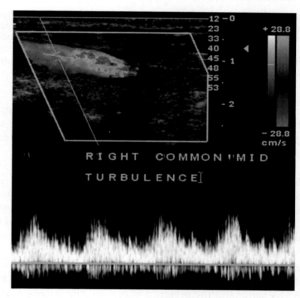

Figure 3.10 This is an example of poststenotic turbulence (documented in the CCA) demonstrated on both pulsed Doppler and color Doppler. There is a proximal CCA high-grade stenosis. Spectral broadening is also present.

flow may be present in the contralateral carotid artery. Although the distal ICA typically dives away from the transducer or is tortuous, it is important to image the ICA as distal as possible since some diseases, such as fibromuscular dysplasia, may develop in this location. If the signal in the distal ICA has a high resistive appearance, a siphon lesion, intracranial stenosis, or distal dissection may be present. A significant elevation in the EDV compared with the contralateral ICA suggests decreased resistance of distal vascular bed, for example, as seen with arteriovenous malformations. If the ICA is occluded, imaging the region just proximal to it will reveal an audible "thump" that is visually represented as a very low velocity, dampened waveform that has brief flow reversal that occurs when blood flow reaches the occlusion.

The vertebral artery is often difficult to examine due to its location, course as it runs through the vertebrae, small size, and frequent tortuosity. Similar to the ICA, the normal vertebral artery has a low resistive signal. Not only is it important to assess the presence of flow and waveform morphology to detect stenosis,

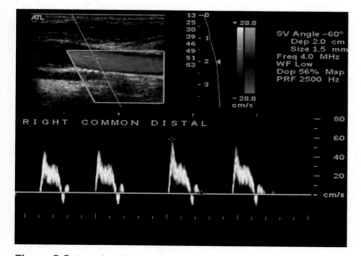

Figure 3.8 A triphasic high-resistive signal is seen in the distal CCA and has a similar appearance to the ECA (see Fig. 3.3). The ICA is occluded.

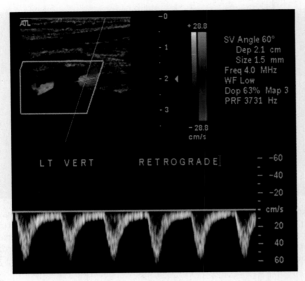

Figure 3.11 By convention, the left side of the screen is cephalad. Vertebral arterial flow should be toward the head, and in this image, to the left of the screen and away from the probe (negative velocity). However, blood is flowing toward the probe and hence, away from the head. This finding is consistent with subclavian steal due to a subclavian artery occlusion.

but also to document flow direction. Bidirectional or retrograde flow often results when there is proximal vertebral artery or subclavian artery (or innominate artery if imaging the right vertebral artery) stenosis or occlusion (Fig. 3.11).

2.5. Interpretation

Criteria for the determination of CCA, ECA, and vertebral artery stenosis have not been validated, but abnormalities in flow velocity, waveform morphology, and appearance should be documented and described in the study report. Centers may choose to use one of several published criteria or use criteria generated and validated at that facility to determine the degree of ICA stenosis. The key parameters employed are the ICA PSV, ICA EDV, the ICA/CCA PSV ratio, and the presence of plaque. The Society of Radiologists in Ultrasound published the following criteria in a 2003 consensus statement[8]:

1. There is <50% stenosis if the ICA PSV is <125 cm/s with plaque (secondary findings ICA/CCA ratio <2 and ICA EDV <40 cm/s); if no plaque is present the vessel is "normal."
2. There is 50% to 69% stenosis if the ICA PSV is 125 to 230 cm/s with plaque (secondary findings ICA/CCA ratio 2 to 4 and ICA EDV 40 to 100 cm/s).
3. There is >70% stenosis if the ICA PSV is >230 cm/s with plaque (secondary findings ICA/CCA ratio is >4 and ICA EDV is >100 cm/s).
4. There is 100% occlusion when there is no flow in the ICA with evidence of plaque (secondary finding ICA/CCA < 1).

Interpretation may be challenging in certain circumstances. Arrhythmias may cause inconsistent PSV measurement. Each laboratory should have a standard approach to study interpretation (e.g., use the highest PSV, average the PSVs). Heavily calcified plaque results in acoustic shadowing (Fig. 3.6). This prohibits penetration of the ultrasound wave and results in the inability to assess that segment of the artery. Velocity elevation naturally occurs due to vessel tortuosity or may result when a contralateral occlusion is present, resulting in overestimation of the degree of

TABLE 3.3
CHARACTERISTICS OF CAROTID IN-STENT RESTENOSIS

1. Focal increase in PSV and EDV
2. Increase in ICA/CCA ratio
3. Poststenotic turbulence
4. Diffuse spectral broadening
5. Diminished poststenotic velocities, often found within the stent
6. Luminal narrowing at site of a velocity shift and/or color bruit on color Doppler
7. Change in the audible Doppler signal at the area of stenosis and in region of poststenotic turbulence
8. Measurable change in PSV, EDV, and ICA/CCA ratio when compared with prior examinations

stenosis. Poor cardiac output will also affect the utility of ICA PSV velocity criteria. The ICA/CCA PSV ratio should preferentially be used in these cases. Lastly, generation of high velocities may not occur despite a high-grade arterial stenosis when tandem lesions or a long plaque is present. Interpretation of the study should comment on this finding.

The Doppler waveform within a stented carotid artery will have a similar morphology to the one seen in a native vessel. However, velocity elevations may be detected due to the placement of the stent (e.g., vessel angulation) or changes in vessel compliance in the absence of in-stent restenosis. Traditional ultrasound criteria may overestimate the degree of stenosis. Universally validated and reliable criteria are not available, but some centers have published site-specific criteria.[9,10] Several findings on examination are helpful in detecting stenosis in these cases (Table 3.3).[11]

3. AORTIC EXAMINATION

3.1. Patient preparation

The patient should be advised to fast beginning at midnight prior to the examination. Morning medications may be taken with a small amount of water. Often laboratories will specifically instruct the patient to avoid consuming gas-producing foods the day before the test and/or take an over-the-counter medication to reduce abdominal gas. For these reasons, it is preferred that these studies are scheduled earlier in the day. The patient should lie supine on the examination table. Minimal elevation of the head is permitted for comfort. Due to the depth of the aorta, a low-frequency transducer (e.g., 3 MHz) is best for obtaining images. Limitations to optimal imaging include recent abdominal surgery, abdominal fluid, bowel gas, and a large body habitus.

3.2. B-mode imaging

The abdominal aorta is generally uniform in size although it may taper just distal to the renal arteries. The aorta is located left of midline in the abdomen and runs along the spine, bifurcating into the iliac arteries at the level of the fourth lumbar vertebrae. A general survey using a longitudinal view permits rapid identification of an aneurysm, including its size (length) and shape (fusiform, saccular, or cylindrical). Next, using a transverse plane, a scan sweep is performed starting at the xiphoid process and the transducer is then slowly moved distally through the level of the common iliac arteries. The sonographer should inspect for evidence of any aneurysm (with or without thrombus), dissection, plaque, or other anomalies.

Once the survey is completed, the aorta at the level of the renal arteries and proximal, mid, and distal segments, including any enlarged area, are measured. The anteroposterior and lateral (transverse) measurements from outer wall to outer wall are recorded from the transverse plane (Fig. 3.12). Any change in the transducer angle from 90° with respect to the aortic wall will result in overestimation of the aortic diameter. Therefore, measurements are repeated from the longitudinal plane. Measurements of the iliac arteries obtained at their origin and proximal segments are recorded using a similar approach. Images of any plaque and/or mural thrombus are recorded. A dissection flap, if present, will appear as an echogenic, linear, mobile structure. Aortic stent grafts are moderately echogenic and may be visualized as well as any thrombus between the stent graft and vessel wall, if present. Fractures or kinking of the stent graft may also be seen.

3.3. Color Doppler examination

A general survey of the aorta and proximal iliac arteries conducted using color Doppler helps identify areas of stenosis with associated color flow disturbance, absence of flow if the aorta is occluded, layered mural thrombus in an aneurysm, and bidirectional flow in an area of a dissection. The aortic dimensions should never be measured from color Doppler. Color "bleeding," also known as a "blooming" effect, occurs with signal amplification and results in overestimation of aortic size. Although ultrasound cannot reliably detect the presence of a stent endoleak or its source, occasionally an endoleak may be identified.

3.4. Pulsed Doppler examination

Flow velocities are recorded using the sweeping technique at a 60° angle. The waveform should appear biphasic within the proximal aorta and triphasic distal to origin of the renal arteries. If a velocity shift is noted, the segments proximal and distal to it should be imaged. A drop in velocity can occur within an aneurysmal segment. Normal or elevated velocities may be detected within the true lumen of a dissection, while low velocities or absence of flow may be noted within the false lumen.

3.5. Interpretation

The normal abdominal aortic diameter varies based upon gender, age, and body size, but on average, it is approximately 2 cm (range 1.1 to 2.4 cm).[12] The anteroposterior aortic diameter is the most reliable measurement. An aneurysm is present if the aortic diameter is 1.5 times its normal size (a proximal, unaffected segment can be used as reference) or >3 cm (Fig. 3.12).[12] An ectatic aorta is one that appears enlarged but does not meet the definition of an aneurysm. The location of the aneurysm (suprarenal, juxtarenal, and infrarenal) should be documented. A dissection must be suspected when true and false lumens are seen during examination as noted previously. Infrequently, significant stenosis of the aorta occurs. It is diagnosed when there is a doubling in the PSV compared with a proximal normal segment, with distal turbulence, and evidence of plaque.

4. RENAL, CELIAC, AND MESENTERIC ARTERY EXAMINATION

4.1. Patient preparation

The patient should be advised to fast beginning at midnight prior to the examination. Preparation is similar as for the aortic examination. The patient should lie supine on the examination table. Minimal elevation of the head is permitted for comfort. Due to

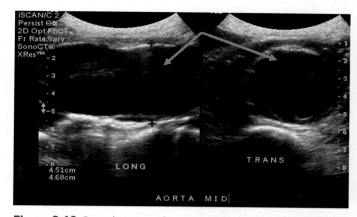

Figure 3.12 B-mode image of an abdominal aorta aneurysm in longitudinal (**left screen**) and transverse (**right screen**). There is significant mural thrombus (*arrows*) narrowing the flow channel.

the depth of the mesenteric and renal vessels, a low frequency transducer (e.g., 3 MHz) is best for obtaining images. Limitations to optimal imaging include recent abdominal surgery, abdominal fluid, bowel gas, a large body habitus, and respiratory disorders, which prohibit the patient from holding his/her breath or comfortably lying flat.

4.2. B-mode imaging

As with all vascular ultrasound examinations, the study begins by conducting a general survey of the vessels. Starting at the xiphoid process, the initial artery to come off the aorta is the celiac artery, which within several centimeters, bifurcates into the splenic and common hepatic arteries (the left gastric artery is rarely seen). Just distal to the origin of the celiac artery, the superior mesenteric artery (SMA) comes off the aorta and runs distally along its anterior surface (Fig. 3.13). As one continues to move the transducer toward the pelvis, first the right renal artery with its anterolateral takeoff followed by the left renal artery with its inferolateral takeoff are visualized before both arteries course posteriorly. The inferior mesenteric artery (IMA), which also arises from the anterior aorta, is typically diminutive in size and due to its location, may not be visualized in many patients unless the SMA is occluded.

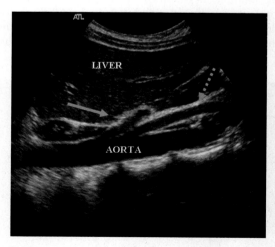

Figure 3.13 B-mode imaging is useful to identify vessels to be examined. The initial artery originating from the aorta is the celiac artery (*solid arrow*) and just distal to it, the SMA (*dotted arrow*), both off the anterior surface of the aorta. There is no clear evidence of plaque in either vessel and the aorta does not appear aneurysmal.

This survey should be conducted with both longitudinal and transverse views to identify the arteries and assess the aorta, mesenteric, and renal vessels for evidence of a dissection, aneurysm, or plaque. Additionally, accessory renal arteries may be found. During vessel identification and assessment, the patient should be imaged in a lateral decubitus position if segments of the vessels and/or the kidneys are difficult to visualize.

The renal artery ultrasound examination should include imaging of both kidneys. The average or the largest of at least three pole-to-pole measurements is recorded, depending upon the specific laboratory's protocol (normal is 9 to 12 cm). Evidence of hydronephrosis, cysts, calculi, masses, and necrosis may require a formal examination by a technologist and physician with expertise in abdominal imaging (Fig. 3.14). A transplanted kidney is typically found in the iliac fossa and when imaged is parallel to and in the same plane as the iliac vessels to which the renal vessels have been anastomosed.

4.3. Color Doppler examination

Color Doppler will assist in confirming vessel anatomy (e.g., differentiating between an artery and a vein and detecting anatomic variants) and identifying areas of stenosis. Bowel gas can produce a color bruit and should not be confused with color turbulence due to arterial disease. Retrograde flow in the hepatic artery suggests severe stenosis or occlusion of the celiac artery. Color Doppler examination is useful to evaluate renal parenchymal flow, especially when infarct of part or the entire kidney is suspected. A low velocity range (similar to a venous study) should be used with an increased sample volume to image the kidney. If no flow is detected in the kidney, power Doppler may detect tissue perfusion if present. Documentation of inferior vena cava (IVC) patency and renal vein patency (or iliac vein in the case of a renal transplant) should be recorded.

4.4. Pulsed Doppler examination

Abdominal imaging often requires breath holding to limit motion during imaging. When assessing the mesenteric and renal arteries, Doppler interrogation in the aorta is performed continuously recording velocities as one enters the branch vessels. This will ensure the detection of ostial stenosis. With a single continuous motion, velocities are recorded throughout each artery documenting multiple measurements to avoid missing focal disease. As in other studies, if a velocity shift is detected the velocity prior to and just distal to this shift must be recorded. Again, imaging with the patient in a lateral decubitus may improve results, as is

often the case when evaluating the distal renal artery and kidney. Complete and accurate measurements may be challenging; the use of angle correction should be documented if required to obtain velocities. Documentation of the velocity in the aorta at or just above the level of the renal arteries is needed to diagnosis renal artery stenosis (see Section 4.5).

Normally, the celiac artery, its branches (e.g., hepatic and splenic arteries), and the renal arteries have a low resistance flow pattern. The SMA and IMA arteries exhibit a high resistance flow pattern. If a low resistive signal is noted in these two arteries it is important to determine when the patient last consumed food. If the patient has fasted, mesenteric arterial disease should be suspected. Changes in renal artery waveform morphology may be due to renal artery disease or renal parenchymal disease. The patient should be asked to take a deep breath and/or sit up if a velocity shift is detected in the celiac artery. Persistently elevated velocities suggest a fixed stenosis. However, the patient likely has median arcuate ligament syndrome if velocities return to normal with inspiration.

Finally, a renal artery examination also includes assessment of renal parenchymal flow in the upper, mid, and lower poles using a 0° angle. Absence of flow suggests tissue infarction. The AT (time to PSV) and the resistive index (RI) [(PSV – EDV)/PSV] in each pole (Fig. 3.15) should be recorded. Intrinsic kidney disease, vessel occlusion, or accessory arteries supplying collateral flow can cause a high resistive, biphasic signal.

4.5. Interpretation

Velocity criteria vary by laboratory and most often are only validated for the celiac and superior mesenteric arteries. General agreement exists that significant stenosis, or a 70% to 99% diameter reduction, is present in the celiac artery when the PSV is at least 200 cm/s with an EDV of at least 55 cm/s and in the SMA when the PSV is at least 275 cm/s with an EDV of at least 45 cm/s in a fasting state.[13,14] Evidence of poststenotic turbulence should be present. Although criteria for IMA stenosis are not available, some laboratories apply SMA velocity criteria to interpret IMA velocities. The vessel is occluded when an artery is clearly visualized and color flow, as well as a Doppler signal, is absent.

A renal to aortic PSV ratio (RAR) is calculated using the PSV obtained within the aorta at the level of the renal arteries and the highest PSV within the renal artery. The RAR, in combination with the absolute PSV, is used to classify the degree of renal artery stenosis.[15]

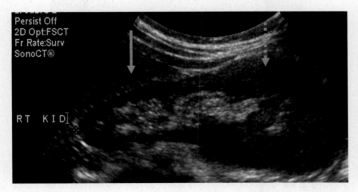

Figure 3.14 A B-mode examination to measure kidney size revealed that approximately half of it has atrophied (*solid arrow*; normal parenchyma is indicated by the *dotted arrow*). Confirmation of the absence of parenchymal flow should be performed with power Doppler and the ipsilateral renal artery examined for evidence of renal artery stenosis.

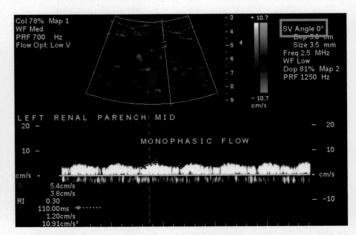

Figure 3.15 Assessment of renal parenchymal flow is performed with a 0° angle (*box*) and the RI and AT (*dotted arrow*) are calculated. Monophasic flow is detected with an AT of 110 ms. These findings are consistent with significant renal artery stenosis.

1. There is 0% to 59% stenosis of the renal artery if the RAR is <3.5 and the PSV is <200 cm/s.
2. There is 60% to 99% stenosis of the renal artery if the RAR is 3.5 or more, the PSV is >200 cm/s, or both are present.
3. There is 100% occlusion if the flow signal is absent and there is a low-amplitude parenchymal signal.

Additionally, an EDV of 150 cm/s or more is suggestive, but not diagnostic, of a high-grade (80% to 99%) stenosis.[15] These criteria may be applied to stented renal arteries. It is important to recognize that alterations in aortic flow velocity will affect the RAR measurement and hence, accuracy of stenosis assessment. When the aorta PSV is <40 cm/s (e.g., due to an aneurysm) or >100 cm/s (e.g., due to focal stenosis within the aorta), the likelihood of significant renal artery stenosis remains high if the PSV is >200 cm/s with evidence of turbulence on color flow. Similarly, this alternative criterion must be applied to the assessment of a transplanted renal artery since the vessel is anastomosed to the iliac artery, not the aorta.[16]

The RI in the renal parenchyma is normally 0.53 to 0.70. The RI increases in the presence of intrinsic renal disease or vessel obstruction, reaching 1 when end-diastolic flow is not detected (the waveform will have a high resistive signal). AT, measured off a single waveform from the onset of systolic blood flow to its peak, is normally <100 ms. An AT of 100 ms or more should increase one's suspicion that there is renal artery stenosis or that the kidney is perfused via collaterals (Fig. 3.15).

A kidney measuring <8 cm pole-to-pole or a 1.5 cm difference in size between the two kidneys suggests that the smaller of the two is diseased, possibly due to poor perfusion resulting from renal artery stenosis. Large kidneys may be seen in patients with diabetes and/or due to an error in measurement, for example when a cyst is present.

5. LOWER EXTREMITY ARTERIAL EXAMINATION

5.1. Patient preparation

The patient should be positioned supine on the examination table. Elevation of the head is permitted for comfort. Slight external rotation of the limb undergoing evaluation will facilitate performance of the examination. A 5 to 7.5 MHz linear transducer is most appropriate for this study. Any lower extremity duplex ultrasound performed for the assessment of peripheral arterial disease must be accompanied by the measurement of the ankle-brachial index (ABI).[17] Imaging may be limited due to a large body habitus, fresh surgical incisions, ulcers, trauma, staples, sutures, bandages, and casts.

5.2. B-mode imaging

The examination begins at the level of the distal external iliac artery (EIA) advancing the transducer distally toward the ankle. The transducer head must often be angled cephalad to visualize this segment. The common femoral artery (FA), origin of the profunda FA, the FA, and popliteal artery are then imaged. As one approaches Hunter canal the artery takes a deeper course. A patient may need to be placed in the prone position to view the distal superficial femoral artery (SFA) and popliteal artery. The origin of the anterior tibial (AT) and tibioperoneal trunk are then imaged. If it becomes difficult to identify these smaller vessels, the transducer should be positioned at the ankle and moved proximally up the leg. The posterior tibial (PT) artery is located posterior to the medial malleolus and the peroneal artery is located posterior to the lateral malleolus. The AT artery is found anterior to ankle along the tibia. During the examination the sonographer should look for evidence of vascular anomalies, plaque, dissection, stents, aneurysms, and bypass grafts.

5.3. Color Doppler examination

Color Doppler enables proper identification of the arteries. Detection of color flow disturbances suggests the presence of a stenosis. It is also a useful tool for following the course of a bypass graft.

5.4. Pulsed Doppler examination

Flow velocities are interrogated using the sweeping technique and a 60° angle in the longitudinal plane from multiple segments within each artery. Normally a high resistive, triphasic waveform will be present and PSVs will decrease as one moves from proximal to distal arteries (normal PSV ranging from 119.3 ± 21.7 cm/s in the EIA down to 68.8 ± 13.5 cm/s in the popliteal artery) (Fig. 3.1).[18] An increase in the PSV and the presence of spectral broadening are consistent with arterial stenosis (Fig. 3.2). Arterial calcification is present in many patients and may prevent adequate visualization of the arterial segment. This finding and its location should be recorded. When imaging arterial bypass grafts, note the PSV in the proximal native artery, at the proximal anastomosis, at multiple segments throughout the graft, at the distal anastomosis, and in the distal native vessel.[19]

5.5. Continuous wave Doppler examination

CW Doppler examination is conducted in isolation infrequently. More commonly, CW Doppler (e.g., 5 MHz) is used to measure the ABI in conjunction with a standard pneumatic blood pressure cuff. After the patient has rested for 5 to 10 min, the cuff is placed on the arm over the brachial artery and inflated. Using the CW Doppler the arterial pressure at which the signal is first audible is recorded. Measurements of the systolic pressure in the contralateral arm are then obtained. The cuff is then placed on the ankle and the CW Doppler over the AT artery and again, the pressure at which the signal is first audible is recorded. This process is repeated for the ipsilateral PT artery and contralateral AT and PT arteries. The ABI is calculated by dividing the highest ankle blood pressure by the highest brachial blood pressure for each limb, recording out to two decimal places (Table 3.4). The same brachial blood pressure should be used as the denominator for each leg.

5.6. Interpretation

Vascular ultrasound provides information regarding the anatomic location and severity of arterial stenosis. The latter is determined using the absolute PSV, PSV ratios within the artery (PSV distal/PSV proximal), and waveform morphology. As previously noted, a normal arterial signal is triphasic with a PSV within the normal range. A total occlusion is present when no flow (on color or pulsed Doppler) is detected. Proximal to the occlusion, flow may be monophasic with an audible "thump." Beyond the occlusion,

TABLE 3.4
CALCULATION OF THE ABI

Resting ABI	Right (mm Hg)	Left (mm Hg)
Brachial artery	130	120
Posterior tibial artery	120	70
Anterior tibial artery	110	90

Right ABI = 120 mm Hg/130 mm Hg = 0.92.
Left ABI = 90 mm Hg/130 mm Hg = 0.69.

diminished velocities and monophasic waveforms are typical. Recommended diagnostic criteria include[19]:

1. There is 1% to 19% stenosis when the PSV ratio is <2:1, the waveform is triphasic, and spectral broadening is present.
2. There is 20% to 49% stenosis when the PSV ratio is <2:1, the waveform is biphasic, and spectral broadening is present.
3. There is 50% to 99% stenosis when the PSV ratio is >2:1 (in other words, there is more than a 100% increase when compared with the proximal arterial segment), the waveform is monophasic, and spectral broadening is present (Fig. 3.2).

More than a 4:1 ratio suggests that there is >75% stenosis and more than a 7:1 ratio suggests that there is >90% stenosis.[19] Specific criteria to evaluate a stented artery have not been published so apply the general principles of velocity and waveform assessment. A variation of these criteria applies to grafts, although with several caveats. An extensive review of arterial bypass graft imaging and its interpretation is beyond the scope of this book.

The method for calculating the ABI is described in Section 5.5. In healthy individuals, the ankle pressure is normally 10 to 15 mm Hg higher than the brachial pressure due to pulse wave reflection. This results in normal ABIs that are >1.00. ABI interpretation is as follows[20]:

    1.30 Noncompressible
    1.00 to 1.29 Normal
    0.91 to 0.99 Borderline (equivocal)
    0.41 to 0.90 Mild-to-moderate arterial disease
    0.00 to 0.40 Severe arterial disease

Noncompressible vessels are due to medial calcification and most commonly occur in diabetic patients. This finding may be present in elderly patients and in individuals with chronic renal disease or who are on chronic steroid therapy.

6. VENOUS EXAMINATION

6.1. Patient preparation

The patient should be positioned supine on the examination table. The leg to be evaluated is slightly rotated and the patient is asked to slightly bend his knee. The table is placed in reverse Trendelenburg. Examination of the upper extremity requires that the table remains flat. The use of a 5 to 7.5 MHz linear transducer is recommended. Adequate venous assessment may be limited in the presence of trauma, open wounds, a large body habitus, casts or braces, and severe edema. Significant arthritis and other diseases may affect proper patient positioning. The clavicle and the presence of a central venous catheter are additional challenges to performing an adequate upper extremity evaluation.

6.2. B-mode imaging

Imaging in B-mode is essential to the diagnosis of a superficial or deep vein thrombosis (DVT). Vessels are imaged using a transverse scan plane. The lower extremity examination begins at the groin by angling the transducer cephalad to image the distal external iliac vein (EIV). The sonographer applies light pressure, enough to readily collapse the vein (Fig. 3.16), and continues down the medial thigh to image the common femoral vein (CFV), profunda femoral vein, femoral vein, and popliteal vein. As one approaches the distal thigh the vein will enter Hunter canal. To visualize the distal femoral vein and popliteal vein, a posterior approach may be required. It is important to look for anatomic variants to avoid

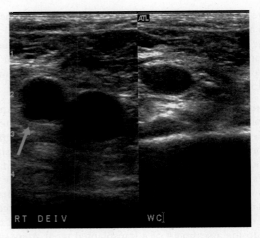

Figure 3.16 The EIA (*arrow*) and vein are visualized on the left frame. In the absence of a DVT, light pressure will collapse the EIV as demonstrated on the right frame.

missing a DVT since approximately one third of individuals have a duplicated femoral vein.[21]

Continuing behind the knee crease the examination proceeds down toward the ankle. It is important to recognize that the PT and peroneal veins are paired. Both must be imaged in order to avoid missing a DVT. The PT veins are found within the space between the Achilles tendon and medial malleolus; the peroneal veins are superficial to the fibula and are best viewed from a medial approach. AT veins, also paired, tend to be diminutive in size and, due to their location along the tibia, easily collapse and are rarely seen. The one or more pairs of gastrocnemial veins and one or more soleal veins should also be examined for thrombus. Compress the veins every 1 to 2 cm. Additionally, the small saphenous vein (drains into the popliteal vein) and the great saphenous vein (drains into the femoral vein) should be imaged along their courses to detect superficial venous thrombosis (SVT). When identified, the proximity of the SVT to the popliteal and femoral veins should be reported.

Similarly, imaging of the upper extremity veins is performed using a transverse scan plane, applying gentle pressure to collapse the vein segment, and recoding compression pictures every 1 to 2 cm. One may use a transducer with a smaller footprint if unable to image and compress the upper extremity veins in the chest due to the clavicle. The examination begins with the IJV and then proceeds down into the chest to image the brachiocephalic vein (due to the sternum it may only be seen in segments) before moving down the arm to the subclavian, axillary, and finally brachial vein. Abduction of the arm may improve visualization of the proximal axillary vein, while placing the arm in pledge position may assist with the assessment of the brachial and basilic veins. The cephalic vein (drains into the subclavian vein) and the basilic vein (drains into the brachial vein), like the superficial lower extremity veins, should be imaged. If a SVT is detected, its proximity to the deep vein into which it drains is then recorded.

6.3. Color Doppler examination

Color Doppler has a limited role in the assessment of the venous system. It is best employed to differentiate an artery from a vein and smaller veins, especially in the calf, from surrounding soft tissue. Color Doppler may help determine if a thrombus is partially or totally occlusive if the gain is set correctly.

6.4. Pulsed Doppler examination

Imaging of the venous system using pulsed Doppler is performed from a longitudinal view. The sonographer should listen and look for evidence of phasic (increases with expiration and decreases with inspiration), spontaneous flow without augmentation (Fig. 3.5). Distal limb compression should result in flow augmentation. If flow is not spontaneous or detectable, an obstruction may be present. Continuous monophasic flow suggests a partial proximal obstruction due to intrinsic disease (e.g., thrombus) or external compression (e.g., tumor, hematoma) (Fig. 3.17). Partial obstruction may be present distal to the probe if flow does not augment with limb compression. Cessation of flow with the performance of a Valsalva maneuver and/or proximal manual compression demonstrates valve competency. Increased flow pulsatility is seen when central venous pressure is increased. It is important to recognize that the Doppler signal may be normal if there is a nonocclusive thrombus. Finally, if a unilateral examination is performed, a Doppler waveform in the contralateral CFV or subclavian vein must be obtained.[22] For example, monophasic waveforms in both CFVs suggest disease in the IVC or proximal bilateral iliac veins.

6.5. Interpretation

Normal veins have smooth, thin walls, are echo free, and collapse with light pressure (Fig. 3.16). Loss of vein compressibility is the single most important ultrasound criterion for the detection of venous thrombosis (Fig. 3.18).[23] Echogenic material within the vein may be visualized when present (Fig. 3.18).

There is no accurate way to determine the age of a DVT on ultrasound although there are findings that are more consistent with acute thrombosis. These include venous dilation, free-floating thrombus (the proximal end of the thrombus does not adhere to the vein wall), and visible collaterals, especially when the thrombus is occlusive. Thrombus may be hypoechoic, or in some cases, anechoic. Older thrombus is more echogenic, adherent to and/or results in thickening of the vein wall, and the vein has a normal diameter or occasionally is atrophied. However, due to significant overlap in vein diameter, size alone cannot be used to determine the age of a thrombus and considerable interobserver variability assessing the aforementioned characteristics exists.[24,25]

Duplex ultrasound is not the ideal imaging modality to detect thrombus in the IVC, proximal iliac veins, and brachiocephalic veins due to the inability to compress these vessels because of their location.

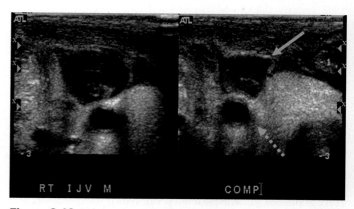

Figure 3.18 Echogenic material is seen within the IJV. Attempts to compress the vein are unsuccessful (*solid arrow*, **right frame**). This patient has a DVT. The other structure shown is the CCA (*dotted arrow*).

7. FUTURE DIRECTIONS

7.1. Carotid intima-media thickness

Carotid intima-media thickness (CIMT) measurements use B-mode imaging to identify and quantify subclinical vascular disease for the assessment of one's risk of cardiovascular disease (CVD; see Chapter 22). An imaging protocol, guidelines for study interpretation, and clinical applications of CIMT were recently published by the American Society of Echocardiography Carotid Intima-Media Thickness Task Force.[26] The patient should lie supine on the examination table. A towel roll is placed beneath the neck and the patient is asked to hyperextend and rotate his neck away from the side to be scanned. To standardize measurements, a 45° angle wedge for lateral neck rotation and a Meijer arc for the transducer angle are used. A high frequency transducer (e.g., at least 7 MHz) is required and the Task Force recommends using a scanning protocol from one of the large epidemiological studies reporting CIMT values by percentiles for gender, race/ethnicity, and age.

Current technology does not allow isolated measurement of true intima thickness. Therefore, a leading edge-to-leading edge technique is used to measure the far wall blood-intima and media-adventitia interface producing a "double line" pattern (Fig. 3.19).[27] An electrocardiogram captures R-wave gated frames with a longitudinal view of the distal 1 cm of the CCA for measurements to be performed. Repeated measurements at three different angles (anterior,

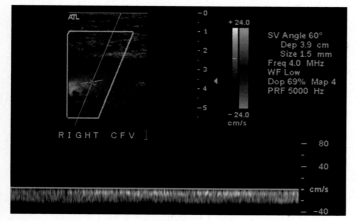

Figure 3.17 Continuous, monophasic flow in the CFV is consistent with proximal disease, either intrinsic (e.g., due to a DVT) or extrinsic (e.g., due to a tumor or large hematoma).

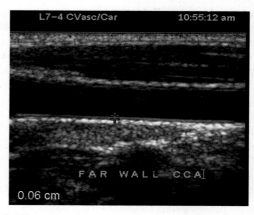

Figure 3.19 A CIMT is calculated with a leading edge-to-leading edge technique measuring the far wall blood-intima and media-adventitia interface. Note the "double line" pattern.

optimal angle of incidence or lateral, and posterior) bilaterally are obtained. Results are compared with normative tables. CIMT values less than or equal to the 25th age–gender-adjusted percentile are associated with lower CVD risk, values in the 25th to 75th percentile are average or unchanged CVD risk, and values in the 75th percentile or greater are considered increased CVD risk.[26] Currently, the number of centers with experienced vascular technologists and physicians to perform and interpret this examination remains limited.

7.2. Flow-mediated dilation in the brachial artery

The use of ultrasound to measure flow-mediated dilation (FMD) in the brachial artery for assessment of endothelial function was first described in 1989.[28] The International Brachial Artery Reactivity Task Force published guidelines for the performance, interpretation, and application of FMD.[29] Briefly, the patient must fast for 8 to 12 h and refrain from cigarette smoking on the day of the test. The patient should lie supine on the examination table in a room at ambient temperature for at least 15 min before beginning the test. A blood pressure cuff is placed on the proximal or mid-forearm. Using a high-frequency transducer (e.g., 7 to 12 MHz) and a 20° angle, measurements of arterial diameter and flow velocity are recorded. The use of electrocardiogram gating ensures that measurements are obtained at the same time during the cardiac cycle.

The cuff is inflated to at least 50 mm Hg above the individual's systolic pressure for 5 min, causing ischemia (the patient should be informed that he/she may feel discomfort prior to inflation). Measurements from the near to far wall of the intima-media surface are recorded at multiple time points once the cuff is deflated. Brachial artery diameter and flow should increase at least 6% and fivefold to sixfold respectively due to vessel dilation (reactive hyperemia).[30] Often the test is repeated with the administration of sublingual nitroglycerin to document endothelium-independent vasodilation. This study is technically challenging to perform, requiring a highly skilled ultrasound technologist and a dedicated laboratory. For now, FMD assessment remains a research tool.

7.3. Contrast-enhanced carotid ultrasound imaging

Contrast agents are approved by the Food and Drug Administration to image the heart. Physicians using these agents off-label for the performance of carotid ultrasound report improved visualization of the arterial lumen and plaque morphology (allowing detection of ulcers), enhanced visualization of the CIMT, and the ability to directly image the adventitial vasa vasorum (demonstrating that arterial nutrient flow emanates from it) and plaque neovascularization (a predictor of a vulnerable lesion).[31] The contrast agent is injected intravenously and circulates freely due to the small size of the microbubbles. As these microbubbles pass through capillary vessels within tissues they have a unique acoustic response to the ultrasound's harmonic frequencies and are easily detected.[32] If properly validated in the future, this imaging method may be used to detect preclinical atherosclerosis and monitor disease progression.

REFERENCES

1. Strandness DE Jr, McCutcheon EP, Rushmer RF. Application of a transcutaneous Doppler flowmeter in evaluation of occlusive arterial disease. *Surg Gynecol Obstet.* 1966;122:1039–1045.
2. Nippa JH, Hokanson DE, Lee DR, et al. Phase rotation for separating forward and reverse blood velocity signals. *IEEE Trans Sonics Ultrasonics.* 1975;22(suppl):340–346.
3. Baker DSW. Pulsed ultrasonic Doppler blood flow sensing. *IEEE Trans Biomed Eng.* 1970;17:170–185.
4. Philips DJ, Powers JE, Eyer MK, et al. Detection of peripheral vascular disease using the duplex scanner III. *Ultrasound Med Biol.* 1980;6:205–218.
5. Brandestini MA, Forster FK. Blood flow imaging using a discrete-time frequency analyzer. *Ultrasonics Symp Proc IEEE.* 1978;1344(suppl):287–293.
6. http://www.icavl.org/icavl/apply/standards.htm
7. Yesenko SL, Whitelaw SM, Gornik HL. Testing in the noninvasive vascular laboratory. *Circulation.* 2007;115:e624–e626.
8. Grant EG, Benson CB, Moneta GL, et al. Carotid artery stenosis: Gray-scale and Doppler US diagnosis—Society of Radiologists in Ultrasound Consensus Conference. *Radiology.* 2003;229:340–346.
9. AbuRahma AF, Abu-Halimah S, Bensenhaver J, et al. Optimal carotid duplex velocity criteria for defining the severity of carotid in-stent restenosis. *J Vasc Surg.* 2008;48:589–594.
10. Cumbie T, Rosero EB, Valentine RJ, et al. Utility and accuracy of duplex ultrasonography in evaluating in-stent restenosis after carotid stenting. *Am J Surg.* 2008;196:623–628.
11. Jaff MR, Goldmakher GV, Lev MH, et al. Imaging of the carotid arteries: The role of duplex ultrasonography, magnetic resonance arteriography, and computerized tomography arteriography. *Vasc Med.* 2008;13:281–292.
12. Johnston KW, Rutherford RB, Tilson MD, et al. Suggested standards for reporting on arterial aneurysms. Subcommittee on Reporting Standards for Arterial Aneurysms, Ad Hoc Committee on Reporting Standards, Society for Vascular Surgery and North American Chapter, International Society for Cardiovascular Surgery. *J Vasc Surg.* 1991;13:452–458.
13. Moneta GL, Lee RW, Yeager RA, et al. Mesenteric duplex scanning: A blinded prospective study. *J Vasc Surg.* 1993;17:79–84.
14. Zwolak RM, Fillinger MF, Walsh DB, et al. Mesenteric and celiac duplex scanning: A validation study. *J Vasc Surg.* 1998;27:1078–1087.
15. Olin JW, Piedmont MR, Young JR, et al. The utility of duplex ultrasound scanning of the renal arteries for diagnosing significant renal artery stenosis. *Ann Intern Med.* 1995;122:833–838.
16. Goel MC, LaPerna L, Whitelaw L, et al. Current management of transplant renal artery stenosis: Clinical utility of duplex Doppler ultrasonography. *Urology.* 2005;66:59–64.
17. http://www.icavl.org/icavl/pdfs/arterial2007.pdf.
18. Jager KA, Ricketts HJ, Strandness DE Jr. Duplex scanning for the evaluation of lower limb arterial disease. In: Bernstein EF, ed. *Noninvasive Diagnostic Techniques in Vascular Disease.* 4th Ed. St. Louis, Mo: CV Mosby; 1985:619–631.
19. Gerhard-Herman M, Gardin JM, Jaff M, et al. Guidelines for noninvasive vascular laboratory testing: A report from the American Society of Echocardiography and the Society for Vascular Medicine and Biology. *Vasc Med.* 2006;11:183–200.
20. Hirsch AT, Haskal ZJ, Hertzer NR, et al. ACC/AHA 2005 Practice Guidelines for the management of patients with peripheral arterial disease (lower extremity, renal, mesenteric, and abdominal aortic): A collaborative report from the American Association for Vascular Surgery/Society for Vascular Surgery, Society for Cardiovascular Angiography and Interventions, Society for Vascular Medicine and Biology, Society of Interventional Radiology, and the ACC/AHA Task Force on Practice Guidelines (Writing Committee to Develop Guidelines for the Management of Patients with Peripheral Arterial Disease): Endorsed by the American Association of Cardiovascular and Pulmonary Rehabilitation; National Heart, Lung, and Blood Institute; Society for Vascular Nursing; Trans-Atlantic Inter-Society Consensus; and Vascular Disease Foundation. *Circulation.* 2006;113:e463–e465.
21. Quinlan DJ, Alikhan R, Gishen P, et al. Variations in lower limb venous anatomy: Implications for US diagnosis of deep vein thrombosis. *Radiology.* 2003;228:443–448.
22. http://www.icavl.org/icavl/pdfs/venous2007.pdf.
23. Lensing AW, Prandoni P, Brandjes D, et al. Detection of deep-vein thrombosis by real-time B-mode ultrasonography. *N Engl J Med.* 1989;320:342–445.
24. Hertzberg BS, Kliewer MA, DeLong DM, et al. Sonographic assessment of lower limb vein diameters: Implications for the diagnosis and characterization of deep venous thrombosis. *Am J Roentgenol.* 1997;168:1253–1257.
25. Linkins LA, Stretton R, Probyn L, et al. Interobserver agreement on ultrasound measurements of residual vein diameter, thrombus echogenicity and Doppler venous flow in patients with previous venous thrombosis. *Thromb Res.* 2006;117:241–247.
26. Stein JH, Korcarz CE, Hurst RT, et al. Use of carotid ultrasound to identify subclinical vascular disease and evaluate cardiovascular disease risk: A consensus statement from the American Society of Echocardiography Carotid Intima-Media Thickness Task Force. Endorsed by the Society for Vascular Medicine. *J Am Soc Enchocardiogr.* 2008;21:93–111.
27. de Groot E, van Leuven SI, Duivenvoorden R, et al. Measurement of carotid intima-media thickness to assess progression and regression of atherosclerosis. *Nat Clin Pract Cardiovasc Med.* 2008;5:280–288.
28. Anderson EA, Mark AL. Flow-mediated and reflex changes in large peripheral artery tone in humans. *Circulation.* 1989;79:93–100.
29. Corretti MC, Anderson TJ, Benjamin EJ, et al. Guidelines for the ultrasound assessment of endothelial-dependent flow-mediated vasodilation of the brachial artery: A report of the International Brachial Artery Reactivity Task Force. *J Am Coll Cardiol.* 2002;39:257–265.
30. Vogel RA. Measurement of endothelial function by brachial artery flow-mediated vasodilation. *Am J Cardiol.* 2001;88:31–34.
31. Feinstein SB. Contrast ultrasound imaging of the carotid artery vasa vasorum and atherosclerotic plaque neovascularization. *J Am Coll Cardiol.* 2006;48:236–243.
32. Granada JF, Feinstein SB. Imaging of the vasa vasorum. *Nat Clin Pract Cardiovasc Med.* 2008;5(suppl 2):S18–S25.

Nuclear Imaging Physics and Instrumentation

4

Ernest V. Garcia
James R. Galt
Tracy L. Faber
Ji Chen

1. INTRODUCTION

Nuclear cardiology imaging is solidly based on many branches of science and engineering, including nuclear, optical and mathematical physics, electrical and mechanical engineering, chemistry, and biology. This chapter uses principles from these scientific fields to provide an understanding of both the signals used and the imaging system that captures these signals. These principles have been simplified to fit the scope of this book.

Nuclear cardiology's signal is a radioactive tracer and its imaging systems are either single-photon emission computed tomography (SPECT) or positron emission tomography (PET) cameras described herein. This combination has met with remarkable success in clinical cardiology. This success is due to the combination of sophisticated electronic nuclear instruments with a highly specific and thus powerful signal. The signal is as important as or more important than the imaging system.

There is a misconception that cardiac magnetic resonance (CMR), cardiac computed tomography (CCT), and echocardiography are superior to nuclear cardiology imaging because of their superior spatial resolution. Yet, in detecting perfusion defects what is really necessary is superior contrast resolution. It is this superior contrast resolution that allows us to differentiate between normal and hypoperfused myocardium facilitating the visual analysis of nuclear cardiology perfusion images. Because these objects are bright compared to the background computer algorithms that allow us to automatically and objectively process and quantify our images have been developed, a feat yet to be successfully performed by these other modalities.

This chapter explains the many important scientific principles necessary to understand nuclear cardiology imaging in general, starting from how radiation is emitted from a nucleus to how these sophisticated imaging systems detect this radiation. These principles are explained at a simple but highly applied level so the nuclear cardiologist can understand them and apply them in routine clinical practice. The better the understanding of how our images are formed and what can go wrong in their formation, the higher should be the accuracy of interpreting clinical studies and the more successful clinical practice should be.

2. RADIONUCLIDES

2.1. Stability of the nucleus

The stability of the nucleus for emitting radiation depends on the ratio of neutrons to protons and on the nuclide's atomic number (Z). Figure 4.1 illustrates this principle. Only nuclides with low proton numbers fall on the line with a neutron–proton ratio of

1. Note that as the number of protons increases, more neutrons are required to keep the nucleus stable. Nuclides with neutron–proton ratios, which are not on the stable nuclei curve, are unstable and thus radioactive. These radioactive nuclides are known as radionuclides. The type of radioactivity emitted depends on which side of the line the radionuclide is found. Isotopes are family of nuclides that all have the same number of protons, or atomic number (Z), and are not necessarily radioactive. Isotones are nuclides with the same number of neutrons (N) and isobars are the nuclides with the same mass number (A) or number of mass particles in the nucleus ($A = Z + N$).

2.2. Modes of radioactive decay

The different modes of radiation from nuclei can be identified by the deviation of their path by a magnetic field perpendicular to the page (Fig. 4.2). The direction of the deflection depends on the charge of the radioactive particle. The least penetrating radiation is deflected to the right and corresponds to the heaviest radiation called an alpha particle (α). An α particle is actually the nuclei of a helium atom (2 protons + 2 neutrons) with positive charge. The moderately penetrating radiation deflected in the opposite direction to an α particle consists of negative particles called beta (β) particles. Because these particles are more strongly bent they are lighter than the α particles. β particles are actually electrons emitted from the nucleus. Showing the same degree of penetration but bending in the opposite direction to the β particles are positron particles or positive electrons (β^+). These are particles made of antimatter and emitted by positron tracers. The radioactive particles that go straight and are not deflected do not consist of charged particles. They are called gamma (γ) rays and have been shown to be identical to particles emitted from an X-ray tube.[1] Both X-rays and γ rays are called photons and are used in nuclear cardiology imaging.

SPECT versus PET radionuclides. The radionuclides, such as technetium-99m (^{99m}Tc) and fluorine-18 (^{18}F), used in SPECT and PET imaging vary significantly. Figure 4.3 demonstrates their differences. ^{99m}Tc is a large radionuclide that emits a single photon or γ ray per radioactive decay that is used in SPECT to create images. The energy of the emitted photon is 140,000 eV or 140 keV. The m in ^{99m}Tc means that the nuclear is meta-stable (almost stable but really unstable). F^{18} is a much smaller radionuclide that emits a positron (β^+) antiparticle. This ionized antiparticle travels through a medium interacting with it, losing energy and slowing down until it interacts with an electron, usually from some atom. Because the electron and the positron are antiparticles of each other, i.e., same mass but opposite charge, they undergo a phenomenon called pair annihilation. In pair annihilation the mass of both particles disintegrates and is converted into energy

45

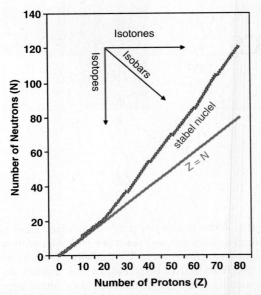

Figure 4.1 Stability of the nucleus. This graph plots as a blue band the number of neutrons versus the number of protons for stable nuclei. The solid red line indicates a neutron–proton ratio of 1. The blue curve indicates the neutron–proton ratio required to keep a nucleus stable.

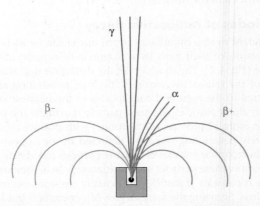

Figure 4.2 Types of radiation. The types of radiation, alpha (α), beta (β), positrons (β^+), or gamma (γ) rays, are separated into different paths by submitting these particles to a magnetic field.

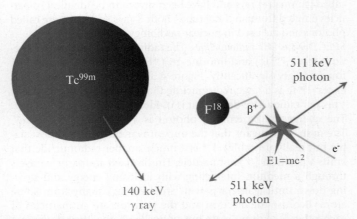

Figure 4.3 SPECT versus PET radionuclides. This figure shows two very different types of radionuclides, technetium-99m (^{99m}Tc) used in SPECT imaging, and fluorine-18 (^{18}F) used in PET imaging. Note the difference in size of the nuclide and mode of decay.

as explained by Einstein's famous equation $E = mc^2$, where E is the emitted energy, m is the mass of the two particles, and c is the speed of light in a vacuum. Because of the nature of the interaction, most of the time the energy is emitted in the form of two photons traveling in exactly opposite direction to each other and each having the same energy, 511 keV, which is the energy equivalent to the rest mass of an electron. It is these two photons that are used to create images in PET.

2.3. Radioactive decay law: Concept of half-life

The concept of half- life can be visualized in Figure 4.4 by considering decay curves for three different radionuclides, ^{99m}Tc, ^{18}F, and thallium-201 (^{201}Tl). The decay curves express the amount of radioactive nuclides that have not decayed as a function of time. The shorter the interval between emissions for a specific radionuclide, the faster the radioactivity is depleted. It is practical to express the rate of radioactive transformations (disintegrations) by specifying the period during which half of all the atoms initially present will disintegrate. This period of time is known as the half life or $T_{\frac{1}{2}}$. The amount of radioactive nuclide is specified in terms of disintegration rate or its activity.

This relationship is provided by the radioactive decay law:

$$A(t) = A_0 e^{-(0.693t)/T_{\frac{1}{2}}} \qquad \text{(Eq. 4.1)}$$

where $A(t)$ is the radioactivity remaining at time t; A_0 is the activity at time 0; and $T_{\frac{1}{2}}$ is the half life of the radionuclide.

A common unit of activity is the curie (Ci), which is 3.7×10^{10} disintegration per seconds. Another common unit of radioactivity used is the Becquerel, which is one disintegration per second. Rates one-thousands of the curie is a millicurie (mCi) corresponding to 3.7×10^7 disintegration per second. Note from the graph that if a 40 mCi dose of a ^{99m}Tc radiopharmaceutical (radioactive pharmaceutical) is delivered to an imaging clinic at 6 AM, 6 h later, at noon, only half or 20 mCi remain, and at 6 PM only half of that or 10 mCi remain.

2.4. Interaction of radiation with matter

Photons. High energy photons, such as γ rays and X-rays, interact with matter in three ways that are relevant to nuclear medicine:

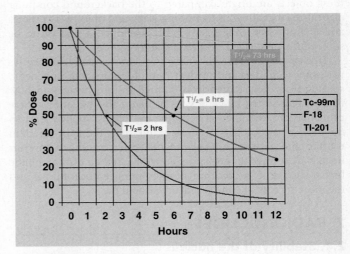

Figure 4.4 Concept of half-life or $T_{\frac{1}{2}}$. This diagram shows decay curves for three different radionuclides. Note that the ^{18}F curve is disintegrating the fastest of the three radionuclides and that it reaches a level of 50% of original activity at 2h. So the half-life of ^{18}F is 2h compared to the half-life of ^{201}Tl, which is 73h, and the half-life of ^{99m}Tc, which is 6h.

Photoelectric effect, Compton scatter, and pair production.[2] Each of these processes results in the emission of charged particles (electrons or positrons) that produce much more ionization than the original event. Thus high energy photons are classified as secondary ionizing radiation.

The photoelectric effect (or photoelectric absorption) occurs when a photon (γ or X-ray) is completely absorbed as it interacts with an innershell electron. All of the energy is lost to the electron, now called a photo-electron, which is emitted from the atom with an energy equivalent to the photon energy (E_0) less than the binding energy of the electron ($E_{Binding}$). After photoelectric absorption the atom has a vacancy in an inner electron shell that will be filled by an outer shell electron, resulting in the emission of characteristic X-rays and possibly auger electrons.

Compton scattering occurs when a photon interacts with an outer shell electron, changing direction and losing some energy (Fig. 4.5). The amount of energy of the photon after scattering depends on the angle of scatter (θ) according to the formula:

$$E_{sc} = 1 + (E_0/511 \text{ keV})*(1-\cos(\theta)) \qquad \text{(Eq. 4.2)}$$

where E_0 is the energy of the photon before scattering; E_{sc} is the energy of the photon after scattering; and θ is the angle between the photon's original path and its new one. The larger the angle the more energy lost. Maximum energy is lost when the photon reverses course ($\theta = 180°$) and backscatters. All of the energy lost to the γ ray ($E_0 - E_{sc}$) is transferred to the electron, which upon ejection from the atom is called a recoil electron (the binding energy of the outer shell electron is negligible). Energies of Compton scattered photons as a function of scatter angle are shown in Table 4.1.

Pair production occurs when a photon passes near a charged particle (usually the nucleus of an atom). The photon is destroyed and a positron-electron pair (β^+, β^-) is created. According to the

TABLE 4.1
ENERGIES OF COMPTON SCATTERED PHOTONS IN KeV

Radionuclide	E_0	Scattering angle			
	(keV)	30°	60°	90°	180°
^{201}Tl	72	71	67	63	56
^{99m}Tc	140	135	123	110	90
Positron annihilation	511	451	341	256	170

This table shows the relationship between the photopeak energy of common radionuclides used in nuclear cardiology, the scattering angle of the Compton scattered photon, and the resulting energy of that photon. Note that in many instances the originally emitted photon can undergo a large scatter angle and still be counted by a 20% energy window in a camera's PHA.

formula $E = mc^2$ the mass of the electron is equivalent to 511 keV, thus the photon has to have at least 1,022 keV for pair production to occur. Energy in excess of 1,022 keV is shared by the positron and the electron as kinetic energy. Because of the high energy required for the process it is of little importance in clinical nuclear medicine laboratories.

Photon attenuation. As photons are absorbed through the photoelectric effect or scattered away from the detector through Compton scatter their loss is called attenuation. The percentage of photons lost depends on the energy of the photons, the density of the material, and the material's thickness. The dependence on thickness is straightforward: the thicker the material, the more photons will be absorbed. The thickness at which half of the photons are absorbed is called a half value layer (HVL). In the example N_0 photons pass through a material, after one HVL, half of photons have been lost; after two HVLs, only one fourth of the photons are left. In practice the attenuation of a beam of photons is usually calculated using the linear attenuation coefficient ($\mu = \ln2/\text{HVL}$) in the equation:

$$I = I_0 e^{-\mu x} \qquad \text{(Eq. 4.3)}$$

where I_0 is the initial beam intensity and I is the intensity after traveling through thickness x. The values of linear attenuation coefficients depend on the energy of the photon and the composition of the material. The denser the material and the higher the energy of the photon the less attenuation and the lower the value of μ. Linear attenuation coefficients and HVLs for radionuclides and materials of interest to nuclear cardiology are given in Table 4.2.

Charged particles. High energy charged particles, such are alpha particles (α), beta particles (β), and the photoelectrons and recoil electrons, discussed earlier slow down and lose energy as they pass through matter. This loss is a result of the forces their charge exerts on the electrons (and to a lesser extent the nuclei) of the material. These interactions are called collisions. The loss of energy is termed collisional losses (even though they do not actually involve a collision between the two particles) or radiation losses depending on the nature of the encounter.

β particles have the same mass as electrons and as they pass through the material the electrical forces of the electrons (attractive for β^+ and repulsive for β^-) cause them to change course with each interaction. These collisions transfer some of the β particles energy to the orbital electrons causing them to escape the orbit (the ejected electron is called a delta ray) or to be raised to a higher energy state (excitation). Because of their tortuous path

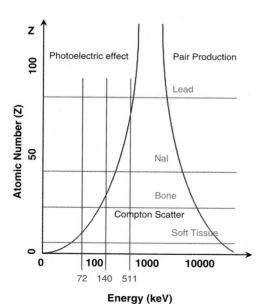

Figure 4.5 Interaction of photon radiation with matter. This graph shows how the most probable interactions between high-energy photons and matter depend on the energy of the photons and the density of the material. Compton scatter is by far the most common interaction within the patient from the photons produced by clinical radiopharmaceuticals. The photoelectric effect is more likely to take place in lead shielding of the collimator

TABLE 4.2
LINEAR ATTENUATION COEFFICIENTS AND HALF VALUE LAYERS

Radionuclide	Energy (keV)	Soft tissue (1.0 gm/cm³)		Bone (1.9 gm/cm³)		Lead (11.3 gm/cm³)	
		μ (1/cm)	HLV (cm)	μ (1/cm)	HLV (cm)	μ (1/cm)	HLV (cm)
^{201}Tl	72	0.191	3.62	0.493	1.40	39.1	0.018
^{99m}Tc	140	0.153	4.52	0.295	2.35	30.7	0.225
Positron annihilation	511	0.952	7.28	0.170	4.08	1.78	0.390

This table shows the relationship between the photopeak energy of common radionuclides used in nuclear cardiology, their corresponding linear attenuation coefficient (μ), and HVL in soft tissue, bone, and lead. Note that the denser the material the smaller the HVL has to be in order to reduce the photon beam by 50%.
Source: Hubble JH, Seltzer SM. *Tables of X-ray Mass Attenuation Coefficients, and Mass Energy-absorption Coefficients*. National Institute of Standards and Technology. 1996. Available at: http://physics.nist.gov/PhysRefData/XrayMassCoef/cover.html.

the depth that β particles will penetrate a material (range) varies between different β particles of the same energy, a process called straggling. Two measures of the depth of penetration of β particles are the extrapolated range (an estimation of the maximum positron penetration) and the average range (the mean penetration). A short positron range is desirable for PET imaging because PET determines the origin of the electron-positron annihilation event, not the actual site of the positron emission. Table 4.3 presents extrapolated and average ranges for several PET radionuclides.

α particles are much more massive than electrons. As collisions occur between α particle and electrons, the electrons are excited or swept from the orbit but the encounter has little effect on the direction of the α particle. As a result, α particles of the same energy have the same range with very little straggling. The range is also very small, so that α particles present very little danger as an external radiation source since they are stopped by a few cm of air or a few μm of tissue.

TABLE 4.3
POSITRON PARTICLE RANGE

Radionuclide	Maximum energy (MeV)	Extrapolated range (cm)		Average range (cm)
		Air	Water	Water
^{11}C	0.961	302	0.39	0.103
^{13}N	1.19	395	0.51	0.132
^{15}O	1.723	617	0.80	0.201w
^{18}F	0.635	176	0.23	0.064
^{82}Rb	3.35	1280	1.65	0.429

This table shows the relationship between the maximum energy of the emitted positron and the distance range that these particles travel in air and water. Note that the lower the energy and the denser the medium the less that it travels and thus the higher the resulting spatial resolution.
Source: Cherry SR, Sorenson JA, Phelps ME. *Physics in Nuclear Medicine*. Philadelphia, PA: Saunders; 2003, Table 6-1, p. 76.

2.5. Formation of radionuclides

Nuclear reactors. The radionuclides used in nuclear cardiology do not occur naturally and must be manufactured. This may be done by extracting them from the spent fuel of a nuclear reactor, bombarding a target nuclide with high energy neutrons to make a nuclide that is neutron rich (too many neutrons to be stable), or bombarding a target with high energy positively charged particles such as protons using a cyclotron or other particle accelerator to make proton rich nuclides (Table 4.4). Generators are devices that allow separation of a daughter radionuclide from the parent in a shielded container that may be transported long distances from the manufacturing site (reactor or accelerator).

Nuclear reactors are an important source of radionuclides for nuclear medicine including iodine-131 and xenon-133. Most importantly, molybdenum-99 (^{99}Mo) the parent of ^{99m}Tc is produced in a nuclear reactor. The heart of a nuclear reactor is a core of fissionable material (usually U-235 and U-238). Fission splits the uranium nucleus into two lighter nuclei and produces two or three fission neutrons. Some of these neutrons strike other U-125 nuclei, converting them to U-236. U-236 quickly undergoes fission and produces many more fission neutrons, which stimulate even more fission events. The uranium in the core is surrounded by a moderator ("heavy water" and graphite), which slows down the fission neutrons to an energy that is more likely to produce further reactions. The ensuing nuclear chain reaction is regulated by control rods, which absorb neutrons made of boron or cadmium. Fission products usually have an excess of neutrons and decay further with β-emission. Over 100 nuclides are created in the fission process. These fragments can be extracted by chemical means from material removed from the core. Another way to use a nuclear reactor to produce radionuclides, neutron activation, is to place a target into the high neutron flux of the core, while keeping it isolated from the core itself. ^{99}Mo can be produced by either process but most is extracted as a fission fragment.

Cyclotrons. Cyclotrons are charged particle accelerators that are used to produce radionuclides by bombarding a target with particles or ions that have been accelerated to high rates of speed (Fig. 4.6). The two basic components of a cyclotron are a large electromagnet and semicircular, hollow electrodes called "dees" because of their shape. Ions are injected into the center of the

TABLE 4.4.
COMMON SPECT RADIONUCLIDES USED IN NUCLEAR CARDIOLOGY

SINGLE PHOTON (SPECT)

Radionuclide	Production	Decay	Emission	Half-life ($T_{1/2}$)
^{123}I (Iodine-123)	Cyclotron	EC	γ 159 keV	13.21 h
201Tl (Thallium-201)	Cyclotron	EC	X 68–0 keV, γ 167 keV (10%)	73 h
99mTc (Technetium-99m)	Generator	IT	γ 140 keV	6 h

Side View **Top View**

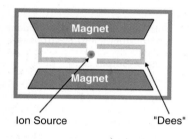

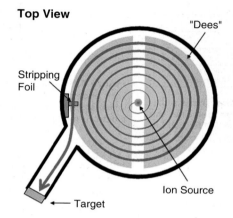

Figure 4.6 Formation of radionuclides by cyclotrons. Positive ion cyclotrons accelerate α particles or protons and use an electrostatic deflector to direct the ion beam to the target. Negative ion cyclotrons, as shown in the figure, accelerate negative hydrogen (H^-) ions, a proton with two electrons. A stripping foil, made of carbon, strips off the two electrons from the ion, leaving a proton. The positive charge of the proton causes it to arch in the opposite direction, causing the beam to exit the cyclotron and strike the target.

device between the dees. An alternating current applied to the dees causes the ions to be attracted to one side. Once inside the dee the ion will travel in a curve because any charged particle moving in a magnetic field (supplied by the electromagnet) moves in a circular path. Though there is no electric field inside the dee the current is carefully timed so that the polarization of the dees changes as the particles emerge from one side. This accelerates the ions and their arc of travel becomes larger as they move faster and faster, picking up speed each time they cross the gap between the dees. At the maximum radius the ions are deflected out of the cyclotron and strike a target, creating new nuclides. An example of this is the use of a cyclotron to bombard an oxygen-18 target with protons, resulting in conversion of the nucleus to fluorine-18 (after emission of a neutron). Several cyclotron-produced radionuclides used in nuclear cardiology are listed in Table 4.5. Most hospital and community based cyclotrons are negative ion cyclotrons because they require less shielding and are more compact than positive ion cyclotrons.

Generators. Generators are devices that allow separation of a radionuclide from relatively long-lived parent. This allows the production of short-lived radionuclides at a location remote from a reactor or cyclotron (such as a hospital, clinic, or local radiopharmacy). The daughter is continuously replenished by the parent inside the generator, which shields both radionuclides while allowing the daughter to be extracted repeatedly.[3]

The most common generator used in nuclear medicine is the ^{99}Mo–^{99m}Tc generator, which produces technetium-99m (^{99m}Tc, half-life of 6 h) from the β decay of molybdenum-99 (^{99}Mo, half-life 66 h) (Fig. 4.7). The ^{99}Mo is produced in a nuclear reactor. The heart of the generator is an alumina column impregnated with ^{99}Mo. A vacuum vial is used to pull saline out of a second

vial through the porous column. Technetium (both ^{99m}Tc and ^{99}Tc) is washed out of the column by the saline and collected in the vacuum vial, leaving the ^{99}Mo behind. The generator must be well shielded because ^{99}Mo emits both β particles and 740 to 780 keV γ rays. The process of extracting ^{99m}Tc from the generator is called milking or elution, and the extracted ^{99}Tc-saline solution is called eluate. After milking, the ^{99m}Tc solution must be tested

TABLE 4.5
COMMON PET RADIONUCLIDES USED IN NUCLEAR CARDIOLOGY

POSITRON EMITTING (PET)

Radionuclide	Production	Positron energy	Half-life ($T_{1/2}$)
^{15}O° (Oxygen-15)	Cyclotron	735 keV	122 s
^{13}N (Nitrogen-13)	Cyclotron	491 keV	9.96 min
11C (Carbon-11)	Cyclotron	385 keV	20.3 min
18F (Fluorine-18)	Cyclotron	248 keV	110 min
82Rb (Rubidium-82)	Generator	1,523 keV	1.3 min

This table compares the energy of the radiation, half-life, and mode of production of PET radionuclides commonly used in nuclear cardiology procedures. Note that due to the short half-life of most cyclotron produced PET tracers a cyclotron must be located nearby. Only ^{18}F is routinely distributed commercially.
Source: Beller GA, Bergmann SR. Myocardial perfusion imaging agents: SPECT and PET. *J Nucl Cardiol.* 2004;11(1):71–86.

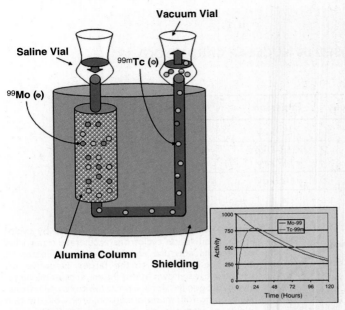

Figure 4.7 Formation of radionuclides by generators. This is a diagram of the most common generator used in nuclear medicine, the ^{99}Mo–^{99m}Tc generator that produces technetium-99m (^{99m}Tc, half-life of 6 h) from the β decay of molybdenum-99 (^{99}Mo, half-life 66 h). The graph insert demonstrates the ^{99m}Tc produced by β decay of ^{99}Mo in the alumina column if the generator is undisturbed.

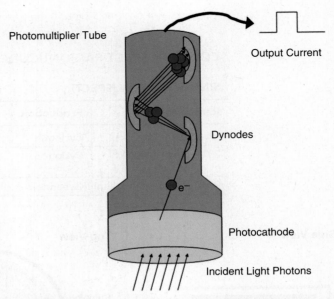

Figure 4.8 Operation of the PMT. This figure illustrates how incident light photons are converted in the photocathode into electrons (e⁻), which are then accelerated to the metal dynodes to extract even more electrons multiplying the signal to create an output current pulse.

for ^{99}Mo and aluminum. ^{99}Mo is detected using a dose calibrator and a shield that blocks the low energy photon from ^{99m}Tc. The maximum amount of ^{99}Mo allowed under Nuclear Regulatory Commission regulations is 0.15 Bq ^{99}Mo per kBq ^{99m}Tc (0.15 μCi ^{99}Mo per mCi ^{99m}Tc) Aluminum is detected chemically which a maximum permissible level of 10 μg/ mL of eluate.

The graph insert in Figure 4.7 represents the ^{99m}Tc produced by β decay of ^{99}Mo in the alumina column when the generator is undisturbed. This is an example of transient equilibrium where the parent $T_{1/2}$ is somewhat longer than the daughter $T_{1/2}$. After a few hours the daughter activity is almost equal (actually slightly higher) to the parent activity. Fortunately the optimal frequency for milking the generator is at intervals slightly less than 24 h. ^{99}Mo–^{99m}Tc generators are designed to last at least two weeks in the nuclear pharmacy.

Another generator of importance to nuclear cardiology is the ^{82}Sr–^{82}Rb generator. ^{82}Rb ($T_{1/2}$ = 1.3 min) is produced by β decay of ^{82}Sr ($T_{1/2}$ = 25 days, manufactured using an accelerator). The daughter activity equals the parent activity very soon after elution and allows elution every hour. This is an example of secular equilibrium where the parent's half-life is a great deal longer than the daughter half-life. The short half-life of ^{82}Rb ($T_{1/2}$ = 1.3 min) makes it impractical to transport the dose to the patient. The generator is designed to deliver the dose directly into an IV line. ^{82}Rb generators are designed to last about a month in the clinic. ^{82}Sr and ^{85}Sr may be low-level contaminants and are found in routine quality control (QC) by assaying the eluent after complete decay of the ^{82}Rb.

3. THE GAMMA CAMERA

3.1. Detector systems

Photomultiplier tubes (PMT) convert energy from visible light into an electric signal. Figure 4.8 illustrates how light interacting with the material in the photocathode causes it to release electrons. These are accelerated along the tube by a high voltage differential. As they travel through the tube, they strike metal electrodes called dynodes, at which point even more electrons are ejected. This cascade of multiplication continues until the electrons are output as current at the other end. The voltage (height) of the pulse generated by the PMT is directly proportional to the amount of visible light that strikes the photocathode.

Scintillating crystals are used to convert γ rays into visible light. A γ ray travels through the collimator and interacts with one of the atoms in the crystal, ejecting an electron, called the primary electron, through the photo-electric effect. This ejected electron continues traveling through the crystal and excites a large number of secondary electrons, which lose their excitation energy by emitting visible light. The glow of the scintillation is converted into electrical signals by the PMTs. The location of the scintillation event is determined by the positioning circuitry based on the relative signals from the different PMTs. The brightness of the scintillation is proportional to the energy of the photon, measured by the pulse height analyzer (PHA).

Note from Figure 4.9 that the γ ray travels some distance through the crystal before it interacts with a crystal atom. If the crystal is very thin, a γ ray may travel through the entire width of the crystal with no interaction. Therefore, a thicker crystal results in a higher sensitivity for the detection of γ rays. Conversely, note that the primary electron travels in an irregular path and may excite atoms far away from its point of origin. The thicker the crystal is, the farther the electron may travel before it exits the crystal. Thus, a thick crystal implies that the scintillation may be more spread out, and this essentially reduces the resolution of the detector. So, just as with collimators, there is a trade-off between sensitivity and resolution with the size and shape of the crystal.

3.2. Image collimation

Because γ rays are emitted uniformly in all directions from a source, a photon from any area of the body can theoretically strike any area of the detector. Instrumentation is needed to determine the

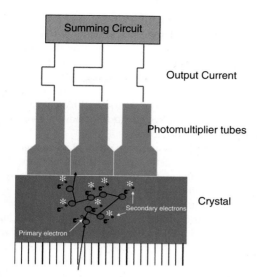

Figure 4.9 Operation of the scintillating crystal. The crystal is used to convert γ rays into visible light. See text for an explanation of how this is done.

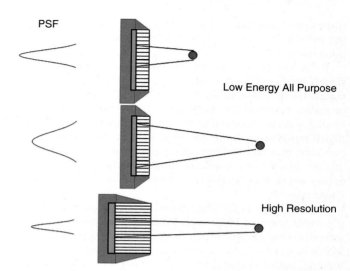

Figure 4.10 Collimation principle. This diagram shows how the γ rays emitted from a radioactive point source (*red sphere*) are "seen" by the collimator. The top row shows that when the point source is closer to the collimator the system generates a sharper response seen by the spread of the counts plotted as a PSF. The middle panel row shows how when the distance from the radioactive point to the collimator increases the PSF spreads more and thus resolution is lost. The bottom row shows how a HRES collimator can be built with long bores (holes) further limiting the angle of photons imaged and thus a sharper PSF.

direction of the photon's emission in order to be able to localize the source. This process is called collimation. For nuclear cardiology, collimators generally consist of an array of long narrow (usually) parallel holes that exclude all photons except those that are traveling parallel to the direction of the hole. Collimators are rated by their sensitivity and resolution, where resolution is defined above and sensitivity is the number of photons that travel through the collimator in a certain amount of time (as a fraction of photons emitted from the source); i.e., counts per second or counts per minute. In this instance, image resolution is affected by collimation because some photons not traveling in exactly a parallel path get through the collimator holes. Thus, a single point source will appear fuzzy on the detector. How much the point "spreads out," that is, the width of its point-spread function (PSF), is related to the spatial resolution and depends upon the length and width of the holes. More specifically, spatial resolution is given by the full width of the PSF at half its maximum or the FWHM. Low energy all purpose (LEAP) and general purpose (GAP) collimators have relatively short, wide holes that accept more photons than (HRES) collimators with long narrow and/or smaller holes. Increasing the length of the hole increases the resolution by decreasing the angle subtended by the hole, and thus, eliminates more γ rays traveling at angles not parallel to the hole. So, a higher resolution is achieved at the cost of sensitivity. In general, the sensitivity and resolution of a collimator are inversely related. A very high sensitivity collimator will have low resolution, and a very HRES collimator will have low sensitivity. In Figure 4.10, the PSF for different shaped collimators are shown at the left of the figure. Note that the width of the PSF curve is broader for LEAP collimators, indicating a lower resolution, but the total area underneath this PSF is higher than that of the HRES collimator, indicating higher sensitivity related to resolution, and the area underneath the curve is related to sensitivity. This figure also demonstrates that the resolution of the collimator, as seen by the PSF curves on the left, depends on the distance between the source and the collimator. This is discussed in more detail in the next figure.

3.3. Digital scintillation camera

The main components of SPECT systems are the scintillation camera, the gantry (the frame that supports and moves the heads),

and the computer systems (hardware and software). Each of these components work together to acquire and reconstruct the tomographic images.

As previously described, the basic components of a scintillation camera shown in Figure 4.11 are the collimator, a sodium iodide (NaI) crystal, PMT, and an analog or a digital computer designed to determine the location and energy of a photon striking the crystal. γ rays (photons) pass through the collimator and cause a scintillation event (a short burst of visible light) to occur in the crystal. The glow of the scintillation is converted into electrical signals by the PMTs. The location of the scintillation event is determined based on the relative signals from the different PMTs. The brightness of the scintillation is proportional to the energy of the photon. Scintillation cameras were developed in the late 1950s and early 1960s. These cameras used PHA and spatial positioning circuitry invented by Hal Anger of the University of California at Berkeley to determine the location and energy of the incident photon.[4] Early cameras were completely analog devices where the output was sent to an oscilloscope, creating a flash on the screen. A lens focused the screen on a piece of X-ray film that

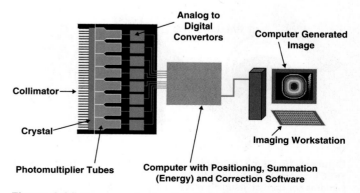

Figure 4.11 Components of a digital scintillation camera.

was exposed, one flash at a time. This allowed for planar imaging but for SPECT the images must be made available to the computer digitally.

Today, camera systems convert the position and pulse height signals generated from analog circuitry in the camera to digital signals using analog to digital converters. The signals may then be further corrected for energy and position through digital processing. Camera designs that convert the output of each PMT to a digital signal as shown in the figure have become common. The computer may then perform all the positioning and pulse height analysis instead of complicated analog circuitry. This results in greater processing flexibility, spatial resolution, and in higher count rates.

Another step in the digitization of scintillation cameras is the replacement of PMTs with solid-state detectors called photodiodes. One camera with this design uses individual cesium iodide (CsI) scintillation crystals, each backed with a silicon photodiode. Each CsI crystal is 3 mm^2, giving similar resolution to conventional camera without the need for positioning circuitry. Elimination of the PMTs greatly reduces the size and weight of the scintillation camera with some trade off in cost and energy resolution. These type of cameras are usually known as solid-state cameras.

Multi-headed SPECT cameras. Multidetector SPECT systems have more than one scintillation camera attached to the gantry (Fig. 4.12). The most obvious benefit of adding more detectors to a scintillation camera system is the increase in sensitivity. Doubling the number of heads doubles the number of photons that may be acquired in the same amount of time. The user may take advantage of the increase in sensitivity by acquiring more counts, by adding HRES collimation, or by increasing throughput.

Two large field of view rectangular cameras may be mounted opposite each other, 180° apart. This configuration may speed 360° SPECT imaging by halving imaging time while collecting the same number of counts since a full 360° of projections can be acquired by rotating the gantry 180°. For cardiac SPECT, where a 180° orbit is recommended, SPECT systems with two detectors mounted next to each other (at 90°) on the gantry allow a full

180° orbit to be acquired while only rotating the gantry through 90° (Fig. 4.12C). Triple detector cameras, shown in Figure 4.12D, are usually dedicated to SPECT imaging. The three heads, as discussed for double headed systems, will result in increased sensitivity that may be used to increase throughput, counts, or resolution. If the three detectors, however, are mounted rigidly at 120° from each other the system must rotate through 120° to obtain 180° of data. Thus, these systems do not have a great impact on cardiac imaging with 180° orbits.

For any multiheaded system, the primary advantage is increase in throughput, since the acquisition will take less time. However, the gain in sensitivity may be traded off to give more precise images by allowing the use of HRES collimators.

Drawbacks of multiple-headed cameras include the increase in QC required by the addition of the additional heads and some loss of flexibility. Double detector systems do not allow the same flexibility of movement that is enjoyed with many single headed systems. This may prevent them from being easily used for some types of planar imaging (such as gated blood pool) where it is often difficult to position the camera correctly. One unique SPECT system acquires planar projections by rotating the patient in an upright position while the camera(s) remain fixed.

180° versus 360° data acquisition. While 360° orbits are generally preferred for body SPECT, 180° orbits may be better for cardiac SPECT. The heart is located forward and to one side of the center of the thorax, resulting in a great deal of attenuation when the camera is behind the patient. The angles chosen for the 180° are those closest to the heart, from 45° right anterior oblique (RAO) to 45° left posterior oblique (LPO). These projections are those that suffer least from attenuation, scatter, and detector response, because they are the ones that get the camera head as close as possible to the heart. Projections taken from the posterior aspect of the body are generally noisier with lower resolution than those taken from the anterior angles. This is easily seen by comparing the 45° LAO projection shown in Figure 4.13 with the 45° LPO projection. Reconstructions from 180° acquisitions have higher resolution and contrast than those from 360° acquisitions; this is particularly true for ^{201}Tl images.[5–7] However, because 180°

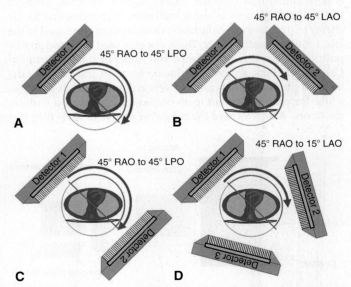

Figure 4.12 Single (**A**), double (**B, C**), and triple (**D**) detector (head) SPECT cameras. Note that to increase the sensitivity of dual head cameras for cardiac imaging more gain is obtained from positioning the two detectors 90° apart (**Panel B**) rather than 180° apart.

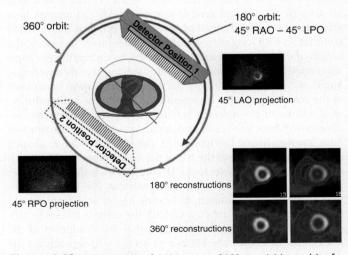

Figure 4.13 Comparison of 180° versus 360° acquisition orbits for SPECT cameras. Note from the planar LAO projection shown as compared to the planar RPO projection the higher contrast and resolution of the LV myocardium. This increased planar resolution is translated to increased LV image contrast for the 180° acquisition versus the 360° orbit as shown on the panel in the lower right. The LV myocardium from the 360° orbit does appear to be more uniform.

reconstructions are not truly complete; that is, new information is available from the other 180° of projections, there are occasional artifacts seen with 180° reconstructions that can be avoided with 360° reconstructions. In particular, 360° reconstructions are generally more uniform than 180° reconstructions. Both of these effects can be seen on the reconstructions included in the bottom right of Figure 4.13.

3.4. Resolution, signal to noise, and efficiency

Resolution. The most common measurements of image quality are spatial resolution and contrast resolution. Spatial resolution refers to how well objects can be separated in space (as opposed to blurring them together), and contrast resolution refers to how well different levels of brightness (representing radionuclide concentration in a scintigram) can be seen.

Spatial resolution is the measure of how close two point sources of activity can come together and still be distinguished as separate. Because no medical imaging modality is perfect, a point source never appears as a single bright pixel, but instead as a blurred distribution. Two blurry points eventually smear together into a single spot when they are moved close enough to each other. Spatial resolution is measured by taking a profile (a graph of counts encountered along a line drawn through a region of interest in the image) through a point source and analyzing the resulting curve. A profile through a perfect point source would look like a sharp single spike rising above the flat background. A profile through a real point source appears as a Gaussian-shaped curve. As previously discussed, this curve is called the point spread function (PSF). When the two Gaussian curves of two point sources get close enough together, they cannot be distinguished as separate. This distance is a measure of image resolution. Figure 4.14A shows an example of this. Two brain tumors are imaged, and a profile is taken through the resulting reconstruction. As the tumors move closer together, the discrete peaks of the profile start to merge into a single peak.

Contrast resolution in nuclear cardiology images can be defined as the measure of counts (or intensity) in the target (the object we are trying to image) compared to the intensity in a background region. High counts in the target increase contrast resolution; high counts in the background region, for example, lung uptake, decrease contrast resolution. Low contrast resolution can make the target fade into the background. Contrast resolution is also easily measured using a profile. Figure 4.14B shows a count profile taken through a decreased area of a myocardial perfusion image. In this case, the "target" counts are those in the perfusion abnormality, and the "background" counts are those in the normal myocardium. The depth of the valley in the profile, compared with the overall height of the rest of the curve, is a measure of contrast resolution.

Resolution versus sensitivity. In air, recall that the amount of radiation from a point source falling on a plane decreases as $1/r^2$. However, if a collimator is placed between the source and the detector, this relationship no longer holds. The same number of γ rays will travel through the collimator no matter how far the source is from the detector. This is because γ rays that travel too obliquely from the line of the collimator holes will not pass through any collimator, no matter how close it is to the source. However, a ray that is near enough to parallel to a collimator hole will be able to pass through a collimator no matter how distant it is to the source. The primary difference between a collimator placed near the source and one placed far away from the source is which collimator hole a γ ray will pass through. A γ ray traveling exactly parallel to the collimator will pass through the hole that is directly "aimed" at the source. If the γ ray is slightly oblique to the collimator, it may pass through a hole not exactly in line with the source. How far away that hole is from the "correct" hole depends upon how far the source is from the collimator. Notice in Figure 4.15 that when the collimator is close to the source (A) most of the γ rays travel through the collimator holes that are nearly in line with that source, even when those γ rays are slightly oblique to the holes. However, if the detector is far away from the source (B), the same number of γ rays travel through the collimator, but more of the oblique rays travel through holes farther away from the one directly in line with the source. This causes a blurring or loss of resolution, which is seen in the PSF shown for each of

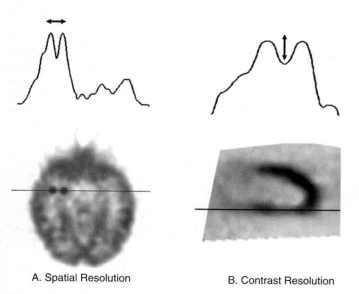

A. Spatial Resolution   B. Contrast Resolution

Figure 4.14 Principle of spatial and contrast resolution. **Panel A** illustrates how spatial resolution relates to the ability to separate as distinct two radioactive distributions, which are close to each other, in this case two brain tumors. **Panel B** illustrates how contrast resolution relates to the ability to separate as distinct two different concentrations, which are close to each other in value, in this case hypoperfused from normal myocardium. It is contrast resolution that is more important in myocardial perfusion imaging.

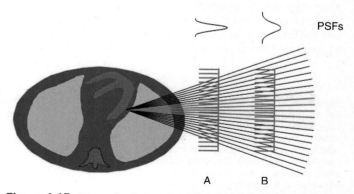

Figure 4.15 Comparing image resolution versus sensitivity with parallel hole collimators. Note that as the collimator is moved from location A to location B the radiation (*red lines*) from a specific region of the myocardium, which pass through the holes and hit the detector, spread more and thus reduce the resolution. Note that the same red lines are collimated at location B; thus, the number of detected counts from this myocardial location remains constant. Thus the area under the graph of each PSF stays the same since it reflects the total number of counts detected.

the collimator positions in the top of this figure. Note that the farther away the detector is from the source, the lower and more spread out the PSF; however, the area underneath these curves does not change. Therefore, the number of photons detected stays the same with collimator-source distance, but the image resolution decreases as the distance increases. This resolution decrease with source-to-detector distance is termed "detector response" or "geometric response."

Nuclear imaging acquires photons emitted from the patient and digitizes the data into a matrix (image). Each matrix position corresponds to a pixel, and the pixel value (total counts) corresponds to the number of accepted photons at that position. The pixel value is proportional to the radiotracer concentration, the length of the acquisition, and square of the pixel size. If the image is 3D (for example, reconstructed tomographic image), each element of the image is cubic instead of square and is called "voxel". The voxel value (total counts) is proportional to the radiotracer concentration, the length of the acquisition, and cubic (not square) of the voxel size.

Statistics, noise level versus total counts. Nuclear imaging measures radioactive decay, which is a random process, and follows the Poisson distribution. The standard deviation of a measured pixel value (counts) from a planar image projection is the square root of the pixel value. A low-count study has a bigger standard deviation and higher noise-to-signal ratio such that the image appears to be noisier than a high-count study. This example shows that if a pixel contains 100 counts it corresponds to a 10% error and if another pixel contains 10,000 counts it corresponds to a 1% error.

3.5. ECG-gated acquisition and display

ECG-gated SPECT myocardial perfusion imaging (MPI) acquisition: Similar to un-gated SPECT MPI acquisition, ECG-gated SPECT MPI acquisition collects projection images at equally spaced angles along a 180° or 360° arc during the camera rotation. This acquisition is depicted in Figure 4.16. At each angle, instead of acquiring only one projection in the un-gated acquisition mode, the camera acquires several (8, 16, or 32) projection images, each of which corresponds to a specific phase of the cardiac cycle. This is done by synchronizing the computer acquisition with the R-wave from the patient's ECG. If 8 frames per heart beat are used and the heart rate is, for example, 1 beat per second, the computer algorithm assigns each 1/8 of a second time interval to each frame. Once the first R wave is detected, all counts are acquired into the first frame; as 1/8 of a second elapses, the counts are now acquired into the second frame, and so on until the first second

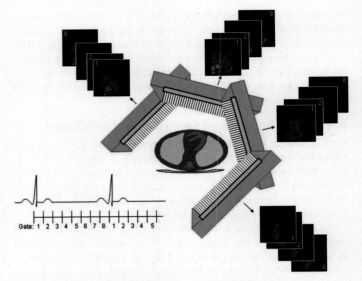

Figure 4.16 ECG-gated SPECT myocardial perfusion imaging acquisition. At each angle, the camera acquires several (8, 16, or 32) projection images, each of which corresponds to a specific phase of the cardiac cycle. This is done by synchronizing the computer acquisition to the R-wave from the patient's EKG. In this figure the cardiac cycle is divided into eight separate frames.

has elapsed or a new R-wave is detected starting the same procedure over again. This technique produces 4D image volumes (3D in space plus time) and allows clinicians to assess not only myocardial perfusion but also myocardial motion and contraction.

Temporal resolution: In this context, temporal resolution is usually expressed in the number of frames per cardiac cycle. The volume–time curve shown in Figure 4.17 plots the value of the left-ventricular cavity volume as a function of the gated SPECT time interval. The smaller the time interval (the more the number of frames acquired during a cardiac cycle), the higher is the temporal resolution and the volume–time curve is closer to the "truth" and thus the more accurate volume and ejection fraction measurements. It is generally agreed that some commonly used 8-frame gated SPECT approach produces errors in measurement of diastolic events, and it has been suggested that 16-frame imaging is quite effective.[8] There are techniques that use a mathematical algorithm (Fourier transform) to replace the discrete eight samples with a continuous curve on a segment-by-segment basis and thus are less dependent on higher temporal resolution to obtain accurate parameters.

Figure 4.17 Principle of temporal resolution. This figure shows two LV volume–time curves acquired from the same patient, the left panel at 16 frames/cardiac cycle and the right panel at 8. The *red curve* represents the gold standard while the blue curves represent the curve obtained at a specific sampling rate. It is generally accepted that the more frames per cardiac cycle the higher the temporal resolution. Note how the blue curve approximates best the true red curve in the left panel as compared to the right panel.

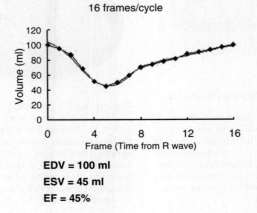

EDV = 100 ml
ESV = 45 ml
EF = 45%

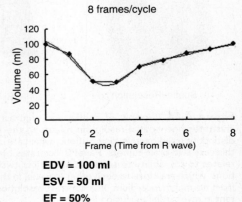

EDV = 100 ml
ESV = 50 ml
EF = 50%

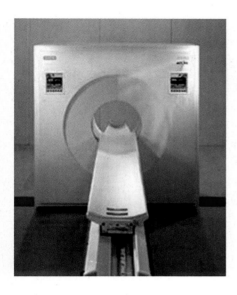

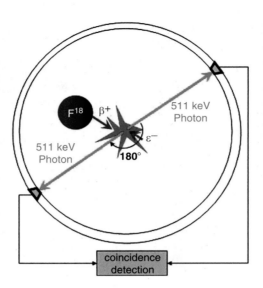

Figure 4.18 Principle of electronic collimation used in PET scanners. The left panel shows a typical PET scanner. The right panel illustrates how an emitted positron (β^+) interacts with an orbital electron resulting in a pair annihilation and the emission of two 511 keV photons traveling in opposite direction. When the system detects one of the photons it waits for a very short time to sense the second photon; when both are detected within this time window they are said to be in coincidence and during reconstruction a straight line is drawn between the two detected locations.

4. POSITRON EMISSION TOMOGRAPHY

Electronic collimation. PET cameras detect paired photons (511 keV of energy each), produced by the positron annihilation effect. The paired 511 keV photons travel in opposite directions at a 180° angle from each other (Fig. 4.18). Thus, positron decay can be localized without collimation with the use of the principle of coincidence detection since if two detectors acquire a count within a short time window it is assumed that they came from the same pair annihilation and thus the event is positioned by drawing a straight line between the two detectors. Since PET cameras do not require collimators, these systems have a much higher sensitivity than SPECT systems.

2D versus 3D PET systems. 2D PET systems, equipped with lead septa, only accept coincidences from crystals in the same ring of detectors. 3D PET systems, by removing the septa, accept coincidences in any ring and greatly increase count rate and sensitivity. However, the difficulties associated with removing the septa are (i) it greatly increases scatter; (ii) it greatly increases random events; and (iii) it greatly increases count rate, and so greatly increases dead-time.[9] These problems must be effectively compensated for the use of 3D PET in cardiac imaging.

PET versus SPECT attenuation correction. PET imaging measures 511 keV photons. Since the two photons must be detected to record the event the entire path length influences the attenuation. In SPECT imaging, even though the energy of the photon is lower its path length to the detector is much shorter and thus is less affected by attenuation. Thus the two PET photons undergo higher attenuation when they travel through the body than the single photons measured in SPECT imaging. These differences in photon attenuation are shown in Figure 4.19. Therefore, there is more attenuation in PET studies than SPECT making PET more susceptible to attenuation artifacts. Only attenuation corrected cardiac images should be used in clinical interpretation.[10] Unlike SPECT, PET data can be accurately corrected for attenuation by simply multiplying each projection line with the appropriate attenuation correction factor. For both PET and SPECT, measurement of the patient-specific attenuation map is required for accurate attenuation correction (AC) and can be done either by radionuclide imaging or by X-ray CT.

Types of attenuation correction. Accurate AC requires two acquisitions from a single study: emission and transmission. The two acquisitions can be done sequentially, one following the other; however, registration between the two acquisitions challenges QC of this approach in practice. To reduce the risk of emission/transmission misalignment the two acquisitions can be done in an interleave mode, where the camera acquires emission and transmission projection images sequentially at each stop and rotates around the patient only once in one study. A simultaneous mode completely solves the problem and reduces the length of the acquisition; however, crosstalk between the emission and transmission photons degrades at least one of the two acquisitions and should be properly compensated for accurate AC.

5. IMAGE PROCESSING

5.1. Filtered backprojection reconstruction

Filtered-backprojection is an analytic method of image reconstruction. Filtered-backprojection is, as its name implies, a combination of filtering and backprojection. The principle of backprojection is shown in the top row of Figure 4.20. When a projection image is acquired, each row of the projection contains

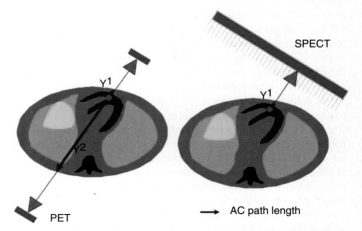

Figure 4.19 Comparison of the radiations' attenuated path length from a PET emission to that of a SPECT emission. Note that in SPECT imaging, even though the energy of the photon is lower its path length to the detector is much shorter and thus is less affected by attenuation.

Figure 4.20 Principles of back projection (**top row**) and filtered back-projection reconstructions (**bottom row**). Each row shows the progression from image acquisition, reprojection, transverse axial reconstruction from a limited 8 projection study, and reconstruction from a complete angular 64 projection study. Note the higher spatial and contrast resolution of the reconstructed point source for the filtered back-projection example.

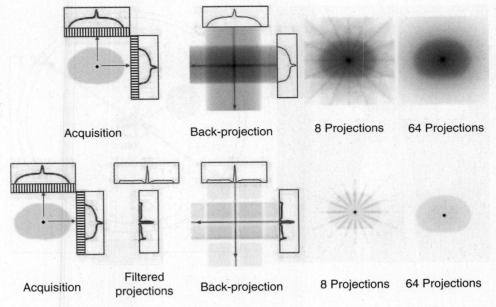

counts that emanate from the entire transverse plane. When projection images are obtained from many angles about the body, enough information is available in each row of the set of angular projections to reconstruct the original corresponding transverse slice. Backprojection assigns the values in the projection to all points along the line of acquisition through the image plane from which they were acquired. This operation is repeated for all pixels and all angles, adding the new values with the previous, in what is termed a superposition operation. As the number of angles increases, the backprojection improves.

Although simple backprojection is useful for illustrative purposes, it is never used in practice without the step of filtering. Note that the backprojection from the top row of Figure 4.20 is quite blurred as compared to the original distribution from which it was created. Also, the reconstructions created from eight projections show instances of the "star artifact," which consist of radial lines near the edges of the object. This artifact is a natural result of backprojection applied without filtering. In clinical practice, the projections are filtered prior to backprojection; filtered backprojection is shown in the bottom row of Figure 4.20. After the projections are acquired, a ramp filter is applied to each of them prior to backprojection. The ramp-filtered projections are characterized by enhancement of edge information and the introduction of negative values (or lobes) into the filtered projections. During the backprojection process, these negative values cancel portions of the other angular contributions, and in effect, help eliminate the star artifact. However, enough projections must be acquired to ensure that proper cancellation is obtained. Radial blurring or streaking toward the periphery of the image often indicates that too few projections were acquired. Finally, a noise-reducing filter such as a Butterworth or Hanning is usually applied before, during, or after the backprojection operation. Such filters are discussed in more detail in following sections.

Image filtering. Filtering is the process by which images are smoothed, sharpened, reduced in noise, or used in reconstruction such as the ramp filter in filtered backprojection. Filtering digital images is accomplished by transforming the images that are used to frequency space from the spatial domain.[11,12] This transformation is usually performed using a mathematical process called a Fourier transform. This transform represents images in terms of cycles per cm or variations of counts over distance. In this representation, smaller objects, edges of objects that abruptly change in counts, and image noise are all associated with high frequencies. Larger smooth organs are associated with lower frequencies. A filter works by defining a curve that specifies how much of each frequency should be modified. If the filter value is one at a specific frequency then it is not modified; if it is less than one, it is reduced by that amount; and if it is more than one it is enhanced by that amount.

Because the filtered backprojection reconstruction process uses a ramp filter that enhances image noise, smoothing must be applied to the reconstructed images to reduce the image noise. The most common filters used for smoothing cardiac perfusion images are the Hanning and Butterworth filters. Both the Hanning and Butterworth filters are known as low-pass filters because they tend to leave the lower frequencies alone while reducing the higher frequencies. The Butterworth filter is defined by two parameters. These parameters are the critical frequency and the order of the filter. The critical frequency is used to define when the filter begins to drop to zero (known as the cut-off frequency for a Hanning filter). The order of the filter determines the steepness of the function's downward slope.

Figure 4.21 illustrates three examples of critical frequencies for the Butterworth filter. The four transaxial cardiac images in the upper panel are examples of that same transaxial image with the various critical frequencies of the Butterworth filter applied. The left-most transaxial image (in the gray square) has had the gray filter applied. Note that the gray filter is one for every frequency and thus no smoothing is performed. This is the original noisy image that results from the filtered backprojection process. The next image, in the purple square, has had the purple filter applied with a critical frequency of 0.6 cycles per cm. Note that this image appears slightly smoother than the one with no smoothing. As the other two filters are applied with increasingly lower critical frequencies the image becomes smoother.

5.2. Iterative reconstruction

Iterative reconstruction techniques require many more calculations and thus much more computer time to create a transaxial image than does filtered-backprojection. However, their great

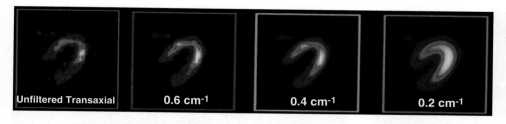

Figure 4.21 Effect of image smoothness as a function of cutoff (critical) frequency. Note in the images surrounded by a square color coded to the filter functions in the bottom panel that as the cut-off frequency is decreased the image increases in smoothness, reducing resolution but also image noise.

Increasing Smoothness = Decreasing cutoff/critical frequency

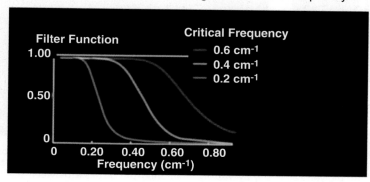

advantage is their ability to incorporate corrections for the factors that degrade SPECT images into the reconstruction process. Iterative techniques use the original projections and models of the acquisition process to predict a reconstruction. The predicted reconstruction is then used again with the models to recreate new predicted projections. If the predicted projections are different from the actual projections, these differences are used to modify the reconstruction. This process is continued until the reconstruction is such that the predicted projections match the actual projections. The primary differences between various iterative methods are how the predicted reconstructions and projections are created and how they are modified at each step. Practically speaking, the more theoretically accurate the iterative technique, the more time-consuming the process. Maximum likelihood methods allow the noise to be modeled, while least squares techniques such as the conjugate gradient method generally ignore noise.

The most widely used iterative reconstruction method is maximum likelihood expectation maximization (MLEM).[13] The MLEM algorithm attempts to determine the tracer distribution that would "most likely" yield the measured projections given the imaging model and a map of attenuation coefficients if available. An example of the reconstruction of the myocardium with the MLEM algorithm is shown in the bottom of this figure. The point of convergence of this algorithm and related number of iterations for clinical use is a source of debate. To date, there is no common rule for stopping the algorithms after an optimal number of iterations on clinical data and protocols; describing the optimal number of iterations will be largely empirically based. As can be seen in the reconstructions at the bottom of this figure, as iteration number increases, the images generally get less blurry but more noisy.

Another approach to the MLEM algorithm for iterative reconstruction is the ordered-subsets expectation maximization (OSEM) approach.[14] This approach performs an ordering of the projection data into subsets. The subsets are used in the iterative steps of the reconstruction to greatly speed up the reconstruction.

The advantage of the OSEM is that an order of magnitude increase in computational speed can be obtained.

5.3. Image display

Nuclear cardiology images are inherently quantitative. This is because the pixel (or voxel) count value is proportional to the tracer concentration at that location. In myocardial perfusion tomographic images, the count value of the voxels over the left ventricle is related to the concentration of the tracer and thus to myocardial blood flow.

Oblique images. The natural products of rotational tomography are images that represent cross-sectional slices of the body, perpendicular to the imaging table (or long axis of the body). These images are called transverse or transaxial slices. We are not restricted to the natural x, y, and z directions, however, for the extraction of images. The computer may be used to extract images at any orientation, and these images are called oblique images. Due to the variation in the heart orientation of different patients it is important that oblique slices are adjusted to try to match the same anatomy from patient to patient. The important oblique sections used for viewing cardiac images are defined thusly:

The 3D set of transaxial sections, some of which are shown in Figure 4.22A, is resliced parallel to the long axis and perpendicular through the transaxial slices. Each of the resulting oblique images is called a vertical long axis (VLA) slice, as shown in Figure 4.22B. They are displayed with the base of the left ventricle toward the left side of the image and the apex toward the right. Serial slices are displayed from medial (septal) to lateral, left to right. The 3D block of VLA slices is recut parallel to the denoted long axis and perpendicular to the stack. The resulting oblique cuts are called horizontal long axis slices, seen in Figure 4.22C. They contain the left ventricle with its base toward the bottom of the image and its apex toward the top. The right ventricle appears on the left side of the image. Serial horizontal long axis slices are displayed from inferior to anterior, from left to right. Slices perpendicular to the denoted long axis and perpendicular to the VLA slices are also cut from the stack. These are termed short axis (SA)

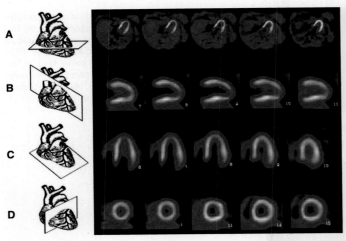

Figure 4.22 Image display of oblique angle reoriented tomograms. **Panel A** shows the transaxial images reconstructed perpendicular to the long axis of the patient's body. **Panel B** shows how trigonometry is used to reorient the transaxial images into VLA images, usually displayed progressively from the septum to the lateral wall. **Panel C** shows how the VLA images are reoriented into horizontal long axis images, usually displayed from inferior to anterior wall. **Panel D** shows how SA tomograms are reoriented perpendicular to both the vertical and horizontal long axis, displayed progressively from apex to base.

slices; they contain the left ventricle with its anterior wall toward the top, its inferior wall toward the bottom, and its septal wall toward the left. Serial SA slices are displayed from apex to base, from left to right, in Figure 4.22D.

5.4. Motion correction

Patient motion can be detected by cine displays, sinograms, and summed planar images. Cine displays of the planar projections are perhaps the simplest and best way to detect patient motion. Watching the heart as it moves from right to left in the planar projections can be used to detect all types of motions. The clinician should watch the movie of the planar projections at a fairly rapid cine rate and observe any up- and down-motion of the heart, particularly in relation to a fixed horizontal line just below the heart. The best way to detect and correct motion is for the technologist to observe the patient and repeat the scan if sufficient motion occurs. Immediately repeating the scan might prevent the patient from having to return for a repeated scan due to the original acquisition being technically impossible to interpret. The projections at the top of each of the two panels in Figure 4.23 illustrate how patient motion might be detected using a cine display. If the distance between the heart and the horizontal line is compared in each of these planar projections, the top images show no variation in the distance between the inferior wall of the left ventricle and the line, whereas, in the bottom panel, the heart is seen to move vertically away from the line starting with the projection where the arrow points. Note that the SA and VLA images in the bottom panel show regions of decreased counts as compared to those in the upper panel of the same patient with no motion. Even a slight amount of motion (3 mm) can result in an artifact in the SPECT images. If this motion is not detected by the clinician before interpretation of the images, a false positive report might result.

A sinogram is another way to detect patient motion. A sinogram is an image comprised of one line of pixels through the planar projections plotted vertically for each of the angular projection views. Thus, the x-axis of the sinogram represents pixels

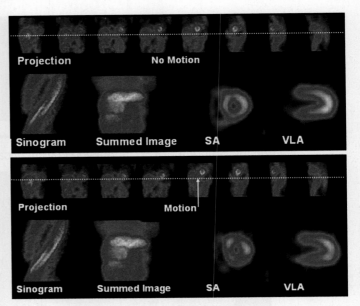

Figure 4.23 Methods for detecting patient motion. Each panel shows how patient motion may be detected by one of three methods: (a) by visually monitoring the distance between the LV and a fixed line as the planar images are dynamically rotated, (b) by reviewing a sonogram, and (c) by reviewing a summed image of all projections. Note that the top panel shows no patient motion while the bottom panel shows patient motion as pointed by the arrow. Also compare the effects of motion on the myocardial perfusion distribution seen on a SA and a VLA images.

across the camera face, and the y-axis represents different planar projections, with the first planar projection at the top. The heart can be seen as a bright stripe from the top right to the lower left of the sinogram. The clinician looks for a break in this stripe that would represent the patient moving to the left or right. Thus, sinograms are best for detecting horizontal motion across the table. Sinograms can also show vertical motion, but not quite as well as they show the horizontal motion.

Patient motion can also be detected by using summed projections. The summed projection is formed by adding all of the planar projections for the SPECT acquisition. The heart can be traced as a blurry horizontal line across the center of the image. To evaluate patient motion, the clinician should look for a change in the height of the heart that would indicate movement during the acquisition. This is best used for detecting vertical motion, that is, motion of the patient along the table.

There are a number of software algorithms both manual and automatic for correcting patient motion.[28] These algorithms work best when the motion is vertical along the table and no twisting motion has occurred. As with any algorithm, although in general they correct for the motion quite well they may sometimes fail. Sometimes when these algorithms are applied to patients that have not moved during acquisition, the software might get confused and detects and corrects for nonexistent motion. It is advisable to always visually confirm that the motion correction software has performed appropriately.

6. IMAGING ARTIFACTS

6.1. Physical factors that may affect SPECT image formation

Accurate reconstructions of the radionuclide distribution in the body depend upon accurate detection of the emitted γ rays.

However, not all of the γ rays emitted by a radionuclide emerge from the body, and those that do are not all detected in the right place. These complicating factors degrade the resulting image. The three factors that cause degradations in SPECT are attenuation, scatter, and distance-dependent resolution or blur of collimation. Attenuation is the absorption of γ rays by other materials and includes photons lost due to both the photoelectric effect and Compton scatter. The probability that a γ ray is absorbed increases with the density of the material through which it must pass, but decreases with increasing energy of the photon.

Other γ rays may interact with electrons in the material through which they are passing, causing them to change direction and lose energy. These γ rays may still emerge from the body, but from a direction other than their original path. If these γ rays are detected by the γ camera, they appear to be originating from the wrong place. Finally, γ rays traveling in paths other than parallel to a collimator hole may still travel through that hole and be detected by the camera. This becomes more likely as the source gets farther and farther away from the collimator. The result is a blurring in the final image that is dependent upon the distance between the source and collimator, called the detector response, which was discussed in Figure 4.21.

SPECT MPI uses transmission-scan-based AC. The transmission scan measures the distribution of attenuation coefficients (attenuation map) of the patient, which is used in iterative reconstruction to correct the decrease in counts resulting from photon attenuation. SPECT scatter correction uses the Compton window subtraction method.[16] In this method, an image that consists of scattered photons is acquired by a second energy window placed below the photopeak window, and this image is multiplied with a scaling factor and then subtracted from the acquired photopeak window image to produce a scatter-corrected image. Another energy-window-based approach uses two energy windows, one above and one below the photopeak window, to estimate the portion of scattered photons in the photopeak window.[17]

6.2. Partial volume effect

The inherent limitation of the resolution of nuclear imaging systems makes the image of a point source appear as a Gaussian curve. Therefore, the image of an object made up of multiple points appears as overlapping Gaussian curves, which have higher value for the center point than that for periphery point even when the object has uniform distribution of the radiotracer. As a result of this phenomenon, myocardial brightness increases when myocardial thickness increases[12] up to twice the resolution of the system (FWHM) as shown in Figure 4.24. If the object is thicker than $2 \times$ FWHM the resulting count profile will reach a plateau representative of the true expected counts. This effect is used quite successfully to assess left-ventricular regional myocardial thickness and thickening, but care must be taken when interpreting gated SPECT images since the myocardium appears brighter in areas where it is thicker and dimmer in areas where it is thinner.

The limited resolution of nuclear imaging systems makes the image of a point source appear as a Gaussian curve (PSF, top panel). The PSF of a nuclear imaging system increases in width with distance away from the surface of the collimator. Measurement of the PSF of the system at various distances allows the development of a resolution recovery algorithm, which deblurs the image and improves the defect contrast. Two types of resolution recovery algorithms are now commercially available: inverse filtering based on frequency-distance principle[18] and 3D modeling of the distance-dependent collimator response in iterative reconstruction.[19] The main idea of resolution recovery is to apply a mathematical algorithm to transform the blurred image response to become a sharp response.

6.3. Attenuation correction artifact due to misregistration

Attenuation correction requires that the emission scan and the transmission scan that is used to correct for photon attenuation must be perfectly registered with each other. Figure 4.25 illustrates the artifact caused by misregistration between the emission and transmission scans due to patient motion. Simultaneous acquisitions of both emission and transmission scans ensure that these two are registered. But when these two acquisitions are performed sequentially and the patient moves in-between the two acquisitions, artifacts are created.

The top left panel shows a diagram of a transaxial emission cardiac image superimposed on the corresponding transaxial transmission image. Note that the entire cardiac silhouette lies in the pericardium not touching the lung area represented in dark blue. The top right image shows an actual attenuated corrected emission cardiac image when correctly registered with the transmission image. The bottom right panel shows a diagram of

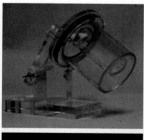
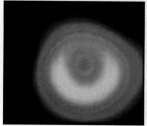
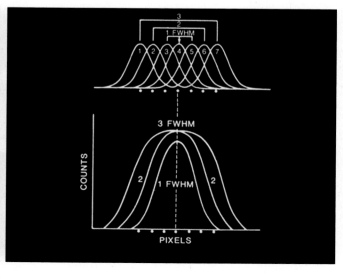

Figure 4.24 Principle of the partial volume effect. This figure shows a study where a phantom representing an eccentric myocardial chamber is filled with a constant concentration of Tl-201. Note the thinner anterior wall appears to be hypoperfused in comparison to the inferior wall. This can be a cause of misinterpretation when, for example, the patient might have a hypertrophic thickened septum making the left ventricular lateral wall of normal thickness and perfusion appear hypoperfused. As described in the text, the right panel illustrates that the partial volume effect is strictly a physics phenomenon explained by the relationship of the superimposition of the PSF, their resolution expressed as the full width at half maximum (FWHM), and the thickness of the radioactive distribution.

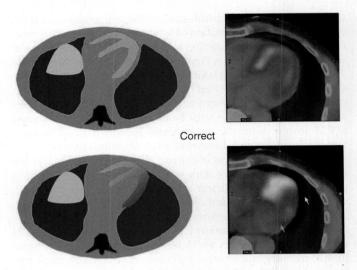

Correct

Misregistration resulting in under-correction

Figure 4.25 Attenuation correction artifact due to misregistration of the emission and transmission images. Note in the bottom panel that when the emission image is misregistered in reference to the transmission image such as it appears that the lateral wall is inside the lung, this wall is under-corrected making it look hypoperfused as compared to the correct registration in the top panel.

a transaxial emission cardiac image superimposed on the corresponding transaxial transmission image. Note that the two images are misregistered and that the free left-ventricular lateral myocardial wall overlaps a portion of the lung. The bottom right image shows an actual attenuated corrected emission cardiac image that is similarly misregistered in relation to the transmission image. Note that the left ventricular free wall overlaps a portion of the lung. This misregistration causes that the lateral wall is under-corrected and thus it appears as though it is hypoperfused.

7. EQUIPMENT MAINTENANCE AND QUALITY CONTROL

7.1. Camera uniformity

The joint commission on the accreditation of hospitals organizations (JCAHO) requires that a uniformity flood be acquired on each scintillation camera before clinical studies are done for any given day. These three million count floods can be used to detect uniformity defects. In Figure 4.26, Panel A, there are two example floods, one using a camera without a uniformity defect on the left, and one with a uniformity defect that might be caused by a poor PMT on the right. Panel B shows, in the same patient, corresponding thallium planar projections acquired with these cameras. Note that the planar image on the right shows decreased counts as compared to the one on the left. The problem is that even if cine displays of the planar images are viewed, it will be very difficult to detect that the decreased counts in the inferior myocardial wall were due to a camera uniformity problem as opposed to a true physiological perfusion abnormality. Correspondingly, when the transaxial slices are reconstructed (Panel C) the basolateral wall is decreased in counts. Although a ring artifact is caused by this uniformity problem and can be seen in transaxial images when imaging a uniform source, in this patient it is difficult to detect. Therefore, just by looking at the images it is difficult to detect this uniformity problem if the QC step is not performed. The VLA images (Panel D) make it even harder to detect when a decrease in counts might be due to a uniformity defect. It is very important that floods be performed on a daily basis in order to detect uniformity problems before they affect clinical images. Differences in positioning the patient between rest and stress scans may cause uniformity artifacts to appear in different locations in the two images, possibly mimicking ischemia.[11]

7.2. Quality control procedures for planar imaging

These are the QC procedures that are necessary to ensure images of diagnostic quality. These procedures are pertinent to guarantee both the quality of studies when performing planar imaging and the quality of the planar projections used in SPECT imaging.

Energy peaking consists of either manually or automatically placing the correct PHA's energy window over the photopeak energy of the radionuclide to be used. This process is usually performed with a radioactive point source imaged a distance away by an uncollimated camera or an extended sheet source on the collimated camera. Either way the entire field of view should be illuminated by the radioactive source. This process should be performed daily even in camera systems that perform this function automatically and that track the shift of the window. A photograph of the spectrum with the window superimposed is used to record these results.[20]

Figure 4.26 Effect of defective PMT on camera uniformity. The left column of each of the panels corresponds to a system with acceptable uniformity. **Panel A** shows the uniform flood field, **Panel B** shows a planar projection acquired with this system, **Panel C** shows a resulting transaxial perfusion image, and **Panel D,** a reoriented VLA image. The right column depicts the same results but now on a system with one defective PMT. Note how difficult it is to detect the artifact in the corresponding planar or transaxial images. Also note in **Panel D** how the inferior wall from the defective system appears to be hypoperfused due to this artifact.

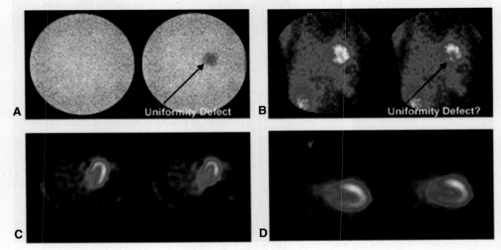

Intrinsic uniformity flood field is another QC procedure that should be performed daily to document the camera uniformity. These are also done using a radioactive point source and without a collimator. This acquisition should be performed using a source of low radioactivity (~100 μCi) in a small volume (~0.5 mL) to mimic a point source positioned at least five diameters of the camera's crystal, directly over the center of the detector. If this process proves difficult or time consuming it can be replaced with an extrinsic uniformity flood measurement. Extrinsic uniformity is measured with an extended radioactive sheet source that covers the entire collimated camera face.[21]

Sensitivity QC tests that the device is consistently counting the same radioactive source and should be performed weekly. This can be done at the same time the intrinsic (or extrinsic) uniformity tests are done by recording the number of counts acquired for a given time period adjusted to the magnitude of radiation used to create the image.

Resolution and linearity test is performed to document spatial resolution and its change over time as well as how the camera reproduces straight lines. This test consists of imaging an extended radioactive sheet flood source through a spatial resolution test phantom known as a bar phantom. Images of the phantom should be photographed to record the camera's performance and QC procedure. These images are assessed for how straight the bar lines are imaged and for intrinsic spatial resolution. Change in resolution is assessed by documenting the smallest bars that are discerned.[20]

7.3. Uniformity artifacts

Uniformity artifacts occur when one area of the camera face has decreased sensitivity compared to the other areas. This can occur when a PMT begins to work improperly or if the collimator is damaged. For example, if an acquisition is performed of an elliptical QC phantom that was filled with a uniform distribution of technetium, it can generate the two count profiles on the left

side of the figure. These count profiles should be steep on the sides and fairly flat across the top depending on the shape of the phantom. In case of uniformity problems, regions of decreased sensitivity are seen in each of these curves that are represented by a small dip at one point. The small dip will correspond to the same location on the camera in all of the projection views. When the images are reconstructed, this small dip is backprojected, as shown in the top right, and with more and more projections it will scribe out a circle in the transaxial image, as shown in the lower image. This kind of artifact may occur when the collimator is damaged and one or a few of the holes in the lead septa have been closed. To correct for small variations across the face of a collimator, 30 million count floods are used. These high count floods should be acquired at least once a month and are applied to images acquired with the same collimator being used by the same camera.[11]

7.4. Center-of-rotation

Center of rotation (COR) is a calibration performed frequently to ensure that the frame of reference used by the computer in reconstructing images is aligned with the mechanical axis of rotation of the SPECT camera system. If the center-of-rotation is properly calibrated, a radioactive point source placed in the center of the camera orbit should project to the center of the computer matrix. These results are seen in the middle panels in Figure 4.27.

Center-of-rotation errors are easy to detect with radioactive point sources. However, these errors can be very difficult to detect with a clinical distribution of activity. In the bottom panels, the center-of-rotation errors that correspond to the images of point sources directly above them can be seen. The center-of-rotation error manifests itself in the myocardial perfusion horizontal long axis images as an area of reduced counts on either side of the myocardium (often surrounding an area of higher counts). It is sometimes difficult to distinguish between the center-of-rotation errors demonstrated here and true clinical defects. This makes it

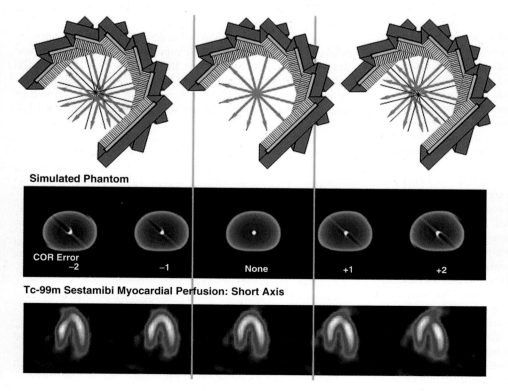

Simulated Phantom

COR Error
−2   −1   None   +1   +2

Tc-99m Sestamibi Myocardial Perfusion: Short Axis

Figure 4.27 Artifacts caused by COR misalignment. For most cardiac SPECT, a 180° orbit is used. When a radioactive point source is used with this orbit, a point source should also be reconstructed as a point in the image. With a COR error, however, the reconstruction no longer yields a point, instead, the point is smeared to make it appear as a tuning fork. This tuning fork artifact is so-named because the shape forms two lines in one direction and something that looks like a stem in the opposite direction. If the COR calibration errs by a negative amount, the images seen in the left panels are seen. In the middle left panels the smeared radioactive point sources reconstructed with this error are seen. If the error is in the positive direction then the images shown in the top right are seen. Note the larger the COR misalignment the more severe the image artifact. The camera processes that generated these errors are seen in the top diagrams.

extremely important that the technologists who perform the QC procedures properly calibrate the center-of-rotation for the camera.[11] There are several excellent reviews published[15,22] of how to detect and account for imaging SPECT artifacts.

8. RADIATION DOSIMETRY AND SAFETY

The type of radiation used in nuclear cardiology imaging is called ionizing radiation. Ionizing radiation refers to the breaking of electron bonds from atoms as the radiation travels through matter causing large number of positive and negative ion pairs, in this case in either the patient or the laboratory personnel. As the amount of ionization increases it increases the likelihood of damage to the living tissue.

8.1. Internal radiation dosimetry

The amount of radiation absorbed by an organ is the most important factor in determining the effects of radiation. Calculation of the radiation energy absorbed is the subject of internal radiation dosimetry. The traditional unit used to measure this energy is the radiation absorbed dose or *rad*, which is equivalent to 100 ergs of energy deposited per gram of absorber. When the relative biological damage absorbed by a specific type of tissue is taken into account it allows comparison of potential radiation damage between organs and is referred as the equivalent dose. Traditionally, the equivalent dose is measured using units of the roentgen-equivalent-man or *rem*.

In 1960 an international system of scientific units called the SI units was adopted. Although use of these units is more popular in Europe it is becoming more common to see these used in the scientific literature. Radiation absorbed dose in SI units is measured in *Gray* (Gy) where 1 Gy is equal to 100 rad. Similarly, the SI units for the equivalent dose is the *Sievert* (Sv) where 1 Sv is equal to 100 rem.

8.2. Radiation safety

Radiation safety is the analysis of issues related to the handling of radiation sources and the development of safe handling practices. It is important to understand the radiation dose received by the public from natural radiation to bring into context the radiation exposure of nuclear personnel and patients. Typical doses to individual from natural sources are approximately 3 mSv per year.[23] A nuclear medicine technologist receives at work roughly the same amount of radiation per year and a patient undergoing a rest/stress myocardial perfusion SPECT study would be receiving equivalent to roughly 5 years of natural radiation. *Exposure* has traditionally been used to describe the radiation levels in any environment. The traditional unit of exposure is the *Roentgen* (R).

Dose-modifying factors. These are factors that must be considered in addition to the knowledge that the more exposure to radiation, the higher the potential risk of radiation injury. These factors include[23] (a) the part of the body exposed; (b) the time span over which the radiation is delivered; (c) the age of the exposed individual; and (d) the type of radiation involved.

Reduction of radiation doses. The main rules to reduce radiation doses from external sources are to decrease the time of exposure, decrease the distance to the source, and use shielding when necessary. The effect of shielding on radiation is evident from our discussion of the attenuation and the half-value-layer concept. The issue of decreasing the time of exposure dictates that the personnel reduce their time working close to the external radiation source like a patient. Although this is a well known fact for radiation workers it can affect even more other personnel. For example

an echocardiographer who scans patients just after the patient's nuclear study can be exposed to significant radiation.

The last rule is to keep as much distance away from the external radiation source. This is because radiation obeys the inverse square law. The intensity of a radioactive point source at a distance from the source obeys the same law as for visible light. If the amount of radioactivity at the point source (S) remains constant, then the intensity of the radioactivity (number of photons) passing through a flat surface is inversely proportional to the square of the distance from the source. At a distance from 1 m, the diverging radioactive beam covers an area A represented by the square with each side of dimension x, or an area of x^2. At 2 m the diverging beam covers a square B in which now each side is twice as long as A ($2x$) and the area is $4x^2$, which is four times the area at 1 m. Since the amount of radioactivity remains constant, the number of photons falling on square A must spread out over four times as large by the time it reaches square B. Thus the activity per unit area at B, which is twice as far as A from the source, is one fourth of the activity passing through A[24] The value of this principle to radiation workers is that they can significantly reduce their radiation burden just by increasing the distance between them and a radioactive source such as patient already injected with a radioactive dose.

9. FUTURE DIRECTIONS

It is reassuring to know that the scientific principles discussed in this chapter have withstood the test of time and are not expected to change anytime soon. Instrumentation, on the other hand, can change at a quick pace. Although the basic Anger γ camera technology used in SPECT imaging had not changed for over 50 years now totally new designs are being commercialized, which focus all the available detectors on the heart increasing the count sensitivity, spatial resolution, or both. Cardiac PET is also migrating to a 3D configuration, which also yields significantly higher count sensitivity. Both PET and SPECT systems are also being coupled with high-end CT systems to create hybrid systems that can image both form and function.

This renaissance in new advanced SPECT and PET technology is due, in part, to the remarkable expansion in utilization of these techniques for imaging the heart. But this interest is also in anticipation of the realization of the promise of cardiovascular molecular imaging,[25] where molecular concepts are coupled to imaging principles to best understand, prevent, diagnose, and treat cardiac disease.

REFERENCES

1. Chandra R. *Introductory Physics of Nuclear Medicine.* Philadelphia, PA: Lea and Febiger; 1992.
2. Powsner RA, Powsner ER. *Essentials of Nuclear Medicine Physics.* Malden, MA: Blackwell Science; 1998.
3. Saha GB. *Fundamentals of Nuclear Pharmacy.* New York, NY: Springer-Verlag; 2003.
4. Anger HO. Scintillation camera with multichannel collimators. *J Nucl Med.* 1964;5:515–531.
5. Maublant JC, Peycelon P, Kwiatkowski F, et al. Comparison between 180° and 360° data collection in technetium-99m MIBI SPECT of the myocardium. *J Nucl Med.* 1989;30:295–300.
6. Hoffman EJ. 180° compared to 360° sampling in SPECT. *J Nucl Med.* 1982;23:745–746.
7. Knesaurek K, King MA, Glick SJ, et al. Investigation of causes of geometric distortion in 180° and 360° angular sampling in SPECT. *J Nucl Med.* 1989;30:1666–1675.
8. Smith WH, Kastner RJ, Calnon DA, et al. Quantitative gated single-photon emission computed tomography imaging: A counts-based method for display and measurement of regional and global ventricular systolic function. *J Nucl Cardiol.* 1997;4:451–463.
9. Machac J, Chen H, Almeida OD, et al. Comparison of 2D and high dose and low dose 3D gated myocardial Rb-82 PET imaging. *J Nucl Med.* 2002;43:777.

10. Schelbert HR, Beanlands R, Bengel F, et al. ASNC PET myocardial glucose metabolism and perfusion imaging guidelines: Part II guideline for interpretation and reporting. *J Nucl Cardiol.* 2003;10:557–571.
11. Garcia EV, Galt JR, Cullom SJ, et al. *Principles of Myocardial Perfusion SPECT Imaging.* North Billerica, MA: Du Pont Pharma; 1994:30.
12. Galt JR, Garcia EV, Robbins WL. Effects of myocardial wall thickness on SPECT quantification. *IEEE Trans Med Imag.* 1990;9:144–150
13. Shepp LA, Vardi Y. Maximum likelihood reconstruction for emission tomography, *IEEE Trans Med Imag.* 1982;1:113–122.
14. Hudson HM, Larkin RS. Accelerated image reconstruction using ordered subsets of projection data. *IEEE Trans Med Imag.* 1994;13:601–609.
15. DePuey EG, Garcia EV. Optimal specificity of thallium-201 SPECT through recognition of imaging artifacts. *J Nucl Med.* 1989;30(4):441–449.
16. Jaszczak RJ, Greer KL, Floyd CE Jr, et al. Improved SPECT quantification using compensation for scattered photons. *J Nucl Med.* 1984;25:893.
17. Ogawa K, Ichihara T, Kubo A. Accurate scatter correction in single photon emission CT. *Ann Nucl Med Sci.* 1994;7:145.
18. Glick SJ, Penney BC, King MA, et al. Noniterative compensation for the distance-dependent detector response and photon attenuation in SPECT imaging. *IEEE Trans Med Imag.* 1994;13:363.
19. Zeng GL, Gullberg GT, Tsui BMW, et al. Three-dimensional iterative reconstruction algorithms with attenuation and geometric point response correction. *IEEE Trans Med Imag.* 1990;38:693.
20. DePuey EG, Garcia EV. Updated imaging guidelines for nuclear cardiology procedures (Part 1). *J Nucl Cardiol.* 2001;8:G1–G58.
21. Nichols KJ, Galt JR. Quality control for SPECT imaging. In: DePuey EG, Garcia EV, Berman DS, eds. *Cardiac SPECT Imaging.* 2nd Ed. New York, NY: Lippincott Williams and Wilkins; 2001:17–39.
22. DePuey EG. Artifacts in SPECT myocardial perfusion imaging. In: DePuey EG, Garcia EV, Berman DS, eds. *Cardiac SPECT Imaging.* 2nd Ed. New York, NY: Lippincott Williams and Wilkins; 2001:17–39.
23. Cherry SR, Sorenson JA, Phelps ME. *Physics in Nuclear Medicine.* Philadelphia, PA: Saunders; 2003.
24. Christensen EE, Curry TS, Dowdey JE. *An Introduction to the Physics of Diagnostic Radiology.* 2nd Ed. Philadelphia, PA: Lea and Febiger; 1978:159.
25. Gropler RJ, Glover DK, Sinusas AJ. *Cardiovascular Molecular Imaging.* New York, NY: Informa Healthcare USA, Inc.; 2007.
26. Hubble JH, Seltzer SM. Tables of x-ray mass attenuation coefficients, and mass energy-absorption coefficients. National Institute of Standards and Technology; 1996. Available at: http://physics.nist.gov/PhysRefData/XrayMassCoef/cover.html
27. Beller GA, Bergmann SR. Myocardial perfusion imaging agents: SPECT and PET. *J Nucl Cardiol.* 2004;11(1):71–86.
28. Geckle WJ, Frank YL, Links JM, et al. Correction for patient motion and organ movement in SPECT: Application to exercise thallium-201 cardiac imaging. *J Nucl Med.* 1988;29:441–450.

5

Nuclear Cardiology Examination and Imaging Protocols

Milena J. Henzlova

1. INTRODUCTION

The discipline of nuclear cardiology evolved from the "tracer" concept of Georg Hevesy (1913; Nobel Prize, 1943), measurements of circulation time in humans using Radon by Blumgart (1925), development of the molybdenum–technetium generator (1951–1953), introduction of commercial Anger camera (Nuclear Chicago Company, 1964) to attempts to image myocardial perfusion at rest (1971) and during stress (1973) using potassium-43. Perhaps, the use of planar thallium-201 imaging of an acute myocardial infarction in 1975 qualifies as the real "birth" of the subspecialty, as we experience it today. Further milestones include the development of Single Photon Emission Computerized Tomography (SPECT, 1977) and dual head SPECT imaging (1979); the introduction of Technetium-based tracers (^{99m}Tc sestamibi, 1990), gated acquisition (1991), attenuation correction (1992); and more recently the introduction of hybrid systems (CT/PET, CT/SPECT), which added anatomic information to physiological (flow) data.[1]

Positron emission tomography (PET), despite its earlier technological development, has much shorter history as a clinical tool for noninvasive evaluation of coronary perfusion and for metabolic (molecular) imaging. Clinical utilization of Rb-82 PET perfusion studies started in 1995. Currently, there are >1,000 PET and PET/CT cameras installed in the United States, mostly used for both clinical oncology and cardiology applications.

The introduction of pharmacological stressors enlarged the pool of patients who could be evaluated for ischemic heart disease. Intravenous dipyridamole was introduced in 1979, dobutamine in 1984, adenosine in 1990 and regadenoson in 2008. In the United States, pharmacological stress is used in most PET studies and in close to 50% of SPECT stress studies.

2. APPLICATIONS

2.1. Myocardial perfusion imaging

The primary role of myocardial perfusion imaging (MPI) is the detection of flow-limiting coronary artery stenoses. The presence of a significant coronary obstruction leads to uneven distribution of resting coronary blood flow or blood flow reserve. The limitation of flow is manifested best with increased demand. Adequacy of coronary flow is, therefore, studied during physical stress (treadmill or bicycle exercise). A surrogate, but not preferred, mode of stress is the visualization of coronary flow distribution after coronary vasodilation (pharmacological stress). Indications for MPI studies are well defined in the ASNC Guidelines[2] and ACCF/ASNC[3] Appropriateness Criteria. Both documents are periodically updated and revised. MPI is used for (a) diagnosis of suspected

coronary artery disease (CAD), (b) assessment of progression of known CAD, both in symptomatic and asymptomatic subjects, and (c) evaluation of myocardial viability in patients with significant left ventricular dysfunction. Effective risk stratification is based on the evaluation of stress data, perfusion and metabolic patterns, and assessment of ventricular function. MPI is currently one of the most extensively validated noninvasive cardiac imaging modalities for both diagnosis and prognosis in patients with known or suspected CAD.

2.1.1. Diagnosis of suspected coronary artery disease

Indication for testing in **symptomatic (chest pain or chest equivalent)** patients is based on "pre test probability" of CAD, which can be assessed by numerous validated scores. Most scores include gender, age, characterization of symptoms,[4] and presence/absence of known risk factors for CAD: smoking, diabetes, hyperlipidemia, hypertension, and family history of premature coronary atherosclerosis (e.g., Framingham risk score). Appropriate indication for MPI is the presence of intermediate or high pretest probability for the presence of CAD. Low pretest probability is an inappropriate reason for testing even in the presence of symptoms. Low CAD risk is defined as below average age-specific risk, i.e., a 10-year absolute risk <10% of an adverse cardiac event, moderate risk is defined as a 10-year absolute risk between 10% to 20%; high risk as 10-year absolute risk of >20%.

A large number of patients present (most often to the Emergency Departments) with acute chest pain syndromes. The role of MPI is well established for **rest imaging** in patients with intermediate CAD probability, no ST elevation, and normal initial serum troponin levels.[5] Stress imaging protocols for this patient population are the same as for ambulatory symptomatic patients (after myocardial necrosis was excluded by serial marker measurements).

Indications for testing of **asymptomatic** patients are also well defined. It is appropriate to test patients free of chest pain, who present with new onset of congestive heart failure, or ventricular tachycardia, and have moderate Framingham risk score for CAD. Another accepted indication is new onset of atrial fibrillation (in patients with high Framingham risk score). It has been documented that the prevalence of perfusion abnormalities in asymptomatic patients with atrial fibrillation is no different from the prevalence in asymptomatic patients in sinus rhythm. However, atrial fibrillation independently increases the risk of cardiac events; thus, prognosis of detected perfusion defects is worse than in patients in sinus rhythm.[6,7] Testing is also recommended in asymptomatic subjects who have high-risk occupations (e.g., commercial airplane pilots) and have moderate to high CAD risk.

Inclusion of additional groups of asymptomatic patients evolves as the concept of detection of **preclinical disease** evolves. Development of imaging techniques, which visualize vascular wall, detect nonobstructive disease, and assess global plaque burden, shift the emphasis from detection of flow-limiting lesions and estimation of short-term risk of cardiac events, to long- term, lifelong estimation of risk with appropriate preventive consequences. Such thinking led to the identification of high-risk asymptomatic patient groups (as opposed to mass-screening) with so called **CAD equivalent**[8]: Known vascular disease (peripheral or cerebrovascular), diabetes mellitus, chronic kidney disease, elderly, functionally impaired, and those with intermediated Framingham score and detected calcium score of >400 U.

2.1.2. Testing in patients with known disease

MPI is appropriate in patients who have documented CAD (by catheterization, rest ECG, history of MI or other noninvasive imaging) and stable symptoms (every 2 years for detection of progression of the disease), or in patients with worsening symptoms (with or without history of mechanical revascularization). Asymptomatic patients after revascularization [coronary artery bypass surgery (CABG) and/or percutaneous interventions

(PCI)] should not be tested more often than every 5 years. MPI after acute coronary syndromes [(unstable angina, non-ST elevation myocardial infarction (NSTEMI) or ST elevation myocardial infarction (STEMI)] is indicated if there are no plans for coronary catetherization (for risk stratification), or for physiological evaluation of significance of a moderate stenosis detected by invasive or noninvasive coronary angiography (CTA).

The role of stress testing in the perioperative cardiovascular evaluation before noncardiac surgery was recently updated,[9] and will be reviewed annually. The need for stress testing depends on surgical urgency and on surgical risk. Urgent (emergency) surgery proceeds without further evaluation. Active cardiac conditions, which include unstable coronary syndromes, decompensated congestive heart failure, significant arrhythmia, and severe stenotic valvular disease, require further evaluation and treatment. The evaluation of patients without active cardiac conditions depends on anticipated surgical risk (Fig. 5.1). The mode of testing depends on patient's ability to exercise (exercise stress test versus MPI or stress echo) and rest ECG (e.g., LBBB, paced rhythm).

The evaluation of **myocardial viability** in the context of known CAD attempts to predict restoration of systolic function after

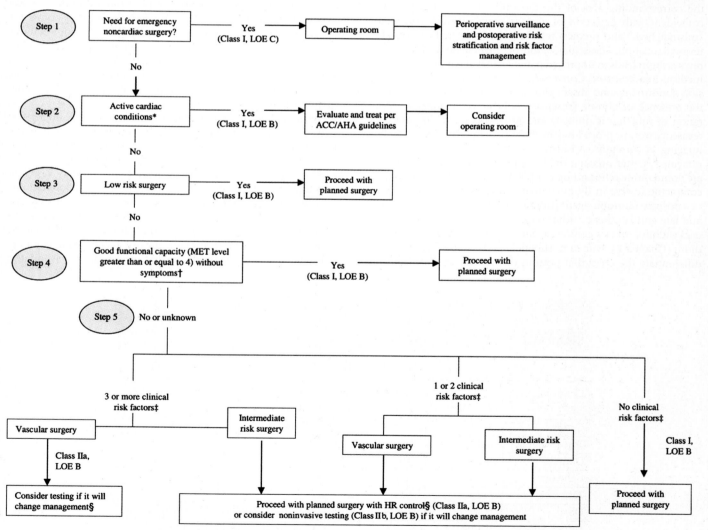

Figure 5.1 Cardiac evaluation and care algorithm prior to noncardiac surgery. (Reproduced from Fleisher LA, Beckman JA, Brown KA, et al. ACC/AHA 2007 Guidelines on Perioperative Cardiovascular Evaluation and Care for Noncardiac Surgery: Executive Summary: A Report of the American College of Cardiology/American Heart Association Task Force on Practice Guidelines. *J Am Coll Cardiol.* 2007;50(17):1707–1732.)

revascularization (surgical or transcutaneous) in patients with severe left ventricular dysfunction (typically defined as left ventricular ejection fraction [LVEF] ≤ 35%). Nuclear methods depend on visualization of viable myocytes in the dysfunctional myocardial segments using **flow** (Tl-201, ^{99m}Tc or Rb-82) or **metabolic tracers** (F16 FDG): The prevailing free fatty acid metabolism in nonischemic myocardium is replaced due to ischemia by glucose metabolism. Visualization of the glucose analog, deoxyglucose, radiolabeled with F16, confirms the presence of functional myocytes.

When flow agents are used, visualization of the myocardium is proof of "viability," since active membrane transport is required for Tl-201 retention in the myocardium. Improved systolic function has been documented after revascularization in dysfunctional segments, which are able to retain Tl-201 during stress or rest imaging or after Tl-201 reinjection. ^{99m}Tc-based agents are retained intracellulary (attached to the mitochondria). Again, visualization of perfusion in dysfunctional segments is predictive of functional improvement after restoration of coronary blood flow. PET metabolic imaging requires documentation of a perfusion deficit using either PET flow agents (Rb-82 or N-13 ammonia) or SPECT flow agents, and visualization of preserved metabolic activity using a glucose analog (Fluorodeoxyglucose FDG labeled with F16) in the corresponding area of the myocardium. A perfusion defect coincident with detection of glucose metabolism is considered "mismatched," and predicts restoration of systolic function after revascularization. Revascularization of "mismatched" areas of the myocardium leads to improved patient survival when compared to medical management. Conversely, "matched" defects with perfusion abnormality and absent glucose metabolism are indicative of the presence of fibrotic (scar) tissue. Postrevascularization restoration of function is unlikely and prognosis is not improved by revascularization procedures in these patients. The F16 FDG PET imaging is currently considered a "gold standard" for viability imaging.[10] Other imaging methods used for the same indication are dobutamine echocardiography, which relies on visualization of contractile reserve in dysfunctional segments after short infusion of a positive inotropic agent (Intravenous Dobutamine, Chapter 2) and late enhancement cardiac magnetic resonance (CMR), which uses gadolinium as a contrast agent to detect areas of scar myocardium (Chapter 7). Due to its superior spatial resolution, CMR can differentiate the epicardial portion of the myocardium from the endocardium, i.e., transmural and subendocardial infarction can be diagnosed. Nevertheless, the superior spatial resolution of CMR is matched by the superior contrast resolution of nuclear scintigraphic methods (Chapter 4).

2.1.3. Stressors

The preferred modality for stressing the myocardium is physical **exercise** (treadmill or stationary bicycle).[11] Prerequisite for successful testing is patient's ability to exercise for a meaningful period of time: Optimal exercise should last at least 6 min and be symptom limited; achieved peak heart rate should be at least 85% of the predicted maximal heart rate adjusted for age (220-age), which guarantees adequate increase in coronary flow for detection of obstructive disease. Standardized exercise protocols need to be used (e.g., Bruce, modified Bruce, and Naughton) to allow comparison of exercise capacity with patient's peers and also comparisons in case of serial testing. Exercise capacity is a very robust prognostic marker of future cardiac events. Various scores have been developed for prognostication (such as the Duke or VA scores). Predictive variables include exercise capacity (length of exercise), ST changes (horizontal and down sloping depressions being diagnostic of ischemia), exercise-induced chest pain, and heart rate recovery. Exercise testing is extremely safe (expected major complications occur in 1/10,000 patients) when contraindications for testing and end points for exercise are adhered to. Exercise combined with MPI requires tracer injection at peak exercise with continuation of exercise for another minute, particularly with ^{99m}Tc based tracers: First pass uptake into the myocardium is incomplete, thus two to four circulation times are desirable to achieve optimal tracer uptake, prior to commencing of imaging (Table 5.1).

Pharmacological stress (Table 5.2) is an acceptable alternative in patients who are unable to exercise adequately or have baseline ECG abnormalities which are known to decrease specificity of MPI results: LBBB, W-P-W pattern and ventricular pacing. Currently approved agents for pharmacological stress are coronary vasodilators: Dipyridamole, adenosine, and regadenoson; and dobutamine, which is a positive inotropic and chronotropic agent, as well as a coronary vasodilator. Most of the PET perfusion studies use pharmacological stress because of very short half-life of the PET tracers.

Dipyridamole (Persantine) was the first agent used in conjunction with MPI. Dipyridamole, an indirect coronary vasodilator,

TABLE 5.1
CHARACTERISTICS OF STRESSORS

	Exercise	Dipyridamole	Adenosine	Dobutamine
Chemical	N/A	Pyridine derivative	Endogenous	Synth. catechol.
CBF	1–2x	3–4x	3–5x	2x
Onset	3–5 min	4–6 min	1–2 min	2–4 min
Tracer injection	Before peak	7–9 min	3 min	At peak
Duration	2–5 min	30–40 min	30–60 s	4–6 min
Ischemia	Yes	Rare	Rare	Yes
AV block	No	Rare	Yes	No
Dose	N/A	0.56/kg	140 mcg/kg/min	5–40 mcg/kg/min
HR/BP effect	Up/up	Up/down	Up/down	Up/up
Antidote	N/A	Aminophylline	Stop infusion	β-blocker

CBF, coronary blood flow.

TABLE 5.2
CHARACTERISTICS OF SPECT AND PET TRACERS

	99mTc sestamibi	99mTc tetrofosmin	Thallium-201	Rubidium-82	N-13 (ammonia)	F-18 (FDG)	Iodine-123 (BMIPP)
Class	Isonitrile	Diphosphine	Element	Element	Element	Element	Element
Dose	20–40 mCi	20–40 mCi	2–4 mCi	30–60 mCi	10–20 mCi	10 mCi	15–20 mCi
Energy	140 keV	140 keV	69–83 keV	511 keV	511 keV	511 keV	159 keV
Half-life	6 h	6 h	73 h	75 s	9.96 min	110 min	13.21 h
Gating	Yes	Yes	Possible	Yes	Yes	Yes	Yes
Viability	Yes	Yes	Yes	Yes	Yes	Yes	Yes
Source	Generator	Generator	Cyclotron	Generator	Cyclotron	Cyclotron	Cyclotron
Redistribution	Negligible	Negligible	Yes	No	No	No	No
SPECT/PET	SPECT	SPECT	SPECT	PET	PET	PET/SPECT	SPECT

prevents rapid break down and re-uptake of endogenous adenosine, and thus increases intravascular concentration of adenosine. A competetive inhibitor of adenosine is theophylline and other methylxantines such as metabolites of caffeine. The recommended i.v. dose of dipyridamole is 0.56 mg/kg infused over 4 min. Expected hemodynamic effects include mild systemic blood pressure drop and reactive heart rate increase. Contraindications to its use are similar to contraindication to exercise and additionally, history of bronchospasm, particularly presence of active wheezing at the time of testing. Recent (12 to 24 h) ingestion of caffeine containing beverages or caffeine containing medicines leads to competitive occupation of adenosine receptors (A2) and subsequent attenuation of expected coronary vasodilation, therefore diagnostic sensitivity of the test is decreased. Aminophilline (125 to 250 mg i.v.) is a selective inhibitor of dipyridamole and could be used to abolish not only unpleasant side effects (such as headache), but also infrequent manifestations of myocardial ischemia (ST depression, chest pain).

Adenosine (Adenoscan) induces coronary vasodilation directly by activation of the A2A receptor. Due to its very short half-life, continuous infusion (140 mcg/kg/min × 6 min) is needed; at 3 min the tracer is injected without interruption of the adenosine infusion. Indications and contraindications for use of adenosine are similar to those of dipyridamole. By nonselective activation of A1, A2b, and A3 receptors, adenosine may induce infrequent but undesirable and self-limiting side effects: Bronchospasm and high degree AV block.

Regadenoson (Lexiscan) is the first "selective adenosine analog" approved for use with MPI. Regadenoson has higher affinity of the A2A adenosine receptor (leading to coronary vasodilation) and lower affinity for the A1, A2b, and A3 receptors. In premarketing testing (in two identical randomized, double blind studies, regadenoson was compared to adenosine in 2,015 patients. P-R prolongation (first degree AV block) was observed in 3% of the patients (compared to 7% after Adenoscan), second degree AV block was observed in one patient. In two separate studies, 49 and 48 patients, respectively, with chronic obstructive pulmonary disease (COPD) or asthma were studied. Incidence of bronchoconstriction in COPD patients was 12% with regadenosone and 6% with placebo. In the asthma group, the incidence was 4% in both regadenosone and placebo groups. The drug is injected as a bolus (0.4 mg or 5 mL), followed by saline flush and then tracer injection. Diagnostic noninferiority of regadenosone compared

to Adenoscan has been documented.[12] Abstinence from caffeine prior to testing is the same as for other coronary vasodilators. Aminophylline can be used as an antidote similarly to the use of dipyridamole. Regadenosone has renal clearance. Caution needs to be exerted in patients with advanced renal failure. No data is currently available in patients requiring hemodialysis.

A second selective adenosine analog (Binodenoson, King Pharmaceuticals, Inc), not yet approved for clinical use, is also administered as an i.v. bolus. Noninferiority with respect to adenosine and fewer adverse events were reported in a multicenter trial (VISION).

Dobutamine, a preferred pharmacological agent for stress echocardiography, is least often used for MPI. Its use is limited to patients who are unable to exercise adequately and have prohibitive bronchospastic disease. Dobutamine is an unsuitable agent for patients with LBBB and W-P-W ECG patterns. Dobutamine, a direct β1 and β2 stimulator, is infused in incremental fashion (from 10 up to 40 mcg/kg/min). Expected effect includes heart rate increase, blood pressure increase, and at higher concentrations coronary vasodilatory effect. Intravenous dobutamine half-life is about 2 min, tracer injection should be followed by additional 2 min of dobutamine infusion. The direct antidotes, in case of severe side effects, such as ischemia or tachyarrhythmia, are short acting β-blockers (e.g., esmolol 0.5 mg/kg over 1 min).

The combined use of i.v. adenosine and low level exercise[13] is safe, may quantify exercise capacity limitation, decreases severity of adenosine side effects, and may improve image quality (by lesser gastrointestinal accumulation of 99mTc-based tracers).

2.1.4. Radiotracers
SPECT: Thallium-201 (Tl-201) and two technetium-99 (99mTc) based tracers (sestamibi—Cardiolite and tetrofosmin—Myoview) are currently available for MPI (Table 5.3). Tl-201 (a potassium analog) has a 73 h physical half-life, peak gamma energy of 80 keV, renal excretion and monoexponential washout (redistribution) from the myocyte. A single injection of 2.5 to 4.0 mCi is used for SPECT imaging. Tl-201 was the first tracer used for MPI, currently it is used for stress imaging less often compared to Tc99m-based agents. However, Tl-201 is a preferred tracer for SPECT "viability" studies. Radiation dose to the patients is the highest of all perfusion tracers.[14] 99mTc sestamibi and 99mTc tetrofosmin have 6 h physical half-life, peak gamma energy of

TABLE 5.3
DIAGNOSTIC PERFORMANCE OF 13 NH3 AND 82 RB PET (COMPARED TO CORONARY ANGIOGRAPHY)

Author	Year	Number	Stress	Tracer	Reference CAG	Sensitivity			Specificity		
						Positive test	Pt. w. CAD	%	Negative test	Pt. w.o. CAD	%
Schelbert HR	1982	45	Dipyridamole	$^{13}NH_3$	>50%	31	32	97	13	13	100
Tamaki N	1985	25	Exercise	$^{13}NH_3$	N/R	18	19	95	6	6	100
Yonekura Y	1987	50	Exercise	$^{13}NH_3$	>75%	37	38	97	12	12	100
Tamaki N	1988	51	Exercise	$^{13}NH_3$	>50%	47	48	98	3	3	100
Gould L [a]	1986	50	Dipyridamole	$^{12}Rb\backslash^{13}NH_3$	QCA SFR <3	21	22	95	9	9	100
Demer L [a]	1989	193	Dipyridamole	$^{12}Rb\backslash^{13}NH_3$	QCA SFR <4	126	152	83	39	41	95
Go RT	1990	202	Dipyridamole	^{12}Rb	>50%	142	152	93	39	50	78
Stewart RE	1991	81	Dipyridamole	^{12}Rb	QCA >50%[b]	50	60	83	18	21	86
Marwick T	1992	74	Dipyridamole	^{12}Rb	>50%	63	70	90	4	4	100
Grover McKay	1992	31	Dipyridamole	^{12}Rb	>50%	16	16	100	11	15	73
Laubenbacher	1993	34	Dipyridamole/adenosine	$^{13}NH_3$	QCA >50%[b]	14	16	88	15	18	83
Bateman TM[c]	2006	112	Dipyridamole	^{12}Rb	>50%[c]	64	74	86	38	38	100
Williams BR[d]	1994	287	Dipyridamole	^{12}Rb	>67%	88	101[d]	87	99[d]	112[d]	88
Simone GL[d]	1992	225	Dipyridamole	^{12}Rb	>67%	[d]	[d]	83	[d]	[d]	91
Totals†		1460				696	778		297	333	
Weighted Mean								89%			89
Weighted Mean excluding R/S						544	603	90%	160	183	87
Nonweighted Mean								91%			91

[a]Study reported than 50pts in Gould et al. (1988) were included. Thus Gould et al not included in mean calculations.
[b]Other cut-offs reported; >50% noted here
[c]Electronic database, matched cohort design; values derived from reported population, sensitivity and specificity.
[d]Retrospective study. MPI influenced CAG decision: mixed patient and region method for sensitivity/specificity, patients with disease could not be easily determined in one study.
N/R, not reported;
R/S, retrospective;
CAG, coronary angiogram;
QCA, quantitative coronary angiography;
SFR, stenosis flow reserve based on QCA Data.
Source: From Beanlands RS, et al. CCS/CAR/CANM/CNCS/CanSCMR joint position statement on advanced noninvasive cardiac imaging using positron emission tomography, magnetic resonance imaging and multidetector computed tomographic angiography in the diagnosis and evaluation of ischemic heart disease—executive summary. Can J Cardiol. 2007;23:107–119. With permission.

140 keV, hepatobiliary excretion, and negligible washout; two tracer injections are needed for rest—stress or stress–reset studies. Due to higher photon flux (higher peak energy, higher tracer dose permissible due to shorter half-life), 99mTc cardiac imaging has lesser soft tissue attenuation (compared to Tl-201) and allows for better quality of gated imaging. Absence of redistribution allows for higher flexibility of imaging: sequence of rest–stress imaging can be reversed or performed on separate days, time to imaging is more flexible. Also, radiation dose to the patients is lower, when compared to Tl-201.

Rubidium-82 **(Rb-82)** is an analog of potassium with a half-life of 75 s. An on-site Strontium-82 (Sr-82) generator is needed (and needs to be replaced every 4 weeks). Myocardial extraction of Rb-82 is similar to Tl-201 (i.e., exceeds extraction of 99mTc-based tracers, Chapter 10). **N-13 ammonia** has half-life of 10 min, an on-site cyclotron is needed. First pass extraction of N-13 ammonia is high (approximately 95%). Both agents allow for gating of the images and calculation of LVEF at rest and during coronary vasodilation. Rb-82 and N-13 ammonia are the most commonly used PET perfusion tracers. F-16 FDG, a glucose analog, is the most commonly used metabolic tracer, has a half-life of 109.8 min, and also needs a cyclotron for production. The physical properties of other radiotracers are discussed at greater extent in Chapter 10. PET tracers energy is 517 keV.[15]

2.1.5. Protocols[16]

A single dose (2.5 to 4.0 mCi) of thallium-201 is injected at peak stress, and stress SPECT imaging is started 10 to 15 min later. A second set of SPECT images is acquired 2.5 to 4 h later. A reversible perfusion abnormality is consistent with diagnosis of stress-induced ischemia. The mechanism of Tl-201 "redistribution" is differential washout of the tracer: Washout is faster from the myocardium with highest stress coronary flow with subsequent highest flow-dependent tracer uptake in the myocytes. Nonreversible, "fixed" perfusion defects may represent fibrotic tissue (a scar). Partial or complete reversibility (i.e., viability) can be assessed with rest imaging after longer interval between the tracer injection and imaging (up to 24 h), or after an additional 1 mCi dose of Tl-201 (reinjection).

99mTc tracers require administration of two tracer doses (rest–stress or stress–rest). A 2-day protocol avoids residual contamination from the first dose. Two day imaging is preferred in overweight patients (BMI > 30) in whom poor quality, low dose rest images are anticipated. Using a 2-day strategy, it is possible to eliminate the rest part of the test (second day rest imaging) in some patients, if all reviewed aspects of the stress test and stress imaging are normal. One-day rest–stress protocol is used most often: Low dose (one third of the total dose) is administered at rest, high dose (two thirds of the total dose) is administered at

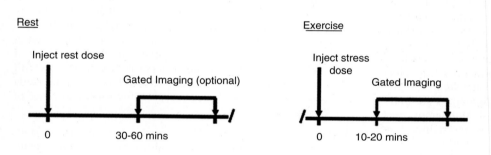

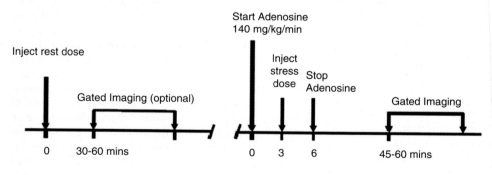

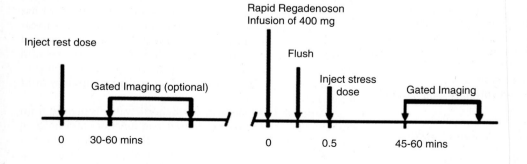

Figure 5.2. Tc99m rest–stress, 1-day or 2-day exercise and pharmacological protocols. (Reproduced from Henzlova MJ, Cerqueira MD, Mahmarian JJ, et al. Stress protocols and tracers. *J Nucl Cardiol.* 2009;13(6):e80–90 (www.asnc.org accessed 7/9/2008, with permission.))

peak stress. Optimal time between rest tracer injection and imaging is 30 to 60 min, 10 to 20 min for exercise stress and 45 to 60 min for pharmacological stress (Fig. 5.2). Dual isotope imaging (Tl-201 rest imaging, ^{99m}Tc stress imaging) allows for somewhat shorter duration of the test and in appropriate patients, evaluation of myocardial viability. However, the downside of dual isotope imaging is markedly higher radiation dose to the patient.

For PET perfusion imaging, similar to SPECT, a rest–stress sequence is used, 30 to 40 mCi of Rb-82 are used for each acquisition. A scout scan (10 to 20 mCi) is used for proper positioning. With PET/CT systems, CT scout is used instead and CT is also used for attenuation correction. Similarly to SPECT, gating is feasible, LVEF can be measured at rest and during pharmacological stress. With an integrated CT scanner with at least 16-slices acquisition and calculation of a calcium score could be performed.

2.1.6. Interpretation and reporting

A result of a completed MPI study needs to be effectively and timely communicated to the referring physician, who is expected to use the findings for best evidence-based therapeutic decisions. ASNC guidelines[17] propose a format which includes INDICATION, CLINICAL INFORMATION, PROCEDURE, FINDINGS and IMPRESSION. PROCEDURES include observations accumulated during the stress part of the test. Adequacy of the stress, ECG ST changes, arrhythmia, provoked symptoms—all contribute to final interpretation of each study. Findings (results) include assessment of study quality (e.g., motion, subdiaphragmatic tracer activity, and attenuation artifacts), perfusion defect description (including localization, severity, extent, and reversibility), evaluation of biventricular size and function (including transient ischemic dilation, lung activity) and extracardiac abnormalities (e.g., pleural or pericardial effusion, ascites, focal tracer uptake in the breast or lungs, splenomegaly). IMPRESSION summarizes all findings and categorizes them as normal or abnormal. Ambiguous conclusions should be discouraged and diagnostic uncertainty should not occur in more than 10% of the studies. Complete study interpretation is expected in 1 business day, final reporting to the requesting physician is required in two business days. Structured and timely reporting as recommended by ASNC is now embraced by ICANL (Intersocietal Commission for Accreditation of Nuclear Laboratories) and thus, needs to be followed as a prerequisite for laboratory accreditation.

MPI is a unique diagnostic method for the evaluation of physiological consequences of inadequate myocardial perfusion due to obstructive CAD. Intuitive correlation with anatomical localization of coronary atherosclerosis let to numerous correlations with selective coronary angiography. The best correlations report >90% sensitivity and specificity for detection of significant (>75% luminal stenosis of epicardial coronary arteries). Both sensitivity and specificity values can be expressed either per patient or per vessel. Correlation is highest for detection of LAD disease, whereas for detection of circumflex artery disease it is the lowest. The highest correlation is achieved in patients with multivessel disease. Those findings have accepted limitations. More data is available for SPECT studies than for PET perfusion studies. However, there is no reason to doubt good correlations between PET MPI and coronary angiography (Table 5.3).

2.1.7. Limitations of myocardial perfusion imaging

(1) MPI depicts coronary flow physiology, not anatomy—coronary anatomy altered by vessel occlusion, collateral development and/or implantation of venous or arterial grafts may at times prevent concordant correlation with coronary anatomy.

(2) Attenuation artifacts create illusion of perfusion defects and lead to false positive studies.

(3) Noncoronary myocardial disease, such as hypertrophy, infiltrative disorders or presence of a LBBB, alter even distribution of the coronary blood flow and mimic the presence of CAD.

(4) Inadequate stress, either due to inadequate exercise or incomplete response to coronary vasodilation, may cause underestimation of CAD severity.

(5) MPI depicts relative distribution of the coronary flow, the most significant stenosis is apparent and less severe disease is underdiagnosed.

2.1.8. Limitations of coronary angiography

(1) Extent of coronary atherosclerosis may be underestimated particularly when the disease is diffuse. This phenomenon is well documented in patients with post-transplant vasculopathy.

(2) Functional significance of imaged stenosis may be overestimated or underestimated using anatomical image.

(3) With the advent of intravascular ultrasound and CTA, it has become clear that the extent of vascular wall pathology exceeds the diagnostic power of the luminogram.

(4) Correlation between a noninvasive test (SPECT) and an invasive test (coronary angiography) is often affected by "referral bias": prevalence of obstructive disease is higher in those referred for coronary angiography than those who are referred for a noninvasive test. Conversely, those with a normal noninvasive test are rarely referred for an invasive test. A category of "normalcy" was suggested to eliminate some of the bias. Normalcy is defined as percentage of patients with a normal study, who were expected to have a normal study based on low (<5%) pretest probability for the presence of obstructive CAD.

Each imaging study needs to be reviewed in systemic manner starting with assessment of the study quality (patient motion, attenuation artifacts, noncardiac findings, reconstruction artifacts, lung uptake, and right ventricular uptake). Perfusion defects need to be evaluated for localization, severity, extent, and reversibility. Semiquantitative evaluation requires use of multisegmental models: A 17-segment model is most commonly used. The use of segmental models allows for quantification of perfusion abnormalities. Sum of segmental perfusion defects during stress (none, mild, moderate, severe, and absent uptake) is called stress sum score, sum of rest values is called rest sum score. Positive values indicate presence of reversibility, i.e., ischemia (and viability). An almost linear correlation between sum scores and prognosis of future events has been well documented. Prolonged survival has been documented after mechanical therapy of obstructive CAD (CABG or PCI) only in patients with high sum scores.[18] To the contrary, a normal study (both the imaging portion and stress part of the test) has an excellent short-term (1.5 to 2 years) prognosis: <1% per year (0.6%) incidence of adverse cardiac events.[19,20] Caution is needed in following patient groups: older patients, diabetics, patients with chronic renal failure, and those with known CAD. Benign prognosis of a normal perfusion study in those patient groups may be of lesser duration.

Additional information and prognostic value is derived from evaluation of the left ventricular size and function. MPI imaging allows for quantification of left ventricular volumes and LVEF—both parameters have known independent prognostic values in patients with left ventricular systolic dysfunction.

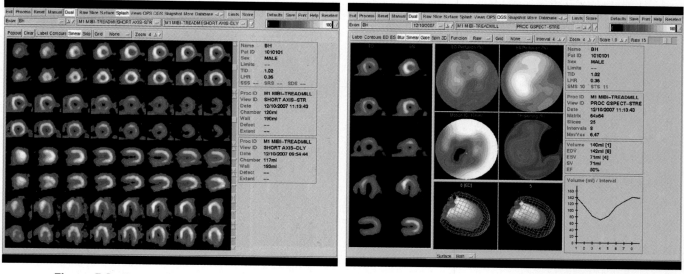

Figure 5.3. ^{99m}Tc exercise stress test in a 72 year old male with chest pain and horizontal ST depressions in multiple ECG leads during exercise. Extensive reversible (ischemic) perfusion defects and transient ischemic dilation (TID) of the left ventricle are present. Post exercise left ventricular ejection fraction was 49%. Subsequent coronary angiography revealed significant three-vessel CAD.
CAD, coronary artery disease.

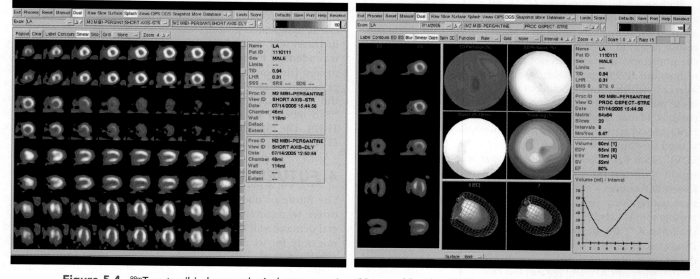

Figure 5.4. ^{99m}Tc setamibi pharmacological stress test in a 98-year old male with history of arterial hypertension and shortness of breath. No perfusion defects were detected; left ventricular size and function were normal.

Examples of MPI studies with ^{99m}Tc tracers are depicted in Figures 5.3–5.5: result of a normal MPI study (Fig. 5.4), result of a study with characteristics of extensive ischemia (Fig. 5.3), and result of a study with evidence of nonreversibilty (scaring, nonviability; Fig. 5.5).

2.2. Assesment of ventricular function

Quantification of LV function is decisive for diagnosis and prognosis, both in coronary (ischemic) and nonischemic cardiomyopathies. Transthoracic echocardiography is a primary imaging method because of availability, portability, cost effectiveness, and ability to assess pericardial disease and valvular function. However, nuclear methods allow for accurate evaluation of ventricular size, global and segmental systolic function.

Gated SPECT and **PET** perfusion studies (Figs. 5.3–5.5) can be easily gated (most often into eight frames per cardiac cycle). Using a calibration factor it is possible to express ventricular volumes in absolute values (ESV and EDV in cc/m^2) and calculated LVEF (LVEDV – LVESV/LVEDV). Both rest and poststress images can be gated. However, gated rest images after a low tracer dose may be noisy due to low counts. Images gated relatively shortly after stress may not represent a true resting state, particularly in patients with extensive stress-induced ischemia, where the effect of stunning may lead to underestimation of true rest LVEF. Gated SPECT derived LVEF has been correlated with other imaging modalities. Correlations are consistently high. Difficult gating, most often due to frequent ectopy or very irregular atrial fibrillation, may rarely preclude ECG gating.[21]

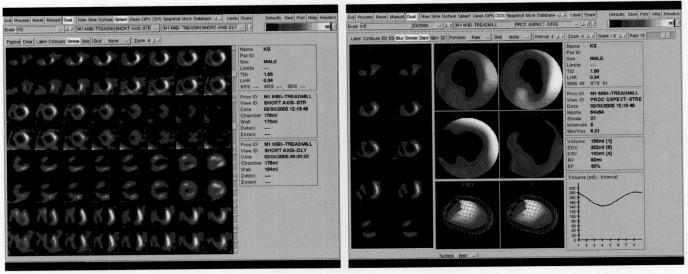

Figure 5.5. ^{99m}Tc sestamibi exercise stress test in a 30-year-old male with history of an anterior Q wave myocardial infarction. Large irreversible (fixed) perfusion defects in the anterior, apical, and septal segments suggest presence of scarring (nonviability) in the LAD territory. Left ventricular ejection fraction was 30%.
LAD, left anterior descending artery disease.

Radionuclide angiography (RNA, MUGA, and GBP) remains an easily obtainable and highly reproducible method for the evaluation of left ventricular function.[22] Main indications include congestive heart failure of any etiology and monitoring of cardiotoxic chemotherapy. The test does not require any patient preparation, technetium Tc-99m pyrophosphate (PYP) injection preceeds ^{99m}Tc injection, which allows labeling of red blood cells. In vivo labeling is the preferred method, which is safe and highly effective in most patients. Planar imaging (anterior, lateral, and long axial oblique [LAO] views) are standard; the LAO (or best septal separation) view is used for count-based quantification of LVEF (LVEDV – LVESV/EDV). Since RNA uses three-dimensional count estimate in the region of interest (ROI) (highest counts in the ROI = end-diastole, lowest ROI counts = end-systole), calculation is devoid of geometrical assumptions used for planimetric methods (such as contrast angiography). Labeling of RBC remains effective for at least 6 h (half-life of ^{99m}Tc), thus ventricular function can be studied under condition other than rest conditions such as exercise. Exercise-induced segmental and global changes in LV function have been used for detection of CAD, and are still used for timing of valve surgery.

A third method for LV evaluation is **first pass**[23]—the method imitates contrast ventriculography, it requires an uninterrupted bolus of ^{99m}Tc injected either at rest or at peak of stress. Additionally, as the tracer travels from a peripheral vein through the right atrium and ventricle, right ventricular function can be assessed without count contamination from the left atria and the left ventricle. The limitations of a successful study include need for a large proximal i.v., uninterrupted i.v. bolus and absence of ectopy, atrial fibrillation and severe tricuspid regurgitation at the time of injection.

3. RADIATION DOSE

With enormous growth in the volume of diverse cardiac imaging methods, many of them delivering radiation to the patient (CT, SPECT, and PET), there is acute awareness of possible long-term effect of cumulative radiation doses.[24] Dose estimates are estimates in statistical sense and are made with numerous assumptions, which continuously evolve. Therefore, any prognostication

of possible future adverse effects of radiation currently depends on modeling and not on true long-term observations. Stochastic effects of radiation postulate that probability of cancer occurrence increases with accumulated dose. With our current knowledge it is prudent to follow As Low As Reasonably Achievable (ALARA) maxim (the lowest possible tracer dose should be used—ALARA principle). Also, the younger the patient, the more important is the minimalization of the radiation dose. For cardiac studies, ^{99m}Tc labeled tracers have preferable dosimetry compared to Tl-201. The highest radiation dose is delivered with dual isotope (Tl-201/^{99m}Tc) protocols (Fig. 5.6).

4. FUTURE DIRECTIONS

The future of nuclear methods for myocardial imaging will be driven by technological progress and therapeutic advances. Societal demand will require that each new technology will be tested not only for its technical feasibility, but also for its diagnostic effectiveness, therapeutic consequences, and effect on clinical outcomes and cost. Maintenance of highest quality of imaging and image interpretation is currently rudimentarily tested by ICANL and by physicians certification boards (CBNC). Both efforts seek to eliminate flagrant outliers, but do not guarantee continuous maintenance and improvement of quality. Adherance to guideliness and appropriateness criteria, elimination of unnecessary studies, awareness of radiation doses and related risks, stability of reimbursement, and elimination of administrative barriers to testing—all remain imperfect and therefore, open to continuous improvement.[25,26]

The objectives of cardiac imaging are similar for both invasive and noninvasive imaging: detection of obstructive CAD, evaluation of ventricular function, detection of viability in patients with severe ventricular dysfunction and evaluation of valvular function. Since none of the available methods represent the elusive "one stop shopping," hybrid devices have become available: PET–CT, SPECT–CT, and perhaps MR–PET.[27] A surrogate for economically unfeasible combinations is the use of fusion technology—as images are acquired sequentially by different techniques and

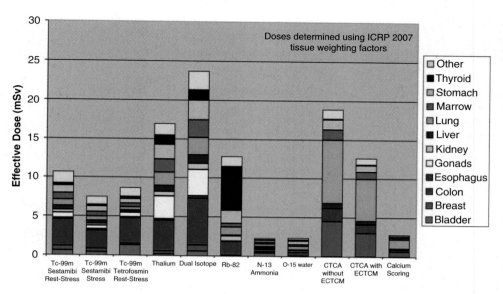

Figure 5.6. Estimated effective and organ doses from standard cardiac imaging studies. (Reproduced from Einstein, et al. *Circulation.* 2007;116:1290–1305, with permission.)

later superimposed. Need for faster acquisition of SPECT studies is being addressed by new reconstruction algorithms using traditional Anger camera as well as by novel solid-state acquisition technologies (Chapter 4).[28,29]

On the horizon is detection of preclinical disease or detection of its markers (such as endothelial dysfunction, vascular wall calcification) particularly in high risk asymptomatic patient groups (e.g., patients with diabetes, autoimmune disease, chronic renal disease, and strong family history). This development will go hand in hand with therapeutic advances—only effective intervention will justify diagnosis in asymptomatic subjects. Study of disease activity (currently mostly with F-16 FDG) may be used in the future for risk stratification of patients at risk for acute coronary syndromes, as well as for evaluation of drug effect on the activity of atherosclerosis.

Utility of neuroimaging using guanidine analog (MIBG—[123]I) for risk stratification of patients with end-stage cardiomyopathies has a long history, and is clinically used in Japan. A large multi-center study is now closed to completing enrollment, and after completion of the follow-up, its role in heart failure patients will be clarified.[30]

No new SPECT tracer has been introduced for over 15 years (^{99m}Tc teboroxime was approved for use, but its production was discontinued). The latest candidate, now in final stages of clinical testing, is a "memory agent." Pentadecanoic acid (BMIPP), an analog of free fatty acid (prevailing substrate of aerobic myocardial metabolism), labeled with ^{123}I was shown to depict ischemic myocardium with up to 30 h latency. The potential is obvious for patients with acute chest pain, who arrive to the ED—immediate rest imaging could potentially shorten the evaluation time, since wait for negative necrosis markers could be avoided. Another indication could be its injection after positive exercise stress testing (either symptomatic or accompanied by ECG changes). The long "memory time" would allow for great flexibility for injection and imaging.[31]

Identification of metabolically active ("vulnerable") atherosclerotic plaques prone to rapture or erosion and subsequent intravascular thrombosis, extends early diagnosis beyond identification of flow obstructing lesions. PET radionuclide molecular imaging[32] appears to be the most suitable method for detection of metabolic activity, apoptosis, thrombogenicity, and angiogenesis (Table 5.4).

TABLE 5.4
VISUALIZATION OF ATHEROSCLEROSIS BY RADIONUCLIDE IMAGING

Underlying Plaque Biology	Radionuclide Tracer	Experimental Setting	Reference
Inflammation	^{99m}Tc-LDL	Human carotid/ileofemoral artery	Lees et al. (1988)[48]
Lipoprotein accumulation	^{123}I-LDL	Human carotid artery	Virgolini et al. (1991)[53]
	^{125}I-LDL	Rabbit aorta	Virgolini et al. (1991)[54]
	^{99m}Tc-ox-LDL	Human carotid artery	Iuliano et al. (1996)[57]
	^{123}I-MDA2 (Ab to ox-LDL epitope)	Rabbit arteries	Tsimikas et al. (1999)[49]
	^{125}I-IK17 (Ab to ox-LDL epitope)	Mouse aorta	Shaw et al. (2001)[50]
	^{123}I-SP4 (apoliprotein B fragment)	Rabbit aorta	Hardoff et al. (1993)[51]
	^{125}I-SP4	Rabbit aorta	Lu et al. (1996)[52]
Chemotaxis	^{125}I-MCP-1 (chemotactic molecule)	Rabbit aorta	Ohtsuki et al. (2001)[9]
Angiogenesis	^{125}I-c(RGD(I)yV) (peptide binding $\alpha_1\beta_3$)	Murine ischemic hindlimbs/ HUVECs	Lee et al. (2005)[33]
	^{99m}Tc-(NC100692) (peptide binding $\alpha_2\beta_3$)	Murine ischemic hindlimbs	Hua et al. (2006)[47]

(Continued)

TABLE 5.4
VISUALIZATION OF ATHEROSCLEROSIS BY RADIONUCLIDE IMAGING (Continued).

Underlying Plaque Diology	Radionuclide Tracer	Experimental Setting	Reference
Monocyte recruitment/ activity	^{111}In-monocytes	Human arteries	Virgolini et al. (1990)[17]
	^{18}F-FDG (metabolic activity)	Rabbit iliac artery	Lederman et al. (2001)[18]
	^{18}F-FDG	Human carotid artery	Rudd et al. (2002)[20]
	^{18}F-FDG	Human arteries	Ben Haim et al. (2004)[19]
	^{18}F-FDG in comparison with ^{18}F-FCH	Mouse aorta	Matter et al. (2007)[24]
	VHSPNKK-modified magnetofluorescent nanoparticle (VNP) (VCAM-1 expression)	Mouse carotid artery	Kelly et al. (2005)[31]
Apoptosis	^{99m}Tc-annexin V (phosphatidylserine expression)	Rabbit aorta	Kolodgie et al. (2003)[72]
	^{99m}Tc-annexin V	Human carotid artery	Kietselaer et al. (2004)[70]
	^{99m}Tc-annexin V	Swine coronary artery	Johnson et al. (2005)[71]
	^{99m}Tc-annexin V	Mouse aorta	Isobe et al. (2006)[75]
Proteolysis	^{123}I-HO-CGS27023 A (MMP inhibitor)	Mouse carotid artery	Schäfers et al. (2004)[10]
	GHPGGPQKC-NH2 (cathepsin K substrate)—NIRF probe	Mouse aorta and human carotid arteries	Jaffer et al. (2007)[66]
Thrombogenicity and cell recruitment	^{111}In platelets	Human carotid artery	Minar et al. (1989)[76]
	^{111}In-platelets	Human carotid artery	Moriwaki et al. (1995)[77]
	^{125}I-GPVI/^{123}I-GPVI (platelet collagen receptor)	Mouse carotid artery	Gawaz et al. (2005)[11]
	^{99m}Tc-DMP-444 (GPIIb-IIa Inhibitor)	Canine coronary artery	Mitchel et al. (2000)[78]
	^{99m}Tc-T2G1s Fab (fibrinogen binding)	Canine femoral/carotid artery	Cerqueira et al. (1992)[79]
	^{125}I-L19 (fibronectin binding)	Mouse aorta	Matter et al. (2004)[82]

Source: From Langer HF, et al. Radionuclide Imaging. A molecular key to the atherosclerotic plaque. *J Am Coll Cardiol.* 2008;52:1–12. With permission. FCH, fluorocholine; FDG, fluorodeoxyglucose; GP, glycoprotein; HUVEC, human umbilical vein endothelial cell; LDL, low-density lipoprotein; MCP, monocyte chemoattractant protein; MDA2, malondialdehyde epitope on oxidized low-density lipoprotein; MMP, matrix metalloproteinase; NIRF, near-infrared fluorescent; ox-LDL, oxidized low-density lipoprotein; RGD, protein sequence "arginine-glycine-aspartic": VCAM, vascular cell adhesion molecule.

REFERENCES

1. Wagner NH. *A Personal History of Nuclear Medicine.* New York: Springer New York; 2006.
2. Imaging guidelines for nuclear cardiology procedures. A Report of The American Society of Nuclear Cardiology Quality Assurance Committee. *J Nucl Cardiol.* 2006;13:e21–e171.
3. ACCF/ASNC Appropriateness Criteria for Single-Photon Emission Computed Tomography Myocardial Perfusion Imaging (SPECT MPI). A Report of the American College of Cardiology Foundation. Quality Strategic Directions Committee Appropriateness Criteria Working Group and the American Society of Nuclear Cardiology. *J Am Coll Cardiol.* 2005;46:1587–1605.
4. ACC/AHA 2002 Guideline Update for Exercise Testing. A Report of the American College of Cardiology/American Heart Association.Task Force on Practice Guidelines (Committee on Exercise Testing). www.acc.org, www.americanheart.org (accessed 7/5/2008).
5. Wackers FJTh, Brown KA, Heller GV, et al. American Society of Nuclear Cardiology position statement on radionuclide imaging in patients with suspected acute ischemic syndromes in the emergency department or chest pain center. *J Nucl Cardiol.* 2002;9:246–250.
6. Abidov A, Hachamovitch R, Rozanski A, et al. Prognostic implication of atrial fibrillation in patients undergoing myocardial perfusion single-photon emission computed tomography. *J Am Coll Cardiol.* 2004;44:1062–1070.
7. Askew JW, Miller TD, Hodge DO, et al. The value of myocardial perfusion single-photon emission computed tomography in screening asymptomatic patients with atrial fibrillation for coronary artery disease. *J Am Coll Cardiol.* 2007;50:1080–1085.
8. Shaw LJ, Berman DS, Blumenthal RS, et al. Clinical imaging for prevention: Directed strategies for improved detection of presymptomatic patients with undetected atherosclerosis - Part I: Clinical imaging for prevention. *J Nucl Cardiol.* 2008;15:e6–e19.
9. ACC/AHA 2007 Guidelines on Perioperative Cardiovascular Evaluation and Care for Noncardiac Surgery. A Report of the American College of Cardiology/American Heart Association Task Force on Practice Guidelines (Writing Committee to Revise the 2002 Guidelines on Perioperative Cardiovascular Evaluation for Noncardiac Surgery). *J Am Coll Cardiol.* 2007;50:e150–e241.
10. Allman KC, Shaw LJ, Hachamovitch R, et al. Myocardial viability testing and impact of revascularization on prognosis in patients with coronary artery disease and left ventricular dysfunction: A meta-analysis. *J Am Coll Cardiol.* 2002;39:1151–1158.
11. Gibbons RJ, Balady GJ, Brficker JT. American College of Cardiology/America Heart Association task force of practice guidelines (Committee to update the 1997 exercise testing guidelines). *Circulation.* 2002;106:1883–1892.
12. Iskandrian AE, Bateman TM, Belardenelli L, et al. On behalf of the ADVANCE MPI investigators: Adenosine versus regadenoson comparative evaluation in myocardial perfusion imaging. Results of the ADVANCE phase 3 multicenter international trial. *J Nucl Cardiol.* 2007;14:645–658.
13. Elliot MD, Holly TA, Leonard SM, et al. Impact of an abbreviated adenosine protocol incorporating adjunctive treadmill exercise on adverse effects and image quality in patient undergoing stress myocardial perfusion imaging. *J Nucl Cardiol.* 2007;7:584–589.
14. Einstein AJ, Moser KW, Thompson RC, et al. Radiation dose to patients from cardiac diagnostic imaging. *Circulation.* 2007;116:1290–1305.
15. Machac J, Bacharach SL, Bateman TM, et al. Positron emission tomography myocardial perfusion and glucose metabolism imaging. *J Nucl Cardiol.* 2006;13:e121–e151.
16. Henzlova MJ, Cerqueira MD, Mahmarian JJ, et al. Stress protocols and tracers. *J Nucl Cardiol.* 2006;13:e80–e90.
17. Hendel RC, Wackers FJTh, Berman DS, et al. American Society of Nuclear Cardiology Consensus. Statement: Reporting of radionuclide myocardial perfusion imaging studies. *J Nucl Cardiol.* 2003;10:705–708.
18. Hachamovitch R, Berman DS, Shaw LJ, et al. Incremental prognostic value of myocardial perfusion single photon emission computed tomography for the prediction of cardiac death. Differential stratification for risk of cardiac death and myocardial infarction. *Circulation.* 1998;97:535–543.
19. Hachamovitch R, Hayes S, Friedman JD, et al. Determinants of risk and its temporal variation in patients with normal stress myocardial perfusion scans. What is the warranty period of a normal scan? *J Am Coll Cardiol.* 2003:41;1329–1340.
20. Yoshinage K, Chow BJ, Williams K, et al. What is the prognostic value of myocardial perfusion imaging using rubidium-82 positron emission tomography? *J Am Coll Cardiol.* 2006;48:1029–1039.

21. Germano G, Berman D. Gated single-photon emission computed tomography. In: Iskandrian IA, Verani MS, eds. *Nuclear Cardiac Imaging: Principles and Applications.* 3rd Ed. New York: Oxford University Press; 2003:121–136.
22. Corbett JR, Akinboboye OO, Bacharach SL, et al. Equilibrium radionuclide angiocardiography. *J Nucl Cardiol.* 2006;13:56–79.
23. Friedman JD, Berman DS, Borges-Neto S, et al. First-pass radionuclide angiography. *J Nucl Cardiol.* 2006;13:e42–e55.
24. Einstein AJ, Sanz J, Dellegrottaglie S, et al. Radiation dose and cancer risk estimates in 16-slice computed tomography coronary angiography. *J Nucl Cardiol.* 2008;15:232–240.
25. Douglas P, Iskandrian AE, Krumholz Gillam L, et al. Achieving quality in cardiovascular imaging: proceedings from the American College of Cardiology-Duke University Medical Center Think Tank on Quality in Cardiovascular Imaging. *J Am Coll Cardiol.* 2006;48(10):2141–2151.
26. Heller GV, Katanick SL, Sloper T, et al. Accreditation for cardiovascular imaging. Setting quality standards for patient care. *JACC Cardiovasc Imaging.* 2008;3: 390–397.
27. Beanlands RS, Chow BJ, Dick A, et al. CCS/CAR/CANM/CNCS/CanSCMR joint position statement on advanced noninvasive cardiac imaging using positron emission tomography, magnetic resonance imaging and multidetector computed tomographic angiography in the diagnosis and evaluation of ischemic heart disease—executive summary. *Can J Cardiol.* 2007;23:107–119.
28. Patton JA, Slomka P, Germano G, et al. Recent technologic advances in nuclear cardiology. *J Nucl Cardiol.* 2007;14:501–513.
29. Einstein AJ, Sanz J, Santo Dellegrottaglie S, et al. Radiation dose and cancer risk estimates in 16-slice computed tomography coronary angiography. *Nucl Cardiol.* 2008;15:232–240.
30. Verberne HJ, Brewster LM, Somsen GA, et al. Prognostic value of myocardial ^{123}I-metaiodobenzylguanidine (MIBG) parameters in patients with heart failure: A systematic review. *Eur Heart J.* 2008;29:1147–1159.
31. Inaba Y, Bergman R. Diagnostic accuracy of b-methyl-p(^{123}I)-iodophenyl-pentadecanoic acid (BMIPP) imaging: A meta-analysis. *J Nucl Cardiol.* 2008; 15:345–352.
32. Langer HF, Haubner R, Pichler BJ, et al. Radionuclide imaging. A molecular key to the atherosclerotic plaque. *J Am Coll Cardiol.* 2008;52:1–12.

Magnetic Resonance Imaging Physical Principles and Instrumentation

6

Randolph M. Setser

George P. Chatzimavroudis

1. INTRODUCTION

Magnetic resonance imaging (MRI) is one of the most widely used diagnostic imaging techniques worldwide, with established applications in neurological, musculoskeletal, abdominal, and oncological imaging, among others. Although cardiovascular MRI (CMR) represents only a small fraction of the examinations performed each year overall, it still remains a powerful tool for assessment of cardiovascular anatomy and function.[1] The strength of MRI lies in its unique ability to produce high resolution tomographic images of the human body in any arbitrary orientation, with soft tissue contrast that is superior to competing imaging modalities such as ultrasound or computed tomography (CT). Furthermore, this is accomplished without the use of ionizing radiation; instead, MRI utilizes radio waves and a large, spatially and time varying magnetic field to create images.

The basis for MRI lies in the physics of nuclear magnetic resonance (NMR) described in 1946 by Purcell et al. and by Bloch,[2,3] who, in 1952, were awarded the Nobel Prize in Physics for their work. NMR has applications in physics and chemistry and can be used to analyze the atomic composition and structure of molecules. Most of MR imaging relies on the fact that NMR physics are applicable to hydrogen (^{1}H, also referred to as protons), an atom found ubiquitously in the body, which of course is composed predominately of water molecules.

The first in vitro MR images were published in 1973,[4] and the first in vivo human study was performed soon after in 1977. Commercial MRI scanners became available in the early 1980s, and by 2002, approximately 22,000 scanners were in use worldwide.[5] Development of CMR, however, began in earnest in the mid-1980s, once initial solutions to the problems of cardiac and respiratory motion had been developed.[6-8]

This chapter contains an introduction to the physics of MRI, with particular attention to the principles relevant to imaging the cardiovascular system. However, for a more complete description of the theoretical basis of MRI, the interested reader is directed to texts dedicated to the subject.[9-11]

2. THE PHYSICS OF MAGNETIC RESONANCE

2.1. Introduction

Magnetism is the result of the movement of electrical charge. All objects in nature have magnetic properties, although in magnets, these properties are strong. Passing an electric current through a loop of wire will create a magnetic field perpendicular to the loop. To create a homogeneous magnetic field with the magnetic field lines parallel to each other in a large region of interest, such as that inside an MRI scanner, a solenoid configuration can be used (Fig. 6.1). Any temporal changes in the strength of the electric field will induce corresponding temporal changes in the strength of the magnetic field and vice versa. This principle is fundamental to the ability to acquire magnetic resonance images.

Before describing how a magnetic resonance image is constructed, it is necessary to first focus on the nucleus of an atom from where the acquired signal actually originates.

2.2. Nuclear spin and magnetization

Any element whose nucleus has an odd number of neutrons or protons has the ability to be imaged using the principles of NMR. Among these elements, hydrogen is by far the most abundant in the human body, since the body contains more than 70% water. The nucleus of a hydrogen atom is a single positively charged proton. From quantum mechanics, it is known that the hydrogen nucleus (proton) has an angular momentum as a result of a property that is called *spin*. The combination of the electric charge and the angular momentum of the proton results in the formation of a magnetic field, making the proton a magnetic dipole (Fig. 6.2) with a magnetic moment μ.

In the absence of a strong magnetic field, the orientation of the vector of the magnetic moment μ of each proton is essentially random because the atom has enough kinetic energy to overcome the effect of earth's relatively weak magnetic field. However, a strong external magnetic field (such as that of an MRI scanner) with strength B_0 will affect the direction of the magnetic moment μ of each hydrogen nucleus. Based on the spin of the hydrogen nucleus (1/2), there are two directions in which μ will be oriented: parallel or anti-parallel to the direction of B_0 (Fig. 6.3). The parallel orientation corresponds to the low energy state and the antiparallel orientation corresponds to the high-energy state of the proton. Without this—even slight—preference, acquisition of MRI images would not be possible.

2.3. Precession and net magnetization

As mentioned above, the presence of a strong external magnetic field B_0 aligns the protons either parallel or antiparallel to B_0. A hypothetical closer look at each individual proton reveals that, in fact, the magnetic moment μ does not have a static alignment with B_0, but it rather wobbles around the direction of B_0 in a manner similar to the wobbling of a spinning top around the vertical

76

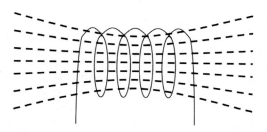

Figure 6.1 When electric current passes through a solenoid wire, a magnetic field is formed with parallel magnetic field lines at the center.

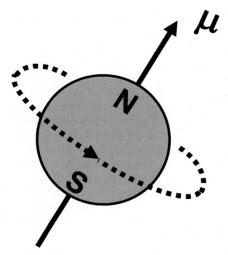

Figure 6.2 The combination of the spin (angular momentum) and the presence of the electric charge in a proton results in the formation of a magnetic field with a magnetic moment μ.

axis (Fig. 6.4). In the case of the top, the wobbling results from the combination of gravity and the angular momentum of the top. Similarly, the wobbling motion of μ results from the combination of B_0 and the angular momentum (due to the spin) of the proton. This wobbling motion is called *precession* and it takes place at a frequency which depends on the element and the strength of B_0, according to the following *Larmor* equation:

$$\omega_0 = \gamma B_0 \qquad (6.1)$$

where ω_0 is the *Larmor* frequency of precession and γ is a constant called the gyromagnetic ratio (42.58 MHz/T for hydrogen). The significance of the precession phenomenon and the *Larmor* frequency to the ability to acquire images will be clearly shown in the next sections.

The magnetic moment μ of each proton can be decomposed into two perpendicular components, referred to as the longitudinal and transverse components (Fig. 6.4). When one considers a mass of nuclei together (Fig. 6.5), all of the transverse components cancel out statistically; the sum of all longitudinal components from the parallel and antiparallel oriented protons equals what is called the *net magnetization M*.

2.4. Radiofrequency excitation and free induction decay

In order to construct an image, signal from the specific tissues and organs has to be acquired. To make the tissues emit a signal (energy), one should first provide excessive energy to the tissues in order to excite them. Based on quantum mechanics, exciting the protons means increasing the number of transitions from the lower energy state (parallel orientation) to the higher energy state (antiparallel orientation). To achieve this, the transmitting signal must have a frequency equal to the Larmor frequency of precession. This is the reason for which the phenomenon is called magnetic **resonance**.

The excitation signal is actually provided by very briefly applying a second external magnetic field, B_1 (Fig. 6.6). The direction of B_1 is perpendicular to that of B_0. Each field separately causes a precession along the axis of application of that field. The result is a composite rotation (Fig. 6.6), which flips the magnetization vector from the z-axis to the transverse plane XY. The component of the magnetization vector that lies on the z-axis is called *longitudinal magnetization* M_Z whereas the component that lies on the XY plane is called *transverse magnetization* M_{XY}. In MRI, the receiver detects only the M_{XY}; nevertheless, the features of M_Z are directly or indirectly contained into M_{XY}, making the behavior of the longitudinal magnetization of great importance in image contrast formation.

The degree of the flip of M_Z into the transverse plan depends on the strength of B_1 and the duration of its application. Flip angles of 90° or 180° are very common in MRI, although other angles are being used depending on the technique of image data acquisition as it will be shown in the next sections. Because the excitation signal is in the radiofrequency (RF) range and has a short duration, it is called *RF pulse*.

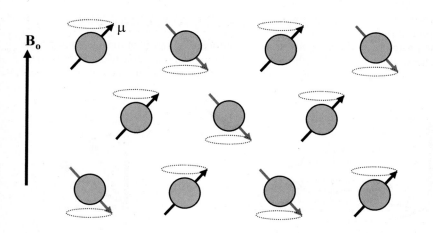

Figure 6.3 When protons (hydrogen nuclei) are subjected to a strong static magnetic field (B_0), they become oriented such that their magnetic moment is either parallel or antiparallel to the direction of B_0.

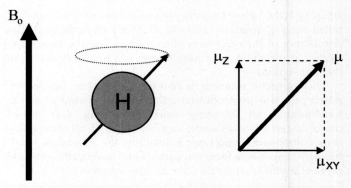

Figure 6.4 The combination of the angular momentum and the external magnetic field B_0 results in a composite motion, called precession. The magnetic moment μ can be analyzed into a longitudinal (Z) and a transverse (XY) component.

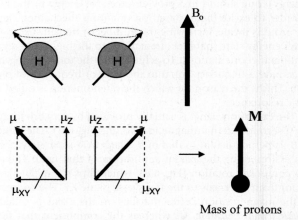

Figure 6.5 When a large mass of protons is considered inside a magnetic field B_0, the transverse component of μ cancels out (due to randomness in orientation), leaving only the longitudinal component. Summation of the longitudinal component of all protons results in the net magnetization, M.

After the end of the application of the RF pulse, if nothing else would have happened, the excessive excitation energy would be emitted back from the protons to the surroundings through relaxation mechanisms, which will be described in the next paragraph. This would result in a decay of M_{XY} and a recovery of M_Z. Since the acquired signal is the M_{XY} component, it would appear as a decreasing amplitude sinusoidal wave, with a frequency equal to the *Larmor* frequency (Fig. 6.7). This signal is called a *Free Induction Decay* (*FID*). In real MRI acquisitions, many processes—which will be described in later sections—follow the application of the RF pulse, in order to encode the positions of the protons into the acquired signal and, thus, to reconstruct an image of the real tissue.

Figure 6.6 The application of an RF pulse through a second magnetic field B_1 applied very briefly, combined with B_0, causes a composite motion of the net magnetization from the longitudinal direction Z toward the transverse plane XY. The strength of B_1 and the duration of its application determine the extent of flipping (described via the flip angle α) of M_Z.

2.5. Spin relaxation

The return of the protons from the excited state (higher energy state) to the equilibrium state (lower energy state) takes place by absorption of the excessive energy from the surroundings of the excited protons, or *lattice*. This process is called *spin–lattice relaxation* or *T1 relaxation* and it describes the recovery of the longitudinal magnetization M_Z. T1 is the time it takes for 63.2% of the original M_Z to recover (Fig. 6.8). Due to the resonance phenomenon, the speed of T1 relaxation depends on the ability of the lattice to absorb the energy from the protons. A lattice that has a magnetic field (as a result of motion of the lattice nuclei) fluctuating with the *Larmor* frequency of the excited protons will speed up the relaxation process. Therefore, the molecular structure, the physical state, and the temperature of the lattice will affect T1 relaxation significantly. In addition, because the Larmor frequency is a function of B_0, the strength of the external magnetic field will also affect T1. For example, large molecules have long T1, because they move at frequencies which are too low (<Larmor) for the energy to transfer to the lattice. However, the presence of end-groups in macromolecules shortens T1, because the end-groups can rotate at frequencies reaching the *Larmor* frequency levels. Medium-sized molecules show short T1, as the rotational frequencies are at the level of the *Larmor* frequency. Pure liquids have long T1 because small molecules have translational frequencies too high to allow energy transfer.

In the same way that T1 (spin–lattice) relaxation describes the recovery of the longitudinal magnetization, T2 (spin–spin) relaxation describes the decay of the transverse magnetization. As two protons interact, the magnetic field of one proton locally changes the total magnetic field strength experienced by the other, temporarily changing the frequency of precession. After the interaction, the Larmor frequency returns to the original value, but now the transverse magnetization vectors of the two protons are out of phase. This dephasing causes a decrease in the total vector of M_{XY} and the phenomenon is called T2 relaxation. T2 is the time it takes for 63.2% of the initial M_{XY} to disappear (Fig. 6.9). T2 relaxation is affected by the molecular size and the physical state of the medium that contains the excited protons; however, in contrast to T1 relaxation, the strength of the external magnetic field does not affect T2. Large molecules and solids have short T2 (fixed molecular structure promotes spin–spin interaction) whereas small molecules (e.g., free water) have long T2. However, in practice, transverse magnetization will always decrease at a rate faster than that predicted by the T2 of a tissue, due to local magnetic field inhomogeneities which cause spins to lose phase coherence more rapidly. The actual rate of transverse magnetization decay is called T2* relaxation and its exponential curve is the envelope of the FID (Fig. 6.7).

3. MAGNETIC RESONANCE IMAGING

The previous section described the physics of magnetic resonance, including the generation of a measurable signal using RF pulses and how this signal decays with time. This section describes how these

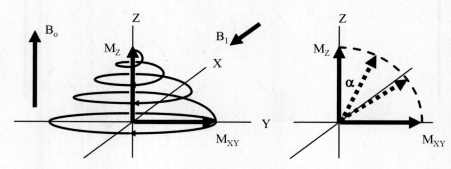

Free Induction Decay (FID)

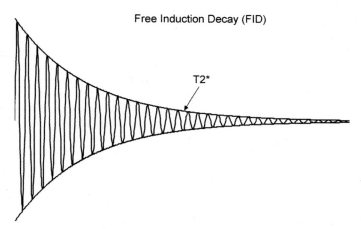

Figure 6.7 The free induction decay (see text for details).

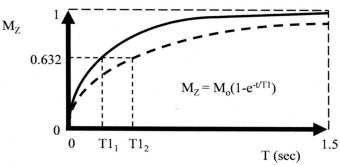

$$M_Z = M_o(1-e^{-t/T1})$$

Figure 6.8 After the application of a 90° RF pulse, M_z starts to recover following the T1 relaxation phenomenon as described by the equation shown in the graph. M_z recovers at a different rate for different tissues, as demonstrated by the solid (shorter T1 tissue) and the dashed (longer T1 tissue) lines. Notice that the greatest relative contrast in T1 between the two tissues (M_z) occurs relatively early. Thus, T1 contrast can be generated by selecting a short TR and a short TE.

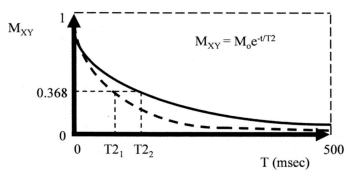

$$M_{XY} = M_o e^{-t/T2}$$

Figure 6.9 After the application of an RF pulse, M_{XY} decays according to the T2 relaxation phenomenon as described by the equation shown in the graph. M_{XY} decays at a different rate in different tissues as shown by the solid (longer T2 tissue) and the dashed (shorter T2 tissue) lines. Notice that the greatest relative contrast in T1 between the two tissues (M_{XY}) occurs relatively early. Thus, T2 contrast can be generated by selecting a relatively long TR and a long TE.

physical principles can be applied to creating an image, including how to spatially encode the MR signal in three dimensions.

4. MAGNETIC FIELD GRADIENTS AND IMAGE LOCALIZATION

Following an RF pulse, the resulting MRI signal is not encoded with any spatial information; in other words, signal emanating from the

brain is indistinguishable from that of the feet and the left arm is indistinguishable from the right arm. Spatial localization of the MRI signal is accomplished in three separate steps, commonly denoted as slice selection, frequency encoding, and phase encoding. The first step (slice selection) occurs simultaneously with excitation (RF pulse) while the second step (frequency encoding) is coincident with data acquisition (readout). Each of these steps is accomplished by spatially varying the magnetic field within the tissue being imaged, using magnetic field gradients that are superimposed on the main magnetic field. The Larmor equation (described above) dictates that the frequency of precession of protons in a tissue sample is proportional to the magnetic field in which the tissue resides. Because it is possible to measure the frequency of precession of these protons, spatially varying the frequencies can be used for localizing the signal (at least in two directions).

To create a two-dimensional (2D) image, the first step is slice selection. This is accomplished by superimposing a gradient on the magnetic field simultaneously with application of the RF pulse, which can be designed to excite only those frequencies that are within the slice of interest, as shown in Figure 6.10.

Once an appropriate slice has been selected, the task of spatial localization is reduced to two dimensions in the plane of the image. Frequency encoding in the excited slice is accomplished in an identical manner to slice selection by varying the precessional frequencies across the slice using a magnetic field gradient, this time applied orthogonal to the slice selection direction. The frequency encoding gradient is applied coincidently with data acquisition. In this way, it is possible, for instance, to differentiate the right arm from the left, in the case of an axial slice.

Unfortunately, it is mathematically impossible to spatially encode proton locations in three orthogonal directions using frequency differences alone. Thus, the last step in spatial localization, phase encoding, relies on creating phase differences between protons in the third spatial direction. Similar to the first two localization steps, phase encoding is accomplished by turning on a magnetic field gradient; however, in this case, the gradient is then turned off after a specified time interval, which creates a phase difference between protons along the gradient direction (Fig. 6.11). The magnitude of this phase difference between protons is dependent on the strength and duration of the magnetic field gradient.

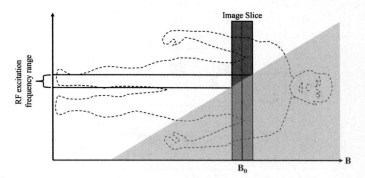

Figure 6.10 Slice selection. An axial slice is excited by spatially varying the magnetic field in the foot–head direction. In this example, the magnetic field (and thus, the frequency of precession) is greater at the head than at the feet. The RF pulse is designed to excite only a certain range of frequencies, encompassing the region of interest within the patient (in this case, the axial slice). The thickness of the slice can be changed by varying either the range of frequencies included in the RF pulse, or by varying the strength of the magnetic field. In practice, the user specifies the slice thickness and the scanner makes the necessary computations to excite only that tissue. By changing the orientation of the magnetic field gradient, a differently oriented slice can be selected (e.g., right–left gradient for a sagittal slice, anterior–posterior gradient for a coronal slice).

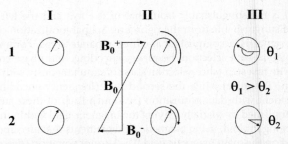

Figure 6.11 Two protons are shown precessing in a homogeneous magnetic field (I). Once a magnetic field gradient is applied (II), proton 2 precesses faster than proton 2 because it experiences a larger magnetic field. After the gradient is removed, the protons revert back to their original (and identical) precessional frequency (III). However, the protons have rotated different amounts during the time the gradient was applied; thus, they have accumulated a phase difference. The magnitude of this phase difference depends on both the strength and duration of the applied magnetic field gradient.

An MR image is created by repetitive application of the various components described above: RF pulse, application of magnetic field gradients applied in three orthogonal directions (slice selection, frequency encoding, and phase encoding), and followed by data acquisition. The order of these components and their relative timing is called a pulse sequence (Fig. 6.12); these components will be discussed in greater detail below.

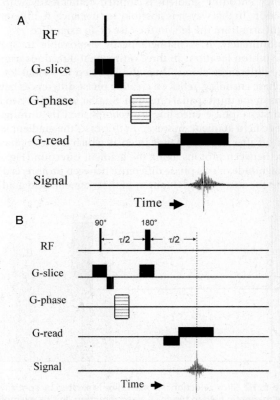

Figure 6.12 The various pulse sequence components, and their typical relative order, are depicted in these pulse sequence diagrams. The two basic pulse sequence types are shown here: gradient echo **(A)** and spin echo **(B)**. By convention, RF pulse components are shown on the top line, followed by magnetic field gradients in three orthogonal directions, shown on three separate lines. Gradients are depicted as rectangles, the height and length of which indicate their strength and duration, respectively. On the last line is shown the timing of the resultant MR signal (echo) at the time of data acquisition.

4.1. Echo formation

Immediately after an RF pulse, all of the spins that have been affected by the pulse are in phase. However, the resulting signal decays rapidly, following the envelope of the FID (as described in the previous section). This decay represents the loss of transverse magnetization due to the combined effects of inherent tissue properties (T2) as well as local magnetic field inhomogeneities (T2*). Much of the signal loss results from the spins losing phase coherence. A pulse sequence is designed to control the phase of the spins, so that they can be brought back into phase during data acquisition—yielding a measurable signal, called an echo. MRI pulse sequences can be grouped into two broad categories depending on their mechanism of echo generation: *Spin echo* pulse sequences use two successive RF pulses to create an echo; *Gradient echo* pulse sequences use one RF pulse and a magnetic field gradient to create an echo.

Spin echo images are created through the action of two separate RF pulses, typically a 90° pulse, which flips all the longitudinal magnetization into the transverse plane, followed by a 180° pulse, which inverts the magnetization. A spin echo pulse sequence diagram is shown in Figure 6.12B, with the two RF pulses separated by a time $\tau/2$ and the echo formed at time τ after the 90° pulse. The 180° pulse compensates for the loss of phase coherence which occurs in the time between the two pulses, causing the spins to come into phase, thus creating an echo at time τ. The principle of spin echo imaging is described in Figure 6.13. It is important to note that the 180° pulse compensates for phase dispersion caused by static magnetic field inhomogeneities; thus, the signal in spin echo images is proportional to the tissue T2.

As its name suggests, the gradient echo pulse sequence utilizes magnetic field gradients to rephase the spins and create an echo. As illustrated in Figure 6.11, magnetic field gradients cause spins to dephase. In gradient echo imaging (Fig. 6.12A), the negative gradient just prior to the frequency encoding (readout) gradient causes phase dispersion that is compensated by the first half of the readout gradient, creating an echo at the midpoint of

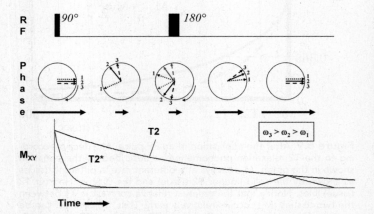

Figure 6.13 Principle of spin echo imaging. The top line designates the two RF pulses characteristic of spin echo imaging. The second line displays the phase of three representative spins that are in phase following the 90° RF pulse, but which then quickly lose phase due to T2* effects. Just prior to the second RF pulse, spin 3 has traversed farther than spin 2, and spin 2 farther than spin 1, due to the existence of small local magnetic field inhomogeneities. The 180° pulse causes the spins to flip (about a horizontal axis, in this example) but does not affect their frequency of precession. Thus, spin 3 now "catches up" with spin 2; likewise, spin 2 "catches up" with spin 1, resulting in an echo, as shown on the bottom line.

this gradient. Thus, the readout gradient is used for both spatial localization and rephasing of the spins. In contrast to spin echo imaging, the signal in gradient echo imaging is proportional to the T2* of the tissue(s) being imaged. Thus, a gradient echo pulse sequence will have less signal than a spin echo sequence with comparable echo time. However, because the gradient echo pulse sequence uses a single RF pulse, it is more amenable to fast imaging and is more widely utilized in cardiovascular imaging.

4.2. K-space

As described above, during creation of an MRI image, spatial locations within the body are encoded using magnetic field gradients. By this process, each spatial location within the tissue has a unique frequency and phase combination. However, locations within the resulting image do not have a unique frequency and phase. This is because as data are acquired, they are placed in an intermediate image space, called k-space, which is then transformed into an image through a mathematical process called the Fourier Transform.

Each k-space "image" contains all the data acquired during each echo and each horizontal line in k-space represents a single echo (Note that there are more advanced k-space filling techniques for which this latter statement does not apply; however, it is a useful starting point for understanding k-space). Therefore, to create a 256 × 256 image, the pulse sequence (Fig. 6.12) must be repeated 256 times to collect enough data to create the image. However, k-space is symmetrical and it is possible to exploit this symmetry in order to reduce the amount of data (i.e., number of lines) required to create an image.[12] In addition, the center of k-space contains low frequency information, related to image contrast, while the periphery contains high frequency information, such as edges and image details (Fig. 6.14). These properties are often exploited during image acquisition. For instance, image acquisition can be sped up by acquiring only a portion of k-space and relying on this symmetry to populate the remainder.

4.3. Pulse sequence (parameters)

Image contrast is defined as the difference in image intensity between two (or more) tissue types and determined by a combination of tissue and hardware (scanner) parameters. Tissue parameters are, by definition, dictated by the tissue(s) being imaged and include the density of protons within the tissue(s) as well as the tissue T1, T2, and T2*.

Hardware parameters are user defined and include the type of pulse sequence used (spin or gradient echo) as well as the prescribed pulse sequence parameters, the most fundamental of which are the repetition time (TR), echo time (TE) and flip angle. TR is the time between successive RF excitation pulses, and TE is the time between the RF excitation pulse and the resulting echo. For spin echo imaging, both TR and TE are defined relative to the 90° RF pulse. Lastly, the flip angle refers to the degree to which longitudinal magnetization is converted into transverse magnetization by the RF pulse (the angle by which the net magnetization vector is rotated).

These hardware parameters can be modified in order to control the contrast between two (or more) tissues in the image. For instance, T1 contrast can be generated by selecting a short TR and a short TE which will accentuate T1 differences between tissues while minimizing T2 differences (Fig. 6.8). Similarly, T2 contrast can be generated by selecting both a long TR and long TE to accentuate the T2 differences between tissues while minimizing T1 differences (Fig. 6.9). A more complete discussion of T1 and T2 weighting can be found elsewhere.[9] However, in many CMR applications, image contrast is dominated by blood moving in and out of the imaging plane. This will be discussed further in subsequent sections.

4.4. Three-dimensional imaging

So far, the discussion of MRI has focused on 2D image acquisition. Applying this method, the inherently three-dimensional (3D) anatomy can be completely covered by acquiring multiple, parallel 2D images. However, it is equally feasible, and often advantageous, to acquire true 3D image data with MRI. The difference lies in the way the data are acquired.

For 3D imaging, the localization steps that were outlined for 2D imaging (Section 3.2) still apply. However, instead of a thin slice, a slab of variable thickness is excited by an RF pulse. Then, an additional set of phase encoding steps is applied in the slice selection direction to partition the slab into thin slices. In general, for 2D imaging, localization is performed by frequency encoding twice and phase encoding once per TR; for 3D imaging, localization requires both frequency and phase encoding to be performed twice per TR.

Some advantages of a 3D acquisition include that thinner slices are typically possible, with relatively greater signal-to-noise, than a comparable 2D acquisition. Disadvantages include increased scan time and/or decreased spatial resolution.

5. CARDIOVASCULAR MAGNETIC RESONANCE IMAGING

5.1. Cardiac motion compensation

The preceding sections have described the general principles behind MRI which can be applied equally well to imaging any anatomical location. However, when specifically imaging the heart

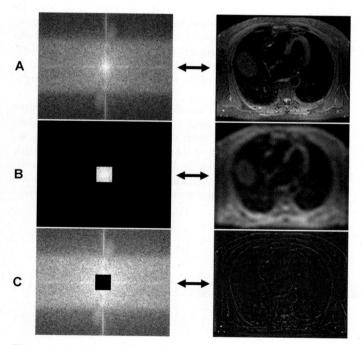

Figure 6.14 Effects of k-space on image reconstruction. Axial image of the heart and the corresponding k-space (**A**). If the same image is reconstructed only using the center portion of k-space (**B**), a low resolution version is produced. Alternatively, if the center portion is omitted, the resulting image contains only edge information, with little contrast.

and blood vessels, CMR is further complicated by the motion of the tissue being imaged (cardiac and respiratory). Thus, image acquisition must be synchronized to this periodic motion, which has significant implications for how the image data are acquired.

There are two main approaches to effectively compensate for cardiac motion in CMR. One approach is to divide the image acquisition over several heart beats, acquiring small chunks of data at comparable points in the cardiac cycle. This technique is called segmented acquisition. Alternatively, the image can often be acquired quickly enough so that cardiac motion does not significantly degrade the image using a technique called single shot acquisition (or real-time acquisition). However, this latter technique typically requires significant compromises in terms of spatial and temporal resolution and is, thus, most often utilized only when a segmented approach has failed.

Using the segmented technique, it is necessary to synchronize image acquisition with the cardiac cycle. This is most commonly accomplished using the patient's electrocardiogram (ECG), although other physiologic signals, such as pulse oxygenation, are suitable as well. Typically, the R-wave of the ECG is detected in real time and is used to trigger image acquisition. However, the ECG signal is often degraded by noise, caused by the RF pulses and magnetic field gradients. In addition, it has been shown that ions in flowing blood can create an electrical signal, which will be superimposed on the ECG, called the magnetohydrodynamic effect.[13] This effect typically coincides with the T-wave and can often cause problems for conventional R-wave detection algorithms. Therefore, several manufacturers have implemented algorithms based on vectorcardiography, which has proven to be a more robust method for detecting the R-wave during CMR examinations.[14]

5.2. Single-frame imaging

Anatomic images of the heart and great vessels are typically single-frame images (i.e., the CMR acquisition results in a single image). With this acquisition scheme, the user selects a suitable trigger delay, defined as the time delay between the R-wave and the point in the cardiac cycle where data are acquired, and the image is acquired at that time point (Fig. 6.15). The trigger delay is usually specified so that image acquisition occurs during mid-to-late diastole when cardiac motion is least. However, this is highly heart rate dependent. At higher heart rates, the period of least cardiac motion often occurs earlier, coinciding with isovolumic relaxation. Of course, images can be acquired during any time of the cardiac cycle (for instance, to obtain an image of the open aortic valve) but, at resting heart rates, these images are typically more susceptible to motion artifacts.

In addition to the trigger delay, the user also defines an acquisition window in single-frame imaging, which represents the amount of data to be acquired per cardiac cycle (Fig. 6.15). Spe-

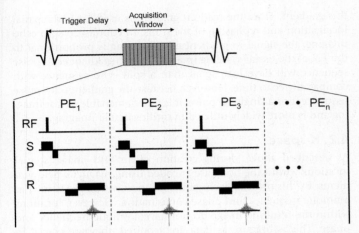

Figure 6.15 Relevant features of single frame MR imaging. A trigger delay is defined by the operator which specifies where data are acquired relative to the preceding R-wave. An acquisition window is also defined which specifies how much data (the number of k-space lines, or phase encoding steps) is acquired per heart beat. Also shown are three representative phase encoding steps. Note that the only difference between each pulse sequence repetition is the strength of the phase encoding gradient (P).

cifically, the acquisition window specifies how many k-space lines are to be acquired during each heart beat (thus, this is a segmented acquisition). As the acquisition window duration is increased, the amount of cardiac motion in the image will increase as well; however, the number of heart beats required for the image to be acquired (total scan duration) will decrease.

5.3. Cine imaging

A cine image acquisition results in a series of images distributed at regular intervals throughout the cardiac cycle. To accomplish this, the cardiac cycle is divided into segments of equal duration, where each segment is associated with a separate image, and the image data acquired during each segment are associated with the corresponding image (Fig. 6.16). Thus, a movie is produced which displays the motion of the structure being imaged throughout the cardiac cycle.

Similar to a single-frame acquisition, it is possible for the user to specify the amount of data acquired for each segment during each cardiac cycle. As more data are acquired per segment, the total acquisition duration decreases but the segment length increases; thus, more cardiac motion is allowed during acquisition. In addition, if a specific frame rate is desired, this can be accomplished by modifying the amount of data acquired per segment as well.

Figure 6.16 In cine imaging, the cardiac cycle is divided into segments, resulting in a movie of cardiac motion. A separate image is associated with each segment. During each cardiac cycle, a portion of each image is acquired. The amount of data acquired per segment per cardiac cycle is controlled by the user. This impacts the total number of phases possible as well as the amount of motion present in the images.

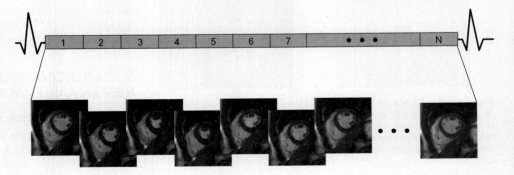

Traditionally, cine images have been acquired using prospective triggering where the cardiac cycle is divided into segments a priori using the ECG R-wave as the trigger (most commonly). However, images during late diastole are not usually acquired when prospective triggering is employed to ensure that the last defined segment does not overlap into the next cardiac cycle due to normal R–R interval fluctuations.

With retrospective gating, however, image data are acquired continuously throughout the cardiac cycle; thus, late diastolic images are also produced. The location of the ECG R-wave is recorded during acquisition and is used to sort the data into suitable segments after acquisition is complete (each segment still corresponds to a separate image).

5.4. Single shot/real-time imaging

In single shot imaging, an entire image is acquired in one continuous stream, or "shot," i.e., image acquisition is not divided over multiple cardiac cycles. However, compromises in both spatial and temporal resolution are required in order to accomplish this without significant blurring due to tissue motion. For CMR, single shot imaging is used most commonly when acquiring scout images that are used to survey the anatomy and plan subsequent image planes. However, HASTE (Half Fourier single shot turbo spin echo) images are another commonly used single shot technique.[9]

In addition, real-time cine images can also be acquired where each image in the cine series is acquired as a single shot.[15] Real-time cine imaging is useful for patients with significant arrhythmias or in whom physiologic triggering fails. Each image can be acquired in as little as 60 to 80 ms.

5.5. Respiratory compensation

Breathing is another significant source of motion during CMR examinations. Common solutions to compensate for respiratory motion include signal averaging, breath-holding, and navigator echo techniques. The simplest and earliest form of respiratory motion compensation was signal averaging in which the same image is acquired multiple times (typically 2 to 4) and the images averaged together. Accordingly, this leads to an increase in image acquisition time which is directly proportional to the number of averages. However, this technique is still widely used, especially when imaging structures less susceptible to respiratory motion or when alternative respiratory motion compensation techniques fail.

Currently, the most commonly used respiratory motion compensation technique is breath-holding. Patients are requested to suspend respiration as each set of images is acquired, and most patients are able to tolerate the 6 to 15 s breath-holds that are required. However, to ensure patient cooperation, each image acquisition must remain within this range. Thus, compromises in spatial and temporal resolution are often required.

Navigator echo techniques are performed during free breathing and represent a one-dimensional (1D) MR acquisition performed just prior and/or following image acquisition within each cardiac cycle.[16] The navigator is a small cylinder, which is typically placed over the dome of the right hemidiaphragm (Fig. 6.17). The result of the navigator acquisition is a line "image" with pixel values showing a clear transition between the dark lungs and the bright liver. An acceptance window is defined at the patient's end-expiratory diaphragm position. Any time the navigator signal indicates that the patient's diaphragm is within this window, the CMR data acquired during that heart beat are accepted; otherwise, they are discarded. As expected, navigator echo techniques can be

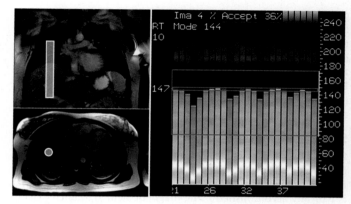

Figure 6.17 Relevant features of the navigator echo technique for respiratory compensation. The user places the navigator over the dome of the right hemidiaphragm (as shown at left). The navigator represents a 1D MR acquisition, the results of which are shown at right. Each column represents the navigator output during one cardiac cycle. The dark region at top is the lungs; the bright region at bottom is the liver. The smaller rectangle represents the user-specified acceptance window; whenever the diaphragm falls within this window, the data from that cardiac cycle are accepted.

quite time consuming since common acceptance rates are 35% to 50% of heart beats. Navigator techniques are most commonly employed when image acquisition prohibits breath-holding or signal averaging. An example is coronary artery imaging[17] where a high spatial resolution is required, in order to visualize the arteries as well as a high temporal resolution to freeze the cardiac motion, therefore requiring long acquisition times.

5.6. Preparatory pulses

In addition to the RF pulses used for image acquisition, additional RF pulses are often utilized to manipulate the tissue magnetization prior to image acquisition. Two common MRI acquisition techniques using preparatory pulses are saturation recovery and inversion recovery.

The saturation recovery technique uses a 90° RF pulse just prior to the imaging pulse. The effect of this pulse is to destroy (or saturate) the magnetization available to the subsequent imaging RF pulse(s). Thus, the tissue affected by the saturation pulse has no signal in the resulting image and, thus, appears dark. Common applications of saturation recovery include MRI perfusion imaging[18] and saturation bands,[9] which are volumes typically placed over the chest wall to saturate the signal from subcutaneous fat or to reduce artifacts arising from respiratory motion. In addition, saturation bands can be placed parallel and adjacent to the imaging plane, in order to null the signal from in-flowing blood.

Inversion recovery utilizes a 180° RF pulse to invert the magnetization in a selected region. Following this pulse, magnetization in the affected tissues will recover according to their T1 relaxation. The delay between the 180° pulse and the subsequent imaging RF pulse is called the inversion time (TI). Typically, an appropriate TI is selected so that the longitudinal magnetization from a specific tissue will be zero during imaging. In this way, T1 differences between tissues can be exploited to null the signal from a specific tissue. A common CMR application of inversion recovery is delayed enhancement imaging.[9,19]

Tissue tagging is a specialized application of preparatory pulses which was proposed separately by Zerhouni et al.[20] and Axel and Dougherty.[21] A train of preparatory pulses is applied perpendicular to the imaging plane in order to saturate bands of tissue in a grid or radial pattern. This is followed by a cine imaging protocol to visualize the grid (or radial lines) as it deforms with the tissue during the cardiac cycle. Because MRI with tissue tagging enables direct visualization of intramyocardial deformation, it can be used to compute myocardial strain in three orthogonal directions, or LV torsion.[22] However, despite the recent advent of semiautomatic postprocessing techniques,[23] tissue tagging remains predominantly a research technique with limited clinical application.

5.7. Parallel imaging

Parallel imaging refers to a class of image reconstruction techniques that utilize spatial information from multiple coil elements, in a phased array coil, to perform the spatial encoding that is typically accomplished using magnetic field gradients.[24] Using these techniques, the number of phase encoding steps required to produce an image can be reduced by factors of two or more. Thus, parallel imaging can be used to reduce scan time by a comparable factor. Alternatively, these techniques can be used to increase spatial resolution while maintaining consistent scan time.

The two best known parallel imaging techniques are SMASH (SiMultaneous Acquisition of Spatial Harmonics)[25] and SENSE (SENSitivity Encoding).[26] Each of these techniques relies on prior knowledge of differences in the sensitivities of individual coil elements in the phased-array. This information can be used to replace phase encoding steps, thus saving time during image acquisition. A practical difference between the techniques is that SMASH is performed in the frequency domain (k-space) while SENSE is performed in the image domain. Parallel imaging has quickly made a great impact on CMR, as it is one of the applications that benefits most from increased imaging speed.

5.8. Balanced steady state free precession imaging

Balanced steady-state free precession (bSSFP) imaging has become increasingly popular over the past decade as gradient system performance has improved, which has allowed the short echo times and repetition times necessary for this technique. Within that time span, however, bSSFP has become the clinical standard for cine imaging of the cardiovascular system because of its superior signal-to-noise and blood-myocardial contrast relative to a comparable gradient echo cine.[27] The increased signal-to-noise in bSSFP imaging results from the fact that the gradients along each axis (e.g., readout) are balanced, meaning that for every positive gradient, there is a negative gradient of equal area along that same axis (Note that the gradients in the pulse sequences shown in Fig. 6.12 are not balanced). bSSFP images do not exhibit either T2 or T1 contrast; rather, image contrast is dependent on the T2/T1 ratio of tissue, so that tissues with high proton content (blood and fat) exhibit relatively higher signal than other tissues. This leads to the high blood-myocardial contrast seen in bSSFP images. Note that bSSFP imaging is more commonly known by the manufacturer-specific names such as True FISP (Siemens), balanced FFE (Philips), or FIESTA (GE).

5.9. Phase-contrast velocity mapping

The signal measured during an MRI image acquisition has two components, magnitude and phase. In traditional MRI imaging, only the magnitude of the acquired signal is used to reconstruct the images. However, the phase of the signal can also be used to provide information about the velocity of moving protons. To achieve velocity-encoded acquisitions, the proton velocity is encoded into the phase of the received signal by using a bipolar magnetic field gradient in the direction of interest (Fig. 6.18). One, two, or all

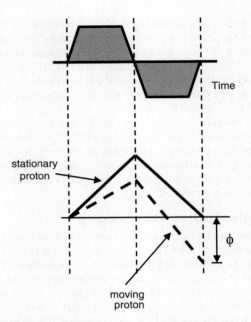

Figure 6.18 The effect of a bipolar gradient in the accumulation of phase in moving protons.

three spatial velocity components can be acquired during a single acquisition by using a single, two, or three bipolar gradients in the three slice axes.

The principle of the phase-contrast velocity mapping technique is shown in Figure 6.18. For stationary protons, no phase is accumulated at the end of the application of the bipolar gradient. However, moving protons experience the effect of the bipolar gradient differently than stationary protons because at different times, they are at different locations. As a result, there is phase accumulation at the end of the gradient. This accumulated phase is proportional to the velocity as given by

$$v = \frac{\varphi}{\gamma T A} \tag{6.2}$$

where T is the time interval between the centers of each lobe of the bipolar gradient and A is the area of each lobe. Knowledge of the characteristics of the bipolar gradient easily provides the proportionality factor to convert the phase values to velocity values. Incorporation of the bipolar gradient into a traditional gradient echo, or any of the newer and faster cine pulse sequences, allows for the measurement, for example, of the velocity of blood throughout the cardiac cycle.

One potential pitfall to consider with phase-contrast MRI is aliasing, which occurs when the maximum velocity of spins being imaged exceeds the maximum encoding velocity (VENC), which is set by the operator. Aliased pixels in the image will appear to have a velocity that is in the opposite direction of their true velocity. Thus, it is important to keep the VENC greater than the maximum velocity expected in the image, but not so high as to reduce the dynamic range of the image.[28]

6. MAGNETIC RESONANCE IMAGING INSTRUMENTATION

The MRI system consists of three primary components: the magnet, RF system, and magnetic field gradients. A schematic showing some of the scanner components is shown in Figure 6.19. In addition to these components, the system also includes com-

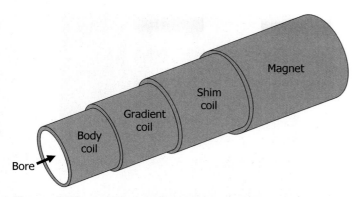

Figure 6.19 A simplistic schematic demonstrating the concentrically placed components in a typical MRI scanner: the bore where the patient is placed, body coil, gradient coils (for applying gradients in three orthogonal directions), shim coil, and superconducting magnet.

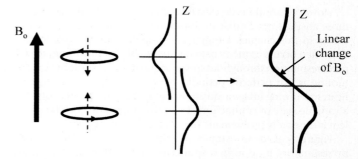

Figure 6.20 Creation of a linear magnetic field gradient in the Z-direction of an MRI scanner by combining two coils with opposing electric current direction.

puters, which control the various scanner components as well as store the images, and dedicated MRI-compatible physiological monitoring equipment. This instrumentation is typically distributed between three rooms: A scanner room, a control room, and an equipment room.

6.1. The magnet

The main purpose of the magnet is to generate a stationary, homogeneous magnetic field. MRI scanners are typically categorized according to the type of the magnet used to generate this magnetic field, i.e., permanent, resistive, or superconducting. Because both permanent and resistive magnets are capable of producing only relatively low field strengths (typically <1 T), CMR is performed almost exclusively on superconducting systems. Note that the strength of a magnetic field (B) is typically measured in units of Tesla or Gauss, where 1 T = 10,000 G. The earth's magnetic field is approximately 0.5 G; as a result, the field inside a 1.5 T MRI scanner is 30,000 times stronger than that of the earth.

Superconducting magnets are solenoids made of niobium–titanium alloy wire, which becomes a perfect conductor when cooled by liquid helium to temperatures of only a few Kelvin and is, thus, able to carry large electric currents with minimal power consumption. Currently, the majority of clinical CMR is performed on 1.5 T systems, although 3 T systems are becoming more prevalent.

A homogeneous magnetic field is essential for good image quality. However, all magnets are inhomogeneous to some extent. In addition, placing an object within the scanner bore introduces additional inhomogeneity. Therefore, the magnetic field must be adjusted (shimmed) to compensate for these factors. Passive shimming typically occurs when the MRI system is installed and is accomplished by placing thin metal bars around the periphery of the magnet in precise locations. Active shimming, however, is accomplished by shim coils, which are situated inside the scanner bore (Fig. 6.19) and generate additional magnetic fields that are externally controlled to compensate for local field inhomogeneities.

6.2. Radiofrequency system

The MRI scanner's RF system consists of a transmitter, a receiver, and various coil(s). The transmitter is used to generate the RF pulse that excites the protons in the imaged object (as described above in Section 2.4) while the receiver is used to receive the signal emanating from the object being imaged. The coils, meanwhile, act as antennae for both the transmitter and the receiver.

Some coils are capable of both transmit and receive functions and are therefore referred to as transmit/receive coils. The body coil, which is built directly into the scanner bore (Fig. 6.19), is an example of this type. Other coils are able to receive only, such as local coils which are placed directly on the body, in close proximity to the tissue being imaged. The advantage of local coils is that they maximize the measured signal, because of their proximity, while minimizing the noise, because of their small size (relative to the body coil). In addition, most of the receive coils used for CMR imaging are a type referred to as phased-array coils. These are comprised of multiple small coil elements, the use of which results in additional signal-to-noise advantages while still maintaining a large field of view. Note that the primary transmit coil for CMR is the body coil, even when local phased-array receiver coils are used.

6.3. Gradient coils

As described above, to spatially encode the MRI signal, a linearly varying magnetic field (gradient) is temporarily superimposed on the main magnetic field. This linear gradient is formed by using gradient coils, as shown in Figure 6.20. Sets of such coils are configured inside the scanner to create linear magnetic field gradients in all three spatial directions (x, y, and z). To create a gradient in an oblique direction, two or even all three gradient coils can be activated simultaneously. Gradient performance is typically characterized by the following measures: Maximum gradient strength, given in units of milli-Tesla per meter (mT/m), and slew rate, which defines how quickly the gradient can be turned on.

7. ARTIFACTS

An artifact is defined as any feature in an image which does not exist in the original object. Artifacts are typically classified according to their source and may be related to technical issues with the scanner, to differences in the magnetic properties of adjacent (or nearby) tissues, or to motion of the patient during imaging. This section will focus on those artifacts found most commonly in CMR, namely, motion, susceptibility (caused by local distortions in the magnetic field), and aliasing. A more complete treatment of artifacts in MRI can be found elsewhere.[9,29]

7.1. Motion artifacts

Motion is a constant issue in CMR. The source of motion is often a singular event, which is impossible to anticipate (e.g., gross patient movement due to discomfort and coughing). In these cases, the only recourse is to repeat the acquisition of any affected images.

However, solutions do exist for repetitive motion artifacts such as those arising from cardiac or respiratory motion, as were discussed earlier in this chapter. Despite this, imperfect motion compensation often occurs as many patients are unable (or unwilling) to suspend respiration throughout image acquisition. In addition, cardiac motion is not perfectly periodic. Normal beat-to-beat changes in heart rate during image acquisition can result in the heart existing in a variable state of contraction at identical trigger delays. This problem is especially problematic in patients with arrhythmias.

Figure 6.21 demonstrates repetitive motion artifacts caused by respiratory motion in a spin echo image. This type of artifact appears in the form of repetitions of the moving structure, called ghosts. The brightness of the moving tissue, as well as the amplitude and frequency of the motion, will affect the appearance of the artifact. Ghosting results from the tissue moving to a different location between successive phase encoding steps. Thus, ghosting only occurs in the phase encoding direction. The time scale for phase encoding is relatively long, on the order of the sequence TR; by comparison, data in the frequency encoding direction are acquired much more rapidly (<1 ms), so ghosting does not occur.

Pulsatile blood flow in an artery can also cause ghosting artifacts (Fig. 6.22). These artifacts are due to the wash-in and wash-out effects as well as the phase dispersion due to the nonuniform blood velocity profiles. Artifact suppression techniques in this case include presaturation of the signal upstream of the imaging slice location, so that protons that enter the slice of interest do not contribute to the image (and thus there is no artifact produced).

7.2. Susceptibility artifacts

Susceptibility is a property of materials that describes how magnetized they become when placed in a magnetic field. Artifacts can occur when materials with different susceptibilities come in close proximity, which can cause local inhomogeneities in the magnetic field (Fig. 6.23). Metals typically have much higher susceptibilities than tissue; thus, they can cause relatively large disruptions in the magnetic field which show up as signal voids in the image (Fig. 6.24). Sternal wires, metallic stents, and artificial valves are common sources of this type of susceptibility artifact. Because they are caused by local magnetic field inhomogeneities, susceptibility artifacts are more severe in gradient echo images than in spin echo images.

7.3. Aliasing artifacts

Also referred to as "foldover" or "wrap" artifacts, aliasing occurs whenever the size of the object being imaged exceeds the field of

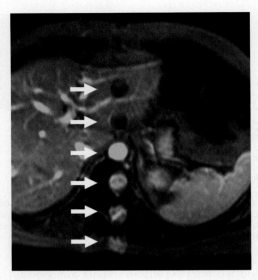

Figure 6.22 Ghosting artifact resulting from pulsations of the aorta (denoted by *arrows*). Phase encoding direction is in the anterior–posterior direction.

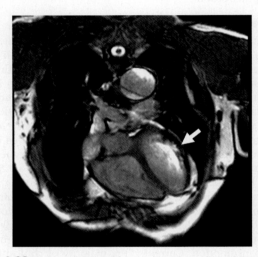

Figure 6.23 Susceptibility artifact in the myocardium at 3 T (denoted by *arrow*) resulting from susceptibility differences between the lung (air) and tissue.

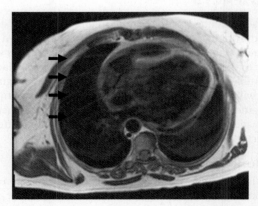

Figure 6.21 Ghosting artifact due to motion of the chest wall during acquisition of a spin echo image (denoted by *arrows*). Phase encoding direction is in the anterior–posterior direction.

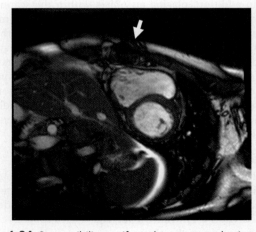

Figure 6.24 Susceptibility artifact due to sternal wires at 1.5 T (*arrow*).

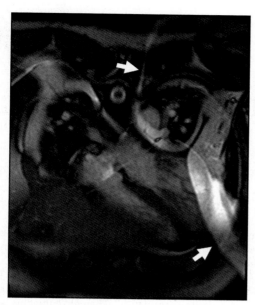

Figure 6.25 Foldover artifact (denoted by *arrows*) resulting from the phase encoding direction specified as right–left. Artifact was removed by switching phase encoding to anterior–posterior.

view in the phase encoding direction. The result is that the part of the object outside the field of view is folded over (or wrapped) back into the image (Fig. 6.25). Depending on the severity, the aliased anatomy may overlap and obscure the real anatomy.

Because aliasing occurs in the phase encoding direction, it is most practical to define the phase encoding direction to coincide with the smallest anatomic dimension. Additional solutions to aliasing artifacts include increasing the field of view (which is usually undesirable because it decreases spatial resolution), using phase oversampling (in which extra phase encoding lines are acquired), or placing a saturation band over the aliased anatomy (thus removing or reducing the effect of aliasing).

8. FUTURE DIRECTIONS

Undoubtedly, CMR is the most versatile of the cardiac imaging modalities, capable of producing stationary and cine anatomical images of the cardiovascular structures with high temporal, spatial, and contrast resolution, functional hemodynamic information, and "virtual histology." This versatility, however, comes at a price. The complex and delicate instrumentation, high technical skills, and long time of acquisition required have limited the wider acceptance of CMR, which by volume, represents a small fraction of the cardiac imaging studies performed in the United States. These issues are currently being addressed by the industry and by the scientific community in the field. Meanwhile, to utilize CMR efficiently, the role of the cardiovascular imaging specialist is to prescribe specific imaging protocols to answer the clinical

questions that are relevant to each patient being studied. This requires detailed knowledge of the patient's clinical history and results of other imaging studies.

REFERENCES

1. Constantine G, Shan K, Flamm SD, et al. Role of MRI in clinical cardiology. *Lancet.* 2004;363(9427):2162–2171.
2. Purcell EM, Torrey HC, Pound RV. Resonance absorption by nuclear magnetic moments in a solid. *Phys Rev.* 1946;69:37–38.
3. Bloch F. Nuclear induction. *Phys Rev.* 1946;70:460–473.
4. Lauterbur PC. Image formation by induced local interactions: Examples of employing nuclear magnetic resonance. *Nature.* 1973;242:190–191.
5. Nobel Foundation. "Press release: The 2003 Nobel prize in physiology or medicine." 6 October 2003. <http://nobelprize.org/nobel_prizes/medicine/laureates/2003/press.html>
6. Lieberman JM, Botti RE, Nelson AD. Magnetic resonance imaging of the heart. *Radiol Clin North Am.* 1984;22:847–858.
7. Waterton JC, Jenkins JP, Zhu XP, et al. Magnetic resonance (MR) cine imaging of the human heart. *Br J Radiol.* 1985;58:711–716.
8. Alfidi RJ, Masaryk TJ, Haacke EM, et al. MR angiography of peripheral, carotid, and coronary arteries. *Am J Roentgenol.* 1987;149:1097–1109.
9. Lee VS. *Cardiovascular MRI: Physical Principles to Practical Protocols.* 1st Ed. Philadelphia, PA: Lippincott Williams & Wilkins, 2005.
10. Edelman RR, Hesselink JR, Zlatkin MB. *Clinical Magnetic Resonance Imaging.* 3rd Ed. Philadelphia, PA: Saunders, 2005.
11. McRobbie DW, et al. *MRI: From Picture to Proton.* 1st Ed. UK: Cambridge University Press, 2003.
12. Paschal CB, Morris HD. K-space in the clinic. *J Magn Reson Imag.* 2004;19:145–159.
13. Fischer SE, Wickline SA, Lorenz CH. Novel real-time R-wave detection algorithm based on the vectorcardiogram for accurate gated magnetic resonance acquisitions. *Magn Reson Med.* 1999;42(2):361–370.
14. Chia JM, Fischer SE, Wickline SA, et al. Performance of QRS detection for cardiac magnetic resonance imaging with novel vectorcardiographic triggering method. *J Magn Reson Imag.* 2000;12(5):678–688.
15. Setser RM, Fischer SE, Lorenz CH. Quantification of left ventricular function with magnetic resonance images acquired in real time. *J Magn Reson Imag.* 2000;12(3):430–438.
16. Firmin D, Keegan J. Navigator echoes in cardiac magnetic resonance. *J Cardiovasc Magn Reson.* 2001;3(3):183–193.
17. Appelbaum E, Botnar RM, Yeon SB, et al. Coronary magnetic resonance imaging: Current state-of-the-art. *Coron Artery Dis.* 2005;16(6):345–353.
18. Gerber BL, Raman SV, Nayak K, et al. Myocardial first-pass perfusion cardiovascular magnetic resonance: History, theory, and current state of the art. *J Cardiovasc Magn Reson.* 2008;10(1):18
19. Saraste A, Nekolla S, Schwaiger M. Contrast-enhanced magnetic resonance imaging in the assessment of myocardial infarction and viability. *J Nucl Cardiol.* 2008;15(1):105–117.
20. Zerhouni EA, Parish DM, Rogers WJ, et al. Human heart: Tagging with MR imaging—a method for noninvasive assessment of myocardial motion. *Radiology.* 1988;169:59–63.
21. Axel L, Dougherty L. MR imaging of motion with spatial modulation of magnetization. *Radiology.* 1989;171:841–845.
22. Reichek N. MRI myocardial tagging. *J Magn Reson Imag.* 1999;10:609–616.
23. Osman NF, Kerwin WS, McVeigh ER, et al. Cardiac motion tracking using CINE harmonic phase (HARP) magnetic resonance imaging. *Magn Reson Med.* 1999;42:1048–1060.
24. Glockner AJ, Hu HH, Stanley DW, et al. Parallel imaging: A user's guide. *Radiographics.* 2005;25:1279–1297.
25. Sodickson DK, Manning WJ. Simultaneous acquisition of spatial harmonics: Fast imaging with radiofrequency coil arrays. *Magn Reson Med.* 1997;38:591–603.
26. Pruessmann KP, Weiger M, Scheidegger MB, et al. SENSE: Sensitivity encoding for fast MRI. *Magn Reson Med.* 1999;42:952–962.
27. Scheffler K, Lehnhardt S. Principles and applications of balanced SSFP techniques. *Eur Radiol.* 2003;13:2409–2418.
28. Chai P, Mohiaddin R. How we perform cardiovascular magnetic resonance flow assessment using phase-contrast velocity mapping. *J Cardiovasc Magn Reson.* 2005;7:705–716.
29. Mirowitz SA. MR imaging artifacts: Challenges and solutions. *MRI Clin N Am.* 1999;7(4):717–732.

Cardiac Magnetic Resonance Examination and Imaging Protocols

Javier Sanz

7

1. INTRODUCTION

1.1. Historical perspective

In 1971, Dr Raymond Damadian reported the potential application of analyzing 1D nuclear magnetic resonance (MR) signals to identify disease.[1] This was followed by the Nobel prize winning work of Drs Paul Lauterbaur and Peter Mansfield on the derivation of spatial information from MR experiments,[2,3] which constituted the basis for MR imaging (MRI). In 1980 it was already possible to acquire (over several minutes) images of the body,[4] but evaluation of the heart remained elusive due to cardiac motion. This limitation was largely overcome with the development of gated MRI in 1984.[5] Subsequent innovation in the 80s and early 90s included flow quantification,[6] cine imaging,[7] coronary angiography,[8] and the application of contrast agents in the assessment of myocardial scar[9] and perfusion.[10] As we will review in the following pages, cardiac MRI (CMR) has evolved from an experimental procedure to a robust modality with extensive clinical applicability in <25 years. The technique has experienced an impressive growth during the last decade, and today CMR examinations are performed on a routine basis throughout the world.

1.2. Cardiac magnetic resonance imaging overview

CMR can evaluate multiple indexes of cardiac status: function, morphology, flow, tissue characterization, perfusion, angiography, and/or metabolism. This versatility relies on the availability of imaging sequences that depict different tissue properties and that therefore provide complementary information. As reviewed in Chapter 6, MR pulse sequences are variations of two basic designs: spin-echo (SE) and gradient-echo (GRE) techniques. These original sequences require long acquisition times and have been improved over the past decades to enable fast assessment of different cardiac parameters. In many cases, the information required to reconstruct an image is divided into *segments* that are collected in different cardiac cycles. These are known as *segmented* sequences. Further modifications in MR equipment and sequence design have enabled the acquisition of whole images in a single heartbeat, approaches often referred to as *single-shot* techniques. The vast majority of sequences, although not all, require compensation of cardiac motion by synchronization of image acquisition to the heart cycle. While image quality is superior if respiratory motion is also eliminated by breath-holding, most applications can be adapted to free-breathing acquisition. Many sequences employed to evaluate the cardiovascular system are also broadly categorized according to the appearance of flowing blood as *black-blood* (generally SE) or *bright-blood* (usually GRE)

techniques. A simplified list of the most common MR sequences employed in cardiac studies and their main applications is presented in Table 7.1.

Despite the advances in image acquisition speed, it is not yet possible to evaluate all the aforementioned cardiac parameters within a single examination. Therefore, imaging protocols are tailored according to the specific indication. Some suggested approaches are shown in Figure 7.1; the Society of Cardiovascular Magnetic Resonance has also recently proposed specific standardized CMR protocols.[11] The duration of a typical CMR study ranges from 30 to 60 min. The order of acquisition of different sequences is partly determined by the influence of contrast agents on image quality, which may be beneficial or detrimental. Although with exceptions, cine images, coronary angiography, and black-blood sequences are typically acquired before contrast, contrast agents are needed for perfusion, noncoronary angiography, and viability assessment. *Phase contrast* (PC) imaging, also known as *velocity encoded* imaging, can be performed either before or after contrast.

2. MAGNETIC RESONANCE CONTRAST AGENTS

2.1. Overview

MR contrast agents alter the magnetic properties of the surrounding water molecules. Specifically, they enhance the relaxation rates of nearby protons; that is, they shorten the T1, T2, and T2* times. Depending on the contrast molecule and the imaging sequence, this results in selective augmentation or reduction of local signal intensity. T1 shortening causes signal increase using T1-weighted sequences; conversely, T2/T2* shortening leads to signal drop on T2-weighted images. Compounds that result in higher signal intensity are often referred to as *positive* contrast agents, whereas those associated with signal loss are denominated *negative* contrast agents. This terminology is, however, misleading because the same compounds may act as positive or negative agents depending on the imaging sequence employed or the dose administered. MR contrast agents contain a metal as an active element with paramagnetic or superparamagnetic properties. Manganese- and iron-based compounds are employed mostly for liver imaging. Because superparamagnetic iron oxides are selectively taken up by the reticuloendothelial system, there is growing interest in the use of these agents for the visualization of macrophages (i.e., in atherosclerotic lesions). However, this application is largely investigational at the present time. In clinical practice, the agents employed for clinical cardiovascular imaging are nonspecific gadolinium (Gd)-based compounds that are administered intravenously.

TABLE 7.1

COMMON MR SEQUENCES EMPLOYED IN CARDIAC STUDIES

	Vendor acronyms				
	Siemens Medical Solutions®	General Electric Healthcare®	Philips Medical Systems®	Toshiba®	Common application(s)
Fast spin-echo	Turbo spin-echo (TSE)	Fast spin-echo (FSE)	Turbo spin-echo (TSE)	Fast spin-echo (FSE)	Anatomy Tissue characterization
Single-shot fast spin-echo	Half Fourier acquisition turbo spin-echo (HASTE)	Single-shot fast spin-echo (SS-FSE)	Single-shot turbo spin-echo (SS-TSE)	Fast asymmetric spin-echo (FASE)	Anatomy Tissue characterization
Ultra fast gradient-echo	Turbo fast low angle shot (TurboFLASH)	Fast gradient recalled echo (Fast GRE)	Turbo field echo (TFE)	Fast field eco (Fast FE)	Perfusion Viability Angiography Tissue characterization Function
Echo planar imaging	Echo planar imaging (EPI)	Echo planar imaging (EPI)	Echo planar imaging (EPI)	Echo planar imaging (EPI)	Perfusion Function
Steady state free precession	True fast imaging with steady-state precession (True-FISP)	Fast imaging employing steady state acquisition (FIESTA)	Balanced fast field echo (Balanced FFE)	True steady state free precession (True SSFP)	Function Anatomy Angiography
Phase contrast	Phase contrast (PC)	Phase contrast (PC)	Phase contrast (PC)	Phase contrast (PC)	Flow quantification

FSE, fast spin-echo; TSE, turbo spin-echo; SS-FSE, single-shot fast spin-echo; HASTE, half Fourier acquisition turbo spin-echo; SS-TSE, single-shot turbo spin-echo; FASE, fast asymmetric spin-echo; FLASH; fast low angle shot; GRE, gradient recalled echo; TFE, turbo field echo; FE, field echo; EPI, echo planar imaging; SSFP, steady-state free precession; FISP, fast imaging with steady-state precession; FIESTA, fast imaging employing steady-state acquisition; FFE, fast field echo; PC, phase contrast.

2.2. Gadolinium-based contrast agents

Gd is a rare metal with strong paramagnetic properties conferred by the presence of seven unpaired electrons and a slow electronic relaxation rate. At commonly employed doses, the T1-shortening properties (*T1 relaxivity*) predominate; therefore, Gd-based compounds are usually employed as positive contrast agents on T1-weighted images. At high doses and/or injection rates, T2* effects may prevail and paradoxically lead to signal loss. A standard dose of Gd is 0.1 mmol/kg, although in clinical practice 0.2 mmol/kg or, less commonly, 0.3 mmol/kg (*double* or *triple* dose, respectively) is frequently administered. Most CMR examinations require doses ≤0.2 mmol/kg. There are several commercially available Gd-based contrast agents, five of which have received approval by Food and Drug Administration (FDA) in the United States (Table 7.2). Of note is that none of these compounds have been approved specifically for cardiac imaging. Most of the first generation agents have similar T1 relaxivity, an extracellular distribution, and are eliminated almost exclusively through the kidneys. Gadobenate dimeglumine (Multihance) has a higher T1 relaxivity, which in clinical practice translates into the possibility of using smaller doses. In addition, gadofosveset (Vasovist) is a novel agent that binds reversibly to albumin and therefore has a predominantly intravascular distribution.

2.2.1. Overall safety profile

Free Gd exists mostly as a highly toxic ion (Gd^{3+}) that is eliminated slowly; therefore, it needs to be chelated with an organic ligand before administration. Current chelates demonstrate an excellent safety profile at commonly employed doses. Acute adverse effects are uncommon (<1%) and are usually transient and minor (flushing, headache, nausea, taste alteration, etc.). Allergic-like reactions are rare (<0.05%), but severe anaphylaxis has been reported.[12,13] At conventional doses there is usually no clinically relevant nephrotoxicity; however, acute renal failure may develop with large doses (usually >0.3 mmol/kg), particularly in patients with diabetes or baseline renal function impairment.[14,15] Although MR contrast agents have been shown to be teratogenic in animal models, there is no evidence of adverse effects to the fetus in humans. The current recommendation is to avoid routine administration in pregnant women, although if contrast is felt to be necessary, decisions should be made on an individualized basis.[16] Similarly, in nursing women who have received Gd there is no data suggesting adverse effects to the infants, but it is common practice to withhold lactation for 24 to 72 h. Most agents are also approved for administration in children >2 years old, and some at an even younger age. The immaturity of the renal system should be considered when contemplating contrast administration in neonates.[14,15]

2.2.2. Nephrogenic systemic fibrosis

In 2006, the FDA issued a warning regarding a potential link between the administration of Gd-based contrast agents and the development of nephrogenic systemic fibrosis (NSF) in patients with advanced renal failure. NSF is a debilitating and potentially lethal disorder in which fibrosis develops in the skin and other internal organs. Although the pathogenic role of Gd is not definitively established, it is hypothesized that persistence of

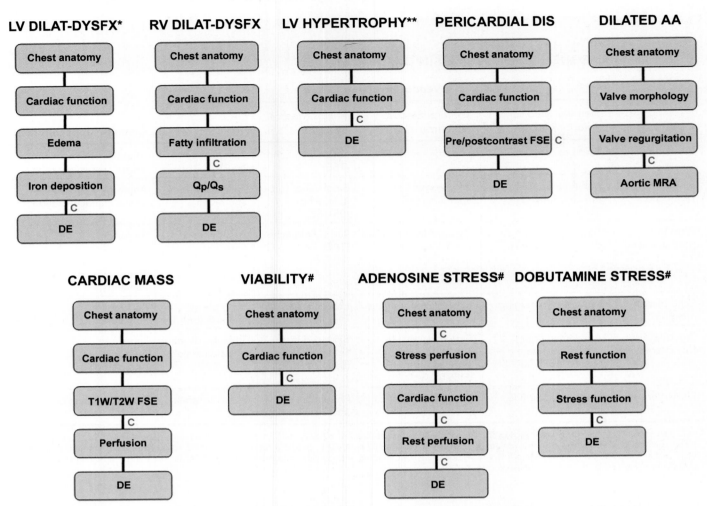

Figure 7.1 Proposed CMR protocols according to common indications. C indicates the timing of contrast administration. *PC imaging of the ascending aorta for the quantification of mitral regurgitation may be added. **T1W/T2W FSE for tissue characterization may be added. #Coronary MRA may be added. AA, ascending aorta; DE, delayed enhancement; Dilat, dilatation; Dis, disease; Dysfx, dysfunction; FSE, fast spin-echo; LV, left ventricle; MRA, magnetic resonance angiography; T1W, T1-weighted; T2W, T2-weighted.

the contrast agent in the body may allow continuous dissociation of the metal from the chelate, resulting in increased concentrations of free Gd^{3+}. The chemical structure of the different compounds influences the stability of the chelate and the probability of Gd^{3+} release, so different agents may portend different risk of NSF. Factors that have been proposed as determinants of lower stability constants and higher toxicity include linear and ionic structure, as well as limited excess chelate in the formulation.[12] At the time of preparation of this chapter, the recommendations regarding the use of Gd-based contrast agents in patients with renal disease are summarized in Table 7.3.

3. MAGNETIC RESONANCE IMAGING SAFETY

3.1. Risks related to the magnetic field/radiofrequency pulses

MRI is an extremely safe modality when minimal precautions are followed. MRI does not require ionizing radiation and the biologic effects of the exposure to a strong magnetic field are negligible. Radiofrequency (RF) pulses may occasionally cause peripheral nerve stimulation that some patients perceive as a tingling sensation or, rarely, as pain. To date, there is no evidence of fetal deleterious effects related to MRI examinations performed at any time during pregnancy. Nonetheless, there remains a theoretical concern that the static magnetic field, magnetic gradients, or RF pulses might have some undesired effect on the fetus. Therefore, the current standard of practice is to proceed only after evaluating the risk–benefit ratio on a case-by-case basis and if the requested information cannot be obtained with other modalities such as ultrasonography.[16]

Despite this excellent safety profile, there exists the possibility for serious adverse events (including death) as a consequence of interactions between the magnetic field and metallic or electronic devices present on or inside the patient. There are several potential mechanisms for such potential hazards.[16] The static magnetic field may exert mechanical forces on external or internal ferromagnetic objects. If these objects are relatively mobile (i.e., brain vascular clips or orbital foreign bodies) there exists a risk for serious injury. Rapid motion near the magnetic field may induce mechanical forces even in nonferromagnetic metallic objects, particularly if large. Fast changes in the magnetic field associated with magnetic gradients and RF pulses may also induce electrical currents and heating in electrically conducting materials (such as wires, leads

TABLE 7.2
MR CONTRAST AGENTS

Molecule	Commercial name	Approval year	FDA-approved	Concentration (mmol/mL)	Structure	Ionicity	T1 Relaxivity (L/mmol/s)[a]	Thermodynamic stability constant	Conditional stability constant[b]	Elimination half-life (h)	Predominant elimination	Cardiac experience
Gadopentetate demiglumine	Magnevist	1988	Yes	0.5	Linear	Ionic	4.3	22.5	17.7	1.6	Renal	Yes
Gadoterate meglumine	Dotarem	1989	No	0.5	Cyclic	Ionic	4.2	25.8	19	1.5	Renal	Yes
Gadoteridol	ProHance	1992	Yes	0.5	Cyclic	Nonionic	4.4	23.8	17.1	1.6	Renal	Yes
Gadodiamide	Omniscan	1993	Yes	0.5	Linear	Nonionic	4.6	16.9	14.9	1.3	Renal	Yes
Gadobenate dimeglumine	MutiHance	1997	Yes	0.5	Linear	Ionic	6.7	22.6	18.4	1.6	Renal (and hepatic)	Yes
Gadobutrol	Gadovist	1999	No	1.0	Cyclic	Nonionic	5.3	21.8	14.7	1.5	Renal	Yes
Gadoversetamide	OptiMARK	1999	Yes	0.5	Linear	Nonionic	5.2	16.6	15	1.7	Renal	Yes
Gadofosveset trisodium	Vasovist	2005	No	0.25	Linear	Ionic	19	22.1	18.9	18.5	Renal (and hepatic)	Yes
Gadoxetate disodium	Primovist	2004	No	0.25	Linear	Ionic	7.3	23.5	18.7	1.0	Renal and hepatic	No

[a]Measured in blood, at 1.5 T and 37°C.
[b]Measured at pH = 7.4
Modified from Lin SP, Brown JJ. MR contrast agents: Physical and pharmacologic basics. *J Magn Reson Imaging.* 2007;25:884–899; Bellin MF, Van Der Molen AJ. Extracellular gadolinium-based contrast media: An overview. *Eur J Radiol.* 2008;66:160–167.

TABLE 7.3

RECOMMENDATIONS FOR THE PREVENTION OF NSF

Screen all patients for renal dysfunction by clinical history and/or laboratory tests[a]

Avoid the use of Gd contrast in patients with:

   Severe acute or chronic renal insufficiency (GFR < 30/mL/min/1.73 m²)

   Acute renal failure (of any severity) due to hepato-renal syndrome or in the perioperative liver transplantation period

If the contrast administration is deemed necessary, use the minimal possible dose

For patients on hemodialysis, consider prompt hemodialysis following contrast administration

[a]Likelihood of renal dysfunction is higher in patients with known renal disease or kidney surgery, aged >65, history of arterial hypertension or diabetes, or severe hepatic disease/liver transplant.
GFR, glomerular filtration rate.
Modified from U.S. Food and Drug Administration (http://www.fda.gov/cder/drug/infopage/gcca/default.htm).

or metallic components in some tattoos and cosmetics), which could in turn result in tissue thermal injury. In addition, the magnetic field/RF gradients may interfere with the programming of electronic systems. Numerous medical implants/devices are MR-compatible, whereas many constitute a formal contraindication, typically brain surgical clips, infusion pumps, neurostimulators, pacemakers, defibrillators (see also below), and others. No metallic implant should be considered MR-safe unless it has been specifically tested as such. Importantly, MR compatibility at a specific magnetic field (i.e., 1.5 T) is not synonymous with safety at higher fields. MR physicians/technologists should consult available references for detailed specifications of individual devices (e.g., www.mrisafety.com) before proceeding with the test. It is mandatory to complete a thorough pretest screening of the patient for possible contraindications. An uneventful prior MRI does not rule out the presence of serious risks. It is also important to remember that any metallic device, even if MR-safe, may create imaging artifacts that interfere with the examination.

Several issues of potential concern are commonly encountered in patients undergoing CMR examinations.[17] Some cutaneous drug-delivery patches (i.e., nitroglycerine) contain metallic foil and may need to be removed before the scan. MRI is safe in patients with sternotomy wires, which are firmly attached to the chest wall. Most prosthetic heart valves and annuloplasty rings experience in each heart beat mechanical forces several orders of magnitude higher than those induced by the magnetic field, so they do not constitute a contraindication for CMR. Similarly, imaging all current coronary stents at magnetic fields up to 3 T, even immediately after implantation, is safe. Short- and long-term follow-up studies have not shown increased incidence of early or late stent thrombosis or other complications. Most peripheral vascular stents, cardiac occluder devices, embolization coils, and inferior vena cava filters are nonferromagnetic and can also be scanned immediately after implantation. For those devices displaying weak ferromagnetism, decisions should be individualized and it may be prudent to postpone the examination for 6 weeks after implantation. Patients with retained epicardial pacing wires can safely undergo MR procedures; however, those with intravenous electri-

cally conducting materials (such as Swan–Ganz catheters and, particularly, retained pacing leads) should not be scanned. Pacemakers and defibrillators have traditionally been considered absolute contraindications for CMR. More recently, the feasibility of safely imaging patients with these devices, particularly pacemakers, has been reported. Nevertheless, these preliminary results should not be interpreted as evidence that the concerns about potential hazards are unfounded. MRI-related deaths in patients with pacemakers/defibrillators have occurred, and potential adverse interactions include changes in programming, mode switch, device movement or heating, pacing inhibition, increases in pacing thresholds, activation of antitachycardia therapies, and others. Therefore, performing CMR examinations in these patients should still be firmly discouraged. In the presence of a strong clinical indication, proceeding with the test might be considered in patients whose device has been specifically tested in vivo, and following a strict protocol that would include informed consent, programming of the device to sense-only or asynchronous pacing modes, modification of the CMR protocol to minimize specific absorption rate, continuous patient monitoring during the procedure, and full device interrogation by an experienced electrophysiologist both before and immediately after the test.[17] These limitations may be solved in the near future, as MR-compatible pacemakers and defibrillators are at various stages of development.

3.2. Other risks/relative contraindications

Contrast-specific issues are discussed in Section 2.2. In order to undergo a CMR examination, subjects need to remain still and follow simple breathing instructions. Consequently, a minimal ability to cooperate is needed, and a severe alteration of mental status can constitute a relative contraindication. Similarly, patients with severe heart failure may be unable to tolerate decubitus. Obesity per se is not a contraindication, but some large patients may not fit inside the bore or exceed vendor-specific limitations regarding the maximal permissible weight for the scanning table (usually 150 to 200 kg).

Some individuals may experience anxiety related to the narrow space of the bore. The incidence of claustrophobic reactions during cardiovascular MRI examinations is 2% to 4%.[18] Anxiety can be minimized by careful explanation to the patient of the steps involved in the procedure, as well as simple measures such as verbal communication, covering the eyes, or playing relaxing music during the test. The patient can also be offered a "panic button" to press if needed. In addition, mild sedation enables more than half of claustrophobic patients to complete the examination successfully.[18] Common sedation approaches usually involve small doses of oral or intravenous benzodiazepines administered a few minutes before the test. Sedation should only be partial, in order to decrease anxiety but to still enable the patient to follow instructions and perform breath-holds when required. As with sedation in any procedure, standard precautions and monitoring are mandatory.

4. PATIENT PREPARATION

In addition to completing the aforementioned screening questionnaire, the patients are asked to remove any clothes that may contain metal, as well as jewelry, dentures, hearing aids, eyeglasses, or other carry-on items (i.e., cell phones or credit cards). The absence of any metallic objects should be confirmed again by adequately trained personnel before entering the magnet room, verbally in the case of conscious, oriented patients, or otherwise by physical examination, ferromagnetic detection systems, and/or plain X-rays. The patient is also instructed about the test and its estimated duration.

Once on the scanning table, MR-compatible electrodes are placed on the chest and connected to the monitoring system for electrocardiographic (ECG) gating. The induction of small voltages on flowing blood by the magnetic field (*magnetohydrodynamic effect*) creates alterations in the ECG signal that may interfere with proper gating. In addition, the MR gradients and RF pulses can induce further artifacts. Most modern magnets include filtering systems to minimize these effects. The majority of cardiac sequences rely on proper ECG gating; therefore, it is essential to obtain a robust ECG signal before proceeding with the study. Testing several electrode configurations if signal is suboptimal may save considerable time during the examination. Signal may be improved by shaving the chest and/or cleaning the skin with water or appropriate gels. When positioning the leads, care should be taken to avoid the formation of loops that may favor the induction of electrical currents. If an adequate ECG signal is not achieved, gating from the peripheral pulse signal can be used as an alternative.

In contrast studies, an intravenous access needs to be obtained and connected to the infusion pump. For stress testing, an MRI-compatible blood pressure cuff is also positioned in the arm. Subsequently, the surface coil is placed on the chest wall and secured appropriately (an additional coil may also lie underneath the patient on the scanning table). Correct positioning on the precordial region will ensure adequate signal reception from cardiac structures. The rapidly changing magnetic gradients generate loud tapping noises, so hearing protection is provided with headphones that additionally allow communicating with the patient during the procedure (visual contact is maintained through glass windows and/or video cameras). The table is finally advanced into the bore so that the cardiac region is in the isocenter, where the magnetic field is most homogeneous and image quality is optimal. Movement of the patient in and out of the bore should be done slowly and carefully to decrease field-induced forces and avoid injury.

5. CHEST EXAMINATION

A CMR study begins with localizer images, low-resolution pictures of the chest that enable the operator to determine the location of the heart. Localizer images are typically a combination of axial, sagittal, and coronal planes obtained with single-shot steady-state free precession (SSFP) imaging or a similar fast sequence. Although few images are enough for depicting the heart's position and orientation, it is common practice in many centers to perform an initial survey of the whole thorax. This can be done with axial, sagittal, and/or coronal single-shot fast SE (FSE) and/or SSFP imaging during free-breathing. One image is acquired every one to two heartbeats, allowing for complete coverage of the chest usually in <1 min. Although not indispensable, it is advisable to perform this approach routinely to rule out gross

abnormalities in extracardiac structures (aortic aneurysm/dissection, pleural effusions, lung masses, congenital abnormalities, etc.) that might be missed in selective cardiac imaging (Fig. 7.2). It must be realized, however, that MRI is suboptimal for detailed evaluation of parenchymal lung disease. Imaging of the complete chest offers the additional advantage of better depiction of the cardiac anatomic relationships that may be helpful for planning subsequent acquisitions.

6. VENTRICULAR ASSESSMENT

6.1. Ventricular morphology and function

Morphology and function are usually evaluated simultaneously from cine images. Cine imaging was initially performed with segmented fast GRE sequences, but these have been largely replaced with segmented SSFP imaging. Because the contrast in SSFP is determined by the tissue T2/T1 ratio, this sequence is less dependent on inflowing blood and provides better delineation of the endocardial border. In addition, temporal resolution, overall image quality, and reproducibility are higher with SSFP.[19] As mentioned before, a segment of the k space is acquired in every heartbeat to complete an image. The temporal resolution is determined by the number of k space lines acquired per segment (or heartbeat) and the repetition time (TR) of the sequence, which represents the time between two consecutive k space lines. As an example, using a segmented sequence with a TR of 3.5 ms and acquiring 10 lines per segment, the temporal resolution would be 35 ms. Temporal resolution can be improved further by using more recent implementations, such as parallel imaging. For accurate cardiac function evaluation temporal resolution should be ≤45 ms, which is easily achieved with current scanners. Spatial resolution is determined by the size of the field-of-view and the imaging matrix and should be kept <2 mm in the x- and y-dimensions.[20] A typical cine image acquisition requires a period of apnea of 5 to 10 s that expands for 8 to 12 heartbeats. ECG gating can be done prospectively or retrospectively. With prospective gating image acquisition is started after the trigger (QRS complex) and stopped before the next anticipated QRS complex; therefore, the final portion of the cardiac cycle is disregarded. Retrospective gating is the method of choice for cardiac function evaluation because it provides images throughout the cardiac cycle. Acquisition of at least 11 cardiac phases is recommended.[21] For patients with limited breath-holding capacity, imaging with multiple (three or four) averages or with respiratory navigators during free-breathing usually provides adequate quality at the expense of longer scanning times. In addition, commercially available sequences can display cardiac function in real time even without apnea/gating, although with lower temporal and spatial resolutions.[22] These approaches (usually variations of SSFP or echo planar imaging [EPI]) are particularly useful in cases with severe arrhythmia, inadequate gating signal, or inability to perform apnea.

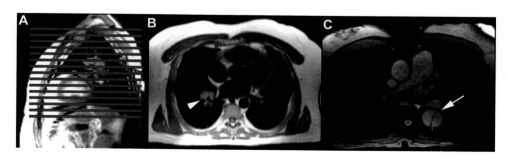

Figure 7.2 Chest imaging with consecutive axial images (blue lines) planned from a sagittal localizer view **(A)**. **(B)** demonstrates an example of axial single-shot FSE imaging in a patient with pulmonary sarcoidosis and enlarged hilar lymph nodes (*arrowhead*). **(C)** displays a type-B aortic dissection visualized with single-shot SSFP imaging.

Figure 7.3 (Movie 7.1). Evaluation of cardiac function with MRI. Multiple contiguous planes (*pink lines*) are prescribed from low-resolution four-chamber and two-chamber localizer images (**left panel**) covering both ventricles from base to apex. High-resolution images are obtained in the short-axis views using cine SSFP imaging (**right panel**).

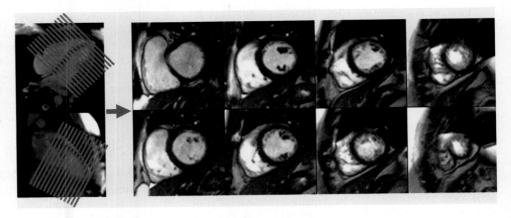

The most common approach for function evaluation is to image both ventricles with multiple cine short-axis slices extending from the bases to the apices (Fig. 7.3 and Movie 7.1). These slices are usually 6 to 10 mm thick and may be contiguous or separated by <5 mm gap. Additionally, cine images may be obtained in any desired orientation, such as axial planes or standard four-, three-, and two-chamber echocardiographic views, as well as long-axis images of the right ventricle (Fig. 7.4 and Movie 7.2). The possibility of imaging in any plane and with large field-of-views results in excellent depiction of size, shape, and wall thickness of both ventricles. Moreover, it is possible to evaluate all myocardial segments and accurately detect focal abnormalities such as regional dyskinesis (Movie 7.2), local remodeling, or myocardial structural anomalies (i.e., segmental hypertrophy or noncompaction). Novel cine 3D sequences that provide complete ventricular coverage in a single-breath-hold have become recently available.[23]

6.2. Quantification of ventricular volumes, function, and mass

Simplified approaches that use geometric formulae (area-length method, biplane ellipsoid method, etc.) can be applied to combinations of long- and short-axis views. However, the most accurate

approach is to avoid geometrical assumptions by applying the Simpson rule to a stack of short-axis images. With the use of dedicated software, the endocardial and epicardial contours of either ventricle can be traced in each short-axis view at the phases of maximal and minimal ventricular dimensions (Fig. 7.5). The volume of ventricular cavity per slice is calculated as the product of the area enclosed within the endocardial contour multiplied by the slice thickness. An equivalent approach is applied to the area between the endocardial and epicardial contours to derive myocardial volume. True end-diastolic and end-systolic volumes (EDV and ESV, respectively) are obtained by adding the cavity volumes of individual slices. Stroke volume (SV) equals EDV–ESV, and ejection fraction equals SV/EDV. Similarly, tracing of the contours in all cardiac phases, although time consuming, enables determination of ejection and filling rates. Ventricular mass is calculated by multiplying the total myocardial volume by the density of the myocardium (1.05 g/mL). Papillary muscles should in principle be considered part of ventricular mass, although inclusion in the cavity facilitates analysis and leads to relatively small inaccuracies.[24] Today, CMR is considered the standard of reference for the quantification of biventricular volumes, ejection fractions, and mass, offering also excellent reproducibility.[25] Normal reference values are reported in Table 7.4.

For regional function assessment, radial thickening is graded visually (1 = normal, 2 = hypokinesis, 3 = akinesis, and 4 = dyskinesis) or objectively from endocardial and epicardial contours. A standard 17-segment model of the left ventricle (LV) is used for reporting purposes.[26] A more sophisticated approach for functional evaluation is the use of myocardial *tagging*.[27] In this technique, special RF pulses are administered immediately after

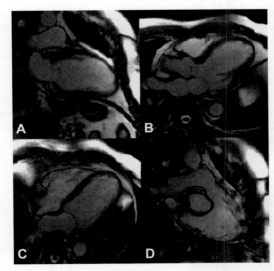

Figure 7.4 (Movie 7.2). Cine SSFP long-axis views. **A:** Standard two-chamber view of the LV; **B:** Standard three-chamber view of the LV; **C:** Standard four-chamber view; and **D:** Three-chamber view of the right ventricle. A large area of anteroapical akinesis can be noted in the LV (movie).

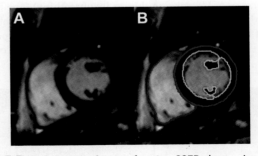

Figure 7.5 End-diastolic frame of a cine SSFP short-axis view (**A**). For quantification of volumes and mass, the epicardial and endocardial contours are traced (**B**) as explained in the text. The example shows the contours for the LV endocardium (yellow), LV epicardium (red), and right ventricular endocardium (blue). The same approach is repeated at all ventricular levels and in end systole (not shown).

TABLE 7.4

NORMAL REFERENCE VALUES OF BIVENTRICULAR VOLUMES, EJECTION FRACTION, AND MASS FOR ADULTS

	Men	Women
LVEDV (mL)	160 ± 29 (102–218)	135 ± 26 (83–187)
LVEDVI (mL/m²)	82 ± 13 (56–108)	78 ± 12 (54–102)
LVESV (mL)	50 ± 16 (18–82)	42 ± 12 (18–66)
LVESVI (mL/m²)	25 ± 8 (9–41)	24 ± 6 (12–36)
LVEF	69 ± 6 (57–81)	69 ± 6 (57–81)
LVM (g)	123 ± 21 (81–165)	96 ± 27 (42–150)
LVMI (g/m²)	63 ± 9.0 (45–81)	55 ± 12 (31–79)
RVEDV (mL)	190 ± 33 (124–256)	148 ± 35 (78–218)
RVEDVI (mL/m²)	96 ± 15 (66–126)	84 ± 17 (50–118)
RVESV (mL)	78 ± 20 (38–118)	56 ± 18 (20–92)
RVESVI (mL/m²)	39 ± 10 (19–59)	32 ± 10 (12–52)
RVEF	59 ± 6 (47–71)	63 ± 5 (53–73)
RVM (g)	41 ± 8 (25–57)	35 ± 7 (21–49)
RVMI (g/m²)	21 ± 3.7 (13–28)	20 ± 3.5 (13–27)

Values are expressed as mean ± standard deviation (normal limits). Normal limits are calculated as mean ± 2 standard deviations. LVEDV, left ventricular end-diastolic volume; LVEDVI, left ventricular end-diastolic volume index; LVESV, left ventricular end-systolic volume; LVESVI, left ventricular end-systolic volume index; LVEF, left ventricular ejection fraction; LVM, left ventricular mass; LVMI, left ventricular mass index; RVEDV, right ventricular end-diastolic volume; RVEDVI, right ventricular end-diastolic volume index; RVESV, right ventricular end-systolic volume; RVESVI, right ventricular end-systolic volume index; RVEF, right ventricular ejection fraction; RVM, right ventricular mass; RVMI, right ventricular mass index.
Data from Hudsmith LE, Petersen SE, Francis JM, et al. Normal human left and right ventricular and left atrial dimensions using steady state free precession magnetic resonance imaging. *J Cardiovasc Magn Reson.* 2005;7:775–782.

the QRS complex to eliminate signal in planes perpendicular to the image. This generates dark lines (tags) in the image, typically displayed as a grid, that can be visualized and tracked during a variable portion of the cardiac cycle (Fig. 7.6 and Movie 7.3). The changes in the tags reflect the deformation and displacement of the myocardium, which can be objectively quantified. Tagging

provides accurate quantifications of global and regional systolic and diastolic functions by determining radial, longitudinal and circumferential strains, strain rates, or ventricular torsion. Novel analysis methods such as harmonic phase analysis have largely reduced postprocessing times and promise to expand the clinical applications of this modality. An alternative approach for regional function evaluation is the pixel-by-pixel measurement of myocardial tissue velocities with PC.[28] Finally, high spatial and temporal resolution strain quantification can be obtained using phase displacement encoding.[29]

6.3. Tissue characterization

The magnetic properties of different tissues vary according to their composition and histological architecture. These differences can be highlighted using CMR sequences that provide specific image weightings. Common applications of these capabilities are the evaluation of cardiac masses or characterization of the myocardium. Black-blood sequences are most frequently employed, particularly double inversion-recovery (IR) FSE. Images are usually obtained before contrast in order to exploit intrinsic tissue differences. Further myocardial characterization can be obtained with the use of Gd, as discussed in Sections 10 and 11.

Adipose tissue is characterized by a short longitudinal relaxation time, which translates into bright signal intensity on T1-weighted images and constitutes the basis for the detection of myocardial fatty infiltration with CMR. T1-weighted, double IR FSE, typically in axial and/or short-axis views, is employed in patients with suspected arrhythmogenic right ventricular cardiomyopathy (Fig. 7.7A).[30] Fat-suppression techniques can be useful to increase diagnostic confidence regarding the presence of adipose tissue. Increased free water content in the myocardium causes a prolongation of transverse relaxation time that can be exploited to detect myocardial edema as areas of bright signal intensity on T2-weighted images (Fig. 7.7B). The most common approach is the use of a T2-weighted triple IR FSE sequence, where the third inversion pulse is applied for fat saturation.[31] FSE sequences are segmented and require a regular heart rhythm and good breath-hold capability for appropriate image quality. In cases of severe arrhythmia or breathing difficulties, single-shot FSE sequences can be employed as an alternative, although spatial resolution is limited and may be insufficient for accurate right ventricular wall evaluation. While focal edema can be detected visually, global increases in myocardial water content may require comparisons of myocardial and skeletal muscle signal intensity. A signal intensity ratio >1.9 has been proposed in the evaluation of myocarditis.[32] Similarly, a relative myocardial signal increase >4 in comparison with skeletal muscle on T1-weighted FSE after Gd administration may indicate diffuse inflammation.[32]

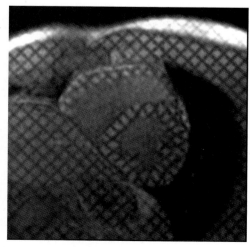

Figure 7.6 (Movie 7.3). Visualization of myocardial deformation with myocardial tagging in a mid-ventricular short-axis slice.

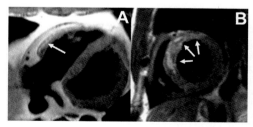

Figure 7.7 A: Axial T1-weighted FSE image demonstrating the presence of fat as areas of bright signal in the right ventricular free wall (*arrow*). **B:** Short-axis T2-weighted FSE image revealing the presence of edema (hyperintense myocardium) in the anterior and anteroseptal segments (*arrows*).

These ratios are dependent on the imaging and contrast protocol and require using signal intensity correction algorithms with surface coils or, alternatively, the body coil.

Apart from the evaluation of postcontrast enhancement, the most common use of bright-blood imaging for myocardial characterization is the detection of iron overload with T2*-weighted fast GRE sequences. Because the T2* of the tissue is shortened by the inhomogeneities in local magnetic field induced by iron deposition, T2* quantifications are closely correlated with myocardial iron content. T2* is calculated from an exponential function that relates changes in myocardial signal intensity to increasing echo times (TE), typically in a short-axis mid-ventricular slice. For a 1.5 T magnet, the normal value of myocardial T2* is generally accepted to be >20 ms.[33]

Finally, MR spectroscopy is based on the detection of signals from nuclei different from water or fat protons. These include [31]P (evaluation of myocardial contents of adenosine triphosphate, phosphocreatine, or inorganic phosphate), [1]H (in molecules other than water, to detect creatine, lactate, or myocardial lipids), [23]Na, and [39]K (for the determination of sodium/potassium levels).[34] These techniques can be applied to study cardiac metabolism in different cardiac diseases, although they are currently restricted to highly specialized centers and are not suitable to generate images.

7. INTRACARDIAC SHUNT CALCULATION

In patients with systemic-to-pulmonary shunts, CMR can provide detailed evaluation of cardiac and extracardiac congenital abnormalities. The Q_p/Q_s can be calculated from the ratio of right SV to left SV obtained from cine volumetric calculations, although this is only accurate in the absence of regurgitant valvular lesions and/or ventricular septal defects. Thus, the most common approach is to obtain PC images perpendicular to the ascending aorta and the pulmonary trunk. Because PC CMR allows for quantification of

blood velocity across the imaging plane in every voxel, the integration of arterial cross-sectional areas and velocities throughout the cardiac cycle provides accurate determinations of flow (Fig. 7.8). The Q_p/Q_s derived in this way is highly precise when compared with invasive measurements.[35] For best accuracy, the limit of velocity detection should be set as close as possible to the expected peak velocity, although slightly higher to avoid aliasing. In most cases, velocity encoding settings of 150 and 100 cm/s for the ascending aorta and main pulmonary artery, respectively, provide good results. Limits need to be set higher, however, in patients with valvular stenosis or increased cardiac output states. The imaging planes should not be too close to the valves to avoid measurement imprecision related to flow turbulence.

8. VALVE EVALUATION

Most valvular abnormalities can be evaluated accurately with echocardiography. The role of CMR is usually reserved for selected cases in which the accuracy of Doppler echocardiographic data is in question.

8.1. Valve morphology

The main advantage of CMR for valve morphology assessment is the possibility of imaging in any desired plane without restrictions in tissue penetration. Applications include noninvasive evaluation of the pulmonary valve, of patients with poor acoustic windows, and of supravalvular or subvalvular disease (i.e., membranes). However, the higher temporal and spatial resolution of echocardiography (particularly, transesophageal) in real time usually results in superior depiction of small and/or highly mobile structures such as vegetations, ruptured chordae, or leaflet abnormalities. SSFP imaging is usually the technique of choice (Fig. 7.9A), although fast GRE sequences may produce fewer artifacts in regions of pulsatile flow.

Figure 7.8 (Movie 7.4). Q_p/Q_s calculation in a patient with an atrial septal defect. PC images are obtained perpendicular to the pulmonary artery (**A:** Magnitude image; **C:** Velocity map) and the ascending aorta (**B:** Magnitude image; **D:** Velocity map). The contours of the arterial cross sections are traced to calculate flow (**E**). The flow curves reveal substantially different SVs with a calculated $Q_p/Q_s = 1.92$.

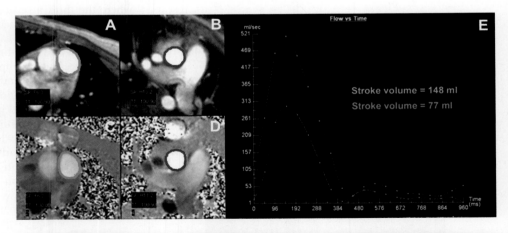

Figure 7.9 (Movie 7.5). Evaluation of aortic valve disease with MRI. (**A**) shows the severely reduced opening of a stenotic bicuspid valve as seen in a peak-systolic frame with cine SSFP imaging (movie). The valvular area can be measured by planimetry (**B**). (**C**) illustrates the quantification of regurgitant fraction from a flow curve obtained from PC imaging of the ascending aorta. The regurgitant fraction in this case is 47%, indicating severe regurgitation.

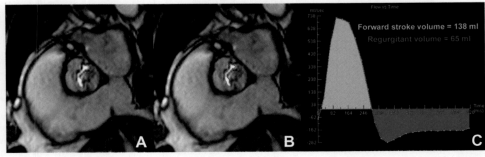

8.2. Flow visualization

Flow turbulence associated with regurgitant and stenotic jets can be detected with bright-blood sequences as areas of signal void (caused by spin dephasing). SSFP and fast GRE imaging can be used for jet visualization, with the size of the signal void being somewhat smaller for SSFP sequences because of their shorter TE.[36] Abnormal jets can also be depicted with PC.

8.3. Quantification of valve disease severity

8.3.1. Stenotic valve disease

There are several MRI approaches for the assessment of valvular stenoses, all similar to those employed in echocardiography. Measurement of velocities with PC can be used to derive peak and mean gradients with the modified Bernoulli equation ($\Delta P = 4V^2$). A combination of in-plane and through-plane PC imaging is useful to detect the point of maximal velocity. Another approach is to measure flow at the tip of the aortic leaflets and at the LV outflow tract (LVOT, 1 to 1.5 cm proximally to the valvular plane) and derive velocity–time integrals (VTI). In combination with LVOT area measurements, the effective aortic valve area can be calculated from the continuity equation: Area$_{valve}$ = Area$_{LVOT}$[VTI$_{LVOT}$/VTI$_{valve}$].[37] One of the most common approaches for the evaluation of stenoses in any valve is direct orifice planimetry on cine images, usually SSFP (Fig. 7.9B).[38] Because of the through-plane motion of the valve during acquisition, the tip of the leaflets may not be captured in one single acquisition. It is, thus, useful to obtain several, thin (i.e., 5 mm), contiguous images oriented parallel to the annulus and extending across the valve. The valvular orifice is traced at the phase of maximal opening in the most distal slice displaying the leaflets. Regions of signal void secondary to calcification are typically considered part of the leaflet tissue.

8.3.2. Regurgitant valve disease

Measurement of the size of signal void in regurgitant valves constitutes a way to semiquantify disease severity. However, similar to Doppler ultrasound, the size of the signal defect is highly dependent on imaging parameters and on the degree of velocity and dispersion of the flow through the valve orifice. Thus, regurgitant flow severity may be underestimated across large regurgitant orifices when flow remains mostly laminar. The main strength of CMR is the ability to provide quantitative measurements. Regurgitant volumes can be determined from the difference in left and right ventricular SV calculated from cine images (Section 6.2), although this method is only accurate for isolated regurgitant lesions. The most widely employed approach for the evaluation of insufficiency of semilunar valves uses PC imaging at the pulmonary trunk or ascending aorta. The slice should be positioned close to the valve but avoiding the leaflets. Motion-corrected techniques have been proposed to increase accuracy.[39] The regurgitant volume can be directly quantified, and the regurgitant fraction is calculated as the ratio of regurgitant volume to forward SV (Fig. 7.9C). For atrioventricular valves, regurgitant volume is determined from the difference between total right or left ventricular SV (calculated from cine images) and forward SV (calculated from PC imaging at the pulmonary trunk or ascending aorta). The regurgitant fraction equals regurgitant volume divided by total SV. Reference regurgitant fraction values for aortic and mitral insufficiency are shown in Table 7.5.[40]

9. CORONARY IMAGING

9.1. Image acquisition

Imaging of the coronary arteries is one of the most challenging CMR applications due to their tortuous course, small size,

TABLE 7.5

CMR CRITERIA OF SEVERITY FOR MITRAL AND AORTIC REGURGITATION

Severity of regurgitation	Regurgitant fraction (%)
Mild	≤15
Moderate	16–25
Moderate-to-severe	26–48
Severe	>48

Data from Gelfand EV, Hughes S, Hauser TH, et al. Severity of mitral and aortic regurgitation as assessed by cardiovascular magnetic resonance: Optimizing correlation with Doppler echocardiography. *J Cardiovasc Magn Reson.* 2006;8:503–507.

and continuous motion. Many different sequences (black- or bright-blood) and acquisition approaches (various k space filling schemes, during apnea or free respiration, with or without contrast agents) have been attempted and can be reviewed elsewhere.[41] The most common approach has been the use of 3D, segmented GRE techniques. These sequences are optimized to improve the contrast between the bright appearance of the blood, the fat surrounding epicardial coronary vessels, and the myocardium. This is usually achieved by a fat saturation pulse to null the signal from adipose tissue and a T2 preparation pulse to decrease myocardial signal, both administered before image acquisition. To compensate for cardiac motion, ECG gating is employed and a temporal resolution <100 ms is desirable. Data is collected at phases of the heart cycle where coronary motion is expected to be minimal, typically mid-diastole and end-systole for slow and fast heart rates, respectively. The period of least coronary motion can be ascertained from cine images. Because the right coronary artery often displays the largest displacement and motion artifacts, four-chamber or mid-ventricular axial cine loops are commonly employed. To compensate for breathing motion, prospective respiratory gating combined with slice correction is used. Respiratory gating is usually accomplished with navigator echoes prescribed perpendicular to the right hemidiaphragm that track the displacement of the diaphragm–lung interface in real time. Image acquisition is performed at end-expiration, because this diaphragmatic position is usually more consistent and has a longer duration. Thus, data is collected at the prespecified phase of the cardiac cycle over multiple heartbeats while the patient is breathing normally, but only data from those cycles where the diaphragm is at the desired location (usually a 3 to 5 mm window) is finally accepted. Traditionally, a 3D slab containing 10 to 20 slices is oriented along the expected course of each main artery, as determined from previous localizer images obtained also during free breathing. Therefore, two to three slabs are prescribed per patient, using double oblique planes that cover broadly the anterior interventricular groove, the anterolateral LV wall, and the atrioventricular grooves. Spatial resolution should be enough to provide discrimination of potential stenosis with sufficient signal-to-noise ratio (SNR) and ideally comparable in all 3D (isotropic). Most 3D GRE approaches require imaging times of 5 to 10 min per slab and yield through-plane resolutions of 1.5 to 3 mm and in-plane resolutions of approximately 1 mm. The "slab" method has been progressively replaced in the last few years with a "whole-heart" approach that combines SSFP and parallel imaging and that provides 3D acquisitions in a manner comparable to computed tomography (CT). Preparatory pulses and motion correction are performed as described above, and the complete cardiac volume is imaged during a single acquisition of approximately 15 min with near-isotropic spatial resolution.[42]

9.2. Image analysis

Datasets can be manipulated to optimize vessel depiction using different 3D postprocessing tools (Fig. 7.10). Luminal stenoses are often quantified visually as significant or nonsignificant (luminal diameter narrowing ≥50% or <50%, respectively), although quantitative analysis tools have also been used. In general, accuracy at the present time is inferior to that of CT, although reasonable for proximal and middle coronary segments. Calcium in the vessel wall creates areas of signal drop that may impede stenosis assessment to some extent. However, this limitation usually is more marked for CT, and MRI may be advantageous in patients with severe coronary calcification.[43]

10. MYOCARDIAL PERFUSION

10.1. Technical considerations

Perfusion is most commonly evaluated by imaging the first pass of conventional extracellular contrast agents through the myocardium. Alternative approaches include the use of intravascular agents[44] or noncontrast techniques such as blood-oxygen level-dependent imaging,[45] which will not be addressed here. The contrast is injected intravenously and multiple ECG-gated images are acquired to visualize its arrival into the right heart side, left cardiac chambers, and, subsequently, the myocardium (Fig. 7.11). The evaluation of the contrast first pass requires imaging for a sufficient number of heartbeats, typically 40 to 60. This is beyond most patients' ability to suspend respiration so there will likely be breathing artifacts at some point during the study. A useful approach is to begin image acquisition and contrast injection simultaneously, reviewing images in real time while the patient is breathing. When the contrast arrives at the right ventricle, the patient is instructed to stop breathing for as long as possible. This will ensure absence of motion at the time of contrast myocardial wash-in, the most important phase for both visual and objective analyses. Then the patient may take another breath and stop breathing again, or resume respiration with slow, shallow breaths.

Evaluation of myocardial perfusion is another technically demanding application. Imaging needs to be performed rapidly in order to capture the dynamic changes and regional differences of myocardial signal intensity. Temporal resolution has to be high so as to obtain a complete image in one heartbeat with minimal motion artifacts. For most current sequences, temporal resolution ranges between 100 and 250 ms; this

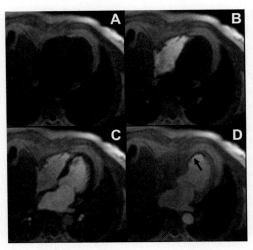

Figure 7.11 (Movie 7.6). Myocardial first-pass perfusion imaging. The figure displays a four-chamber view at different time during the first pass of the contrast agent: Preinjection (**A**), arrival at the right heart chambers (**B**), arrival at the left heart chambers (**C**), and passage through the myocardium (**D**). A perfusion defect can be noted in the mid-apical septum (*arrow*).

enables the acquisition of more than one image per heartbeat. Depending on the heart rate, three to five images are obtained per cycle, each at a different level of the LV. However, temporal resolution is usually insufficient to cover the whole heart in every beat so the most common approach is to image limited views. Alternatively, complete cardiac coverage can be achieved by acquiring part of the slices in one heartbeat and the remaining in the following cycle. This approach can be used also for the visualization of microvascular obstruction (see Section 11.1), but imaging every heartbeat is usually preferred for stress/rest perfusion (see also Section 12.1). Different slices are obtained at different phases of the cardiac cycle, but each specific slice is always acquired after the same delay from the QRS complex, so the resulting cine loop displays a motionless LV where only the signal intensity varies amongst frames (Fig. 7.11 and Movie 7.6). Slice thickness is usually 5 to 10 mm, and in-plane resolution is in the order of 1.5 to 3 mm, sufficient to differentiate subendocardial from transmural abnormalities.[46] Preparation pulses are given before image acquisition to null tissue signal before contrast arrival. Options include nonselective saturation recovery (SR; the most common), "notched" SR, or IR pulses. It is unclear at this point which sequence is preferable for the evaluation of perfusion imaging. SSFP offers higher contrast-to-noise ratio (CNR) but requires longer imaging times and is more prone to field inhomogeneity. Hybrid GRE–EPI techniques have a higher temporal resolution, intermediate CNR, and susceptibility to off-resonance artifacts. Fast GRE sequences usually display an intermediate temporal resolution and lower CNR.[47]

Another unresolved issue is the optimal contrast infusion protocol. Ideally, myocardial signal intensity should parallel contrast concentration, which in turn should reflect perfusion. In reality, because conventional contrast distributes also into the interstitium, signal intensity changes reflect both perfusion and diffusion. In addition, the relationship between contrast dose and signal intensity is only linear at small contrast concentrations of approximately ≤0.05 mmol/kg for the myocardium and ≤0.01 mmol/kg for the blood pool,[48] although this also depends

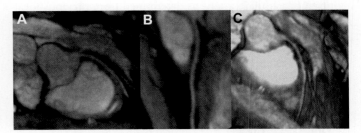

Figure 7.10 Coronary MRA of the left main and left anterior descending coronary arteries obtained with a 3D SSFP sequence. **A:** Maximum intensity projection; **B:** Curved multiplanar reformation; and **C:** 3D volume-rendered reconstruction.

on imaging parameters. Further increases in dose do not lead to corresponding changes in signal intensity due to T2* effects. This is particularly important for objective quantification of perfusion (see below) so small doses are frequently employed, but this may result in limited CNR. Two recent multicenter trials have compared the diagnostic performance of three different doses: 0.05, 0.1, and 0.15 mmol/kg. The first study reported comparable accuracy, slightly superior for the lower dose, by using visual analysis of perfusion.[49] The second study reported improved accuracy for the higher doses and employed a semiquantitative analysis method.[50] A common protocol in many centers is to administer 0.05 mmol/kg at 4 to 6 mL/s, followed by a saline bolus of 10 to 20 mL at the same rate.

10.2. Quantification of myocardial perfusion

The most common approach in clinical practice for the evaluation of myocardial perfusion is visual interpretation. Perfusion deficits can be noted as areas of delayed and/or decreased myocardial enhancement (Fig. 7.11 and Movie 7.6). The main limitation of visual interpretation is the frequent presence of subendocardial *dark rim* artifacts or areas of hypointensity in the blood–myocardium interface that need to be differentiated from true perfusion defects. Reasons for these artifacts are complex and include insufficient k space sampling, contrast-related magnetic susceptibility, and motion or partial volume effects. They occur more commonly with SSFP sequences and with higher contrast doses or injection rates.[46] Dark rim artifacts tend to have sharply defined borders, last only for a few heartbeats (true perfusion deficits usually persist longer), and are occasionally visible even before myocardial perfusion occurs (when the contrast has reached the LV cavity but the myocardium has not enhanced yet). However, the most reliable way to interpret the meaning of potential perfusion deficits is to compare rest and stress perfusion as well as delayed postcontrast images (see Section 12.1).

Objective indexes of perfusion can also be obtained from quantifying myocardial signal intensity in different myocardial segments.[51] This generates signal versus time curves and subsequently a gamma-variate function is fitted to isolate the component corresponding to the contrast first pass. Myocardial signal intensity is usually corrected for baseline signal, background noise, and blood pool signal (regarded as the arterial input function). The nonlinearity between signal intensity and contrast dose is particularly important for an accurate input function measurement, so small doses are recommended. Alternative new methods that include a dual-bolus injection protocols or combination of different sequences have been proposed to overcome this limitation.[46] Analysis of perfusion requires time-consuming postprocessing and has not gained generalized acceptance in routine practice. Numerous semiquantitative indexes of perfusion can be measured from the curves, including time to contrast arrival, peak signal intensity, time to peak, upslope of the signal enhancement, time to maximal upslope, mean transit time, or area under the curve (Fig. 7.12). These indexes can be used to compare myocardial segments amongst themselves or, more commonly, perfusion during stress versus rest. The signal intensity upslope, typically normalized to the upslope of the input function, is measured in the initial portion of the curve and is relatively insensitive to diffusion. A myocardial perfusion reserve index based on the stress/rest upslope ratio has been widely used in clinical research. Absolute quantifications of blood flow are also possible with complex mathematical analysis.[51]

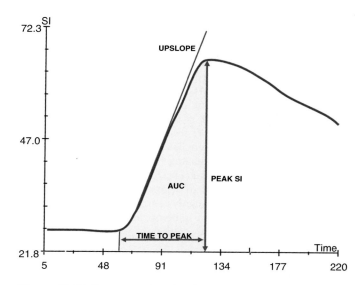

Figure 7.12 Representative signal intensity (SI) versus time curve derived from first-pass myocardial perfusion images. The figure also illustrates some semiquantitative indexes of perfusion. AUC, area under the curve.

11. MYOCARDIAL VIABILITY

11.1. Postcontrast delayed enhancement imaging

Myocardial viability with CMR can be studied measuring maximal ventricular wall thickness, assessing contractile response to dobutamine (Section 12.2), or using spectroscopy (Section 6.3). However, *delayed enhancement* (DE) imaging has become the standard for the evaluation of viability in most laboratories. DE is the result of the accumulation of extracellular contrast agents in infarcted myocardium, both in the acute and the chronic phase. This leads to depiction of the infarct as a bright area, whereas normal, viable myocardium appears dark (Fig. 7.13). The mechanisms for accumulation include delayed wash-in and wash-out of the contrast agent, as well as increased volume of distribution. In the acute phase, the loss of integrity of myocyte membranes allows the contrast to gain access to the intracellular space. In the chronic setting, the volume of distribution increases because of an enlarged interstitium in the presence of extensive fibrosis.[52] In some areas with severe ischemic insult and largely reduced perfusion, it may take longer for the contrast to accumulate than in the remaining infarcted tissue. These appear as dark, typically subendocardial regions completely surrounded by DE and correspond histologically to microvascular obstruction.[52] Microvascular obstruction is best visualized in the first few minutes after contrast administration, either with first-pass perfusion or DE sequences.

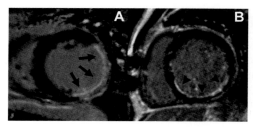

Figure 7.13 Examples of DE imaging of myocardial infarction. **A:** Short-axis view demonstrating transmural lateral scarring (*arrows*). **B:** Short-axis view showing a subendocardial inferior infarct (*arrowheads*).

The standard sequence for DE imaging is a segmented, IR-prepared fast GRE technique that provides the best differentiation between normal and infarcted tissue.[53] The timing of image acquisition after the IR pulse (inversion time; TI) is optimized so that normal myocardium has minimal signal and is clearly delineated from the infarct. Using this technique, the extent of DE matches precisely the true infarct size as demonstrated by pathology.[54] The optimal TI is usually determined from fast, single-shot SSFP or from a *TI scout* (a sequence where several images are acquired at different TIs in a single breath-hold). An important strength of DE imaging is the ability to resolve the transmural extent of infarction (Fig. 7.13), which is the basis for the prediction of likelihood of segmental functional recovery. In addition, DE imaging is highly reproducible. After its initial development for the study of ischemic heart disease, DE applications have extended to the evaluation of fibrosis in multiple cardiomyopathies.[55]

DE imaging is performed 5 to 30 min after the administration of an extracellular Gd contrast agent. Doses of 0.1 to 0.2 mmol/kg provide comparable results in terms of infarct sizing.[56] With smaller doses and with longer times after contrast administration, higher TIs are required to null normal myocardium and therefore to preserve the accuracy of the technique. TIs typically range from 200 to 400 ms. Imaging is performed during apnea for 8 to 10 s. Data is normally collected every other heartbeat to allow for recovery of longitudinal magnetization after the IR pulse. In patients with faster heart rates, the interval is increased to three to four heartbeats. Multiple short-axis as well as long-axis views are prescribed, typically matching the slice positions of the cine images in order to correlate contractility and infarct extent. Slice thickness is usually 6 to 8 mm, and in-plane resolution <2 mm. During the last few years, several improvements in pulse sequences for DE imaging have been developed. Phase-sensitive techniques are more robust to variations in TI and therefore less operator dependent.[57] Single-shot IR-SSFP sequences allow for the acquisition of a complete image in one heartbeat and are well suited for rapid imaging during free breathing.[58] More recently, 3D techniques for complete heart coverage in a single breath-hold have also been proposed.[59]

11.2. Delayed enhancement analysis

DE presence and extent is most frequently assessed visually. A common semiquantitative method estimates the percent area of a segment demonstrating DE (none, 1% to 25%, 26% to 50%, 51% to 75%, and 76% to 100%). Alternatively, objective analysis tools have been developed. These usually require tracing of the endocardial and epicardial contours and the determination of a signal intensity threshold that differentiates enhanced from normal myocardial voxels. Several analytic approaches have been proposed,[60] but to date there is no consensus on which method is optimal.

12. STRESS PROTOCOLS

The most common CMR stress protocols are based on a pharmacologic challenge and evaluation of myocardial function and/or perfusion. Changes in blood flow and cardiac metabolism can also be assessed with PC or spectroscopic techniques. There is also some experience with exercise stress testing, although limited to very few laboratories. Approaches have included handgrip exercise, supine exercise with MR-compatible cycle ergometers, or imaging of patients immediately after upright exercise on an MR-compatible treadmill.[61]

Stress protocols are largely comparable to those employed with other imaging techniques, including general contraindications for stress or to specific drugs and indications for termination (see Chapter 10). However, there are some particularities specific to CMR. Because of the magnetohydrodynamic effect, the ECG cannot be used to monitor the ST segments. Therefore, early detection of ischemia relies on the evaluation of perfusion and/or wall motion abnormalities that, according to the "ischemic cascade," are expected to precede ECG changes. A complete 12-lead ECG is nonetheless obtained both at baseline and after termination of the test. One of the most common concerns is the challenge of responding to potential emergencies within the constraints of the magnetic environment. Should any life-threatening situation occur (i.e., cardiac arrest), the patient needs to be swiftly removed out of the magnet and provided assistance in a safe environment. As reviewed in Section 3, only MR-compatible equipment should be brought inside the scanning room. The study needs to be supervised by a physician knowledgeable in CMR, and personnel trained in advanced resuscitation and MR safety procedures need to be readily available. A fully equipped resuscitation cart should be present outside the scanning room. Heart rate and rhythm (and optionally pulse oxymetry) are monitored continuously throughout the procedure, and blood pressure is measured every minute. Additionally, visual and verbal contact with the patient is maintained at all times. Following these recommendations, stress CMR has demonstrated a safety profile comparable to other imaging modalities.[62]

12.1. Stress perfusion (see also Section 10.1)

Myocardial stress perfusion is usually studied with vasodilator drugs such as dipyridamole or adenosine.[46,62] Dipyridamole is typically administered at a dose of 0.56 mg/kg/min for 4 min, whereas the dose for adenosine is 0.14 mg/kg/min over 4 to 6 min. Both drugs act by stimulation of smooth muscle adenosine receptors and cause vasodilatation of the microcirculation and myocardial hyperemia. Flow increase is limited in areas supplied by stenotic coronary arteries, so perfusion is lower than in normal segments. Because perfusion is rarely reduced below resting levels, both agents are very safe and widely employed for stress MRI. In addition, perfusion protocols are usually shorter than dobutamine stress function studies. Mild adverse effects are common, and some patients tolerate the test better if they remain partially outside of the magnet during the first few minutes of the infusion. The rate of major complications is <0.1%.[62] In addition, the relatively small increase in heart rate associated with these drugs is advantageous for maintaining sufficient heart coverage during perfusion imaging at peak stress. Caffeinated substances, theophylline, and nitrates should be stopped for 24 h and food intake for 6 to 8 h before the procedure.

As mentioned before, perfusion evaluation usually involves comparison of stress and rest acquisitions, as well as DE imaging (Table 7.6, Fig. 7.14 and Movie 7.7). A suggested protocol is shown in Figure 7.1, administering 0.05 mmol/kg of contrast agent for each perfusion acquisition and an additional dose of 0.1 mmol/kg immediately after rest perfusion evaluation, for a total dose of 0.2 mmol/kg. We usually obtain three short axis slices (at the basal, mid, and apical levels) plus additional long-axis views depending on the heart rate. If the heart rate increases markedly with adenosine, the long-axis views can be eliminated. An additional series of cine images at peak stress may be added to the protocol, particularly if ischemia is noted. Perfusion acquisitions should be performed at least 15 min apart to allow for adequate wash-out of the contrast agent. Some contrast may still

TABLE 7.6

INTERPRETATION OF MYOCARDIAL PERFUSION DEFECTS

Stress perfusion defect	Rest perfusion defect	Delayed enhancement	Interpretation
Absent	Absent	Absent	Normal
Present	Absent	Absent	Ischemia
Present	Present	Absent	Artifact
Present	Present	Present (similar to perfusion defect)	Infarct
Present	Present	Present (smaller than perfusion defect)	Infarct with peri-infarct ischemia

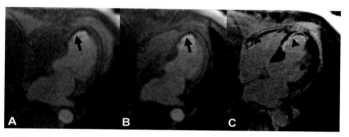

Figure 7.14 (Movie 7.7). The figure shows the stress perfusion (**A**, left panel in the movie), rest perfusion (**B**, right panel in the movie), and DE images (**C**) for the same patient as Figure 7.12. There is a perfusion defect in both first-pass acquisitions (*arrows*), slightly more prominent at stress. The DE images reveal an approximately 50% transmural scar in this area (*arrowhead*).

remain in the myocardium for the second acquisition and could mask a perfusion deficit, so ideally stress imaging should be performed first. This can be done with adenosine because of its short half-life (<10 s), an additionally attractive feature in case adverse reactions occur. A disadvantage of adenosine is that, at the end of the stress portion, the contrast and drug are administered simultaneously, so a second intravenous access is needed for the contrast. Dipyridamole has a longer half-life (~30 min), so the study should begin with the evaluation of rest perfusion. In the stress portion, the drug can be stopped after the end of the infusion and before contrast injection.

12.2. Stress function

A continuous infusion of intravenous dobutamine is the most common pharmacologic challenge for the analysis of stress function. Dobutamine is a sympathomimetic drug with a half-life of approximately 2 min that increases myocardial oxygen requirements through its positive inotropic and chronotropic effects. Dobutamine has the potential to induce significant ischemia and is pro-arrhythmogenic, so the safety profile is slightly worse than that of adenosine/dipyridamole. The rate of severe complications with dobutamine stress CMR is approximately 0.2%.[62,63] Antianginal medications are usually stopped before the test for 24 h and food intake for 6 to 8 h.

Protocols employed with CMR resemble those used with other modalities, although DE imaging is frequently included in the

study (Fig. 7.1). Dobutamine dose is started at a dose of 5 µg/kg/min and escalated every 3 min. For viability assessment, contractile reserve is evaluated at doses of 5 and 10 µg/kg/min. For the detection of ischemia, infusion rates are titrated up (5, 10, 20, 30, and 40 to 50 µg/kg/min) until the target heart rate is achieved or the maximal dose is reached. If necessary, atropine (0.25 mg intravenous boluses to a maximal dose of 1 mg) and/or handgrip exercise are added to peak dobutamine dose to increase heart rate. Cine images are acquired at baseline and at the end of each dosing step and are reviewed for wall motion abnormalities before increasing the dose. Therefore, the magnet should have online "real-time" (or near "real-time") image display capabilities. Both the development of new wall motion abnormalities and the lack of expected improvement in contractility are considered pathologic findings. Three short-axis slices (base, mid, and apex) plus one or two long-axis views are normally acquired using cine SSFP imaging. Because the heart rate increases with dobutamine, it is necessary to improve the temporal resolution of the sequence as the exam proceeds. This is done by progressively reducing the number of k space lines acquired per heartbeat. As a simple approximation, a temporal resolution ≤5% of the RR interval may be used (e.g., if the RR interval is 600 ms, the temporal resolution should be ≤30 ms). Improving temporal resolution implies acquiring images over a higher number of heartbeats; however, because of the increase in heart rate, the duration of the breath-hold remains basically constant. If imaging is performed only at the end of each stage, ischemia may be missed for a significant period of time. It is therefore a routine practice to monitor function at additional intervals, either with standard SSFP or with real-time cine sequences.[64] If wall motion remains normal at peak stress, perfusion imaging may be added in an attempt to detect an earlier stage of ischemia. It must be realized that the faster heart rate may contribute to artifacts and hinder interpretation as well as adequate coverage.

13. FUTURE DIRECTIONS

As reviewed in the introduction, CMR technology and its clinical utilization have expanded exponentially during the last decade. Similar impressive advances are likely to develop in the next few years. From a clinical standpoint, not only novel uses are forthcoming but also the prognostic implications of many current findings are being elucidated as longer follow-up studies become available. Improvements in sequence design, some of them briefly addressed in the preceding sections, promise to enable comprehensive cardiovascular evaluations in shorter imaging times. Together with advances in coil technology and parallel imaging, many current applications are likely to be performed in a single breath-hold, including function, viability, tissue characterization, or even "whole-heart" coronary angiography.[65] The field of high-field imaging (i.e., at 3T) is still evolving but holds promise in further improving CMR capabilities. The increases in SNR and image contrast attainable with higher magnetic fields allow for superior spatial resolution and enhanced exploitation of parallel imaging capabilities, therefore affording faster imaging.[66] Finally, contrast agent design is another area of substantial innovation. Not only compounds displaying different pharmacokinetic properties (i.e., intravascular agents) are being developed, but also many molecules with high affinity for specific ligands (fibrin, cell adhesion molecules, macrophage receptors, etc.). This ability to visualize disease-related processes at a cellular or molecular level in vivo (*molecular imaging*), either with MRI or other modalities, holds an unparalleled potential to improve our understanding of cardiovascular disease.[67]

REFERENCES

1. Damadian R. Tumor detection by nuclear magnetic resonance. *Science.* 1971;171:1151–1153.
2. Lauterbur PC. Image formation by induced local interactions: Examples employing nuclear magnetic resonance. *Nature.* 1973;242:190–191.
3. Mansfield P, Grannell PK. NMR 'diffraction' in solids? *J Phys C: Solid State Phys.* 1973;6:L422–L426.
4. Edelstein WA, Hutchison JM, Johnson G, et al. Spin warp NMR imaging and applications to human whole-body imaging. *Phys Med Biol.* 1980;25:751–756.
5. Lanzer P, Botvinick EH, Schiller NB, et al. Cardiac imaging using gated magnetic resonance. *Radiology.* 1984;150:121–127.
6. Bryant DJ, Payne JA, Firmin DN, et al. Measurement of flow with NMR imaging using a gradient pulse and phase difference technique. *J Comput Assist Tomogr.* 1984;8:588–593.
7. Waterton JC, Jenkins JP, Zhu XP, et al. Magnetic resonance (MR) cine imaging of the human heart. *Br J Radiol.* 1985;58:711–716.
8. Edelman RR, Manning WJ, Burstein D, et al. Coronary arteries: Breath-hold MR angiography. *Radiology.* 1991;181:641–643.
9. McNamara MT, Higgins CB, Schechtmann N, et al. Detection and characterization of acute myocardial infarction in man with use of gated magnetic resonance. *Circulation.* 1985;71:717–724.
10. Atkinson DJ, Burstein D, Edelman RR. First-pass cardiac perfusion: Evaluation with ultrafast MR imaging. *Radiology.* 1990;174:757–762.
11. Kramer CM, Barkhausen J, Flamm SD, et al. Standardized cardiovascular magnetic resonance imaging (CMR) protocols, society for cardiovascular magnetic resonance: Board of trustees task force on standardized protocols. *J Cardiovasc Magn Reson.* 2008;10:35.
12. Ersoy H, Rybicki FJ. Biochemical safety profiles of gadolinium-based extracellular contrast agents and nephrogenic systemic fibrosis. *J Magn Reson Imaging.* 2007;26:1190–1197.
13. Dillman JR, Ellis JH, Cohan RH, et al. Frequency and severity of acute allergic-like reactions to gadolinium-containing i.v. contrast media in children and adults. *Am J Roentgenol.* 2007;189:1533–1538.
14. Lin SP, Brown JJ. MR contrast agents: Physical and pharmacologic basics. *J Magn Reson Imaging.* 2007;25:884–899.
15. Bellin MF, Van Der Molen AJ. Extracellular gadolinium-based contrast media: An overview. *Eur J Radiol.* 2008;66:160–167.
16. Kanal E, Barkovich AJ, Bell C, et al. ACR guidance document for safe MR practices: 2007. *Am J Roentgenol.* 2007;188:1447–1474.
17. Levine GN, Gomes AS, Arai AE, et al. Safety of magnetic resonance imaging in patients with cardiovascular devices: An American Heart Association scientific statement from the Committee on Diagnostic and Interventional Cardiac Catheterization, Council on Clinical Cardiology, and the Council on Cardiovascular Radiology and Intervention: Endorsed by the American College of Cardiology Foundation, the North American Society for Cardiac Imaging, and the Society for Cardiovascular Magnetic Resonance. *Circulation.* 2007;116:2878–2891.
18. Francis JM, Pennell DJ. Treatment of claustrophobia for cardiovascular magnetic resonance: Use and effectiveness of mild sedation. *J Cardiovasc Magn Reson.* 2000;2:139–141.
19. Plein S, Bloomer TN, Ridgway JP, et al. Steady-state free precession magnetic resonance imaging of the heart: Comparison with segmented k-space gradient-echo imaging. *J Magn Reson Imaging.* 2001;14:230–236.
20. Miller S, Simonetti OP, Carr J, et al. MR imaging of the heart with cine true fast imaging with steady-state precession: Influence of spatial and temporal resolutions on left ventricular functional parameters. *Radiology.* 2002;223:263–269.
21. Roussakis A, Baras P, Seimenis I, et al. Relationship of number of phases per cardiac cycle and accuracy of measurement of left ventricular volumes, ejection fraction, and mass. *J Cardiovasc Magn Reson.* 2004;6:837–844.
22. Nagel E, Schneider U, Schalla S, et al. Magnetic resonance real-time imaging for the evaluation of left ventricular function. *J Cardiovasc Magn Reson.* 2000;2:7–14.
23. Jahnke C, Nagel E, Gebker R, et al. Four-dimensional single breathhold magnetic resonance imaging using kt-BLAST enables reliable assessment of left- and right-ventricular volumes and mass. *J Magn Reson Imaging.* 2007;25:737–742.
24. Sievers B, Kirchberg S, Bakan A, et al. Impact of papillary muscles in ventricular volume and ejection fraction assessment by cardiovascular magnetic resonance. *J Cardiovasc Magn Reson.* 2004;6:9–16.
25. Pujadas S, Reddy GP, Weber O, et al. MR imaging assessment of cardiac function. *J Magn Reson Imaging.* 2004;19:789–799.
26. Cerqueira MD, Weissman NJ, Dilsizian V, et al. Standardized myocardial segmentation and nomenclature for tomographic imaging of the heart: A statement for healthcare professionals from the Cardiac Imaging Committee of the Council on Clinical Cardiology of the American Heart Association. *Circulation.* 2002;105:539–542.
27. Gotte MJ, Germans T, Russel IK, et al. Myocardial strain and torsion quantified by cardiovascular magnetic resonance tissue tagging: Studies in normal and impaired left ventricular function. *J Am Coll Cardiol.* 2006;48:2002–2011.
28. Paelinck BP, de Roos A, Bax JJ, et al. Feasibility of tissue magnetic resonance imaging: A pilot study in comparison with tissue Doppler imaging and invasive measurement. *J Am Coll Cardiol.* 2005;45:1109–1116.
29. Kim D, Gilson WD, Kramer CM, et al. Myocardial tissue tracking with two-dimensional cine displacement-encoded MR imaging: Development and initial evaluation. *Radiology.* 2004;230:862–871.
30. Castillo E, Tandri H, Rodriguez ER, et al. Arrhythmogenic right ventricular dysplasia: Ex vivo and in vivo fat detection with black-blood MR imaging. *Radiology.* 2004;232:38–48.
31. Simonetti OP, Finn JP, White RD, et al. "Black blood" T2-weighted inversion-recovery MR imaging of the heart. *Radiology.* 1996;199:49–57.
32. Abdel-Aty H, Boye P, Zagrosek A, et al. Diagnostic performance of cardiovascular magnetic resonance in patients with suspected acute myocarditis: Comparison of different approaches. *J Am Coll Cardiol.* 2005;45:1815–1822.
33. Anderson LJ, Holden S, Davis B, et al. Cardiovascular T2-star (T2*) magnetic resonance for the early diagnosis of myocardial iron overload. *Eur Heart J.* 2001;22:2171–2179.
34. Neubauer S. Cardiac magnetic resonance spectroscopy: Potential clinical applications. *Herz.* 2000;25:452–460.
35. Hundley WG, Li HF, Lange RA, et al. Assessment of left-to-right intracardiac shunting by velocity-encoded, phase-difference magnetic resonance imaging: A comparison with oximetric and indicator dilution techniques. *Circulation.* 1995;91:2955–2960.
36. Krombach GA, Kuhl H, Bucker A, et al. Cine MR imaging of heart valve dysfunction with segmented true fast imaging with steady state free precession. *J Magn Reson Imaging.* 2004;19:59–67.
37. Caruthers SD, Lin SJ, Brown P, et al. Practical value of cardiac magnetic resonance imaging for clinical quantification of aortic valve stenosis: Comparison with echocardiography. *Circulation.* 2003;108:2236–2243.
38. Kupfahl C, Honold M, Meinhardt G, et al. Evaluation of aortic stenosis by cardiovascular magnetic resonance imaging: Comparison with established routine clinical techniques. *Heart.* 2004;90:893–901.
39. Kozerke S, Scheidegger MB, Pedersen EM, et al. Heart motion adapted cine phase-contrast flow measurements through the aortic valve. *Magn Reson Med.* 1999;42:970–978.
40. Gelfand EV, Hughes S, Hauser TH, et al. Severity of mitral and aortic regurgitation as assessed by cardiovascular magnetic resonance: Optimizing correlation with Doppler echocardiography. *J Cardiovasc Magn Reson.* 2006;8:503–507.
41. Manning WJ, Stuber M, Danias PG, et al. Coronary magnetic resonance imaging: Current status. *Curr Probl Cardiol.* 2002;27:275–333.
42. Weber OM, Martin AJ, Higgins CB. Whole-heart steady-state free precession coronary artery magnetic resonance angiography. *Magn Reson Med.* 2003;50:1223–1228.
43. Liu X, Zhao X, Huang J, et al. Comparison of 3D free-breathing coronary MR angiography and 64-MDCT angiography for detection of coronary stenosis in patients with high calcium scores. *Am J Roentgenol.* 2007;189:1326–1332.
44. Kraitchman DL, Chin BB, Heldman AW, et al. MRI detection of myocardial perfusion defects due to coronary artery stenosis with MS-325. *J Magn Reson Imaging.* 2002;15:149–158.
45. Fieno DS, Shea SM, Li Y, et al. Myocardial perfusion imaging based on the blood oxygen level-dependent effect using T2-prepared steady-state free-precession magnetic resonance imaging. *Circulation.* 2004;110:1284–1290.
46. Gerber BL, Raman SV, Nayak K, et al. Myocardial first-pass perfusion cardiovascular magnetic resonance: History, theory, and current state of the art. *J Cardiovasc Magn Reson.* 2008;10:18.
47. Kellman P, Arai AE. Imaging sequences for first pass perfusion—a review. *J Cardiovasc Magn Reson.* 2007;9:525–537.
48. Utz W, Niendorf T, Wassmuth R, et al. Contrast-dose relation in first-pass myocardial MR perfusion imaging. *J Magn Reson Imaging.* 2007;25:1131–1135.
49. Wolff SD, Schwitter J, Coulden R, et al. Myocardial first-pass perfusion magnetic resonance imaging: A multicenter dose-ranging study. *Circulation.* 2004;110:732–737.
50. Giang TH, Nanz D, Coulden R, et al. Detection of coronary artery disease by magnetic resonance myocardial perfusion imaging with various contrast medium doses: First European multi-centre experience. *Eur Heart J.* 2004;25:1657–1665.
51. Jerosch-Herold M, Seethamraju RT, Swingen CM, et al. Analysis of myocardial perfusion MRI. *J Magn Reson Imaging.* 2004;19:758–770.
52. Mahrholdt H, Wagner A, Judd RM, et al. Assessment of myocardial viability by cardiovascular magnetic resonance imaging. *Eur Heart J.* 2002;23:602–619.
53. Simonetti OP, Kim RJ, Fieno DS, et al. An improved MR imaging technique for the visualization of myocardial infarction. *Radiology.* 2001;218:215–223.
54. Fieno DS, Kim RJ, Chen EL, et al. Contrast-enhanced magnetic resonance imaging of myocardium at risk: Distinction between reversible and irreversible injury throughout infarct healing. *J Am Coll Cardiol.* 2000;36:1985–1991.
55. Mahrholdt H, Wagner A, Judd RM, et al. Delayed enhancement cardiovascular magnetic resonance assessment of non-ischaemic cardiomyopathies. *Eur Heart J.* 2005;26:1461–1474.
56. Wagner A, Mahrholdt H, Thomson L, et al. Effects of time, dose, and inversion time for acute myocardial infarct size measurements based on magnetic resonance imaging-delayed contrast enhancement. *J Am Coll Cardiol.* 2006;47:2027–2033.
57. Huber AM, Schoenberg SO, Hayes C, et al. Phase-sensitive inversion-recovery MR imaging in the detection of myocardial infarction. *Radiology.* 2005;237:854–860.
58. Sievers B, Elliott MD, Hurwitz LM, et al. Rapid detection of myocardial infarction by subsecond, free-breathing delayed contrast-enhancement cardiovascular magnetic resonance. *Circulation.* 2007;115:236–244.
59. Dewey M, Laule M, Taupitz M, et al. Myocardial viability: Assessment with three-dimensional MR imaging in pigs and patients. *Radiology.* 2006;239:703–709.
60. Amado LC, Gerber BL, Gupta SN, et al. Accurate and objective infarct sizing by contrast-enhanced magnetic resonance imaging in a canine myocardial infarction model. *J Am Coll Cardiol.* 2004;44:2383–2389.
61. Rerkpattanapipat P, Gandhi SK, Darty SN, et al. Feasibility to detect severe coronary artery stenoses with upright treadmill exercise magnetic resonance imaging. *Am J Cardiol.* 2003;92:603–606.
62. Nagel E, Lorenz C, Baer F, et al. Stress cardiovascular magnetic resonance: Consensus panel report. *J Cardiovasc Magn Reson.* 2001;3:267–281.

63. Wahl A, Paetsch I, Gollesch A, et al. Safety and feasibility of high-dose dobutamine-atropine stress cardiovascular magnetic resonance for diagnosis of myocardial ischaemia: Experience in 1000 consecutive cases. *Eur Heart J.* 2004;25:1230–1236.

64. Schalla S, Klein C, Paetsch I, et al. Real-time MR image acquisition during high-dose dobutamine hydrochloride stress for detecting left ventricular wall-motion abnormalities in patients with coronary arterial disease. *Radiology.* 2002;224:845–851.

65. Niendorf T, Hardy CJ, Giaquinto RO, et al. Toward single breath-hold whole-heart coverage coronary MRA using highly accelerated parallel imaging with a 32-channel MR system. *Magn Reson Med.* 2006;56:167–176.

66. Lee VS, Hecht EM, Taouli B, et al. Body and cardiovascular MR imaging at 3.0 T. *Radiology.* 2007;244:692–705.

67. Sosnovik DE, Nahrendorf M, Weissleder R. Molecular magnetic resonance imaging in cardiovascular medicine. *Circulation.* 2007;115:2076–2086.

8

X-Ray Computed Tomography Physics and Instrumentation

Sandra S. Halliburton

1. INTRODUCTION

1.1. Historical perspective

From its inception, there was a desire to apply the technology of X-ray computed tomography (CT) to imaging of the cardiovascular system because of the potential for acquiring cross-sectional images, differentiating soft tissue, and quantifying structural and functional parameters. However, cardiac imaging with CT requires (i) high temporal resolution to limit cardiac motion artifacts, (ii) high spatial resolution to visualize small cardiac anatomy, (iii) fast anatomic coverage allowing scanning of the heart during a breath-hold to reduce respiratory motion artifacts, and (iv) synchronization of data acquisition or rec onstruction to the cardiac cycle to ensure imaging during a desired cardiac phase.

With initial mechanical or conventional CT technology, the power supply required to rotate the X-ray tube was provided by cables that restricted the rotation of the gantry.[1] This technology permitted only two-dimensional acquisition, termed "axial," "sequential," or "step-and-shoot" scanning, where a single transaxial slice is acquired during one 360° rotation of the gantry and the patient table is incremented to the next slice position. The acquisition time for each image eventually improved from 300s in 1972 down to 2s by 1990[1] but was still too prolonged for cardiac imaging without the introduction of significant motion artifact.

In 1983, a new type of CT scanner was introduced for cardiovascular imaging that eliminated the requirement for mechanical motion of the X-ray source around the patient through the use of electron beam CT (EBCT) technology.[2] Parallel advances in conventional CT included, most notably, the introduction of "helical" or "spiral" scanning in 1989, where data are acquired during continuous rotation of the gantry and continuous movement of the patient table.[3,4] A continuously rotating gantry was achieved using slip ring technology where electrical energy for the X-ray tube was transferred by slip rings instead of electrical cables, eliminating the previously required start–stop motion of the gantry.[1] Although significant improvements in volume coverage were realized, the scan time for each image was still typically 1 s—too long for diagnostic imaging of the heart.

The advent of systems capable of both axial and helical acquisition with sub-second rotation times and electrocardiographic (ECG)-synchronized scanning in 1994 brought conventional CT into the domain of cardiac imaging. Initial results demonstrated the clinical potential of mechanical CT but restrictions in temporal resolution, longitudinal or z-resolution, and anatomic coverage (even for helical acquisition) limited applications for evaluation of the heart primarily to coronary artery calcium scoring.[5–7]

Multidetector row technology did not have a major impact on cardiac imaging with mechanical CT until Multi-detector computed tomography (MDCT) scanners capable of quad-slice imaging were introduced in 1998.[7,8] These scanners permitted the simultaneous acquisition of four slices, rotation times as short as 500 ms, slices as thin as 1.25 mm, and scan times for the coverage of the entire heart equal to 35 to 40s, thereby significantly improving the utility of mechanical CT for cardiac imaging. Additional improvements were observed with the introduction of 8-slice scanners in 2001, 16-slice in 2002,[9,10] 64-slice in 2004,[11] dual source scanners in 2006,[12] and 320-slice in 2007.[13] In addition to the increased number of slices, the evolution of conventional CT scanners has resulted in rotation times as short as 270 ms, slices as thin as 0.5 mm, and scan times for imaging of the coronary arteries ranging from <1 to 10 s.[12,13]

The purpose of this chapter is to review the basic physics and instrumentation of X-ray CT. X-ray generation and transmission, EBCT and MDCT scanners, ECG-referenced acquisition modes, acquisition parameters, image formation and reconstruction, imaging artifacts, radiation dose estimation, equipment maintenance and quality control, and future perspectives will be discussed.

2. X-RAY GENERATION AND TRANSMISSION

X-rays are produced when highly energetic electrons interact with matter. Electrons are accelerated toward a target to gain kinetic energy. For most diagnostic imaging applications, the electrons gain a maximum kinetic energy between 80 and 140 keV. The accelerated electrons interact with the nucleus or orbital electrons of the target atom.[14]

Interaction of an incident electron with the target atomic nucleus causes the electron to lose kinetic energy and change trajectory. The kinetic energy lost by the electron is converted into an X-ray photon. The energy of the X-ray photon is inversely related to the distance of interaction between the incident electron and the target atom's nucleus. The result of interactions at varying distances from the target atomic nucleus is X-ray photons spanning a continuous energy spectrum, termed the Bremsstrahlung spectrum, with the maximum X-ray photon energy equal to the maximum kinetic energy of the incident electron (between 80 and 140 keV for diagnostic imaging). Because of the increased probability of interactions further from the nucleus, the majority of X-ray photons produced have much lower energies. Lower energy X-rays are absorbed by the body before reaching the detector and, subsequently, serve only to increase radiation dose without contributing information to the reconstructed image. Therefore, low energy X-rays are typically filtered before reaching the patient.

Interaction of an incident electron with an orbital electron in the target atom results in ejection of the target electron if its binding energy is less than the energy of the incident electron. An outer shell electron in the target atom then transitions to the lower energy state, releasing an X-ray photon with a discrete energy equal to the difference between the binding energies of the shells and characteristic of the target material. Tungsten is the most widely used target material in diagnostic imaging systems because it provides useful characteristic X-ray energies (~60 to 70 keV) for most body applications.[14]

The discrete, characteristic X-ray energies produced by the interaction of incident electrons with target electrons are super-imposed on the continuous filtered Bremsstrahlung spectrum produced by the interaction of incident electrons with the target atomic nucleus. A typical X-ray spectrum generated for diagnostic imaging is shown in Figure 8.1.

For medical imaging, the generated X-rays are transmitted through the patient and the transmitted X-rays are measured by detectors opposite the X-ray source. X-rays are modified between the X-ray source and X-ray detectors according to the following equation:

$$I_t = I_o e^{-\mu t} \tag{Eq. 8.1}$$

where

I_t = intensity of transmitted X-rays
I_o = intensity of incident X-rays
μ = average linear attenuation coefficient of tissue between X-ray source and X-ray detector
t = thickness of tissue between X-ray source and X-ray detector

The attenuation, or removal, of photons from X-rays passing through tissue depends on both the energy of the X-rays and the physical properties of the tissue. Within the diagnostic energy range, X-rays interact with tissue primarily through three mechanisms: photoelectric effect, Compton scattering, and Rayleigh or coherent scattering.[14] The linear attenuation coefficient, μ, with units of cm^{-1} can therefore be expressed as

$$\mu = \mu_{photoelectric} + \mu_{Compton} + \mu_{coherent} \tag{Eq. 8.2}$$

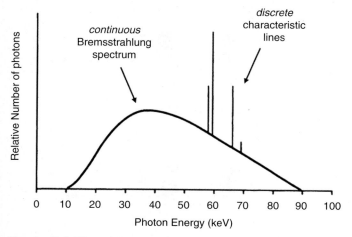

Figure 8.1 Filtered Bremsstrahlung spectrum with characteristic radiation generated from the interaction of incident electrons with a maximum kinetic energy equal to 90 keV and a tungsten target (Modified from Bushberg, et al. *The Essential Physics of Medical Imaging.* 2nd Ed. Philadelphia: Lippincott Williams & Wilkins; 2002.).

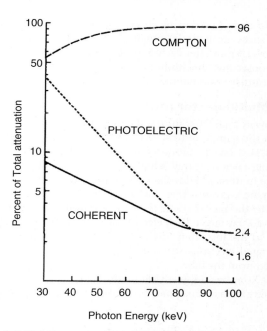

Figure 8.2 Relative percentages of the three X-ray photon/tissue interactions contributing to attenuation in the CT image for international commission on radiation units and measurements (ICRU) muscle. (Modified from McCollough CH, Morin RL. The technical design and performance of ultrafast computed tomography. *Radiol Clin North Am.* 1994;32(3):521–536.).

Photoelectric interactions produce characteristic X-rays and provide excellent tissue contrast while Compton and coherent scattering produce scattered X-rays and provide little tissue contrast.

The relative percentages of the three mechanisms of interaction contributing to attenuation vary with X-ray energy[15] (Fig. 8.2). Attenuation is dominated by the photoelectric effect at lower energies and by Compton scattering at higher energies while the contribution from coherent scattering is negligible at all energies. Further, the contribution of each type of interaction to the total attenuation varies with tissue properties, namely atomic number and density (g/cm^3); $\mu_{photoelectric}$ depends mainly on the atomic number while $\mu_{Compton}$ depends primarily on the tissue density. Most medical imaging occurs in the energy range dominated by Compton scattering such that attenuation in the CT image is governed primarily by the density of the tissue within the scanned region.

3. COMPUTED TOMOGRAPHY SCANNERS

CT scanners use X-rays to produce an image of a three-dimensional object. Measurement of a transmitted X-ray by a single detector at a single time point is termed a ray. Measurement of a group of transmitted X-rays passing through a patient at the same orientation from all detectors at a single time point is termed a projection or view. CT scanners acquire multiple X-ray projections at different orientations around the patient to create a tomographic image.

3.1. Electron beam

EBCT systems house a stationary 210° arc ring of tungsten targets within the system gantry.[16] X-rays are produced by deflecting a magnetically focused electron beam onto the tungsten target ring. Attenuated X-rays are detected on the opposite side of the patient by a stationary ring of detectors. A complete rotation of the electron beam typically takes 100 ms.

Data are acquired using an axial scanning mode. Overlapping 3 mm slices are typically obtained by incrementing the patient table by 1.5 mm after each 360° rotation of the electron beam. Two consecutive breath-holds are required to complete most EBCT cardiac examinations.

3.2. Multidetector row

In conventional CT scanners, the measurement system is housed within the gantry and rotated mechanically around the patient (Fig. 8.3). X-rays are produced in an X-ray tube, which is mounted opposite a detector array. A high voltage generator is used to apply voltage in units of kilovolts (kV) between two electrodes housed within the X-ray tube (Fig. 8.4). Electrons are accelerated from the cathode, the negative source of the electrons, to the anode, the positive X-ray target. Each electron acquires a kinetic energy (keV) equal to the instantaneous voltage (kV) across the tube. When accelerated electrons strike the target, X-rays are produced and emitted from the tube.

The X-ray beam spreads within the scan (x–y) plane in a fanlike geometry from an imaginary pointlike focus. The angle covered by the fan of X-rays within the scan plane is termed the fan angle. As the number of detector rows increases, the geometry of the X-ray beam emerging from the X-ray source changes to a cone shape.[1] The angle covered by the cone of X-rays along the direction of the system axis of rotation (z) is the cone angle.

Attenuated X-rays are detected on the opposite side of the patient by multiple rows of detectors. The X-ray tube is coupled to the detector array, and these components rotate together around the patient. A 360° rotation of the X-ray tube/detector system requires between 270 and 350 ms with state-of-the-art mechanical CT scanners.

Data covering the entire heart are acquired using either axial or helical modes within a single breath-hold. Images are reconstructed with thicknesses ranging from 0.5 to 3 mm depending on the specific cardiac application.

Compared to EBCT, MDCT offers the advantages of increased spatial resolution, increased signal-to-noise ratio (SNR), and decreased scan time. Another major distinction between technologies is user access. EBCT scanners are a highly specialized scanner type used exclusively for cardiac imaging and available at relatively few institutions while MDCT scanners are used for a range of body imaging applications and are much more widely available.

4. ECG-REFERENCED ACQUISITION MODES

An important requirement for cardiac imaging is correlation of data acquisition or reconstruction to the cardiac cycle to obtain images during a desired cardiac phase. The ECG signal is used to reference data to the cardiac cycle. The ECG signal may be used to either prospectively trigger data acquisition or retrospectively gate data reconstruction. The starting position of the acquired or reconstructed data within each cardiac cycle is described in relation to the R wave of the ECG signal using one of the following phase parameters or a combination of these parameters: (i) Relative delay—a relative delay time after the onset of the initial R wave of an RR interval defined as a given percentage of the RR interval and (ii) Absolute delay—a fixed time after the onset of the initial R wave of an RR interval (Fig. 8.5). With prospective referencing of the ECG signal, selection of the cardiac phase is

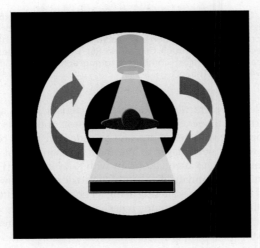

Figure 8.3 Anatomy of the gantry of a multidetector row CT scanner. The X-ray source is mounted 180° from the detector array, both rotating together during image acquisition.

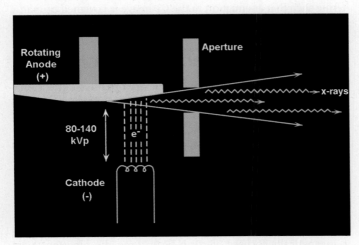

Figure 8.4 Schematic of a typical X-ray tube used in conventional CT scanners. Electrons are accelerated from the cathode, the negative source of the electrons, to the anode, the positive X-ray target. When accelerated electrons strike the target, X-rays are produced and emitted from the tube.

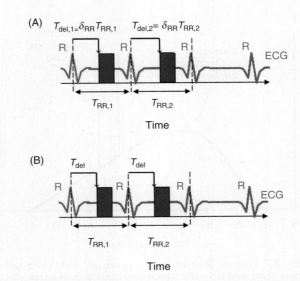

Figure 8.5 Cardiac phase selection strategies for ECG-referenced imaging: (A) relative-delay—variable delay time (T_{del}) after the previous R wave defined as a fraction (δ_{RR}) of the RR interval (T_{RR}); (B) absolute-delay—fixed delay time (T_{del}) after the previous R wave.

based on prospective estimation of the upcoming RR interval based on previous RR interval lengths.

For morphologic evaluation, data are usually selected from the diastolic phase of the cardiac cycle where heart motion is minimized. The precise phase with minimal motion is scanner and heart rate dependent[17-20] and should be optimized to ensure maximum image quality. Data can also be chosen from other cardiac phases (e.g., end-systole) for functional evaluation.

4.1. Axial mode with prospective ECG triggering

In the axial mode of operation, data acquisition is prospectively triggered by the ECG signal during the desired cardiac phase (Fig. 8.6). The patient table is incremented between periods of data acquisition.

The major advantage of the axial technique for cardiac imaging is that X-ray exposure occurs only during imaging of a single cardiac phase. However, this precludes imaging during multiple phases of the cardiac cycle without additional radiation exposure. Furthermore, axial scanning is similarly restricted to the acquisition of nonoverlapping images because of required increases in radiation dose for overlapping data. Other limitations of the axial mode include increased sensitivity to arrhythmia due to prospective referencing of the ECG signal and increased examination times due to the increment of the patient table between data acquisitions.

4.2. Helical mode with retrospective ECG gating

In the helical mode of operation, data are acquired continuously with simultaneous recording of the ECG signal (Fig. 8.7). Data are then retrospectively gated to the ECG signal after acquisition and reconstructed during one or more cardiac phases.

Helical data acquisition provides continuous volume coverage which permits reconstruction of overlapping slices and reconstruction during multiple cardiac phases. Another advantage of the helical technique is faster anatomic coverage. In addition, retrospectively, ECG-gated techniques should be less sensitive to arrhythmia; most scanner software allows the deletion of extrasystolic beats, the insertion of missed beats, and the shifting of R peak locations to adjust for arrhythmia. However, the helical mode requires higher patient radiation doses than the axial mode for comparable SNR.

4.3. ECG-based tube current modulation

Higher patient radiation doses with helical compared to axial techniques are in part the result of continuous X-ray exposure

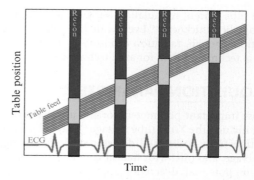

Figure 8.7 Basic spiral technique for cardiac imaging. Data from multiple channels are acquired simultaneously while the patient table is moving. The patient's ECG signal is recorded during data acquisition. Data are retrospectively reconstructed during the specified cardiac phase. Diagonal lines indicate table feed. Trace along bottom represents ECG signal. Vertical rectangles indicate reconstruction periods.

during the entire cardiac cycle. However, only data during a limited portion of the cardiac cycle, the diastolic phase, is typically used for reconstruction. The tube current outside the diastolic phase can, therefore, be reduced for patients with stable sinus rhythm to decrease patient radiation exposure with retrospectively ECG-gated helical imaging.[21-23]

One approach, similar to ECG-triggering, switches X-ray radiation on and off to acquire data from only the target cardiac phase during continuous movement of the patient table.[21] Another more common approach is prospective online modulation of the tube current where the current is at a maximum during imaging of the desired cardiac phase or phases but is reduced (to as much as 4% of the nominal value) outside this region[22,23]; patient radiation exposure is subsequently reduced by up to 50% depending on heart rate (HR). Although data are available during the entire cardiac cycle, image quality during periods of low current is limited (Fig. 8.8). Retrospective reconstruction of the thin slices of helical data necessary for morphologic evaluation is, then, restricted to a smaller portion of the cardiac cycle. However, multiple-phase reconstruction of thicker slices for functional evaluation such as measurement of left ventricular volumes may still be possi-

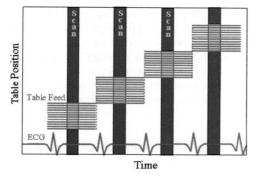

Figure 8.6 Basic axial technique for cardiac imaging. Acquisition is prospectively triggered by the ECG signal during the specified cardiac phase. Data from multiple channels are acquired simultaneously while the patient table is stationary. The patient table is incremented and the process is repeated. Horizontal lines indicate table feed. Vertical rectangles indicate scanning periods. Trace along the bottom represents ECG signal.

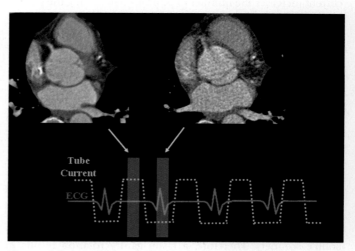

Figure 8.8 Prospective online modulation of the tube current based on the ECG signal. Tube current is at a maximum during imaging of the desired cardiac phase or phases but is reduced outside this region. Data are acquired throughout the entire cardiac cycle but images reconstructed during periods of low tube current contain significant image noise.

ble with tube current modulation because noise decreases with increasing slice thickness.[24] Even with ECG-based tube current modulation, though, radiation exposure is still typically greater for helical techniques than for axial techniques.

5. ACQUISITION PARAMETERS

The most important parameters for the acquisition of cardiac CT data include the X-ray tube voltage, X-ray tube current, gantry rotation time, collimated detector row width, longitudinal or z-coverage, and pitch (for helical data acquisition only). The maximum potential difference applied between the positive and negative electrodes in an X-ray tube is described as the peak X-ray tube voltage (kVp). An increase in the peak tube voltage increases the energy of the electrons striking the target and, subsequently, the energy and number of X-rays produced. Discrete values for peak X-ray tube voltage are selectable on diagnostic CT systems: 80, 100, 120, 135, and 140 kVp. Because of the increase in both the energy and the number of X-ray photons, selection of a higher tube voltage results in increased X-ray penetration and decreased image noise. This benefit, though, comes at the expense of increased radiation exposure to the patient. Additionally, image contrast is compromised with the selection of higher voltage values because, within the diagnostic CT energy range, differences in attenuation among body tissues decrease with increasing X-ray photon energy as a result of a decrease in the number of photoelectric interactions. A peak tube voltage of 120 kVp is standard for cardiac imaging but a lower voltage of 100 kVp may be indicated in patients with a body mass index <30 kg/m^2 to reduce radiation dose.[25,26]

The number of electrons flowing from the negative to the positive electrode in an X-ray tube is described as the X-ray tube current and expressed in units of milliamperes (mA). An increase in the X-ray tube current increases the number of electrons striking the target and, subsequently, the number of X-rays produced per unit time. A range of tube currents are available on clinical CT systems; the specific range available varies with the scan protocol but is typically within 50 to 300 mA. Because an increase in X-ray tube current increases the number of X-ray photons produced per unit time, selection of a higher X-ray tube current increases the number of photons penetrating the patient and reaching the detectors, thereby decreasing image noise. This, however, results in increased radiation exposure to the patient. Therefore, the lowest X-ray tube current that meets the image noise requirements of the clinical application is desired. Lower tube currents are appropriate in smaller patients and for clinical indications requiring reconstruction of only thicker (>1.5 mm) slices.

Another important acquisition parameter is the time required for the X-ray tube/detector system to rotate 360° around the patient. The gantry rotation time determines the temporal resolution, or the time needed to acquire enough data for reconstruction of a single image. Because approximately 180° of projection data are required by cardiac algorithms to reconstruct each image, the temporal resolution is approximated as one-half the gantry rotation time for single X-ray source CT scanners and one-fourth the gantry rotation time for dual X-ray source scanners. Therefore, a faster gantry rotation results in improved temporal resolution. The minimum gantry rotation time depends on the make and model of the CT scanner; values for state-of-the-art scanners range from 270 to 350 ms. A faster gantry rotation time, however, decreases the number of X-ray

photons produced (for a given tube voltage and tube current) and, subsequently, the number of photons interacting with the body, resulting in increased image noise. Therefore, an increase in radiation exposure is required with improvements in temporal resolution to maintain image noise.[27] For cardiac imaging, the dose increase is typically justified by the significant benefit of higher temporal resolution.

The width and number of detector rows are important for image acquisition. The collimated width of one detector row determines the minimum reconstruction slice thickness. State-of-the-art CT systems have 0.5- or 0.625-mm wide detector rows at the center of rotation. Although smaller collimated slice widths offer improved z-axis spatial resolution, fewer X-ray photons contribute to the reconstructed image (for a given tube voltage and tube current), resulting in increased image noise.[14] This increased noise can be overcome by increasing the X-ray tube voltage or, more likely, the tube current. Because of the radiation dose cost, however, the reconstruction of sub-millimeter slices should be reserved for coronary artery imaging. For other cardiovascular applications (e.g., evaluation of pulmonary vein anatomy) that do not demand such high spatial resolution, data acquired using these small detectors can be combined during image reconstruction, so more photons contribute to the reconstructed image (i.e., thicker slices can be reconstructed) and the desired image noise is achieved with decreased radiation exposure.

In addition to the width of the detector rows, the number of detector rows is critical for data acquisition. Increased z-coverage per rotation and, subsequently, decreased scan time are associated with a greater number of detector rows in a multidetector array. It is important to note that the number of detector rows does not necessarily equal the number of slices that can be acquired per rotation; some scanners sample each detector twice per rotation such that the number of slices acquired per rotation is two times the number of detector rows used.[11] The z-coverage at the isocenter with state-of-the-art scanners ranges from approximately 2 to 16 cm per rotation.

Finally, an important parameter meaningful only for helical imaging is pitch. Pitch describes patient table movement with respect to gantry rotation during a helical scan and is defined as:

$$\frac{\text{table movement (mm) per } 360° \text{ rotation of the gantry}}{\text{total beam collimation (mm)}} \quad \text{(Eq. 8.3)}$$

A pitch of 1 indicates acquisition of contiguous data slabs equivalent to axial scanning. A pitch less than 1 indicates acquisition of overlapping data slabs while a pitch greater than 1 indicates gaps in the acquisition of successive data slabs. Pitch values much less than 1, typically 0.2 to 0.5, are required for cardiac data acquisition to insure continuity in z-coverage between image sets reconstructed from consecutive cardiac cycles. Lower pitch values, however, result in increased radiation exposure and increased total scan time.[27]

6. IMAGE FORMATION AND RECONSTRUCTION

Although the method of X-ray production differs with EBCT and mechanical CT, the basic principles governing the creation of the CT image are the same. Projection data are used to reconstruct a two-dimensional array of pixels, or picture elements, corresponding to a three-dimensional section of voxels, or volume elements, within the patient. Each image pixel displays the average attenuation of X-rays within each corresponding patient voxel. The total attenuation coefficient, μ, along a given ray is divided into smaller components representing the individual attenuation coefficients for n voxels along the ray[14] such that

$$\mu = \mu_1 + \mu_2 + \mu_3 + \cdots + \mu_n \qquad \text{(Eq. 8.4)}$$

The coefficient for each voxel of thickness Δt is then computed from a series of equations of the form

$$I_t = I_o e^{(\mu_1 + \mu_2 + \mu_3 + \mu_n)\Delta t} \qquad \text{(Eq. 8.5)}$$

Numerous reconstruction algorithms[1] exist for solving these equations and include both analytic methods, such as filtered back projection, and iterative methods, but detailed description is beyond the scope of this text.

Basic algorithms for cardiac CT require $180 + \delta$ ($\delta <$ fan angle) of projection data to reconstruct each image.[1] Therefore, the gantry must rotate $180°$ around the patient to obtain the necessary data yielding a temporal resolution approximately equal to the gantry rotation time $t_{rot}/2$ for an object sufficiently centered in the scan field. Cardiac CT data are acquired during one or more cardiac cycles. With axial MDCT, data are acquired during a single cardiac cycle and reconstructed using single segment reconstruction algorithms. With helical MDCT, data are acquired throughout the cardiac cycle and reconstructed either from data acquired during a single cardiac cycle using single segment reconstruction algorithms or from multiple cardiac cycles using multisegment algorithms.

Multisegment algorithms are often used for patients with higher HRs (HRs > 65 to 70 beats per minute depending on the scanner and the specific algorithm) to effectively improve temporal resolution.[28-30] Multisegment reconstruction algorithms obtain the required projection data from the same heart phase of N consecutive cardiac cycles to effectively improve the temporal resolution to at best $t_{rot}/(2N)$ for single source systems and $t_{rot}/(4N)$ for dual source systems. However, multisegment reconstruction algorithms only achieve the optimal temporal resolution for certain combinations of HR, t_{rot}, and pitch, and all other combinations fail to reach the optimal value.[28] Because both t_{rot} and pitch are fixed during the scan, the effective temporal resolution is defined dynamically as a function of the HR at each reconstruction position and ranges from $t_{rot}/(2N)$ to $t_{rot}/2$ for single source systems and from $t_{rot}/(4N)$ to $t_{rot}/4$ for dual source systems (Fig. 8.9). Because the improvement in temporal resolution with multisegment reconstruction is achieved at the expense of decreased z-axis spatial resolution[31] and increased sensitivity to arrhythmia, N is typically limited to 2.[28] Recent studies on newer scanners with improved temporal resolution, however, indicate that these

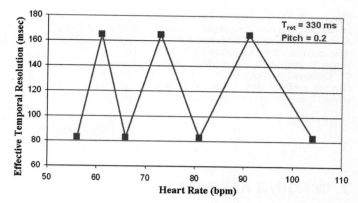

Figure 8.9 Effective temporal resolution achieved at clinically relevant heart rates using dual-segment reconstruction algorithms for a gantry rotation time of 330 ms and a pitch of 0.2. Absolute minimum temporal resolution can only be achieved for certain combinations of heart rate, gantry rotation time, and pitch.

disadvantages of multisegment reconstruction may actually outweigh the benefits of the algorithms even for $N = 2$.[32]

The X-ray attenuation coefficient for a given voxel of tissue is normalized to the attenuation coefficient of water and magnified to a larger integer[14] to define the CT number of the corresponding image pixel:

$$\text{CT number} = [(\mu_{pixel} - \mu_{water}) / \mu_{water}] \times K \qquad \text{(Eq. 8.6)}$$

When $K = 1{,}000$, CT numbers are described in Hounsfield Units (HU) and typically range from $-1{,}000$ to $3{,}000$ HU. Water has a CT number of zero. Tissues with attenuation coefficients less than that of water, such as air spaces or fatty tissues, have negative CT numbers and appear dark on the CT image while tissues with attenuation coefficients greater than water, such as dense soft tissue or bone, appear bright.

For image display, CT numbers are assigned gray levels. To facilitate detection of small changes in CT numbers, viewing is limited to a portion of the available range of CT numbers through a technique called windowing. The specific range of CT numbers displayed depends on the tissue of interest. The CT number assigned to the center of the gray scale, known as the window level or window center, is typically determined by the average CT number of the tissue of interest. A single shade of gray is then assigned to a specified range of CT numbers above and below the center CT number. The complete range of CT numbers above and below the center CT number is the window width. The window level and the window width can be manipulated to change the appearance of the image but do not alter the value of the CT numbers (Fig. 8.10).

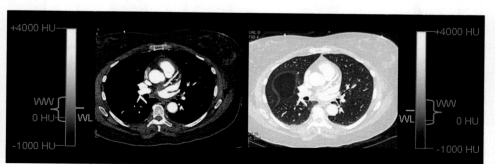

Figure 8.10 CT data are displayed with a typical cardiac window [window width = 600 Hounsfield units (HU), window level = 70 HU] (**left**) and (**right**) typical lung window (window width = 1,500 HU, window level = −600 HU) (**right**). WW, window width; WL, window level.

Figure 8.11 Cardiac motion causes various artifacts in CT images of the heart. **A:** Axial image displays blurred left and right coronary arteries (arrows). **B:** Axial image is degraded by parallel streaks. **C:** Oblique multiplanar reconstruction displays artificial shift (a.k.a. "stair-step-artifact") of left coronary artery (arrow).

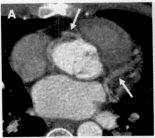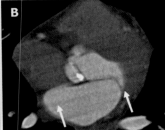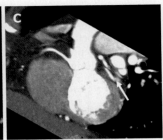

7. IMAGING ARTIFACTS

Cardiovascular CT images are susceptible to common artifacts including cardiac motion artifacts, respiratory motion artifacts, partial volume averaging, beam hardening, and noise. Recognition of these artifacts is critical for accurate image interpretation.

Movement of the heart and great vessels during data acquisition can lead to cardiac motion artifacts. The current temporal resolution of CT scanners is not sufficient to limit the acquisition of data needed for reconstruction to a single cardiac phase, particularly for high heart rates. Cardiac motion can result in misregistration of the reconstructed data and blurriness or streaks in the cross-sectional image (Fig. 8.11A and B). Further, the z-axis coverage of most current scanners requires multiple gantry rotations to image the entire scan range resulting in a three-dimensional volume comprising data from multiple cardiac cycles. Heart beat irregularities can, therefore, cause misregistration of adjacent image sets and a "stair-step" appearance in off-axis orientations (Fig. 8.11C). Cardiac motion artifacts are minimized by improving temporal resolution, adjusting the phase of data acquisition or reconstruction, or lowering patient heart rate.

Inability of the patient to maintain a breath-hold during CT data acquisition can lead to similar artifacts described as respiratory motion artifacts. Image sets reconstructed from data acquired during respiratory motion are shifted through a plane relative to adjacent image sets. Unlike misregistration of data due to cardiac motion, misregistration due to respiratory motion involves the chest wall (Fig. 8.12). Respiratory motion artifacts are eliminated with shorter scan times that permit complete breath-holding.

Highly attenuating tissue components such as calcium and materials such as iodine or surgically implanted objects [e.g., stents, clips, markers (bypass surgery), and wires] can give rise to several types of image artifacts. Overestimation of the extent of very dense objects results from partial volume averaging and is commonly referred to as the "blooming artifact."[33] The attenuation value assigned to each image pixel is a weighted average of the attenuation of all tissues within the corresponding patient voxel. Therefore, the presence of even a small amount of dense material within a voxel will dominate the attenuation value of the pixel. This leads to overestimation of object size when voxels are not sufficiently small (Fig. 8.13). Partial volume averaging is reduced with smaller pixel size and thinner slices.

Artificially lowered CT numbers (i.e., dark spots or streaks) adjacent to highly attenuating objects result from beam hardening.[34] In general, lower energy X-rays are preferentially attenuated so that the X-ray beam exiting the imaged object contains a lower percentage of low energy photons with respect to the incident X-ray beam. The transmitted X-ray beam is described as hardened. X-ray beams passing through highly attenuating objects are excessively hardened. The disproportionally large number of high energy photons in this beam results in such high signal recorded by the detectors that the reconstruction algorithm assumes that the beam passes through a low attenuating object and assigns low CT numbers to pixels adjacent to the dense object (Fig. 8.14).

In addition, streaks of high CT numbers sometimes radiate from dense objects because of severely reduced transmission of X-rays, also known as photon starvation.[34] At some orientations of the X-ray source, the X-ray beam may fail to penetrate a highly attenuating object and reach the detector. The reconstruction algorithm then

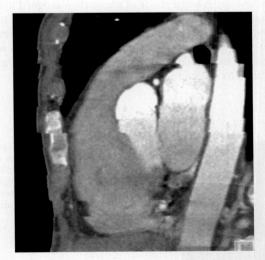

Figure 8.12 Respiratory motion causes artificial shifts of data in CT images in the direction of table movement (z-direction). Sagital multiplanar reconstruction displays shifts involving the chest wall.

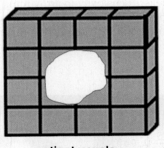

patient voxels

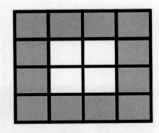

image pixels

Figure 8.13 Diagram illustrating partial volume averaging (a.k.a. blooming artifact). Each image pixel on the right is assigned a value equal to the weighted average of the attenuation of the tissue within the corresponding patient voxel on the left. Dense tissues such as calcium dominate the attenuation value of image pixels if present within the corresponding patient voxel resulting in overestimation of tissue size when voxels are not sufficiently small.

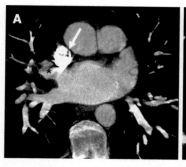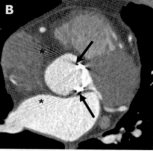

Figure 8.14 Axial images display streak artifacts (asterisk) and beam hardening (arrow) caused by (**A**) highly concentrated contrast material in the superior vena cava and (**B**) a prosthetic aortic valve.

receives incomplete attenuation profiles and assigns high attenuation values at additional locations along the X-ray path. (Fig. 8.14).

CT images sometimes have a grainy appearance and a large variation in pixel values within a homogeneous region as a result of image noise. CT image noise is inversely proportional to the number of photons contributing to the reconstructed image.[27] For some patients, the selected tube voltage and tube current do not allow sufficient X-ray photon penetration, thereby preventing absorption of attenuated photons by the detectors and increasing image noise. In addition, acquisition of projection data during a shorter time duration (i.e., higher temporal resolution) or reconstruction of thinner slices (i.e., higher z-axis spatial resolution) results in fewer photons contributing to the reconstructed image and increased noise for a given tube voltage and tube current compared to longer acquisition times or thicker slices. Image noise can be decreased for larger patients or for faster rotation times and thinner slices but at the expense of increased radiation exposure.

8. RADIATION DOSE ESTIMATION

Radiation dose describes the radiation energy absorbed by a patient's body and is expressed in the standard international (SI) units of Gray (Gy) [conventional units are Roentgen Equivalent in Man (rem) where 1 Gy = 100 rem]. Radiation dose is difficult to measure directly. More often, radiation exposure or the number of ions produced in air by X-ray photons (SI unit: Coulomb/kg; conventional unit: Roentgen) is measured and converted to radiation dose. The preferred measure of radiation exposure in the clinical setting involves scanning an ionization chamber.[35] Typically, the radiation exposure from a single axial scan is integrated over a 100-mm length ionization chamber and the result expressed by the CT dose index (CTDI) parameter $CTDI_{100}$. For body imaging, the ionization chamber is inserted into a 32-cm diameter plexiglass phantom at multiple locations around the periphery (12, 3, 6, and 9 o'clock) and in the center to capture the spatial distribution of the X-ray exposure.[35] The measured exposure can then be converted to absorbed dose in the phantom and used as an approximation of the radiation energy absorbed by a patient's body.

The average radiation dose of a cross section of a patient's body can be approximated by the average absorbed dose over the x and y dimensions of a standard CTDI phantom and expressed by the parameter $CTDI_w$:

$$CTDI_w = [^2/_3\ CTDI_{100}(periphery) + ^1/_3\ CTDI_{100}(center)] \times f \quad (Eq.\ 8.7)$$

where $f = 33.7$ Gy/C/kg and reflects the difference in absorption of radiation in air and another media.[36] $CTDI_w$ however, does not

account for absorbed dose in the z-direction when multiple contiguous or partially overlapping scans are acquired.

The average radiation dose of a three-dimensional slab of a patient's body can be approximated by the average absorbed dose over the x, y, and z dimensions of a standard phantom. The parameter, $CTDI_{vol}$, accounts for the overlap of the radiation dose profiles of adjacent slices and is defined for axial scanning as

$$CTDI_{vol} = \frac{N \times T}{I} \times CTDI_w \quad (Eq.\ 8.8)$$

where N = number of slices, T = nominal width of one slice (mm), I = distance between slices (mm). For helical imaging,

$$CTDI_{vol} = \frac{1}{pitch} \times CTDI_w \quad (Eq.\ 8.9)$$

$CTDI_{vol}$ values estimated from phantoms by scanner manufacturers are displayed on the scanner console for each scan protocol and are useful for assessing radiation dose during the design of CT protocols. $CTDI_{vol}$ values reflect X-ray properties (tube voltage, tube current) and the spatial distribution of scans but not the total number of scans and are, therefore, independent of scan length.

Estimates of the total radiation energy absorbed by a patient's body must be obtained by integrating the $CTDI_{vol}$ along the scan length. The resulting value is the dose–length product (DLP). The DLP is also provided by CT scanners:

$$DLP = CTDI_{vol} \times scan\ length \quad (Eq.\ 8.10)$$

Some scanners provide DLP estimates prior to the scan based on projected scan length. However, DLP values cannot be finalized until data acquisition is complete and the actual scan length is known. It is also important to note that the DLP values currently reported on some scanners do not represent dose savings from tube current modulation and, therefore, overestimate dose for some patients. Still, the DLP is useful for estimating the radiation energy absorbed by a specific patient during a specific CT scan.

Patients and referring physicians are typically most interested, though, in the biologic effects of the radiation dose received. Biologic effects depend not only on the magnitude of the radiation dose but also on the biological sensitivity of the irradiated tissue. Effective dose is a dose descriptor that reflects the radiosensitivity of the tissues within the scan volume. A weighting factor is assigned to each tissue in the body based on its radiosensitivity and relative contribution to radiation risk, and the sum of the weighted absorbed doses in all irradiated tissues is defined as the effective dose. Effective dose can be estimated directly from organ measurement within an anthropomorphic phantom or calculated using Monte Carlo methods to simulate the interaction of X-rays with a virtual phantom.[35] A simpler method for obtaining a reasonable approximation of the effective dose was proposed by the European Working Group for Guidelines on Quality Criteria in Computed Tomography that groups tissues into body regions and assigns a single coefficient to each region based on the radiosensitivies of all tissues within the region.[36] The effective dose, E, for cardiovascular imaging can then be calculated using the equation

$$E = DLP \times k \quad (Eq.\ 8.11)$$

where $k = 0.014$ mSv/mGy/cm for the chest.

All of the methods described for estimating effective dose are limited for an individual patient to the extent the patient differs from the actual or virtual phantom employed in dose estimation. Phantoms, for example, fail to model changes for a given X-ray exposure in the radiation energy absorbed by the most radiosensitive tissues as a result of changes in patient size. Also, tissue weighting factors are assumed to be independent of age despite the inverse relationship between tissue radiosensitivity and age. In addition, the conversion factors used to estimate E from the DLP are the same for men and women despite obvious differences in the type of radiosensitive tissues contained within certain body regions. Therefore, estimates of effective dose describe risk for a specific scan but not for an individual patient and have limited application to a clinical population. Still, effective dose estimates are indicators of biologic risk and provide an opportunity to compare risk among sources of exposure (e.g., nuclear stress test vs. coronary CT angiography) and identify unacceptable imaging practices. Effective dose values ranging from 3 to 44 mSv have been reported for coronary CTA[37,38] based on estimates from DLP and reflect differences in dose-related scan (e.g., tube current, tube voltage, and pitch) and patient (e.g., size and heart rate) parameters.

9. EQUIPMENT MAINTENANCE AND QUALITY CONTROL

Equipment performance and quality standards for CT scanners within the United States are dictated by state and federal regulations as well as American College of Radiology (ACR) requirements for CT accreditation.[39] CT equipment performance should be evaluated by a certified medical physicist annually or when scanner repairs affect radiation exposure. Performance evaluation should include evaluation of scanner hardware accuracy such as alignment light accuracy and table incrementation accuracy as well as assessment of display devices. Evaluation of slice thickness accuracy, CT number accuracy based on scanning of known materials, and image quality parameters such as high-contrast spatial resolution, low-contrast spatial resolution, image uniformity, noise, and image artifacts should also be performed. Dose evaluation should include measurement of the CTDI value for an average adult abdomen, adult head, and a pediatric abdomen. Also, the reproducibility of dose values for representative examinations should be determined. Finally, safety evaluation should include confirmation of properly functioning audio/visual communication systems and measurement of scattered radiation. A complete listing of performance evaluation measures recommended by the ACR is provided in Table 8.1. Quality control programs should also be designed by a certified medical physicist and include preventative maintenance by a qualified service engineer and periodic testing of display devices, alignment light accuracy, slice thickness, CT number accuracy, and image quality measures (Table 8.2).

If the results of an equipment performance or quality test fall outside of acceptable limits, corrective action should be taken by the medical physicist or service engineer. Unresolved issues impacting radiation dose or low-contrast spatial resolution may warrant suspension of patient scanning.

10. FUTURE DIRECTIONS

Recently introduced MDCT scanners offer a range of technical features. All manufacturers have made improvements to varying degrees in the number of detector rows, gantry rotation time, detector element size, and dose saving features.

Still, improving temporal resolution, improving spatial resolution, and lowering radiation dose remain the common goals driving the development of all new CT systems. Gains in temporal

TABLE 8.1

AMERICAN COLLEGE OF RADIOLOGY (ACR) CT EQUIPMENT PERFORMANCE EVALUATION MEASURES

Alignment light accuracy	Display devices
Alignment of table to gantry	Video display
Table/gantry tilt	Hard copy display
Slice localization from scanned projection radiograph (localization image)	Dosimetry
	Computed tomography dosimetry index (CTDI)
Table incrementation accuracy	Patient radiation dose for representative examinations
Slice thickness	Safety evaluation
Image quality	Visual inspection
High-contrast resolution	Audible/visual signals
Low-contrast resolution	Posting requirements
Image uniformity	Scattered radiation measurements
Noise	
Artifact evaluation	
CT number accuracy and linearity	
Other tests as required by state or local regulations	

Source: From ACR requirements for CT accreditation, Morin RL, Gerber TC, McCollough CH. Radiation dose in computed tomography of the heart. *Circulation*. 2003;107:917–922.

TABLE 8.2

AMERICAN COLLEGE OF RADIOLOGY (ACR) QUALITY ASSURANCE TESTING MEASURES

Image quality	Alignment light accuracy
High-contrast resolution	Slice thickness
Low-contrast resolution	CT number accuracy
Image uniformity	Display devices
Noise	
Artifact evaluation	

Source: From ACR requirements for CT accreditation, Morin RL, Gerber TC, McCollough CH. Radiation dose in computed tomography of the heart. *Circulation*. 2003;107:917–922.

resolution are being pursued through decreasing the gantry rotation time and increasing the number of X-ray sources from one to two. Improvements in spatial resolution may be achieved through the development of new detector materials that permit faster conversion of detected X-ray photons to electrical signals processed by scanner software. These new materials may permit the use of thinner detectors without the penalty of increased noise.

Efforts to lower radiation dose include refinement of axial data acquisition and more efficient ECG-based tube current modulation with helical data acquisition. In addition, implementation of computationally intensive iterative reconstruction algorithms widely used in nuclear medicine imaging is being explored for CT imaging. Compared to standard reconstruction of the data acquired using a given amount of radiation, equivalent SNRs can be achieved with iterative reconstruction of the data acquired with less radiation. Therefore, selection of a lower X-ray tube voltage or tube current and, subsequently, a reduction in radiation dose may be possible without a loss in image quality using iterative reconstruction algorithms.

Resources are also being devoted to the application of multiple X-ray energies simultaneously or near simultaneously to obtain multiple image sets from the region-of interest with differing attenuation characteristics. Techniques that use two X-ray tubes to simultaneously acquire data at two different tube voltages (typically 80 and 140 kVp) have already been applied to imaging of the heart.[40] In addition, alternating between two tube voltages during data acquisition and acquiring two complete sets of projections during each gantry rotation has been proposed. A third approach uses layered detectors to capture both a low energy and a high energy set of attenuated X-ray photons; lower energy radiation is absorbed by the top detector and higher energy radiation is absorbed by the bottom detector.

ACKNOWLEDGMENTS

The author would like to thank William Davros, PhD, for his helpful contribution to Section 9, Equipment Maintenance and Quality Control.

REFERENCES

1. Kalendar WA. *Computed Tomography: Fundamentals, System Technology, Image Quality, and Applications.* Germany: Publicis MCD Verlag; 2000.
2. Boyd DP, Lipton MJ. Cardiac computed tomography. *Proc IEEE.* 1983;71: 298–307.
3. Kalendar WA, Seissler W, Klotz E, et al. Spiral volumetric CT. With single-breath-hold technique, continuous transport, and continuous scanner rotation. *Radiology.* 1990;176:181–183.
4. Crawford CR, King KF. Computed tomography scanning with simultaneous patient translation. *Med Phys.* 1990;17(6):967–982.
5. Carr JJ, Crouse JR, Goff DC, et al. Evaluation of subsecond gated helical CT for quantification of coronary artery calcium and comparison with electron beam CT. *Am J Roentgenol.* 2000;174:915–921.
6. Becker CR, Jakobs TF, Aydemir S, et al. Helical and single-slice conventional CT versus electron beam CT for the quantification of coronary artery calcification. *Am J Roentgenol.* 2000;174:543–547.
7. Klingenbeck-Regn K, Schaller S, Flohr T, et al. Subsecond multi-slice computed tomography: Basics and applications. *Eur J Radiol.* 1999;31:110–124.
8. Hu H, He HD, Foley WD, et al. Four multidetector-row helical CT: Image quality and volume coverage speed. *Radiology.* 2000;215:55–62.
9. Flohr T, Stierstorfer K, Bruder H, et al. New technical developments in multislice CT: Approaching isotropic resolution with sub-millimeter 16-slice scanning. *Röfo: Fortschritte auf dem Gebiet der Röntgenstrahlen und der bildgebenden Verfahren.* 2002;s174(7):839–845.
10. Flohr T, Bruder H, Stierstorfer K, et al. New technical developments in multislice CT, part 2: Sub-millimeter 16-slice scanning and increased gantry rotation speed for cardiac imaging. *Röfo: Fortschritte auf dem Gebiet der Röntgenstrahlen und der bildgebenden Verfahren.* 2002;174(8):1022–1027.
11. Flohr T, Stierstorfer K, Raupach R, et al. Performance evaluation of a 64-slice CT system with z-flying focal spot. *Rofo.* 2004; 176(12):1803–1810.
12. Flohr TG, McCollough CH, Bruder H, et al. First performance evaluation of a dual-source (DSCT) system. *Eur Radiol.* 2006;16:256–268.
13. Rybicki FJ, Otero HJ, Steigner ML, et al. Initial evaluation of coronary images from 320-detector row computed tomography. *Int J Cardiovasc Imaging.* 2008;24:535–546.
14. Bushberg JT, Seibert JA, Leidholdt EM, et al. *The Essential Physics of Medical Imaging.* 2nd Ed. Philadelphia: Lippincott Williams & Wilkins; 2002.
15. McCullough EC. Photon attenuation in computed tomography. *Med Phys.* 1975;2(6):307–320.
16. McCollough CH, Morin RL. The technical design and performance of ultrafast computed tomography. *Radiol Clin North Am.* 1994;32(3):521–536.
17. Kopp A, Schoroeder S, Kuettner A, et al. Coronary arteries: Retrospectively ECG-gated multi-detector row CT angiography with selective optimization of the image reconstruction window. *Radiology.* 2001;221:683–688.
18. Nagatani Y, Takahashi M, Takazakura R, et al. Multidetector-row computed tomography coronary angiography: Optimization of image reconstruction phase according to the heart rate. *Circ J.* 2007;71(1):112–121.
19. Wintersperger BJ, Nikolaou K, von Ziegler F, et al. Image quality, motion artifacts, and reconstruction timing of 64-slice coronary computed tomography angiography with 0.33-second rotation speed. *Invest Radiol.* 2006;41(5):436–442.
20. Seifarth H, Wienbeck S, Pusken M, et al. Optimal systolic and diastolic reconstruction windows for coronary CT angiography using dual-source CT. *Am J Roentgenol.* 2007;189:1317–1323.
21. Hiraoka M, Ota T, Taguchi K, et al. Patient dose reduction for volumetric cardiac imaging with multislice helical CT. *Radiology.* 2000;217–487 (abstract).
22. Jakobs T, Becker CR, Ohnesorge B, et al.. Multislice helical CT of the heart with retrospective ECG gating: Reduction of radiation exposure by ECG-controlled tube current modulation. *Eur Radiol.* 2002;12:1081–1086.
23. Leschka S, Scheffel H, Desbiolles L, et al. Image quality and reconstruction intervals of dual-source CT coronary angiography: Recommendations for ECG-pulsing windowing. *Invest Radiol.* 2007;42(8):543–559.
24. Bardo D, Kachenoura N, Newby B, et al. Multidetector computed tomography evaluation of left ventricular volumes: Sources of error and guidelines for their minimization. *J Cardiovasc CT.* 2008;2(4):222–230.
25. Hausleiter J, Meyer T, Hadamitzky M, et al. Radiation dose estimates from cardiac multislice computed tomography in daily practice: Impact of different scanning protocols on effective dose estimates. *Circulation.* 2006;113(10):1305–1310.
26. Gutstein A, Dey D, Cheng V, et al. Algorithm for radiation dose reduction with helical dual source coronary computed tomography angiography in clinical practice. *J Cardiovasc CT.* 2008;2(5):311–322.
27. Primak AN, McCollough CH, Bruesewitz MR, et al. Relationship between noise, dose, and pitch in cardiac multi-detector row CT. *Radiographics.* 2006;26:1785–1794.
28. Halliburton SS, Stillman AE, Flohr T, et al. Do segmented reconstruction algorithms for cardiac multi-slice computed tomography improve image quality? *Herz.* 2003;28(1):20–31.
29. Dewey M, Teige F, Laule M, et al. Influence of heart rate on diagnostic accuracy and image quality of 16-slice CT coronary angiography: Comparison of multi-segment and halfscan reconstruction approaches. *Eur Radiol.* 2007;17(11):2829–2837.
30. Herzog C, Nguyen SA, Savino G, et al. Does two-segment image reconstruction at 64-section CT coronary angiography improve image quality and diagnostic accuracy? *Radiology.* 2007;244:121–129.
31. Flohr T, Ohnesorge B. Heart rate adaptive optimization of spatial and temporal resolution for electrocardiogram-gated multislice spiral CT of the heart. *J Cardiovasc CT.* 2001;25(6):907–923.
32. Leschka S, Alkadhi H, Stolzmann P, et al. Mono- versus bisegment reconstruction algorithms for dual-source computed tomography coronary angiography. *Invest Radiol.* 2008;43(10):703–711.
33. Kroft LJM, de Roos A, Geleijns J. Artifacts in ECG-synchronized MDCT coronary angiography. *Am J Roentgenol.* 2007;189:581–591.
34. Prokop M, Galanski M, Van Der Molen A. *Spiral and Multislice Computed Tomography of the Body: Computed Tomography of the Body.* Germany: Thieme Medical Publishers; 2003.
35. Morin RL, Gerber TC, McCollough CH. Radiation dose in computed tomography of the heart. *Circulation.* 2003;107:917–922.
36. Bongartz G, Golding SJ, Jurik AG, et al. European guidelines for multislice computed tomography 2004. Available at http://www.msct.eu/CT-Quality-Criteria.htm#Download%20th%202004%20CT%20Quality%20Criteria. Accessed 2 Feb 2009.
37. Earls JP, Berman EL, Urban BA, et al. Prospectively gated transverse coronary CVT angiography versus retrospectively gated helical technique; improved image quality and reduced radiation dose. *Radiology.* 2008;246(3):742–753.
38. Hausleiter J, Meyer T, Hermann F, et al. International prospective multicenter study on radiation dose estimates of coronary CT angiography in daily practice: The PROTECTION I study. *J Am Coll Cardiol.* 2008;51(10A):A417, 66(abstract).
39. American College of Radiology: CT Accreditation Program Requirements. Available at http://www.acr.org/accreditation/computed/ct_reqs.aspx. Accessed Octorber 20, 2008.
40. Ruzsics B, Lee H, Zwerner PL, et al. Dual-energy CT of the heart for diagnosing coronary artery stenosis and myocardial ischemia-initial experience. *Eur Radiol.* 2008;18(11):2414–2424.

Cardiac Computed Tomography Examination and Protocols

9

Susanna Prat-Gonzalez

1. INTRODUCTION

Although invasive coronary angiography is the gold standard for the evaluation of coronary artery stenosis, cardiac computed tomography (CCT) constitutes an attractive diagnostic tool for a noninvasive assessment of coronary artery disease (CAD). New advances in CT technology over the past few years have made possible to quantify coronary calcium in atherosclerotic plaques, visualize the lumen of native coronary arteries and bypass grafts, assess ventricular size and function, and evaluate pulmonary vein anatomy and other cardiovascular structures.

Diagnostic quality images in CCT are related to adequate patient selection and preparation, contrast enhancement optimization, optimal scan protocol selection, image display, and visualization tools. This chapter provides guidelines to perform a CCT study for evaluation of the coronary arteries and the rest of the cardiac anatomy.

1.1. Historical perspective

Since the first commercially available CT scanner in 1972, for which Godfrey Hounsfield and Alan Cormack received the Nobel Prize in 1979, the ability to rapidly obtain cross-sectional images of the body with CT has revolutionized medicine as a clinical tool. Initially, CT technology was applied to the brain and later to the whole body, requiring up to 5 s to acquire each single slice.

The increase in morbidity and mortality due to CAD in developed countries urged the necessity to design better diagnostic techniques to detect CAD. The challenge presented by the need to image the heart in motion was overcome when technological advances in electron-beam CT (EBCT) and multidetector CT (MDCT) lead to faster acquisition with higher spatial and temporal resolution. The introduction of ECG-gated scanning made possible to reconstruct images at multiple phases of the cardiac cycle to visualize the beating heart. In the early 1980s clinical cardiac evaluation was performed with EBCT, mostly applied to coronary calcium quantification, cardiac volumes, and function.[1] However, the technology that experienced faster improvement after the introduction of helical scanning was MDCT. Since the introduction of four-row detectors CT in 1999, coronary artery visualization was feasible, but significant number of vessels were nonassessable because of the long acquisition time and relatively low temporal and spatial resolution. Current CT scanners (16- to 64-row detector) with submillimeter spatial resolution and improved temporal resolution have reduced the number of unevaluable segments due to cardiac and respiratory motion artifacts. In the last few years, modern scanners with acquisition of up to 320 slices per rotation and dual X-ray source systems have been developed. These tech-

nologies, besides high-quality contrast-enhanced visualization of the coronary arteries, provide short scan times and significant contrast media volume reduction.

2. PATIENT PREPARATION

For diagnostic assessment of the coronary arteries by CCT high quality images need to be obtained. A necessary step to achieve this goal is an appropriate patient selection and preparation, which includes heart rate control, ECG gating, adequate IV access, patient positioning, and breath-hold instructions.

2.1. Patient selection

Before each procedure, a brief medical history of the patient should be taken. It is important to know what clinical question needs to be addressed and recognize if absolute or relative contraindications for the test apply. Cardiac CT for coronary anatomy requires the use of iodine contrast, which is contraindicated in patients with previous severe anaphylaxis reaction. Also, iodine contrast can be detrimental in patients with renal insufficiency, renal amyloidosis, and multiple myeloma due to the risk of contrast-induced nephropathy. In patients with hyperthyroidism, iodine contrast can trigger a thyroid crisis.

If the patient cannot hold still and follow breathing instructions he/she should not be scanned. Breathing during the scan significantly compromises image quality producing unevaluable segments. Cardiac CT in very obese patients (body mass index [BMI] >40 kg/m²) should be discouraged due to the significant increase in effective dose of radiation needed to maintain image quality. In Table 9.1, absolute and relative contraindications are summarized.

Recently, possible malfunction of electronical devices including pacemakers, defibrillators, neurostimulators, and implanted or externally worn drug infusion pumps caused by CT scanning has been reported.[2,3] If the medical device is in or immediately adjacent to the programmed scan range the current recommendations for the operator should be

- Determine the device type.
- If it is possible, try to move external devices out of scan range or in patients with neurostimulators to shut off the device temporarily.
- Minimize X-ray exposure to the device with the lowest tube current possible for the required image quality and make sure that the X-ray beam does not dwell on the device more than a few seconds.

After the scanning, the medical devices should be turned on or checked for proper functioning.

TABLE 9.1
CONTRAINDICATIONS FOR CONTRAST-ENHANCED CARDIAC CT

Absolute
1. Severe allergy to contrast media (iodine contrast)
2. Pregnancy

Relative
3. Renal insufficiency (creatinine level >1.5 mL/dL)
4. Severe thyroid disease, multiple myeloma
5. Severe dysrrythmia or frequent extrasystole[a]
6. Inability to maintain a breath-hold for >12 s[a]
7. Morbid obesity (BMI >40 kg/m²)

[a]Newer and faster equipments let to scan in shorter time and patients with atrial fibrillation.
Source: Modified from HoffmannU, Ferencik M, Cury RC, et al. *J Nucl Med.* 2006;47:797–806.

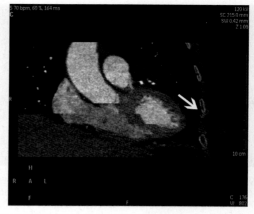

Figure 9.1 Cardiac CT image obtained from a patient who was breathing during image acquisition. Respiratory artifacts are easily visible in a sagittal plane. Notice the "stair-step" artifacts over the myocardium and chest wall (*arrow*). Practicing breathing instructions multiple times can help avoid significant motion artifacts.

2.2. Heart rate control

The image quality of cardiac CT has greatly improved in patients with a stable, low heart rate. Motion artifacts related to movement of the coronary arteries observed in patients with higher heart rates contribute substantially to the degradation of image quality. Most studies have demonstrated that the highest image quality of cardiac CT for the current scans is achieved at heart rates <65 bpm.[4] At slow heart rate the best cardiac phase (free of coronary motion) is centered on 75% of the R–R interval, corresponding mostly to the mid end-diastolic phase of the cardiac cycle. For this reason, data obtained in the diastolic phase is safely used for image reconstruction. One of the advantages of heart rate control is that the images are commonly reconstructed using a single-segment, that is, only data from a single heart beat may be used for image reconstruction of each slice. In patients with faster heart rates, instead, multisegment reconstructions are recommended to improve temporal resolution. In this algorithm, data from two or more consecutive heartbeats is used to reconstruct each slice in order to decrease motion artifact.[5]

Another advantage of slow and stable heart rate is related to total patient radiation exposure. In heart rates <65 bpm, radiation exposure can be reduced up to 30% to 50% using ECG-gated dose modulation. The tube current is delivered during the selected phases of the cardiac cycle and it is reduced for the rest of the cardiac cycle. With the same objective of radiation reduction, most manufactures have developed prospective ECG-gating acquisition on nonhelical mode for coronary artery evaluation. In selected patients with low (<63 bpm) and stable heart rate, some studies suggest that acceptable results can be obtained with significant reduction of radiation.[6]

Consequently, oral and/or intravenous β-blockers with a short half-life (50 to 100 mg of oral metoprolol/12 h to 1 h before the scan or 5 to 20 mg of intravenous metoprolol/immediately before the scan) should be administered aiming for a resting regular heart rate of 50 to 60 bpm. If β-blockers are contraindicated, calcium antagonists may be used as alternative agents, although these drugs are not as effective.

In the newer dual-source scans, patients with higher heart rates and even with irregular heart rates can be scanned with high accuracy for the diagnosis of CAD.[7,8]

In addition to the β-blocker medication, sublingual administration of short-acting nitroglycerin (0.4 mg) immediately before the scan has been used to improve the visualization of the coronary artery lumen due to its vasodilator effect and to avoid coronary artery spasm. Nitroglycerin is contraindicated in subjects taking phosphodiesterase inhibitors, such as sildenafil or vardenafil, and in subjects with hypersensitivity to organic nitrates, increased intracranial pressure, symptomatic hypotension, and severe anemia. In very anxious patients, anxiolytic medications (1 mg of lorazepam) can be administered before the scan.

2.3. Patient position

Patients are in supine position during the scan. Cardiac CT requires ECG-gating, meaning that raw image data acquisition is synchronized to the ECG signal acquisition. Thus, it is important to obtain an adequate ECG tracing from the three ECG leads placed in the patient's thorax. Before starting the test and to avoid motion artifacts, one should (a) inform the patient to lie still, even if he/she experiences a warmth feeling or pelvic tingling due to the contrast injection; (b) repeat test breath-holds to be sure that patient is able to hold the breath for 10 to 15 s and to check the heart rate variability during breath-hold (Fig. 9.1).

3. CHEST TOPOGRAM

Once the patient is correctly prepared, image acquisition begins. The first step is the acquisition of a chest topogram that is used in planning the desired scan depending on the protocol and to establish where the target organs are located. The topogram or scout image appears similar to a chest radiograph and is acquired as a low energy scan at end inspiration (Fig. 9.2).

4. CONTRAST TYPE, DOSE, AND INJECTION PROTOCOLS

In order to visualize the lumen of the coronary arteries the use of iodinated contrast media is required. There are some factors that contribute to optimize and to achieve the highest enhancement in the coronary lumen: type of contrast (iodine concentration), rate and volume of contrast, and technique of delivery.[9]

4.1. Types of contrast

There are various types of iodine contrast media; however, water-soluble iodinated contrast medium is the one used for coronary

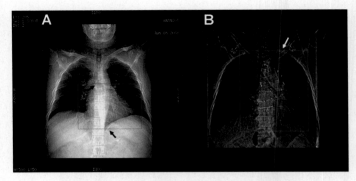

Figure 9.2 The topogram is the first step for image acquisition protocol. In (**A**) an anteroposterior topogram shows the required volume to scan (FOV) in a patient going for coronary arteries evaluation. The FOV starts from the carina to the base of the heart (*pink box and black arrows*). The same scan range is used for a coronary calcium score protocol and for a typical pulmonary vein study. (**B**) shows the topogram of a patient who had previous bypass surgery, one of them, a LIMA. In this scenario the FOV (*pink box*) includes from the level of the clavicles (origin of the LIMA) to the base of the heart. The *white arrow* points the beginning of the scan.

CT. Also, iodinated contrast medium may be either ionic or nonionic. The ionic type tends to create a high osmolality in blood and may cause more contrast media reactions in some individuals. The nonionic forms are nearly isotonic. Therefore, they have significantly less side effects and discomfort (flushing and heat) and less hypersensitivity reactions.[10] These reactions range from mild symptoms such as itching, nausea, or vomiting to severe life-threatening events such as dyspnea, circulatory shock, and even cardiac arrest. In the clinical practice, nonionic contrast media are much more widely used today and agents with higher iodine concentration are recommended for coronary imaging. They include

- Nonionic low-osmolar with high iodine concentration (mgI/mL): Iopamidol-370 mgI/ml (*Isovue*), Iohexol-350 mgI/mL (*Omnipaque*), Iopromide-350 mgI/mL (*Ultravist*), and Iomeprol-400 mgI/mL (*Iomeron*). The latter is commercially available in Europe.
- Nonionic iso-osmolar with less iodine concentration: Iodixanol 320 mgI/mL (*Visipaque*)

In patients with previous anaphylactic reactions to iodine, the use of gadolinium-based contrast agents may be an alternative, although their use can result in lower enhancement of the coronary arteries. Nevertheless, further research needs to validate preliminary data.[11,12]

As mentioned previously, CCT is contraindicated in subjects with previous severe contrast allergy. Those with a history of mild contrast allergy should be premedicated with steroids and antihistaminics prior to the test. Relative risk of contrast-induced nephropathy needs to be considered especially in patients with preexisting renal insufficiency and/or diabetic patients. In the daily practice these patients are pretreated with hydration and acetylcysteine. Diabetic patients taking metformin should discontinue the use of this drug for 2 days following the test to reduce the risk of lactic acidosis. A good tool for the correct use of iodinated contrast media is the guideline provided by the American College of Radiology.[13]

4.2. Rate and volume

A large intravenous line (18 gauge) in the antecubital fossa is preferred to ensure an injection of media contrast at a flow rate of 5 to 6 mL/s, ideally. In difficult vein access patients, a flow rate of 4 mL/s

(20 gauge) is acceptable. If the protocol is to assess coronary bypass and one of the grafts is the left internal mammary artery (LIMA), a right antecubital vein should be chosen to avoid venous contrast streak artifact during evaluation of the origin of the LIMA.

Ideally, the contrast volume should be normalized for body weight but ordinarily a fixed amount of contrast is generally applied. With the newer scanners smaller amounts of contrast are required (from ~120 mL of contrast media with a four-detector scans to 80 mL with 64-detector CT scans). As a rule, the total amount of contrast can be calculated as: scan time (s) by flow rate (mL/s) plus 10 mL to ensure correct opacification. For example, if we have a scan time of 12 s and we inject at 5 mL/s the total amount of contrast medium will be $(12 \times 5) + 10 = 70$ mL.

A remote-control dual-injection system capable of administering iodine contrast and saline separately is used for the contrast-enhanced study. Injection of saline (30 to 50 mL) immediately after contrast injection (known as a bolus chaser) improves image contrast by increasing the amount of contrast media available for image acquisition. Also, bolus chaser reduces the total contrast volume (15% to 20%) and streak artifacts from contrast in the right atrium and ventricle. When the right ventricular (RV) anatomy is the target of the study, a three-phase protocol is applied. For example, a dual-phase injection protocol administering 60 to 70 mL of iodine contrast at a flow rate of 5 mL/s followed by 20 to 30 mL of iodine contrast at 2.5 to 3 mL/s and a saline chaser of 50 mL at 5.0 mL/s is used. The goal is to obtain homogeneous RV enhancement in order to evaluate right-heart pathology and ventricular function.[14]

Contrast agent administration remains one of the most challenging aspects of CCT. The method used to inject contrast media influences image quality. In general there are three techniques for optimal synchronization between the arterial phase of the contrast and scan data acquisition. The fixed delayed technique is mostly used in vascular angiography and is not recommended for coronary studies. The two main strategies to ensure optimal timing of CCT image acquisition with homogeneous contrast enhancement of the entire coronary artery tree are bolus tracking and the timing bolus.

4.3. Bolus-tracking technique

The bolus-tracking technique is based on real-time monitoring of the full contrast bolus during injection with the acquisition of a series of dynamic low-dose monitoring scans (120 kV, 20 mA) in the region of interest (ROI), usually at the level of the ascending aorta (AA). The acquisition of the dynamic monitoring scans starts 10 s after the beginning of the injection of intravenous contrast material. It is possible to start main scanning manually or automatically with a trigger threshold. Once a predefined threshold inside the ROI is met (e.g., 100 to 150 HU above the baseline), the table moves to the cranial start position while the patient is instructed to sustain a breath-hold. During this interval (4 to 8 s delay for instruction) the contrast material concentration increases to the desired level of enhancement and the data acquisition is initiated by the system (Fig. 9.3).[15,16]

4.4. Timing bolus technique

The principle of this technique is that circulation time can be measured for each patient using a small test bolus (10 to 20 mL) of contrast media injected at the same rate that will be used for the scan together with a saline flush, followed by image acquisition through the area of interest every second or every other second. A time–density curve is created by plotting the attenuation values obtained at the ROI (e.g., AA) and the patient's circulation time can be determined by identifying the peak of this curve (image

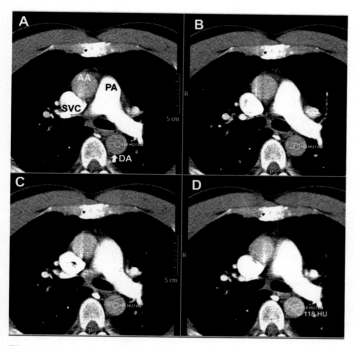

Figure 9.3 Bolus tracking acquisition. Ten seconds after iodine contrast injection low radiation sequential images are acquired every other second. In (**A**), (**B**) and (**C**), contrast is seen in the SVC and pulmonary artery (PA). The ROI is placed in the descending aorta (DA), since this area has less motion and is far from the SVC. When a threshold of >100 HU is detected in the ROI, (**D**), the technologist asks the patient to perform a breath-hold (4 s) and starts the acquisition. AA, ascending aorta.

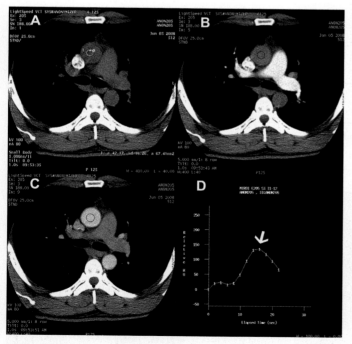

Figure 9.4 Timing bolus image acquisition. A small bolus of iodine contrast (15 to 20 mL) is injected. Axial images are acquired every 2 s. (**A**) to (**C**) show how contrast arrives to the AA. Automatic software calculates the time to the peak enhancement in the AA (ROI). (**D**) shows a calculated delay time of 18 s (*white arrow*) in this patient. The final delay time will be 18 s plus 10 s fixed delay that corresponds to time between the start of the injection and the first monitoring image.

with maximum contrast enhancement). The circulation time is used to select the scan delay, which is the delay between the start of the contrast injection and the start of the scan data acquisition. Then, the full contrast bolus is administered at the same rate and with the same saline flush and the entire heart volume is scanned at the calculated fixed delay within a single breath-hold.[16] Even though bolus-timing allows testing patient breathing performance and intravenous injection, this technique implies an additional 20 mL of contrast and prolongs the total CCT study by a few minutes (Fig. 9.4).

5. CALCIUM SCORE ACQUISITION PROTOCOL

The presence of calcium in the coronary arteries is pathognomonic of atherosclerosis. The coronary artery calcification (CAC) is a robust predictor of adverse cardiovascular events, and the prognostic value of coronary calcium has been clearly established.[17]

5.1. Technology and protocols for calcium scoring

Although fluoroscopy was able to detect calcium in the coronary arteries, the challenge was to quantify the calcium in vessels in constant motion. Newer technologies were introduced in the late 1980s to solve this problem, first with EBCT and more recently with MDCT.

EBCT uses a rapidly steered electron beam that generates X-rays without the need for mechanical rotating parts. A stationary high-voltage electron gun produces a beam of electrons, which is rapidly steered to sweep over tungsten targets, arranged in a semicircular array under the patient table. Thus, a fan of X-rays is created that penetrates the patient. Stationary detector arrays receive the attenuated signal. Cross-sectional images can thus be rapidly acquired without the constraints of mechanical motion. The EBCT uses prospective ECG triggering at a predetermined phase of the R–R, with advancement of the table in a step-and-shoot fashion (sequential). The whole acquisition lasts between 20 and 40 s (depending on the generation of EBCT). While this offers excellent temporal resolution per slice (~50 to 100 ms), the technology is limited by spatial resolution in the z-axis (1 to 2 mm), high cost and slow coverage of large imaging volumes. Radiation exposure is about 1 mSv and ranges between 0.8 to 1.3 mSv. In patients with severe obesity the signal to noise in the EBCT is high, because this system does not have the capability to adjust tube current.

In most institutions, EBCT has been replaced by MDCT technology. For CAC assessment, there are some minimal technical requirements that were postulated in a scientific statement from the American Heart Association.[18] They recommended the use of scanners with four or more detectors, or EBCT C150 with a gantry rotation at least 0.5 s or faster (0.5 to 0.33 s), reconstructed images at 2.5 to 3 mm to compare results with published studies, and the use of prospecting cardiac gating in the early to mid-diastole to reduce radiation. In the prospective scan mode (step-and-shoot), the table is advanced a distant equivalent to the width of the detector panel and then stopped. The X-ray tube is then turned on at the chosen phase of the cardiac cycle for ½ gantry rotation plus fan angle and turned off. The table is advanced again and the process is repeated until complete volume coverage is obtained. This method has the potential to reduce radiation exposure significantly since X-ray is administered only during a small portion of the cardiac cycle. However, with MDCT retrospective gating in helical mode can be used as well for a calcium score, reducing the variability in calcium quantification at the expense of higher radiation exposure (ranging 1 to 5 mSv).[19]

The protocol for CAC is a noncontrast scan. The scan range expands from the carina to the base of the heart (see topogram, Fig. 9.2). CAC scans are usually done using low tube current setting due to the higher attenuation values (Hounsfield Units) of the calcium.

Recommended protocols for CAC in a medium size adult using EBCT and MDCT are shown in Table 9.2.

5.2. Coronary quantification

CAC measurement is performed on dedicated computed workstations where the interpreting physician needs to review which calcifications are in the coronary arteries and which are not to score them correctly. For CAC quantification there are two widely used methods: the Agatston score[20] and the volume score.[21] Recently another measurement has been proposed: calcium mass score.[22]

In the Agatston score, the area of calcium, which is defined as an area ≥3 adjacent pixels (at least 1 mm²) above a threshold of 130 HU, is multiplied by a factor related to CT density. All the areas of calcium are computed, and the total score for the entire coronary system is reported (Fig. 9.5).

In some recent studies the volume score method showed better reproducibility than Agatston score.[23] This method creates small new "voxels" (volume unit) using isotropic interpo-

TABLE 9.2
CAC PROTOCOL

Setup and patient preparation			
Intravenous injection/iodine contrast	No		
ECG leads	Yes		
Medications (beta-blockers)	No if <70 bpm		
Patient instructions	End-inspiration breath-hold		
Calcium scoring scan parameters	*EBCT*	*64-row detector CT scanner*	
Acquisition	Sequential	Sequential	Helical
ECG synchronization	Prospective	Prospective	Retrospective
Scan coverage	From the carina to the base of the heart		
Detector collimation (mm)	1 × 3	0.6	0.6/1.2
Rotation time	0.1	0.33	0.33
Pitch	1	1	0.2
Tube voltage (kV)	130	120	120
Effective mA	63 (fixed)	70	70
Slice thickness (mm)	3	2.5–3	2.5–3
Slice overlap (mm)	No	No	1.5
Kernel	Sharp	Standard/medium	Standard/medium
Effective dose (mSv)	1	0.6–1.7	2.5–5.25

Source: Modified from McCollough CH, Ulzheimer S, Halliburton SS, et al. *Radiology.* 2007;243:527–538.

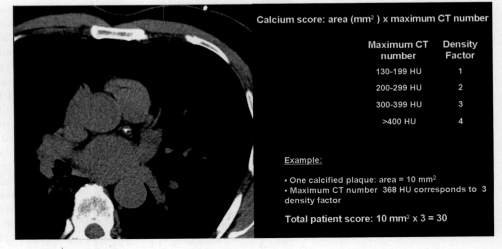

Figure 9.5 Agatston calcium score in a 67-year-old Hispanic male with hypertension and hyperlipemia as cardiovascular risk factors. The patient presented with only one calcified plaque in the distal left main (*circle*). The total calculated calcium score by the Agatson method was 30 that corresponds to the 45th percentile adjusted for the patient's age, gender, and ethnicity (see Section 5).

Calcium score: area (mm²) x maximum CT number

Maximum CT number	Density Factor
130-199 HU	1
200-299 HU	2
300-399 HU	3
>400 HU	4

Example:

• One calcified plaque: area = 10 mm²
• Maximum CT number 368 HU corresponds to 3 density factor

Total patient score: 10 mm² x 3 = 30

lation with a value >130 HU. These voxels are used in the final 3D reconstruction of the calcified plaque by the software. The obtained value is a volume estimated as a fraction of a cubic centimeter, but for the purpose of presenting it as a whole number the measured calcified volume is multiplied by 1,000. The volume score is much less dependent on minor changes in slice thickness[21] but also uses a threshold of >130 HU to define calcification. This value is conventional, and it does not represent a real physical measurement.

Recently the calcium mass score has also been reported.[22] It represents the total mineral content (hydroxyapatite mass) and corresponds to a real physical measure. It has become the best measurement of the amount of CAC.[23,24] To determine the calcium mass score, the mean CT number in the calcification is multiplied by the volume (in mm³) and a calibration constant in order to obtain absolute values. The calibration factor is measured by a CCT thoracic phantom to mimic CAC, and it depends on the scanning protocol and the scanner used.[25]

Currently, in clinical practice the computer software provided by all vendors converts the pixel values to an Agatston score, calcium volume, and, more recently (some manufactures), calcium mass score. In the final report the total patient CAC score and his percentile distribution in the respective age and gender matched population is reported. Studies in large populations showed that CAC is age, gender, and ethnicity dependent as reported in MESA (Multi-Ethnic Study on Atherosclerosis)[26] and HNR (Heinz Nixdorf Recall)[27] studies. Both provide online calculators: www.mesa-nhlbi.org <www.recall-studie.uni-essen.de>.

6. CONTRAST-ENHANCED PROTOCOLS

6.1. Coronary angiogram protocol

With the advance of CT technologies, improvements in temporal and spatial resolution (64-row detectors or dual-source scanners) have markedly improved the evaluation of coronary stenosis. Protocols for coronary anatomy should be optimized to get the best possible compromise between diagnostic quality and radiation exposure for any individual patient. In planning the cardiac CT study, the typical acquisition parameters to consider are gantry rotation speed, collimation section width, pitch, tube current, and voltage.

The imaging speed is determined by the CT gantry rotation time, defined as the time required for the CT gantry to make one full rotation. Temporal resolution corresponds to ½ rotation plus the fan angle, using single-segment reconstruction. As a rule, the fastest gantry rotation time should be selected, except in patients with a very slow heart rate or very obese patients. In the first scenario a slower gantry rotation can avoid gaps in the acquisition data set and in obese patients it can improve the signal to noise ratio.[28] Also, in normal size adults the thinnest possible collimation should be chosen. In a 64-row detector CT it corresponds to 0.5 to 0.625 mm. The tube current should be adjusted based on BMI and in patients with slow and steady heart rates (<65 bpm) tube current modulation should be used.[29] In a 64-row detector CT scanner with 0.6-mm collimation and 330-ms gantry rotation, tube current is usually adjusted to 500 to 900 mA.

A tube voltage of 120 kV is ordinarily employed, but it can be safely lowered to 100 kV in thin patients (BMI <25 kg/m²) or young adults with reasonable results. Only in very obese patients a high tube voltage of 140 kV should be considered, but generally it is not recommendable due to significant increase in effective dose of radiation needed to maintain image quality.

Until recently, coronary studies have been acquired during continuous rotation of the gantry, continuous movement of the patient coach, and retrospective ECG-gating, in the so-called spiral or helical technique. An important scan parameter related to this acquisition method is the pitch, which is defined as the table travel per complete rotation of the gantry divided by the detector width. When helical scan mode is used for a coronary protocol, the pitch should be between 0.2 and 0.35, providing the necessary overlap in the data set for ECG image reconstruction. A pitch >1 implies gaps in the data set, whereas a pitch between 0 and 1 implies data overlap.

In order to decrease radiation exposure, some groups have shown promising results using prospective triggering and using the step-and-shoot scan mode for coronary studies. As previously explained, radiation is administered during a small portion of the cardiac cycle. However, patient selection needs to be very strict, with low and steady heart rates in order to get a diagnostic study.[6]

Typical image protocols for a 64-row detector CCT (prospective and retrospective gating) are listed in Table 9.3.

TABLE 9.3
CORONARY CT PROTOCOL (NATIVE CORONARIES AND BYPASS GRAFTS)

Setup and patient preparation		
IV injection/iodine contrast (mL)	Yes/60–110 mL	
Injection rate	4–5 mL/s	
ECG leads	Yes	
Medications	Beta-blockers if >60 bpm and sublingual nitro-glycerin (NTGsl)	
Patient instructions	End-inspiration breath-hold	
Coronary CT scan parameters	*64-row detector CT scanner*	
Acquisition	Sequential	Helical
ECG synchronization	Prospective	Retrospective
Scan coverage	Carina to base of heart	Carina-base heart[a]
Detector collimation (mm)	0.6	0.6
Rotation time	0.35	0.33 (0.37)[b]
Pitch	1	0.2
Tube voltage (kV)	100/120	100/120
Effective tube current(mA)	400–850	500–900
Slice thickness (mm)	0.625	0.625–0.75
Slice overlap (mm)	35 mm (increment)	0.3–0.6
Kernel	Medium/sharp	Medium/sharp
Effective dose (mSv)	1.1–3.0	7–10[c]

[a]If bypass protocol larger coverage from left clavicle to the base of the heart applies.
[b]If heart rate is <45 bpm slower gantry rotation is used.
[c]If dose modulation is not used estimated radiation doses up to 21 mSv.

6.2. Bypass grafts protocol

One potential indication of cardiac CT includes the evaluation of coronary artery bypass. There is good evidence that this technique has high sensitivity and specificity to detect graft patency and stenosis.[30-32] The protocol used for bypass grafts evaluation is very similar to the one for coronary anatomy assessment, except for a few exceptions. The knowledge of prior surgical procedure is needed (number of grafts, vein, arterial, or both grafts). The presence of a LIMA graft requires extending the scan range from the top of the left clavicle in order to identify the origin of the LIMA to the base of the heart (Fig. 9.2B). Evaluation of saphenous vein graft patency can be performed from the mid-AA to the base of the heart. Furthermore, if patient has a LIMA, the IV catheter should be placed into a right antecubital vein to avoid streaking artifacts from the contrast in the left subclavian vein. These artifacts could interfere with the evaluation of the LIMA origin. Using timing bolus or tracking the contrast, volume is adjusted. As always, practicing breathing instructions (breath-hold will be 20% to 30% longer than for coronary evaluation alone) and lowering the heart rate will increase the quality of the images.

Retrospective ECG gating is used to evaluate grafts and anastomosis patency and the rest of the scan parameters are similar as those used for coronary arteries protocol. Cardiac CT scans are usually performed in the cranio–caudal direction; however, in the presence of coronary artery bypass grafts (large coverage), it is possible to scan in the opposite direction. Caudal–cranial direction compensates for possible involuntary respiratory motion at the end of the scanning (Table 9.3). Increasing pitch may reduce scan time in patients unable to sustain a prolonged breath-hold or when 16-slice scanners are used. However, this will result in lower spatial resolution in the z-axis.

6.3. Pulmonary vein protocol

Presently, with the use of pulmonary vein isolation procedures for atrial fibrillationl CCT imaging allows (a) to evaluate the left atrium (LA), left atrial appendage, and the pulmonary vein anatomy before the procedure; (b) to establish the anatomical position of the esophagus to avoid its perforation during the procedure; and (c) to detect pulmonary vein stenosis following the procedure[33] (Fig. 9.6).

New technological developments allow merging CCT 3D data with electro-mapping systems or with images acquired by fluoroscopy in order to guide the ablation catheter. This translates to a positive impact on the success rate of ablation and reduced fluoroscopy time.[34-36]

Pulmonary vein protocols have been developed by all scanners in the market (4-, 16-, and 64-row detectors), the latter being the most used in many institutions at present. Patients undergoing cardiac CT prior to radiofrequency ablation may be in atrial fibrillation or in a regular sinus rhythm (paroxysmal episodes of atrial fibrillation). Many groups use ECG-gated studies for patients in sinus rhythm and nongated studies for patients in atrial fibrillation or other arrhythmias.[37] If the study is ECG-gated, measurements of cardiac volumes and pulmonary vein measurements are more accurate, and the ability to detect the presence of thrombus in the left atrial appendage improves.

For the timing or tracking bolus technique the ROI is placed in the LA and the complete acquisition is obtained in a single breath-hold after 75 to 125 mL of nonionic contrast media. The entire thorax can be scanned to visualize an aberrant pulmonary venous drainage to the brachiocephalic veins or superior vena cava (SVC) or only the heart starting at the level of the carina.

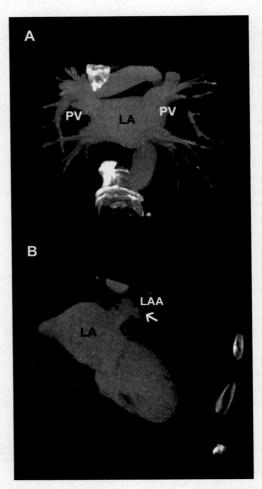

Figure 9.6 A: MIP reconstruction with 30-mm slice thickness shows a posterior view of the LA with normal anatomy of the pulmonary veins (PV), two in the right side and two PV in the left side entering in LA. **B:** Long-axis view (two-chamber view) of the LV and LA. This study was performed with ECG-gating in a patient in sinus rhythm with history of paroxysmal atrial fibrillation. The *arrow* shows the left atrial appendage (LAA) free of thrombus.

In some centers the patient receives an extra oral ingestion of barium sulfate immediately before the breath-hold to image better the esophagus. As some groups reported, a late phase scan (5 min) after the pulmonary vein study with lower radiation and small coverage of LA appendage can help to differentiate blood stasis from thrombi in this location.[38]

Although parameters can differ slightly among vendors and users, Table 9.4 shows a common protocol for the evaluation of the pulmonary vein anatomy.

7. WORKSTATION ANALYSIS

Once the scan is finalized, postprocessing analysis begins with the reconstruction of the raw data set. To reconstruct the large amount of data obtained the appropriate phase of the cardiac cycle is chosen and analyzed in low stable heart rates corresponding to 65% to 75% of the R–R interval. In patients with faster heart rates (>70 bpm) systolic phases, for example 25% to 35% R–R interval, are preferred. Also, when reconstructing images, a kernel is selected. Kernels are computer algorithms that process raw data in an image maintaining a degree of edge enhancement,

TABLE 9.4
PULMONARY VEIN CT PROTOCOL

Setup and patient preparation

Intravenous injection/ iodine contrast (mL)	Yes/60–120 mL
Injection rate	4–5 mL/s
ECG leads	Yes, if sinus rhythm
Medications	None
Patient instructions	End-inspiration breath-hold
Scan parameters	*64-row detector CT scanner*
Acquisition	Helical
ECG synchronization	Retrospective[a]
Scan range	Carina to the base of the heart[b]
Detector collimation (mm)	1.2
Rotation time	0.33–0.35
Pitch	0.2
Tube voltage (kV)	120
Effective tube current (mA)	300–400
Slice thickness (mm)	1.5 mm
Slice overlap (mm)	0.6–1
Kernel	Medium

[a]If the patient is in atrial fibrillation, nongated scan can be used.
[b]Scan entire thorax if anomalous vein drainage needs to be ruled out.

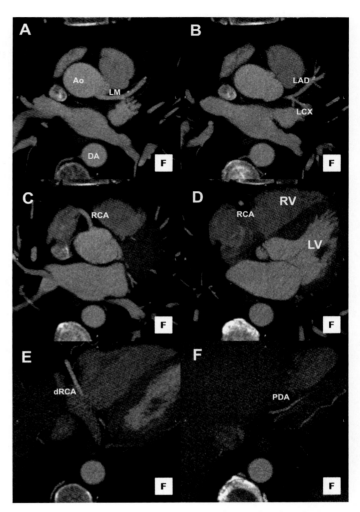

Figure 9.7 The raw axial data is reviewed first in thin slice (0.75 mm). From (**A**) to (**F**) scroll from cranial to caudal direction to assess the coronary arteries and the rest of the thorax (aorta, mediastinum, and pericardium). **A**: Ascending aorta (Ao), descending aorta (DA), and left main coronary artery (LM). **B**: Proximal and mid left anterior descending artery (LAD) and left circumflex artery (LCX). **C**: Right coronary artery (RCA). **D**: RCA, LV, and RV. **E**: Distal RCA (dRCA). **F**: Posterior descending artery (PDA) coming from RCA.

to provide enough vascular detail. For example, "soft" kernels are selected to evaluate coronary anatomy (lower image noise and more smooth contours) and "sharp" kernels are used in presence of stents or calcifications (more noise but more edge detection). Reconstructed images are transferred to workstations that provide several advanced image display methods for coronary and cardiac evaluation.

7.1 Axial plane evaluation

Evaluation of the images in the axial projection is usually done first using a thin slice (0.6 to 0.75 mm), as it represents the data in the form that is acquired and is less prone to reconstruction artifacts. Careful adjustment of image windowing parameters are done to differentiate the iodine-enhanced lumen from calcified and noncalcified plaques. When selecting windowing parameters, there are two important measures: window center that corresponds to the midpoint of the Hounsfield Unit range used and the window width that represents the range of Hounsfield values to set a gray scale (white corresponds to the upper limit and black to the lower limit). Typical windowing for a coronary evaluation is width 1,000 and level 350. Scrolling up and down through the originally acquired cross-sectional images is useful to assess normal anatomy and chamber and vessel relationship (Fig. 9.7).

7.2. Volume-rendered image analysis

Volume rendered (VR) is a technique that uses all the volumetric data acquired in the scan and combines voxels into a 3D image. Each voxel can be assigned a specific color, providing as a final result an anatomic view in an easily understandable format. These images are the most useful to evaluate complex anatomy, bypass grafts, coronary anomaly, and fistulas. Some physicians prefer to use 3D VR as a first step in the evaluation of bypass grafts, regarding types and course. Also, these images can be used in the report

system to help the patient understand better his or her cardiac anatomy (Fig. 9.8).[39]

7.3. Multiplanar reformatting

Multiplanar reformatting (MPR) is a basic tool used to interpret the reconstructed 3D image data sets in any plane (coronal, sagittal, and oblique projections) with the thinnest slice reconstruction. The multiplanar capabilities of the workstation allow images of the heart and coronary arteries to be manually rotated for optimal evaluation of the cardiac anatomy. MPR is used to assess calcified and noncalcified coronary atherosclerotic plaque, lumen patency, and stent patency. Analysis of MPR short-axis view is displayed when a region of stenosis is suspected. Curved MPR is a modification of MPR, where the vessel can be reconstructed on a plane to fit a curve (usually the path of a coronary artery) and allow the display of the entire vessel in a single image. This can be done manually or automatically in some workstations. This reconstruction can be helpful in patients with coronary grafts or tortuous vessels (Fig. 9.9).

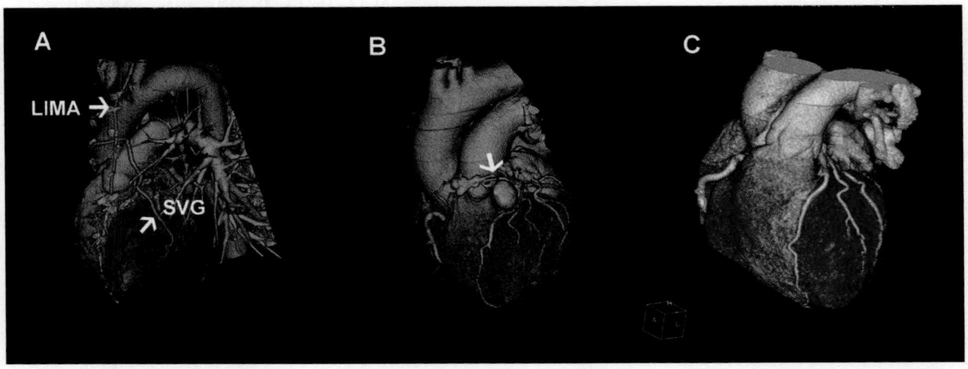

Figure 9.8 VR images. **A:** Contrast enhanced 64-row detector coronary CT angiography in a 68-year-old male referred for evaluation of previous bypass surgery. VR technique shows a LIMA graft to the distal left anterior (LAD), coronary artery (*upper arrow*), and a saphenous vein graft (SVG) anastomosis to the obtuse marginal. **B:** Coronary CT angiography in a 72-year-old female patient with history of chest pain shows an aneurysm in the proximal LAD with a fistulous trajectory to the PA (*arrow*). **C:** Nice 3D VR image of normal coronary arteries for the reporting system, useful for referring physician and patients.

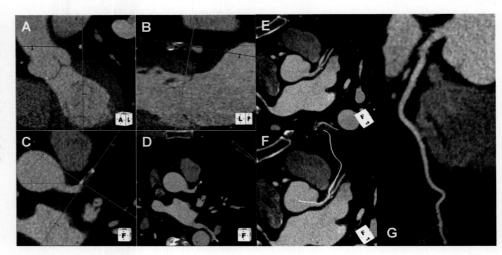

Figure 9.9 (**A**) displays a multiplanar reformation short-axis view of a severe lesion in the proximal left anterior descending coronary artery (LAD) obtained from two orthogonal planes (**B,C**). (**D**) shows an axial view of the severe stenosis in the proximal LAD. Axial views should be the first step to assess coronary arteries anatomy. (**E**) and (**F**) are curved multiplanar reformats that display the entire vessel from axial views. (**F**) shows how the vessel is tracked (manually or most commonly automatically by workstations software) to be displayed in a 2D view.

7.4. Maximum intensity projection

An additional postprocessing technique to evaluate the coronary arteries is the maximum intensity projection (MIP). This is a visualization method for 3D data that projects in the visualization plane the voxels of a slab of data with the highest Hounsfield Unit. The thickness of a MIP can be adjusted and the images are similar to traditional angiograms. This allows following longer vessel paths (Fig. 9.10).

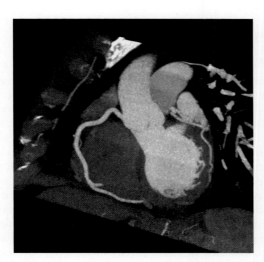

Figure 9.10 MIP image with 10-mm slice thickness of the entire right coronary artery (RCA) imitating the views obtained in an invasive angiography study.

7.5. Multiphase analysis

Retrospective ECG gating in cardiac CT studies allows reconstructing images in any phase of the cardiac cycle. Usually the data set is reconstructed at 10% intervals from 0% to 90% of the R–R interval. Generally, with ten-phases, global and regional left ventricular (LV) function can be accurately evaluated. However, as the number of reconstructions increases, interpretation time and size of the data set increase accordingly. In order to decrease the size of the data set thicker slices can be reconstructed (1.2 mm).

Multiphase reconstruction is also used in certain circumstances. When heart rate is low most of coronary segments can be reviewed with images from mid- to late-diastole reconstructed at 65%, 75%, and 85% of the R–R interval. But if the heart rate is faster it also becomes necessary to reconstruct images from end-systolic phases of the cardiac cycle, 25% to 35% to 45% of the R–R interval. There are coronary segments with subtle motion artifacts where the quantification of the coronary atherosclerotic plaque can be misinterpreted. Reviewing multiphase reconstructions provides the highest confidence in interpretation and should be performed routinely in all studies.

8. ANALYSIS AND CALCULATIONS

8.1. Stenosis calculation

Newer generations of scanners have proven to be reliable to document significant coronary stenosis (Fig. 9.11).[40-43] Most of the published studies defined a significant stenosis as >50% estimated obstruction

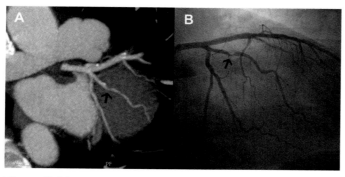

Figure 9.11 A: 67-year-old male with hypertension, hypercholesterolemia, and history of chest pain. Stress echocardiography showed mild ischemia in the anterolateral wall. A cardiac CT angiography demonstrated a significant stenosis (>50% luminal diameter) (*arrow*) in the first oblique marginal (OM1). **B:** Stenosis was confirmed by invasive coronary angiography (*arrow*).

of coronary luminal diameter.[40,42] In the daily practice in cardiac CT studies, coronary stenoses are evaluated using qualitative grading by visual analysis following the segmentation as suggested by The American Heart Association[44]. Despite the absence of a standardized grading protocol for coronary stenosis by CCT, usually in the reporting system they are graded as none or very mild (<30% estimated obstruction of coronary luminal diameter), mild (30% to 49% estimated obstruction of coronary luminal diameter), moderate (50% to 69% estimated obstruction of coronary luminal diameter), or severe (≥70% estimated obstruction of coronary luminal diameter) (Fig. 9.12).[45,46]

Once the atherosclerotic plaque is identified using MPR or MIP reconstructions, one of the best tools to assess the degree of stenosis is a MPR reconstruction. The luminal diameter in a cross-sectional view is compared to the luminal diameter of the normal vessel immediately proximal to the plaque (Fig. 9.9). In calcified plaques or in stents the degree of stenosis can be overestimated.

In addition, recently most available software packages provide semiquantitative evaluation of stenosis severity.[46] Briefly, they display an automatic detection of the centerline through the coronary vessels within the 3D data set and in a cross-sectional view of the vessel, an estimation of the percent diameter stenosis is calculated automatically. However, as with any automated algorithm sometimes manual correction is necessary to better delineate the vessel border (Fig. 9.13).

8.2. Plaque analysis

Unlike conventional angiography, cardiac CT provides visualization of the vessel wall and atherosclerotic plaque. One of the main goals of this technique is to identify the vulnerable plaque, the rupture of which plays a significant role in acute coronary syndromes.[47] This noninvasive method may provide important prognostic information in the near future. Several studies with 16- and, more recently, 64-row detector CT scanners have evaluated the ability of this technique to quantify atherosclerotic coronary plaques and differentiate calcified from noncalcified lesions based in their X-ray attenuation in comparison to IVUS. Their results concluded that, as compared to intravascular ultrasound (IVUS), cardiac CT tends to underestimate noncalcified plaque volume and overestimate calcified plaque. These studies have demonstrated average attenuation values in the range of 30 to 60 HU for "soft" (lipid-rich) plaques in comparison with mean values of 70 to 120 HU for fibrous and >350 HU for calcified plaque.[48–52] However, there is overlap in the attenuation values between soft (lipid-rich) and fibrous plaques

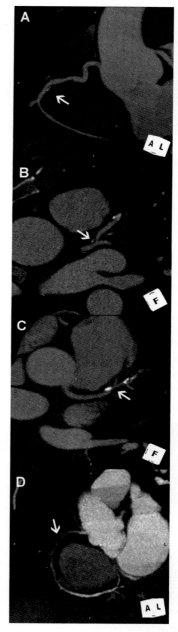

Figure 9.12 A: MIP reconstruction of a mixed plaque (calcified spot and noncalcified plaque) causing mild stenosis (<49% obstruction luminal diameter) in the mid right coronary artery. **B:** MPR image of a moderate stenosis (50% to 69% obstruction luminal diameter) caused by a mixed plaque involving the left main and ostial left anterior descending artery. **C:** Example of a severe stenosis (≥70% obstruction luminal diameter) caused by a noncalcified plaque in the proximal left anterior descending artery. **D:** MIP reconstruction of a total proximal occlusion of the proximal right coronary artery, which is retrogradely filled from collaterals. *Arrows* show coronary artery lesion.

from patient to patient. This problem seems to be related to the vessel wall contrast-enhancement after contrast media.[53] From a practical point of view, then, atherosclerotic plaques can be classified as calcified, noncalcified (soft and fibrous), and mixed plaque (calcified spots and noncalcified spots).

More recently, new software tools are being developed to automatically quantify the coronary plaque volume, even though contour detection delineation usually needs hand correction.

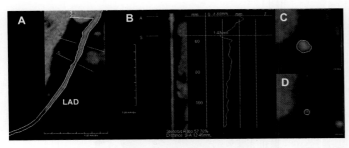

Figure 9.13 A: Automatic detection of the outer border of the left anterior descending artery (LAD) in a curved multiplanar reformatted image. (**B**) shows the degree of stenosis comparing the proximal normal vessel (*A*) as a reference with the stenotic segment (*S*). The total luminal diameter reduction is 58%. **C:** Proximal luminal diameter in normal segment. **D:** Stenotic segment in the proximal LAD with significant reduction of the lumen diameter.

The outer vessel border at the adventitia-fat boundary is not completely well defined on cardiac CT images as a result of insufficient temporal, spatial, and contrast resolution.[54] Also, for plaque composition detection, advanced software tools are being refined to be able to identify and quantify the different components of the atherosclerotic plaque. They depicted different plaque (*soft, fibrous, or calcified*) in different colors according to their corresponding CT Hounsfield Unit ranges.[55] Nevertheless, reliable differentiation of the composition of noncalcified plaques is still limited and more investigation in this direction needs to be done (Fig. 9.14).

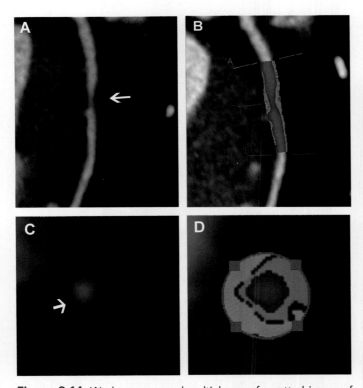

Figure 9.14 (A) shows a curved multiplanar reformatted image of a noncalcified plaque in the proximal left anterior descending artery. **B,C:** When a prototype software for plaque composition is applied, different colors are displayed in the vessel depending on the attenuation measured in Hounsfield Units. In this example, the lumen is blue (170 to 400 HU) and the noncalcified plaque is displayed in color green (60 to 161 HU). The epicardial fat is displayed in yellow (−50 to 50 HU). (**C**) shows a cross-sectional view of the plaque, where white arrow points to the lumen of the vessel and the black arrow indicates fibrous plaque.

For practical purpose, however, a semiquantitative plaque composition in addition to the luminal stenosis evaluation is recommended in the final report for the referring physician.

8.3. Chamber dimension analysis

With the technical improvements of spatial and temporal resolution of CCT studies, LV function assessment can be obtained with a good agreement with established imaging modalities (echocardiography, invasive ventriculography, and cardiac MRI).[56–58] As previously mentioned, for LV function and volumes, the acquired data set usually is reconstructed at 10% intervals from 0% to 90% of the R–R interval with thicker slices (1 to 1.5 mm) to reduce the size of the data set. However, in the literature, reconstructions of 20 phases of the cardiac cycle, starting at early systole (0% of cardiac cycle) to end-diastole (95% of cardiac cycle) in steps of 5% are described.[56] Also, using multisegment image reconstruction can improve image quality and assessment of regional wall motion compared with the standard single-segment reconstruction.[59] When tube current dose modulation is used in the scan protocol, the reconstructed systolic phases will present increased noise but delineation of endocardial borders is still feasible.

If functional information from the right chambers needs to be obtained, the contrast injection protocol should be changed to a three-phase injection protocol or application of diluted contrast (with saline) after the initial contrast bolus.

Cardiac function and wall motion abnormalities can be analyzed visually, playing a cine-loop of the cardiac phases in standard views of the heart (long-axis orientation—two-, three-, four-chambers, and short axis). Wall motion analysis can be evaluated using the 17-segment model recommended by the AHA/ACC[60] with a qualitative grading: normal, mild to moderate hypokinesis, severe hypokinesis, akinesis, or dyskinesis (Fig. 9.15).

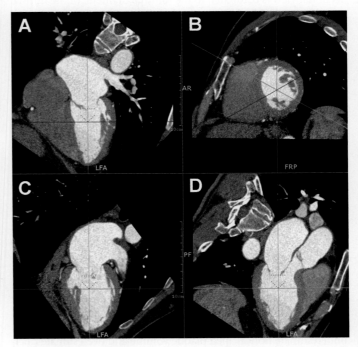

Figure 9.15 Example of standard views of the heart to assess the cardiac function visually playing cine loops. (**A**) shows a long axis, four-chamber view and (**C**) shows a two-chamber view. (**B**) is a true short axis that is created from two orthogonal planes to the previous long axis (*blue line* in (**A**), *red line* in (**B**)). (**D**) is a three-chamber view that is obtained from a basal short axis through the LV outflow tract.

The LV volume can be measured by use of the area-length method (used primarily in echocardiography based on a vertical or horizontal long-axis view), the Simpson method, or a threshold-based 3D volumetric method. Generally, the Simpson method and the threshold-based volumetric method are considered more reliable as they do not rely on geometric assumptions for determination of global LV parameters such as LV volumes or ejection fraction (EF). For the Simpson method, contours of the endocardial and epicardial borders of short-axis images in end-diastolic and end-systolic phases from the base of the heart to the apex are traced manually or automatically using dedicated postprocessing software. Papillary muscles are often considered part of the LV cavity. Then LV end-diastolic (EDV) and end-systolic (ESV) volumes are calculated and subsequently, the EF is calculated with EDV and ESV values.[57,58]

In the threshold-based 3D volume measurement, the total chamber volume is calculated by summing all the voxels that exceed a predefined attenuation threshold once the valvular annulus level is selected. Pixels included in the segmentation are generally displayed with a different color and if the automatic threshold does not accurately correspond with the cavity volume, the contours can be manually corrected. This approach allows a fast and semiautomatic assessment of ventricular volumes, wall thickening, and wall motion[61] (Fig. 9.16).

9. EVALUATION OF EXTRACARDIAC STRUCTURES

When a noncontrast or a cardiac CT is performed the entire mid thorax is irradiated. Because of this, reconstructing images of the heart together with images of the chest as a maximum field of view provide no additional radiation to the patient. In addition to the anatomy of the heart and coronary vessels, these studies also contain information about the lungs, mediastinum, spine, chest wall, and upper abdomen structures. Several studies have shown high prevalence of extra cardiac findings, some of them, clinically relevant emphasizing the importance of reviewing

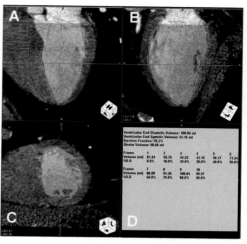

Figure 9.16 Example of EF and LV volumes using a threshold-based 3D volume method in a dedicated cardiac CT scanner software. Standard views of the heart; four-chamber (**A**) view, two-chamber view (**B**), and short-axis view (**C**). **D**: LV volumes are calculated in each of the ten phases reconstructed of the cardiac cycle and total EF and LV volumes are reported.

them.[62,63] The interpreting physician (cardiologist, radiologist, or both in collaboration) should be systematic in the approach to evaluate the lungs, mediastinum, breast tissue, and bones. In Figure 9.17, a flow diagram outlines the typical windows parameters and the most common extracardiac findings in cardiac CT studies. More detailed information about this issue can be found in Chapter 51.

10. FUTURE DIRECTIONS

Cardiac CT is one of the fastest growing noninvasive imaging cardiac modality. CT technology has reached a temporal resolution up to 83 ms with the advent of dual-source systems.[8,64]

Figure 9.17 Extracardiac findings.

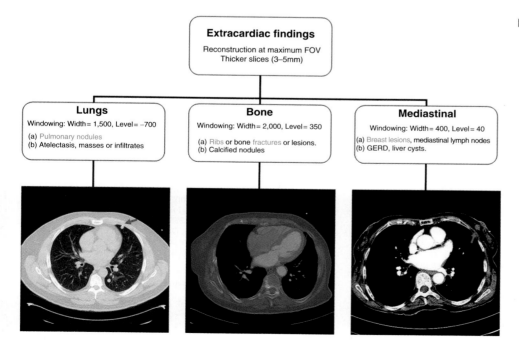

A promising approach with dual-source CT is the use of dual-energy imaging: areas of interest are scanned with different voltages (kV) and can be subsequently subtracted. Because different tissues and contrast agents have distinct energy absorption profiles, this technique could potentially improve tissue differentiation (vascular lumen and wall components).[64]

Scanners with wider coverage per rotation, such as 256-row area detectors, make possible imaging of the heart in a single heartbeat. These systems could make feasible imaging patients with arrhythmias and those who cannot hold their breath. So far, the main limitations of CT technology are (a) insufficient temporal resolution, (b) relatively high radiation exposure, and (c) limited spatial resolution for coronary imaging. It is expected that new generation scanners will improve rotational speed and that dose may be reduced using prospective gating.[65]

CT systems with flat panel detectors (FPD) can achieve a higher spatial resolution than MDCT, but up to now, gantry rotation time is 2 s or longer, and tissue characterization (contrast-noise) is limited. For these reasons, FPD is still under development (new materials for flat-panel detectors) and it is not used nowadays for cardiac imaging.

Merging technologies like PET/CT imaging may help detect inflammatory activity in atherosclerotic plaques.[66] Advances in image acquisition, data analysis, image processing, and workstation applications are in a state of continuous development. A good interaction between engineers, physicists, technologists, and physicians will expand the clinical application of this technology in the near future.

ACKNOWLEDGMENTS

The author is supported by a grant from Fundacion CajaMadrid (Spain).

REFERENCES

1. McCollough CH, Morin RL. The technical design and performance of ultrafast computed tomography. *Radiol Clin North Am.* 1994;32:521–536.
2. Yamaji S, Imai S, Saito F, et al. Does high-power computed tomography scanning equipment affect the operation of pacemakers? *Circ J.* 2006;70:190–197.
3. McCollough CH, Zhang J, Primak AN, et al. Effects of CT irradiation on implantable cardiac rhythm management devices. *Radiology.* 2007;243:766–774.
4. Giesler T, Baum U, Ropers D, et al. Noninvasive visualization of coronary arteries using contrast-enhanced multidetector CT: Influence of heart rate on image quality and stenosis detection. *Am J Roentgenol.* 2002;179: 911–916.
5. Dewey M, Laule M, Krug L. Multisegment and halfscan reconstruction of 16-slice computed tomography for detection of coronary artery stenoses. *Invest Radiol.* 2004;39:6.
6. Husmann L, Valenta I, Gaemperli O, et al. Feasibility of low-dose coronary CT angiography: First experience with prospective ECG-gating. *Eur Heart J.* 2008;29:191–197.
7. Oncel D, Oncel G, Tastan A. Effectiveness of dual-source CT coronary angiography for the evaluation of coronary artery disease in patients with atrial fibrillation: Initial experience. *Radiology.* 2007;245:703–711.
8. Flohr TG, McCollough CH, Bruder H, et al. First performance evaluation of a dual-source CT (DSCT) system. *Eur Radiol.* 2006;16:256–268.
9. Cademartiri F, van der Lugt A, Luccichenti G, et al. Parameters affecting bolus geometry in CTA: A review. *J Comput Assist Tomogr.* 2002;26(4):598–607.
10. Thomsen HS, Morcos SK. Radiographic contrast media. *BJU Int.* 2000;86 (Suppl. 1):1–10.
11. Gul KM, Mao SS, Gao Y, et al. Noninvasive gadolinium-enhanced three dimensional computed tomography coronary angiography. *Acad Radiol.* 2006;13:840–849.
12. Carrascosa PMDP, Merletti PGMD, Capunay CMD, et al. New approach to noninvasive coronary angiography by multidetector computed tomography: Initial experience using gadolinium. *J Comput Assist Tomogr.* 2007;31(3):441–443.
13. American College of Radiology Committee on Drugs and Contrast Media. Manual on contrast media: version 5.0 Reston V, 2004.
14. Koch K, Oellig F, Oberholzer K, et al. Assessment of right ventricular function by 16-detector-row CT: Comparison with magnetic resonance imaging. *Eur Radiol.* 2005;15:312–318.
15. Cademartiri F, Mollet NR, van der Lugt A, et al. Intravenous contrast material administration at helical 16-detector row CT coronary angiography: Effect of iodine concentration on vascular attenuation. *Radiology.* 2005;236:661–665.
16. Cademartiri F, Nieman K, van der Lugt A, et al. Intravenous contrast material administration at 16-detector row helical CT coronary angiography: Test bolus versus bolus-tracking technique. *Radiology.* 2004;233:817–823.
17. Greenland P, LaBree L, Azen SP, et al. Coronary artery calcium score combined with Framingham score for risk prediction in asymptomatic individuals. *JAMA.* 2004;291:210–215.
18. Budoff MJ, Achenbach S, Blumenthal RS, et al. Assessment of coronary artery disease by cardiac computed tomography: A scientific statement from the American Heart Association Committee on Cardiovascular Imaging and Intervention, Council on Cardiovascular Radiology and Intervention, and Committee on Cardiac Imaging, Council on Clinical Cardiology. *Circulation.* 2006;114:1761–1791.
19. Horiguchi J, Yamamoto H, Akiyama Y, et al. Variability of repeated coronary artery calcium measurements in 16-MDCT with retrospective reconstruction. *Am J Roentgenol.* 2005;184:1917–1923.
20. Agatston AS, Janowitz WR, Hildner FJ, et al. Quantification of coronary artery calcium using ultrafast computed tomography. *J Am Coll Cardiol.* 1990;15: 827–832.
21. Callister TQ, Cooil B, Raya SP, et al. Coronary artery disease: Improved reproducibility of calcium scoring with an electron-beam CT volumetric method. *Radiology.* 1998;208:807–814.
22. Ferencik MMD, Ferullo A, Achenbach SMD, et al. Coronary calcium quantification using various calibration phantoms and scoring thresholds. *Invest Radiol.* 2003;38:559–566.
23. Yoon HC, Greaser LE 3rd, Mather R, et al. Coronary artery calcium: Alternate methods for accurate and reproducible quantitation. *Acad Radiol.* 1997;4: 666–673.
24. Halliburton SS, Stillman AE, Lieber M, et al. Potential clinical impact of variability in the measurement of coronary artery calcification with sequential MDCT. *Am J Roentgenol.* 2005;184:643–648.
25. McCollough CH, Ulzheimer S, Halliburton SS, et al. Coronary artery calcium: A multi-institutional, multimanufacturer international standard for quantification at cardiac CT. *Radiology.* 2007;243:527–538.
26. Bild DE, Detrano R, Peterson D, et al. Ethnic differences in coronary calcification: The multi-ethnic study of atherosclerosis (MESA). *Circulation.* 2005;111: 1313–1320.
27. Schmermund A, Möhlenkamp S, Berenbein S, et al. Population-based assessment of subclinical coronary atherosclerosis using electron-beam computed tomography. *Atherosclerosis.* 2006;185:177–182.
28. Hoffmann U, Ferencik M, Cury RC, et al. Coronary CT angiography. *J Nucl Med.* 2006;47:797–806.
29. McCollough CH, Bruesewitz MR, Kofler JM Jr. CT dose reduction and dose management tools: Overview of available options. *Radiographics.* 2006;26:503–512.
30. Burgstahler C, Kuettner A, Kopp AF, et al. Non-invasive evaluation of coronary artery bypass grafts using multi-slice computed tomography: Initial clinical experience. *Int J Cardiol.* 2003;90:275–280.
31. Schlosser T, Konorza T, Hunold P, et al. Noninvasive visualization of coronary artery bypass grafts using 16-detector row computed tomography. *J Am Coll Cardiol.* 2004;44:1224–1229.
32. Malagutti P, Nieman K, Meijboom WB, et al. Use of 64-slice CT in symptomatic patients after coronary bypass surgery: Evaluation of grafts and coronary arteries. *Eur Heart J.* 2007;28:1879–1885.
33. Jongbloed MRM, Dirksen MS, Bax JJ, et al. Atrial fibrillation: Multi-detector row CT of pulmonary vein anatomy prior to radiofrequency catheter ablation—initial experience. *Radiology.* 2005;234:702–709.
34. Feuchtner GM, Dichtl W, DeFrance T, et al. Fusion of multislice computed tomography and electroanatomical mapping data for 3D navigation of left and right atrial catheter ablation. *Eur J Radiol.* 2008; 68(3):456–464.
35. Knecht S, Skali H, O'Neill MD, et al. Computed tomography-fluoroscopy overlay evaluation during catheter ablation of left atrial arrhythmia. *Europace* 2008:eun145.
36. Kistler PM, Rajappan K, Jahngir M, et al. The impact of CT image integration into an electroanatomic mapping system on clinical outcomes of catheter ablation of atrial fibrillation. *J Cardiovasc Electrophysiol.* 2006;17:1093–1101.
37. Lacomis JM, Wigginton W, Fuhrman C, et al. Multi-detector row CT of the left atrium and pulmonary veins before radio-frequency catheter ablation for atrial fibrillation. *RadioGraphics.* 2003;23:S35–S48.
38. Imada M, Funabashi N, Asano M, et al. Anatomical remodeling of left atria in subjects with chronic and paroxysmal atrial fibrillation evaluated by multislice computed tomography. *Int J Cardiol.* 2007;119:384–388.
39. Cody DD. AAPM/RSNA Physics tutorial for residents: Topics in CT: Image processing in CT. *Radiographics.* 2002;22:1255–1268.
40. Leber AW, Knez A, von Ziegler F, et al. Quantification of obstructive and non-obstructive coronary lesions by 64-slice computed tomography: A comparative study with quantitative coronary angiography and intravascular ultrasound. *J Am Coll Cardiol.* 2005;46:147–154.
41. Mollet NR, Cademartiri F, Krestin GP, et al. Improved diagnostic accuracy with 16-row multi-slice computed tomography coronary angiography. *J Am Coll Cardiol.* 2005;45:128–132.
42. Achenbach S, Giesler T, Ropers D, et al. Detection of coronary artery stenoses by contrast-enhanced, retrospectively electrocardiographically-gated, multislice spiral computed tomography. *Circulation.* 2001;103:2535–2538.

43. Dewey MMD, Rutsch WMD, Schnapauff DMD, et al. Coronary artery steno-sis quantification using multislice computed tomography. *Invest Radiol.* 2007;42:78–84.

44. Austen WG, Edwards JE, Frye RL, et al. A reporting system on patients evaluated for coronary artery disease. Report of the Ad Hoc Committee for Grading of Coronary Artery Disease, Council on Cardiovascular Surgery, American Heart Association. *Circulation.* 1975;51:5–40.

45. Min JK, Shaw LJ, Devereux RB, et al. Prognostic value of multidetector coronary computed tomographic angiography for prediction of all-cause mortality. *J Am Coll Cardiol.* 2007;50:1161–1170.

46. Busch S, Johnson T, Nikolaou K, et al. Visual and automatic grading of coronary artery stenoses with 64-slice CT angiography in reference to invasive angiography. *Eur Radiol.* 2007;17:1445–1451.

47. Burke AP, Farb A, Malcom GT, et al. Coronary risk factors and plaque morphology in men with coronary disease who died suddenly. *N Engl J Med.* 1997;336:1276–1282.

48. Schroeder S, Kopp AF, Baumbach A, et al. Noninvasive detection and evaluation of atherosclerotic coronary plaques with multislice computed tomography. *J Am Coll Cardiol.* 2001;37:1430–1435.

49. Leber AW, Knez A, Becker A, et al. Accuracy of multidetector spiral computed tomography in identifying and differentiating the composition of coronary atherosclerotic plaques: A comparative study with intracoronary ultrasound. *J Am Coll Cardiol.* 2004;43:1241–1247.

50. Leber AW, Becker A, Knez A, et al. Accuracy of 64-slice computed tomography to classify and quantify plaque volumes in the proximal coronary system: A comparative study using intravascular ultrasound. *J Am Coll Cardiol.* 2006;47:672–677.

51. Carrascosa PM, Capuñay CM, Garcia-Merletti P, et al. Characterization of coronary atherosclerotic plaques by multidetector computed tomography. *Am J Cardiol.* 2006;97:598–602.

52. Motoyama S, Kondo T, Anno H, et al. Atherosclerotic plaque characterization by 0.5-mm-slice multislice computed tomographic imaging. *Circ J.* 2007;71:363–366.

53. Halliburton SSAB, Schoenhagen PAC, Nair ABE, et al. Contrast enhancement of coronary atherosclerotic plaque: A high-resolution, multidetector-row computed tomography study of pressure-perfused, human ex-vivo coronary arteries. *Coron Artery Dis.* 2006;17:553–560.

54. Otsuka MMD, Bruining NP, Van Pelt NCMD, et al. Quantification of coronary plaque by 64-slice computed tomography: A comparison with quantitative intracoronary ultrasound. *Invest Radiol.* 2008;43:314–321.

55. Sun J, Zhang Z, Lu B, et al. Identification and quantification of coronary atherosclerotic plaques: A comparison of 64-MDCT and intravascular ultrasound. *Am J Roentgenol.* 2008;190:748–754.

56. Henneman MM, Schuijf JD, Jukema JW, et al. Assessment of global and regional left ventricular function and volumes with 64-slice MSCT: A comparison with 2D echocardiography. *J Nucl Cardiol.* 2006;13:480–487.

57. Hundt WMD, Siebert K, Wintersperger BJMD, et al. Assessment of global left ventricular function: Comparison of cardiac multidetector-row computed tomography with angiocardiography. *J Comput Assist Tomogr.* 2005;29(3):373–381.

58. Wu Y-W, Tadamura E, Yamamuro M, et al. Estimation of global and regional cardiac function using 64-slice computed tomography: A comparison study with echocardiography, gated-SPECT and cardiovascular magnetic resonance. *Int J Cardiol.* 2008; 128(1):69–76.

59. Mahnken AHMD, Hohl CMD, Suess CP, et al. Influence of heart rate and temporal resolution on left-ventricular volumes in cardiac multislice spiral computed tomography: A phantom study. *Invest Radiol.* 2006;41:429–435.

60. Cerqueira MD, Weissman NJ, Dilsizian V, et al. Standardized myocardial segmentation and nomenclature for tomographic imaging of the heart: A statement for healthcare professionals from the Cardiac Imaging Committee of the Council on Clinical Cardiology of the American Heart Association. *Circulation.* 2002;105:539–542.

61. Juergens K, Fischbach R. Left ventricular function studied with MDCT. *Eur Radiol.* 2006;16:342–357.

62. Onuma Y, Tanabe K, Nakazawa G, et al. Noncardiac findings in cardiac imaging with multidetector computed tomography. *J Am Coll Cardiol.* 2006;48:402–406.

63. Burt JR, Iribarren C, Fair JM, et al. Incidental findings on cardiac multidetector row computed tomography among healthy older adults: Prevalence and clinical correlates. *Arch Intern Med.* 2008;168:756–761.

64. Achenbach S, Ropers D, Kuettner A, et al. Contrast-enhanced coronary artery visualization by dual-source computed tomography—Initial experience. *Eur J Radiol.* 2006;57:331–335.

65. Motoyama S, Anno H, Sarai M, et al. Noninvasive coronary angiography with a prototype 256-row area detector computed tomography system comparison with conventional invasive coronary angiography. *J Am Coll Cardiol.* 2008;51:773–775.

66. Dunphy MPS, Freiman A, Larson SM, et al. Association of vascular 18F-FDG uptake with vascular calcification. *J Nucl Med.* 2005;46:1278–1284.

10

Vascular Magnetic Resonance and Computed Tomography Examination and Protocols

Emil I. Cohen
Pranay Krishnan
Robert A. Lookstein

1. INTRODUCTION

Magnetic resonance angiography (MRA) and computed tomography angiography (CTA) have seen many advances since their introduction in the 1990s. Both techniques have seen dramatic improvements in image quality and at the same time have seen a reduction in the exam time for most routine clinical inquiries. Continued development of both modalities holds promise not only for improving traditional anatomical diagnosis of disease but also for enabling better functional evaluation of both the normal and diseased vasculatures.

Besides basic indications such as aortic aneurysm and dissection, CT vascular angiographic techniques did not achieve their potential until the spiral multidetector and partial rotational image reconstruction algorithms were implemented in the past decade. With each advance, routine imaging of smaller and more pulsatile vessels became feasible with tolerable radiation exposures and scan times. The administered contrast load has been substantially reduced with the reduction in scan times. MRA has seen improvements from higher field strengths, faster gradient speeds, and innovative imaging sequences, some of which obviate the need for contrast administration.

It is customary for most commercially available CT and MR systems to include a basic set of protocols for routine vascular examinations. It is beyond the scope of this chapter to address the details of all these protocols, let alone provide instructions on the development of new ones. Our main goal is to provide the average physician performing these examinations with knowledge of the important aspects that are universal to all CT and MR equipment so that one may better supervise and when necessary modify imaging protocols in order to answer a specific clinical question.

An important benefit of noninvasive imaging is its ability to exclude patients without significant disease and thereby avoid the need for further invasive examinations such as digital subtraction angiography (DSA). The contrast and spatial resolutions of the current CTA and MRA scanners, however, are an order of magnitude below DSA and therefore cannot always replicate its accuracy in marginal cases when a disease is noted.

2. PATIENT PREPARATION

2.1. Intravenous access

Nearly all routine diagnostic CTA and MRA evaluations require the administration of an intravenous (IV) contrast agent. The preferred location for IV access is the right antecubital fossa to avoid artifact along the aortic arch from dense contrast, as it traverses the left brachiocephalic vein (Fig. 10.1). Since CTA and MRA require different contrast concentrations, in general a larger IV (20 gauge or larger) is required for most CTA studies, while a 22-gauge access is sufficient for most MRA studies.

2.2. Contrast reactions and preparation

2.2.1. Computer tomography (iodinated) contrast

Among all medications routinely used, IV iodinated contrast has one of the lowest rates of complications with the risk of death being <1 in 130,000.[1] Contrast-induced nephropathy (CIN) is a well-known adverse effect of iodinated contrast. The occurrence rate, however, is low (<3% after the administration of nonionic contrast) and is only seen in patients with preexisting renal insufficiency.[2]

Although the pathophysiology of CIN is not completely understood, the mechanism of damage appears to relate to both vasoconstrictive effects and direct renal tubular toxicity of iodinated contrast. In patients with renal insufficiency and particularly those with renal insufficiency and diabetes, the use of nonionic low osmolar contrast agents is associated with a lower risk of CIN, than the ionic high osmolar agents used in the past. Consensus does not exist as to whether newer iso-osmolar agents confer a further reduction in risk. Adequate oral or IV hydration (0.9% saline or 0.45% saline with added sodium bicarbonate) is an important pre-emptive action that can be taken to reduce the risk of CIN.[3-5] Administration of N-acetylcysteine can also be considered as an additional preventive step, although its efficacy is not universally supported.[6] Dialysis-dependent patients with end-stage renal disease (ESRD) are not at risk for further nephrotoxicity and can be given iodinated contrast without the need for prompt postexamination dialysis provided iso-osmolar or low-osmolar contrast media is administered. ESRD patients are, however, particularly sensitive to changes in volume overload, and steps should be taken to limit dose and avoid hypertonic agents. The benefits of contrast-enhanced imaging must be weighed against the risk of CIN on a patient-by-patient basis with appropriate steps taken to decrease risks when possible (Table 10.1).

Metformin, a common medication used in the treatment of diabetes, should be stopped at or prior to the time of iodinated contrast administration and withheld for 48 h in patients with

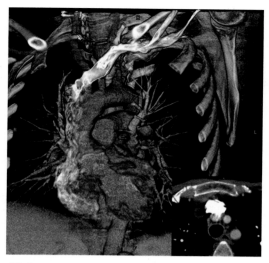

Figure 10.1 Three-dimensional reformatted and inset axial image from a CT angiogram of the chest. Arrow points to streak artifact over the right common carotid artery extending from the dense bolus of contrast in the left brachiocephalic vein.

TABLE 10.2

PREMEDICATION FOR PATIENTS AT HIGH RISK FOR ALLERGIC REACTION

Prednisone: 50 mg po 13, 7, and 1 h prior to examination
Diphenhydramine: 50 mg po 1 h prior to examination

TABLE 10.1

CONTRAST-INDUCED NEPHROPATHY: DETERMINING AND REDUCING RISK

Emergent contrast CT → Perform CT immediately.
(e.g., traumatic injury, dissection). If patient has known renal insufficiency, use lowest dose possible (nonionic, low osmolar).
Nonemergent contrast CT → Measure serum creatinine in following patient groups:

History of renal disease, family history of renal failure, diabetes, paraproteinemia syndromes/diseases (multiple myeloma), collagen vascular disease, medications (metformin, NSAIDS, nephrotoxic antibiotics). Patients with renal insufficiency/failure not on chronic dialysis → Discuss alternative imaging options with patient and referring physician (noncontrast CT or MRI). If contrast enhanced CT → Obtain informed consent deemed necessary Hydration – oral or IV 100 mL/h, 6 to 12 h before and 4 to 12 h after nonionic low osmolar contrast.

Source: "Contrast nephrotoxicity," ACR manual on contrast media, 2008.

conditions that increase the risk of metformin accumulation. No specific cross reactivity exists between the drug and iodinated contrast. Metformin accumulation, however, is known to increase the risk of lactic acidosis. It is the risk of renal dysfunction after iodinated contrast that would thereby lead to metformin accumulation that necessitates the suspension of medication administration in patients with renal insufficiency. Patients with liver dysfunction in whom lactate metabolism may be altered should similarly have the medication stopped prior to contrast administration. In patients with conditions that increase lactate production by promoting anaerobic metabolism, i.e., ischemia and infection, treatment should also be stopped prior to contrast administration.

It has been previously noted that multiple myeloma may be a risk factor for the development of CIN, but more recent studies have shown a stronger link to dehydration which may often be present in this patient population. Iodinated contrast may safely be administered, provided there is adequate hydration and no history of hypercalcemia.[7]

For a known allergy to iodinated contrast, a patient is premedicated using one of the several available protocols. The protocol used at the author's institution is shown in Table 10.2. It is worthwhile to note that no other allergy (including shellfish) is a contraindication for the administration of iodinated contrast or requires the initiation of a premedication regimen prior to contrast administration. The risk of allergic reaction to the currently used nonionic iodinated contrast agents is significantly decreased in comparison to their ionic counterparts of the past. If there is a distant history of contrast allergy prior to 1985 (prior to the use of new contrast agents), nonionic contrast administration can, therefore, be considered without steroid premedication.[8] Patients with history of asthma have an increased risk of bronchospasm after iodinated contrast administration. In such cases when contrast administration is deemed necessary, physician and/or nursing supervision during administration is advised.

2.2.2. Magnetic resonance contrast (Gadolinium chelates)

The overall safety of MR contrast surpasses even that of iodinated contrast in the general population. The rate of a serious adverse event is extremely low for all agents. Recently, the food and drug administration (FDA) has issued a warning about the utilization of these agents in patients with renal insufficiency particularly in patients whose glomerular filtration rate (GFR) is under 30 mL/min for all agents due to the fear of development of nephrogenic systemic fibrosis (NSF). It has since become evident that the incidence of this potentially fatal complication varies by agent and dose administered.[9] At the author's institution, gadobenate dimeglumine (MultiHance, Bracco) is routinely used for all MRA due to its greater T1 relaxivity. The greater T1 relaxivity of this agent allows utilization of lower dose and injection rates in most patients including those with renal insufficiency. A written informed consent is obtained from patients whose GFR is less than the limit set by the FDA, and a reduced dose of 0.05 mol/kg is utilized when alternative testing options are not available or carry greater risks (Table 10.3).

2.3. Lactating and pregnant patients

The evaluation of the pregnant patient has been controversial and reserved for emergent scenarios. In these settings, it is felt that whenever necessary, an answer should be obtained with sonography, MR, and CT in that order. This is no different in the evaluation of vascular emergencies. If at all possible, imaging evaluation with CT and MR should be postponed to the second and third trimesters since this would protect the fetus from stages during which the fetus undergoes organogenesis. If contrast use is necessary, it is felt that CT contrast is safer than MR contrast agents.

In the lactating patient receiving IV contrast, the traditional advice has been to have the mother express or pump her breast

TABLE 10.3
MR CONTRAST ADMINISTRATION IN PATIENTS WITH RENAL INSUFFICIENCY

Estimated GFR should be measured within 6 weeks of anticipated gadolinium-enhanced examination in the following patient groups:

History of renal disease, age >60, hypertension, diabetes, history of liver disease, patients that are acutely ill
eGFR 60 to 119 mL/min/1.73 m^2 → No increased risk of NSF
eGFR 30 to 59 mL/min/1.73 m^2 → Low to no risk of NSF (with dose of 0.1 mol/kg or less)
eGFR <30 mL/min/1.73 m^2 → avoid MR contrast if possible
ESRD on chronic dialysis → avoid MR contrast if possible
Consider contrast enhanced CT
If necessary, performing prompt post-MR dialysis may decrease likelihood of NSF
Discuss with patient and referring physician. Obtain informed consent

Source: "Nephrogenic systemic fibrosis," ACR manual on contrast media, 2008.

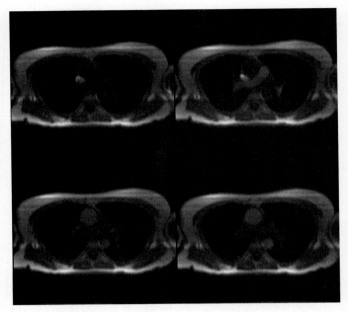

Figure 10.2 Axial images from a T1 weighted postcontrast timing bolus run. Sequential images demonstrate contrast flow through the SVC, pulmonary artery, and ultimately into the aorta.

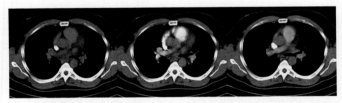

Figure 10.3 Bolus chase images performed prior to CT pulmonary angiogram. Sequential axial images demonstrate contrast flow within the SVC, right atrium, and pulmonary artery. Region of interest is placed over the pulmonary artery to measure Hounsfield units to determine when the level of opacification is sufficient for scanning.

milk for 24 h and discard it before resuming nursing her infant. However, with the recent understanding that the ingested dose of the contrast agent by the infant is much lower than that administered for routine imaging of infants, this fear has been abated. It is now recommended that after receiving IV iodinated contrast, the nursing mother be advised of the above and allowed to choose which option she is most comfortable with. As for MR contrast, since the ingested dose is even lower, no cessation of nursing is felt to be required.[10]

3. CONTRAST TIMING AND DOSING

To ensure the maximum contrast opacification of a selected vessel with the smallest possible dose of contrast, an optimized timing protocol is required. Multiple variables including but not exclusive to IV location, injection rate, cardiac output, and underlying vascular pathology contribute to a variable contrast transit time for each individual patient.[11,12] To accommodate this variability, two techniques are employed: test bolus and bolus chase.

The test bolus technique involves injecting a small amount of contrast while obtaining serial images with relatively low spatial resolution and high temporal resolution. For a CT examination the dose is usually 10 mL while for MR it is from 1 to 2 mL (Fig. 10.2). The amount of time needed for the bolus of contrast to arrive at a predetermined region of interest is measured, and this amount of time is taken into account in the imaging delay for the subsequent diagnostic study. The rate of the injection along with that of the saline flush is calculated based on the expected duration of the imaging study.

In the bolus chase method, the entire dose of contrast is injected and the onset of imaging is triggered by the arrival of the bolus in the region of interest. Serial images of this region of interest measure the amount of opacification and imaging is triggered when a predetermined threshold is reached. The diagnostic test usually begins after a short gap of 3 to 6 s (Fig. 10.3).

These techniques only have minimal advantages over each other. The primary advantage of the bolus chase technique is an overall decreased exam time, while with the test bolus technique the gap between the timing injection and exam is eliminated since the examination is started at the peak of the contrast bolus without potential delay which may occur when the scanner changes modes. This is only important in select applications such as carotid MRA and CTA where a relatively short window exists for imaging.

The dose of the administered contrast will depend on the total scan time and iodine concentration of the contrast agent. An injection rate delivering a total of 1 g of iodine per second is ideal for most cardiac and vascular applications.[13] A simple formula can be used to calculate the total dose of contrast required for an examination:

$$\text{Dose (mL)} = (\text{scan length [s]} + \text{scan delay [s]}) \times \text{injection rate(mL/s)} \quad \text{(Eq. 10.1)}$$

As illustrated in the formula, the overall scan time includes not only the length of the scan but also the delay to the start of the scan as may be encountered in the bolus chase technique.

4. PROTOCOLS

4.1. Neck and computed tomography angiography and magnetic resonance angiography evaluation

Ultrasonography is the mainstay by which the carotid arteries are studied clinically. CT and MRI are predominantly utilized as problem-solving tools. The majority of CT and MR angiographic studies of the neck are performed primarily to further define carotid disease detected by a duplex evaluation. There are two primary challenges for imaging of the carotid arteries. Due to the rapid venous filling from the cerebral circulation, the image acquisition must be completed in <10 s in most instances to avoid venous contamination.[14,15] The second issue is the relatively poor spatial resolutions of CTA and MRA compared to conventional angiography on which the criteria for the treatment of carotid disease is based. This latter issue is significant only in marginal cases.

The choice of CTA versus MRA is physician and institution specific. Although a CTA examination has the advantages of being more rapid and cost-effective, it is limited by the same dense calcifications that hinder accurate sonographic evaluation. In such cases, an MRI may be more capable of deriving an answer due to the inherent absence of signal from calcium. However, most MRA examinations have a lower spatial resolution leading to a higher number of cases in which the precise magnitude of stenosis may be indeterminate, particularly in smaller caliber vessels.

4.1.1. Computed tomography angiography technique

CTA of the carotid arteries is performed in the caudo-craniad direction to "follow" the contrast bolus and minimize the opacification of the adjacent jugular veins. The area imaged includes the aortic arch to the circle of Willis. The total contrast dose can be calculated with the above formula, but in general a small dose of 80 mL of contrast injected at 4 mL/s is adequate for nearly all patients. In plane, resolution should be at least 0.6 mm in order to better quantify the stenosis in the vessels, which range in between 3 and 6 mm in diameter on average.

4.1.2. Magnetic resonance angiography technique

Noncontrast time of flight technique was the most widely used technique until nearly a decade ago. Since then, contrast enhanced MRA has gained increasing acceptance due to fewer imaging artifacts. To minimize the acquisition time, the area imaged should be strictly restricted to the carotid arteries. To this end, a series of rapid 2D axial and coronal images are obtained (single-shot long echo train sequence or time of flight images with low spatial resolution and thick slices). Alternatively, a 3D time of flight scout can be used to perform the same function (Fig. 10.4).

Contrast is injected at 1 to 3 mL/s (depending on the T1 relaxivity of the agent), and imaging is performed either after a test bolus or with a bolus chase technique. More recently, time-resolved imaging with variable k-space sampling has been utilized to eliminate the need for a timing bolus and minimize possible venous contamination. If this technique is employed, then a minimum temporal resolution of 7 s is necessary (Fig. 10.5).

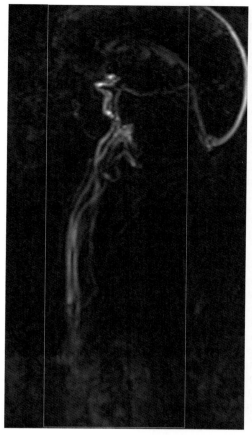

Figure 10.4 Three-dimensional time of flight scout image of the carotid arteries. Rectangular box indicates field of view for subsequent contrast-enhanced imaging.

4.2. Pulmonary angiography

Establishing the diagnosis of pulmonary emboli (PE) is critically important due to the relatively high prevalence in both the ill inpatient population as well as in the healthier outpatient population with acute onset of dyspnea. Before the advent of high speed CTA and MRA, diagnosis often relied on nuclear medicine studies, which are hampered by a myriad of artifacts and confounding variables, which limits their utility in excluding disease in many patients. Ventilation/perfusion testing is also expensive and time consuming, although for nearly a decade it was an improvement over invasive angiographic techniques, which have their own limitations.

Today, CTA remains the dominant technique by which PE are diagnosed, and although initially conventional angiography was

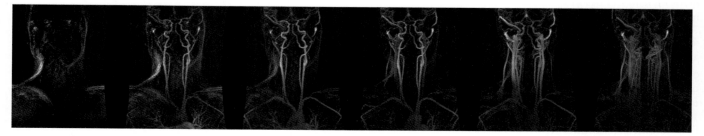

Figure 10.5 Time resolved contrast-enhanced examination of the neck demonstrates sequential enhancement of the arteries and then veins of the neck.

felt to represent the gold standard for this diagnosis, a paradigm shift is underway in support of the former. MRA has gained some acceptance for diagnosing PE; however, its inferior spatial resolution creates the potential for more false negative results. It is important to remember that when performing vessel analysis by MRA, the spatial resolution must be at least a factor of 3 greater than the vessel being evaluated.[16] Overall, MRA has a lower sensitivity for the detection of PE when compared with modern CTA[17,18]; however, if MR perfusion imaging is incorporated, the sensitivity increases to nearly 100% at the expense of a lower specificity.[18]

4.2.1. Computed tomography technique

CTA of the pulmonary arteries is very similar to the evaluation used for the thoracic aorta but with two critical differences. The first involves timing for the examination. When using either a test bolus or a bolus chase technique, the imaging delay after contrast injection must not exceed 6 s. This is in contrast to the normal delay to imaging of 10 s or more when timing for the systemic arteries. A second variation which is most important for slower machines and/or patients who cannot tolerate long breath holds is to image in the caudo-craniad orientation. This will minimize respiratory motion artifact that is most pronounced at the bases by imaging this part of the lungs first when the patient is more likely to maintain a breath-hold. This improved image quality at the bases should also increase sensitivity for detection, as more PE are located in the lung bases due to the increased pulmonary vascular flow. Caudo-craniad imaging can also decrease streak artifact related to dense contrast collection within the superior vena cava (SVC) by allowing more time for contrast to traverse through into the right atrium before this region is imaged. Utilizing the standard technique a small portion of examination will still be suboptimal due to poor contrast opacification of the pulmonary arteries. It is thought that this is most likely due to the deep inspiration the patient takes immediately before the scan begins. This inspiration may increase the venous return from the inferior vena cava and hence dilute the contrast bolus that arrives via the SVC. A solution is asking the patient to simply stop breathing instead of taking a deep inspiration before the scan begins.[19]

4.2.2. Magnetic resonance technique

MR pulmonary angiography is best obtained after a timing bolus or with a time-resolved sequence. The timing bolus acquisition must begin with 6 s of the start of the injection as described above. With both techniques several acquisitions are obtained so that not only can a filling defect be visualized, but an overall assessment of perfusion can also be made. The latter part is analogous to both conventional angiography and ventilation/perfusion imaging. It is again important to remember that a spatial resolution of 1.5 mm or less is required to obtain an adequate sensitivity for the detection of PE.

Steady state free precession (SSFP) imaging has been utilized in the imaging of PE recently[20] and has yielded good initial results; however, further validation with additional studies is required.

4.3. Thoracic aorta

Aortic emergencies demand accurate diagnosis and anatomical evaluation especially with the emergence of endovascular techniques as treatment options that often require precise measurements with respect to vessel origin and extent of pathology (Movie 10.1). Treatment of nonemergent disease similarly requires reproducible and precise measurements for management decisions. Evolving techniques for imaging of the coronary arteries that are often more mobile than the aorta have translated to improved

imaging of the thoracic aorta, which undergoes a similar pulsatile movement. This movement is most pronounced in the ascending aorta and decreases distally. It can change the diameter of the aorta by as much as 11% and can introduce artifacts that limit the sensitivity and specificity of diagnostic images (Figs. 10.6 and 10.7). It is, therefore, important to utilize cardiac gating for the evaluation of the thoracic aorta with either CTA or MRA.

During a cardiac gated CT, continuous ECG tracings are obtained along with image acquisition. Pulsatile motion is corrected for with either prospective or retrospective gating. In retrospective gating, images are obtained throughout the cardiac cycle, but in order to minimize motion artifact, images used for diagnosis are reconstructed from a specific interval during the cardiac cycle. In prospective gating, imaging is primarily obtained during a brief period centered on diastole. The latter technique will deposit less radiation in the patient.

4.3.1. Computed tomography angiography technique

The utilization of a gated technique in CT significantly increases the radiation exposure of the patient. In order to decrease the total dose to the patient, several variables can be adjusted. Since most current CT scanners utilize cardiac gating for evaluation of the coronary arteries, the detector collimation that is typically used is below 1 mm. This technique is not necessary for the evaluation of the aorta, and any collimation under 3 mm will be adequate for diagnostic imaging. As the collimation is increased the total

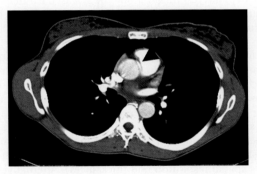

Figure 10.6 Axial image from a nongated CT angiogram of the chest demonstrates motion artifact producing an apparent linear filling defect along the medial aspect of the ascending aorta that could be misinterpreted as a dissection.

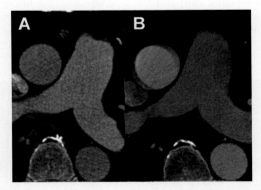

Figure 10.7 Axial images from gated (**A**) and nongated (**B**) CT angiograms of the chest in the same patient. Motion artifact in the nongated exam (**B**) can lead to inaccurate measurement of aortic size as well as false-positive diagnosis of mural thrombus and/or dissection.

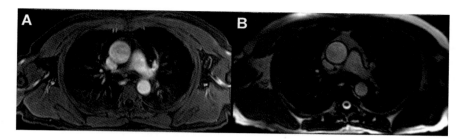

Figure 10.8 Axial images from an MRA of the chest. **A:** T1-weighted postcontrast sequence; **B:** gated noncontrast SSFP sequence.

amount of tube current required to produce a diagnostic image is reduced proportionally. Therefore, the total patient exposure can be reduced by half to one third compared with a conventional coronary CT. Additional factors, which can be modified, are equipment-specific and include beam modulation with the cardiac cycle, examination pitch, and prospective gating.

Nevertheless, nearly always, the total patient exposure is increased when compared to a nongated examination. When evaluating a patient who has had mediastinal surgery for a variety of reasons, gating is not required as the postoperative fibrosis decreases any aortic motion to a negligible level.

4.3.2. Magnetic resonance angiography technique

A routine MRA technique can used to evaluate the thoracic aorta, but it must be supplemented with a gated sequence to evaluate for dissection and/or aortic measurements. A gated balanced SSFP sequence is optimal for this purpose and studies have shown that these sequences have high sensitivity and specificity for diagnosis of acute disease.[21,22] This sequence can also be used alone in patients with renal insufficiency. The limitation of the noncontrast sequences at the current time is their limited spatial resolution and poor depiction of smaller vessels (Fig. 10.8). As with the CTA examination any technique which is utilized must have a cranio-caudad resolution of at least 5 mm and an in-slice resolution of <1 mm.

The contrast-enhanced examination is performed with a breath-hold sequence. A coronal 3D slab is acquired, as this affords the shortest path for acquiring the entire thoracic aorta and therefore offers the best compromise between speed and resolution (Fig. 10.9). Another option is to image the aorta in the "candy-cane" (oblique sagittal) view as this also affords a small slab for acquisition. Although the latter technique can afford a quicker scan time and/or a higher resolution, it requires higher operator skill as the slab must be positioned appropriately. In addition, only the origins of the great vessels are visualized with this technique (Fig. 10.10). Finally, it is theoretically possible to utilize cardiac gating for the contrast-enhanced portion of the

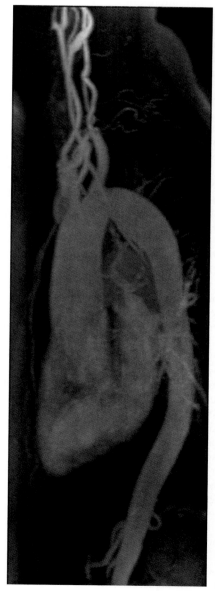

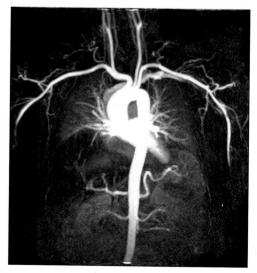

Figure 10.9 Coronal T1 spoiled gradient postcontrast sequence from an MRA of the chest.

Figure 10.10 "Candy cane" view—T1 gated postcontrast spoiled gradient sequence from an MRA of the chest.

examination, but it requires increasing the breath-hold duration and thus is not feasible in all patients.

An MRA examination has the capability of assessing the aortic valve in addition to the aorta, thereby broadening its impact on clinical management by documenting the presence of valvular disease.

4.4. Abdominal aorta

In contrast to the thoracic aorta, imaging of the abdominal aorta is less prone to motion degradation. Again, accurate depiction by either MRA or CTA is necessary both for diagnosis and treatment of aortic and visceral vessel disease such as renal artery stenosis. Due to the variety of the diseases and treatments available, it is in this region that CTA and MRA have their niches.

4.4.1. Computed tomography angiography technique

Evaluation of the abdominal aorta and visceral vessels by CT is a relatively simple matter. Every abdominal CT performed today, no matter the indication, can answer some basic questions such as aortic dimensions and presence of atherosclerotic disease. Accurate study of the visceral vessels, however, requires that more specific protocols are observed. To correctly evaluate the visceral vessels, which have a small diameter ranging between 3 and 6 mm, the slice collimation must be <1 mm.

4.4.2. Magnetic resonance angiography technique

As with CTA, the basic evaluation of the abdominal aorta is routine. Again several routine rapid gradient echo sequences may be used to image the larger vessels without contrast. In contrast-enhanced sequences, the abdominal aorta is imaged in the coronal plane to yield a rapid acquisition time. When evaluating the visceral vessels, velocity sensitive sequences may be used as supplements to attempt to better quantify stenosis. One such sequence is the 3D phase contrast which can be used to aid categorization of marginal cases of renal arterial stenosis.[23]

4.5. Peripheral vasculature

MRA and CTA of the lower extremities can be one of the most challenging noninvasive vascular evaluations. This is mostly due to a combination of two factors. The first is the proximity of the venous structures to their corresponding arteries, particularly in the calf where paired veins accompany all major vessels. The second is that limb ischemia can decrease the available scan time through arteriovenous shunting. On a practical level, a protocol which may work perfectly for a healthy test subject will usually fail secondary to venous contamination in a patient with peripheral vascular disease unless these factors are taken into consideration.

A complete assessment of the vasculature of the lower extremities will, at a minimum, start imaging at the level of the abdominal aorta (Fig. 10.11). For suspected embolic disease, however, the entire thoracoabdominal aorta must be assessed. The injection duration for either CTA or MRA must be at least 35 s,[24] with imaging being completed in 30 s to avoid venous contamination in a patient suffering from ischemic disease.

Current generation CT scanners can achieve high table speeds, which may outpace the contrast bolus. They also have a high spatial resolution that allows for an often adequate assessment of the underlying arterial tree even if there is filling of the adjacent venous structures. As with all CTA examinations, atherosclerotic calcifications can limit assessment of the small caliber vessels distally, and this pathology is often exaggerated in patients suffering from long-standing diabetes. In this situation an MRI examina-

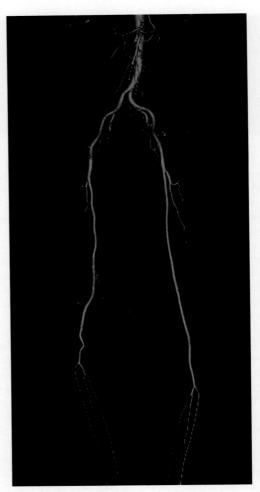

Figure 10.11 Three-dimensional reformatted image of a CT run-off. The area imaged typically includes the abdominal aorta to the level of the feet.

tion may have added value. It has been observed that CTA and MRA have the capability of visualizing more patent segments when compared with DSA.[25-27]

4.5.1. Computed tomography angiography technique

The ability of each individual machine to complete imaging in the above-mentioned 30 s time frame depends on the maximum pitch it can achieve. The pitch, in turn, will directly vary with the available collimation. On a practical level, if a machine is unable to accommodate this time limitation with the thinnest collimation, a higher collimation (i.e., thicker slices) may be used. The drawback is the added volume average artifact, which may hide underlying occlusive disease in a normal appearing vessel and vice versa. Similarly, an increase in pitch will increase blur along the z-axis, but this is of little clinical significance on a practical level.

Pitfalls of this technique are few but are most often seen in patients with large aortic aneurysms. In this group the contrast transit time to the toes is increased and significant dilution is also noted.

4.5.2. Magnetic resonance angiography technique

Most current MR scanners do not have the capability to image the peripheral vasculature in the above mentioned time limitations utilizing a standard cranio-caudad imaging approach as utilized in CT. Furthermore, due to its lower spatial resolution, venous contamination of the distal vessels renders the evaluation nondiagnostic in this region. There are several solutions to this problem but the most practical approach has been the implementation of a hybrid technique in which the distal (calf and foot) vessels are imaged prior to the remaining vessels. To avoid a difficult timing bolus in this segment, a time-resolved imaging technique is also implemented with variable k-space sampling (Fig. 10.12). The key lies in maintaining a temporal resolution of 10 s at this level. A contrast bolus of 5 to 10 mL is adequate to image this region.

Following the imaging of the distal vessels, a two-station bolus chase technique can be used to assess the inflow and femoropopliteal segments which can be completed in the standard 30 s time frame. The increase in available time can then be used to yield improved image quality in these two stations compared with the traditional three-station image technique.

4.6. Aortic stent graft evaluation

Evaluation of a patient who has had an endovascular prosthesis placed for an aortic aneurysm requires special attention due to the frequent rate of endoleaks and their variable treatment. An initial noncontrast examination is required to localize the calcifications on CT and high signal intensity thrombus on MR within the excluded aneurysm. These findings can confound evaluation for an endoleak once contrast is administered. A routine CTA or MRA can then be performed followed by a delayed examination to note any pooling of contrast (Fig. 10.13 and Movie 10.2).

On a practical level, in the absence of aneurysm enlargement, the presence of an endoleak is only important in establishing more frequent follow-up of the patient. Therefore, in the patient who cannot receive contrast, a noncontrast CT is sufficient for determining the aneurysm size. MRA is better at detecting endoleaks than CTA but is a more expensive and time-consuming examination. It is, therefore, utilized as a problem-solving tool in patients with an enlarging aneurysm but unknown or unclear source of endoleak. In this situation time-resolved imaging with variable k-space sampling adds useful information (Fig. 10.14).[28]

4.6.1. Stents and metallic artifacts

Many follow-up examinations require evaluating patients who have had metallic implants placed either as a result of prior endovascular therapy or secondary to other diseases. These devices pose two distinct challenges. The first is the need to assess in-stent patency on follow-up examinations, while the second is the difficulty in evaluating vessels adjacent to dense prostheses secondary to metallic artifact.

4.6.2. Computed tomography technique

There are few variables that can be modified in the acquisition of a CT examination to reduce metallic artifact. The most effective is to increase tube current. The major drawback to this technique is the proportional increase in the deposited radiation. A second

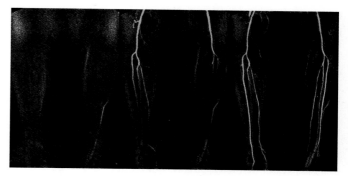

Figure 10.12 Coronal time resolved T1 postcontrast sequences from an MRA of the lower extremities demonstrating the distal popliteal artery as well as the anterior tibial, posterior tibial, and peroneal arteries bilaterally.

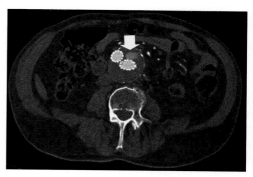

 Figure 10.13 (**Movie 10.2**). CT angiogram of the abdomen and pelvis performed in a patient who had undergone stent graft repair for an abdominal aortic aneurysm. Axial image demonstrates pooling of contrast within the aneurysm sac consistent with an endoleak (*arrow*).

problem is that in order to generate the increased tube current, scan time may need to be prolonged to allow for heat dissipation from the X-ray tube.

Other variables which are not as easily modified but may help reduce artifact include increasing tube voltage and decreasing collimation. The available range of tube voltages on clinically available machines has scarce practical effect in the routine practice. A decrease in collimation may help eliminate a small amount of artifact. Reconstruction of images with thicker slices and smoother kernels will also lead to a decrease in artifact, particularly if related to noise secondary to photon starvation.[29]

4.6.3. Magnetic resonance technique

There are many more variables that can be modified on an MR scanner to deal with metallic artifact than with CT. Unfortunately, despite these modifications, on average an MR examination is more prone to image degradation from metallic artifact than CT. Although spin echo techniques with short echo times (TEs) are

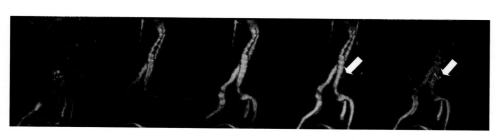

Figure 10.14 Coronal time resolved postcontrast T1 weighted sequences in a patient who had undergone stent graft repair for an abdominal aortic aneurysm demonstrates pooling of contrast within the aneurysm sac consistent with an endoleak (*arrow*).

best at decreasing metallic artifacts, they are not well suited for postcontrast imaging. To decrease the metallic artifact while utilizing a gradient echo sequence a few variables may be modified. The key is to remember to decrease the TE. Since a routine postcontrast study should already be optimized for an ultra-short TE, which also yields the best contrast after administration of a gadolinium chelate, there is usually little room for modification.

An increase in bandwidth may allow for a lower TE. Decreasing voxel size may also aid in decreasing the presence of metallic artifact.[29] As a final measure, when assessing aneurysm size, it may be useful to switch to a spin echo (black-blood) imaging sequence to assess vessel diameter. Finally, despite their many advantages, moving to a higher field strength (i.e., 1.5 to 3 T) will increase the metallic susceptibility artifact.

4.7. Venous examination

Most routine venous evaluation can and should be performed with grayscale and color duplex sonography. When necessary, for instance, in the central venous system or in the patient whose sonographic exam is limited, evaluation of the venous system by CT and MRI is less challenging than most arteriographic examinations. Due to inability of current techniques to achieve a high contrast concentration in the venous system, assessment is limited to the larger caliber veins. Since a lower concentration of contrast is required to alter the signal in MR when compared with CT, in general, MR postcontrast venography will be less prone to artifact and less sensitive to timing issues. Postcontrast imaging with both modalities is similar in that a large dose of contrast is injected rapidly and imaged for 2 to 3 min afterward.

The contrast is injected at a rapid rate (3 to 5 mL/s for CT and 2 to 3 mL/s for MR) to achieve a high venous concentration after the bolus has passed the porous capillary beds and lost a significant fraction of its concentration. MR also offers noncontrast techniques in patients who cannot tolerate IV contrast agents.

4.7.1. Computed tomography venography

Unlike CT arteriography, a large bolus of contrast is required for consistent successful evaluation (120 to 140 mL)[30] with every case regardless of the duration of scan time. Imaging is simply commenced 2 to 3 min after injection has been started to minimize mixing artifact which can simulate venous thrombosis. Lower limb CT venography has been routinely combined with PE studies to elucidate a source of embolus.[31,32]

4.7.2. Magnetic resonance venography

There are three basic methods for assessing veins on MR. The traditional approach, referred to as a time-of-flight technique, utilizes flow dynamics to image veins. In this type of sequence, signal within the slice is nulled and inflowing blood generates signal necessary for imaging. In general, since arteries and veins have opposite directions of flow, an additional saturation band can be added to null out the signal from the arteries. This technique is prone to flow artifacts from either too rapid or slow flow simulating a filling defect. Therefore, the technique has a high negative predictive value but can sometimes simulate thrombus leading to, at a minimum, reporting constraints.

A second, contrast enhanced technique is very similar to CT venography. Contrast at a single or double dose is injected and imaging is begun 2 to 3 min afterward. Recently, a new class of intravascular contrast agents have been introduced which maintain a high intravascular concentration by not diffusing out of the capillary bed. The benefits of such agents for venous imaging are obvious; however, they have yet to gained FDA approval.

A third technique is based on SSFP imaging. This subgroup of techniques relies on the high T2 signal intensity of blood to generate an image. The pitfall of this technique lies in the fact that the signal characteristics of thrombus can vary depending on its age, demonstrating both high T1 and high T2 signal intensities depending on the phase of thrombus formation. Imaging based on these sequences can, therefore, lead to the inadvertent masking of thrombus as these sequences yield images of mixed T2/T1 signal intensity. This drawback has been confirmed in several studies.[33,34]

5. FUTURE DIRECTIONS

There are two goals in vascular imaging which require further development. The first is resolution (both contrast and spatial). Although the spatial resolutions of both CTA and MRA have seen dramatic improvements, the goal of plaque visualization and characterization has only been partially met. We know from pathological studies that there are several stages and pathways through which atherosclerotic plaques develop and potentially regress. To date, most noninvasive imaging modalities do not have the required spatial and contrast resolutions to routinely monitor individual plaques in most locations. The exceptions include superficial regions such as the carotids and/or femoral arteries. Even in these locations special imaging sequences and equipment are required to obtain a reasonably reproducible answer. Reproducibility is mandatory for monitoring the effect of new therapies noninvasively. Experimental studies with MRA and combined PET/CTA have yielded early results which are promising.[35]

Higher field strength magnets such as 3 T scanners can produce images with twice the signal strength. This can then be utilized to increase spatial or temporal resolution at the operator's discretion.

Cardiovascular pulsatility remains a challenge for both CTA and MRA despite advances in the field. Non-Cartesian image acquisition has successfully been applied to neurological applications to reduce motion, and they are being introduced to cardiovascular applications.[36,37]

The idea of atherosclerotic disease as a systemic illness has gained wide acceptance. In the past, focused examination of individual vascular territories has been used to predict cardiovascular risk. With the advent of total body MRA and CTA, it became possible to evaluate the entirety of the vascular system in one examination.[38,39] Whole body vascular evaluation entails combining assessment of the thoracoabdominal aorta as well as the distal vessels. Potential benefits may also be realized from screening patients with atherosclerotic disease due to the frequent coexistence of multiple regions of clinically significant pathology.[40]

Implementation of this examination is easiest with CTA where a modern machine with an adequate pitch can easily complete the examination. The only required modification is the addition of a time interval corresponding to the time it would take to image the thoracic aorta separately to the traditional 30 s allotted for the evaluation of the lower extremities. This will avoid outpacing the contrast in the distal segments. In addition, since most subjects do not have ischemic distal vessel disease the total scan time may be increased to 60 s.

Although MRA evaluation is possible in this setting with multiple coil changes and injections, on a practical level multiple imaging coil inputs are required to perform this examination in a reasonable fashion with a single contrast bolus. Again since ischemic disease rarely coexists in a patient undergoing an initial evaluation for vasculitis, the total time available for imaging is adequate for a traditional multistation bolus chase technique.

When evaluating vasculitis, MRA holds two distinct advantages. The lack of ionizing radiation allows for repeated follow-ups without fear of danger to patients who are often younger than the average patient with atherosclerotic disease. MRA also allows for a more accurate evaluation of the degree of enhancement of lesions and medial thickening which can guide clinical management.[41,42]

Finally, as touched on briefly previously, new contrast agents are under development. Agents, such as MS-325(Vasovist; Schering), that remain largely in the intravascular space promise to allow both first pass steady state imaging with low administered doses. These agents also hold promise for improved venous imaging.

REFERENCES

1. Bettmann MA, Heeren T, Greenfield A, et al. Adverse events with radiographic contrast agents: Results of the SCVIR Contrast Agent Registry. *Radiology.* 1997;203(3):611–620.
2. Rudnick MR, Goldfarb S, Wexler L, et al. Nephrotoxicity of ionic and nonionic contrast media in 1,196 patients: A randomized trial. The Iohexol Cooperative Study. *Kidney Int.* 1995;47(1):254–261.
3. Solomon R, Werner C, Mann D, et al. Effects of saline, mannitol, and furosemide to prevent acute decreases in renal function induced by radiocontrast agents. *N Engl J Med.* 1994;331(21):1416–1420.
4. Mueller C, Buerkle G, Buettner HJ, et al. Prevention of contrast media-associated nephropathy: Randomized comparison of 2 hydration regimens in 1,620 patients undergoing coronary angioplasty. *Arch Intern Med.* 2002;162(3):329–336.
5. Merten GJ, Burgess WP, Rittase RA, et al. Prevention of contrast-induced nephropathy with sodium bicarbonate: An evidence-based protocol. *Crit Pathw Cardiol.* 2004;3(3):138–143.
6. Nallamothu BK, Shojania KG, Saint S, et al. Is acetylcysteine effective in preventing contrast-related nephropathy? A meta-analysis. *Am J Med.* 2004;117(12):938–947.
7. Toprak O. Conflicting and new risk factors for contrast induced nephropathy. *J Urol.* 2007;178(6):2277–2283.
8. Bettmann MA. Frequently asked questions: Iodinated contrast agents. *Radiographics.* 2004;24 (Suppl.1):S3–S10.
9. Martin DR. Nephrogenic system fibrosis: A radiologist's practical perspective. *Eur J Radiol.* 2008;66(2):220–224.
10. Radiology ACo. Manual On Contrast Media (Version 6). American College of Radiology (ACR); 2008.
11. Bae KT, Heiken JP, Brink JA. Aortic and hepatic peak enhancement at CT: Effect of contrast medium injection rate–pharmacokinetic analysis and experimental porcine model. *Radiology.* 1998;206(2):455–464.
12. Bae KT, Heiken JP, Brink JA. Aortic and hepatic contrast medium enhancement at CT. Part II. Effect of reduced cardiac output in a porcine model. *Radiology.* 1998;207(3):657–662.
13. Becker CR, Hong C, Knez A, et al. Optimal contrast application for cardiac 4-detector-row computed tomography. *Invest Radiol.* 2003;38(11):690–694.
14. Kim JK, Farb RI, Wright GA. Test bolus examination in the carotid artery at dynamic gadolinium-enhanced MR angiography. *Radiology.* 1998;206(1):283–289.
15. Herold T, Paetzel C, Volk M, et al. Contrast-enhanced magnetic resonance angiography of the carotid arteries: Influence of injection rates and volumes on arterial-venous transit time. *Invest Radiol.* 2004;39(2):65–72.
16. Westenberg JJ, van der Geest RJ, Wasser MN, et al. Vessel diameter measurements in gadolinium contrast-enhanced three-dimensional MRA of peripheral arteries. *Magn Reson Imaging.* 2000;18(1):13–22.
17. Pleszewski B, Chartrand-Lefebvre C, Qanadli SD, et al. Gadolinium-enhanced pulmonary magnetic resonance angiography in the diagnosis of acute pulmonary embolism: A prospective study on 48 patients. *Clin Imaging.* 2006;30(3):166–172.
18. Kluge A, Luboldt W, Bachmann G. Acute pulmonary embolism to the subsegmental level: Diagnostic accuracy of three MRI techniques compared with 16-MDCT. *Am J Roentgenol.* 2006;187(1):W7–W14.
19. Wittram C, Yoo AJ. Transient interruption of contrast on CT pulmonary angiography: Proof of mechanism. *J Thorac Imaging.* 2007;22(2):125–129.
20. Kluge A, Muller C, Hansel J, et al. Real-time MR with True FISP for the detection of acute pulmonary embolism: Initial clinical experience. *Eur Radiol.* 2004;14(4):709–718.
21. Pereles FS, McCarthy RM, Baskaran V, et al. Thoracic aortic dissection and aneurysm: Evaluation with nonenhanced true FISP MR angiography in less than 4 minutes. *Radiology.* 2002;223(1):270–274.
22. Francois CJ, Tuite D, Deshpande V, et al. Unenhanced MR angiography of the thoracic aorta: Initial clinical evaluation. *Am J Roentgenol.* 2008;190(4):902–906.
23. Schoenberg SO, Knopp MV, Londy F, et al. Morphologic and functional magnetic resonance imaging of renal artery stenosis: A multireader tricenter study. *J Am Soc Nephrol.* 2002;13(1):158–169.
24. Fleischmann D, Rubin GD. Quantification of intravenously administered contrast medium transit through the peripheral arteries: Implications for CT angiography. *Radiology.* 2005 ;236(3):1076–1082.
25. Edwards AJ, Wells IP, Roobottom CA. Multidetector row CT angiography of the lower limb arteries: A prospective comparison of volume-rendered techniques and intra-arterial digital subtraction angiography. *Clin Radiol.* 2005;60(1):85–95.
26. Ota H, Takase K, Igarashi K, et al. MDCT compared with digital subtraction angiography for assessment of lower extremity arterial occlusive disease: Importance of reviewing cross-sectional images. *Am J Roentgenol.* 2004;182(1):201–209.
27. Martin ML, Tay KH, Flak B, et al. Multidetector CT angiography of the aortoiliac system and lower extremities: A prospective comparison with digital subtraction angiography. *Am J Roentgenol.* 2003;180(4):1085–1091.
28. Cohen EI, Weinreb DB, Siegelbaum RH, et al. Time-resolved MR angiography for the classification of endoleaks after endovascular aneurysm repair. *J Magn Reson Imaging.* 2008;27(3):500–503.
29. Lee MJ, Kim S, Lee SA, et al. Overcoming artifacts from metallic orthopedic implants at high-field-strength MR imaging and multi-detector CT. *Radiographics.* 2007;27(3):791–803.
30. Sheth S, Fishman EK. Imaging of the inferior vena cava with MDCT. *Am J Roentgenol.* 2007;189(5):1243–1251.
31. Stein PD, Fowler SE, Goodman LR, et al. Multidetector computed tomography for acute pulmonary embolism. *N Engl J Med.* 2006 ;354(22):2317–2327.
32. Goodman LR, Stein PD, Matta F, et al. CT venography and compression sonography are diagnostically equivalent: Data from PIOPED II. *Am J Roentgenol.* 2007;189(5):1071–1076.
33. Smith CS, Sheehy N, McEniff N, et al. Magnetic resonance portal venography: Use of fast-acquisition true FISP imaging in the detection of portal vein thrombosis. *Clin Radiol.* 2007;62(12):1180–1188.
34. Pedrosa I, Morrin M, Oleaga L, et al. Is true FISP imaging reliable in the evaluation of venous thrombosis? *Am J Roentgenol.* 2005;185(6):1632–1640.
35. Sanz J, Fayad ZA. Imaging of atherosclerotic cardiovascular disease. *Nature.* 2008;451(7181):953–957.
36. Yeh EN, Stuber M, McKenzie CA, et al. Inherently self-calibrating non-Cartesian parallel imaging. *Magn Reson Med.* 2005;54(1):1–8.
37. Bansmann PM, Priest AN, Muellerleile K, et al. MRI of the coronary vessel wall at 3T: Comparison of radial and cartesian k-space sampling. *Am J Roentgenol.* 2007;188(1):70–74.
38. Fenchel M, Scheule AM, Stauder NI, et al. Atherosclerotic disease: Whole-body cardiovascular imaging with MR system with 32 receiver channels and total-body surface coil technology—initial clinical results. *Radiology.* 2005;238(1):280–291.
39. Fenchel M, Scheule AM, Stauder NI, et al. Atherosclerotic disease: Whole-body cardiovascular imaging with MR system with 32 receiver channels and total-body surface coil technology–initial clinical results. *Radiology.* 2006;238(1):280–291.
40. Goyen M, Herborn CU, Kroger K,et al. Total-body 3D magnetic resonance angiography influences the management of patients with peripheral arterial occlusive disease. *Eur Radiol.* 2006;16(3):685–691.
41. Choe YH, Kim DK, Koh EM, et al. Takayasu arteritis: Diagnosis with MR imaging and MR angiography in acute and chronic active stages. *J Magn Reson Imaging.* 1999;10(5):751–757.
42. Steeds RP, Mohiaddin R. Takayasu arteritis: Role of cardiovascular magnetic imaging. *Int J Cardiol.* 2006;109(1):1–6.

Three-Dimensional Echocardiographic Imaging

11

Victor Mor-Avi
Lissa Sugeng
Roberto M. Lang

1. INTRODUCTION

One of the most significant developments of the last decade in ultrasound imaging of the heart was the introduction of three-dimensional (3D) imaging and its evolution from slow and labor-intense off-line reconstruction to real-time volumetric imaging. This imaging modality currently provides valuable clinical information that empowers echocardiography with new levels of confidence in the diagnosis of heart disease.[1] The growing availability of real-time 3D echocardiographic (RT3DE) technology, its ease of use, and its multiple attractive features have sparked significant interest in the research community, resulting in multiple publications, most of which have endorsed RT3DE imaging for clinical use by demonstrating its unique capabilities in different clinical scenarios. One major advantage of seeing the additional dimension is the improvement in the accuracy of the evaluation of cardiac chamber volumes. Another benefit of the 3D imaging is the "surgeon's views" of cardiac valves capable of demonstrating a variety of pathologies in a unique noninvasive manner. The most recent clinically significant addition is matrix array transesophageal echocardiography (TEE), which provides images of unprecedented quality that aid surgeons and interventional cardiologists in planning and guiding procedures and evaluating outcomes. This chapter describes the major technological developments in 3D echocardiography as well as some of the recent literature that has provided the scientific basis for its clinical use.

1.1. Historical perspective

From the day ultrasound imaging technology provided the first insight into the human heart, our diagnostic capabilities increased exponentially as a result of our growing knowledge and developing technology. Nevertheless, the limitations of two-dimensional (2D) echocardiographic imaging in the interrogation of the 3D human heart have been long recognized. Geometric modeling of ventricular volumes from one or two cross-sectional planes proved inaccurate in the presence of aneurysms or asymmetric ventricles.[2,3] In addition, even in symmetric ventricles, the use of foreshortened views to improve endocardial definition turned out to be an additional source of error when measuring ventricular volumes.[4,5] Similarly, despite the major role echocardiography has played in the evaluation of valvular heart disease, its 2D nature has limited the accuracy of the assessment of valve geometry and function. The recognition of these issues has driven developers of ultrasound imaging technology into a journey of relentless search for ways to break through the invisible walls of this seemingly inherent planar world and develop new tools for online 3D visualization of cardiac anatomy.

Initial results of off-line 3D reconstruction from serial ECG-gated acquisitions of multiple 2D planes were reported in the early 1980s.[6,7] This multiplane acquisition strategy was implemented in three different approaches based on parallel linear motion,[8] rotation,[9] and free-hand sectioning with electromagnetic or acoustic locating devices capable of registering transducer position and spatial orientation.[10] While parallel linear motion was found less efficient because of the difficulties in maintaining adequate acoustic windows throughout the scan, rotation of the imaging plane from a fixed transducer position was implemented and widely used with transesophageal imaging. The free-hand scanning method proved to be a useful option for transthoracic imaging, since it used existing transducers and allowed integration of information obtained from multiple acoustic windows from which the structures of interest could be optimally visualized. Importantly, all these multiplane acquisitions required ECG- and respiratory gating to ensure that all planes were acquired at the same phase of the respiratory cycle with the heart in an identical position within the chest, for each consecutive acquisition.

Later, a different approach was pursued in order to eliminate the need for tedious multiplane acquisition and time-consuming 3D reconstruction altogether. This approach is based on real-time volumetric imaging (Fig. 11.1), which utilizes transducers containing arrays of piezoelectric elements capable of scanning pyramidal volumes, rather than the conventional 2D phased-array transducers that scan a fan-shaped sector in a single plane. Initial reports on the use of sparse array transducers date back to the early 1990s.[11,12] Processing the information generated by these transducers required computational power that was beyond what was available at the time. To overcome this limitation, a dedicated system was developed based on parallel processing that allowed for the first time real-time 3D ultrasound imaging of the heart. Such systems were used in several academic centers to demonstrate the additional benefits of real-time 3D imaging in multiple clinical scenarios.[13,14] Importantly, real-time volumetric imaging allowed fast acquisition of pyramidal datasets during a single breath-hold, without the need for off-line reconstruction, thus eliminating radial artifacts known to have adversely affected the rather lengthy multiplane acquisition and reconstruction methodology.

Significant advances in ultrasound, electronic, and computer technology has thrust the field forward toward the development of a fully-sampled matrix array transducer and on-line 3D display of rendered images, as well as software for postprocessing and quantification. The ease of data acquisition, the ability to image the entire heart nearly in real time, as well as the ability

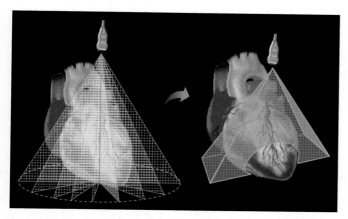

Figure 11.1 At first, 3D echocardiography was performed from a sequential multiplane acquisition approach, gated to ECG and respiration (**left**). This approach was tedious, time-consuming, and prone to radial artifacts. Recently, this approach was replaced by real-time volumetric imaging that allows acquisition of a pyramid of data (**right**) using matrix array transducers.

to focus on a specific structure in a single beat, have brought 3D echocardiography closer to routine clinical use. Within several years of its inception, "realtime" 3D technology has sparked new endeavors in research and is making strides on its way to become part of routine clinical echocardiography.

Most recent advances in ultrasound transducer technology have allowed the miniaturization of matrix array transducers, which was achieved by fitting thousands of piezoelectric elements into the tip of the TEE transducer and using integrated circuits that perform most of the beam forming within the transducer. These technological advances have simplified the connection between the transducer and the imaging system, resulting in a reduction of the size of the connecting cable and significantly lowering power consumption, thus allowing real-time 3D TEE imaging that provides on-line display of unique 3D views of unparalleled quality for optimal visualization of cardiac structures.

2. TECHNICAL CONSIDERATIONS AND LIMITATIONS

With the numerous advantages matrix array transducers offer the clinicians, this technology has its limitations. While some of these limitations can potentially be minimized as computer technology continues evolving, thus allowing higher speeds of processing, others are intrinsic to the nature of ultrasound imaging. For instance, since there is no technological solution to expedite the motion of sound waves in the human body, the spatial resolution of RT3DE images is lower than that of the 2D images generated by state of the art imaging systems. Moreover, because of the finite speed of sound, until recently commercial imaging systems were not fast enough to scan the entire heart throughout the cardiac cycle and create 3D images with high temporal resolution in real time. Two different approaches were implemented to overcome this limitation: (a) narrow-angled acquisition that improves the temporal resolution at the expense of reduced scan volume, which is suitable for targeted zoomed acquisition of anatomic structures such as valves or septal defects, and (b) sequential ECG-gated acquisition of subvolumes over several cardiac cycles, which are then combined into a single "full-volume" dataset that can contain images of the entire left ventricle. Most recently, scanners capable of capturing the entire left ventricle in a single cardiac cycle became commercially available.

Nevertheless, it is important to remember that RT3DE imaging is unique among all cardiac imaging modalities in that it provides dynamic 3D images of the beating human heart virtually on-line, without any off-line postprocessing. In this regard, the relatively low spatial and temporal resolution of RT3DE imaging is a trade-off for its dynamic 3D nature.

3. VENTRICULAR GEOMETRY AND FUNCTIONAL ANALYSIS

3.1. Left ventricular volume and ejection fraction

A well-established advantage of 3D imaging over cross-sectional slices of the heart is the improvement in the accuracy of the evalu-

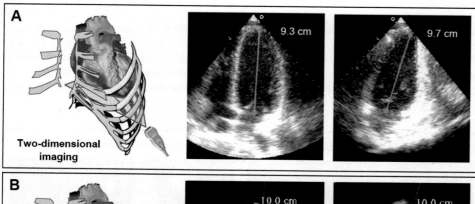

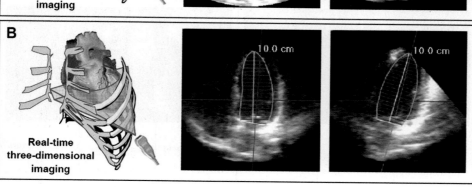

A

Two-dimensional imaging

9.3 cm

9.7 cm

B

Real-time three-dimensional imaging

10.0 cm

10.0 cm

Figure 11.2 Imaging the left ventricle from an apical window frequently results in foreshortened views. This is because imaging plane obtained through the intercostal space nearest to LV apex (**top, left**) may not necessarily contain the true LV apex. Tilting the transducer to improve endocardial visualization can result in even more anatomically oblique views, in which the long-axis dimension of the left ventricle is foreshortened (**top, right**). With 3D imaging from the same transducer position (**bottom, left**), the entire left ventricle is included in the full volume scan, which allows by the use of cropping identification of the anatomically correct, nonforeshortened views for analysis (**bottom, right**). In this example, the long-axis dimension was longer in both apical views when measured from the 3D dataset. LV, left ventricular.

ation of left ventricular (LV) volumes and ejection fraction (EF) by potentially eliminating the need for geometric modeling, which is inaccurate in the presence of aneurysms, asymmetric ventricles or wall motion abnormalities, and the errors caused by foreshortened apical views even in symmetric ventricles (Fig. 11.2). The value of RT3DE imaging in this context has been demonstrated by multiple studies that compared RT3DE volume measurements to widely accepted reference techniques, including radionuclide ventriculography and cardiac magnetic resonance (CMR).[14–18] These studies and others have demonstrated higher levels of agreement between the RT3DE approach and the respective reference technique, when compared to conventional 2DE methodology. Additionally, RT3DE measurements were found to be more reproducible than 2DE,[5,16,17] and in some studies even as reproducible as CMR.[19]

The improved accuracy and reproducibility of RT3DE-based LV volume and EF measurements are of vital importance, because clinical decision making heavily relies on these measurements in multiple clinical scenarios. Also, these findings translate into smaller numbers of patients required to test a hypothesis, promising to result in significant savings in future studies aimed at assessing the effects of new drugs. Indeed, this trend was demonstrated by a recent follow-up study in patients postmyocardial infraction (MI), in which similar to CMR, serial RT3DE measurements had low test–retest variability and were thus able to detect with confidence subtle changes in LV volumes over time that were not detectable by 2D echocardiography.[20] Similar findings were described in another study aimed at risk stratification in patients post MI and patients with heart failure.[21]

Nevertheless, despite the high correlation with the CMR reference values and the high reproducibility, several studies have reported that RT3DE-derived LV volumes were significantly underestimated.[5,19,20,22–26] Different possible explanations have been offered that focused mostly on intertechnique acquisition and analysis differences, but none of the studies were able to conclusively identify the main sources of error. Importantly, the degree of underestimation varied widely between these single-center studies from a few mL to considerable biases as high as 30% of the measured values. One possible explanation for the variable degrees of underestimation is that RT3DE datasets were analyzed differently by different investigators. Indeed, there are two approaches that are commonly used for LV quantification from RT3DE datasets (Fig. 11.3). One approach is based on selecting from a pyramidal RT3DE dataset two anatomically correct nonforeshortened 2D views, from which LV volume is calculated using a biplane approximation,[5,27] same as used with 2D imaging (Fig. 11.3, left). While this 3D-guided biplane technique can min-

imize LV foreshortening, it still relies on geometric modeling to calculate volumes, and is thus likely to be inaccurate in distorted ventricles. In an attempt to minimize this problem, investigators used a larger number of planes to interpolate LV endocardial surface[26, 28] with partial success. A different approach to quantify LV volumes from RT3DE datasets, which was recently implemented in commercial analysis software, is based on semiautomated detection of LV endocardial surface followed by calculation of the volume inside this surface either for selected phases, such as end-systole and end-diastole, or throughout the cardiac cycle[29] (Fig. 11.3, right). Not being affected by LV foreshortening and geometric modeling, not surprisingly this approach was found to be more accurate,[5,17,26] irrespective of wall motion abnormalities[19] and distorted ventricular shape.[26]

Nevertheless, even direct volumetric analysis, which is the more accurate of the two techniques, was found to significantly underestimate LV volumes, threatening to undermine the usefulness of RT3DE evaluation of LV size and function. To investigate this issue in depth, we recently conducted a multicenter study, which was designed to identify the potential sources of error and determine their relative contributions to the underestimation of RT3DE-derived LV volumes.[30] This study demonstrated that the spatial resolution of RT3DE images is not sufficiently high to differentiate between myocardial tissue and endocardial trabeculae, which were as a result excluded from the LV cavity, different to the CMR reference which in most patients clearly depicts the trabeculae and by convention includes them in the LV cavity (Fig. 11.4). The results of this study underscored the need for unified guidelines for tracing LV endocardial boundary in order to obtain RT3DE measurements of LV volumes, comparable to the current standard reference CMR technique.

3.2. Left ventricular mass

As opposed to LV volume measurements that require accurate identification of the endocardial boundaries, LV mass measurements rely on epicardial visualization, which is known to be even more challenging. This difficulty is in addition to inaccurate modeling and foreshortening. Nevertheless, in our initial studies aimed at RT3DE evaluation of LV mass by either the 3D-guided biplane technique[27] or the volumetric analysis,[31] the accuracy and reproducibility of RT3DE estimates were higher than those of the traditional M-mode and 2D techniques. More recently, these observations were confirmed in a large group of patients with concentric LV hypertrophy.[32] Moreover, volumetric measurements of LV mass were found to correlate highly with CMR reference values in patients with wall motion abnormalities,[19] and in patients

Figure 11.3 Comparison chart for two approaches to LV volume measurement from RT3DE datasets: 3D-guided biplane analysis (**left**) and direct volumetric analysis (**right**). See text for details. RT3DE, real-time 3D echocardiographic.

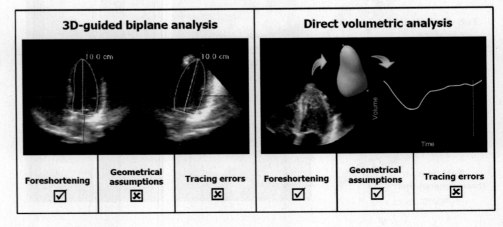

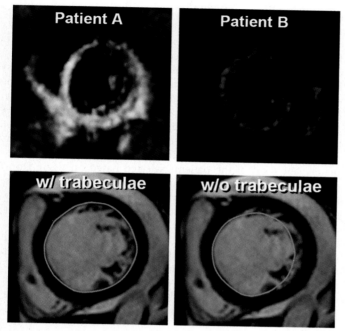

Figure 11.4 Top: Example of short-axis cut-planes extracted from RT3DE datasets, while in one patient (**left**) trabeculae can be well visualized and clearly differentiated from the myocardium, in another patient (**right**) the spatial resolution of the RT3DE image is not sufficient to provide this kind of detail. **Bottom:** Example of a short-axis CMR slice with endocardial surface traced to include trabeculae in the LV cavity (**left**) and, in a separate analysis, to exclude them (**right**) from the LV cavity. CMR, cardiac magnetic resonance. (Modified from Mor-Avi V, Jenkins C, Kuhl HP, et al. Real-time 3D echocardiographic quantification of left ventricular volumes: Multicenter study for validation with magnetic resonance imaging and investigation of sources of error. *J Am Coll Cardiol Imaging.* 2008;1:413–423.)

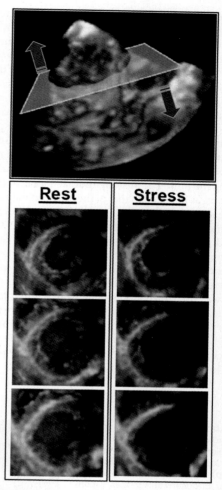

Figure 11.5 Off-line viewing of real-time 3D data obtained during dobutamine stress test. These datasets can be used to extract multiple short-axis views at different levels of the left ventricle (**top**). Example of such views extracted from datasets obtained at rest (**bottom, left**) and during peak dobutamine stress (**bottom, right**).

with abnormally shaped ventricles secondary to congenital heart disease.[33] While the former study described a considerable negative bias, the latter reported only minimal biases. Similar to the inconsistencies with LV volume measurements, these differences are likely to be due to differences in strategies for identifying and tracing the endo- and epicardial boundaries. Nevertheless, as guidelines for the quantification of LV volumes, EF and mass from RT3DE images are better defined, this methodology will become suitable for daily clinical use.

3.3. Assessment of regional LV wall motion

The ability of RT3DE imaging to almost instantaneously capture the entire heart into a dataset that contains the complete dynamic information on LV chamber, from which the ventricle can be viewed in any arbitrary plane, suggested that RT3DE datasets are suitable for simultaneous analysis of regional wall motion in all LV segments. In a recent study,[34] RT3DE-derived regional EF was validated against a CMR reference, and the feasibility of its use as an index of regional LV function was tested for objective detection of wall motion abnormalities. Moreover, the fast volumetric imaging of the entire heart has pointed at its potential usefulness in the context of exercise stress testing where the speed of acquisition of multiple views is crucial.[35,36] More recently, RT3DE imaging was used with dobutamine stress testing.[37] An important advantage of the RT3DE approach in this context is its ability to extract off-line multiple views of the ventricle (Fig. 11.5), which can help in determining the extent of wall motion abnormality as well as in ruling out artifacts frequently noted in standard imaging

planes due to limited endocardial visualization. This study demonstrated that RT3DE datasets contained sufficient information for the interpretation of stress tests, which allowed accurate diagnosis of myocardial ischemia compared to SPECT myocardial perfusion imaging. Another recent study[38] showed high levels of agreement with 2DE-based wall motion scores.

3.4. Assessment of LV dyssynchrony

Tissue Doppler imaging (TDI) is currently considered the standard technique for the selection of patients for CRT based on its ability to quantify intraventricular dyssynchrony. Despite the excellent temporal resolution of TDI, this methodology has several limitations, including: (a) inability to assess multiple myocardial segments in different planes simultaneously, (b) angle dependency that translates into the evaluation of the longitudinal motion only, and (c) inability to reliably depict wall motion in the apical segments. In addition, despite the wealth of TDI-based dyssynchrony research, different investigators have used different analysis techniques to quantify dyssynchrony, resulting in inconsistent conclusions. Since no TDI-based technique has been proven to reliably measure dyssynchrony in large clinical trials, other techniques for the quantification of intraventricular dyssynchrony are required.

With its capability to quickly capture the 3D dynamics of the entire left ventricle, including the timing of regional wall motion independently of its direction, RT3DE imaging has emerged as an alternative approach for the quantification of LV dyssynchrony.[39] Most RT3DE dyssynchrony studies have used the SD of the regional ejection times (interval between the R wave and minimum systolic LV volume) as an index of dyssynchrony. Recent attempts to compare this index against TDI have resulted in disparate results that ranged from fair inter-technique correlation[40] to poor agreement, which was explained by the angle-dependency of TDI[41] and the fact that these two techniques measure different parameters. RT3DE assessment of LV dyssynchrony has the potential advantage of measuring the timing of the longitudinal, radial, and circumferential motions, as opposed to that of the longitudinal motion only, which is measured by TDI. Of note, RT3DE dyssynchrony index was recently compared against phase analysis of gated SPECT images[42] and showed good inter-technique correlation. One limitation of RT3DE compared to TDI for the assessment of dyssynchrony is its lower temporal resolution (25 Hz vs. 200 Hz), which may limit the ability to detect smaller differences in timing.

RT3DE was used in patients with heart failure, low ejection fraction, and wide QRS complex to predict the acute response to CRT: it was shown that approximately two-third of patients with high RT3DE-derived dyssynchrony index responded to biventricular pacing with a decrease in dyssynchrony (Fig. 11.6, left) and acute improvement in global LV function.[43] Recent studies have shown a direct relationship between overall LV performance and synchronicity.[44] In these studies, RT3DE assessment of LV dyssynchrony identified patients with heart failure, low ejection fraction, and asynchronous LV contraction, who could theoretically benefit from CRT but would not be considered candidates based on their narrow QRS duration.[44] Interestingly, contrary to expectations, biventricular pacing did not result in significant long-term benefits in this subgroup of patients with narrow QRS and increased intraventricular dyssynchrony as reflected by tissue Doppler parameters.[45] One of the possible explanations for the failure of CRT to improve long-term outcomes in approximately one-third of the patients selected based on tissue Doppler criteria could be that placement of the pacing electrodes was not optimized because of the lack of sufficiently accurate tools to guide the positioning of the pacing catheter at the site of latest activation. In this regard, RT3DE imaging may also prove useful, because RT3DE-based mapping of the distribution of regional contraction times (Fig. 11.6, right) shows which LV myocardial segments are the latest to contract.[41,46] One of the emerging technological advancements in this context is the fusion of RT3DE-derived dyssynchrony maps with coronary vein CT to guide the placement of the pacing catheter.[47]

3.5. Right ventricular volumes and function

The ability to accurately measure right ventricular (RV) volumes and function is important in the management of congenital heart

Figure 11.6 Assessment of the improvement in synchrony of LV contraction with pacing. Regional volume time curves (**left**) obtained in a patient with LV dyssynchrony without (**top**) and with (**bottom**) biventricular pacing. Endocardial surfaces reconstructed from each dataset are shown with segmentation and color coding according to regional time to end ejection (**right**). Note the changes in colors with pacing reflecting the effects of resynchronization therapy in this parametric display.

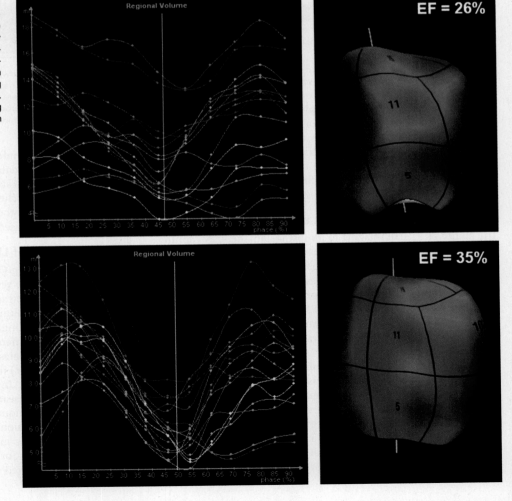

disease and primary pulmonary hypertension. Due to the complex geometrical crescent shape of this chamber, the estimation of RV volumes based on geometric modeling from 2D images has been extremely challenging. As a result, in clinical practice, tricuspid annular plane systolic excursion (TAPSE) has been traditionally used as a surrogate for RV performance. Theoretically, the intrinsic ability of RT3DE imaging to directly measure RV volumes without the need for geometric modeling could be expected to result in improved accuracy and reproducibility compared to traditional 2DE measurements. Surprisingly however, the first study to compare these two techniques side-by-side against CMR reference found that RT3DE measurements offered no significant advantage over the 2D measurements.[48] A subsequent RT3DE study[49] reported only slightly better levels of agreement with CMR. Similar to LV volume measurements, there are probably multiple ways to explain these findings. The major sources of errors, which may be different for the left and right ventricles, have not yet been identified for the right ventricle.[50,51]

Another potential source of intermodality discordance is that the complex 3D shape of the right ventricle may affect the ability of CMR imaging to accurately quantify RV volumes. In particular, the identification of RV boundaries near the RV outflow tract may be quite challenging from short-axis slices perpendicular to the long axis of the left ventricle, which is the standard for CMR image acquisition. It is likely that a different acquisition strategy is necessary for accurate RV volume measurements. Indeed, two more recent studies using new software designed specifically for volumetric analysis of the right ventricle from RT3DE datasets (Fig. 11.7A) as well as from a combination of short- and rotated long-axis CMR views, found high levels of agreement between the two techniques.[52,53] Moreover, the RT3DE measurements were both more accurate and more reproducible than several 2DE-based measurements.[52]

3.6. Real-time three-dimensional echocardiographic evaluation of atrial volumes

Left atrial (LA) enlargement is a marker of both the severity and long-term elevation of LA pressures. It is known to be associated with increased incidence of atrial fibrillation, ischemic stroke, and poor cardiovascular outcomes, including increased risks of overall mortality in patients after MI. When LA size is measured, volume determinations should be preferred over linear dimensions because they allow accurate assessment of the asymmetric remodeling of the left atrium. Consequently, LA volume calculations from 2D cut planes are recommended as a standard technique[54] instead of linear measurements. However, both the proposed area-length technique and the biplane method of disks are dependent on the selection of the location and direction of the LA minor axis and on the ability to clearly visualize and

accurately trace LA boundaries, as well as on geometric modeling. With its independence of geometrical assumptions, RT3DE imaging has the potential to provide more accurate LA volume measurements (Fig. 11.7B). However, there is no consensus on the specific methods that should be used for data acquisition and analysis aimed at LA quantification.

Until recently, most studies have compared RT3DE measurements of LA volume against traditional 2DE measurements and reported good agreement between these[55-57] techniques. Although these results are of limited value in the absence of an independent reference technique, these studies demonstrated several findings that support the superiority of RT3DE imaging for LA volume measurements. First, RT3DE-derived LA volume was more sensitive to volume changes than the 2DE-drived indices.[55] Second, it was demonstrated for the first time that RT3DE-derived maximum LA volume is a major predictor of cardiac events in patients with severe LV dysfunction.[57] Similar to previous 2DE studies, progressive increase in RT3DE-derived maximum LA volume directly correlated with age, LV mass, and LV diastolic function, and inversely correlated with LV systolic function.[58]

The feasibility of RT3DE evaluation of right atrial (RA) volume and its superiority over 2DE measurements were also recently demonstrated.[59] Nevertheless, RT3DE measurements of either LA or RA volumes have yet to be validated against an independent reference technique such as CMR. Importantly, these studies would require CMR acquisition to be specifically targeted to LA or RA quantification, including appropriate imaging planes and sufficient number of slices, in order to provide accurate CMR reference values.

4. VALVE MORPHOLOGY AND FUNCTIONAL ASSESSMENT

4.1. Mitral valve

Initially, 3D visualization of the mitral valve used a wireframe display, which was instrumental in describing the saddle shape of the mitral annulus and redefining the diagnostic criteria for mitral valve prolapse.[60] A variety of mitral valve abnormalities have been demonstrated by 3D reconstructions using gated TEE acquisition and volume-rendered display. The feasibility of obtaining the "surgeon's views" of the mitral valve by real-time volumetric imaging from the transthoracic approach recently demonstrated in 70% of consecutive patients.[61] These views provide optimal visualization of mitral leaflets, commissures, and the orifice. In particular, en-face views of the mitral valve orifice (Fig. 11.8) have contributed toward the improved accuracy of 3D measurements of the mitral valve area in patients with mitral stenosis.[62-64] These

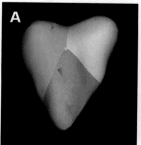
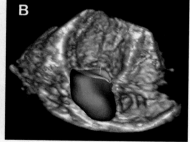

Figure 11.7 Software for volumetric analysis of heart chambers. **A:** cast of the right ventricular cavity showing in different colors the inlet septum (*green*), trabecular septum (*pink*), and infundibular septum (*yellow*) of the ventricle. **B:** 3D surface of the left atrium superimposed on the RT3DE dataset.

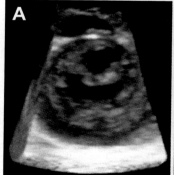
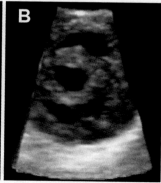

Figure 11.8 Transthoracic RT3DE views of a mitral valve from LA (**left**) and LV (**right**) perspectives obtained in a patient with severe rheumatic mitral stenosis. Note the thickened mitral valve leaflets and fused medial and lateral commissures.

studies and others have demonstrated the robustness of this methodology, suggesting that RT3DE should be the new clinical standard for the measurement of mitral valve area in patients with rheumatic mitral stenosis.[65] In addition, the ease of acquisition and online review of the 3D image allows immediate assessment of the results of percutaneous balloon mitral valvuloplasty in the cardiac catheterization laboratory.

A recent study compared segmental analysis of mitral prolapse from transthoracic RT3DE images against TEE findings and found that these two techniques yield similar comparative accuracy for precise anatomic localization of prolapsing mitral valve segments.[66,67] Interestingly, the study by De Castro and colleagues reported higher concordance between 3D TEE and surgery than 2D TEE in the identification of prolapsing mitral valve scallops.[68] The diagnostic accuracy of RT3DE evaluation of functional anatomy of mitral regurgitation was also recently demonstrated against surgical findings.[69] The more complex the mitral lesion, the more valuable 3D echocardiography is compared to 2D TEE.[70]

An important technological development of the last three years was the development of dedicated software to allow advanced 3D rendering of the valves and quantitative analysis of mitral apparatus geometry (Fig. 11.9). The availability of this software sparked new research aimed at improved characterization of the mechanisms leading to mitral regurgitation.[71–74] Recent studies characterizing the mitral valve apparatus in nonischemic and ischemic cardiomyopathy have demonstrated geometric differences in mitral annular deformation with increased intercommissural and anteroposterior dimensions, compared with healthy individuals, coupled with increased leaflet tenting and cordal tethering.[75–77] Similarly, in patients with MI, the mitral annulus was found to be more dilated and flattened and further deformed in anterior versus posterior infarction.[71] Studies in patients with mitral regurgitation and ischemic cardiomyopathy have demonstrated that the regurgitation occurs in parallel with LV remodeling rather than as an intrinsic valve disorder.[78,79]

Most recently, it was demonstrated that the analysis of RT3DE images of the mitral valve can provide information on dynamic changes in MV annular surface area and annular longitudinal displacement throughout the cardiac cycle, as well as define the position of the papillary muscles in 3D space.[80–82] Specifically, in patients with dilated cardiomyopathy and mitral regurgitation, symmetric papillary muscle displacement with simultaneous enlargement of the mitral annulus leads to progressive cordal tethering and leaflet tenting, resulting in predominantly central mitral regurgitation, as a result of decreased leaflet coaptation.[80–82] These changes were associated with a relatively nonpulsatile mitral annulus, which displaces minimally toward the apex during systole. By contrast, in patients with ischemic mitral regurgitation, LV remodeling caused by abnormal inferior wall motion results in uneven papillary muscle displacement and asymmetric localized tethering associated with eccentric mitral regurgitation.[74,80] In addition, the characteristics of the mitral annular function were compared between patients with hypertrophic cardiomyopathy and LV hypertrophy secondary to hypertension or aortic stenosis.[83] The annular function in the LV hypertrophy group was similar to that of normal subjects, whereas annular apical–basal motion and annular area changes were reduced in hypertrophic cardiomyopathy.[83] All of these observations carry important implications in the planning of mitral valve repair.

The feasibility of visualizing valvular regurgitant jets using RT3DE color flow imaging (Fig. 11.10) has also been demonstrated, and the quantification of mitral regurgitation jet volumes was shown to correlate well with 2D flow convergence methods.[84] RT3DE-derived ratio of mitral regurgitant jet volume over LA volume has been proposed as a new method to assess the severity of regurgitant lesions, although these ratios were smaller than those measured using 2D echocardiography.[84] Having the advantage of volumetric imaging of the geometry of the flow convergence surface, without the assumption of rotational symmetry, RT3DE color flow imaging can quantify mitral regurgitation more reliably than 2D echocardiography.[85] Indeed, it was shown that the

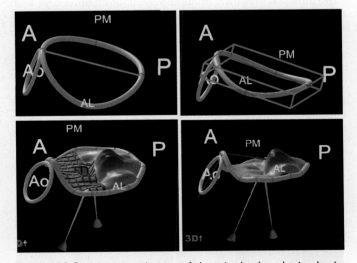

Figure 11.9 Volume renderings of the mitral valve obtained using quantitative analysis software in four patients, showing different mitral apparatus measurements: annular diameter (**top left**, *green line*), the height of the saddle-shaped mitral valve (**top right**, the height of the *green box*), prolapse height and volume as well as leaflet angles, surfaces, and lengths (**bottom left**, the surface of the anterior leaflet represented by the green grid), and the aortic orifice to mitral plane angle as well as the position of the papillary muscles in 3D space (**bottom right**, *green lines*). Ao, aortic valve; A, anterior; P, posterior; PM, posteromedial; AL, anterolateral.

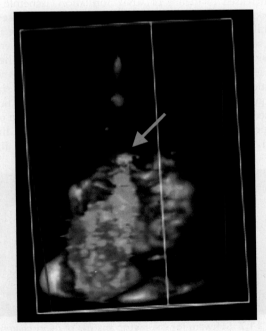

Figure 11.10 Transthoracic RT3DE image of a mitral regurgitant jet in a patient with severe ischemic mitral regurgitation. Please note the area of flow convergence (*arrow*).

true proximal flow convergence region is more hemielliptic than hemispheric, as previously believed.[86] Based on these observations, a hemielliptic approach was proposed for improved 2DE quantification of mitral regurgitation.[86] Direct assessment of the vena contracta using RT3DE imaging revealed significant asymmetry in functional compared to organic mitral regurgitation resulting in poor estimation of the effective regurgitant orifice area during single plane vena contracta measurements.[87]

4.2. Tricuspid valve

The utility of 3D echocardiography in the evaluation of tricuspid valve disease has not been explored in depth. There have been numerous case reports describing tricuspid abnormalities such as tricuspid stenosis, cleft tricuspid valve, and a flail tricuspid leaflet.[88] A recent study has found that RT3DE measurements of the tricuspid annulus are comparable to those obtained from magnetic resonance images,[89] which may have important implications in tricuspid valve surgical planning. Several studies that have subsequently explored the 3D geometry of the normal tricuspid annulus and compared it with the mitral annulus using RT3DE imaging combined with the newly developed quantitative analysis software.[90] The tricuspid annulus was found to have a less nonplanar saddle shape compared to the mitral annulus, with a round or oval shape.[90] In patients with functional tricuspid regurgitation, the annulus is even larger, more planar, and more circular.[91] In patients with tricuspid regurgitation secondary to pulmonary hypertension, in addition to annular dilatation, an enlargement in tenting volume was reported.[92] The severity of tricuspid regurgitation was found to be mainly determined by septal leaflet tethering, septal-lateral annular dilatation, and the severity of pulmonary hypertension.[93] Characterization of the tricuspid annulus and leaflets in patients with rheumatic heart disease with mitral stenosis and severe tricuspid regurgitation was also recently performed using RT3DE imaging, which allowed in addition to tricuspid valve planimetry, separate evaluation of each tricuspid valve leaflet with regard to thickness, mobility, and calcification, as well as the commissural width, at the time of maximal tricuspid valve opening.[94]

4.3. Aortic valve

RT3DE imaging of the aortic valve by either the transthoracic approach (Fig. 11.11) or transesophageal approach is challenging probably due to the oblique angle of incidence of the ultrasound beam combined with the thinner leaflets. RT3DE imaging has been recently used to improve the accuracy of the quantification of aortic stenosis. Planimetry of the aortic valve using RT3DE images showed good agreement with the standard 2D TEE technique, flow derived methods, and cardiac catheterization data,

with the advantage of improved reproducibility.[95] Analysis of RT3DE images in a small group of normal subjects revealed that in half of the subjects, the shape of LV outflow tract cross section is not round but rather elliptical. Incorrectly assuming a round LV outflow tract geometry during assessment of aortic stenosis may significantly underestimate the measurements of the aortic valve area.[96] This hypothesis was subsequently confirmed in an animal model of upper septal hypertrophy, the severity of which correlated with the discrepancy between the traditional 2DE and RT3DE measurements of the aortic valve area.[97] This experimental work also showed that the continuity equation based on RT3DE color Doppler derived estimates of stroke volume correlated better with that based on invasive outflow tract flow measurements than 2DE-based measurements. An alternative approach based on direct volumetric measurements of stroke volume using semi-automated LV endocardial border detection was compared in humans side-by-side with Doppler continuity equation and 2D Simpson technique against invasive Gorlin formula.[98] This study showed that volumetric evaluation from RT3DE images is more accurate than traditional noninvasive techniques.

5. REAL-TIME THREE-DIMENSIONAL TRANSESOPHAGEAL IMAGING

We have recently described our initial experience with matrix TEE imaging and tested its feasibility and clinical utility for real-time 3D imaging of different cardiac structures, including mitral, aortic, and tricuspid valves, interatrial septum, LA appendage, and pulmonic veins.[99] One of the major findings of this study was that real-time 3D TEE consistently provided excellent quality of volume-rendered images of the mitral valve apparatus, including the anterior and posterior leaflets, as well as annulus and subvalvular structures. This finding suggests that matrix TEE imaging may become one of the modalities of choice for perioperative planning of mitral valve surgery (Figs. 11.12 and 11.13). Similar to previous 3D TEE acqui-

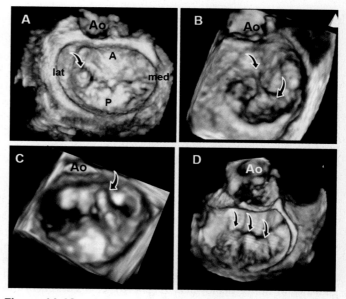

Figure 11.12 Volume rendered images of the mitral valve obtained in the zoom mode with a matrix array TEE transducer, as visualized from the left atrium in four patients: (**A**) prolapse of the P1 scallop, (**B**) prolapse of the P2 scallop with a ruptured chord, (**C**) flail P3 scallop, and (**D**) Barlow syndrome with multisegment prolapse (P1, P2, and P3). The images are oriented with the aortic valve (Ao) on top. A, anterior; P, posterior; lat, lateral; med, medial.

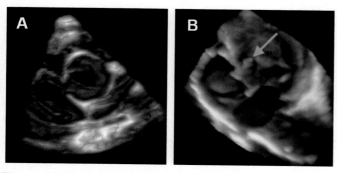

Figure 11.11 Real-time transthoracic zoomed acquisition of: (**A**) bicuspid aortic valve as visualized from the aortic perspective; (**B**) aortic valve in a patient with aortic vegetations (*arrow*).

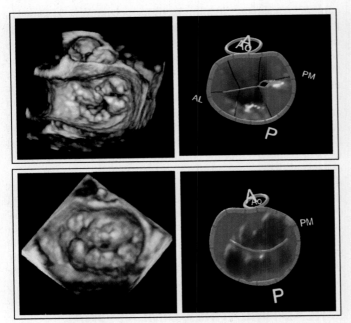

Figure 11.13 Matrix TEE images of the mitral valve, as visualized from the left atrium (**left**) and a volume rendering of the mitral valve obtained using quantitative analysis software (**right**) in two patients: prolapse of the P3 scallop (**top**), and multisegmental prolapse (**bottom**).

sition methods, the views of the mitral valve from both LA and LV perspectives are unique to 3D imaging; but what distinguishes matrix TEE from rotational 3D acquisition is the consistency of superb quality of visualization of the mitral valve, the absence of rotational artifacts, and immediate on-line display of volume-rendered views. With the unparalleled level of anatomic detail, these volume renderings allow detailed volumetric analysis of the geometry and dynamics of the mitral valve (Fig. 11.13, right panels).

6. REAL-TIME THREE-DIMENSIONAL ECHOCARDIOGRAPHIC GUIDANCE AND EVALUATION OF INTRACARDIAC INTERVENTIONS

The recent increase in the use of less invasive interventional therapies for a variety of cardiac disease states created a need for improved image guidance. Both transthoracic and transesophageal RT3DE imaging holds promise in addressing this increasing need because it provides improved visualization of device location and spatial orientation relative to the surrounding anatomic structures.[100] This modality has been used to visualize the LV bioptome along its entire course, as opposed to only partial views with 2D echocardiography, to guide LV endomyocardial biopsies.[101]

Successful transcatheter closure of secundum atrial septal defects (ASD) is dependent on accurate assessment of ASD location and size and the surrounding rim tissue of the atrial septum (Fig. 14A). These ASD features are important to determine the appropriateness of transcatheter closure, device selection, and guidance of device deployment (Fig. 14B). This assessment can be accomplished using RT3DE imaging by either transthoracic or transesophageal approach (Fig. 14A).[102–104] Historically, guidance of ASD closure, device selection and placement has been performed with fluoroscopy and 2D TEE. Intracardiac echocardiography has since emerged as the preferred method in the United States due to shorter procedure times and the lack of need for general anesthesia.

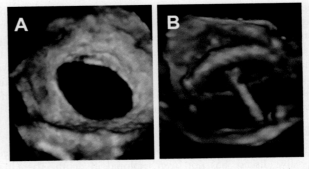

Figure 11.14 Volume renderings of the interatrial septum obtained using 3D-MTEE in a patient with a large oval-shaped atrial septal defect before (**A**) and after (**B**) placement of an Amplatz closure device.

However, because intracardiac transducers are costly and not universally available, RT3DE TEE, which allows dynamic en-face visualization of the atrial septum and related cardiac anatomy in 3D in real time, has been used as an alternative to intracardiac imaging.[102] Similarly, RT3DE imaging has been used to guide transcatheter closure of perimembranous ventricular septal defects (VSDs) with an Amplatzer occluder, where RT3DE provided information on defect size and rims, as well as device position and profile.[105]

Real-time 3D-MTEE has been shown to consistently provide excellent quality volume-rendered images of the mitral valve components including the anterior and posterior leaflets, as well as the annulus and subvalvular structures.[99] Not surprisingly, 3D-MTEE imaging has been used to guide: (a) percutaneous balloon mitral valvuloplasty in patients with rheumatic mitral stenosis (Fig. 11.15), (b) percutaneous closures of mitral and aortic perivalvular leaks, (c) percutaneous mitral valve repair using the edge-to-edge technique in patients with mitral regurgitation, and (d) percutaneous mitral annuloplasty for ischemic mitral regurgitation.[106]

Atrial fibrillation is increasing in prevalence and currently, is a major public health concern. Although the combination of rate control and anticoagulation is an affective treatment for atrial fibrillation, not all patients are candidates for anticoagulation. LA appendage occluder devices constitute a novel treatment option for patients with atrial fibrillation at risk for stroke, who have contraindications to warfarin. Accurate real-time quantification of the LA appendage, which is essential to ensure correct sizing and placement of occluder devices, has been achieved by 3D-MTEE imaging (Fig. 11.16A).[107] The role of 3D-MTEE for the guidance of catheter placement during electrophysiology procedures (Fig. 11.16B) remains to be established. In the future, developments in intracardiac 3D ultrasound may address the challenges of acquiring high quality 3D visualization of the left atrium and pulmonic veins.

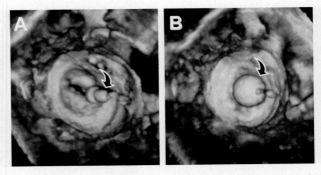

Figure 11.15 Volume renderings of the mitral valve as visualized from the LA perspective during percutaneous valvuloplasty using an Inoue balloon (**A, B**, before and after balloon inflation, *arrows*).

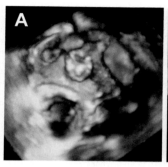
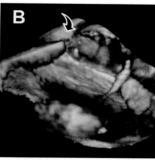

Figure 11.16 Volume renderings of a percutaneous transcatheter LA appendage occluder (*arrow*; Watchman device, Atritech Inc.) in a patient with atrial fibrillation **(A)**. Use of 3D-MTEE imaging to guide the positioning of a Lasso circular mapping catheter (*arrow*, Biosense Webster Inc.) during ablation in a patient with atrial fibrillation **(B)**.

7. FUTURE DIRECTIONS

Currently, many laboratories perform complete 2D echocardiographic studies, which are followed by a focused 3D examination in patients with specific pathologies in which RT3DE imaging could potentially provide additional diagnostic information. It can be anticipated that a full volume acquisition of the left ventricle will be performed in every patient to obtain LV volumes and ejection fraction. The 3D images will likely be stored in a digital archiving system together with the 2D study, to allow integrated interpretation of all images and incorporation of 3D findings into the report.

Future advances in transducer and computer technology will result in several important improvements that will further advance the clinical application of RT3DE imaging. Future improvements in both spatial and temporal resolutions of the transthoracic RT3DE imaging, which are still below those of 2DE, will broaden the spectrum of patients who can be imaged with this modality. Future software developments will allow new types of sophisticated quantitative analysis of the cardiovascular anatomy and function, including the fusion of RT3DE data with other 3D imaging modalities, such as MR andCT.

Further miniaturization of the 3D-MTEE technology will allow 3D TEE imaging in pediatric patients, as well as the development of real-time 3D imaging intracardiac catheters. It is anticipated that with the ability of real-time acquisition, on-line adjustments of rendering and cropping capabilities, 3D TEE imaging will be used routinely in perioperative planning of mitral valve surgery as well as guidance of percutaneous interventions. It is easy to predict that the ease and speed of data acquisition coupled with the ability to display cardiac structures using unique 3D views is likely to result in rapid integration of matrix TEE into clinical practice and have an impact on echocardiographic diagnosis of valve disease.

REFERENCES

1. Lang RM, Mor-Avi V, Sugeng L, et al. Three-dimensional echocardiography: The benefits of the additional dimension. *J Am Coll Cardiol.* 2006;48:2053–2069.
2. Schiller NB, Acquatella H, Ports TA, et al. Left ventricular volume from paired biplane two-dimensional echocardiography. *Circulation.* 1979;60:547–555.
3. Erbel R, Krebs W, Henn G, et al. Comparison of single-plane and biplane volume determination by two-dimensional echocardiography. 1. Asymmetric model hearts. *Eur Heart J.* 1982;3:469–480.
4. Gopal AS, Keller AM, Rigling R, et al. Left ventricular volume and endocardial surface area by three-dimensional echocardiography: Comparison with two-dimensional echocardiography and nuclear magnetic resonance imaging in normal subjects. *J Am Coll Cardiol.* 1993;22:258–270.
5. Jacobs LD, Salgo IS, Goonewardena S, et al. Rapid online quantification of left ventricular volume from real-time three-dimensional echocardiographic data. *Eur Heart J.* 2006;27:460–468.
6. Matsumoto M, Inoue M, Tamura S, et al. Three-dimensional echocardiography for spatial visualization and volume calculation of cardiac structures. *J Clin Ultrasound.* 1981;9:157–165.
7. Stickels KR, Wann LS. An analysis of three-dimensional reconstructive echocardiography. *Ultrasound Med Biol.* 1984;10:575–580.
8. Bartel T, Muller S, Erbel R. Dynamic three-dimensional echocardiography using parallel slicing: A promising diagnostic procedure in adults with congenital heart disease. *Cardiology.* 1998;89:140–147.
9. Roelandt J, Salustri A, Mumm B, et al. Precordial three-dimensional echocardiography with a rotational imaging probe: Methods and initial clinical experience. *Echocardiography.* 1995;12:243–252.
10. Raichlen JS, Trivedi SS, Herman GT, et al. Dynamic three-dimensional reconstruction of the left ventricle from two-dimensional echocardiograms. *J Am Coll Cardiol.* 1986;8:364–370.
11. von Ramm OT, Smith SW. Real time volumetric ultrasound imaging system. *J Digit Imaging.* 1990;3:261–266.
12. Sheikh K, Smith SW, von Ramm OT, et al. Real-time, three-dimensional echocardiography: Feasibility and initial use. *Echocardiography.* 1991;8:119–125.
13. Ota T, Fleishman CE, Strub M, et al. Real-time, three-dimensional echocardiography: Feasibility of dynamic right ventricular volume measurement with saline contrast. *Am Heart J.* 1999;137:958–966.
14. Qin JX, Jones M, Shiota T, et al. Validation of real-time three-dimensional echocardiography for qantifying left ventricular volumes in the presence of a left ventricular aneurysm: In vitro and in vivo studies. *J Am Coll Cardiol.* 2000;36:900–907.
15. Arai K, Hozumi T, Matsumura Y, et al. Accuracy of measurement of left ventricular volume and ejection fraction by new real-time three-dimensional echocardiography in patients with wall motion abnormalities secondary to myocardial infarction. *Am J Cardiol.* 2004;94:552–558.
16. Jenkins C, Bricknell K, Hanekom L, et al. Reproducibility and accuracy of echocardiographic measurements of left ventricular parameters using real-time three-dimensional echocardiography. *J Am Coll Cardiol.* 2004;44:878–886.
17. Nikitin NP, Constantin C, Loh PH, et al. New generation 3-dimensional echocardiography for left ventricular volumetric and functional measurements: Comparison with cardiac magnetic resonance. *Eur J Echocardiogr.* 2006;7:365–372.
18. Tighe DA, Rosetti M, Vinch CS, et al. Influence of image quality on the accuracy of real time three-dimensional echocardiography to measure left ventricular volumes in unselected patients: A comparison with gated-SPECT imaging. *Echocardiography.* 2007;24:1073–1080.
19. Pouleur AC, le Polain de Waroux JB, Pasquet A, et al. Assessment of left ventricular mass and volumes by three-dimensional echocardiography in patients with or without wall motion abnormalities: Comparison against cine magnetic resonance imaging. *Heart.* 2008; 94:1050–1057.
20. Jenkins C, Bricknell K, Chan J, et al. Comparison of two- and three-dimensional echocardiography with sequential magnetic resonance imaging for evaluating left ventricular volume and ejection fraction over time in patients with healed myocardial infarction. *Am J Cardiol.* 2007;99:300–306.
21. Gopal AS, Chukwu EO, Mihalatos DG, et al. Left ventricular structure and function for postmyocardial infarction and heart failure risk stratification by three-dimensional echocardiography. *J Am Soc Echocardiogr.* 2007;20:949–958.
22. Kuhl HP, Schreckenberg M, Rulands D, et al. High-resolution transthoracic real-time three-dimensional echocardiography: Quantitation of cardiac volumes and function using semi-automatic border detection and comparison with cardiac magnetic resonance imaging. *J Am Coll Cardiol.* 2004;43:2083–2090.
23. Sugeng L, Mor-Avi V, Weinert L, et al. Quantitative assessment of left ventricular size and function: Side-by-side comparison of real-time three-dimensional echocardiography and computed tomography with magnetic resonance reference. *Circulation.* 2006;114:654–661.
24. Jenkins C, Chan J, Hanekom L, et al. Accuracy and feasibility of online 3-dimensional echocardiography for measurement of left ventricular parameters. *J Am Soc Echocardiogr.* 2006;19:1119–1128.
25. Krenning BJ, Kirschbaum SW, Soliman OI, et al. Comparison of contrast agent-enhanced versus non-contrast agent-enhanced real-time three-dimensional echocardiography for analysis of left ventricular systolic function. *Am J Cardiol.* 2007;100:1485–1489.
26. Soliman OI, Krenning BJ, Geleijnse ML, et al. Quantification of left ventricular volumes and function in patients with cardiomyopathies by real-time three-dimensional echocardiography: A head-to-head comparison between two different semiautomated endocardial border detection algorithms. *J Am Soc Echocardiogr.* 2007;20:1042–1049.
27. Mor-Avi V, Sugeng L, Weinert L, et al. Fast measurement of left ventricular mass with real-time three-dimensional echocardiography: Comparison with magnetic resonance imaging. *Circulation.* 2004;110:1814–1818.
28. Yao GH, Li F, Zhang C, et al. How many planes are required to get an accurate and timesaving measurement of left ventricular volume and function by real-time three-dimensional echocardiography in acute myocardial infarction? *Ultrasound Med Biol.* 2007;33:1572–1578.
29. Corsi C, Lang RM, Veronesi F, et al. Volumetric quantification of global and regional left ventricular function from real-time three-dimensional echocardiographic images. *Circulation.* 2005;112:1161–1170.
30. Mor-Avi V, Jenkins C, Kuhl HP, et al. Real-time 3D echocardiographic quantification of left ventricular volumes: Multicenter study for validation with magnetic resonance imaging and investigation of sources of error. *J Am Coll Cardiol Imaging.* 2008;1:413–423.
31. Caiani EG, Corsi C, Sugeng L, et al. Improved quantification of left ventricular mass based on endocardial and epicardial surface detection with real time three dimensional echocardiography. *Heart.* 2006;92:213–219.

32. Yap SC, van Geuns RJ, Nemes A, et al. Rapid and accurate measurement of LV mass by biplane real-time 3D echocardiography in patients with concentric LV hypertrophy: Comparison to CMR. *Eur J Echocardiogr.* 2008;9:225–260.

33. van den Bosch AE, Robbers-Visser D, Krenning BJ, et al. Comparison of real-time three-dimensional echocardiography to magnetic resonance imaging for assessment of left ventricular mass. *Am J Cardiol.* 2006;97:113–117.

34. Nesser HJ, Sugeng L, Corsi C, et al. Volumetric analysis of regional left ventricular function with real-time three-dimensional echocardiography: Validation by magnetic resonance and clinical utility testing. *Heart.* 2007;93:572–578.

35. Zwas DR, Takuma S, Mullis-Jansson S, et al. Feasibility of real-time 3-dimensional treadmill stress echocardiography. *J Am Soc Echocardiogr.* 1999;12:285–289.

36. Sugeng L, Kirkpatrick J, Lang RM, et al. Biplane stress echocardiography using a prototype matrix-array transducer. *J Am Soc Echocardiogr.* 2003;16:937–941.

37. Matsumura Y, Hozumi T, Arai K, et al. Non-invasive assessment of myocardial ischaemia using new real-time three-dimensional dobutamine stress echocardiography: Comparison with conventional two-dimensional methods. *Eur Heart J.* 2005;26:1625–1632.

38. Yang HS, Pellikka PA, McCully RB, et al. Role of biplane and biplane echocardiographically guided 3-dimensional echocardiography during dobutamine stress echocardiography. *J Am Soc Echocardiogr.* 2006;19:1136–1143.

39. Gorcsan J, III, Abraham T, Agler DA, et al. Echocardiography for cardiac resynchronization therapy: Recommendations for performance and reporting – A report from the American Society of Echocardiography Dyssynchrony Writing Group endorsed by the Heart Rhythm Society. *J Am Soc Echocardiogr.* 2008;21:191–213.

40. Takeuchi M, Jacobs A, Sugeng L, et al. Assessment of left ventricular dyssynchrony with real-time 3-dimensional echocardiography: Comparison with Doppler tissue imaging. *J Am Soc Echocardiogr.* 2007;20:1321–1329.

41. Burgess MI, Jenkins C, Chan J, et al. Measurement of left ventricular dyssynchrony in patients with ischaemic cardiomyopathy: A comparison of real-time three-dimensional and tissue Doppler echocardiography. *Heart.* 2007;93:1191–1196.

42. Marsan NA, Henneman MM, Chen J, et al. Real-time 3-dimensional echocardiography as a novel approach to quantify left ventricular dyssynchrony: A comparison study with phase analysis of gated myocardial perfusion single photon emission computed tomography. *J Am Soc Echocardiogr.* 2008;21:801–807.

43. Marsan NA, Bleeker GB, Ypenburg C, et al. Real-time three-dimensional echocardiography permits quantification of left ventricular mechanical dyssynchrony and predicts acute response to cardiac resynchronization therapy. *J Cardiovasc Electrophysiol.* 2008;19:392–399.

44. Kapetanakis S, Kearney MT, Siva A, et al. Real-time three-dimensional echocardiography: A novel technique to quantify global left ventricular mechanical dyssynchrony. *Circulation.* 2005;112:992–1000.

45. Beshai JF, Grimm RA, Nagueh SF, et al. Cardiac-resynchronization therapy in heart failure with narrow QRS complexes. *N Engl J Med.* 2007;357:2461–2471.

46. Becker M, Hoffmann R, Schmitz F, et al. Relation of optimal lead positioning as defined by three-dimensional echocardiography to long-term benefit of cardiac resynchronization. *Am J Cardiol.* 2007;100:1671–1676.

47. Van de Veire NR, Marsan NA, Schuijf JD, et al. Noninvasive imaging of cardiac venous anatomy with 64-slice multi-slice computed tomography and noninvasive assessment of left ventricular dyssynchrony by 3-dimensional tissue synchronization imaging in patients with heart failure scheduled for cardiac resynchronization therapy. *Am J Cardiol.* 2008;101:1023–1029.

48. Kjaergaard J, Petersen CL, Kjaer A, et al. Evaluation of right ventricular volume and function by 2D and 3D echocardiography compared to MRI. *Eur J Echocardiogr.* 2005;7:430–438.

49. Prakasa KR, Dalal D, Wang J, et al. Feasibility and variability of three-dimensional echocardiography in arrhythmogenic right ventricular dysplasia/cardiomyopathy. *Am J Cardiol.* 2006;97:703–709.

50. Hoch M, Vasilyev NV, Soriano B, et al. Variables influencing the accuracy of right ventricular volume assessment by real-time 3-dimensional echocardiography: An in vitro validation study. *J Am Soc Echocardiogr.* 2007;20:456–461.

51. Gopal AS, Chukwu EO, Iwuchukwu CJ, et al. Normal values of right ventricular size and function by real-time 3-dimensional echocardiography: Comparison with cardiac magnetic resonance imaging. *J Am Soc Echocardiogr.* 2007;20:445–455.

52. Jenkins C, Chan J, Bricknell K, et al. Reproducibility of right ventricular volumes and ejection fraction using real-time three-dimensional echocardiography: Comparison with cardiac MRI. *Chest.* 2007;131:1844–1851.

53. Niemann PS, Pinho L, Balbach T, et al. Anatomically oriented right ventricular volume measurements with dynamic three-dimensional echocardiography validated by 3-Tesla magnetic resonance imaging. *J Am Coll Cardiol.* 2007;50:1668–1676.

54. Lang RM, Bierig M, Devereux RB, et al. Recommendations for chamber quantification. *Eur J Echocardiogr.* 2006;7:79–108.

55. Anwar AM, Soliman OI, Geleijnse ML, et al. Assessment of left atrial volume and function by real-time three-dimensional echocardiography. *Int J Cardiol.* 2008;123:155–161.

56. Muller H, Burri H, Shah D, et al. Evaluation of left atrial size in patients with atrial arrhythmias: Comparison of standard 2D versus real time 3D echocardiography. *Echocardiography.* 2007;24:960–966.

57. Suh IW, Song JM, Lee EY, et al. Left atrial volume measured by real-time 3-dimensional echocardiography predicts clinical outcomes in patients with severe left ventricular dysfunction and in sinus rhythm. *J Am Soc Echocardiogr.* 2008;21:439–445.

58. de Castro S, Caselli S, Di AE, et al. Relation of left atrial maximal volume measured by real-time 3D echocardiography to demographic, clinical, and Doppler variables. *Am J Cardiol.* 2008;101:1347–1352.

59. Muller H, Burri H, Lerch R. Evaluation of right atrial size in patients with atrial arrhythmias: Comparison of 2D versus real-time 3D echocardiography. *Echocardiography.* 2008;25:617–623.

60. Levine RA, Handschumacher MD, Sanfilippo AJ, et al. Three-dimensional echocardiographic reconstruction of the mitral valve, with implications for the diagnosis of mitral valve prolapse. *Circulation.* 1989;80:589–598.

61. Sugeng L, Coon P, Weinert L, et al. Use of real-time three-dimensional transthoracic echocardiography in the evaluation of mitral valve disease. *J Am Soc Echocardiogr.* 2006;19:413–421.

62. Sugeng L, Weinert L, Lammertin G, et al. Accuracy of mitral valve area measurements using transthoracic rapid freehand 3-dimensional scanning: Comparison with noninvasive and invasive methods. *J Am Soc Echocardiogr.* 2003;16:1292–1300.

63. Zamorano J, Cordeiro P, Sugeng L, et al. Real-time three-dimensional echocardiography for rheumatic mitral valve stenosis evaluation: An accurate and novel approach. *J Am Coll Cardiol.* 2004;43:2091–2096.

64. Mannaerts HF, Kamp O, Visser CA. Should mitral valve area assessment in patients with mitral stenosis be based on anatomical or on functional evaluation? A plea for 3D echocardiography as the new clinical standard. *Eur Heart J.* 2004;25:2073–2074.

65. Mannaerts HF, Kamp O, Visser CA. Should mitral valve area assessment in patients with mitral stenosis be based on anatomical or on functional evaluation? A plea for 3D echocardiography as the new clinical standard. *Eur Heart J.* 2004;25:2073–2074.

66. Sharma R, Mann J, Drummond L, et al. The evaluation of real-time 3dimensional transthoracic echocardiography for the preoperative functional assessment of patients with mitral valve prolapse: A comparison with 2-dimensional transesophageal echocardiography. *J Am Soc Echocardiogr.* 2007;20:934–940.

67. Gutierrez-Chico JL, Zamorano Gomez JL, Rodrigo-Lopez JL, et al. Accuracy of real-time 3-dimensional echocardiography in the assessment of mitral prolapse. Is transesophageal echocardiography still mandatory? *Am Heart J.* 2008;155:694–698.

68. de Castro S, Salandin V, Cartoni D, et al. Qualitative and quantitative evaluation of mitral valve morphology by intraoperative volume-rendered three-dimensional echocardiography. *J Heart Valve Dis.* 2002;11:173–180.

69. Agricola E, Oppizzi M, Pisani M, et al. Accuracy of real-time 3D echocardiography in the evaluation of functional anatomy of mitral regurgitation. *Int J Cardiol.* 2008;127:342–349.

70. Muller S, Muller L, Laufer G, et al. Echocardiography for preoperative evaluation in mitral valve prolapse. *Am J Cardiol.* 2006;98:243–248.

71. Watanabe N, Ogasawara Y, Yamaura Y, et al. Geometric differences of the mitral valve tenting between anterior and inferior myocardial infarction with significant ischemic mitral regurgitation: Quantitation by novel software system with transthoracic real-time three-dimensional echocardiography. *J Am Soc Echocardiogr.* 2006;19:71–75.

72. Song JM, Qin JX, Kongsaerepong V, et al. Determinants of ischemic mitral regurgitation in patients with chronic anterior wall myocardial infarction: A real time three-dimensional echocardiography study. *Echocardiography.* 2006;23:650–657.

73. Ryan L, Jackson B, Parish L, et al. Quantification and localization of mitral valve tenting in ischemic mitral regurgitation using real-time three-dimensional echocardiography. *Eur J Cardiothorac Surg.* 2007;31:839–834.

74. Daimon M, Saracino G, Gillinov AM, et al. Local dysfunction and asymmetrical deformation of mitral annular geometry in ischemic mitral regurgitation: A novel computerized 3D echocardiographic analysis. *Echocardiography.* 2008;25:414–423.

75. Ahmad RM, Gillinov AM, McCarthy PM, et al. Annular geometry and motion in human ischemic mitral regurgitation: Novel assessment with three-dimensional echocardiography and computer reconstruction. *Ann Thorac Surg.* 2004;78:2063–2068.

76. Kwan J, Shiota T, Agler DA, et al. Geometric differences of the mitral apparatus between ischemic and dilated cardiomyopathy with significant mitral regurgitation: Real-time three-dimensional echocardiography study. *Circulation.* 2003;107:1135–1140.

77. Watanabe N, Ogasawara Y, Yamaura Y, et al. Quantitation of mitral valve tenting in ischemic mitral regurgitation by transthoracic real-time three-dimensional echocardiography. *J Am Coll Cardiol.* 2005;45:763–769.

78. Agricola E, Oppizzi M, Maisano F, et al. Echocardiographic classification of chronic ischemic mitral regurgitation caused by restricted motion according to tethering pattern. *Eur J Echocardiogr.* 2004;5:326–334.

79. Otsuji Y, Kumanohoso T, Yoshifuku S, et al. Isolated annular dilation does not usually cause important functional mitral regurgitation: Comparison between patients with lone atrial fibrillation and those with idiopathic or ischemic cardiomyopathy. *J Am Coll Cardiol.* 2002;39:1651–1656.

80. Veronesi F, Corsi C, Sugeng L, et al. Quantification of mitral apparatus dynamics in functional and ischemic mitral regurgitation using real-time 3-dimensional echocardiography. *J Am Soc Echocardiogr.* 2008;21:347–354.

81. Tsukiji M, Watanabe N, Yamaura Y, et al. Three-dimensional quantitation of mitral valve coaptation by a novel software system with transthoracic real-time three-dimensional echocardiography. *J Am Soc Echocardiogr.* 2008;21:43–46.

82. Song JM, Fukuda S, Kihara T, et al. Value of mitral valve tenting volume determined by real-time three-dimensional echocardiography in patients with functional mitral regurgitation. *Am J Cardiol.* 2006;98:1088–1093.

83. Yalcin F, Shiota M, Greenberg N, et al. Real time three-dimensional echocardiography evaluation of mitral annular characteristics in patients with myocardial hypertrophy. *Echocardiography.* 2008;25:424–428.

84. Sugeng L, Weinert L, Lang RM. Real-time 3-dimensional color Doppler flow of mitral and tricuspid regurgitation: Feasibility and initial quantitative comparison with 2-dimensional methods. *J Am Soc Echocardiogr.* 2007;20:1050–1057.
85. Sitges M, Jones M, Shiota T, et al. Real-time three-dimensional color doppler evaluation of the flow convergence zone for quantification of mitral regurgitation: Validation experimental animal study and initial clinical experience. *J Am Soc Echocardiogr.* 2003;16:38–45.
86. Yosefy C, Levine RA, Solis J, et al. Proximal flow convergence region as assessed by real-time 3-dimensional echocardiography: Challenging the hemispheric assumption. *J Am Soc Echocardiogr.* 2007;20:389–396.
87. Kahlert P, Plicht B, Schenk IM, et al. Direct assessment of size and shape of noncircular vena contracta area in functional versus organic mitral regurgitation using real-time three-dimensional echocardiography. *J Am Soc Echocardiogr.* 2008;21:912–921.
88. Faletra F, La MU, Bragato R, et al. Three dimensional transthoracic echocardiography images of tricuspid stenosis. *Heart.* 2005;91:499.
89. Anwar AM, Soliman OI, Nemes A, et al. Value of assessment of tricuspid annulus: Real-time three-dimensional echocardiography and magnetic resonance imaging. *Int J Cardiovasc Imaging.* 2007;23:701–705.
90. Kwan J, Kim GC, Jeon MJ, et al. 3D geometry of a normal tricuspid annulus during systole: A comparison study with the mitral annulus using real-time 3D echocardiography. *Eur J Echocardiogr.* 2007;8:375–383.
91. Ton-Nu TT, Levine RA, Handschumacher MD, et al. Geometric determinants of functional tricuspid regurgitation: Insights from 3-dimensional echocardiography. *Circulation.* 2006;114:143–149.
92. Sukmawan R, Watanabe N, Ogasawara Y, et al. Geometric changes of tricuspid valve tenting in tricuspid regurgitation secondary to pulmonary hypertension quantified by novel system with transthoracic real-time 3-dimensional echocardiography. *J Am Soc Echocardiogr.* 2007;20:470–476.
93. Park YH, Song JM, Lee EY, et al. Geometric and hemodynamic determinants of functional tricuspid regurgitation: A real-time three-dimensional echocardiography study. *Int J Cardiol.* 2008;124:160–165.
94. Anwar AM, Geleijnse ML, Soliman OI, et al. Evaluation of rheumatic tricuspid valve stenosis by real-time three-dimensional echocardiography. *Heart.* 2007;93:363–364.
95. Goland S, Trento A, Iida K, et al. Assessment of aortic stenosis by three-dimensional echocardiography: An accurate and novel approach. *Heart.* 2007;93:801–807.
96. Doddamani S, Bello R, Friedman MA, et al. Demonstration of left ventricular outflow tract eccentricity by real time 3D echocardiography: Implications for the determination of aortic valve area. *Echocardiography.* 2007;24:860–866.
97. Poh KK, Levine RA, Solis J, et al. Assessing aortic valve area in aortic stenosis by continuity equation: A novel approach using real-time three-dimensional echocardiography. *Eur Heart J.* 2008;29(20):2526–2535.
98. Gutierrez-Chico JL, Zamorano JL, Prieto-Moriche E, et al. Real-time three-dimensional echocardiography in aortic stenosis: A novel, simple, and reliable method to improve accuracy in area calculation. *Eur Heart J.* 2007;29(10):1296–1306.
99. Sugeng L, Shernan SK, Salgo IS, et al. Live three-dimensional transesophageal echocardiography: Initial experience using the fully-sampled matrix array probe. *J Am Coll Cardiol.* 2008;52:446–449.
100. Gill EA, Liang DH. Interventional three-dimensional echocardiography: Using real-time three dimensional echocardiography to guide and evaluate intracardiac therapies. *Cardiol Clin.* 2007;25:335–340.
101. Amitai ME, Schnittger I, Popp RL, et al. Comparison of three-dimensional echocardiography to two-dimensional echocardiography and fluoroscopy for monitoring of endomyocardial biopsy. *Am J Cardiol.* 2007;99:864–866.
102. Lodato JA, Cao QL, Weinert L, et al. Feasibility of real-time three-dimensional transesophageal echocardiography for guidance of percutaneous atrial septal defect closure. *Eur J Echocardiogr.* 2009 Jan 29. (Epub ahead of print).
103. Morgan GJ, Casey F, Craig B, et al. Assessing ASDs prior to device closure using 3D echocardiography. Just pretty pictures or a useful clinical tool? *Eur J Echocardiogr.* 2007; 9(4):478–482.
104. van den Bosch AE, Ten Harkel DJ, McGhie JS, et al. Characterization of atrial septal defect assessed by real-time 3-dimensional echocardiography. *J Am Soc Echocardiogr.* 2006;19:815–821.
105. Acar P, Abadir S, Aggoun Y. Transcatheter closure of perimembranous ventricular septal defects with Amplatzer occluder assessed by real-time three-dimensional echocardiography. *Eur J Echocardiogr.* 2007;8:110–115.
106. Daimon M, Gillinov AM, Liddicoat JR, et al. Dynamic change in mitral annular area and motion during percutaneous mitral annuloplasty for ischemic mitral regurgitation: Preliminary animal study with real-time 3-dimensional echocardiography. *J Am Soc Echocardiogr.* 2007;20:381–388.
107. Shah SJ, Bardo DM, Sugeng L, et al. Real-time three-dimensional transesophageal echocardiography of the left atrial appendage: Intial experience in the clinical setting. *J Am Soc Echocardiogr.* 2008;21:1362–1368.

Digital Acquisition, Storage, and Network

Neil Greenberg
Mario J. Garcia

1. INTRODUCTION

Digital imaging offers many advantages over film and videotape media formats, including higher image quality, ease of access and comparison to prior exams, improved quantification as calibration of data is known, more efficient review and interpretation, efficiency advances in workflow and integration with hospital information systems (HISs), facilitation of research efforts in both exchange of information as well as access to rich databases of information, and overall improved accuracy and reproducibility.

Efforts in digital medical imaging began in the late 1970s with traditional radiological static imaging modalities and expanded to cine-X-ray and cine-ultrasound in the 1980s and 1990s. With ultrasound, specialized hardware was first utilized to digitize a few frames during systole of regions of interest within specific echocardiographic views.[1] As computing capabilities advanced, technological advances permitted registration of moving images in digital format, logical data archival, rapid data retrieval, data copy and transfer, off-line quantitative analysis, and side-by-side comparison with superior image resolution.[2] DICOM (digital imaging and communications in medicine) is an application layer network protocol for the transmission of medical images, waveforms, and ancillary information. It was originally developed by the National Electrical Manufacturers Association and the American College of Radiology for computed tomographic (CT) and magnetic resonance (MR) scan images. It is now controlled by the DICOM Standards Committee, and supports a wide range of medical images across the fields of radiology, cardiology, pathology, and dentistry. DICOM uses transmission control protocol (TCP)/internet protocol (IP) as the lower-layer transport protocol. The American Society of Echocardiography later established in 1992 a task force to educate the echocardiographic community on the promise and pitfalls of digital echocardiography and advise DICOM committee on a standard image format for echocardiography.[3,4]

2. ANALOG VERSUS DIGITAL IMAGING

The principal feature of analog representations is that they are continuous. In contrast, digital representations consist of values measured at discrete intervals. Analog technology refers to electronic transmission accomplished by adding signals of varying frequency or amplitude to carrier waves of a given frequency of alternating electromagnetic current. Analog data is typically represented as a series of sine waves. Television, radio, and telephone transmission mostly use analog technology, although more recently, the use of digital technology in these fields is rapidly expanding. A theoretical advantage of analog data is its ability to provide in theory an infinite spectrum of data. This is most easily appreciated when analyzing the fidelity of signals that are "naturally" analog, such as audio or video signals. In order to transform this data into a digital format, an electronic process known as analog-to-digital conversion needs to be implemented. The input to any analog-to-digital converter consists of a signal with a theoretically infinite number of values that has been transformed to an electrical voltage, and the output is a multilevel signal that has defined levels, typically a power of two (e.g., 2, 4, 8, 16, 32, etc.). Thus, the most basic digital signal has only two states, and is called a binary signal, whereas the only possible values are 0 and 1. Any number can then be represented in binary form as sequences of zeros and ones.

For example, in echocardiography, a rectangular image of theoretically unlimited resolution is first limited to a matrix of finite dimensions, e.g., 800 horizontal × 600 vertical lines (Video Graphics Array (VGA) resolution). This matrix then has 480,000 pixels (smallest distinct geographical square zone). In a picture, each pixel may contain color information within a scale. The number of color values is given by a number of bits that are contained in each pixel, and is equal to 2 to the power of the number of bits, e.g., if there are 3 bits per pixel, then 8 different values could be encoded (000, 001, 010, 100, 011, 101, 110, and 111). In a typical grayscale echocardiographic image, there are 256 shades of gray (8-bit per pixel or $2^8 = 256$). Thus, the size of the raw binary digital file that encodes the information contained in this picture is $400 \times 600 \times 8 = 384,000$ bits (or 48,000 bytes, since 1 byte = 8 bits). If higher color definition is required, the number of bits per pixel may be increased. A 32 bit per pixel resolution provides $2^{32} = 4,294,967,296$ colors and will require $400 \times 800 \times 32 = 1,920,000$ bits = 240,000 bytes.

Regardless of its resolution, digital data has a finite limitation, and that is why, in theory, an audio signal recorded in analog format (vinyl record) may be reproduced with higher fidelity than a digital recording (compact disk). If such is the case, what is the advantage of digital media? Digital signals travel more efficiently than analog signals, mainly because digital impulses, which are well-defined, are easier for electronic circuits to distinguish from noise, which is chaotic. Noise can occur naturally or by electrical interference and is incorporated randomly to analog data during transmission, recording, processing, and display. In an audio recording, noise can be appreciated as background "hissing." Once noise is introduced, it cannot be separated from the original signal and is compounded with more noise introduced during each additional process. Thus, every time that analog data is transferred and/or copied, signal-to-noise ratio decreases. For that reason, second copies of video or music analog recordings are

150

never identical to their originals. Here lies one of the main advantages of digital media, which is capable of reproducing identically the original set of data.

3. ELEMENTS OF A DIGITAL IMAGING LABORATORY

The key components of a digital noninvasive imaging laboratory are the acquisition devices, the storage and archive system, data review and analysis tools, the network infrastructure, interfaces to the HIS, and the users and support personnel (Fig. 12.1).

3.1. Acquisition devices

Acquisition devices (CT and MRI scanners, nuclear cameras, ultrasound equipment) have capabilities that allow for great flexibility and usability in a digital imaging laboratory today. While analog options (film, videotape) are still available on many imaging centers, all current acquisition devices are designed and optimized to store digital data. The networked acquisition devices can be configured to connect to a variety of useful devices throughout a hospital if available, including a picture archiving and communication system (PACS). PACSs system to store and archive the exams and a modality worklist server to provide a patient list from which demographic and order information can be downloaded to the modality.

Network configuration of the modality involves setting parameters for the given hospital environment. The common network parameters required include an IP address for the modality and an application entity title, or the name given to the particular device for DICOM communication. In addition, a network gateway and mask are generally required along with proper setting of the network connection speed which may have to be switched from the common auto setting to either 10 or 100 BT speed in either half or full duplex mode. Improper settings can result in a loss of connectivity or reduced performance caused by resulting network errors. It is important to work with the information technology (IT) team to define the capabilities and requirements in a particular setting. At most modern hospitals, various areas have a variety of switched network hardware that requires different network configurations based on the area or building where a part of the laboratory is located. This design can be configured for stationary devices and for mobile imaging units. Given that portability of ultrasound is a key advantage of the technology, the network connectivity approach to address this concern deserves

attention. Dynamic network addressing dynamic host configuration protocol may be useful to allow a network connection in various locations that require different addressing due to network architecture. Standard network connection hardware has also not been designed for cables to be plugged and unplugged into outlets as frequently as used with a lab performing bedside exams. Wireless network capabilities exist for some echocardiographs and permit the echocardiograph to maintain connectivity as the device moves throughout the hospital. There are various wireless protocols and security measures that can be used to allow communication without the need for a network cable and network drop locations throughout the hospital environment. The main disadvantage of wireless connectivity is network transfer speed, but even with wireless bandwidth limitations, exams can be transferred to the PACSs effectively. One useful mode on many modalities is the ability to transfer images during the exam as they are acquired. This transfer should occur as a background task and not interfere with data acquisition. For this strategy to be employed, the user limits their ability to edit the exam during the scan. However, whether in progress transfers are employed wirelessly or with fixed network connections, the positive outcomes include reduced time to complete transfer at the end of the exam to allow access for offline analysis as well as in progress access via PACSs clients to monitor acquisitions remotely for guidance.

Image acquisition devices not only acquire digital image data, but provide extensive tools to maintain a database of the exams performed on the device, assist users in acquisition of exams through protocols, and allow users to perform both basic and advanced measurements directly on the acquisition cart that can be passed to the PACs system. Diagnostic imaging procedures begin with a collection of demographic information including patient name, medical record number (MRN), and date of birth. These parameters can be manually entered, or if available selected from a worklist provided to the modality from the HIS and a worklist server.

Digital medical imaging systems allow for "intelligent" compression of data, or a reduction in the temporal scope of the exam. A single frame echocardiographic image has a resolution of 640 horizontal × 480 vertical pixels × 24-bits per pixel, equaling 922 KB. Thus, at an average frame rate of 30 Hz, a 15 min uncompressed echocardiography study results in ~25 GB of data. As compared to this traditional video tape recording, representative digital acquisitions of limited length, based on ECG triggering for 1 to 3 beats or fixed 1 to 2 s durations can reduce the volume of data to 0.8 GB, achieving 30:1 compression. This selection of representative beats of echocardiographic data works well in most cases, but does have drawbacks in some situations.

Digital compression is a complementary method for increased data reduction. Digital compression is achieved using mathematical algorithms that reduce data redundancy within an image or across a temporal sequence of images. Lossless compression algorithms, such as run length encoding, are generally capable of modest data reductions on the order of 2:1 to 3:1. Lossy compression algorithms have been adopted to achieve 20:1 or greater data reductions. The compression offered by the Joint Photography Expert Group (JPEG) format, although not intended for movies or sequences of images, has provided a means to reduce data size and facilitate data transfer and storage issues. The JPEG compression algorithm uses a frequency-based Discrete Cosine transform, a quantization technique for losing selective information that can be acceptably lost from visual information and Huffman coding, a technique of lossless compression that uses

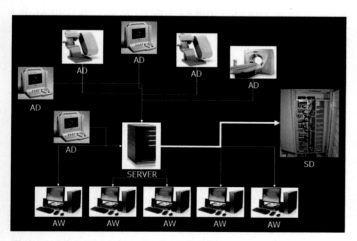

Figure 12.1 Architecture of a digital network. AE, acquisition devices; AW, analysis workstations; SD, long-term storage device.

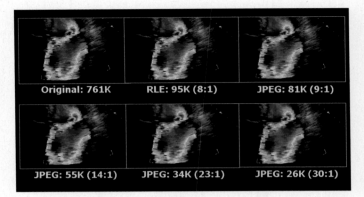

Figure 12.2 Impact of compression of image quality.

code tables based on statistics about the encoded data. The JPEG compression scheme has demonstrated in clinical studies to be usable in echocardiography at compression ratios of 20:1 or higher (Fig. 12.2).[5-7] Additionally, clinical studies have shown that interpretations made by digital acquisitions are accurate in comparison to the traditional videotape review.[8-10]

While the output from cine-imaging modalities was once limited in frame rate capability by the video subsystems which produced images at either 30 fps National Television System Committee (NTSC) or 24 fps Phase Alternating Line (PAL), the ability to digitally generate and store data or "images" at higher frame rates became possible. Today, most modalities offer the ability to store data and generate images at the acquired frame rate. This is a significant advance in digital echocardiography, which now can allow preserved high temporal resolution views of valvular anatomy for example. The ability to store high frame rate data is also critically important for applications where heart rates are faster, including pediatric echocardiography and research investigations on small animals. With these capabilities, however, comes a great increase in data storage. Frames rates of 60 fps, double the size of exams as compared to those originally possible with videotape limitations. Storage itself is not the major issue; however, the ability to work with these larger files presents additional challenges of data transfer and real-time display. While ecine-clips have grown temporally larger in size (higher frame rates and the desire to record longer segments of data), technology to further compress them using temporal data information has not been employed. In addition to the techniques used for JPEG compression, the Moving Picture Experts Group (MPEG) format uses motion compensated predictive coding, in which the differences in what has changed between an image and its preceding image are calculated and only the differences are encoded, as well as bidirectional prediction, in which some images are predicted from the pictures immediately preceding and following the image. MPEG and other video compression algorithms would be ideal candidates for effective file size reduction, but these options are not currently available.

3.2. Storage and archive system

In addition to the hardware necessary to implement a digital noninvasive cardiovascular imaging laboratory, software is needed to manage the transfer, storage, and archival of data as well as the connectivity to HISs including scheduling, reporting and billing. This server software generally runs in the background as a service or services to provide continuous access to the system. The software manages the image transfers from the networked acquisition devices to the local storage and then migrates that data on to the archive.

This software may be part of an integrated hardware–software–network solution or a stand-alone piece of software to be used on third party hardware purchased separately. Integrated solutions are usually more expensive but easier to implement. In general, they are also easier to service, since any problem that may occur falls into the responsibility of a single manufacturer and service contract. Software solutions are less expensive and offer the advantage of allowing unlimited future hardware upgrades, running separate applications within the same hardware. Maintenance issues, however, may become more complex, since problems need to be troubleshot in order to determine if they are caused by software, hardware, or the network itself, which may be covered by separate contracts and manufacturers. Either integrated or a separate software solutions for the digital echo lab can provide similar functionality.

The first main function of the server software is to receive studies acquired on the acquisition devices. The server must be scaled to handle the volume of data that is being simultaneously acquired. In general, the software is configured with connectivity information from each of the modalities that connect to send DICOM images. As the study is received, the images are stored and the exam record is added to a database that includes the patient's name, MRN, date and time of the study and study type, as well as any other desired information, is then available to the review workstations. For each exam, the database maintains the list of all files stored for each exam as well as the location or locations where these files are stored or archived. In more complex environments, the database may be configured to store and match records from various hospitals within an enterprise so that a complete patient record is available.

The second function of the server software is to provide the stored data to the clients or users requesting data. The server software may update the workstation with information about availability of new exams or perhaps details of a change in exam status. Requests for exam images or reports must be processed quickly and delivered to the appropriate client location initiating the request for data. Exams that are in progress may be requested for review, meaning that image data must be forwarded as received by the server to the client that has an exam open for review.

Another function of the server software is data management. The server software can monitor the capacity of the server's redundant array of inexpensive disks (RAID) array and can be automatically set up to erase old studies to accommodate new ones and to transfer studies to the long term archival. These maintenance functions can occur transparently at times when network traffic is lower. If the server is connected with the HIS, it can identify patients that appear in the active hospital list (in-patients or out-patients) and automatically retrieve their pre-existing studies from long-term archival to the RAID array, making them immediately available for review, if desired. This "prefetch" capability can be configured to set limits on the number of prior exams automatically retrieved as well as control the requests based on the period of time for which these prior exams would be desired. These rules could allow, for example, that 3 prior exams from the past 2 years are automatically retrieved to allow quicker access if desired for comparative purposes.

The server software also allows for interfaces with the HIS to receive demographic patient information and electronic exam orders and to transmit reports. Generally, these transactions with the HIS use Health Level Seven standard protocols. With patient demographic and order information, new exams can be verified to ensure that key information was entered properly and matched to orders so that a directly tie between the order and report can be established. Fully integrated reporting ensures accuracy as a link or loop is created through the entire process.

3.3. Network infrastructure

Network transfer is a key component of the digital imaging laboratory as the exchange of data between modalities, servers, and workstations provides the foundation for the use of all components of the system. Computer networks can be characterized in many ways including the distance covered, for example, a local area network (LAN) or a wide area network. A network can be also characterized by the type of data transmission in use (TCP/IP or system network architecture); by the usual nature of its connections (dial-up or switched, dedicated or nonswitched, or virtual connections); and by the types of physical links. All these variables in turn determine data transfer speed.

Ethernet is the most widely installed LAN technology. An Ethernet LAN can use different types of physical links, such as twisted pair wires, coaxial cable, or physical fiber. The most commonly installed Ethernet systems are 100BASE-T and provide transmission speeds up to 100 Mbps (Megabits or million bits per second). "BASE" indicates baseband signaling, which means that only Ethernet signals are carried on the medium, and "T" represents twisted-pair. Gigabit ethernet provides 1 gigabit (or 1 billion bits per second) may also be appropriate. As a network grows in size, areas of increased traffic will benefit from faster connections. The segments might be the connections between the server and archive or storage devices or perhaps between the server and main review workstations.

A network card or adapter is the circuitry designed to provide expanded capability to the workstations, servers, and modalities on the network. The devices are connected to each other through a network switch, which selects the path or circuit for sending a unit of data to its next destination. A switch may also include the function of a router, a device or program that can determine the route and specifically what adjacent network point the data should be sent to. Network switches are also known as layer 3 switches or IP switches and control traffic among LAN devices that have specific IP addresses. A network connection can be used exclusively for a given time interval by two or more LAN devices and then switched for use to another set of parties. This type of all or none "switching" is known as circuit switching and is primarily used for telephone communications. Alternatively, using packet switching, multiple LAN devices can share the same paths at the same time and the particular route a data unit travels can be varied as traffic conditions change in the network. In packet switching, a file is divided into packets, which are units of a certain number of bytes. The network addresses of the sender and of the destination are added to each packet. Packets from the same file may travel different routes and arrive at different times, but at their destination, these are reassembled into the original file. Packet switching is the preferred method implemented in computer network communications.

4. DATA REVIEW AND ANALYSIS TOOLS

Client software at each reviewing station permits query of the server's database. After logging in to establish a connection with the server, the user is presented with a view of information that facilitates workflow. For example, a study list may be displayed showing unread cases for a particular physician or perhaps a work list of new exams for which preliminary assessment is required by the technician (Fig. 12.3). Another common view is a list of exams performed on the current day or for the past several days. In addition to these predefined views, the ability to search the database for a specific patient's exams based on patient name or MRN is common. The view of the information presented to the user should include basic information such as the patient name, MRN, exam date and type, but may also show a second level of detail including performing sonographer and assigned physician

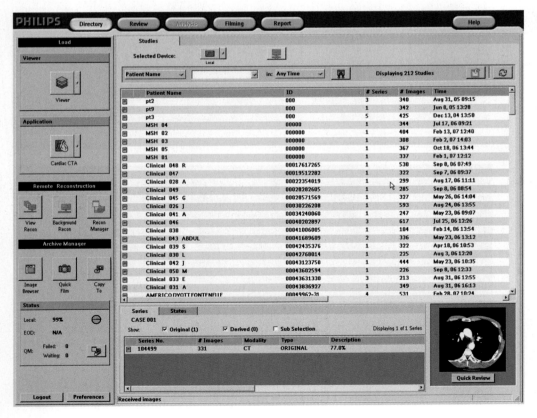

Figure 12.3 Work list display in a typical analysis workstation.

reader, report status (incomplete, unread, verified), exam storage location (local server RAID vs. archived), and HIS verification of matching order and results.

Once single exams or multiple studies are requested for review, they need to be transferred over the network to the client. Upon arrival, they are cached on the client in memory, on disk, or both. The ability to begin a review of the exam without waiting for the entire study to be transferred is advantageous. A series of thumbnails can be displayed on most systems to allow easier navigation through the images and or clips that comprise an exam. The user is able to navigate in order through each image or jump to a desired image by selecting a particular thumbnail. The user can also select a set of thumbnails to bring various images together in a more comprehensive organization. Images acquired with a stress protocol can be displayed in predefined layouts to allow for side-by-side comparison (Fig. 12.4). Once thumbnails are selected, the corresponding images appear in a larger size that

is generally configurable. Multiple controls permit contrast and brightness adjustment, clip play speed control, trimming and magnification. These manipulations may be possible using the mouse buttons or wheel as well as through the use of keyboard shortcuts. Side-by-side comparisons of either different images within a study or between different studies are also extremely useful features. Review of exams during acquisition is also possible and the client software should present new images as they become available. This capability can offer possibilities of guidance from locations away from the acquisition of the exam.

A complete and customizable measurement package is often available, permitting the performance of almost any measurement and calculations that are commonly performed directly in the acquisition device. In contrast to analog media, calibration is not necessary since the calibration information is already included in the digital file (Fig. 12.5). The results of these measurements and calculations can be transferred into a database and use to generate

Figure 12.4 Side-by-side comparison of echocardiography of serial studies obtained on a patient with a pericardial effusion.

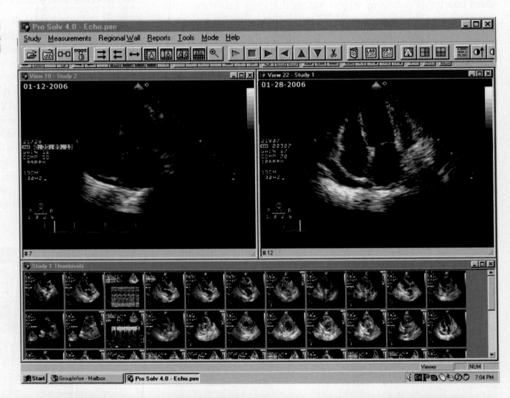

Figure 12.5 Calibration and demographic information included in a DICOM image file.

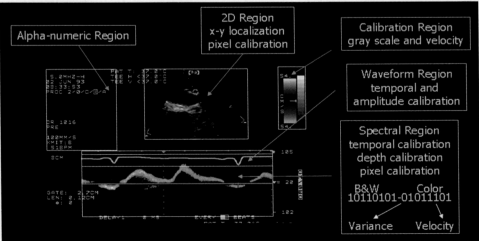

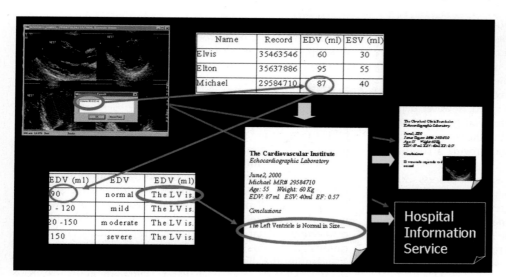

Figure 12.6 Scheme demonstrating the process of analysis, intelligent interpretation, and semiautomated structured report generation.

a report at the end of the review. This feature can save time and eliminate data entry errors. Moreover, measurements can be compared with tables of normalcy, and thus used to generate automatic interpretation (Fig. 12.6). Once a report is completed, it can be electronically signed, transferred to the electronic medical record and perhaps sent to a network printer at a specific location or sent as an e-mail attachment to the referring physician. (Fig. 12.7)

As of to date, most advanced analysis workstations are modality specific. However, common analysis features have been adopted by different imaging modalities and "hybrid" workstations are capable of analyzing data from multiple modalities.

Structured Reporting (see Chapter 13) is terminology that has several meanings. Reports, perhaps even those that are dictated, have structure: Measurements, findings, and conclusions. Reports may also be generated from data entry through a database application where the use selects values from lists in a structured fashion. However, DICOM SR is the ability to pass measurements and calculations performed on the modality to the PACS system for incorporation into the reporting subsystem. This for example can allow a technician to measure end-systolic and end-diastolic volumes directly on the modality and have these values passed to the PACS system for display directly on the report without the need

to re-enter these values from handwritten notes or from copying from images with measurements visible. The process does come with the addition cost in using the modalities measurement tools to identify, by name, each measurement performed, for example, not simply using an area tool to measure left atrial area, but selecting the appropriate label for the measurement such that the PACSs system is able to interpret the value and use it appropriately. The standardization terms for echocardiographic measurements and calculations that can be transmitted as part of a DICOM message.

Propriety imaging data elements are stored by many venders in the DICOM files produced by the acquisition devices. Some of these proprietary elements may be small and contain a parameter that could be used to assist in image postprocessing. Other elements may contain alternative versions of the data, sometimes called raw or native data. These data blocks contain noncompressed or lossless compressed scan-line data that can be used by the vendors' specific analysis workstations to manipulate data to perform post-processing. One example is the ability to perform postacquisition color Doppler gain alterations. Advanced tools like the speckle tracking and three-dimensional (3D) ultrasound volume algorithms also utilize these propriety datasets contained within the DICOM files. The positive aspects of this process is that the DICOM files can be managed by the PACS system allowing access to the raw and native data at any future point in time so that retrospective data analysis can be performed long after the study acquisition date has passed. DICOM file exports or DICOM query-retrieve allows a user access to the raw or native data content. One disadvantage is that these files are often much larger as the data content has in essence doubled.

Remote access capabilities can be very beneficial to allow review of exams away from the laboratory. The limitations of remote access may include network speed, data confidentiality, and reduced review feature capabilities. Data encryption should be implemented for data transmission outside the hospital "firewall" in order to protect patient confidentiality and to comply with State and Federal regulations. Home-based connections to the hospital network are generally possible at fairly low cost using digital subscriber line (DSL) or cable modem solutions. DSL can also provide high-bandwidth data transfer over ordinary telephone lines. A DSL service requires close distance to a telephone that offers the service. With DSL, data can be downloaded from

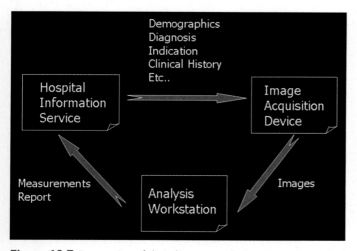

Figure 12.7 Integration of digital images with the electronic medical record.

1 to 6 Mbps, this speed depending on both the physical distance between the provider and the subscriber, and the thickness of the copper wire line in use. On the other hand, data can only be uploaded at about 128 Kbps, Thus DSL is adequate for receiving but not for sending digital imaging studies. Cable modem allows internet access through the cable TV coaxial line, with download speed in average about 1.5 Mbps. Access speed, however, depends on the number of users connected simultaneously, who share the bandwidth. Cable modems are attached to the computer using a 10/100BASE-T ethernet adaptor card and provide a continuous connection.

DICOM media exchange is in theory a simple process whereby an exam is exported in standard format and made available on media for delivery to another user for review. The process however has been complicated by the type media selected, the format of the data used on the media, and the tools included to allow direct viewing of the images. The media types vary from magneto-optical disk (MODs) to CD and DVD, while CDs are now most commonly used. Most imaging exams can be stored on a single CD (~700 MB) with minimal cost as compared to the MODs of the past which not only presented financial issues but access issues as the variety of sizes and densities always presented challenges. Vendor and customers have added viewing software to the basic DICOM export of data on media to allow a simple means to access these data directly from disc without the need to use additional systems. While sometimes convenient, the software choices sometimes mean application installs which at times may fail due to IT restrictions. To overcome some issues seen with this process and perhaps reduce the file size and make for quicker access to the exam, some have selected nonDICOM formatted files for media export, for example windows media formatted clips. While vendors have gone out of their way to find alternative file types for exchange purposes, these CD exams can not be imported into a DICOM system for subsequent storage and review. DICOM files should always be used for data exchange.

Appliances that deliver labeled DICOM media with a selectable viewer can be utilized to allow large quantities of exams to be exported with greater ease and control. These systems are installed on the network as DICOM destinations and data can be transferred to them from the PACs. Once the images are transferred, the process of copying them to media is automatically performed via software and robotic access to CD/DVD cache. Once written, the CD is moved to a printer where a customized label is printed with the source as well as the patient and exam details. Although these systems are currently fairly costly, the ability to create and label exported CDs without a great detail of interaction is attractive.

Web-based and thin-client applications are useful to transfer imaging data remotely at faster speed by applying higher data compression or "streamlining" the processed images for remote viewing. While the data processing capabilities may be limited, these applications are useful for remote consultation and for distribution to referring physicians.

5. FUTURE DIRECTIONS

The digital imaging laboratory is complex and requires a support structure to maintain functionality, train and educate users, troubleshoot issues, and adapt to the changing environment. Maintenance of functionality includes additions of new client installs, configuration of new users, software upgrades, setup of new modalities, and improvements or additions to the reporting component. Troubleshooting can involve PC software issues, network issues (switch/drop configuration, damaged cables, and connections), database issues (correcting patient or exam identifications), and modality acquisition issues such as merged exams.

Adapting the digital laboratory to a multimodality environment will be the newest challenge. Different modalities have unique display and processing features. For example, ultrasound images require color display and fast-cine reproduction, whereas CT requires high spatial resolution display, 3D volume rendering, and wide gray-scale imaging display. Hopefully, adapting analysis workstation to multimodality imaging will reduce the existing space and cost constraints existing in the current environment.

REFERENCES

1. Feigenbaum H. Exercise echocardiography. *J Am Soc Echocardiogr.* 1988;1: 161–166.
2. Feigenbaum H. Digital recording, display, and storage of echocardiograms. *J Am Soc Echocardiogr.* 1988;1:378–383.
3. Thomas JD, Khandheria B. Digital formatting standards in medical imaging: A primer for echocardiographers. *J Am Soc Echocardiogr.* 1994;7:100–104.
4. Thomas J, Adams D, DeVries S, et al. Guidelines and recommendations for digital echocardiography: A report from the digital echocardiography committee of the American Society of Echocardiography. *J Am Soc Echocardiogr.* 2005; 18(3):287–297.
5. Karson TH, Chandra S, Morehead AJ, et al. Compression of digital echocardiographic images: Impact on image quality. *J Am Soc Echocardiogr.* 1995;8:306–318.
6. Thomas JD, Chandra S, Karson TH, et al. Digital compression of echocardiograms: Impact on quantitative interpretation of color Doppler velocity. *J Am Soc Echocardiogr.* 1996;9:606–615.
7. Karson TH, Zepp RC, Chandra S, et al. Digital storage of echocardiograms offers superior image quality to analog storage even with 20:1 digital compression: Results of the Digital ERA (Echo Record Access) study. *J Am Soc Echocardiogr.* 1996;9:769–778.
8. Segar DS, Skolnick D, Sawada SG, et al. A comparison of the interpretation of digitized and videotape recorded echocardiograms. *J Am Soc Echocardiogr.* 1999;12(9):714–719.
9. Lambert AS, Miller JP, Foster E, et al. The diagnostic validity of digitally captured intraoperative transesophageal echocardiography examinations compared with analog recordings: A pilot study. *J Am Soc Echocardiogr.* 1999;12(11):974–980.
10. Haluska B, Wahi S, Mayer-Sabik E, et al. Accuracy and cost- and time-effectiveness of digital clip versus videotape interpretation of echocardiograms in patients with valvular heart disease. *J Am Soc Echocardiogr.* 2001;14:292–298.

Structured Reporting for Noninvasive Cardiology

13

Andrew D. Boyd
Jeffrey S. Soble

1. INTRODUCTION

Historically, computerization in cardiology has been driven by the efficiencies gained from digital imaging, in the form of image availability, image manipulation, and serial comparison. However, in parallel with the use of computers for the acquisition, transmission, and manipulation of digital images, there has been ongoing development and adoption of technology to improve and enhance the clinical reports, which are an integral part of these cardiology procedures. Today, most commercial cardiovascular information systems (CVIS) contain software for digital imaging and the computerized generation of associated procedural reports. Structured Reporting (SR), as used in the context of this review, comprises the use of computerized data input controls to construct this clinical documentation.

The benefits of SR in comparison to free text narrative include (i) potential for integration of information between cardiology devices, image review workstations, and hospital information systems (HISs), (ii) more rapid report generation for commonly encountered clinical scenarios, (iii) consistency in clinical terminology and report layout, (iv) the ability to perform reporting in parallel with image and data review, (v) instantaneous report completion and distribution, and (vi) coded data from procedural reports that can be used for administrative, quality assurance, and research purposes. However, the major challenge of SR is to enhance, rather than detract from the efficiency of physicians, nurses, and technicians, who are often accustomed to and very efficient with reporting by dictation or on paper.

2. HISTORY

As early as the 1960s there were adaptations of generic computer-based medical records focused on cardiac physical findings.[1] In the 1970s digitizers were used in conjunction with standard video echocardiographic output to overlay electronic calipers for measurements performed on a frozen image. In the 1980s the earliest commercial frame grabbers became available and enabled the capture and display of low-resolution echo cineloops.[2] In the 1980s computed tomography, magnetic resonance, and nuclear imaging modalities within radiology adopted the digital imaging and communications (DICOM) standard. In 1992 the American Society for Echocardiography (ASE) formed the Digital Formatting committee to address issues of conversion from analogue to digital echocardiography. The ASE in conjunction with working group 12 of DICOM standard produced supplements specifying formats for echo images and their associated structured reports. These standards promoted the interoperability of echocardiog-

raphy machines with storage devices and imaging workstations, both for echo images and measurement data (Fig. 13.1).[3] In parallel with the implementation of standards and advent of device interoperability, there were numerous academic and commercial efforts to design both modality reporting solutions and comprehensive CVIS. "Iceberg" is an example of one such early departmental SR system built on relational databases.[4] The German Cardiac Society released EchoBefundSystem to promote standardized echocardiography reports across the country.[5]

3. REPORTING METHODS

3.1. Nonstructured reporting

The traditional approach to procedural reporting has been dictation and transcription. In this paradigm the physician reviews all the available data on the procedure, and then dictates a procedural report from start to finish. This dictation is later transcribed by someone on or off site, and the transcribed report is routed back to the physician (either electronically or on paper), who then edits this report and corrects any errors. After the report is retranscribed the final report is then sent back to the physician for final signing and then routed to referring physicians. Over time, the technology has evolved to support transcription and dictation electronically using digital voice capture. Voice files can be sent to transcription services anywhere in the world and the transcribed text routed back to the physician through an electronic document system. In addition, there has been steady improvement in speech recognition systems that are able to transcribe physician speech into text in real time.[6] Hybrid approaches using a speech to text engine with review by a "correctionist" are also in use.

3.2. Structured reporting

SR is generally accomplished using a computer interface integrated with the review of digital images, waveforms, and other data. Procedural reporting entails a workflow that is integrated with the overall operations of the laboratory. This requires that the information system is connected to external sources of data such as the HIS from which patient identifiers (patient name, date of birth, medical record number, etc.) are obtained. DICOM modality worklist provides a standard protocol for importing procedural information directly from the HIS to the device, including the correct patient identifiers and procedures ordered. This eliminates the problems with mistyping patient identifiers that can lead to mismatches between the device output, the hospital, and CVIS.

The acquisition devices themselves provide data about acquisition parameters, measurements and calculations, and specific procedures performed. In addition to effective interfaces between

57

Figure 13.1 DICOM information embedded in a Doppler image.

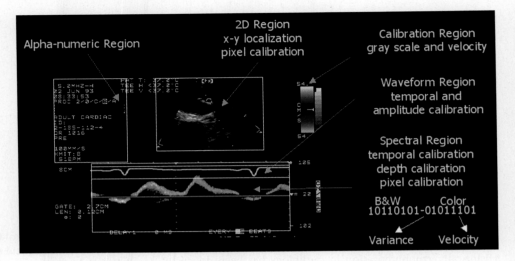

the technical components that make up the system, the system needs to support the workflow of each of the individuals involved in the procedure and their specific laboratory functions. This will typically include the technologist, possibly a nurse or exercise physiologist, and one or more physicians. In academic institutions, cardiology fellows are involved in procedures and the system may support initial interpretation by the fellow followed by over-read by the attending physician. A diagram of a typical SR workflow is shown in Figure 13.2.

A significant benefit of the SR is the consistency of report format and terminology between different reporting physicians. It is certainly possible to achieve this consistency when clinicians are properly trained and oriented to using the system fully. In a study comparing SR interpretation from matched MPEG and VHS echo recordings, there was an 83% exact agreement on specific structured findings and only a 2.7% rate of major discrepancies.[7] In addition, SR can guide or encourage the user to provide a more complete study interpretation; in one study examining SR with cardiologists, the clinical documents generated with SR were more complete and included more clinical concepts than with dictation alone.[8]

However, although uniformity is considered an advantage by administrators and referring physicians, the challenge will be accommodating the reporting styles and preferences of individual reporting physicians. This may be done by allowing user-specific text output for particular coded findings, modification of standard text output on a case-by-case basis, or by allowing the addition of ad hoc free text. In one study[9] examining free text entries and modifications of the standard text output from a SR system, the most common changes were insertions and deletions of normal observations, followed by changes in certainty. Another consideration to review is the contextual nature of medical data.[10] Some report findings may be brought forward from prior reports of the same type; however, the database representation as well as the text output needs to be unambiguous about whether this represents "quotation" of prior results in the current report or new observations that are identical to those from a prior encounter.

The basic technology infrastructure for SR is the same as that required for digital image management and other network data management within the department. This includes generic computer workstations and operating systems connected over a local or wide area network (WAN) or possibly connected to the Internet. Traditionally these systems have been set up in hospital apartments over a local area network. The network is generally protected from the outside world by a firewall and/or other security systems. More recently, there has been a growing emphasis on the wider availability of information retrieval and reporting capabilities over the Internet. This requires a secure WAN using technology such as virtual private networks. A WAN will have technical restrictions related to available bandwidth and the ability for the program to run within standard Internet browsers. In general, however, the software, hardware and network infrastructure required for reporting is much less demanding than that required for digital imaging and is rarely a problem in an environment that can handle the transmission and review of digital images.

3.2.1. Relevant standards

There are a number of important standards and initiatives relevant to SR in cardiology. HL-7 is a global information standard accredited by the American National Standards Institute (ANSI). It specifies a base communication protocol for interchange of data amongst hospital systems. HL-7 is generally used to obtain the correct patient demographic information from the hospital departmental system for the procedure. It is also commonly used to send back the procedural reports in a format that can be imported into a HIS. HL-7 has a cardiology special interest group (SIG), which in part works to harmonize with other relevant standards such as DICOM.

Another important standard is DICOM (digital image communication in medicine). This was initially implemented as a format for the capture and display of digital images and waveforms across modalities (the standard is available for download from ftp://medical.nema.org/medical/dicom/). Over time, it included a supplement for SR (supplement 17). As of this writing, there are relatively complete specifications for structured data in noninvasive vascular, echocardiography, and nuclear cardiology.[3,11] In general, the DICOM standard has evolved from the input of various professional societies in cardiology to describe the interchange of measurements and other key observations. It does not, however, specify the user interface paradigm for the capture of this data, nor does it explicitly describe all of the potential structured data that would be required for complete clinical reporting.

A summary of common standards relevant to SR in cardiology is listed in Table 13.1.

In addition to their involvement in DICOM, relevant professional societies have also been involved in the development of guideline documents outlining the preferred approach to reporting for those modalities.[3,12,13] These official guidelines are extremely useful in delineating the standard approach to modality reporting, although they may not conform to local preferences or change rapidly in response to technological innovations

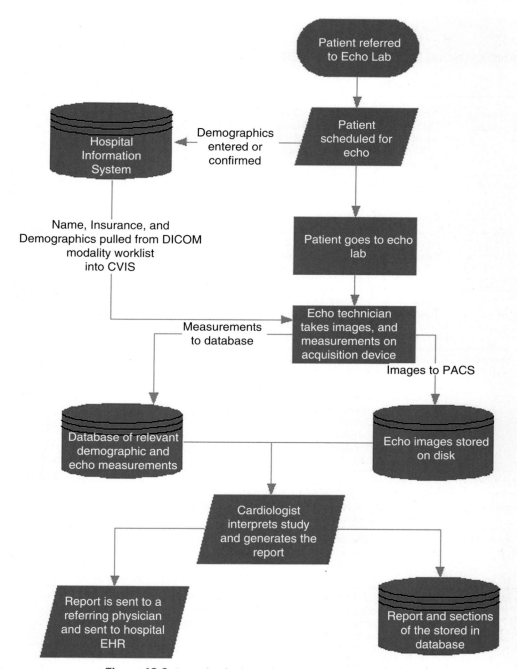

Figure 13.2 Example of echocardiography reporting workflow.

introduced in clinical practice. Over time it is not unlikely that lab accreditation will depend on some level of conformance to these reporting guidelines.

3.2.2. Functional elements
Structural reporting is generally accomplished from within a system that includes a digital image archive, a database for storage and retrieval of patient information and reports, and a series of interfaces to relevant hospital, departmental systems, and devices. The SR system itself is presented to the users through a graphical user interface (GUI). The elements of the structured reported include (i) patient demographics, (ii) patient history and procedural indications, (iii) procedural detail, (iv) detailed procedural findings, and (v) summary and impressions.[14,15]

The graphical interface may allow the user to enter the required procedural data using any number of interface elements, including checkboxes, pick lists, or graphical data entry approaches. Graphical data entry (selecting from anatomic diagrams) often allows a very efficient solution for complex data and can produce output that is clinically intuitive and communicative. An important graphical representation in nuclear and echo imaging is the left ventricular segmentation model. Left ventricular wall motion and perfusion are central to echo and nuclear reports, and the American College of Cardiology has standardized the left ventricular segmentation out of 17 segment model, which has been adopted by the American Society of Echocardiography and the American Society of Nuclear Cardiology.[16] There is more than one graphical representation of the 17 segment model; it can

TABLE 13.1

COMMON STANDARDS RELEVANT TO STRUCTURED REPORTING IN CARDIOLOGY

Standard	Description	Application
ICD-9-CM (International Classification of Diseases)	Published by World Health Organization, CM refers to Clinical Modifications. Rest of the world has transitioned to ICD-10. A version of ICD-10-CM has been published by the federal government	Coding commonly used for billing purposes
CPT (Current Procedural Terminology)	Published by the American Medical Association, updated annually	Coding refers to procedures; complex rules apply to some terms on how the appropriate code is assigned. Primarily used for billing
HL-7 v 2.X	Health Level 7 is a Standards Developing Organizations, who publishes health related standards	Standard used to share data between Clinical Information Systems within a health care enterprise
SNOMED-CT (Systematized Nomenclature of Medicine-Clinical Terms)	Developed by the College of American Pathologists, currently owned by the International Health Terminology Standards Organization	Provides a core terminology for electronic health records. 357,000 concepts; reasonable representation of cardiology concepts could be used to share structured data between systems
IHE (Intergrating the Health care Enterprise)	International organization designed to enable interoperability of clinical information systems across health care domains. Primary sponsors are ACC, RSNA, and HIMSS. IHE Cardiology Technical Framework is focusing on EKG, echocardiography, and Cardiac Catheterization. No standards are developed, but profiles are developed that select appropriate standard implementations for specific clinical work flows	
DICOM SR (Digital Imaging and Communications in Medicine Structured Reporting)	DICOM is an international standards development organization administered by National Electrical Manufacturers Association (NEMA), Medical Imaging, and Technology Alliance	Standard used to create specialized reports that are interoperable between clinical information systems.
LOINC (Logical Observation Identifiers Names and Codes)	Published by the Regenstrief Institute	Terminology designed for laboratory values and other clinical observations to be shared between information systems, including cardiac echo, EKG, etc.
HL-7 Cardiology SIG	Health Level 7 is a Standards Developing Organizations. Cardiology SIG is a forum in which data specific to cardiology is identified and appropriate standards are developed	
RADLEX	Created by the Radiological Society of North America (RSNA)	A lexicon for indexing and retrieval of radiological resources, expanding into cardiology imaging

be displayed in a series of standard cardiac short axis and long axis tomographic images or in a bull's-eye model (Figs. 13.3 and 13.4). The bull's-eye model is a more compact representation, is consistent between modalities, and is optimal for representing data across multiple stages of a procedure (such as wall motion or perfusion). However, it is more abstract than a tomographic representation, and the latter may be a more intuitive for a particular modality. The representations can be used interchangeably, and different representations can even be used for data input and data output, depending on user preference.

From a physician perspective, the study generally begins by review of existing data from different sources such as measure-

ments and calculations by technicians and data from devices. The user is then presented with the most appropriate GUI to complete data entry for the procedure in concert with additional image and waveform or data review. This is generally accomplished by using side-by-side display (Fig. 13.5), often in a multimonitor environment. There are two basic approaches to data entry: forward chaining and backward chaining. Forward chaining of structured data entry involves adding data about the patient on a one-by-one basis as it is interpreted. Backward chaining (sometimes called "reporting by exception") involves the use of standard templates (or macros) from which the individual patient report is constructed. The template allows the

Left Ventricular Segmentation

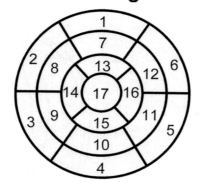

1. basal anterior
2. basal anteroseptal
3. basal inferoseptal
4. basal inferior
5. basal inferolateral
6. basal anterolateral
7. mid anterior
8. mid anteroseptal
9. mid inferoseptal
10. mid inferior
11. mid inferolateral
12. mid anterolateral
13. apical anterior
14. apical septal
15. apical inferior
16. apical lateral
17. apex

Figure 13.3 Left ventricular segmentation, Bull's-eye display. (Reproduced from Cerqueira MD, Weissman NJ, Dilsizian V, et al. Standardized myocardial segmentation and nomenclature for tomographic imaging of the heart: A statement for healthcare professionals from the cardiac imaging committee of the council on clinical cardiology of the American Heart Association. *Circulation.* 2002 Jan;105(4):539–542, with permission.)

report to be populated with "prototypical data," which then needs to be reviewed and edited to conform to the findings of the particular study. Backward chaining has the significant advantages in the rapidity of data entry but requires meticulous review by the operator to make sure that all of the components of the template are appropriate for the individual patient. Data entry is generally completed simultaneously with image and waveform review, and the operator has been able to review a completed, formatted report.

An important step in interpretation is comparison to previous studies. Comparison of serial measurements or quantitative analysis (such as nuclear perfusion) is obviously more amenable to automated or semiautomated computer analysis but is still subject to issues of measurement technique and reproducibility, as well as biologic variability.[17] Subjective interpretations make up the bulk of noninvasive cardiovascular reports, and appropriate serial comparison depends on the availability and integration of both prior images and reports into the physician reporting workflow. Automated comparison of qualitative findings is a logical direction for SR systems but is yet to be utilized in routine clinical practice.

An electronic signature is generally applied using a password protected sign-off, and the procedural report is automatically routed. It is generally the function of the departmental or information system to route the report back to the hospital system through an HL-7 interface and to all referring physicians, most commonly, through automated fax routing. An important part of the reporting system is the ability to handle an addendum, so a user can reopen a study to add corrections and modifications after signing

3.2.3. Software components
Knowledge base—This is the data representation of the clinical knowledge that drives the system. The knowledge base contains the clinical data elements, the metadata that governs the display,

and other behavior of this data in the GUI, as well as the lexical output that creates the text of the report and the formatting elements that govern the visual look and display of the report.

Software component—This is the software that is operated by the user through the GUI based on the knowledge-based data element and constructs the final report.

Database—This is the persistent data storage, in the form of structured documents and/or individual structured data elements. A relational database stores information in tables, while an object database stores individual data elements.

Interfaces—These are the communication mechanisms with other hospital and departmental systems and devices that allow the bidirectional communication of data required to construct and distribute the report.

Web Server—This can be used to provide access to reports using a standard Internet browser (rather than a specialized application), typically either as standard HTML (HyperText Markup Language) pages or in PDF (Portable Document Format).

Fax router—This is used to fax completed reports to referring physicians.

3.2.4. Analysis, calculations, and intelligent interpretation
Cardiology procedures use complex data and reports are dependent on accurate measurements and calculations. In echocardiography, there are a wide range of measurements and calculations in routine clinical practice. Many of these have been encoded in the DICOM Supplement for Structural Reporting. However, more than one equation may exist for a single calculation (for instance, body surface area). It is important that the system is explicit about the calculations used and the references upon which these calculations are based. In addition, cardiology procedures are the results of measurements and calculations often compared to normal databases to determine whether the results are normal or abnormal. Normal ranges may be available in the literature, but can vary from study to study. In addition, degrees of abnormality (mild, moderate, and severe) are less well standardized in the literature.

Calculations often need to be normalized to body size, and this can also be done in a variety of ways, including normalization to body height, body surface area, or body mass index. To make things more complicated, measurements and calculations are often done on the acquisition device and imported into the information system. There can be multiple instances of any particular measurement, and the system needs to be able to display the raw data as well as any calculated means so that the physician can review these data and make sure only the most appropriate information is included in the report.

A more recent area of interest is the use of measurements and calculations to trigger automated interpretations (Fig. 13.6). This has inherit clinical appeal in at least two ways—the time to complete a report may be reduced as much of the report might be automatically generated from measurement data, and the resulting report is more likely to enforce consistency between measurements and interpretations. However there is a potential pitfall to this approach, which can be summarized as "garbage in–garbage out." Any measurement errors will be amplified since not only the measurement itself will be wrong, but the resulting interpretation will also be erroneous. Automated interpretations require meticulous physician review prior to sign-off. Another approach would be to have computer systems enforce this review step, by presenting interpretations to the physician for review prior to inclusion in the report if appropriate.

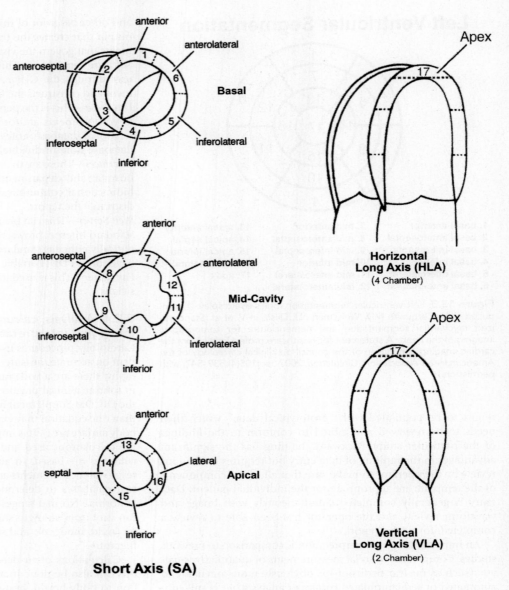

Figure 13.4 Diagram of vertical long-axis, horizontal long-axis, and short-axis planes of the left and right ventricles. (Reproduced from Cerqueira MD, Weissman NJ, Dilsizian V, et al. Standardized myocardial segmentation and nomenclature for tomographic imaging of the heart: A statement for healthcare professionals from the cardiac imaging committee of the council on clinical cardiology of the American Heart Association. *Circulation.* 2002 Jan;105(4):539–542, with permission.)

A related form of reporting intelligence is to have the system apply clinical rules or algorithms to automatically check for reporting consistencies, such as inconsistencies between measurements/calculations and their respective interpretations, as well as inconsistencies within the interpretive data itself. The latter may consist of logically or clinically mutually exclusive data items (such as the statement that there is severe mitral regurgitation and that the mitral valve is normal).

3.2.5. Integration of images
The Holy Grail of cardiology and radiology reporting has been the tight integration of digital imaging with image interpretation. The basis upon which interpretations are made could be much more readily presented to referring physicians and care providers, and serial comparison would be facilitated. The DICOM standard provides a mechanism for linking regions of interest on an image to structural reporting elements, but this has not yet been widely implemented. The primary barrier is physician efficiency and ease of use; clinicians need to be able to easily link together image regions of interest with calculations and interpretations without adding to the time required to do reports.

3.2.6. Report distribution
An important part of clinical reporting is the timely delivery of reports to the point of care. One of the major advantages to SR is that reports are completed in real time during image review;however, these reports need to be routed efficiently to the referring physician to capitalize on this benefit. It is also important that the report (including any graphical elements) be formatted in a way that is appropriate for all modes of distribution. Web access to the report in the browser generally will support colors, flexible layouts, and graphical images; however, HL-7 reports do not support graphical images. Also, reports are still very commonly faxed to referring physicians. This means that all of the report elements including graphics need to be displayed, legible and easily readable in black and white format.

3.2.7. Critical results
An important performance metric for the Joint Commission for Hospital Accreditation is the timely reporting of stat procedures and critical results to the provider(s) caring for the patient. It is important not only to define what constitutes a critical result for any procedure, but also to document the transmission of critical

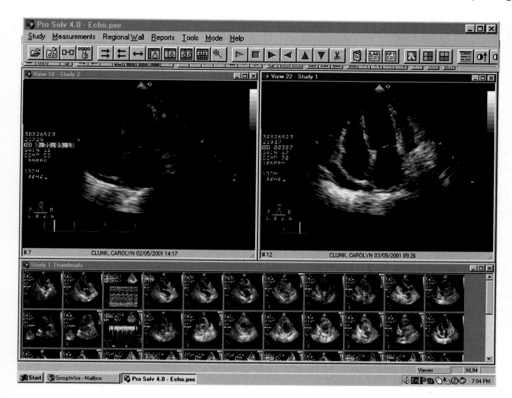

Figure 13.5 Side-by-side comparison of serial studies in a patient with a pericardial effusion.

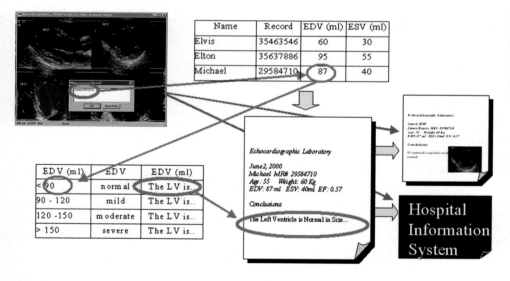

Figure 13.6 Diagram illustrating the process of "intelligent interpretation." A measurement performed in a calibrated image is transferred into a database containing demographic information. The value is related to a table to generate a descriptive statement in the report.

results, including the timing of events and individuals involved. The reporting system should facilitate critical results reporting and tracking.

3.2.8. Data merging, migration, and queries

One of the important benefits of SR is the clinical data elements that are created as a byproduct of the process of care. These data elements can be stored in any number of formats, including XML (extensible markup language), or relational database tables. Advanced database capabilities have allowed for the principal query of information of multiple formats. An important consideration, however, is the clinical terminology that is used in the structured data. This can include proprietary coding formats or standard terminology such as ICD-9/10, Current Procedural Ter-

minology (CPT), DICOM SR, and Systematized Nomenclature of Medicine (SNOMED). Each of these terminologies has its own advantages and particular uses. ICD-9 and CPT codes are used for diagnosis and procedure codes primarily for billing. DICOM SR codes incorporate parts of SNOMED and allow for the transition of data through the DICOM standard. SNOMED is an international standard for clinical terminology that has been used to create interoperability amongst clinical data from disparate systems.

Most cardiologists are familiar with the limitations of ICD-9 and CPT codes. Neither code set represents the complete clinical picture of a patient. A study examining billing data[18] versus the data stored in the clinical information system for patients with ischemic heart disease, demonstrated that the billing data failed to identify more than one half of the patients with conditions that would affect prognosis. Few physicians would make clinical care decisions from just billing data.

SNOMED-CT was created by the College of American Pathologists. Through extensive refinement the terminology has been expanded to cover multiple medical disciplines. SNOMED-CT provides the finest detail over the largest clinical domains compared to other medical terminologies. However, like all structured terminologies, perfect representation of medical concepts is allusive. Mapping clinical data to SNOMED-CT can produce ambiguity and missing concepts.[19] Trying to electronically track the AHA/ACC guidelines for chronic heart failure with structured terminology covered only 86% of the concepts.[20] This ambiguity needs to be resolved by professional coders and clinicians searching for the appropriate representations.

No matter what the coding system, the SR system must be combined with the tools required for users to produce administrative, quality assurance, and research reports. This may include stock reports, as well as the ability to perform ad hoc queries. SQL (standard query language) is a commonly used approach to learning the data query from standard SQL tables and relational databases. Other types of visual data query tools can be constructed from relational, objective, or XML databases.

3.2.9. Quality assurance
An important function of the coded clinical data for structured reports is to enable quality assurance within the laboratory and department. This would include (i) monitoring and documenting the communication of stat procedural findings and clinical results, (ii) identification and investigation of sentinel events and their root cause analysis, (iii) monitoring of best practices amongst the users, (iv) the potential ability to look at the clinical variables and their effect on patient outcomes, and (v) tracking quality indicators over time.

The specific quality assurance parameters and methods implemented by the laboratory and department will vary. However, the SR system should provide the requisite data, in a usable database format, and have the data query at retrieval tools to support these ongoing processes. A recent consensus statement regarding quality in cardiovascular imaging, confirmed the need for SR.[21] The American Society for Nuclear Cardiology (ASNC) consensus statement also supports the use of structure reporting for myocardial perfusion imaging.[12]

4. FUTURE DIRECTIONS

Hybrid reporting attempts to utilize the best attributes of GUI elements, speech recognition engines, and natural language processing (NLP). NLP is the ability to derive semantic meaning from free text statements. The advantage of free text is that users can simply report findings in their own language through speech, which is very efficient. NLP attempts to derive coded data from this text, primarily for use in billing or quality assurance. However, the limitations of NLP have been detailed extensively.[22]

Another potential direction will be the distribution of report elements throughout the enterprise. This may include having procedure reporting capabilities on devices themselves, in addition to laboratory and departmental workstations. There needs to be a seamless flow of information through the work flow chain, and distribution of information components through web-based technologies is now practical.

Harmonization of society recommendations for SR with coded terminologies such as SNOMED will be an important direction for SR. In addition, institutions are gradually recognizing the advantages of integrating cardiology and radiology functions. "Enterprise image management" will provide an impetus to the integration of clinical reporting as well. A new radiology lexicon was released in November 2006. RADLEX is a lexicon for radiological images developed by the Radiological Society of North America (RSNA). There is a commitment to map available SNOMED-CT terms to RADLEX. However, in the first release of RADLEX coverage of cardiology terms was sparse. A more complete integration of RADLEX, SNOMED, and DICOM SR would facilitate the development of more interoperable SR systems based on standardized terminologies.

REFERENCES

1. Juergens JL, Kiely JM. Physician entry of cardiac physical findings into a computer-based medical record. *Mayo Clin Proc.* 1969 Jun;44(6):361–366.
2. Feigenbaum H. Digital recording, display, and storage of echocardiograms. *J Am Soc Echocardiogr.* 1988 Sep–Oct;1(5):378–383.
3. Thomas JD, Adams DB, Devries S, et al. Guidelines and recommendations for digital echocardiography. *J Am Soc Echocardiogr.* 2005 Mar;18(3):287–297.
4. Bandini A, Balestra G, Simoni C, et al. Comprehensive computer-assisted management of a cardiology department. *G Ital Cardiol.* 1991 Mar;21(3):281–289.
5. Schweikart O, Metzger F. Standardized findings in echocardiography using WWW: echobefundsystem. *Z Kardiol.* 2001 Jan;90(1):12–20.
6. Kauppinen T, Koivikko MP, Ahovuo J. Improvement of report workflow and productivity using speech recognition—a follow-up study. *J Digit Imaging.* 2008;21(4):378–382.
7. Soble JS, Yurow G, Brar R, et al. Comparison of MPEG digital video with super VHS tape for diagnostic echocardiographic readings. *J Am Soc Echocardiogr.* 1998 Aug;11(8):819–825.
8. Rosenbloom ST, Kiepek W, Belletti J, et al. Generating complex clinical documents using structured entry and reporting. *Medinfo.* 2004;11(Pt 1):683–687.
9. Wilcox AB, Narus SP, Bowes WA, III. Using natural language processing to analyze physician modifications to data entry templates. *Proc AMIA Symp.* 2002:899–903.
10. Berg M. Patient care information systems and health care work: A sociotechnical approach. *Int J Med Inform.* 1999 Aug;55(2):87–101.
11. Port SC. Imaging guidelines for nuclear cardiology procedures. *J Nucl Cardiol.* 1999;6(2):G47–G84.
12. Hendel RC, Wackers FJ, Berman DS, et al. American society of nuclear cardiology consensus statement: Reporting of radionuclide myocardial perfusion imaging studies. *J Nucl Cardiol.* 2003 Nov–Dec;10(6):705–708.
13. Gerhard-Herman M, Gardin JM, Jaff M, et al. Guidelines for noninvasive vascular laboratory testing: A report from the American Society of Echocardiography and the Society for Vascular Medicine and Biology. *Vasc Med.* 2006 August;11(3):183–200.
14. Clunie DA. *DICOM Structured Reporting.* Bangor, PA: PixelMed Publishing; 2000.
15. Hussein R, Engelmann U, Schroeter A, et al. DICOM structured reporting: Part 1. overview and characteristics. *Radiographics.* 2004 May;24(3):891–896.
16. Cerqueira MD, Weissman NJ, Dilsizian V, et al. Standardized myocardial segmentation and nomenclature for tomographic imaging of the heart: A statement for healthcare professionals from the cardiac imaging committee of the council on clinical cardiology of the american heart association. *Circulation.* 2002 Jan;105(4):539–542.
17. Iskandrian AE, Garcia EV, Faber T. Analysis of serial images: A challenge and an opportunity. *J Nucl Cardiol.* 2008 Jan–Feb;15(1):23–26.
18. Jollis JG, Ancukiewicz M, DeLong ER, et al. Discordance of databases designed for claims payment versus clinical information systems. Implications for outcomes research. *Ann Intern Med.* 1993 Oct;119(8):844–850.
19. Hunscher D, Boyd A, Green LA, et al. Representing natural-language case report form terminology using health level 7 common document architecture, LOINC, and SNOMED-CT: Lessons learned. *AMIA Annu Symp Proc.* 2006:961.
20. Dykes PC, Currie LM, Cimino JJ. Adequacy of evolving national standardized terminologies for interdisciplinary coded concepts in an automated clinical pathway. *J Biomed Inform.* 2003;36(4–5):313–325.
21. Douglas P, Iskandrian AE, Krumholz HM, et al. Achieving quality in cardiovascular imaging: proceedings from the American College of Cardiology–Duke University medical center think tank on quality in cardiovascular imaging. *J Am Coll Cardiol.* 2006 11/21;48(10):2141–2151.
22. van Ginneken AM. Structured data entry in ORCA: The strengths of two models combined. *Proc AMIA Annu Fall Symp.* 1996:797–801.

Image Fusion

14

Raj Shekhar

1. INTRODUCTION

The motivation for fusing cardiac images parallels that for image fusion in noncardiac applications: simultaneous presentation of complementary anatomic and functional information. No single imaging modality gathers complete information on the underlying cardiac anatomy and physiology, whether normal or pathological. External means are therefore needed to register (spatially align) and then fuse data from two or more different imaging modalities.

From the perspective of image fusion, cardiac imaging modalities can be classified as structural or functional. Computed tomography (CT), magnetic resonance (MR) imaging, and echocardiography belong to the former category, whereas nuclear medicine modalities—positron emission tomography (PET) and single-photon emission CT (SPECT)—fall in the latter category. Although both MR imaging and echocardiography show the potential for gathering functional information, these capabilities remain in the early stages of development. It is unlikely that in the near term they can match the unique functional imaging capabilities of radionuclide imaging. The need for multimodality cardiac image fusion is thus expected to persist well into the foreseeable future.

The majority of past and present cardiac image fusion attempts have combined an imaging modality from the structural group with an imaging modality from the functional group. This combination is clinically valuable because of the relative strengths and weaknesses of the anatomic and functional imaging modalities. Nuclear medicine techniques offer higher sensitivity and an ability to detect even subtle changes resulting from disease or in response to therapy, often before corresponding anatomic changes can be detected by structural imaging techniques.

Because of their poor spatial resolution, lack of anatomic detail, and propensity for nonspecific uptakes even in healthy tissues, nuclear medicine techniques cannot optimally perform these tasks alone. Their fusion with CT, MR imaging, and echocardiography provides anatomic reference to functional and metabolic abnormalities, while simultaneously ruling out disease in healthy tissues with abnormal uptakes.[1] The higher spatial resolution of CT and MR imaging has been used to mitigate both image noise and the partial volume effect in PET and SPECT.[2,3]

Cardiac image fusion improves on the diagnostic accuracy of a single imaging modality. It is also a key to making disease diagnosis at an earlier stage and performing timely post-therapy assessment.[1,4] The emergence of hybrid PET/CT and SPECT/CT (and, more recently, PET/MR) scanners is clearly playing a significant role in bringing out these advantages and driving new applications. Cardiac image fusion tasks involving echocardiography remain limited clinically at present, but their novel applications in both diagnostics and in real-time procedure guidance are emerging. This chapter attempts to survey notable multimodality cardiac imaging attempts to date, beginning with a historical perspective.

1.1. Historical perspective

Multimodality image fusion, for obvious reasons, followed the development of individual modalities. The desire to combine dual-modality images, however, dates back to the beginning of tomographic imaging. Early attempts at emission and transmission tomographic imaging began in the early 1960s. The first example of multimodality imaging has been attributed to the work of Kuhl et al.,[5] who in 1966 reported acquisition of an axial scan of the thorax using a SPECT prototype. It was not until the late 1980s that the field saw more systematic multimodality image fusion attempts after the commercial introduction and growth of CT and SPECT in the 1970s and MR and PET imaging in the 1980s. Although ultrasound predates tomographic imaging modalities, with the first use in the heart reported in 1951, the 1980s also saw maturation and wider use of echocardiography, building on the development of M-mode ultrasound in the 1960s and two-dimensional (2D) ultrasound in the 1970s.

Early image registration attempts, developed primarily for brain images, relied on either manual, fiducial-based, or feature-based methods to register images collected on separate scanners and often during separate visits.[6,7] Although applying these to the brain (which does not deform between imaging sessions) was relatively easy and produced good accuracy, comparative attempts with cardiac images were complicated by respiratory and heart motion and the fact that the heart offered few landmarks or features that could be reliably identified. Nevertheless, several software-based techniques were applied to cardiac images.[8] These techniques and their specific applications are described in more detail in Section 3.

Even with the recent emergence of hybrid imaging devices, software-based methods continue to grow and have a definite role to play, especially in cardiac image fusion. First, this is because software-based approaches are the only option when no appropriate hybrid imaging technique exists and at facilities with no hybrid imaging capability. Because cardiac imaging involves significant voluntary and involuntary (breathing and heart) motion, dual-modality scans from hybrid scanners still need refinement for accurate spatial matching, a task possible only with manual or software-based techniques.[1,9] These methods continue to gain sophistication and increasingly account for nonrigid elastic changes beyond correcting for simply rigid changes resulting from translation and rotation.

As a result of the pioneering work of Hasegawa and colleagues at the University of California, San Francisco (UCSF) in the 1990s, a new approach to image fusion emerged, which is often referred to as the hardware approach. Software-based methods combine separately acquired images, but these investigators envisioned a system that could produce dual-modality images simultaneously, eliminating the need for postacquisition image alignment.[1,4,10] The prototype system they developed could simultaneously acquire a radionuclide image and a low-dose CT image of the anatomy of interest. The original system was suitable for preclinical phantom and animal imaging only, and with it these investigators showed the first fusion scan that overlaid a perfusion image of swine myocardium acquired with ^{99m}Tc-sestamibi SPECT onto a grayscale CT image. The group also pioneered and implemented CT-based attenuation correction of SPECT using this prototype. A novel and defining feature of this system was a common detector sensitive to both X-ray photons and photons from the radioisotope. Although this afforded perfect registration between the two component images, it came at the expense of small detector array size and, therefore, long acquisition times. Despite the use of low-dose X-ray, the high photon count of the X-ray beam created a challenge for the photon-counting detector. Attempts to alternate between the detection of CT and SPECT scans were not successful either. Although conceptually attractive, this initial design proved impractical and too expensive for routine clinical use.

The Hasegawa team is also credited with conceiving the first modern-day SPECT/CT scanner. The impracticality of their earlier prototype led the group to think of the now familiar design in which CT and SPECT gantries are arranged in tandem with a common couch that extends far enough so that both scans can be performed during a single session, without the patient leaving the couch between scans.[1,4,10] In the mid-1990s, the group combined a GE 9,800 Quick CT scanner and a GE XR/T SPECT and demonstrated clinical studies with this approach. The CT data, as in the earlier prototype, were used for SPECT attenuation correction.

The first PET/CT scanner, along the lines of the UCSF SPECT/CT prototype, was independently proposed by Townsend.[4] in the early 1990s. The first prototype was built by CTI PET Systems (now Siemens Molecular Imaging) in 1998 and combined a single-slice Siemens Somatom CT scanner with a rotating CTI ECAT ART PET scanner, using a common couch. The PET detectors were mounted on the back of the CT support and rotated with the CT as a single unit. The CT data were used for attenuation correction of PET photons. This prototype scanner was installed at the University of Pittsburg (PA) Medical Center and a number of clinical oncology studies were conducted using this prototype. It was replaced in 2001 with a commercial PET/CT system (described in more detail later in this chapter).

2. HYBRID IMAGING SYSTEMS

2.1. Introduction

Two types of hybrid imaging systems—PET/CT and SPECT/CT—are currently available commercially for clinical use and are offered by most medical imaging vendors. These systems follow the common couch design of the earlier prototypes and combine a latest-version CT scanner with a latest-version PET or SPECT scanner. In all current SPECT/CT designs, the gamma camera is in front of the CT gantry and, in all current PET/CT designs, the CT gantry is in front of the PET gantry. The two types of scans are performed sequentially with minimal time delay during a single session. Often the CT scan is performed before sliding the patient either up or down for SPECT or PET scanning. Because of the geometry of these scanners, only an axial translation separates the two coordinate systems in which the two scans are recorded. Spatial registration is thus achieved by simply sliding one scan with respect to another by the axial distance between the two gantries.

Both types of hybrid scanners are enjoying great success and seeing growing clinical acceptance. Several factors are responsible for this success. First, hybrid scanning, by virtue of being performed by a single system and during a single visit, ensures colocation of the two datasets that are readily available for fusion. Similar scans from standalone scanners may be brought to a single medical workstation for fusion purposes, but doing so remains inconvenient and labor intensive. Hybrid scanning further ensures that the same body position and orientation are maintained during the two scans, thereby removing the most obvious sources of geometric misalignments (patient repositioning, different couch shapes, variable filling status of internal organs, etc.) between the two scans and greatly facilitating the anatomic location of functional findings. Some patient motion, however, is unavoidable during the sequential scanning, especially because of the different scan protocols and scan durations. Although CT can be performed in a single breath-hold on most multislice systems, the slower PET and SPECT scan may last from 10 min up to an hour, depending on the protocol. In cardiac imaging, breathing-induced misregistration between the two component images is even more pronounced. Strategies to reduce motion artifacts are discussed later in this chapter.

The ability to use CT for attenuation correction of both PET and SPECT images is another strength of the hybrid systems. Although a transmission scan for attenuation correction could be acquired before the advent of hybrid devices by using a standalone PET or SPECT scanner, SPECT images acquired on a standalone SPECT scanner are seldom corrected for attenuation in most clinical centers. The importance of attenuation correction can be appreciated by disappearance of an apparent perfusion defect in cardiac SPECT following attenuation correction (Fig. 14.1). Technical details of CT-based attenuation correction are reviewed later in this section.

Yet another advantage of modern hybrid scanners is that they are a "loose" integration of two standalone scanners. This design intrinsically offers the flexibility to choose any configuration of the CT scanner (from low-end to high-end) for the hybrid device, offering a broad range of hybrid systems in terms of technical and clinical capabilities. Practical considerations such as cost can influence the type of CT used, as in SPECT/CT, where the highest-end CT currently offered is a 16-slice CT scanner even when scanners with 64 or more slices exist. This design flexibility also affords future upgrade capabilities without the need to replace the whole system.

Finally, although a prototype of a hybrid PET/MR device has recently emerged,[11] its early applications remain limited to brain imaging and so will not be discussed here. A limited number of small animal hybrid PET/MR scanners are in use at research centers around the world, and initial preclinical work has been reported on imaging of rat hearts.[12] These efforts, too, are outside the scope of this chapter. In the following two sections, we describe hybrid SPECT/CT and PET/CT systems, as well as technical aspects common to both and special considerations for cardiac imaging.

2.2. SPECT/CT

The first commercial SPECT/CT system—the GE Hawkeye—was introduced in 1999.[1,10] This system used a dual-head GE Discovery VG SPECT system capable of planar scintigraphy, SPECT, and

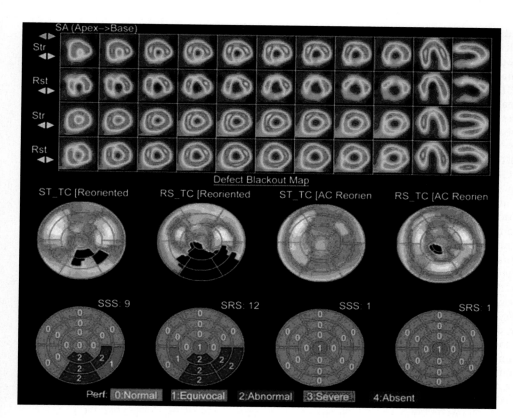

Figure 14.1 An apparent perfusion defect is visible in cardiac SPECT images before attenuation correction (*top two rows*). Following attenuation correction (*next two rows*), the defect disappears. The disappearance of defect following attenuation correction can be seen in the corresponding bull's-eye views at the bottom. (Reproduced from Bybel B, Brunken RC, DiFilippo FP, et al. SPECT/CT imaging: Clinical utility of an emerging technology. *Radiographics.* 2008 Jul–Aug;28(4):1097–1113, with permission.)

coincident ^{18}F-FDG PET imaging. Integrated with this system was a low-dose CT system that operated at 140-kV tube voltage and 2.5-mA tube current and could rotate around the patient's body continuously—although quite slowly (rotation time of ~20 s) because of the heavy detector assembly. The resulting CT images had an in-plane resolution of 2.5 and 10-mm slice thickness. Acquired at a significantly lower dose than the diagnostic dose (2.5 and 100 mA or greater, respectively), the CT images provided adequate information for attenuation correction in a cost-effective manner, but the anatomic information available for fusion was of very low resolution. This model was followed with the Infinia Hawkeye-4, still featuring a low-power X-ray tube (120/140 kV tube voltage; 2.5 mA tube current) but capable of collecting thinner 2.5-mm slices.

The other two major vendors, Siemens and Philips, began offering hybrid SPECT/CT in 2004.[4] Much like PET/CT systems, these vendors offer SPECT/CT with modern CT systems capable of diagnostic quality imaging. Both Siemens Symbia and Philips Precedence series SPECT/CT scanners combine dual-head gamma cameras with multislice CT scanners (up to 16 slices for both Philips Precedence and Siemens Symbia) and with subsecond rotation speeds. Both systems, much like the GE Hawkeye series, are also offered with a low-power CT system capable of basic anatomic localization and attenuation correction. Advanced CT capabilities offered as part of SPECT/CT systems have the advantage of offering high-resolution images with greater soft tissue contrast for anatomic correlation, improved accuracy for the quantification of radiotracer uptake, and the ability to perform contrast-enhanced perfusion studies. An important emerging application of hybrid systems with multislice CT is correlating myocardial perfusion data from SPECT with coronary anatomy from CT angiography (CTA) for more accurate diagnosis of coronary artery disease (CAD) (discussed in Section 4.1).

2.3. PET/CT

The first commercial PET/CT system (GE Discovery LS) was announced in early 2001. It was soon followed by the Biograph model by Siemens and the Gemini model by Philips. These systems have evolved rapidly since their introduction. Thanks to its significance in oncologic imaging and the availability of reimbursement, PET/CT, in fact, has been the fastest growing clinical imaging modality over the past decade. The CT subsystem is available in up to a 64-slice configuration in systems offered by all three major vendors. The PET subsystem uses vendor-specific detector technologies, most taking advantages of the latest advances in the PET technology, such as septaless three-dimensional (3D) data acquisition that maximizes photon counts and has been shown to produce higher sensitivity images. The Siemens Biograph and Philips Gemini models acquire data only in the 3D mode, whereas the GE Discovery models offer both 2D and 3D image acquisition. Although all systems offer a radionuclide-based transmission source for creating a transmission scan for attention correction, CT-based attention correction is the de facto standard now for hybrid PET/CT. From the attention correction perspective, the fields of view of PET and CT systems are of particular importance. A smaller CT field of view is a source of artifacts, as discussed below.

2.4. Technical considerations

2.4.1. Attenuation correction

In both PET and SPECT, the source of radiation is the gamma photons emitted by the radioisotopes distributed nonuniformly throughout the patient's body. Depending on the location of these radioisotopes, the gamma photons travel different distances inside the body and are attenuated (absorbed by the tissue) to varying degrees. For example, in cardiac SPECT, photons originating from the inferior wall of the left ventricle must travel though much denser tissues (heart, blood, etc.) than photons from the lateral wall and, therefore, are more likely to be absorbed before reaching the detector. This varying attenuation of photons must be accounted for in the reconstruction process. If no correction is made, the result is well-known artifacts in the inferior wall, affecting the diagnostic outcome.[13]

Attenuation correction requires a map of linear attenuation coefficients, which is exactly what a CT image represents. The ready availability of a registered CT image along with a SPECT or PET scan from hybrid imaging devices makes attenuation correction convenient. The process of CT-based attenuation correction is well described in the literature.[1,4,10,13] Before the advent of hybrid imaging devices, standalone SPECT and PET scanners provided a radionuclide source to create a CT-like transmission scan for the express purpose of attenuation correction. The lengthy acquisition of this transmission scan affected throughput and all but discouraged attenuation correction for SPECT images at most centers. Using CT for attenuation correction has several advantages. CT acquisition on modern multislice scanners is fast, and CT images are less noisy. Unlike a radionuclide source with decreasing activity during scanning, the X-ray source maintains consistent beam intensity throughout CT acquisition.

A CT image represents a map of linear attenuation coefficients at the mean energy of the polychromatic X-ray beam. Because the linear attenuation coefficient is energy dependent and different radionuclides emit photons of different energies, linear attenuation coefficients measured by CT at the mean photon energy of ~70 KeV must be converted to the energy of the emission photons, which for SPECT varies by the radiotracer used (e.g., 140 KeV) and is 511 KeV for the positron-emitting radiotracers used in PET. The scaling factors that convert CT intensity (measured in Hounsfield units) to linear attenuation coefficients have been determined by scanning phantoms with varying concentrations of biologically equivalent materials. The typical shape of these conversion plots is bilinear (Fig. 14.2): one linear segment for tissues representing mixtures of air and water and another representing mixtures of water and bone. Once corrected for energy, the CT image is down-sampled to match the lower spatial resolution of SPECT and PET, forward projected, and used during PET/SPECT image reconstruction. Image reconstruction is increasingly performed using iterative techniques. The original CT image continues to be used for the fusion of anatomy and function.

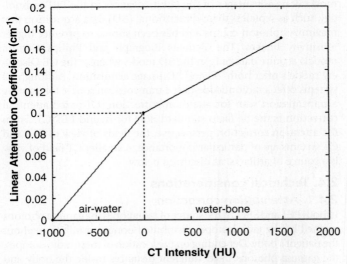

Figure 14.2 Bilinear scaling curve to convert CT intensity of linear attenuation coefficient at PET photon energy (511 KeV) for CT-based attenuation correction of PET. A similar relationship exists at other photon energies for use with SPECT. (Redrawn from Townsend DW. Multimodality imaging of structure and function. *Phys Med Biol.* 2008; 53(4):R1–R39.)

2.4.2. Motion-induced attenuation correction artifacts and correction strategies

CT-based attenuation correction is sensitive to spatial misalignment between the CT and emission scans as a result of a number of factors: breathing, cardiac contraction, patient movement between sequential scans, and table sag (less problematic in newer hybrid imaging systems). Figure 14.3 shows examples of correct attenuation correction as well as artifacts introduced in cardiac PET/CT as a result of misalignment. Although the severity of artifacts is patient dependent, even a single-pixel shift (~7 mm in SPECT) can cause overcorrection or undercorrection of attenuation when cardiac and lung tissues are misaligned.[10]

The CT subsystem in the modern hybrid scanners is sufficiently fast to image the entire heart in a single breathhold. No respiratory gating is needed, but cardiac gating (either retrospective or, more recently, prospective) is used to reconstruct artifact-free images of the heart. A cardiac CT scan thus represents a snapshot of the thorax for a given breathing and cardiac phase. SPECT or PET scans, on the other hand, are reconstructed from data collected over tens of minutes and over numerous cycles of shallow breathing and cardiac contraction and represent a motion-averaged heart and thorax. This difference in scan procedures is a significant contributor to the anatomic mismatch between CT and PET or SPECT scans and a source of artifacts in CT-based attenuation. Gould et al.[14] have reported false-positive results in cardiac PET/CT arising from improper attenuation correction in up to 40% of patients. Goetze and Wahl.[15] have observed a similar rate of misalignment artifacts in cardiac SPECT/CT.

Addressing this problem remains an area of active research.[13,14,16] Almost all solutions attempt to match breathing patterns between the two scans, and one of the easiest approaches is to do so by "blurring" the CT scan while leaving PET or SPECT unchanged, so that the CT image represents a motion-averaged anatomy as well. This is achieved by acquiring a slow CT scan that averages measurements from several breathing and cardiac cycles (although not as many as in PET or SPECT). The resulting CT is, however, not of diagnostic quality. When a diagnostic-quality CT (with breath hold) is clinically indicated, the acquisition of a separate low-dose slow CT scan for attenuation correction only is often recommended. An alternate technique is to acquire CT in multiple phases of the breathing cycle through respiratory gating. An average of all the phases is then presumed to depict roughly the same thoracic and cardiac anatomy as that in the PET or SPECT images. Although any of the phases can be used as a diagnostic scan, respiratory gating of CT remains uncommon outside radiotherapy applications. Both these techniques result in longer CT acquisition times and higher radiation doses to patients.

An alternative to blurring CT is to "deblur" PET or SPECT to make them equivalent to breathhold CT.[13] An emerging technique is to acquire respiratory-gated PET and perform attenuation correction of only those PET images with phases that match the phases of the CT. In other words, if the CT was acquired in end-inspiration, perform attenuation correction on end-inspiration PET. An obvious disadvantage of this technique is lower signal-to-noise ratio in the PET image as a result of lower photon count. This problem may be overcome by using sophisticated nonrigid image registration algorithms (in software) to consolidate gated PET to a simulated breathhold PET. This would mean creating an end-inspiration PET and using the end-inspiration CT for both attention correction and anatomic correlation.

These approaches, although attractive, do not guarantee perfect alignment between emission and transmission scans. A quality control step to ensure accurate spatial alignment before moving on with

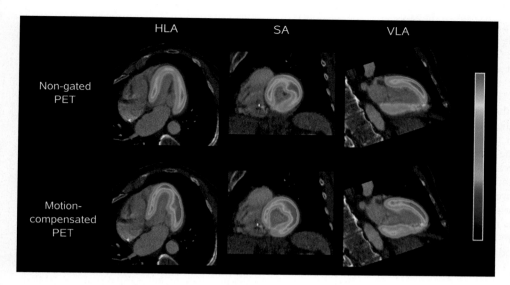

Figure 14.3 The results of CT-based attenuation correction in cardiac PET/CT. Fusion images in horizontal long axis (HLA), short axis (SA) and vertical long axis (VLA) orientations show an underestimation of radiotracer uptake when inspiration CT is used for attenuation correction of motion-averaged PET (top row). The apparent artifact dissappears when motion-averaged PET is replaced with inspiration PET (bottom row) following motion compensation. (Courtesy of Dr. Klaus Schäfers, European Institute of Molecular Imaging, University of Münster.)

attenuation correction is recommended in most clinical settings.[17] This step may involve manually refining any residual mismatch.

2.4.3. Other sources of attenuation correction artifacts

Metals, calcifications, and oral and intravenous contrast agents in the imaging field of view can also cause artifacts in attenuation correction.[4] By properly adjusting attenuation correction coefficients at the voxel locations of these confounding elements, their harmful effects can be mitigated. The issue of intravenous contrast is particularly important for cardiac imaging as dual-modality PET/CTA and SPECT/CTA are emerging as new clinical applications. Although highly attenuating at X-ray photon energies, iodine causes only about 2% attenuation at the PET energy. Using a contrast CT for attenuation correction directly has been shown to yield a very low rate of artifacts, yet a suppression of contrast intensity in CT (identified through image segmentation) for attenuation correction is warranted. Another common approach to avoid artifacts in the case of CTA is to acquire an additional noncontrast CT (often low-dose) for the purpose of attention correction.

The smaller axial field-of-view of CT compared to that of SPECT and PET could also cause artifacts in attenuation correction because the CT scan may fail to image the patient, especially those who are obese, completely. Extrapolation techniques that extend the CT scan to generate an attenuation map have been suggested to overcome this problem and have produced satisfactory results.

3. MULTIPLE-PLATFORM INTEGRATION

At the same time that SPECT/CT and PET/CT hybrid imaging devices are seeing growing clinical acceptance because of their convenient approaches to multimodality imaging, many other modality combinations are also of clinical interest. For many of these combinations no hybrid imaging option currently exists (and, in some cases, may never exist) because of technical challenges complicating development and because of a lack of projected clinical demand. Software-based techniques are expected to "fill the gap" when a specific hybrid imaging option is not available. Software-based techniques continue to have a significant role to play in conjunction with hybrid imaging devices in refining spatial alignment between component scans. These could also prove cost effective if, for example, instead of initially referring a patient for a dual-modality scan, the provider chooses

a sequential approach to prescribing imaging tests.[9] Sequential tests can then be combined using software methods. Most vendors offer some or all of these registration approaches on their medical workstations, including manual editing tools. In the next section, technical aspects of software-based image registration are discussed, followed by specific examples of multiple-platform integration using software-based techniques.

3.1. Technical considerations

Several review papers have focused on medical image registration, but Makela et al.[8] present the most comprehensive review of software-based cardiac image registration techniques. Software-based techniques can be classified into three categories: point-based, edge- or surface-based, and image similarity-based. These were developed initially in the context of brain imaging but have been extended to registration of cardiac images.

In point-based algorithms, the "points" can be external markers or fiducials placed on the thorax prior to imaging. However, because the heart moves with respect to the body, the utility of skin markers in cardiac image registration can be highly inaccurate and is limited mainly to phantom studies. Methods that use internal cardiac landmarks (e.g., apex of the left ventricle, papillary muscles, etc.) as points have been reported[18] and can be more accurate. Whereas landmark-based registration is easy to compute, the number of landmarks that can be accurately identified in a heart is small. This reality conflicts with the requirement that a large number of landmarks be available if image registration is to successfully account for nonrigid deformation of the heart. Note that three markers are sufficient to register brain images rigidly (i.e., no change in shape and size), but nonrigid registration requires more than three landmarks. Another complication with cardiac images is that landmarks could be affected by the presence of any disease and may not represent the exact same anatomical location in multimodality images.

Edge- and surface-based techniques rely on aligning matching surfaces in a pair of images. In certain cases, one of the surfaces may be described by a dense set of points with the goal of aligning this point set with the given surface. Overall, the techniques used are the familiar chamfer matching, iterative closest point, and head-and-hat algorithms, details of which are presented in standard texts.[19] In the case of cardiac image registration, a number of initial methods achieved registration by matching thorax and lung surfaces. Although it poses a harder segmentation task, a more accurate approach is to perform registration using heart surfaces.[20,21] These methods typically identify endocardial and epicardial surfaces using deformable model segmentation or another approach prior to registration.

Image similarity-based methods that use the complete voxel intensity information currently provide the best framework for robust and accurate image registration. These methods define an intensity-based cost function such that the maximum of the cost function corresponds to perfect spatial alignment between the two images in question. The transformation that maximizes the cost function is found iteratively by attempting a sequence of candidate transformations using standard search techniques. The approach is retrospective, in that no extra steps at the time of imaging are needed, and the process is fully automatic. Moreover, no limit on the nature of transformation (rigid or nonrigid) is imposed, making it suitable for cardiac image registration. Various cost functions have been proposed and used, but mutual information[22] has emerged as the most accurate and robust measure for multimodality applications.

3.2. SPECT/CT

Before hybrid SPECT/CT emerged, software-based registration of standalone CT and SPECT was suggested for the purposes of CT-based attenuation correction of SPECT.[23] Examples of the actual application of this technique remained few and far between and found little clinical use. More recently, in the posthybrid imaging era, software-based techniques have found two specific applications: (i) improvement of spatial alignment between SPECT and CT scans from a hybrid scanner before attenuation correction,[24] and (ii) integration of 64-slice CT and SPECT studies from separate scanners.[25] The interest in the first application comes from the introduction of artifacts and potential shadowing of diagnostically important perfusion defect from using a misaligned CT for attenuation correction. The second application is motivated by the lack of fast-rotation-speed, 64-slice CT as part of marketed hybrid SPECT/CT scanners. The 64-slice CT, it should be noted, is ideally suited for many cardiac exams such as CTA and coronary calcification imaging.

3.3. PET/CT

Many attempts to register thoracic CT and PET through software methods have been presented.[26,27] Studies showing comparable performance of hybrid imaging and software methods for PET and CT have been reported. In the majority of these software methods, the transmission PET is used as an intermediary and registered with the CT. The deformation needed to align transmission PET with CT is then applied to emission CT for PET/CT registration. The most prominent current application of software-based PET/CT registration is in refining the alignment of component PET and CT before attenuation correction.[14,28]

3.4. SPECT/MR imaging and PET/MR imaging

The interest in registering cardiac MR imaging with radionuclide imaging goes as far back as the early 1990s, when Faber et al.[20] demonstrated spatial and temporal registration of gated SPECT and MR images and Sinha et al.[21] reported a similar study for fusing cardiac MR imaging and PET. The temporally matched images were rigidly registered by minimizing the distance between automatically detected left ventricular endocardial surfaces. Such fusion allowed localization of perfusion defects with left ventricular wall motion and thickness. The latter study involving PET permitted correlation of both myocardial perfusion and metabolism with contractile function. In a similar approach, Makela et al.[29] presented a surface model-based technique to register PET with MR images. PET, which was not gated, was registered to the end-diastolic MR image. Figure 14.4 shows the results, in which PET activity was projected on the biventricular heart model (from registered MR data). Such visualization complements the traditional bull's-eye view and allows a direct correlation of metabolic abnormalities and ventricular anatomy. More recently, using mostly manual tools available on commercial software, Misko et al.[30] reported registering cine MR, delayed enhancement MR, and gated SPECT images for simultaneous assessment of myocardial perfusion, function, and viability.

3.5. SPECT-ultrasound and PET-ultrasound

Only a very few attempts to register echocardiography with radionuclide imaging have been reported. Rakotobe et al.[31] registered 2D, end-diastolic, and apical two- and four-chamber images of the heart with the closest (in orientation) sagittal or frontal 2D slice of SPECT images by matching up myocardial borders, traced manually in ultrasound images. Savi et al.[18] reported on the application of a geometric transformation to the 3D PET image so that the user-selected anatomic landmarks (papillary muscles and inferior junction of the right ventricle) in the PET image corresponded with their counterparts in the 2D ultrasound image. Walimbe et al.[32] presented one of the most advanced and validated methods to register 2D and 3D echocardiography images with gated SPECT, both acquired at rest. The method is intensity-based and relies on the maximization of mutual information. Spatial registration is applied to temporally matched ultrasound and SPECT image pairs. An example of this SPECT-echocardiography fusion is shown in Figure 14.5. Diagnosis based on such multimodality fused images promises to be more accurate than that based on either echocardiography or SPECT alone.

3.6. MR imaging-ultrasound

The fusion of echocardiography and cardiac MR imaging is promising, because high spatial resolution MR images can complement lower spatial resolution but higher temporal resolution ultra-

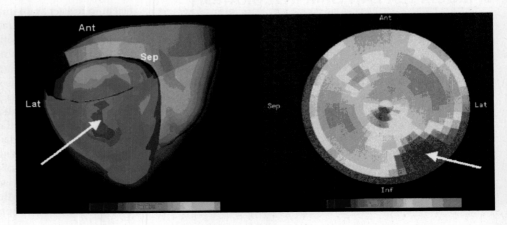

Figure 14.4 Fusion of cardiac PET and MR Imaging. Registered PET activity shown over a biventricular heart model from MR imaging **(left)** and the corresponding bull's-eye view **(right)**. The *arrow* indicates the region of low FDG uptake. (Reproduced from Makela T, Pham QC, Clarysse P, et al. A 3-D model-based registration approach for the PET, MR and MCG cardiac data fusion. *Med Image Anal.* 2003 Sep;7(3):377–389, with permission.)

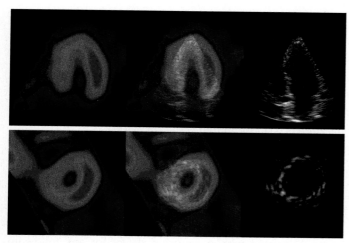

Figure 14.5 Long- and short-axis views of the heart showing SPECT image **(left)**, real-time 3D echocardiogram **(right)** and their fusion **(center)**. Note the correspondence of left ventricular wall in the two images upon registration.

sound images. Such fusion efforts, however, are in their infancy and remain mainly focused on the development of appropriate registration techniques. No large-scale clinical study on echocardiography-MR imaging fusion has been reported to date. Some early work in MR-ultrasound fusion[33,34] have also involved real-time 3D echocardiography as opposed to conventional 2D echocardiography because of the relative ease of 3D-to-3D registration compared with 2D-to-3D registration. The first step in this process is echocardiograph-based temporal registration to create multimodality image pairs belonging to the same phase. The phase-matched image pairs are then registered using an intensity-based measure of mutual information and either a rigid transformation model[33] or a nonrigid model.[34] Figure 14.6 is an example of such registration and shows three planes for a specific cardiac phase. An interesting study along similar lines demonstrated the feasibility of fusing ultrasound myocardial elastography with tagged MR images in an effort to compare and correlate myocardial strain derived from the two modalities.[35]

4. CLINICAL APPLICATIONS

Most clinical applications of cardiac image fusion remain in development and can be characterized as emerging applications. Additional research will be needed to precisely quantify their specific advantages and roles in the clinical management of cardiac patients. Described here are some leading emerging applications with the potential to enter the mainstream of clinical practice in the next decade.

4.1. Improved diagnosis of coronary artery disease

A leading cardiac application of multimodality imaging, especially integrating CT with either SPECT or PET, is improved diagnosis of CAD. Hybrid PET/CT and SPECT/CT scanners are a natural choice as imaging platforms and are serving as catalysts for increasing interest in such fusion studies. A software approach to combine standalone examinations[25] is also a viable alternative, especially for SPECT and CT, because cost considerations have thus far prevented hybrid SPECT/CT scanners from being offered with faster, higher-performance 64-slice CT, shown to be more suitable for artifact-free imaging of coronary arteries.

Although the technologies have many parallels, we separate the discussions of CT-SPECT and CT-PET fusion. In the context of SPECT/CT, CT used for attenuation correction of SPECT alone, without anatomic-functional overlay, has been shown to yield superior diagnostic results. In a multicenter trial involving 118 patients and 4 blinded readers, Masood et al.[36] compared the diagnostic performance of SPECT myocardial perfusion imaging with and without attenuation correction against angiographic findings. The outcome was an improvement in the diagnostic performance, especially normal calls, of all four readers. The improvement in sensitivity and specificity were reader dependent; however, an important finding was that the sensitivity increased without a simultaneous decrease in specificity, and vice versa.

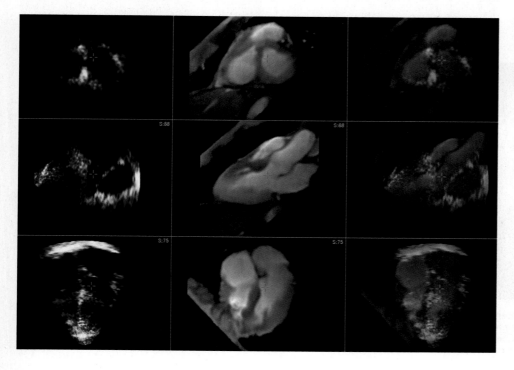

Figure 14.6 Fusion of cardiac MR with real-time 3D echocardiography. Only a single phase of a fused spatiotemporal data is shown. (Courtesy of Drs Edward Huang and Terry Peters, Robarts Research Institute, University of Western Ontario.)

In addition to attenuation correction, CT affords the opportunity for noninvasive CTA and thereby direct visualization of coronary lumens. Combining SPECT and CTA thus has implications for a direct correlation of function and anatomic findings and simultaneous assessment of myocardial ischemia and atherosclerosis.[1,4,9,13,17,37] It is well known that not all coronary artery stenoses are hemodynamically significant. Fusion of coronary lumen information with myocardial perfusion, as shown in Figure 14.7, helps identify narrowed but physiologically normal coronary segments, thus facilitating therapeutic decision-making. This fusion is also significant in identifying artifactual perfusion defects when they are not presented with a simultaneous occlusion of the coronary lumen. In a study involving 170 coronary segments, Rispler et al.[38] showed significant improvement in specificity (from 63% to 95%) and positive predictive value (31% to 77%) between diagnoses of CAD made using CTA alone and using SPECT/CTA, treating invasive coronary angiography findings as gold standard. The sensitivity (96%) and negative predictive value (99%), already high for CTA, stayed the same following fusion.

As in SPECT/CT, attenuation-corrected PET (using a [82]Rb perfusion tracer) obtained from hybrid PET/CT scanners is associated with high sensitivity and overall accuracy for detecting CAD.[39] Compared with SPECT, an advantage of attenuation-corrected

PET is that it lends itself well to quantification of myocardial perfusion and flow reserve and has been shown to be more accurate than SPECT in diagnosis of CAD.[37,40] If respiration and cardiac contraction-induced motion artifacts are properly addressed, hybrid PET/CT has the added advantage of concurrent assessment of the structure of coronary arteries from CTA by adding function from myocardial perfusion PET.[4,40,41] Figure 14.8 shows fusion of CTA and [82]Rb myocardial perfusion images and also shows identification of a stress-induced perfusion defect.

Both SPECT/CT and PET/CT, whether hybrid or software supported, are emerging as more accurate alternatives to any single modality in diagnosing CAD and as useful tools for risk stratification. Perfusion data from SPECT and PET help identify hemodynamically significant CAD, whereas structure information from CTA rules out any artifactual perfusion observed in radionuclide imaging and also identifies the culprit coronary lesion associated with a perfusion defect for any follow-up revascularization procedure.

4.2. Improved prognosis of coronary artery disease

Advances in CT technology have enabled precise noninvasive measurement of coronary artery calcium (CAC), and there is a

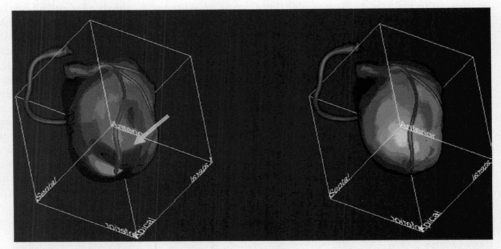

Figure 14.7 Combined presentation of coronaries from CTA and color-mapped perfusion data from SPECT at stress **(left)** and rest **(right)**. Whereas perfusion is normal at rest, it is reduced at stress in the apex and antero-apical wall. The fused image is helpful in correlating the perfusion defect to the left anterior descending artery. (Reproduced with permission from Rispler S, Keidar Z, Ghersin E, et al. Integrated single-photon emission computed tomography and computed tomography coronary angiography for the assessment of hemodynamically significant coronary artery lesions. *J Am Coll Cardiol.* 2007 Mar 13;49(10):1059–1067.)

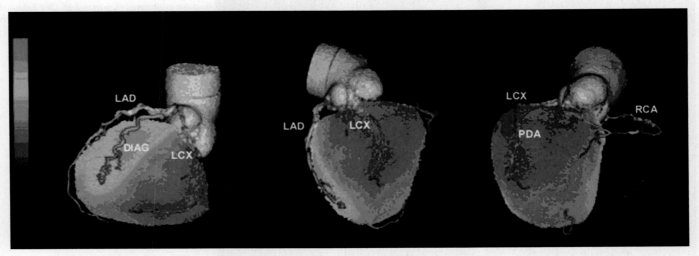

Figure 14.8 Combined presentation of coronaries from CTA and color-mapped perfusion data from PET at stress. CTA showed a three-vessel disease, whereas only the left circumflex artery territory showed stress-induced perfusion abnormality. (Reproduced from Di Carli MF, Dorbala S, Meserve J, et al. Clinical myocardial perfusion PET/CT. *J Nucl Med.* 2007 May;48(5):783–793, with permission.)

growing interest in using CAC score as a predictor of adverse cardiac events. Numerous studies have illustrated correlations between CAC score, size of atheresclerotic plaque burden, and the presence of ischemia in myocardial perfusion imaging.[42] This correlation, however, remains modest and is influenced by other risk factors. This is evidenced by a wide range of CAC scores in patients with or without ischemia and the fact that the absence of calcification has a mere 84% negative predictive value in ruling out ischemia. Prior studies, however, have made two clear associations: (i) a higher risk of ischemia with higher CAC score; and (ii) in patients with similar CAC scores, a higher risk of adverse cardiac events in those with ischemia than in those without.

The use of SPECT/CT and PET/CT hybrid devices that can combine CAC score with any findings of myocardial ischemia is emerging as a potentially more accurate noninvasive tool than any single modality alone for assessing the risk of CAD. Such fusion will permit a new risk assessment strategy, as proposed by Schenker et al.[43] for combined PET myocardial perfusion imaging and CT. As shown in Figure 14.9, this strategy categorizes risk by the absence or presence of ischemia first and then by a threshold CAC score.

4.3. Electrophysiologic guidance

One new and promising application for cardiac image fusion is in intervention guidance, a specific example of which is ventricular tachycardia (VT) ablation. The current practice is to use a steering catheter to build an endocardial voltage map point-by-point during the procedure to define scar and then ablate the entry and exit channels on the scar border to disrupt reentrant tachycardia. Preprocedural PET/CT, either through a hybrid device or through software registration, has the potential to provide an independent and well-accepted definition of scar (region with PET tracer uptake) within a detailed anatomic context (from CT). The availability of such data in the form of a 3D heart model during the procedure has the potential to guide the operator to the site of scar and relieve the operator from the tedious and lengthy task of gathering endocardial voltage data. The initial feasibility of this application has been studied by Dickfeld and Kocher.[44] (Fig. 14.10). Given the growing incidence of VT and the increasing need for VT ablation, combined imaging-guided ablation presents an attractive and novel approach to abbreviate the duration of procedures and improve outcomes.

4.4. Other emerging applications

Research continues into many diagnostic and interventional applications of cardiac image fusion. One such diagnostic application is multimodality stress testing that combines real-time 3D echocardiography and gated SPECT.[45] Gated SPECT allows evaluation of myocardial perfusion data and only resting wall motion. In contrast, fused images provide the potential for diagnosis based on the availability of complete prestress and poststress myocardial wall motion and perfusion information: wall motion data from real-time 3D echocardiography together with the spatially and temporally correlated perfusion data from SPECT. The application has the potential to simultaneously improve the sensitivity and specificity of stress-induced ischemia detection.

An example of an emerging interventional application is registration of real-time intracardiac echocardiography with preop-

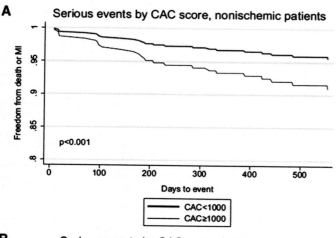

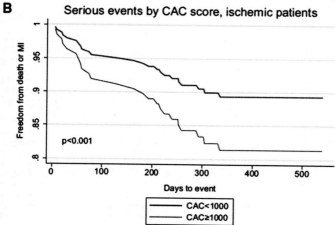

Figure 14.9 Freedom from death or myocardial infarction (MI), adjusted for typical risk factors (age, sex, etc.), versus CAC score in nonischemic and ischemic patients. (Reproduced from Schenker MP, Dorbala S, Hong EC, et al. Interrelation of coronary calcification, myocardial ischemia, and outcomes in patients with intermediate likelihood of coronary artery disease: A combined positron emission tomography/computed tomography study. *Circulation.* 2008 Apr;117(13):1693–1700, with permission.)

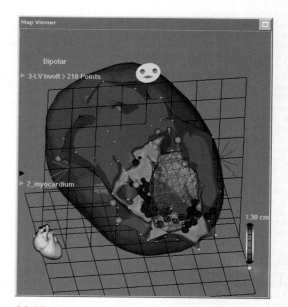

Figure 14.10 Three-dimensional model of the left ventricular endocardium from PET with superimposed voltage map. Shown in brown is the PET-defined scar, which matched well with the voltage-defined scar. (Courtesy of Dr Timm Dickfeld, Department of Cardiology, University of Maryland)

erative CT/MR images or even procedure-room C-arm CT images in electrophysiology applications.[46] Such registration can be accomplished semiautomatically using intensity-based registration and matching ultrasound, so that a CT/MR image slice can be presented to the surgeon. Higher spatial resolution CT or MR images with a larger field of view compared with that of ultrasound has the potential to provide additional visual aids in carrying out the procedure and may shorten the procedure time and improve outcomes.

5. FUTURE DIRECTIONS

We are currently in a period of tremendous promise and exploration in cardiac imaging as instrumentation and techniques develop rapidly and as modalities are tested in ever-evolving combinations, both as hybrid systems and through software-directed registration. Although CT fused with PET or SPECT now play dominant clinical roles, it is clear that MR, ultrasound, and even bioluminescence and optical imaging fusion techniques may be used routinely in the next decade. For cardiac diagnosis and treatment, these techniques promise to provide novel approaches that will doubtless be significant adjuncts to contributions from other disciplines, including monitoring of stem cell and nanotechnology-based therapies and enhancement of image-guided procedures.

REFERENCES

1. Seo Y, Mari C, Hasegawa BH. Technological development and advances in single-photon emission computed tomography/computed tomography. *Semin Nucl Med.* 2008 May;38(3):177–198.
2. Laurette I, Zeng GL, Welch A, et al. A three-dimensional ray-driven attenuation, scatter and geometric response correction technique for SPECT in inhomogeneous media. *Phys Med Biol.* 2000 Nov;45(11):3459–3480.
3. Seo Y, Wong KH, Sun M, et al. Correction of photon attenuation and collimator response for a body-contouring SPECT/CT imaging system. *J Nucl Med.* 2005 May;46(5):868–877.
4. Townsend DW. Multimodality imaging of structure and function. *Phys Med Biol.* 2008 Feb 21;53(4):R1–R39.
5. Kuhl DE, Hale J, Eaton WL. Transmission scanning: A useful adjunct to conventional emission scanning for accurately keying isotope deposition to radiographic anatomy. *Radiology.* 1966 Aug;87(2):278–284.
6. Pietrzyk U, Herholz K, Heiss WD. Three-dimensional alignment of functional and morphological tomograms. *J Comput Assist Tomogr.* 1990 Jan–Feb;14(1):51–59.
7. Viergever MA, Maintz JB, Stokking R. Integration of functional and anatomical brain images. *Biophys Chem.* 1997 Oct;68(1–3):207–219.
8. Makela T, Clarysse P, Sipila O, et al. A review of cardiac image registration methods. *IEEE Trans Med Imaging.* 2002 Sep;21(9):1011–1021.
9. Slomka PJ, Berman DS, Germano G. Applications and software techniques for integrated cardiac multimodality imaging. *Expert Rev Cardiovasc Ther.* 2008 Jan;6(1):27–41.
10. O'Connor MK, Kemp BJ. Single-photon emission computed tomography/computed tomography: Basic instrumentation and innovations. *Semin Nucl Med.* 2006 Oct;36(4):258–266.
11. Pichler BJ, Judenhofer MS, Wehrl HF. PET/MRI hybrid imaging: Devices and initial results. *Eur Radiol.* 2008 Jun;18(6):1077–1086.
12. Garlick PB, Marsden PK, Cave AC, et al. PET and NMR dual acquisition (PANDA): Applications to isolated, perfused rat hearts. *NMR Biomed.* 1997 May;10(3):138–142.
13. Schafers KP, Stegger L. Combined imaging of molecular function and morphology with PET/CT and SPECT/CT: Image fusion and motion correction. *Basic Res Cardiol.* 2008 Mar;103(2):191–199.
14. Gould KL, Pan T, Loghin C, et al. Frequent diagnostic errors in cardiac PET/CT due to misregistration of CT attenuation and emission PET images: A definitive analysis of causes, consequences, and corrections. *J Nucl Med.* 2007 Jul;48(7):1112–1121.
15. Goetze S, Wahl RL. Prevalence of misregistration between SPECT and CT for attenuation-corrected myocardial perfusion SPECT. *J Nucl Cardiol.* 2007 Apr;14(2):200–206.
16. Nehmeh SA, Erdi YE. Respiratory motion in positron emission tomography/computed tomography: a review. *Semin Nucl Med.* 2008 May;38(3):167–176.
17. Bybel B, Brunken RC, DiFilippo FP, et al. SPECT/CT imaging: Clinical utility of an emerging technology. *Radiographics.* 2008 Jul–Aug;28(4):1097–1113.
18. Savi A, Gilardi MC, Rizzo G, et al. Spatial registration of echocardiographic and positron emission tomographic heart studies. *Eur J Nucl Med.* 1995 Mar;22(3):243–247.
19. Hajnal JV, Hill DLG, Hawkes DJ, eds. *Medical Image Registration.* Boca Raton, FL: CRC Press; 2001.
20. Faber TL, McColl RW, Opperman RM, et al. Spatial and temporal registration of cardiac SPECT and MR images: Methods and evaluation. *Radiology.* 1991 Jun;179(3):857–861.
21. Sinha S, Sinha U, Czernin J. Noninvasive assessment of myocardial perfusion and metabolism: Feasibility of registering gated MR and PET images. *AJR Am J Roentgenol.* 1995 Feb;164(2):301–307.
22. Maes F, Collignon A, Vandermeulen D, et al. Multimodality image registration by maximization of mutual information. *IEEE Trans Med Imaging.* 1997 Apr;16(2):187–198.
23. Dey D, Slomka PJ, Hahn LJ, et al. Automatic three-dimensional multimodality registration using radionuclide transmission CT attenuation maps: A phantom study. *J Nucl Med.* 1999 Mar;40(3):448–455.
24. Fricke H, Fricke E, Weise R, et al. A method to remove artifacts in attenuation-corrected myocardial perfusion SPECT introduced by misalignment between emission scan and CT-derived attenuation maps. *J Nucl Med.* 2004 Oct;45(10):1619–1625.
25. Gaemperli O, Schepis T, Kalff V, et al. Validation of a new cardiac image fusion software for three-dimensional integration of myocardial perfusion SPECT and stand-alone 64-slice CT angiography. *Eur J Nucl Med Mol Imaging.* 2007 Jul;34(7):1097–1106.
26. Shekhar R, Walimbe V, Raja S, et al. Automated 3-dimensional elastic registration of whole-body PET and CT from separate or combined scanners. *J Nucl Med.* 2005 Sep;46(9):1488–1496.
27. Slomka PJ, Dey D, Przetak C, et al. Automated 3-dimensional registration of stand-alone (18)F-FDG whole-body PET with CT. *J Nucl Med.* 2003 Jul;44(7):1156–1167.
28. Khurshid K, McGough RJ, Berger K. Automated cardiac motion compensation in PET/CT for accurate reconstruction of PET myocardial perfusion images. *Phys Med Biol.* 2008 Oct 21;53(20):5705–5718.
29. Makela T, Pham QC, Clarysse P, et al. A 3-D model-based registration approach for the PET, MR and MCG cardiac data fusion. *Med Image Anal.* 2003 Sep;7(3):377–389.
30. Misko J, Dziuk M, Skrobowska E, et al. Co-registration of cardiac MRI and rest gated SPECT in the assessment of myocardial perfusion, function and viability. *J Cardiovasc Magn Reson.* 2006;8(2):389–397.
31. Rakotobe RH, Marek A, Langevin F, et al. Echography and Tl-201 SPECT cardiac images registration using elliptical models. *Annual International Conference of the IEEE Engineering in Medicine and Biology Society--Proceedings 1994,* 1994;604–605.
32. Walimbe V, Zagrodsky V, Raja S, et al. Mutual information-based multimodality registration of cardiac ultrasound and SPECT images: A preliminary investigation. *Int J Cardiovasc Imaging.* 2003 Dec;19(6):483–494.
33. Huang X, Hill NA, Ren J, et al. Dynamic 3D ultrasound and MR image registration of the beating heart. *Med Image Comput Comput Assist Interv Int Conf Med Image Comput Comput Assist Interv.* 2005;8(Pt 2):171–178.
34. Zhang W, Noble JA, Brady JM. Spatio-temporal registration of real time 3D ultrasound to cardiovascular MR sequences. *Med Image Comput Comput Assist Interv Int Conf Med Image Comput Comput Assist Interv.* 2007;10(Pt 1):343–350.
35. Qian Z, Lee WN, Konofagou EE, et al. Ultrasound myocardial elastography and registered 3D tagged MRI: quantitative strain comparison. *Med Image Comput Comput Assist Interv Int Conf Med Image Comput Comput Assist Interv.* 2007;10(Pt 1):800–808.
36. Masood Y, Liu YH, Depuey G, et al. Clinical validation of SPECT attenuation correction using x-ray computed tomography-derived attenuation maps: Multicenter clinical trial with angiographic correlation. *J Nucl Cardiol.* 2005 Nov–Dec;12(6):676–686.
37. Buck AK, Nekolla S, Ziegler S, et al. Spect/Ct. *J Nucl Med.* 2008 Aug;49(8):1305–1319.
38. Rispler S, Keidar Z, Ghersin E, et al. Integrated single-photon emission computed tomography and computed tomography coronary angiography for the assessment of hemodynamically significant coronary artery lesions. *J Am Coll Cardiol.* 2007 Mar 13;49(10):1059–1067.
39. Sampson UK, Dorbala S, Limaye A, et al. Diagnostic accuracy of rubidium-82 myocardial perfusion imaging with hybrid positron emission tomography/computed tomography in the detection of coronary artery disease. *J Am Coll Cardiol.* 2007 Mar;49(10):1052–1058.
40. Di Carli MF, Dorbala S, Meserve J, et al. Clinical myocardial perfusion PET/CT. *J Nucl Med.* 2007 May;48(5):783–793.
41. Smith MF. Advances in rubidium PET and integrated imaging with CT angiography. *Curr Cardiol Rep.* 2008 Mar;10(2):135–141.
42. Raggi P, Berman DS. Computed tomography coronary calcium screening and myocardial perfusion imaging. *J Nucl Cardiol.* 2005 Jan–Feb;12(1):96–103.
43. Schenker MP, Dorbala S, Hong EC, et al. Interrelation of coronary calcification, myocardial ischemia, and outcomes in patients with intermediate likelihood of coronary artery disease: A combined positron emission tomography/computed tomography study. *Circulation.* 2008 Apr;117(13):1693–1700.
44. Dickfeld T, Kocher C. The role of integrated PET-CT scar maps for guiding ventricular tachycardia ablations. *Curr Cardiol Rep.* 2008 Mar;10(2):149–157.
45. Walimbe V, Jaber WA, Garcia MJ, et al. Multimodality cardiac stress testing: combining real-time 3-dimensional echocardiography and myocardial perfusion SPECT. *J Nucl Med.* 2009;50(2):226–230.
46. Sun Y, Kadoury S, Li Y, et al. Image guidance of intracardiac ultrasound with fusion of pre-operative images. *Med Image Comput Comput Assist Interv Int Conf Med Image Comput Comput Assist Interv.* 2007;10(Pt 1):60–67.

Evaluation of Acute Chest Pain

15

Michael Shen
Deepa Sangani

1. INTRODUCTION

1.1. General epidemiology

The current system to triage patients with acute chest pain (ACP) in the United States is time consuming and expensive due to its low specificity and sensitivity. There are 6 million chest pain-related emergency department (ED) visits annually. Approximately, up to 72% of these patients are admitted to the hospital with a low yield of about 15% of patients who are ultimately diagnosed as having a true acute coronary syndrome (ACS). The cost of chest pain triage and management has been estimated to be as high as $8 billion dollars annually.[1] Moreover, up to 8% of patients are discharged from the ED and later diagnosed as having ACS.[2] The mortality rate for these patients is approximately 25%, which is twice as high as those who are admitted.[3] Healthcare is in demand of a streamlined and accurate system to evaluate up to 80% of patients with ACP in the low to intermediate risk of ACS.

Based on recent consensus statement of ACP from the North American Society of Cardiac Imaging and the European Society of Cardiac Radiology, common life threatening potential causes of nontraumatic chest pain include ACS, pulmonary embolism, and acute aortic disease (aortic dissection, aneurysm/rupture, intramural hematoma, or penetrating ulcer, Table 15.1).[4]

Majority of the patients admitted to the hospital are at low risk for ongoing ACS. The challenge remains in separating these patients from the patients that present with actual but not obvious ACS. The concept of chest pain units is becoming widely accepted in the United States over the last decade. It involves a team of physicians, nurses, and technologists and the laboratory.

Chest pain units have been shown to be a safe, effective, and cost-saving means of ensuring appropriate care to patients with unstable angina and at intermediate risk of cardiovascular events.[5] From an economic standpoint for hospitals, the introduction of these units has been shown to decrease the length of hospitalization by one to two days.

The Protocols for chest pain units may vary; however, majority of them consist of the following:

1. Event monitoring and continuous ST-segment monitoring;
2. Measurement of troponins I or T and/ or creatinine kinase-muscle and brain (CK-MB) at admission and 6 to 8 h after admission;
3. A ratio of four patients staffed by one full-time nurse;
4. Admission to the cardiac care unit or a telemetry bed on the cardiology service for patients with elevated cardiac enzyme levels, recurrent chest pain consistent with unstable angina, or significant ventricular arrhythmias;

5. An exercise treadmill test for patients without abnormal findings on the initial tests, or a nuclear stress test or echocardiographic stress test;
6. Admission of patients with equivocal or positive results.

1.2. Clinical assessment and patient characteristics

Derived and validated to predict 14-day outcomes in trials of patients with unstable angina and non-ST-segment elevation MI, the TIMI (thrombosis in myocardial infarction) Risk Score uses seven variables to risk-stratify patients with respect to outcomes. The TIMI score has been proven a reliable and valid means for risk-stratifying ED patients with chest pain of all causes[6] as well as helping to guide the treatment of those patients with readily identified ACS,[7,8] even when applied at the time of ED presentation.

However, the clinical features have a limited role to play in triage decision making for individual patient care. In a recently published large prospective, observational cohort study, Goodacre et al.[9] demonstrated low positive predictive value of 13.9% (10.5, 18.1) in patients with a nondiagnostic echocardiogram (ECG) (Table 15.2).

1.3. Acute myocardial infarction: Evolving definition and strategies

1.3.1. Historical definition

Historically, the definition of an acute myocardial infarction (AMI) was made by the WHO in the 1970s. The previously defined acute MI has a combination of at least two of the following three components: symptoms consistent with an acute MI, ECG changes diagnostic of an acute MI, and a temporal pattern of enzyme creatinine kinase (CK) and its muscle and brain (MB) subfraction rise and fall consistent with myocardial cell death.

Revision of the current WHO definition for AMI occurred in 2001. This redefinition made blood troponin determination a critical component in the identification of myocardial cell death, despite normal blood determinations for CK and CK-MB.[10]

1.3.2. Universal definition

In October 2008, the European Society of Cardiology, American Heart Association, American College of Cardiology Foundation, and the World Heart Foundation established a new Universal Definition of AMI. In addition to the elevated troponin levels (the 99th percentile of the upper reference limit), AMI diagnosis is made with one of the following:

■ Symptoms of ischemia
■ ECG changes indicative of new ischemia [new ST-T changes or new left bundle branch block (LBBB)]

TABLE 15.1
COMMON POTENTIAL CAUSES OF NONTRAUMATIC CHEST PAIN

Life threatening	Nonlife threatening
Acute coronary syndrome	Pneumonia/pulmonary parenchymal disease
Pulmonary embolism	Pulmonary, mediastinal, or pleural neoplasm
Aortic dissection	Musculoskeletal injury or inflammation
Intramural hematoma	Cholecystitis
Penetrating aortic ulcer	Pancreatitis
Aortic aneurysm /rupture	Herpes zoster
Esophageal rupture	Hiatus hernia/GERD/ esophageal spasm
Pericardial tamponade	Pericarditis/myocarditis
Tension pneumothorax	Simple pneumothorax

Source: Lee TH, Goldman L. Evaluation of the patient with acute chest pain. *N Engl J Med.* 2000;342(16):1187–1195.

TABLE 15.2
TIMI RISK SCORE FOR UNSTABLE ANGINA AND NSTEMI

- Age ≥ 65 years
- History of known CAD (documented prior coronary artery stenosis >50%)
- ≥3 conventional cardiac risk factors (age, male sex, family history, hyperlipidemia, diabetes mellitus, smoking, obesity, etc.)
- Use of aspirin in the past 7 days
- ST-segment deviation (persistent depression or transient elevation)
- Increased cardiac biomarkers (troponins)
- ≥2 anginal events in the preceding 24 h

TIMI, thrombosis in myocardial infarction; CAD, coronary artery disease; Score, sum of number of above characteristics.
Source: Sabatine MS, Antman EM. The thrombolysis in myocardial infarction risk score in unstable angina/non-ST-segment elevation myocardial infarction. *J Am Coll Cardiol.* 2003;41(4 Suppl S): 89S–95S.

- Development of pathologic Q waves in the ECG
- Imaging evidence of new loss of viable myocardium or new regional wall motion abnormality

It is the very first time that cardiac imaging is considered as one of the standards to diagnose AMI.

1.3.3. The electrocardiogram: Initial diagnostic tool

A resting 12-lead ECG is performed virtually on every patient who presents for the evaluation of ACP. The ECG is extremely high yielding in the diagnosis of patients with ST elevation MIs and high-risk unstable angina. The prevalence of acute MI is 80% among patients with 1 mm or more of new ST segment elevation but only 20% among patients with new ST segment depression or

T wave inversion. In the low to moderate risk patients, the ECG can often be normal up to 50% of the time.[11] A normal resting ECG does not exclude the presence of severe coronary artery disease (CAD), especially certain ECG patterns that may "mimic" ACS, such as left ventricular hypertrophy (LVH) with strain pattern, pericarditis, hypertrophic obstructive cardiomyopathy, medical conditions causing right heart strain, hypothermia, and electrolyte imbalance.

1.3.4. Cardiac enzymes: The current "Gold Standard" with limitations

Cardiac biomarkers are an integral part in the diagnosis and risk stratification of patients presenting with ACP. Troponin T and troponin I, myoglobin, and CK-MB are most often used. Measurements of troponin T or I has been shown to be a more sensitive and more specific marker of AMI than CK-MB.[12,13] The ACC/AHA guidelines recommend cTnI or cTnT as the preferred first-line markers.

However, using combinations of clinical criteria including CK-MB data, cardiac troponins have sensitivity approximately 85% for detecting acute MIs. Results should be interpreted in the context of the patient's overall probability of having CAD. Thus, a normal result on a test or series of tests in a patient with a high clinical probability of ACS does not exclude this diagnosis, although it raises the question of whether any myocardial injury may have occurred several days previously. Similarly, an abnormal test result in a patient with a low probability of coronary disease does not necessarily mean that the patient has had myocardial injury but should prompt a reassessment of the patient's clinical data. Many common cardiac conditions can cause "false-positive" troponin elevations (Table 15.3).

TABLE 15.3
ELEVATIONS OF TROPONIN IN THE ABSENCE OF OVERT ISCHEMIC HEART DISEASE

- Cardiac contusion or other trauma including surgery, ablation, pacing, etc.
- Congestive heart failure—acute and chronic
- Aortic dissection
- Aortic valve disease
- Hypertrophic cardiomyopathy
- Tachy- or bradyarrhythmias, or heart block
- Apical ballooning syndrome
- Rhabdomyolysis with cardiac injury
- Pulmonary embolism, severe pulmonary hypertension
- Renal failure
- Acute neurologic disease, including stroke or subarachnoid hemorrhage
- Infiltrative diseases, e.g., Amyloidosis, haemochromatosis, sarcoidosis, and scleroderma. Inflammatory disease, e.g., myocarditis or myocardial extension of endo- or pericarditis
- Drug toxicity or toxins
- Critically ill patients, especially with respiratory failure or sepsis
- Burns, especially if affecting >30% of body surface area
- Extreme exertion

Source: Jaffee AS, Babuin L, Apple FS. Biomarkers in acute cardiac disease. *J Am Coll Cardiol.* 2006;48:1–11.

1.3.5. Cardiac imaging: The new comer with significant potentials

The current diagnostic paradigm has limitations with low sensitivity and specificity based on clinical presentation and ECG. In essence, the cardiac enzymes are a biochemical marker, which can also be positive in many other clinical conditions. It dose not reflect specific pathological information on coronary status at the time of evaluation. Moreover, it may take up to 12 to 24 h to establish a diagnosis. Immediate diagnosis at the time of ACP presentation is necessary for prompt action with coronary intervention. In comparison, cardiac imaging can be taken immediately at the presentation of chest pain in patients with nondiagnostic ECG and cardiac enzymes. Cardiac imaging can provide *direct and specific* information on cardiac function, myocardial metabolism, perfusion, coronary anatomy, and plaque characterization. The critical clinical decision can be made immediately based on the information for prompt action for patient management. The introduction of imaging as a criterion in the "Universal definition of AMI" opens a new opportunity for clinical applications of imaging to evaluate patients with ACP.

This chapter focuses on the analysis of outcomes in diagnosis, prognosis, service, and finance in ACP syndromes comparing a variety of imaging modalities.

2. DIAGNOSTIC EVALUATION

2.1. Chest X-ray

The chest roentgenogram is often normal in patients presenting with ACP. Its usefulness as a routine test is not well established. However, it is one of the most readily available tests in the emergency room setting.

There is no direct evidence of AMI seen on chest X-ray. However, indirect evidence such as atherosclerotic calcification may be present. The actual sensitivity of detection of coronary calcifications is <50%. The usual location of coronary artery calcifications is in the coronary triangle in the mid upper part of the left heart corresponding to the proximal portions of the left coronary arteries. Fluoroscopic studies show that evident coronary calcification is associated with higher likelihood of significant coronary stenosis.

Chest X-ray may also show cardiac enlargement that may be attributable to previous MI, acute LV failure, pericardial effusion, or chronic volume overload of the LV such as occurs with aortic or mitral regurgitation.

It is ultimately most helpful to the emergency room physician to exclude life-threatening conditions like an aortic dissection, tension pneumothorax, and large pericardial effusion. Abnormal physical findings, associated chest X-ray findings (e.g., pulmonary venous congestion), and abnormalities detected by noninvasive testing (echocardiography) may indicate the correct etiology. Enlargement of the upper mediastinum often results from an ascending aortic aneurysm with or without dissection (Figure 15.1).

2.2. Echocardiography

Over the last two to three decades, two-dimensional (2D)-echocardiography has been a long-standing imaging modality available to assist in the evaluation of patients presenting to the emergency room with chest pain, especially when the ECG and serum biomarkers are nonconclusive. Over the last 10 years, many new techniques have been developed to further enhance the accuracy of 2D-echocardiography, including the introduction of harmonic imaging. The artifacts related with chest wall, location nearest the transducer, and side lobes have been significantly improved by tissue harmonic echocardiography.[14,15] Contrast

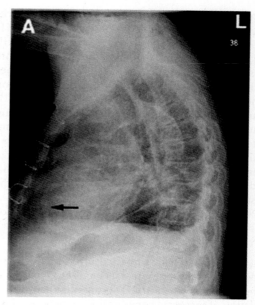

Figure 15.1 Lateral CXR showing coronary calcification *(arrow)* over anterior cardiac silhouette. (From Kuo D, Dilsizian V, Prasad R, et al. Emergency cardiac imaging: State of the art. *Cardiol Clin.* 2006;24:53–65.)

echocardiography using microbubbles is able to improve imaging quality by enhancing the detection of endomyocardial borders as well as assessing myocardial perfusion.[16] The recent advances in 2D- and three-dimensional (3D)-echocardiography have dramatically reduced the acquisition for stress echo to few single heart beats, allowing assessment of wall motion abnormalities and left ventricular (LV) function at the true peak of stress.

2.2.1. Resting echocardiogram

Regional wall motion is apparent almost immediately after the onset of acute myocardial ischemia and has been documented to precede electrocardiographic changes.[17] Echocardiography in patients with angina provides a great amount of incremental value when ECG and clinical findings are nondiagnostic. The regional wall motion abnormalities detected by resting echocardiography provide an excellent confirmatory evidence of CAD as a likely cause of the patients' chest pain. The segmental distribution of the wall motion abnormality correlates well with the distribution of CAD. In these high-risk patients who have segmental wall motion abnormalities, the sensitivity of an ECG used to diagnose myocardial ischemia is 94%, but the specificity is modest at 57%. The absence of a wall motion abnormality has a high negative predictive value of 98% for MI. However, in low-risk rule out MI populations, the positive predictive value of a resting wall motion abnormality on echo is only 31%.[18]

Studies in animals have demonstrated that wall motion abnormalities may not be detected when infarction involves <20% of ventricular wall thickness[19] or <12% of LV circumference.[20] Therefore, patients who have non-ST elevation MI (NSTEMI) and unstable angina may have no discernible abnormalities of wall motion. Echocardiography provides no information on the age of a wall motion abnormality, reducing its usefulness in patients who have known CAD or cardiomyopathies. Finally, wall motion abnormalities may be seen in patients who have left bundle branch block and right ventricular volume or pressure overload that complicate interpretation of the ECG for ischemic wall motion abnormalities.

In summary, resting echocardiography may lack sufficient sensitivity to be of clinical usefulness in the patient who has low-risk chest pain in the ED. The National Heart Attack Alert Program Working Group concluded that "false negative rates in the prospective studies are too high to be safe."[21] In addition, the American College of Cardiology/American Heart Association 2002 Guideline Update for the Management of Patients with Unstable Angina and Non-ST Segment Elevation Myocardial Infarction does not include echocardiography in the initial evaluation and management of patients.[22] By contrast, another viewpoint is offered by the American College of Cardiology/American Heart Association/American Society of Echocardiography that states that "early echocardiography is particularly useful in patients with a high clinical suspicion of AMI but a nondiagnostic ECG."[23]

The 2007 ACCF/ASE/ACEP Appropriateness Criteria for transthoracic echocardiography in the setting of ACP provide a score of 8 and 9 respectively for the following indications.[24]

1. Evaluation of ACP with suspected myocardial ischemia with nondiagnostic laboratory markers and ECG and in whom a resting ECG can be performed during chest pain.
2. Evaluation of suspected complication of myocardial ischemia/infarction including mitral regurgitation (MR), hypoxemia, abnormal chest X-ray (CXR), ventricular septal defect (VSD), free-wall rupture/tamponade, shock, right ventricular involvement, heart failure, or thrombus.

Thus, it is very acceptable to perform a 2D ECG under these circumstances.

2.2.2. Stress echocardiography

In patients who have ACP and resting 2D ECG, ECG and clinical findings continue to be nondiagnostic; stress testing can often provide further diagnostic information because resting echocardiography lacks sufficient sensitivity to clinically rule out the presence of CAD in low-risk chest pain patients. Based on the patients overall clinical status, it can be performed with exercise or pharmacologic stress.

Ideally, an exercise stress test should be performed because it provides physiologic information including functional capacity. However, a pharmacological stress test can be used in patients who are unable to exercise because of deconditioning, neurological, or orthopaedic limitations. Two categories of pharmacological agents can be used to simulate stress. These are inotropic agents (dobutamine, arbutamine), which increase adrenergic response and contractility, or vasodilatory agents (adenosine, dipyrimadole), which cause heterogeneous myocardial perfusion that may or may not induce ischemia.

Stress echocardiography primarily depends upon imaging the endomyocardial border and LV segmental wall motion and thickening.[25] A decrease in wall motion or thickening at stress in a specific coronary distribution is highly suggestive of CAD. The overall sensitivity and specificity reported by the ACC/AHA practice guidelines in patients with chronic stable angina is 85% and 86%, respectively.[26] However, in a study performed by Bholasingh and colleagues in low-risk rule out myocardial ischemia population, dobutamine stress echo had positive and negative predictive values of 31% and 96%.[27] A normal exercise and a normal stress ECG confer excellent prognosis.

2.2.3. Prognostic value

In the low-risk rule out MI population, the overall cardiac event rate is 0.9% to 1.1% per year.[28] An abnormal study increases the risk of a cardiac event by three to four times.[29] In addition, left anterior descending (LAD) territory ischemia on resting echocardiography has a fivefold higher cardiac event rate at 5 years than all other wall motion abnormalities.

The positive predictive value (PPV) and negative predictive value (NPV) of resting echo for cardiac events in patients with ACP are better than clinical variables and ECG. However, the PPV of a resting wall motion abnormality is low, varying between 31% and 57%. In many studies, the patients who had false negative echocardiographic findings had NSTEMI or unstable angina, reflecting the limited sensitivity of wall motion abnormalities for identification of this population. Patients with diabetes and hypertension, despite normal stress ECGs, have significantly higher cardiac event rates, 6% and 1.8%, respectively, than general population.[30]

More portable and relatively inexpensive hand-held echocardiographic (HHE) devices are becoming more widely available and may allow ED physicians' greater accessibility to cardiac ultrasound scanning. Although the negative predictive value of hand-held echo was 91%, the incidence of either AMI or ischemia was 7.6% (6/78) in the normal HHE group and 14.6% (6/30) in the abnormal HHE group ($p = 0.11$).[31] These results suggested its limited role in the examination of patients with a low likelihood of myocardial ischemia or infarction and symptoms suggestive of ACS.

New technologies with tissue harmonic and contrast echocardiography may further improve the positive and negative predictive values when compared with clinical history and the electrocardiogram. However, focusing on the group diagnosed as having unstable angina without troponin elevation, the sensitivity of resting wall motion abnormality is 17% and the sensitivity of myocardial contrast echocardiography is 66%, suggesting one of three patients who has unstable angina without troponin elevation will go undetected using myocardial contrast echocardiography.[32]

Comparing myocardial contrast echocardiography to resting single photon emission computed tomographic (SPECT) imaging, Kaul et al.[33] found in 203 patients with ACP that myocardial contrast echocardiography perfusion was superior to SPECT myocardial perfusion in predicting events. However, SPECT myocardial regional function was superior to echocardiographic regional function in predicting events, resulting in SPECT having a greater overall predictive value compared with myocardial contrast echocardiography.

Recently, the Stress Pharmacological Echocardiography in Emergency Department (SPEED) trial in 502 patients using high dose dipyridamole (up to 0.84 mg/kg) and high dose dobutamine (up to 40 mcg/kg/min, plus atropine up to 1 mg) showed high negative predictive value of stress echocardiography, 98.8% for all events and 99.6% for hard events. However, the results of stress echo with dipyridamole are inconsistent and rarely performed in the United States, especially at the acute setting. Martin et al[101]. showed that dobutamine stress echocardiography was more sensitive and better tolerated than adenosine and dipyridamole. However, the European Society of Echocardiography argues that they are equally potent ischemic stressors for inducing wall motion abnormalities in presence of critical CAD.[34]

Further studies are warranted to investigate the diagnostic and prognostic value of pharmacological stress echo in the low and intermediate risk population.

With the advantages of convenience, availability, and portability, resting and stress echocardiography can be used to assess ACP patients and identify patients who are at low enough risk to be discharged home and those who are at high risk and require admission.

The most important limitation for echocardiography is the need for skilled, experienced technicians for adequate data acquisition. Especially stress echocardiography requires experienced personnel to perform and interpret test results. Access to skilled technicians and cardiologists for interpretation may not be available after hours or outside tertiary referral centers. Even with skilled personnel, image quality may not be interpretable. Poor image quality primarily seen in obese patients has always been a limiting factor for echocardiography. Another limitation may occur in patients with known CAD with wall motion abnormalities. Without knowledge of this patients' prior history, it may be very difficult to determine the age of the wall motion abnormality seen.

2.2.4. Cost/benefits

The cost of echocardiography is low compared with other imaging modalities. To compare with SPECT imaging, Shaw et al.[35] examined prognosis and cost-effectiveness of exercise echocardiography ($n = 4,884$) versus SPECT ($n = 4,637$) imaging in stable, intermediate risk, chest pain patients. When cardiac event rates were <2%, stress echo was superior to SPECT. However, when yearly cardiac event rates were ≥2%, cost-effectiveness ratios for echocardiography became inferior. The study suggests using echocardiography in low-risk patients with suspected coronary disease whereas high-risk patients may benefit from referral to SPECT imaging.

A study from Kuntz et al.[36] studied the cost-effectiveness of diagnostic strategies for patients with chest pain. They determined that in patients with moderate risk for CAD, the use of noninvasive diagnostic testing, particularly exercise echocardiography, was associated with reasonable cost-effectiveness. However, in patients with a very low probability, the cost-effectiveness ratios of all testing strategies were higher than those of most well accepted medical interventions.

2.3. SPECT myocardial perfusion imaging

Over the past 30 years, nuclear cardiology has made significant advances in both instrumentation and radiopharmaceuticals suitable for acute imaging. In 1979, Wackers et al.[37] in the Netherlands first demonstrated the feasibility of ^{201}Tl myocardial perfusion imaging (MPI) by using planar techniques to assess patients with ACP. The rapid redistribution characteristics of ^{201}Tl, its limited acute availability, and the need for portable camera systems made its widespread use impractical. In addition, the inherent limitations of planar imaging with low sensitivity for detecting small areas of ischemia and for detecting ischemia in the posterior distribution prevented widespread adoption of the technique in the clinical management of ACS.

Many of these impediments to application of imaging in this setting were overcome by the introduction of the ^{99m}Tc based agents, sestamibi and tetrofosmin. With their relative lack of redistribution, images may be acquired up to several hours after injection and reflect myocardial blood flow at the time of injection. In addition, high quality SPECT imaging has been widely used in the nuclear medicine departments. The most recent development of rapid imaging technologies has cut down the imaging time from traditional 10 to 12 min to 2 to 3 min, making it more feasible to assess ACP.[38] The ability to perform simultaneously wall motion and perfusion significantly improves specificity[39,40] and is particularly valuable in the acute setting where serial images are not available.

2.3.1. Resting perfusion imaging

Rest MPI with ^{99m}Tc-sestamibi or ^{99m}Tc-tetrofosmin has a high sensitivity and NPV for diagnosing AMI in low-risk patient population. Studies have also demonstrated that acute ED MPI does offer incremental value over traditional risk factors and ECG. Bilodeau et al. performed rest SPECT sestamibi imaging in patients already hospitalized for suspected unstable angina (UA), injecting them with tracer at the time of an episode of spontaneous chest pain while also recording an ECG. The sensitivity of the SPECT sestamibi images for determining the presence of a severe coronary stenosis on subsequent angiography was 96% while the sensitivity of ECG was only 35%. In patients with AMI, a perfusion defect involving as much as 20% of the left ventricle can exist on acute rest sestamibi imaging in the presence of a normal or nondiagnostic ECG. A high negative predictive value for ruling out MI is greater than or equal to 99% in all published series.[41–44] Patients with positive results have a substantially higher risk of untoward cardiac events during the index hospitalization as well as during follow up. Such data suggest that MPI provides important information to assist triage decisions (admit or not admit) in the ED using resting MPI (Table 15.4[45] and Fig. 15.2).

However, there are many issues related with patient selection, standard used to define AMI, as well as technical and logistic limitations of MPI for its wide spread clinical use.

1. Patient selection bias. Because acute MPI is performed predominantly in low-risk patients, the absolute numbers of patients who have MI in any individual study is small, resulting in an imprecise measurement of sensitivity. Another confounding

---

TABLE 15.4

DIAGNOSTIC ACCURACY OF REST MYOCARDIAL PERFUSION IMAGING IN PATIENTS WHO HAVE ACUTE CHEST PAIN SYNDROME AND NORMAL OR NONISCHEMIC REST ELECTROCARDIOGRAMS

	Year	N	Tracer	Sensitivity, %	Specificity, %	NPV, %	End point
Wackers (et al.)[37]	1979	203	[201]Tl	100	72	100	AMI
Varetto (et al.)[41]	1993	64	Tc-mibi	100	92	100	CAD
Hilton (et al.)[42]	1994	102	Tc-mibi	94	83	99	CAD/AMI
Tatum (et al.)[43]	1997	438	Tc-mibi	100	78	100	AMI
Kontos (et al.)[46]	1997	532	Tc-mibi	93	71	99	AMI
Heller (et al.)[44]	1998	357	Tc-tetro	90	60	99	AMI
Kontos (et al.)[46]	1999	620	Tc-mibi	92	67	99	AMI
Udelson (et al.)[77]	2002	1215	Tc-mibi	96	NR	99	AMI

AMI, acute myocardial infarction; CAD, angiographic coronary artery disease; NPV, negative predictive value; NR, not reported; Tc-mibi, ^{99m}Tc-sestamibi; Tc-tetro, ^{99m}Tc-tetrofosmin; ^{201}Tl, thallium-201.
Source: Kontos MC, Tatum JL. Imaging in the evaluation of the patient with suspected acute coronary syndrome. *Cardiol Clin.* 2005;23:517–530.

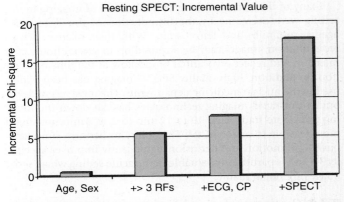

Figure 15.2 Analysis of the incremental value of resting perfusion imaging data to predict cardiac events in ED patients. (Adapted from Heller GV, Stowers SA, Hendel RC, et al. Clinical value of acute rest technetium-99 m tetrofosmin tomographic myocardial perfusion imaging in patients with acute chest pain and nondiagnostic electrocardiograms. *J Am Coll Cardiol.* 1998;31:1011–1017.)

issue with these studies is that most of the healthcare providers used elevations in either CK or CK-MB as the diagnostic standard for MI rather than current standard troponin. Although the sensitivity of MPI was high, it was significantly lower than that of troponin-I or troponin-T.[46,47] In a larger study, Konto et al.[48] analyzed diagnostic outcomes in 319 patients who were initially considered low risk for MI and underwent acute rest MPI as part of standard chest pain evaluation protocol and were subsequently found to have elevated TnI values, thus meeting the new definition for MI[13].Seventy-seven patients had negative MPI, giving a sensitivity of only 76%; much lower than when CK or CK-MB was used as the diagnostic standard for MI.

2. Limitations of imaging resolution. An experimental study demonstrated that approximately 3% to 4% of the left ventricle must be ischemic to allow detection by MPI.[49] In a cohort of 357 patients imaged acutely as part of an ED triage protocol, Heller et al.[44] reported normal images at rest in 12 of 35 patients (34%) who were ultimately diagnosed with ACS, including two with acute MI. Normal images were acquired in 7 of 32 patients with ACS (22%) in a cohort of 1,000 patients with chest pain. In a multicenter trial of 102 ED patients with typical angina but nondiagnostic ECG, only 3 of 15 patients with unstable angina had abnormal sestamibi studies.

3. Prior history of CAD. The defects with acute imaging do not distinguish among acute ischemia, acute infarction, or previous infarction. Although serial changes on follow-up perfusion imaging may suggest an acute process myocardium at risk and final infarct size assessed, which is the area initially at risk minus the final infarct size, technically it cannot definitely distinguish ischemia from infarction.

4. Logistics in operation. The operation of acute radionuclide imaging is difficult. This includes isotope preparation, decay and licensing issues, a preponderance of small nuclear medicine laboratories with insufficient support to provide imaging 24 h/day, and the difficulties associated with single-image interpretation without the customary second image for comparison. Other limitations include low spatial resolution, limited temporal resolution, and high frequency of artifacts due to gastrointestinal (GI) activity overlapping inferior wall without appropriate patient prep and fasting.

Despite the relatively long period for which acute imaging with radionuclide has been available, the technique has not been embraced on a large scale at present.

2.3.2. Resting imaging using "memory" agents

With myocardial ischemia, a reduced coronary blood flow and subsequent reduction in the supply of oxygen, fatty acids, and other energy substrates can cause a shift from fatty acid (aerobic) to glucose (anaerobic) oxidation. If the ischemia is transient, myocardial injury is most likely reversible. Despite restoration of blood flow, persistent reduction of fatty acid metabolism within the same vascular distribution has been described, termed *metabolic stunning*.[50] The use of fatty acid radiotracers, therefore, can elucidate these metabolic alterations at rest without the need for a stress examination, also called *ischemic memory*, to reflect the ischemia changes even after blood flow has been restored.

Beta-methyl-p-[(123)I]-iodophenyl-pentadecanoic acid (BMIPP) uptake within the myocardium following myocardial ischemia is a dynamic process. During the acute phase (1 to 6 h) of ischemia, the size of the intracellular nonoxidized fatty acid pool increases.[51] It has been shown in animal models that during the acute phase of ischemia, BMIPP uptake is enhanced significantly in the vascular distribution at risk and is usually higher than perfusion tracers, ^{201}Tl and ^{99m}Tc-tetrofosmin.[52,53] When the same animal models were imaged in the subacute phase (>6 h), a BMIPP defect was evident. When BMIPP is used with a perfusion tracer, discordant BMIPP and thallium uptake values were noticeable in the acute and subacute phases. The higher ratio of BMIPP to thallium in the acute phase was inverted in the subacute phase. In the chronic phase, uptake of BMIPP recovered back to the baseline value and was similar to that of thallium. Similar to the observations in animal models, in patients with stunned myocardium (prolonged but reversible post ischemic LV dysfunction after a period of ischemia and coronary reperfusion), BMIPP accumulation changed dynamically over the acute and subacute phases. BMIPP accumulation within stunned myocardium did not decrease in the acute phase; however, there was a BMIPP defect in the subacute phase.[54]

Among patients presenting to the ED with ACS and no prior MI, the clinical utility of BMIPP for identifying myocardial ischemia was examined in 111 consecutive patients.[55] All the patients were admitted and underwent rest myocardial perfusion SPECT study within 24 h of chest pain, rest BMIPP metabolic images within 48 h after the perfusion SPECT, and coronary angiography within 1 to 4 days of admission. BMIPP defects at rest were present in 74% of patients with documented coronary artery stenosis or vasospasm (on ergonovine provocation) whereas only 38% of patients showed myocardial perfusion defects at rest ($p < 0.001$). Both BMIPP and perfusion studies were normal in nearly 90% of patients without coronary artery stenosis or vasospasm. These early observations among patients with ACS were subsequently extended to patients experiencing myocardial ischemia during treadmill exercise (Fig. 15.3).

However, there are limitations for BMIPP use:

1. Regulatory issues. The only clinical indication that has received U.S. Food and Drug Administration approval for the assessment of cardiac metabolism is in myocardial viability. BMIPP has not been approved for diagnosing CAD at acute and stable chronic setting yet at this point.

2. Logistic in operation. [123]I is difficult to prepare, requiring special trained personnel to handle the isotope. It makes the widespread use at the acute setting impractical.

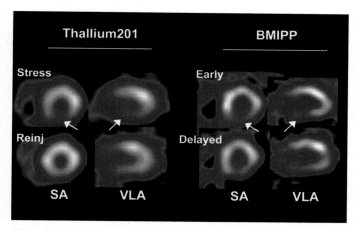

Figure 15.3 201-Tl stress and reinjection (Reinj) images after treadmill exercise in the short-axis (SA) and vertical long-axis (VLA) SPETC (**left**). Thallium images demonstrate a severe reversible inferior defect (*arrows*), consistent with exercise stress-induced ischemia. A similar defect is seen on the early β-Methyl-p-^{123}I-iodophenyl pentadecanoic acid (BMIPP) images (**right**) in the same tomographic cuts (*arrows*), with BMIPP injected 22h after the stress-induced ischemia. (Adapted from Dilsizian V, Bateman TM, Bergmann SR, et al. Metabolic imaging with beta-methyl-p-[(123)I]-iodophenyl-pentadecanoic acid identifies ischemic memory after demand ischemia. *Circulation.* 2005;112:2169–2174.)

3. The difference in tissue attenuation between ^{123}I and ^{201}Tl and the downscatter from [123]I 159 KeV to [201]Tl 79 KeV often makes the imaging interpretation difficult. The correction mechanism has not been well established. It is even more difficult to differentiate from 140 KeV ^{99m}Tc based agents, if it is used with BMIPP, since it is more commonly used in the acute setting.

4. Radiation. The combination of ^{201}Tl and ^{123}I makes the radiation dose significantly higher given both the agents' half-lives are longer than ^{99m}Tc-based agents.

2.3.3. Stress MPI

Normal rest perfusion imaging in patients with chest pain confers an excellent short-term prognosis. However, these patients are generally referred for further outpatient cardiac evaluation upon discharge, which often entails a regular stress perfusion imaging or exercise treadmill ECG. This constitutes an essential part of the evaluation

process because it is considered inadequate to exclude infarction only and discharge a patient who may still have unstable angina or critical CAD.[56] Patients with chest pain, who show normal rest perfusion imaging, can safely undergo further stress perfusion imaging in the ED to determine the presence of any inducible ischemia.[57]

Stress SPECT MPI has been used routinely in patients who have suspected ACS with nondiagnostic ECG and negative serial cardiac enzymes over 6 to 24h. Among patients who are considered clinically to be at very low risk, stress myocardial perfusion SPECT study can be performed rather early. SPECT MPI in this setting can potentially allow earlier patient triage decisions than serial enzyme evaluation. The current data suggest that if stress myocardial perfusion studies are normal, the risk of ACS or unfavorable cardiac events is low, and therefore early discharge from the ED may be considered. On the other hand, if the stress imaging results are abnormal (ischemia or infarction), rapid admission and entry into an appropriate evidence-based treatment pathway for ACS are in order.

The accuracy of stress SPECT MPI has been well established over the last two decades. The commonly acknowledged sensitivity and specificity for MPI are 87% and 73% for exercise and 89% and 75% for pharmacological studies, respectively, based on 50 large clinical studies[58] (Fig. 15.4).

Although resting followed by stress MPI has been considered as a standard care, and it may replace hospitalization in patients with nondiagnostic ECG and negative biomarkers in low to intermediate risk patient population, it still has significant limitations in clinical care:

1. Time consuming. It can take up to 16 to 24h to complete both resting and stress testing, especially delivery of isotope after hours can be a major delay.

2. High cost.

3. Imaging quality. Many patients are not adequately prepared for SPECT imaging. Imaging quality can be significantly decreased in patients without fasting. Stress images can also be false negative if patients are on beta-blockers or nitrates.

2.3.4. Prognostic value

MPI has been shown to be particularly useful in the predischarge risk stratification of patients with ACP. In a study by Brown[59] 52 patients with medically stabilized unstable angina underwent exercise planar ^{201}Tl imaging within 1 week of admission. At an

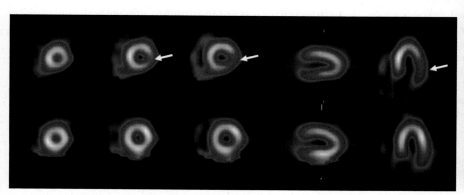

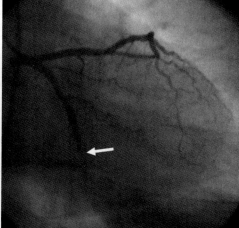

Figure 15.4 Stress MPI (left panel) showing moderate ischemia in the lateral wall of a 49-year-old man presenting to the ED with chest pain. ECG and cardiac enzymes were negative. Coronary angiography (right panel) revealed an occluded circumflex.

average follow-up of 39 months, cardiac death or nonfatal MI occurred in 6 of 23 (26%) patients with positive thallium redistribution versus 1 of 29 (3%) of those without redistribution. The number of segments with thallium redistribution and a history of prior MI were the only significant predictors of all events. However, thallium redistribution was the only predictor of cardiac death or nonfatal MI on follow-up. In this study, coronary anatomy was not a good predictor of future events. In a similar study, patients with unstable angina stabilized on medical therapy underwent a symptom-limited exercise thallium SPECT.[60] Reversible thallium defects occurred in 20 of 22 patients (91%) who developed cardiac events versus 5 of 17 patients (29%) of those who did not develop events, over a mean follow-up of 39 months.

In another study by Strattman et al.,[61] patients underwent a sestamibi stress myocardial perfusion SPECT study before hospital discharge. The event-free survival was approximately 90% over a follow-up of 18 months in patients with normal scans versus 55% in those with abnormal scans. Patients with reversible defects in this study had a less favorable prognosis, with an event-free survival of only 30% over 18 months. Death or MI in this study was rare in patients with a normal scan but occurred in 20% of those with abnormal scans and in 40% of those with reversible defects over 18 month follow-up. Several other studies give support to the use of MPI either with ^{201}Tl, ^{99m}Tc-sestamibi, exercise, or dipyridamole imaging in patients with unstable angina.[62–65]

The predictive value of a negative acute MPI also extends beyond the immediate setting in identifying patients at low risk for short- and long-term cardiac complications. For example, Hilton et al.[66] found that patients who had normal perfusion imaging had an excellent prognosis, with no late events at 90-day follow-up. Similarly, Kontos reported that patients who had negative acute MPI had a cardiac event rate of only 3% during the subsequent year. In one center experience over the last 9 years, low-risk patients discharged from the ED after undergoing acute ED rest MPI (*n* = 10,775) demonstrated a 30-day cardiac mortality of only 0.08%.

An important prognostic parameter provided by acute MPI is that it not only identifies patients who have ACS but also provides a validated measurement of the ischemic risk area. The size of a perfusion defect is of significant clinical importance as patients who have larger defects have a worse long-term prognosis.[67,68] The most important determinant of infarct size is the ischemic risk zone or the amount of myocardium in jeopardy.[69] MPI is the only technique among those commonly available that can determine the ischemic risk zone.[70,71] In studies in which post-MI patients had MPI before discharge, defect size correlated well with other outcome predictors including LV ejection fraction, regional wall motion index, end systolic volume, and peak CK levels.[72–74]

In an earlier study, Hilton and colleagues used ^{99m}Tc-sestamibi SPECT imaging to study 102 patients presenting to the ED with typical angina and either a normal or nondiagnostic ECG. Seventy patients had a normal perfusion scan; only one of them had a cardiac event. In comparison, 2 of the 15 (13%) patients who had equivocal scans and 12 of the 17 (71%) patients who had perfusion defects had cardiac events. When equivocal scans were classified as abnormal, the sensitivity and specificity of an abnormal study for predicting adverse cardiac events were 94% and 83%, respectively. Similarly, Kontos et al.[75] found that abnormal MPI was the most important independent predictor of MI or revascularization in 532 patients who underwent acute ED MPI (Fig. 15.5). Finally, Heller et al.[44] found that abnormal SPECT was the most important multivariate predictor of MI in 357 patients who underwent acute MPI.

In an interesting intent-to-treat survey study, Knott et al.[76] performed acute MPI on 120 patients in the ED. The requesting

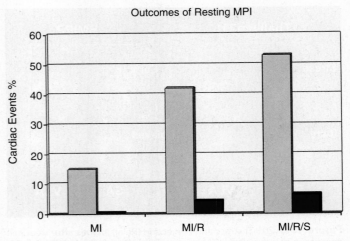

Figure 15.5 Outcomes associated with results of acute rest MPI. Patients who had positive rest MPI *(dark bars)* have greater risk pf MI, revascularization (R) or >70% stenosis (S). (Reproduced from Kontos MC, Jesse RL, Schmidt KL, et al. Value of acute rest sestamibi perfusion imaging for evaluation of patients admitted to the emergency department with chest pain. *J Am Coll Cardiol.* 1997;30:976–982, with permission.)

physician completed a questionnaire before imaging, asking what the proposed management would be had the test not been available. They found a 34% reduction in overall hospital admissions and a 59% reduction in planned CCU admissions. Overall, CCU admissions were not reduced because 17 patients initially considered low risk were admitted to the CCU after MPI was found to be abnormal. Similar data from several observational studies were confirmed in the Emergency Room Assessment of Sestamibi for Evaluating Chest Pain (ERASE) study, a large prospective randomized controlled study. This study demonstrated that acute MPI was effective when compared with standard management of low-risk chest pain patients.[77] In this study, 2,475 patients were randomized to routine care or ED MPI, in which patients were injected with sestamibi in the ED and subsequently underwent acute imaging, with the results called back to the ED physician. All patients, whether admitted or discharged, underwent marker analysis and diagnostic evaluation. There was no difference in the percentage of patients who had ACS and either MI (97% vs. 96%) or unstable angina (83% vs. 81%), who were admitted, with one patient who had MI from each group discharged from the ED. However, there was a significantly lower admission rate and a higher rate of direct discharge from the ED in the ED MPI arm compared with the standardized care arm.

However, the logistics of setting up an acute perfusion imaging service in the ED are formidable and the cost of providing such a service around the clock is significant. The ED physicians should be able to identify accurately those patients who will benefit most from an acute MPI strategy (Fig. 15.6). Continuous availability of doses of the ^{99m}Tc-labelled perfusion agents is an essential prerequisite for the smooth running of this service in the ED. The nuclear cardiology department must be able to accommodate the addition of patients with little advance notice. Emergency room nurses or physicians should be trained to inject patients during ACP. The logistics and costs can increase if nuclear technologists are on call 24 h a day to come to the ED to inject patients with doses of the imaging agent and then image them. Most importantly, trained nuclear cardiologists must be available to interpret the MPI with many such reporting undertaken out of hours. The availability of remote reading has improved out-of-hours with advancement of web-based workstation systems.

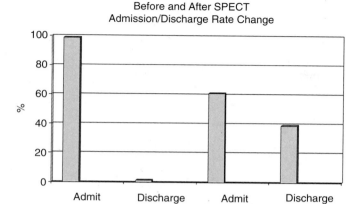

Before and After SPECT
Admission/Discharge Rate Change

Figure 15.6 Change in admission and discharge rates for patients with chest pain and nondiagnostic ECGs before sestamibi (control group) and after sestamibi (acute sestamibi group). (Adapted from Heller GV, Stowers SA, Hendel RC, et al. Clinical value of acute rest technetium-99m tetrofosmin tomographic myocardial perfusion imaging in patients with acute chest pain and nondiagnostic electrocardiograms. *J Am Coll Cardiol.* 1998; 31: 1011–1017.

2.3.5. Cost/benefits

The potential for reduction of inappropriate hospital admissions by the use of acute rest MPI in the ED may offset the additional costs of MPI (Table 15.5). There are several studies that evaluated the economic implications of the use of early risk stratification with MPI for assessment of chest pain in the ED. Weissman et al.[78] used a survey method of decision making by physicians before and after the MPI results were available. They found that 68% of the physicians' decisions were affected by the MPI results and estimated potential cost savings of $786 per patient.

2.4. Cardiac MR

Over the last decade, cardiac magnetic resonance (CMR) imaging has emerged as a powerful imaging modality for the assessment of a wide spectrum of cardiovascular diseases in patients with ACP. Rapid developments in CMR technology has helped transition the use from research applications to routine clinical practice. The inplane spatial resolution achievable in CMR perfusion studies has

reached the order of 1 to 2 mm and has therefore been shown to be superior to SPECT perfusion imaging, particularly for the detection of subendocardial ischemia. It is expected that the ongoing technological advances in CMR imaging will have a marked impact on the diagnostic paradigm of cardiovascular disease management. CMR imaging techniques are routinely being used for the assessment of cardiovascular anatomy, ventricular function, valvular status, stress function, perfusion, and myocardial viability in a single imaging setting. CMR coronary angiography is evolving and current techniques permit limited evaluation of the proximal and mid coronary artery segments. Clinical application of CMR in the ED for chest pain evaluation has been slowly evolving over the last 10 years.

Compared to Multi-detector computed tomography (MDCT), CMR does not involve exposure to ionizing radiation or iodinated contrast agents. However, similar to MDCT, CMR is very susceptible to artifacts caused by irregular heart rhythm and erratic respiratory patterns.

2.4.1. Coronary MRA

Over the past two decades, CMR coronary angiography has continued to evolve[79] with the development and implementation of enhanced pulse sequences. The images were typically obtained with steady-state free precession (SSFP) bright blood pulse sequences. The most recent improvement to CMR coronary angiography was development of whole-heart imaging. With this approach, instead of individually localizing each coronary artery for imaging, a single axial prescription covering the entire heart is acquired and the 3D image stack is (similar to MDCT) postprocessed at later times to visualize the coronary arteries. This approach significantly simplifies the difficult localization and prescription phase which used to be extremely time consuming and required significant user experience. The 3D approach reduces the total image scanning time from more than 50 min to under 20 min. In addition, it allows better visualization of the smaller branch vessels. Presently, the challenges of magnetic resonance coronary angiography (MRCA) remains in limited signal-to-noise ratio as well as spatial resolution with voxel size of 1.0 × 1.0 × 1.5 mm³.

The diagnostic accuracy of CMR coronary angiography has improved over time (Table 15.6), but is still inferior to MDCT. According to the most recent studies, whole-heart CMR coronary angiography[80] currently allows interpretation of about 80% of segments with sensitivies between 78% and 82% and specificities of 90% to 92%. Direct comparison of MDCT versus CMR coronary angiography has been performed with older CMR imaging sequences and CT technology (4-slice and 16-slice MDCT) in small group of patients. The accuracy of both MR and CT was in the range of 78% to 80%.[81,82]

However, the current challenge to use CMR for the anatomical assessment of coronary arteries is the need for acquisition to be averaged over several cardiac and respiratory cycles, with many patients been unable to sustain a stable respiratory pattern. This limitation is particularly challenging in patients with ACP through ED. The use of navigators that compensate for the breathing cycle may attenuate the problem with diagnostic accuracy of 89%.[83]

2.4.2. Stress CMR perfusion and function

Several studies have evaluated the role of CMR for the assessment of chest pain in patients with suspected or known CAD. Unlike other imaging modalities, very few studies were performed with CMR in the ED setting among patients presenting with ACP, which makes it difficult to compare the modalities in this scenario. Kwong et al.[84] evaluated the feasibility and diagnostic performance of CMR in a prospective study of 161 consecutive patients

---

TABLE 15.5

COST EFFECTIVENESS OF REST MYOCARDIAL PERFUSION IMAGING IN THE ASSESSMENT OF ACUTE CHEST PAIN

Study	Number of patients	Cost saving ($) per patient
Stowers et al.[148]	46	1,843
Weissman et al.[78]	50	786
Radensky et al.[149]	209	796
Stowers et al.[150]	180	923
Heller et al.[44]	357	4,258
Kontos et al.[75]	874	1,014
Ziffer et al.[151]	6,548	1,900

Source: Gani F, Jain D, Lahiri A. The role of cardiovascular imaging techniques in the assessment of patients with acute chest pain. *Nucl Med Commun.* 28:441–449.

TABLE 15.6

DIAGNOSTIC ACCURACY OF CMR CORONARY ANGIOGRAPHY

Study	MR	Patients, n	Evaluable segments (%)	Sensitivity (%)	Specificity (%)
Kim et al.[153]	3D-TGE DIR-NAV	109	84	93	42
Bogaert et al.[86]	3D-SSFP DIR-NAV	21	71	44–55	84–95
Sommer et al.[154]	3D-SSFP DIR-NAV	18	86	82	88
Jahnke et al.[83]	3D-SSFP WH-NAV	55	83	78	91
Sakuma et al.[16]	3D-SSFP WH-NAV	38	92	82	91
All		241	84	84	69

DIR, directional; NAV, navigator gating; SSFP, steady-state free precession; TGE, turbo-gradient-echo; WH, whole-heart.

presenting to the ED with 30 min of ischemic chest pain but no ECG evidence of AMI. Patients were followed for 8 weeks after hospitalization for major adverse cardiac events (MACE). CMR scans were performed as early as feasible after resolution of chest pain and stabilization in the ED, including LV regional and global function, perfusion, and gadolinium enhanced MI detection. CMR was compared with conventional care chosen by the attending physician. The CMR scan lasted 38 min and patients were away from the ED for 58 min. CMR provided 84% sensitivity and 85% specificity for the diagnosis of ACS. An abnormal ECG had similar sensitivity (80%) but lower specificity (61%). Troponin-I, either initial or peak, was not as sensitive for ACS as CMR, but an abnormal troponin was more specific, while TIMI risk score had 48% sensitivity and 85% specificity for ACS. Multivariate logistic regression analysis showed that CMR was the strongest predictor of ACS and added diagnostic value over clinical parameters. This single center study clearly demonstrated that CMR is feasible among selected ED chest pain patients with improved detection of ACS compared to conventional care because of its ability to detect unstable angina and MI. These promising data need to be confirmed within larger, multicenter trials.

One of the most challenging areas for existing imaging modalities in the assessment of myocardial injury in patients with ACP is to differentiate acute from chronic irreversible myocardial injury for clinical decision-making. Both patterns of injury present as a regional wall motion abnormality in echocardiography, and although wall thinning is a feature of chronic infarct,[85] this finding is not observed in acute or nontransmural infarcts.[86] In the absence of viable myocardial cells, both AMI and chronic MI fail to uptake radioactive tracers in radionuclide imaging and thus appear as fixed defects.[87] Finally, although delayed enhancement on CMR accurately detects irreversible myocardial injury, both acute MI and chronic MI exhibit delayed enhancement regardless of their age.[88–91] Recently developed T2-weighted CMR provided information about infarct age.[92] In the new infarct area, myocardial edema is further intensified and then gradually resolves as the infarct heals. The old scar, however, manifests only as delayed enhancement. This approach of combining delayed enhancement (DE) and T2-weighted CMR is a clinically reliable tool to differentiate acute from chronic MI (Fig. 15.7).

CMR has also been effective in diagnosis of other etiologies of ACP, such as aortic pathology, myocarditis, and pericardial diseases.[93–95]

2.4.3. Prognostic value

The prognostic value of CMR has been well documented to detect the infarct size, location, and trasmural extent.[96] In patients with a clinical suspicion of CAD but without a known MI, the presence and extent of unrecognized myocardial scar by CMR provide strong prognostic value. The presence of delayed enhancement by CMR is a better multivariable predictor of MACE and cardiac mortality compared with common clinical, ECG, and LV functional variables. There is a primary "threshold effect," wherein even a very small myocardial scar by delayed enhancement (≤2% mean LV mass) is associated with a ≥ sevenfold increase in MACE hazards. The delayed enhancement provides complementary and incremental associations with MACE and cardiac mortality beyond clinical predictors alone or combined with angiographic or LV function predictors. Because the prognosis of patients with an unrecognized MI is comparable to or worse than that of patients with a recognized MI,[97,98] contrast enhanced CMR can improve the current risk assessment of patients without a prior known MI and who are presenting with possible CAD.

Ingkanisorn et al.[99] evaluated the diagnostic value of adenosine stress CMR on 135 patients who presented to the ED with chest pain and had AMI excluded by serial troponin. The imaging protocol included regional and global function, adenosine stress perfusion, and delayed enhancement infarct imaging (Fig. 15.8). Patients were followed for one year for adverse outcomes defined as interval diagnosis of 50% stenoses on coronary angiography, abnormal correlative stress test, new MI, or death. On a median follow-up of 1.3 years, 20 patients (14.8%) experienced an endpoint event. Adenosine perfusion abnormalities had 100% sensitivity and 93% specificity and were the most accurate component of the CMR examination. Combining all CMR results to label a CMR study as normal or as abnormal only reduced specificity to 91%. None of the patients with a normal adenosine CMR study had a subsequent diagnosis of CAD or an adverse outcome. Therefore, in patients with chest pain who had MI excluded by troponin and nondiagnostic electrocardiograms, an adenosine

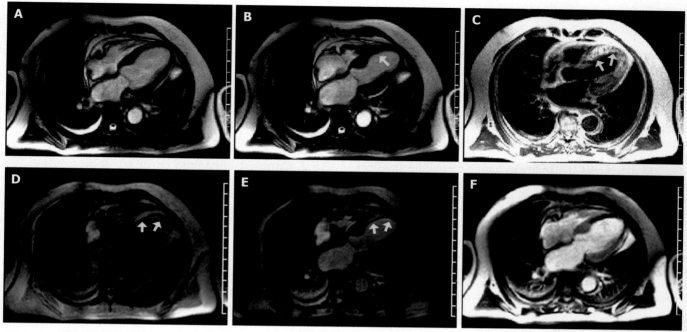

Figure 15.7 Cine SSFP end-diastolic (**A**) and end-systolic (**B**) images obtained from a patient with a recent anteroseptal infarct showing midseptal and apical akinesis (**Movie 15.1**); (**C**) T2 weighted image showing increased signal intensity in the septum and apex, indicating myocardial edema; (**D, E, F, Movie 15.2**) TI-scout images obtained after gadolinium injection with progressively longer inversion time (TI); (**D, E**) show the area of gadolinium delayed enhancement; (**F**) shows the smaller area of subendocardial microvascular obstruction.

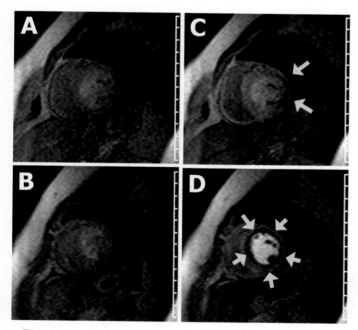

Figure 15.8 First-pass gadolinium perfusion images obtained at basal and mid ventricular level at rest (**A, B, Movies 15.3 and 15.4**) and after adenosine stress (**C, D, Movies 15.5 and 15.6**) indicating basal lateral and global midventricular subendocardial ischemia in a patient with three-vessel obstructive CAD.

CMR examination was highly accurate in predicting significant CAD and MACE during 1-year follow-up.

The study from Plein et al.[100] also suggested comprehensive CMR analysis (function, rest and adenosine-stress perfusion, delayed enhancement, and coronary artery anatomy) that yielded a sensitivity of 96% and a specificity of 83% to predict the presence of significant coronary stenosis and it was more accurate than the analysis of any individual CMR method predicting revascularization in patients with NSTEMI.

2.4.4. Cost/benefits

CMR is very safe and no long-term side effects have been demonstrated. Claustrophobia may be problematic in about 2% of patients, but mild anxiolytics (lorazepam or diazepam) are often effective. One of the most important safety issues for CMR is the prevention of ferromagnetic objects in the scanner, which can become projectile. Permanent metallic implants such as hip prostheses, prosthetic heart valves, coronary stents, and sternal sutures present no hazard since the materials used are weakly ferromagnetic. Care is required in patients with cerebrovascular clips, and specialist advice is needed for such patients. Patients with pacemakers, implanted cardioverter defibrillators (ICD), retained permanent pacemaker leads, and other electronic implants are generally excluded from MRI, although some reports of success do exist.[101,102] A definite or possible pregnancy must be identified prior to permitting the patient into the MR environment and an MR procedure should only be performed to address important clinical questions. Patients with advanced renal disease (GFR 30 ml/min/1.73 m²) should not undergo gadolinium enhanced MRI due to potential for a serious side effect of nephrogenic systemic fibrosis.

Patients with chest pain in the ED need continuous close observation and management and taking these patients to the MR scanner may interrupt this important observation. Therefore, patients with ongoing chest pain, hemodynamic instability, arrhythmias, heart failure, or ischemic ECG changes should not be removed from a monitored setting to undergo CMR. The availability of around-the-clock MRI scanners staffed with CMR trained personnel and safety concerns related to longer imaging times (average 30 min) during which patients are removed from the ED have been limiting factors. There is no large clinical trial to assess the impact of CMR on the cost and financial outcomes in triaging patients with ACP in the ED.

2.5. Cardiac computed tomography

Computed tomography (CT) has been an important tool for evaluation of emergency and trauma patients since the 1970s. Cardiac CT (CCT) is the fastest evolving technology with the advent of multislice CT (MSCT) starting from 4-slice in the year of 2000 to 256 or 320 slice scanners in the year of 2008. Comparing other imaging techniques, CT has the advantages of high spatial resolution (0.4 to 0.5 mm), fast acquisition time in a single breath hold (5 to 10 s), and widespread availability, including community hospitals in the United States. Its true 3D volumetric acquisition permits virtually unlimited views for image projections post processing, making CT the fastest screening tool for the entire thorax in life threatening cardiovascular diseases with a wide spectrum of complexities in anatomy, physiology, and pathology.[103,104] In patients with suspected coronary disease, CTA can provide simultaneous assessment of coronary artery anatomy, myocardial perfusion, and ventricular function. The high-resolution 64-slice scanners have become standard for CCT in current cardiac imaging services.

2.5.1. Calcium scoring

The utility of electron-beam CT-based detection of coronary artery calcification for predicting the likelihood of ACSs in patients with ACP has been studied.[105-107] Georgiou et al.[106] assessed the prognostic value of negative predictive value of normal EBCT in a prospective observational study of 192 patients admitted to ED with suspected ACS. They followed this group of patients for 7 years for subsequent cardiac events. The presence of coronary artery calcium and increasing score quartiles were strongly related to the occurrence of hard cardiac events including MI and death and all cardiovascular events. The results of these studies using calcium scoring demonstrate a high negative predictive value of the absence of coronary calcifications for ACSs. However, the diagnostic value of a finding of coronary calcification in patients with ACP is significantly challenged. Calcification was present in only approximately 50% of culprit lesions in the coronary arteries of people who experienced sudden death from cardiac causes.[108] In a study by Greenland et al.,[109] 14% of events (MI and death) were observed in patients in whom no evidence of coronary calcification was found at CT. Thus, the absence of coronary calcification does not exclude the presence of noncalcified coronary atherosclerotic plaques, especially in young patients. Thus, calcium scoring may be of limited value for the triage of patients with ACP.

However, coronary artery calcium scoring by MDCT may be useful in the acute CP setting prior to CTA since the quality of the CTA is likely to be impaired or nondiagnostic if large quantities of coronary calcium are found. A decision not to proceed with CTA must then be made if the calcium score is very high. Moreover, the calcium score can be compared to existing age and gender benchmarks to guide primary prevention as an outpatient if the patient is not admitted. Clearly, there is a need for more research to define the relative roles of both coronary artery calcium (CAC) and CTA for ACP patients.

2.5.2. Contrast-enhanced coronary angiography

Within a short interval of 4 years, over 30 published studies have compared cardiac computed tomographic angiography (CCTA) to quantitative invasive coronary angiography, encompassing over 2,000 patients.[110-116] Among the 18 studies in which per-patient analyses are available (involving 1,329 patients, using either 16- or 64-slice CT), the mean subject-weighted sensitivity and specificity for the detection of significant CAD (i.e., ≥50% luminal stenosis) was 97% and 84%, respectively. Analysis of just the 64-slice studies revealed a sensitivity and specificity of 99% and 93%, respectively (Table 15.1).[117] Although 10% to 20% of coronary artery segments cannot be assessed by CTA because of motion artifacts or severe calcifications, the combined results from all 18 studies demonstrated a mean per-patient negative predictive value of 97%, rendering CT a reliable method to rule out CAD if the study can be performed successfully.

A recent metaanalysis on CTA in patients with ACP (nine studies, 566 patients) showed pooled sensitivity and specificity of 0.95 (95%CI, 0.90–0.98) and 0.90 (95%CI, 0.87–0.93).[118] These data support that a normal CCTA may obviate the need for invasive angiography in properly selected clinical circumstances. The notably high sensitivity and negative predictive value of coronary CTA for the detection and exclusion of CAD makes it uniquely suited to be an effective triage tool in the ED for low- to intermediate-risk patients without pre-existing coronary disease (Table 15.7).

The positive predictive value to detect obstructive coronary disease compared to catheterization has been reported around 75%. Although it is much higher than current conventional stress testing, there is a tendency of CTA to overestimate the degree of coronary artery stenoses. One of the reasons for overestimation may be the presence of heavily calcified plaques that appear to narrow the lumen, if adjacent widening of the outer lumen (positive remodeling) is not taken into account. Underestimation of the degree of stenosis due to eccentric stenosis and suboptimal angulation is presumably another cause.

TABLE 15.7

SENSITIVITY AND SPECIFICITY OF CT CORONARY ANGIOGRAPHY FOR THE DETECTION OF CORONARY STENOSIS IN COMPARISON TO INVASIVE CORONARY ANGIOGRAPHY

Scanner type	Studies, n	Per-segment analysis		Per-patient analysis	
		Sensitivity (%)	Specificity (%)	Sensitivity (%)	Specificity (%)
4-slice CT	22	84	93	91	83
16-slice CT	26	83	96	97	81
64-slice CT	6	93	96	99	93

Metaanalysis of pooled data from Vanhoenacker PK, Heijenbrok-Kal MH, Van Heste R, et al. Diagnostic performance of multidetector CT angiography for assessment of coronary artery disease: Meta-analysis. *Radiology*. 2007;244:419–428.

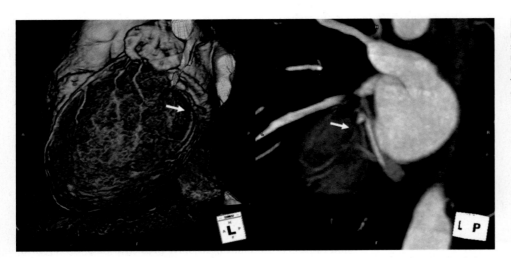

Figure 15.9 Volume-rendered 3D and maximum-intensity projections images showing occluded OM1 in a 63-year-old man presenting to the ED with chest pain, nondiagnostic ECG, and borderline positive creatine phosphokinase (CPK) after chest trauma.

Caution must be used in patients with pre-existing CAD because such patients often have extensive coronary calcifications, a multitude of intermediate severity coronary lesions, and/or coronary stents with resultant metal artifacts. All these factors tend to reduce the diagnostic accuracy of CCTA. Similarly, patients with prior coronary bypass grafting often have extensively calcified native vessels and small caliber distal coronary arteries. Although CCTA is very accurate for defining coronary bypass graft patency and stenosis, stress testing is often required to meaningfully evaluate the native vessel circulation in such patients.

The ability of CCTA to quantitatively estimate coronary artery lesion severity has also been studied.[119,120] In general, there is good correlation with invasive coronary angiography (Pearson correlation, r = 0.72). The considerable standard deviation, however, limits its quantitative accuracy. This suggests that patients at the opposite ends of the disease spectrum (i.e., those with <25% vs. >70% maximal luminal stenoses) can be accurately triaged by CCTA alone while patients with lesions of intermediate severity (25% to 70% stenosis) may need further evaluation with physiologic stress testing.

Plaque characterization. There is growing evidence that the presence, amount, and composition of noncalcified coronary atherosclerotic plaque and the degree of coronary remodeling can be assessed with multidetector CT with a level of accuracy comparable to that achievable with intravascular ultrasound (IVUS). The characterization of other features associated with plaque vulnerability, such as positive coronary remodeling (growth of atherosclerotic plaque into the vessel wall rather than the vessel lumen), is feasible and may be important for the short- and long-term risk stratification of patients with ACP.[121]

2.5.3. Assessment of function, resting, and adenosine stress myocardial perfusion

Coronary CTA may be used to assess global and regional LV function (Figs. 15.9–15.11)[122–125] and to obtain information about myocardial perfusion.[126–128] Many studies have demonstrated that regional wall motion and LV function can be accurately assessed by CTA, comparable with CMR.

Recent animal studies[129] have suggested that CTA perfusion imaging at rest may identify and characterize morphologic features of acute and healed MI, including infarct size, transmurality, and the presence of microvascular obstruction and scar. Infarcted myocardial tissue by MDCT is characterized by well-delineated hyperenhanced regions that reach peak intensity 5 min after contrast

END-DIASTOLE **END-SYSTOLE**

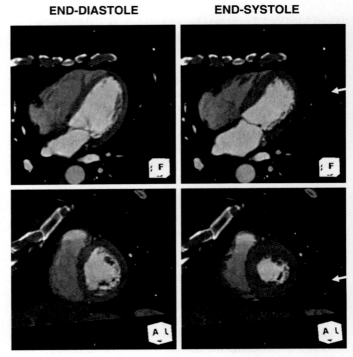

Figure 15.10 Multiplanar reconstructions showing decreased perfusion and wall motion abnormality observed on the lateral wall, consistent with coronary CTA findings of Figure 15.9.

injection whereas regions of microvascular obstruction or fibrofatty replacement in chronic MI by MDCT are characterized by hypoenhancement on early imaging. MDCT MPI was able to detect LAD territory flow deficit during adenosine stress, correlating well with microsphere-derived absolute myocardial blood flow.[130]

2.5.4. Evaluating other life threatening chest pain etiologies: "Triple Rule-Out"

Given the robust clinical performance of CCTA for exclusion of ACS in ED patients, as well as the widespread use and proven clinical accuracy of CT angiography for diagnosis of acute aortic dissection[131–133] and pulmonary embolism,[134–137] a "triple rule-out" scan protocol to simultaneously exclude all three potentially fatal causes of ACP with a single scan is an attractive option.

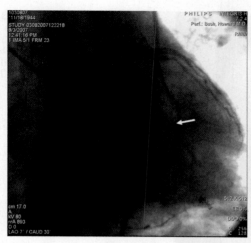

Figure 15.11 Invasive coronary angiogram showing the occluded marginal branch, consistent with CTA findings of Figure 15.9.

When 64-slice CT scanners became widely available, the technical limitations of combined simultaneous evaluation of all three vascular areas have been largely overcome. The wider anatomic coverage of the 64-slice scanner allows much faster movement of the patient through the scan plane. This has reduced the "triple rule-out" scan duration to under 20 s in most cases comparing over 30 s using a 16-slice scanner.

Combined simultaneous evaluation of the pulmonary, coronary, and thoracic aorta requires a carefully tailored imaging and injection protocol by catering the contrast volume, injection rate, and timing. The goal is to provide maximal and consistent enhancement of the coronary arteries/LV structures, high enhancement of the right ventricle (RV)/pulmonary arteries (PA), and low enhancement of right atrium (RA) to avoid streak artifacts from dense contrast in the RA to the right coronary artery (RCA).

A "tri-phasic" injection protocol may deliver the standard 100 mL of iodinated contrast at 5 mL/s, followed by an additional 30 mL at 3 mL/s to maintain PA opacification, followed by a standard saline flush injection. Mean coronary artery, PA, and aortic enhancement values can be consistently higher than 250 Hounsfield Units, and right atrial enhancement does not interfere with interpretation of the coronary arteries. Although feasibility studies of this and similar protocols are promising, large-scale clinical trials assessing the clinical accuracy of such "triple rule-out" protocols are not yet available.

2.5.5. Prognostic value

Patient safety and prognostic outcomes in 197 low-risk ACP patients were evaluated in a single center randomized trial by either early CCTA or a standard diagnostic protocol.[138] Patients randomized to immediate CCTA were eligible for discharge with normal or minimally abnormal results (<25% stenosis), patients with severe stenosis (>70%) were referred for immediate invasive angiography, whereas patients with intermediate-grade stenosis underwent additional stress testing. Among patients randomized to CCTA, 75% had decisive triage by CCTA alone (67% immediately discharged and 8% referred for immediate catheterization, which revealed significant disease in seven of eight cases). Among the patients discharged immediately, none had a major cardiac event or subsequent diagnosis of CAD over a 6-month follow-up period. The overall diagnostic accuracy of CCTA was 94%, and the negative predictive value was 100%. None of the patients discharged from the ED in the MDCT-based

strategy and only one in the conventional strategy experienced MACE at 30 days.

ACP patients from ED with a low to intermediate pretest likelihood of coronary disease and negative cardiac biomarkers and electrocardiograms are best suited for CCTA based triage. At least six recent studies have evaluated the safety and diagnostic accuracy of 64-slice CCTA for triage of ED patients with ACP.[139–144] In aggregate, 376 ED patients (predominantly low to intermediate pretest coronary risk) with ACP were prospectively followed over a 30-day to 15-month follow up period after diagnosis by CCTA. All six studies excluded patients with abnormal cardiac biomarkers or ischemic electrocardiographic changes, and two of the six studies excluded patients with pre-existing CAD. Overall, an adjudicated diagnosis of ACS occurred in 72 (19.1%) of the 376 study patients. The absence of significant coronary artery stenosis by CCTA accurately excluded the presence of ACS in 373 of the 376 patients, resulting in a combined study mean negative predictive value of 99%. This suggests that CCTA can identify a subset of ED chest pain patients who can be safely discharged home on the basis of CT findings.

Over the last two decades, CT in general is considered as test of the choice in patients that require acute imaging due to its speed, availability, and imaging quality. Application of MDCT as part of the initial diagnostic approach for patients presenting with ACP to the ED is safe, efficient, and reduces avoidable admissions in patients with an intermediate risk for ACS. In most cases, MDCT could be successfully performed within 2 to 3 h after arrival to the ED. The MDCT-based strategy had fewer avoidable admissions predominantly in intermediate-risk patients who also had a borderline significantly decreased ED length of stay.

Coronary CTA has several important limitations that affect its usefulness in the triage of ED patients with ACP.

1. Controlling heart rate. It has been convincingly shown that the heart rate and regularity of heart rhythm are closely related to image quality and accuracy of coronary stenosis estimation. It is common practice to premedicate patients who have resting heart rates >65 beats per min with beta blocking drugs and to administer sublingual nitroglycerin to all patients to enhance image quality. Up to 15% of ED patients have some contraindication to beta antagonists. At this time, only patients with a normal sinus rhythm should undergo CCTA in most facilities. Recent hardware and software improvements, however, show promise for patients with irregular rhythms including atrial fibrillation.
2. Contrast use. It is essential to screen patients in the ED for a history of iodine allergy and to avoid administration of contrast in patients with diminished creatinine clearance.
3. Calcified lesion and artifacts. Coronary CTA has reduced accuracy in patients with very high coronary calcium scores, although this is highly dependent on the location of calcification in a given patient.
4. Functional significance of intermediate lesion. CCTA presently provides data regarding anatomical lesions only, not their physiologic impact on coronary blood flow. For this reason, about 15% of ED patients with ACP require additional noninvasive stress imaging owing to the intermediate severity lesions detected on CCTA.
5. Equipment and networking requirements. Accurate assessment of coronary stenosis as well as perfusion and wall motion abnormalities require advanced software on workstations. Recent advances in thin-client server have significantly improved remote access. Physicians can remotely process large data set (up to 2 Gigabyte per patient) and

review images using advanced four-dimensional software. However, the bandwidth is quite limited between regular physician office or home and radiology departments at hospitals, except dedicated lines in place.

6. Service availability. Operationally, it is also challenging to have trained technologists and physicians provide 24/7 coverage, considering cardiac CTA is still a new technology.

2.5.6. Cost/benefits

Diagnostic efficiency, defined as time from randomization to definitive diagnosis, showed that the CCTA approach was more rapid (3.4 vs. 15.0 h) and reduced costs by 15%, compared to MPI. In addition, the cost saving due to improving outcomes and decreasing mortality/morbidity and hospital stay of patients with true ACS is also substantial, although quantification of the cost is difficult.

The cost saving may be more significant in women, who have high incidence of chest pain with normal coronary arteries, where CCTA-based triage will generally lead to their discharge because of the high negative predictive accuracy of this test (Fig 15.12). However, the imbursement for CTA has been challenging, especially with private payers.[145]

2.5.7. Limitations and evolution of the technology

Important radiation safety concerns should limit indiscriminate application of a "triple rule-out" scan protocol. The effective

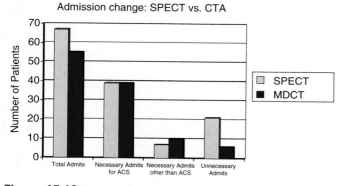

Figure 15.12 Impact of MDCT in the evaluation of patients with chest pain in the ED.

radiation dose of "triple rule-out" scan is often increased by 50% because of the increased field of view. Further, among patients who undergo CCTA as a primary triage test in the ED, there is a subset that also requires a noninvasive stress test (often a radionuclide test), followed in some cases by diagnostic and interventional invasive angiographic procedures. This combined radiation dose is a cause for concern, particularly in younger patients. Thus, unless there is a high index of suspicion, the "triple rule-out" should be avoided.

CT is the fastest evolving technology in medical imaging related to cardiology. In the spatial resolution, the improved detector and collimator hardware can provide submillimeter image resolution (0.4 to 0.5 mm). In the acquisition time, the new generation of CT scanner with 256 and 320 slices can minimize scan time to one heart beat[146]; these new scanners can decrease current radiation levels from 15 to 20 mSv to 2 to 3 mSv with prospective scanning. In patients with arrhythmias, dual-source scanners with improved temporal resolution of 75 to 83 ms or single-beat coverage (256 to 320 slices) may improve image quality significantly. With above mentioned developments, CTA can potentially provide "one-stop-shop" to imaging coronary, perfusion, and function at rest and stress with radiation levels of 5 to 6 mSv in 10 to 15 min. In the near future, CT may overcome the challenges of radiation, artifacts form motion, and calcification to become the test of the choice for patients with ACP presented in the ED.

3. FUTURE DIRECTIONS

Over the last three decades, multiple strategies and imaging modalities have become available to evaluate patients presenting to the ED with ACP. To better select an initial test for risk stratification, one needs to integrate information on pathophysiology, patient risk, technological limitations, as well as local expertise and availability. If the initial test results are suboptimal or clinical questions are still needed to be clarified, subsequent test might be considered for additional clinical value (Fig. 15.13). Ultimately, we need to understand the outcomes of imaging modality to serve our patients.

3.1. Anatomy versus physiology

Choosing an imaging modality to assess patients with ACP is based on the sequential cascade and the stage of patient presentation in

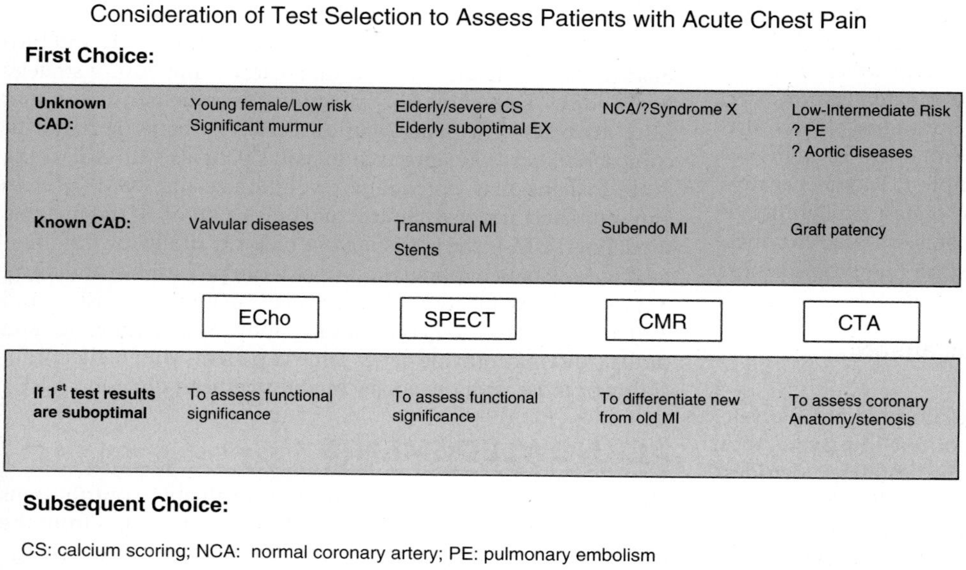

Figure 15.13 Sequential cascade of events during ischemia caused by CAD.

Consideration of Test Selection to Assess Patients with Acute Chest Pain

First Choice:

Unknown CAD:	Young female/Low risk Significant murmur	Elderly/severe CS Elderly suboptimal EX	NCA/?Syndrome X	Low-Intermediate Risk ? PE ? Aortic diseases
Known CAD:	Valvular diseases	Transmural MI Stents	Subendo MI	Graft patency
	ECho	SPECT	CMR	CTA
If 1st test results are suboptimal	To assess functional significance	To assess functional significance	To differentiate new from old MI	To assess coronary Anatomy/stenosis

Subsequent Choice:

CS: calcium scoring; NCA: normal coronary artery; PE: pulmonary embolism

Figure 15.14 Considerations of initial and subsequent test selections to assess patients with ACP.

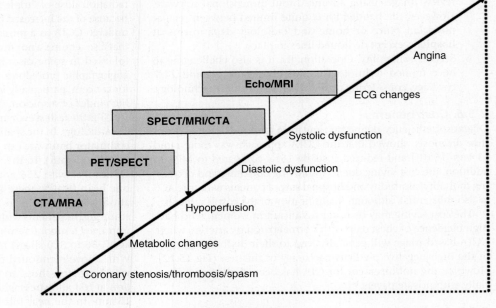

Duration of Ischemia

the process. The rationale for using stress SPECT as the current standard care in the low- to intermediate-risk population with nondiagnostic ECG and cardiac biomarkers is that flow heterogeneity during an insult of myocardial ischemia occurs much earlier than contraction abnormalities on ECG or ECG changes. However, hypoperfusion and ventricular dysfunction are the results of the coronary stenosis, spasm, or thrombosis. Thus, coronary CTA may be more sensitive than SPECT or Echo to rule-out ACSs. However, in some circumstances, coronary abnormalities might not reveal the extent of severity at the time of the scan, especially in patients with resolution of spasm or thrombosis; the consequences of coronary pathophysiology might be more prominent with hypoperfusion or contractile dysfunction (Fig. 15.14).

3.2. Appropriateness criteria: Patient selection

The American College of Cardiology, in collaboration with several other professional societies, has recently released appropriateness criteria to help guide usage of cardiac imaging for diagnosis and management of cardiovascular diseases.

In ACP patients classified as intermediate pretest probability of CAD with uninterpretable ECG and negative cardiac enzymes, Stress Echo, SPECT, and MDCT were considered appropriate, and CMR stress testing was considered uncertain. CTA is also considered as uncertain in patients with either low or high pretest probability of CAD with uninterruptible ECG and negative cardiac enzymes. In patients with a high pretest probability of CAD and ST-segment elevation and/or positive cardiac enzymes, all imaging modalities received a rating of inappropriateness (Table 15.8).

3.3. Challenges and opportunities ahead: Changing the process of ROMI

Ruling out AMI (ROMI) with admission to hospital or CP observation unit has been part of the standard of care in patients with chest pain without ECG changes over the last three decades. Although chemical biomarkers and electrocardiogram remain the most important tools in the assessment of patients with ACS, most patients without diagnostic ECG and negative enzymes have

TABLE 15.8
APPROPRIATENESS CRITERIA TO ASSESS ACUTE CHEST PAIN

	Pretest probability of CAD[a]		
	Low	*Intermediate*	*High*
Stress Echo	–	Appropriate (8)	–
SPECT	–	Appropriate (9)	–
MR	–	Uncertain (6)	–
CTA	Uncertain (5)	Appropriate (7)	Uncertain (6)

[a] No ECG changes and negative serial enzymes.

to wait and observe in the acute period. Due to lack of accuracy of these diagnostic tests, often it leads to a delay in the diagnosis of myocardial injury until MI is ruled in.

In essence, waiting for AMI in patients without ECG and biomarker changes is the standard care. Clearly, this *passive* strategy is not ideal since many clinical studies have demonstrated that early establishment of reperfusion correlates better survival. In comparison, *proactive* approach to assess patients with ACP using acute imaging may potentially revolutionize the ROMI process and ultimately improve clinical outcomes. Out of all the imaging modalities, CTA is the best suited in majority of the low- to intermediate-risk patient population since it can provide fast and direct noninvasive visualization of the coronary anatomy, perfusion, and wall motion. However, echocardiography, SPECT imaging, and cardiac MRI may provide better value in patients with higher probability or those with previously established heart disease.

ACKNOWLEDGMENTS

The authors would like to thank the invaluable contributions from Dr. Tudor Scridon and Dr. Neal Saxena, as well as from the attendings and fellows in the Dept of Cardiology and Radiology.

REFERENCES

1. Fineberg HV, Scadden G, Goldman L. Care of patients with a low probability of acute myocardial infarction. Cost effectiveness of alternatives to coronary care unit admission. N Engl J Med. 1984;310(20):1301–1307.
2. Lee TH, Goldman L. Evaluation of the patient with acute chest pain. N Engl J Med. 2000;342(16):1187–1195.
3. Lee TH, Rouan GW, Weisberg MC, et al. Clinical characteristics and natural history if patients with acute myocardial infarction sent home from the emergency room. Am J Cardiol. 1987;60(4):219–224.
4. Stillman A, Odukerk M, Ackerman M, et al. Use of multidetector computed tomography for the assessment of acute chest pain: A consensus statement of the North American Society of Cardiac Imaging and European Society of Cardiac Radiology. Int J Cardiovasc Imaging. 2007;23:415–427.
5. Arnold J, Goodcare S, Morris F. Structure, process and outcomes of chest pain units established in ESCAPE Trial. Emerg Med J. 2007;24:462–466.
6. Bartholomew BA, Sheps DS, Monroe S, et al. A population-based evaluation of the thrombolysis in myocardial infarction risk score for unstable angina and non-ST elevation myocardial infarction. Clin Cardiol. 2004;(2):74–78.
7. Sabatine MS, Antman EM. The thrombolysis in myocardial infarction risk score in unstable angina/non-ST-segment elevation myocardial infarction. J Am Coll Cardiol. 2003;41(4 Suppl S):89S–95S.
8. Antman EM, Cohen M, Bernink PJ, et al. The TIMI risk score for unstable angina/non-ST elevation MI: A method fro prognostication and therapeutic decision making. JAMA. 2000;284(7):835–842.
9. Goodacre S, Cross E, Lewis C, et al. Effectiveness and safety of chest pain assessment to prevent emergency admissions: ESCAPE cluster randomized trial. BMJ. 2007;ver2:1–6.
10. Thygesen K, Alpert J, White H, et al. Joint ESC/ACCF/AHA/WHF task force for redefinition of myocardial infarction. J Am Coll Cardiol. 2007;50:2173–2195.
11. Connolly DC, Elveback LR, Oxman HA. Coronary heart disease in residents of Rochester, Minnesota, IV. Prognostic value of the resting electrocardiogram at the time of initial diagnosis of angina pectoris. Mayo Clin Proc. 1984;59:247–250.
12. Jaffee AS, Babuin L, Apple FS. Biomarkers in acute cardiac disease. J Am Coll Cardiol. 2006;48:1–11.
13. Jaffee AS, Ravkilde J, Roberts R, et al. It's time for a change to a troponin standard. Circulation. 2000;102:1216–1220.
14. Lewis W. Echocardiography in the evaluation of patients in chest pain units. Cardiol Clin. 2005;23:531–539.
15. Rubin DN, Yazbek N, Garcia MJ, et al. Qualitative and quantitative effects of harmonic echocardiographic imaging on endocardial edge definition and side-lobe artifacts. J Am Soc Echocardiogr. 2000;13(11):1012–1018.
16. Sakuma T, Hayashi Y, Shimohara A, et al. Usefulness of myocardial contrast echocardiography for the assessment of serial changes in the risk areas in patients with acute myocardial infarction. Am J Cardiol. 1996;78:1273–1277.
17. Hauser AM, Gangadharan V, Ramos RG, et al. Sequence of mechanical, electrocardiographic observations during coronary angioplasty. Am J Cardiol. 1990;65:1071–1077.
18. Sabia P, Afrookteh A, Touchstone DA, et al. Value of regional wall motion abnormality in the emergency room diagnosis of acute myocardial infarction. A prospective study using two-dimensional echocardiography. Circulation. 1991;84:I85–I92.
19. Liberman AN, Weiss JL, Jugdutt BL, et al. Two dimensional echocardiography and infarct size: Relationship of regional wall motion and thickening to the extent of myocardial infarction in the dog. Circulation. 1981;63:739.
20. Kaul S. Echocardiography in coronary artery disease. Curr Probl Cardiol. 1990;15:233.
21. Sleker HP, Zalenski RJ, Antman EM, et al. An evaluation of technologies for identifying acute cardiac ischemia in the emergency department: A report for a National Heart Attack Program Working Group. Ann Emerg Med. 199;29:13–87.
22. ACC/AHA 2002 Guideline Update for the management of Patients with Unstable Angina and Non-ST segment Elevation Myocardial Infarction. A report of the American College of Cardiology/American Heart Association Task Force on Practice Guidelines.
23. Cheitlin MD, Armstrong WF, Aurigemma GP, et al. ACC/AHA/ASE 2003 Guideline update for the Clinical Application of Echocardiography. A report of the American College of Cardiology/American Heart Association Task Force on Practice Guidelines. J Am Coll Cardiol. 2003;42:954–970.
24. ACCF/ASE/ACEP/ASNC/SCAI/SCCT/SCMR 2007 Appropriateness Criteria for Transthoracic and Transesophageal Echocardiography. J Am Coll Cardiol. 2007.
25. Koch R, Lang RM, Garcia MJ. Objective evaluation of regional left ventricular wall motion during dobutamine stress echocardiographic studies using segmental analysis of color kinesis images. J Am Coll Cardiol. 1999;34(2):409–419.
26. Gibbons RJ, Abrams J, Chaterjee K, et al. ACC/AHA 2002 guidelines update for the management of patients with chronic stable angina: A report of the American College of Cardiology/American Heart Association Task Force on Practice Guidelines (Committee to Update the 1999 Guidelines for the Management of Patients with Chronic Stable Angina). 2002. Available at www.acc.prg/clinical/guidelines/stable/stable.pdf.
27. Bholasingh R, Cornel JH, Kamp O, et al. Prognostic value of predischarge dobutamine stress echocardiography in chest pain patients with a negative cardiac troponin T. J Am Coll Cardiol. 2003;41(4):596–602.
28. Marwick TH, Case C, Short L, et al. Prediction of mortality in patients without angina: Use of an exercise score and exercise echocardiography. Eur Heart J. 2003;24(13):1223–1230.
29. Kuo D, Vasken D, Prasad R, et al. Emergency cardiac imaging: State of the art. Cardiol Clin. 2006;24:53–65.
30. Kamalesh M, Matorin R, Sawada S. Prognostic value of a negative stress echocardiographic study in diabetic patients. Am Heart J. 2002;143(1):163–168.
31. Weston P, Alexander J, Wagner G, et al. Hand-held echocardiographic examination of patients with symptoms of acute coronary syndromes in the emergency department: The 30-day outcome associated with normal left ventricular wall motion. Am Heart J. 2004;148:1096–1101.
32. Korosoglou G. Usefulness of real-time myocardial perfusion imaging in the evaluation of patients with first time chest pain. Am J Cardiol. 2004;94(10);1225–1231.
33. Kaul S, Sneior R, Firschke C, et al. Incremental value of cardiac imaging in patients with chest pain and without ST segment elevation: A multicenter study. Am Heart J. 2004;148(1):129–136.
34. Koch R, Lang RM, Garcia MJ. Objective evaluation of regional left ventricular wall motion during dobutamine stress echocardiographic studies using segmental analysis of color kinesis images. J Am Coll Cardiol. 1999;34(2):409–419.
35. Shaw L, Marwick T, Berman D, et al. Incremental cost effectiveness of exercise echocardiography vs. SPECT imaging for the evaluation of stable chest pain. Eur Heart J. 2006;27:2448–2458.
36. Kuntz KM, Fleischmann KE, Hunink MG, et al. Cost effectiveness of diagnostic strategies for patients with chest pain. Ann Int Med. 1999;130(9):709–718.
37. Wackers FJ, Lie KI, Liem KL, et al. Potential value of thallium-201 scintigraphy as a means of selecting patients for the coronary care unit. Br Heart J. 1979;41:111–117.
38. Madsen MT. Recent advances in SPECT imaging. J Nucl Med. 2007;48:661–673.
39. Bilodeau L, Theroux P, Gregoire J, et al. Technetium-99 m sestamibi tomography in patients with spontaneous chest pain: Correlations with clinical, electrocardiographic and angiographic findings. J Am Coll Cardiol. 1991;18:1684–1691.
40. Nicholson CS, Tatum JL, Jesse RL, et al. The value of gated tomographic Tc-99 m-sestamibi perfusion imaging in acute ischemic syndromes. J Nucl Cardiol. 1995;2:S57.
41. Varetto T, Cantalupi D, Altieri A, et al. Emergency room technetium-99 m sestamibi imaging to rule out acute myocardial ischemic events in patients with nondiagnostic electrocardiograms. J Am Coll Cardiol. 1993;22:1804–1808.
42. Hilton TC, Thompson RC, Williams HJ, et al. Technetium-99 m sestamibi myocardial perfusion imaging in the emergency room evaluation of chest pain. J Am Coll Cardiol. 1994;23:1016–1022.
43. Tatum JL, Jesse RL, Kontos MC, et al. Comprehensive strategy for the evaluation and triage of the chest pain patient. Ann Emerg Med. 1997;29:116–123.
44. Heller GV, Stowers SA, Hendel RC, et al. Clinical value of acute rest technetium-99 m tetrofosmin tomographic myocardial perfusion imaging in patients with acute chest pain and nondiagnostic electrocardiograms. J Am Coll Cardiol. 1998;31:1011–1017.
45. Kontos MC, Tatum JL. Imaging in the evaluation of the patient with suspected acute coronary syndrome. Cardiol Clin. 2005;23:517–530.
46. Kontos MC, Jesse RL, Anderson FP, et al. Comparison of myocardial perfusion imaging and cardiac troponin I in patients admitted to the emergency department with chest pain. Circulation. 1999;99:2073–2078.
47. Duca MD, Giri S, Wu AH, et al. Comparison of acute rest myocardial perfusion imaging and serum markers of myocardial injury in patients with chest pain syndromes. J Nucl Cardiol. 1999;6:570–576.
48. Kontos MC, Fratkin MJ, Jesse RL, et al. Sensitivity of acute rest myocardial perfusion imaging for identifying patients with myocardial infarction based on a troponin definition. J Nucl Cardiol. 2004;11:12–19.
49. O'Connor MK, Hammell T, Gibbons RJ. In vitro validation of a simple tomographic technique for estimation of percentage myocardium at risk using methoxyisobutyl isonitrile technetium 99 m (sestamibi). Eur J Nucl Med. 1990;17:69–76.
50. Dilsizian V, Bateman TM, Bergmann SR, et al. Metabolic imaging with beta-methyl-p-[(123)I]-iodophenyl-pentadecanoic acid identifies ischemic memory after demand ischemia. Circulation. 2005;112:2169–2174.
51. Straeter-Knowlen IM, Evanochko WT, den Hollander JA, et al. 1H NMR spectroscopic imaging of myocardial triglycerides in excised dog hearts subjected to 24 hours of coronary occlusion. Circulation. 1996;93:1464–1470.
52. Noriyasu K, Mabuchi M, Kuge Y, et al. Serial changes in BMIPP uptake in relation to thallium uptake in the rat myocardium after ischemia. Eur J Nucl Med Mol Imaging. 2003;30:1644–1650.
53. Hosokawa R, Nohara R, Fujibayashi Y, et al. Myocardial metabolism of 123I-BMIPP in a canine model with ischemia: Implications of perfusion-metabolism mismatch on SPECT images in patients with ischemic heart disease. J Nucl Med. 1999;40:471–478.
54. Kawai Y, Morita K, Nozaki Y, et al. Diagnostic value of 123I-betamethyl-p-iodophenyl-pentadecanoic acid (BMIPP) single photon emission computed tomography (SPECT) in patients with chest pain. Comparison with rest–stress 99mTc-tetrofosmin SPECT and coronary angiography. Circ J. 2004;68:547–552.
55. Kawai Y, Morita K, Nozaki Y, et al. Diagnostic value of 123I-betamethyl-p-iodophenyl-pentadecanoic acid (BMIPP) single photon emission computed tomography (SPECT) in patients with chest pain. Comparison with rest–stress 99mTc-tetrofosmin SPECT and coronary angiography. Circ J. 2004;68:547–552.
56. Abbott BG, Jain D. Nuclear cardiology in the evaluation of acute chest pain in the emergency department. Echocardiography. 2000;17:597–604.
57. Abbott BG, Jain D. Symposium on myocardial perfusion imaging in acute coronary syndromes: Impact of myocardial perfusion imaging on clinical

management and the utilization of hospital resources in suspected acute coronary syndromes. *Nucl Med Commun.* 2003;24:1061–1069.

58. ACC/AHA/ASNC guidelines for the clinical use of cardiac radionuclide imaging: A report of the American College of Cardiology/American Heart Association Task Force on practice guidelines (ACC/AHA/ASNC Committee to revise the 1995 guidelines [trunc]. Bethesda (MD): American College of Cardiology Foundation. *Circulation.* 2003;108(11):1404–1418.

59. Brown KA. Prognostic value of thallium-201 myocardial perfusion imaging in patients with unstable angina who respond to medical treatment. *J Am Coll Cardiol.* 1991;17:1053–1057.

60. Amanullah AM, Lindvall K. Prevalence and significance of transient–predominantly asymptomatic–myocardial ischemia on Holter monitoring in unstable angina pectoris, and correlation with exercise test and thallium-201 myocardial perfusion imaging. *Am J Cardiol.* 1993;72:144–148.

61. Stratmann HG, Younis LT, Wittry MD, et al. Exercise technetium-99 m myocardial tomography for the risk stratification of men with medically treated unstable angina pectoris. *Am J Cardiol.* 1995;76:236–240.

62. Madsen JK, Stubgaard M, Utne HE, et al. Prognosis and thallium-201 scintigraphy in patients admitted with chest pain without confirmed acute myocardial infarction. *Br Heart J.* 1988;59:184–189.

63. Kroll D, Farah W, McKendall GR, et al. Prognostic value of stress-gated Tc-99 m sestamibi SPECT after acute myocardial infarction. *Am J Cardiol.* 2001;87:381–386.

64. Bodenheimer MM, Wackers FJ, Schwartz RG, et al. Prognostic significance of a fixed thallium defect one to six months after onset of acute myocardial infarction or unstable angina: Multicenter myocardial ischemia research group. *Am J Cardiol.* 1994;74:1196–1200.

65. Freeman MR, Chisholm RJ, Armstrong PW. Usefulness of exercise electrocardiography and thallium scintigraphy in unstable angina pectoris in predicting the extent and severity of coronary artery disease. *Am J Cardiol.* 1988;62:1164–1170.

66. Hilton TC, Fulmer H, Abuan T, et al. Ninety-day follow-up of patients in the emergency department with chest pain who undergo initial single-photon emission computed tomography perfusion scintigraphy with technetium 99 m-labeled sestamibi. *J Nucl Cardiol.* 1996;3:308–311.

67. Miller TD, Christian TF, Hopfenspirger MR, et al. Infarct size after acute myocardial infarction measured by quantitative tomography 99mTc sestamibi imaging predicts subsequent mortality. *Circulation.* 1995;92:334–341.

68. Miller TD, Hodge DO, Sutton JM, et al. Usefulness of technetium-99 m sestamibi infarct size in predicting posthospital mortality following acute myocardial infarction. *Am J Cardiol.* 1998;81:1491–1493.

69. Reimer KA, Jennings RB, Cobb FR, et al. Animal models for protecting ischemic myocardium: Results of the NHLBI Cooperative Study. Comparison of unconscious and conscious dog models. *Circ Res.* 1985;56:651–665.

70. De Coster PM, Wijns W, Cauwe F, et al. Area at-risk determination by technetium-99 m-hexakis-2-methoxyisobutyl isonitrile in experimental reperfused myocardial infarction. *Circulation.* 1990;82:2152–2162.

71. Sinusas AJ, Trautman KA, Bergin JD, et al. Quantification of area at risk during coronary occlusion and degree of myocardial salvage after reperfusion with technetium-99 m methoxyisobutyl isonitrile. *Circulation.* 1990;82:1424–1437.

72. Christian TF, Behrenbeck T, Gersh BJ, et al. Relation of left ventricular volume and function over one year after acute myocardial infarction to infarct size determined by technetium-99 m sestamibi. *Am J Cardiol.* 1991;68:21–26.

73. Christian TF, Behrenbeck T, Pellikka PA, et al. Mismatch of left ventricular function and infarct size demonstrated by technetium-99 m isonitrile imaging after reperfusion therapy for acute myocardial infarction: Identification of myocardial stunning and hyperkinesia. *J Am Coll Cardiol.* 1990;16:1632–1638.

74. Behrenbeck T, Pellikka PA, Huber KC, et al. Primary angioplasty in myocardial infarction: Assessment of improved myocardial perfusion with technetium-99 m isonitrile. *J Am Coll Cardiol.* 1991;17:365–372.

75. Kontos MC, Jesse RL, Schmidt KL, et al. Value of acute rest sestamibi perfusion imaging for evaluation of patients admitted to the emergency department with chest pain. *J Am Coll Cardiol.* 1997;30:976–982.

76. Knott JC, Baldey AC, Grigg LE, et al. Impact of acute chest pain Tc-99 m sestamibi myocardial perfusion imaging on clinical management. *J Nucl Cardiol.* 2002;9:257–262.

77. Udelson JE, Beshansky JR, Ballin DS, et al. Myocardial perfusion imaging for evaluation and triage of patients with suspected acute cardiac ischemia: A randomized controlled trial. *JAMA.* 2002;288:2693–2700.

78. Weissman IA, Dickinson CZ, Dworkin HJ, et al. Costeffectiveness of myocardial perfusion imaging with SPECT in the emergency department evaluation of patients with unexplained chest pain. *Radiology.* 1996;199:353–357.

79. Gerber BL. MRI versus CT for the detection of coronary artery disease: Current state and future promises. *Curr Cardiol Rep.* 2007;9:72–78.

80. Weber OM, Martin AJ, Higgins CB. Whole-heart steadystate free precession coronary artery magnetic resonance angiography. *Magn Reson Med.* 2003;50:1223–1228.

81. Gerber BL, Coche E, Pasquet A, et al. Coronary artery stenosis: Direct comparison of four-section multi-detector row CT and 3D navigator MR imaging for detection—initial results. *Radiology.* 2005;234:98–108.

82. Kefer J, Coche E, Pasquet A, et al. Head to head comparison of multislice coronary CT and 3D navigator MRI for the detection of coronary artery stenosis. *J Am Coll Cardiol.* 2005;46:92–100.

83. Jahnke C, Paetsch I, Nehrke K, et al. Rapid and complete coronary arterial tree visualization with magnetic resonance imaging: Feasibility and diagnostic performance. *Eur Heart J.* 2005;26:2313–2319.

84. Kwong R, Schussheim A, Rekhraj S, et al. Detecting acute coronary syndrome in the emergency department with cardiac magnetic resonance imaging. *Circulation.* 2003;107:531–537.

85. Baer FM, Smolarz K, Jungehulsing M, et al. Chronic myocardial infarction: Assessment of morphology, function, and perfusion by gradient echo magnetic resonance imaging and 99mTc-methoxyisobutyl-isonitrile SPECT. *Am Heart J.* 1992;123:636–645.

86. Bogaert J, Kuzo R, Dymarkowski S, et al. Coronary artery imaging with real-time navigator three-dimensional turbofield-echo MR coronary angiography: Initial experience. *Radiology.* 2003;226:707–716.

87. Sechtem U, Baer F, Voth E. Myocardial viability. In: Manning W, Pennell D, eds. *Cardiovascular Magnetic Resonance.* 1st Ed. New York, NY: Churchill Livingstone; 2002:167–185.

88. Thornhill RE, Prato FS, Wisenberg G. The assessment of myocardial viability: A review of current diagnostic imaging approaches. *J Cardiovasc Magn Reson.* 2002;4:381–410.

89. Choi KM, Kim RJ, Gubernikoff G, et al. Transmural extent of acute myocardial infarction predicts long-term improvement in contractile function. *Circulation.* 2001;104:1101–1107.

90. Wu E, Judd RM, Vargas JD, et al. Visualisation of presence, location, and transmural extent of healed Q- wave and non-Q-wave myocardial infarction. *Lancet.* 2001;357:21–28.

91. Mahrholdt H, Wagner A, Holly TA, et al. Reproducibility of chronic infarct size measurement by contrast-enhanced magnetic resonance imaging. *Circulation.* 2002;106:2322–2327.

92. Abdel-Aty H, Zagrosek A, Shulz-Menger J, et al. Delayed enhancement and T2-weighted cardiovascular magnetic resonance imaging differentiate acute from chronic myocardial infarction. *Circulation.* 2004;109:2411–2416.

93. Lohan DG, Krishnam M, Saleh R, et al. MR imaging of the thoracic aorta. *Magn Reson Imaging Clin N Am.* 2008;16(2):213–234.

94. Maksimovic R, Dill T, Seferovic PM, et al. Magnetic resonance imaging in pericardial diseases. Indications and diagnostic value. *Herz.* 2006;31(7):708–714.

95. Masci PG, Dymarkowski S, Bogaert J. The role of cardiovascular magnetic resonance in the diagnosis and management of cardiomyopathies. *J Cardiovasc Med.* 2008;9:435–449.

96. Kwong RY, Chan AK, Brown KA, et al. Impact of unrecognized myocardial scar detected by cardiac magnetic resonance imaging on event-free survival in patients presenting with signs or symptoms of coronary artery disease. *Circulation.* 2006;113:2733–2743.

97. Yano K, MacLean CJ. The incidence and prognosis of unrecognized myocardial infarction in the Honolulu, Hawaii, Heart Program. *Arch Intern Med.* 1989;149:1528–1532.

98. Rosenman RH, Friedman M, Jenkins CD, et al. Clinically unrecognized myocardial infarction in the Western Collaborative Group Study. *Am J Cardiol.* 1967;19:776–782.

99. Ingkanisorn WP, Kwong RY, Bohme NS, et al. Prognosis of negative adenosine stress magnetic resonance in patients presenting to an emergency department with chest pain. *J Am Coll Cardiol.* 2006;47:1427–1432.

100. Plein S, Greenwood JP, Ridgway JP, et al. Assessment of non-ST-segment elevation acute coronary syndromes with cardiac magnetic resonance imaging. *J Am Coll Cardiol.* 2004;44:2173–2181.

101. Martin ET, Coman JA, Shellock FG, et al. Magnetic resonance imaging and cardiac pacemaker safety at 1.5-Tesla. *J Am Coll Cardiol.* 2004;43:1315–1324.

102. Roguin A, Zviman MM, Meininger GR, et al. Modern pacemaker and implantable cardioverter/defibrillator systems can be magnetic resonance imaging safe. In vitro and in vivo assessment of safety and function at 1.5 T. *Circulation.* 2004;110:475–482.

103. Gallagher MJ, Raff GL, Use of multislice CT for the evaluation of emergency room patients with chest pain: The so-called "Triple Rule-Out." *Catheter Cardiovasc Interv.* 2008;71:92–99.

104. Gotway MB, Dawn SK. Thoracic aorta imaging with multislice CT. *Radiol Clin N Am.* 2003;41(3):521–543.

105. Laudon DA, Vukov LF, Breen JF, et al. Use of electron-beam computed tomography in the evaluation of chest pain patients in the emergency department. *Ann Emerg Med.* 1999;33:15–21.

106. Georgiou D, Budoff MJ, Kaufer E, et al. Screening patients with chest pain in the emergency department using electron beam tomography: A follow-up study. *J Am Coll Cardiol.* 2001;38:105–110.

107. McLaughlin VV, Balogh T, Rich S. Utility of electron beam computed tomography to stratify patients presenting to the emergency room with chest pain. *Am J Cardiol.* 1999;84:327–328.

108. Burke AP, Taylor A, Farb A, et al. Coronary calcification: Insights from sudden coronary death victims. *Z Kardiol.* 2000;89(suppl 2):49–53.

109. Greenland P, LaBree L, Azen SP, et al. Coronary artery calcium score combined with Framingham score for risk prediction in asymptomatic individuals. *JAMA.* 2004;291:210–215.

110. Leschka S, Alkadhi H, Plass A, et al. Accuracy of MSCT coronary angiography with 64-slice technology: First experience. *Eur Heart J.* 2005;26:1482–1487.

111. Raff GL, Gallagher MJ, O'Neill WW, et al. Diagnostic accuracy of noninvasive coronary angiography using 64-slice spiral computed tomography. *J Am Coll Cardiol.* 2005;46:552–557.

112. Mollet NR, Cademartiri F, van Mieghem CA, et al. High-resolution spiral computed tomography coronary angiography in patients referred for diagnostic conventional angiography. *Circulation.* 2005;112:2318–2323.

113. Pugliese F, Mollet NR, Runza G, et al. Diagnostic accuracy of non-invasive 64-slice CT coronary angiography in patients with stable angina pectoris. *Eur Radiol.* 2006;16:575–582.

114. Ropers D, Rixe J, Anders K, et al. Usefulness of multidetector row spiral computed tomography with 64- 3 0.6 mm collimation and 330-ms rotation for the noninvasive detection of significant coronary artery stenoses. *Am J Cardiol.* 2006;97:343–348.

115. Hamon M, Biondi-Zoccai GGL, Malagutti P, et al. Diagnostic performance of multislice spiral computed tomography of coronary arteries as compared with conventional invasive coronary angiography. A meta analysis. *J Am Coll Cardiol.* 2006;48:1896–1910.

116. Raff GL, Goldstein JA. Coronary angiography by computed tomography: Coronary imaging evolves. *J Am Coll Cardiol.* 2007;49:1830–1833.

117. Vanhoenacker PK, Heijenbrok-Kal MH, Van Heste R, et al. Diagnostic performance of multidetector CT angiography for assessment of coronary artery disease: Meta-analysis. *Radiology.* 2007;244:419–428.

118. Vanhoenacker PK, Decramer I, Olivier Bladt O, et al. Detection of non-ST-elevation myocardial infarction and unstable angina in the acute setting: Meta-analysis of diagnostic performance of multi-detector computed tomographic angiography. *BMC Cardiovasc Disord.* 2007;7:39

119. Caussin C, Larchez C, Saïd Ghostine S, et al. Comparison of coronary minimal lumen area quantification by sixty-four–slice computed tomography versus intravascular ultrasound for intermediate stenosis. *Am J Cardiol.* 2006;98:871–876.

120. Schoenhagen P, Stillman AE, Sandy S. et al. Non-invasive coronary angiography with multi-detector computed tomography: Comparison to conventional X-ray angiography. *Int J Cardiovasc Imaging.* 2005;21:63–72.

121. Achenbach S, Ropers D, Hoffmann U, et al. Assessment of coronary remodeling in stenotic and nonstenotic coronary atherosclerotic lesions by multidetector spiral computed tomography. *J Am Coll Cardiol.* 2004;43:842–847.

122. Shen MYH, Bush H, Ortiz L, et al. Simultaneous assessment of coronary stenosis, myocardial perfusion and ventricular function in a patient with acute MI. *J Cardiovasc Comput Tomogr.* 2008;2:123.

123. Dirksen MS, Bax JJ, de Roos A, et al. Usefulness of dynamic multislice computed tomography of left ventricular function in unstable angina pectoris and comparison with echocardiography. *Am J Cardiol.* 2002;90:1157–1160.

124. Mohlenkamp S, Lerman LO, Lerman A, et al. Minimally invasive evaluation of coronary microvascular function by electron beam computed tomography. *Circulation.* 2000;102:2411–2416.

125. Juergens KU, Grude M, Maintz D, et al. Multidetector row CT of left ventricular function with dedicated analysis software versus MR imaging: Initial experience. *Radiology.* 2004;230:403–410.

126. Paul JF, Dambrin G, Caussin C, et al. Sixteen-slice computed tomography after acute myocardial infarction: From perfusion defect to the culprit lesion. *Circulation.* 2003;108:373–374.

127. Budoff MJ, Gillespie R, Georgiou D, et al. Comparison of exercise electron beam computed tomography and sestamibi in the evaluation of coronary artery disease. *Am J Cardiol.* 1998;81:682–687.

128. Hoffmann U, Millea R, Enzweiler C, et al. Acute myocardial infarction: Contrast-enhanced multidetector row CT in a porcine model. *Radiology.* 2004;231:697–701.

129. Lardo AC, Cordeiro MAS, Silva S. Contrast-enhanced multidetector computed tomography viability imaging after myocardial infarction: Characterization of myocyte death, microvascular obstruction, and chronic scar. *Circulation.* 2006;113;394–404.

130. Richard T, George RT, Caterina Silva C, et al. Multidetector computed tomography myocardial perfusion imaging during adenosine stress. *J Am Coll Cardiol.* 2006;48:153–160.

131. Willoteaux S, Lions C, Gaxotte V, et al. Imaging of aortic dissection by helical computed tomography (CT). *Eur Radiol.* 2004;14:1999–2008.

132. Sebastia C, Pallisa E, Quiroga S, et al. Aortic dissection: Diagnosis and follow-up with helical CT. *Radiographics.* 1999;19:45–60.

133. Shiga T, Wajima Z, Apfel CC, et al. Diagnostic accuracy of transesophageal echocardiography, helical computed tomography, and magnetic resonance imaging for suspected thoracic aortic dissection. *Arch Intern Med.* 2006;166:1350–1356.

134. Ghaye B, Remy J, Remy-Jardin M. Non-traumatic thoracic emergencies: CT diagnosis of acute pulmonary embolism: The first 10 years. *Eur Radiol.* 2002;12:1886–1905.

135. Prologo JD, Gilkeson RC, Diaz M, et al. CT pulmonary angiography: A comparative analysis of the utilization patterns in emergency department and hospitalized patients between 1998 and 2003. *Am J Roentgenol.* 2004;183:1093–1096.

136. Ghanima W, Almaas V, Aballi S, et al. Management of suspected pulmonary embolism (PE) by D-dimer and multi-slice computed tomography in outpatients: An outcome study. *J Thromb Haemost.* 2005;3:1926–1932.

137. Quiroz R, Kucher N, Zou KH. Clinical validity of a negative computed tomography scan in patients with suspected pulmonary embolism. A systematic review. *JAMA.* 2005;293:2012–2017.

138. Goldstein JA, Gallagher MJ, O'Neill WW, et al. A randomized controlled trial of multi-slice coronary computed tomography for evaluation of acute chest pain patients. *J Am Coll Cardiol.* 2007;49:863–871.

139. Sato Y, Matsumoto N, Ichikawa M, et al. Efficacy of multislice computed tomography for the detection of acute coronary syndrome in the emergency department. *Circ J.* 2005;69:1047–1051.

140. White CS, Kuo D, Kelemen M, et al. Chest pain evaluation in the emergency department: Can MDCT provide a comprehensive evaluation? *AJR Am J Roentgenol.* 2005;185:533–540.

141. Gallagher MJ, Ross MA, Raff GL, et al. The diagnostic accuracy of 64-slice computed tomography coronary angiography compared with stress nuclear imaging in emergency department low-risk chest pain patients. *Ann Emerg Med.* 2007;49:125–136.

142. Rubinshtein R, Halon DA, Gaspar T, et al. Usefulness of 64- slice cardiac computed tomographic angiography for diagnosing acute coronary syndromes and predicting clinical outcome in emergency department patients with chest pain of uncertain origin. *Circulation.* 2007;115:1762–1768.

143. Johnson TR, Nikolaou K, Wintersperger BJ, et al. ECG-gated 64- MDCT angiography in the differential diagnosis of acute chest pain. *Am J Roentgenol.* 2007;188:76–82.

144. White CS, Kuo D, Kelemen M, et al. Chest pain evaluation in the emergency department: Can MDCT provide a comprehensive evaluation? *Am J Roentgenol.* 2005;185:533–540.

145. Shen MYH, Saxena, N, Thomas GS. Indications & reimbursement of cardiac CTA: History, present & future perspectives. *J Cardiovasc Comput Tomogr.* 2008;2:3.

146. Kido T, Kurata A, Higashino H, et al. Cardiac imaging using 256-detector row four-dimensional CT: Preliminary clinical report. *Radiat Med.* 2007;25:38–44.

147. Kuo D, Dilsizian V, Prasad R, et al. Emergency cardiac imaging: State of the art. *Cardiol Clin.* 2006;24:53–65.

148. Stowers SA, Eisenstein EL, Wackers F, et al. An economic analysis of an aggressive diagnostic strategy with photon emission computed tomography myocardial perfusion imaging and early exercise stress testing in emergency department patients who present with chest pain but nondiagnostic electrocardiograms: results from a randomized trial. *Ann Emerg Med.* 2000;35:17–25.

149. Radensky PW, Hilton TC, Fulmer H, et al. Potential cost effectiveness of initial myocardial perfusion imaging for assessment of emergency department patients with chest pain. *Am J Cardiol.* 1997;79:595–599.

150. Stowers SA. Myocardial perfusion scintigraphy for assessment of acute ischemic syndromes: can we seize the moment? *J Nucl Cardiol.* 1995;3:274–277.

151. Kontos MC, Schmidt KL, McCue M, et al. A comprehensive strategy for the evaluation and triage of the chest pain patient: A cost comparison study. *J Nucl Cardiol.* 2003;10:284–290.

152. Ziffer J, Nateman D, Janowitz WR, et al. Improved patient outcomes and cost effectiveness of utilizing nuclear cardiology protocols in an emergency department chest pain center: Two year results in 6548 patients [Abstract]. *J Nucl Med.* 1998;39:13.

153. Kim WY, Danias PG, Stuber M, et al. Coronary magnetic resonance angiography for the detection of coronary stenoses. *N Engl J Med.* 2001 Dec 27;345(26):1863–1869.

154. Sommer T, Hackenbroch M, Hofer U, et al. Coronary MR angiography at 3.0 T versus that at 1.5 T: initial results in patients suspected of having coronary artery disease. *Radiology.* 2005;234(3):718–725.

Dyspnea, Heart Failure, and Myocardial Dysfunction

16

Mario J. Garcia

1. INTRODUCTION

1.1. Epidemiology

Dyspnea is one of the most common complaints from patients referred for cardiovascular evaluation. The incident peaks between the fifth and the seventh decades of life.[1] Its differential diagnosis is broad, including a myriad of cardiovascular, pulmonary, and systemic diseases (Table 16.1). Approximately, two thirds of the cases are attributed to a pulmonary or a cardiac disorder.[2] The clinical history and physical examination identify the cause of dyspnea 50% of the time. In those cases where the etiology remains unclear after history, physical examination, chest X-ray, and spirometry, the most common causes are chronic obstructive pulmonary disease (COPD), congestive heart failure (CHF), psychogenic dyspnea, and physical deconditioning.[3] The etiology may be multifactorial in up to one third of the patients.

CHF is a highly prevalent condition and a common cause of dyspnea. In the United States alone, 5 million people carry the diagnosis and more than 500,000 new cases are diagnosed each year. Even though new therapies for ischemic and nonischemic cardiomyopathies continue to extend the survival, it is expected that the prevalence of heart failure will continue to increase.

CHF may be associated with systolic dysfunction, diastolic dysfunction, or both. Diastolic dysfunction is very prevalent in the general population. In 2,042 subjects >45 years of age referred for echocardiographic studies in Olmsted County, Minnesota, 28% had diastolic dysfunction (20.8%, mild; 6.6%, moderate; and 0.7%, severe).[4] In comparison, only 6% had an ejection fraction (EF) ≤0.50 and 2% had an EF ≤0.40 in the same group. In this study, the prevalence of diastolic dysfunction increased with age, and it was more commonly found in patients with hypertension, diabetes, coronary artery disease, and obesity.

1.2. Clinical presentation

1.2.1. Symptoms

Dyspnea is defined as a subjective experience of breathing discomfort that consists of qualitatively distinct sensations that vary in intensity. Dyspnea is considered to be chronic when symptoms last longer than one month. Dyspnea may vary in severity for a given degree of functional impairment. The sensation of dyspnea is controlled by multiple centers in the brain stem and cerebral cortex, reacting to afferent stimuli from upper airways, lungs, and chest wall. The quality and severity of symptoms are also influenced by environmental, social, and psychological factors. There is a poor association between the quality or intensity of symptoms and the underlying cause.[5] Patients with dyspnea secondary to lung disease or CHF may adjust their level of activity to limit

their symptoms. In others, inactivity leads to physical deconditioning that worsens the symptoms relative to their disease severity. Therefore, clinical history is a poor correlate of disease severity and specific diagnostic testing may be required. However, specific symptoms may help to establish the etiology in up to 50% of the cases. For example, chronic productive cough, sputum production, and dyspnea that is exacerbated by respiratory infections or exposure to smoke or dust are consistent with the diagnosis of COPD.[6] On the other hand, dyspnea on exertion, particularly accompanied by orthopnea and paroxysmal nocturnal dyspnea, is more typical of CHF. A loud murmur could lead to the diagnosis of severe valvular stenosis or regurgitation. The detection of an S3 gallop, a laterally displaced apical impulse and jugular venous distension (JVD), increases the probability of CHF to >80%. On the other hand, the presence of persistent inspiratory crackles that do not clear with cough or respond to diuretics and the presence of clubbing suggest the diagnosis of pulmonary fibrosis. Patients with asthma may have exertional dyspnea. However, a careful history often reveals episodic flare-ups and association to allergen exposure. Profound anemia, thyroid disease, and neuromuscular disorders such as myasthenia gravis are uncommon causes of dyspnea. Other specific symptoms and respiratory findings often lead to their diagnosis. A list of symptoms and physical findings associated to specific causes of dyspnea is presented in Table 16.2.

2. PATHOPHYSIOLOGY

In the following section we will review the most commonly measured hemodynamic parameters of myocardial performance. The pathophysiology of valvular heart disease is discussed in detail in other chapters of this textbook. Readers should refer to other specialty textbooks for a description of the role of neurohormonal activation and other mechanisms involved in non-cardiac causes of dyspnea.

CHF may be defined as the inability to provide an adequate cardiac output under normal filling pressures. This imbalance may result from an excess in demand, such as in hypermetabolic states, or from a decrease in supply due to a decrease in hemoglobin carrying capacity, an intrinsic inability to eject blood (systolic heart failure), or an inability to fill the heart under normal filling pressures (diastolic heart failure). Valvular diseases that result in severe obstruction to flow and/or regurgitant flow to or from the left ventricle are also causes of CHF. These are discussed in detail in other chapters of this book.

When CHF is associated with a reduced left ventricular (LV) EF, the pathological state is typically defined as systolic CHF. When CHF occurs in the absence of a reduced LV EF, the pathological state may be called diastolic HF. However, most patients with

TABLE 16.1
DIFFERENTIAL DIAGNOSIS OF CHRONIC DYSPNEA

Cardiac
Congestive heart failure
Coronary artery disease
Cardiac arrhythmias
Pericardial disease
Valvular heart disease

Pulmonary
Chronic obstructive pulmonary disease
Asthma
Interstitial lung disease
Pleural effusion
Malignancy (primary or metastatic)
Bronchiectasis

Noncardiac or nonpulmonary (less common)
Thromboembolic disease
Psychogenic causes (GAD, PTSD, and panic disorders)
Deconditioning
Pulmonary hypertension
Obesity (massive)
Severe anemia
Gastroesophageal reflux disease
Metabolic conditions (acidosis, uremia, etc.)
Liver cirrhosis
Thyroid disease
Neuromuscular disorders (myasthenia gravis, amyotrophic lateral sclerosis, etc.)
Chest wall deformities (kyphoscoliosis)
Upper airway obstruction (laryngeal disease, tracheal stenosis)

GAD, generalized anxiety disorder; PTSD, posttraumatic stress disorder.
Source: Adapted from Morgan WC, Hodge HL. Diagnostic evaluation of dyspnea. *Am Fam Physician*. 1998;57:712, with permission.

CHF have abnormal systolic and diastolic dysfunction. Patients with systolic CHF have abnormalities of diastolic function and those with diastolic CHF may have abnormalities of contractility, which are not detected by simple measurement of LV EF.[7]

It is important to recognize that CHF, whether it results from systolic or diastolic dysfunction, is a clinical syndrome with diverse etiologies, which may produce different alterations in the cardiovascular system.

2.1. Left ventricular systolic dysfunction

LV systolic performance is the ability of the LV to empty. This ability of LV can be quantified as a stroke volume or as a LV EF (a ratio of stroke volume to end-diastolic volume).

2.1.1. Left ventricular stroke volume
The LV stroke volume is defined as the volume of blood ejected in a single heart beat into the systemic circulation (across the aortic valve). In the presence of significant left-sided valvular regurgitation or a left-to-right shunt (ventricular septal defect or patent ductus arteriosus), the LV stroke volume may be high, while the effective or forward stroke volume (stroke volume minus regurgitant volume or shunt volume) is lower. Forward stroke volume multiplied by heart rate gives the systemic cardiac output.

Stroke volume may be obtained by echocardiography as the product of the pulsed Doppler velocity time integral (VTI) recorded in the LV outflow tract (LVOT) multiplied by its cross-sectional area (see Chapter 2). By cardiac magnetic resonance

(CMR), stroke volume is measured by the product of the average velocity obtained by phase encoding either at the ascending aorta or LVOT multiplied by its cross-sectional area (see Chapter 7). In the presence of significant aortic regurgitation, the regurgitant volume must be subtracted to obtain the effective stroke volume. Stroke volume may also be determined by echocardiography, CMR, or cardiac computed tomography (CCT) as the difference of end-diastolic and end-systolic volumes. By this method, both aortic and mitral regurgitation will result in overestimation of the effective stroke volume. This is an important limitation in CCT since regurgitant flow cannot be determined by this modality.

2.1.2. Left ventricular ejection fraction
In common clinical practice, LV systolic dysfunction is usually defined as a decreased EF. The EF can be obtained by determining the LV volume by the use of 2-dimensional (2D) or 3-dimensional (3D) echocardiography with or without contrast, radionuclide ventriculography, CCT, or CMR.

Although the EF is the most commonly used index of myocardial contractility, it is also influenced by LV preload and afterload. In the presence of severely increased afterload, such as in hypertensive crisis or aortic stenosis, the EF may be reduced in the presence of normal LV contractility. On the other hand, in the presence of left-sided valvular regurgitation or a left-to-right shunt (ventricular septal defect or patent ductus arteriosus), the LV EF may be normal, but the forward stroke volume (stroke volume minus regurgitant volume or shunt volume) may be reduced. The effective EF is defined as the forward stroke volume divided by end-diastolic volume. Normal values for EF are defined above 0.54 by different modalities (Table 16.3).

2.1.3. Left ventricular stroke work
The systolic performance of LV is best described by its ability to eject a volume of blood (stroke volume) against resistance (afterload). The LV stroke work is defined as the product of developed pressure and total stroke volume. Stroke work may be increased in hypertensive patients or decreased in patients with a small LV chamber. Although this index is not commonly measured in clinical practice, its principle forms the pathophysiologic basis for the interpretation of stress echocardiography when an abnormal response in stroke and end-systolic volume at peak exercise may be physiologically normal in the setting of an exaggerated blood pressure response.

A ventricular function curve (Frank–Starling) can be constructed by plotting stroke work against preload (end-diastolic volume) to define preload-recruitable stroke work. This curve is shifted upward when LV contractility is increased and downward when LV contractility is decreased.

2.1.4. Left ventricular (+) dP/dt
To reduce the influence of loading conditions, indices of LV performance measured during isovolumic contractility have been proposed. One of such indices is the first derivative of LV pressure rise (+ dP/dt). Although its main determinant is LV contractility, (+) dP/dt may be altered by acute changes in preload.

2.1.5. Left ventricular end-systolic elastance
This index, considered by many as the "gold standard" of LV contractility, represents the slope of the end-systolic pressure–volume

TABLE 16.2
HISTORY AND PHYSICAL EXAMINATION CLUES TO CAUSES OF DYSPNEA

Findings	Clinical conditions
Intermittent breathlessness; triggering factors; allergic rhinitis; nasal polyps; prolonged expiration; wheezing	Asthma
Significant tobacco; barrel chest; prolonged expiration; wheezing	Chronic obstructive pulmonary disease
History of hypertension, coronary artery disease, or diabetes mellitus; orthopnea; paroxysmal nocturnal dyspnea; pedal ederna; jugular vein distention; S_3 gallop; bibasilar rales; wheezing	Congestive heart failure
History of generalized anxiety disorder, posttraumatic stress disorder, obsessive-compulsive disorder, and panic disorder; intermittent symptoms; sighing breathing	Anxiety disorder; hyperventilation
Postprandial dyspnea	Gastroesophageal reflux disease; aspiration; food allergy
Hemoptysis	Lung neoplasm; pneumonia; bronchiectasis; mitral stenosis; arteriovenous malformation
Recurrent pneumonia	Lung cancer; bronchiectasis; aspiration
Drug exposure	Beta blockers aggravating obstructive airway disease
	Amiodarone (Cordarone)/nitrofurantoin (Furadantin): Pneumonitis
	Methotrexate (Rheumatrex): Lung fibrosis
	Illicit drugs (e.g., heroin): Talcosis
History of immunosuppressive disease or therapy; acquired immunodeficiency syndrome	Opportunistic infections: Protozoal (*Pneumocystis carinii* pneumonia); bacterial (tuberculosis; *Legionella*); viral (cytomegalovirus); fungal (*Aspergillus*)
Exposure to inorganic dust, asbestos, or volatile chemicals	Pneumoconiosis; silicosis; berylliosis; coal workers lung; asbestosis
Organic exposure to dust (birds, mushrooms, etc.)	Hypersensitivity pneumonitis (bird fancier's lung)
Accentuated P_2; right ventricular heave; murmurs	Pulmonary hypertension
Abnormal inspiratory or expiratory sounds; heard best over the trachea	Central airway obstruction; vocal cord paralysis; laryngeal tumor; tracheal stenosis
Localized, decreased, or absent breath sounds	Pleural effusion; atelectasis; pneumothorax

Source: Adapted from Morgan WC, Hodge. Diagnostic evaluation of dyspnea. *Am Fam Physician*. 1998;57:713, with permission.

TABLE 16.3
NORMAL ECHOCARDIOGRAPHIC VALUES FOR CARDIAC CHAMBER QUANTIFICATION

	Male				Female			
	Normal range	Mildly abnormal	Moderately abnormal	Severely abnormal	Normal range	Mildly abnormal	Moderately abnormal	Severely abnormal
LVEDV (mL)	67–155	156–178	179–201	>201	56–104	105–117	118–130	>130
LVESV (mL)	22–58	59–70	71–82	>82	19–49	50–59	60–69	>69
LV mass (gm)	96–200	201–227	228–254	>254	66–150	151–171	172–182	>182
LV EF (%)	>54	45–54	30–44	<30	>54	45–54	30–44	<30
RVEDA (cm^2)[a]	11–28	29–32	33–37	>37	11–28	29–32	33–37	>37
RVESA (cm^2)[a]	7.5–16	17–19	20–22	>22	7.5–16	17–19	20–22	>22
RV FAC (%)[a]	32–60	25–31	18–24	<18	32–60	25–31	18–24	<18
LAV$_{MAX}$ (mL)	18–58	59–68	69–78	>78	22–52	53–62	63–72	>72

[a] measured by area–length method in the four-chamber view.
LV, left ventricle; RV, right ventricle; EDV, end-diastolic volume; ESV, end-systolic volume; EF, ejection fraction; EDA, end-diastolic area; ESA, end-systolic area; FAC, fractional area change; and LAV$_{MAX}$, maximum left atrial volume.
Source: Adapted from Lang R, Bierig M, Deveraux RB, et al. Recommendations for chamber quantification. *Eur J Echocardiogr*. 2006;7:79–108.

relationship. To be calculated, this slope requires acute preload reduction and/or volume loading to obtain the end-systolic pressure–volume relationship at different loading points.[8] The most accepted methodology used requires simultaneous invasive acquisition of high-fidelity intraventricular pressures and volumes from a calibrated conductance catheter. The defined slope of end-systolic elastance (Ees) is reduced when contractility is impaired (Fig. 16.1). Some investigators have proposed indices that estimate Ees from a single static end-systolic pressure–volume relationship point assuming a fixed asymptote, replacing conductance volumes by echocardiographic determinations of LV area, and replacing invasive LV pressures by calibrated peripheral pulsed pressure tracings obtained by tonometry to make this index more practical for clinical applications. However, the validation of all these alternative methods has so far been limited. Ees may be affected by chronic changes in LV mass/volume ratio.[9]

2.1.6. Left ventricular strain (ε), strain rate, and left ventricular torsion

While all the indices described above are useful to characterize global LV performance, many patients with CHF have regional alterations in systolic function. Regional myocardial performance may be assessed qualitatively or quantitatively by echocardiography or CMR. Measurements of the extent and velocity of regional myocardial length transients (both shortening and lengthening) can be made using a variety of techniques, including high-frame rate 2-D echocardiographic speckle tracking, tissue Doppler imaging (TDI), CMR tagging, and CMR myocardial velocity encoding. Echocardiography can also be used to define circumferential shortening at the LV endocardial surface or at the midwall, given its higher spatial resolution. To be interpreted appropriately, the measurements must be normalized to produce regional strain and strain rate (SR); these parameters are dimensionless and are expressed as percent change and inverse seconds, respectively. The spiral architecture of the myocardial fiber bundles determines strain deformation in multiple directions. Thus, changes in LV geometry during LV systole relate primarily to radial (short axis), longitudinal (long axis), and meridional (LV torsion) strain.

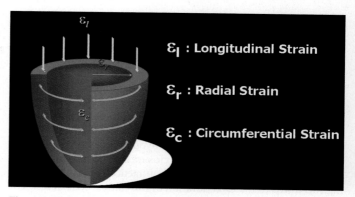

Figure 16.2 Main vectors of LV strain.

Figure 16.2 illustrates the directions of LV longitudinal, circumferential, and radial strain (ε). Systolic strain or shortening may be expressed as the ratio of (end-diastolic length–end-systolic length)/end-diastolic length, whereas SR represents the instantaneous velocity of fiber shortening. Experimental studies have suggested that ε correlates with global indices of LV ejection (stroke volume, EF) whereas SR correlates best with global indices of LV contractility (Ees, (+) dP/dt).[10,11]

In addition to radial and longitudinal deformation, there is torsional deformation of the LV during the cardiac cycle due to the helical orientation of the myocardial fibers.[12–19] During systole, the basal segments of the LV myocardium rotate or twist in counterclockwise direction whereas the apical segments twist in clockwise direction. During diastole, untwisting occurs in the opposite direction. Systolic torsion represents the net effect of basal and apical twist. Apical twisting is the main component of global LV systolic torsion, whereas basal rotation is of less importance. CMR tagging, high-frame rate 2-D echocardiographic speckle tracking, or TDI may quantify torsional deformation.

Systolic LV torsion tends to equalize sarcomere shortening between endocardial and epicardial layers of the LV and is a possible mechanism by which potential energy can be stored during ejection and then released during early diastole to generate suction and rapid filling by "elastic recoil." LV untwisting has been shown to be dissociated from filling and accentuated by catecholamines, with the untwisting rate related to LV pressure decay. The magnitude of the restoring force appears to be inversely related to end-systolic volume.[20,21] Epicardial contraction dominates the direction of torsion because these fibers are at larger radii and therefore produce greater torque than do those in the inner layers. The process can be viewed as a global LV spring between the epicardium and endocardium that is stretched during systole, storing potential energy for release in early diastole.

2.2. Left ventricular diastolic dysfunction

Diastolic dysfunction refers to an abnormality of LV relaxation, distensibility, or filling. The spectrum of clinical presentation ranges from asymptomatic diastolic dysfunction[22] and exercise intolerance to overt CHF.[23] In the absence of significant valvular disease or a reduced EF, such patients with clinical evidence of CHF meet published criteria for diastolic heart failure.

Cardiac structural abnormalities in patients with diastolic dysfunction differ from those with systolic CHF. The LV cavity is typically normal or small while LV wall thickness may be normal or increased, regardless of the etiology. In about 85% of patients with diastolic heart failure, systemic hypertension is the only identifiable cause. Most of these patients exhibit a concentric pattern

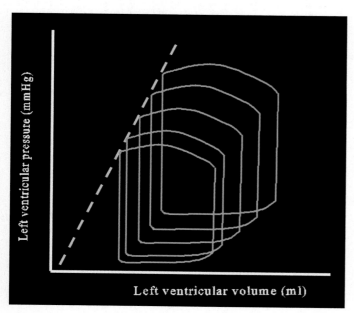

Figure 16.1 Determination of end-systolic elastance (slope of the end-systolic pressure–volume relationship) from pressure–volume loops obtained during preload altering maneuvers.

of LV remodeling and increased wall thickness with a high ratio of mass to volume and a high ratio of wall thickness to chamber radius. Histologically, the myocyte exhibits an increased diameter, and there is an increase in the amount of collagen surrounding it. Abnormal passive elastic properties are caused largely by increased myocardial mass and alterations in the extramyocardial collagen network, but changes in intramyocardial components (e.g., titin) also contribute to an increase in passive stiffness.[24] These features may vary of course in other less common causes of diastolic heart failure, such as the restrictive cardiomyopathies (see Chapter 34).

Diastole starts after aortic valve closure and extends until mitral valve closure with the onset of LV contraction, typically comprising two thirds of the total duration of the cardiac cycle at rest. The different periods of diastole are represented in Figure 16.3. Various hemodynamic parameters can affect LV diastolic function. These parameters interact to maintain LV filling under relatively low atrial pressure, including LV relaxation, LV stiffness, left atrial (LA) contractility, atrioventricular and intraventricular electrical conduction, neurohormonal activation, and pericardial constraint. Alterations in preload, afterload, contractility, and heart rate may affect several of these parameters simultaneously, making it often difficult to determine their individual contribution.[25-27]

2.2.1. Left ventricular relaxation

Active relaxation of the LV is one of the most fundamental determinants of diastolic function. Relaxation is an energy dependent process that starts with the reuptake of Ca^{2+} by the sarcoplasmic reticulum, which in turn inactivates the troponin–tropomyosin complex,[28] allowing the myocardial fiber to enlarge. Rapid relaxation of the LV myocytes generates a force that rapidly decreases the LV intracavitary pressure during early diastole and generates a pressure gradient across the mitral valve drawing blood from the left atrium (LA). Investigators have shown that the onset of active relaxation is asynchronous, starting earlier in the most apical myocardial segments. Early apical relaxation creates an intracavitary pressure gradient within the LV that generates a suction force. Experimental studies have demonstrated that these intraventricular gradients result from active myocardial events.[29] They suggested that the apex serves as a prominent source of recoil during early diastole, contributing to the process of filling by actively drawing blood from the mid and basal levels of the heart into the

apical region. In ischemia and cardiomyopathy, these gradients are markedly reduced.[30] Since LV relaxation is energy dependent, this parameter is very sensitive to ischemia. Increased cardiac mass and conduction abnormalities can also reduce the rate of LV relaxation by slowing the transmission of the depolarizing current. The composition of the cardiac skeleton can also affect the velocity of relaxation in proportion to the ratio of elastic to collagen fibers. Using high-fidelity pressure recordings, LV relaxation can be estimated from the rate of intracavitary pressure decay during isovolumic relaxation, the period comprised between aortic valve closure and mitral opening. The time constant of isovolumic relaxation (τ) is considered the gold standard that defines LV relaxation. The fall in intraventricular pressure follows an exponential curve and is used to determine τ assuming either zero ($p_0 e^{-t/}\tau$) or nonzero ($p_0 e^{-t/}\tau + p_b$) asymptote.[31] A small value of τ indicates rapid relaxation and is directly related to the duration of isovolumic relaxation, while inversely related to the magnitude of the difference between LV pressure at aortic closure and LV pressure at mitral opening.

2.2.2. Left ventricular distensibility

When a myocardial fiber is subjected to a given load (stress), it responds by stretching to a given length (strain). The distensibility (strain/stress relationship) of a muscle fiber is typically nonlinear. The forced required to stretch a muscle fiber increases geometrically as the fiber is stretched.[32] This property determines a curvilinear relationship between volume and pressure in the ventricle. As the volume of LV increases during diastole, the intracavitary pressure also increases. The magnitude of pressure change (dP) over a given change in volume (dV) defines the operating stiffness of the LV ($S = dp/dV$). Compliance is the reciprocal of LV stiffness. Therefore, with increasing LV filling volume (preload), there is a proportionally larger increase in LV pressure and S. Paradoxically, a slow LV relaxation rate decreases S during early filling since the myocardium continues to relax during this period,[33] which tends to decrease LV cavity pressure. LV relaxation usually does not affect S during late diastole, when it is mostly determined by passive properties.

The curvilinear slope of the ventricular pressure–volume curve can vary according to myocardial fiber distensibility, elasticity of the connective tissue, LV cavity diameter and wall thickness, duration of active relaxation, and the effect of pericardial constraint. This slope may be represented as the relative dp/dV for a given LV pressure (p), defining the LV diastolic stiffness constant (K). A higher proportion of collagen to elastic fibers as seen with aging, hypertensive heart disease, and cardiomyopathies and following myocardial infarction results in increased K.[34-36] The external constraining effect of the pericardium increases K, a phenomenon that becomes clinically relevant in constrictive pericarditis.

Figure 16.4 illustrates the changes in dP and S (dp/dV) that occur when preload is augmented in a normal ventricle (from A to B) and in a patient with diastolic dysfunction and increased K. For the same increase in preload, dp increases more in the patient with diastolic dysfunction (from C to D).

2.2.3. Left atrial contribution to Left ventricular filling

The left atrium has three important functions. It acts as a reservoir of blood, as a passive conduit during early LV filling, and as an active pump at end-diastole.[37] In young and healthy subjects, its role as a pump is insignificant, contributing to <20% of the total filling volume. In the presence of impaired LV relaxation, the atrial contribution to LV filling increases significantly, at times over 50%. This is an adaptive mechanism governed by the Frank–Starling law: As the volume and pressure in the LA prior to its contraction increase, LA contractility also increases. In these patients,

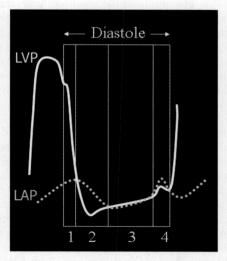

Figure 16.3 Phases of diastole: (1) isovolumic relaxation; (2) early filling; (3) diastasis; (4) atrial contraction. LAP, left atrial pressure; LVP, left ventricular pressure.

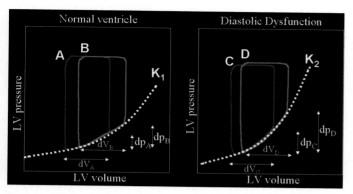

Figure 16.4 Normal (K1) and abnormal (K2) end-diastolic stiffness curves. After a volume infusion, the pressure–volume loops shift from A to B and C to D. Both LV end-diastolic pressure as well as operating stiffness (dP/dV) increase, but the increase is greater in the diastolic function patients.

LV end-diastolic pressure is elevated but mean atrial pressure remains relatively normal at rest. Symptoms are usually absent or minimal unless atrial fibrillation occurs. With worsening LV diastolic function and elevation of LV filling pressure, the LA size increases, losing its mechanical efficiency eventually in advanced stages. Left atrial mechanical function may be also decreased after cardioversion of atrial fibrillation.[38]

2.2.4. Other parameters

As mentioned above, the pericardium plays an important role in diastolic function. In constrictive pericarditis, the LV pressure–volume curve is shifted upward and to the left (increased K) due to the abnormal external pericardial constraint. The intact pericardium is a major contributor to ventricular interdependence. For example, in acute right ventricle (RV) volume or pressure overload resulting in severe RV dilation, LV filling may be impaired due to the increased intrapericardial pressure. Neurohormonal activation affects several parameters of diastolic function. Catecholamines increase LV relaxation and heart rate, decreasing the duration of diastole. Conduction abnormalities may reduce the rate of LV relaxation by inducing segmental asynchrony. This may contribute to decreased exercise tolerance in patients with left-bundle branch block or right ventricular paced rhythms.

2.3. Right ventricular dysfunction

The RV acts as a pump to maintain adequate circulation through the lungs while maintaining a relatively low central venous pressure. Many patients with RV dysfunction or even those without a functioning RV, such as in complex congenital disease post-Fontan surgery, may have relatively normal functional capacity. However, once the pulmonary vascular resistance is elevated, RV plays an important role to maintain adequate pulmonary blood flow. In this case, RV failure is characterized by symptoms of venous congestion, such as hepatomegaly, ascites, edema, and/or low cardiac output by limiting flow to the systemic circulation. RV failure may affect LV function, not only by limiting LV preload but also by limiting LV filling due to the ventricular interdependence imposed by the pericardium. RV dysfunction may occur as a primary entity, such as in RV dysplasia or RV infarction, or secondary to LV failure. RV function has been shown to be a major independent determinant of clinical outcome in patients with cardiovascular disease.[39–41]

The RV muscle mass approximately accounts for 15% of the total cardiac muscle mass under normal loading conditions. The lower muscle mass is explained by the low pulmonary vascular resistance. Under normal loading conditions, the RV wall is thin (<5 mm) and the LV cavity is crescent shaped.[42] The RV is structurally and functionally divided into an inflow and and an outflow tract separated by a thick intracavitary muscle band, the crista supraventricularis.[43] The inflow tract is mainly composed of circumferential fibers in the subepicardium and longitudinal fibers in the subendocardium, whereas at the outflow tract, both subendocardial and subepicardial fibers run longitudinally. During systole, there is a longitudinal shortening of the RV from base to apex and a radial motion toward the common septum. Additional circumferential motion provides a small rotational component or a squeeze of the ventricle.[44] Longitudinal motion appears to provide the largest contribution to ejection; thus, many indices of RV function are based on the longitudinal motion of the RV free wall. Most indices of LV systolic and diastolic function may be applied for the evaluation of RV performance.

2.3.1. Right ventricular stroke volume

Unless there is a regurgitant valve lesion or an intracardiac shunt, the stroke volume of RV will be equal to the LV stroke volume. Stroke volume may be obtained by echocardiography as the product of the pulsed Doppler VTI recorded in the RV outflow tract multiplied by its cross-sectional area (see Chapter 2). By CMR, the RV stroke volume is measured by the product of the average velocity obtained by phase encoding in the proximal pulmonary artery, also multiplied by its cross-sectional area (see Chapter 7). In the presence of significant pulmonic regurgitation, the regurgitant volume must be subtracted to obtain the effective stroke volume. Stroke volume may also be determined by echocardiography, CMR, or CCT as the difference of RV end-diastolic and end-systolic volumes. By this method, both pulmonic and tricuspid regurgitation will result in overestimation of the effective stroke volume.

2.3.2. Right ventricular ejection fraction

The RV EF can be obtained by determining the RV volumes by 2- or 3-D echocardiography, radionuclide ventriculography, CCT, or CMR. The RV EF is also influenced by preload and afterload. In the presence of severe pulmonary hypertension, the RV EF may be reduced in the presence of normal RV contractility. On the other hand, in the presence of severe tricuspid regurgitation, the RV EF may be normal, but the forward stroke volume and RV contractility may be reduced. This is clinically evident by the noted decline in RV EF following tricuspid valve repair or replacement in these patients. Normal values for RV EF are lower than those for RV EF due to the normally larger RV end-diastolic and end-systolic volumes.

2.3.3. Right ventricular stroke work

The systolic performance of RV is best described by its ability to eject a volume of blood (stroke volume) against resistance (afterload). The RV stroke work is defined as the product of developed pressure and total stroke volume. Stroke work may be normal in patients with pulmonary hypertension with a reduced RV EF. If pulmonary vascular resistance is decreased in response to therapy, the RV EF usually improves while RV stroke work remains unchanged.

2.3.4. Right ventricular (+) dP/dt

Although less validated than LV (+) dP/dt, this index may be estimated in patients with tricuspid regurgitation using continuous wave Doppler.

2.3.5. Right ventricular end-systolic elastance

This index may be obtained by simultaneous invasive acquisition of high-fidelity intraventricular pressures and volumes from a calibrated conductance catheter or substituting the conductance volumes by echocardiographic determinations of RV area. However, the complex geometry of RV makes the determination of volumes less reliable than in the LV.

2.3.6. Right ventricular strain (ε) and strain rate

Regional RV myocardial performance may be assessed qualitatively or quantitatively by echocardiography or CMR using the same methods and principles as in the LV.

2.4. Left atrial dysfunction

The LA is an oval-shaped chamber with thin, muscular walls. The LA chamber changes its size during a cardiac cycle, being largest at ventricular systole and smallest at atrial systole. During ventricular systole, LA functions as a reservoir that collects pulmonary venous (PV) flow. During early diastole, it functions as a conduit allowing the passage of stored blood from the LA to the LV and during atrial contraction, LA acts as a contractile pump contributing to LV filling. Atrial contraction makes a significant contribution to maintaining

cardiac output, especially in patients with LV dysfunction.[45] Atrial contractility increases in response to moderate increase in LA volume (preload), according to the Frank–Starling law.

Chronic elevation of LA pressure, as seen in patients with LV dysfunction or mitral valve disease, increases LA volume. By this mechanism, LA distensibility also increases, mitigating the transfer of acute changes in LA pressure into the pulmonary veins. However, in advanced heart failure, the overstretching of the LA myocytes leads to reduced LA contractility and LA mechanical failure.

The LA size is a powerful predictor of adverse events in various cardiovascular diseases, including atrial fibrillation,[46–48] after myocardial infarction,[49,50] and in patients with cardiomyopathies.[51,52]

The LA volume may be determined by echocardiography, CCT, biplane contrast ventriculography, and CMR.[53–55]

3. DIAGNOSTIC EVALUATION

A diagnostic algorithm for the evaluation of patients with dyspnea is presented in Figure 16.5.

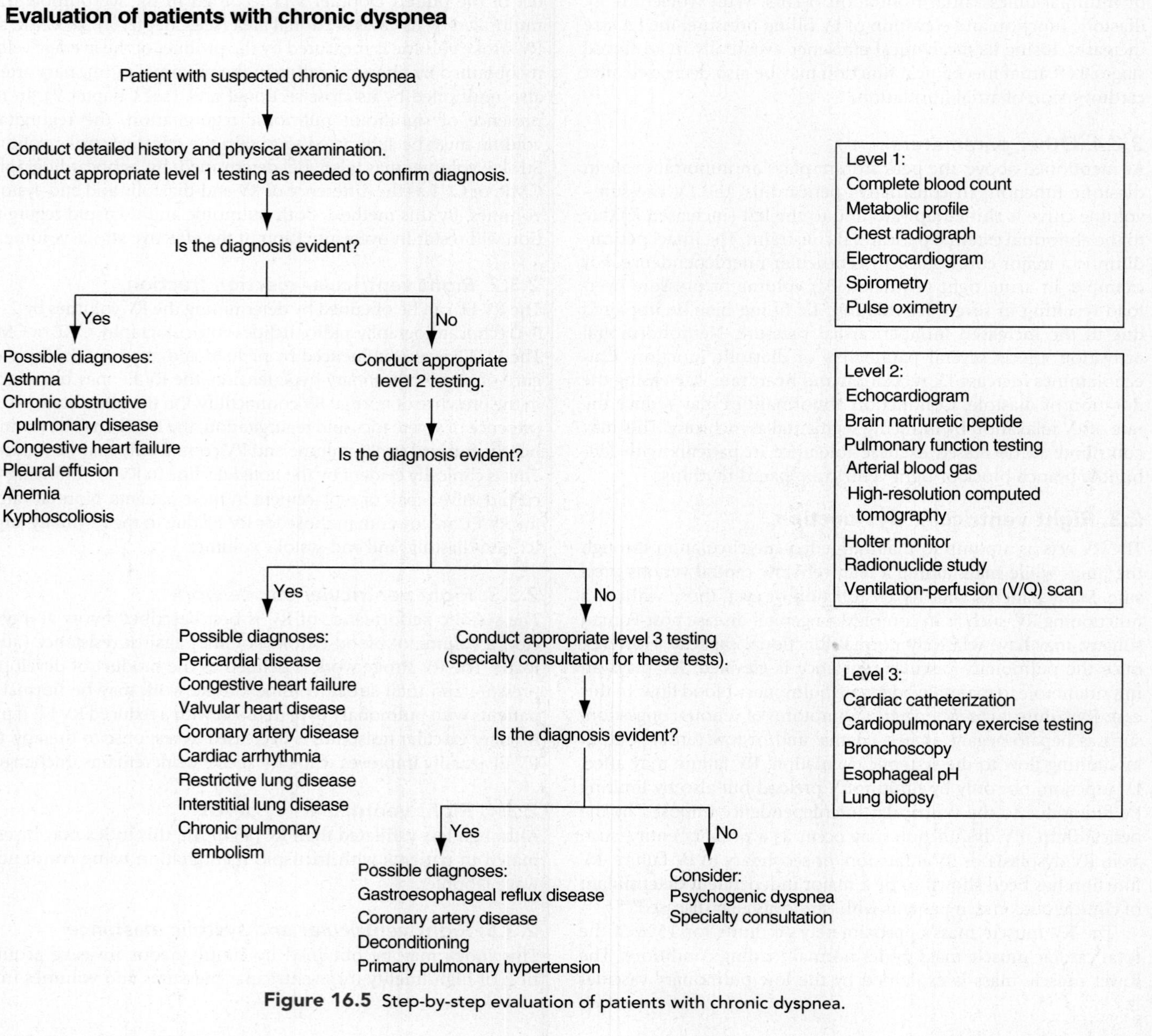

Figure 16.5 Step-by-step evaluation of patients with chronic dyspnea.

3.1. Laboratory testing

Initial laboratory testing should include a complete blood count, metabolic panel, and thyroid stimulating hormone (TSH). Anemia and thyroid disease are uncommon causes of dyspnea but can be easily corrected. The metabolic panel may be useful to identify respiratory acidosis and compensatory metabolic alkalosis in patients with severe lung disease, neuromuscular disorders, or hyponatremia and prerenal azotemia in patients with advanced CHF. A brain natriuretic peptide (BNP) assay may be useful to differentiate heart failure from other causes of dyspnea. Using a threshold of 100 pg/mL, this test is 82% sensitive and 99% specific to establish the diagnosis of CHF.[56] BNP is released in proportion to LV wall stress; accordingly, it is more likely to be significantly elevated in patients with systolic heart failure and cardiomegaly, but it may be only marginally elevated or normal in patients with diastolic heart failure.[57]

3.2. Chest X-Ray

The chest X-ray may reveal chest wall deformities, parenchymal lung disease, cardiomegaly, or an elevated hemidiaphragm. To measure accurately the cardiothoracic ratio, a full anteroposterior film obtained at end-inspiration must be obtained. Lateral films are also important to evaluate specific chamber enlargement.

3.3. Electrocardiogram

The electrocardiogram (ECG) is a useful initial test to screen for a cardiac origin of dyspnea. Tachyarrhythmias and, less commonly, bradyarrhythmias may be the direct cause or an aggravating factor in CHF patients. The ECG may reveal the diagnosis of previous myocardial infarction or a wide QRS that may lead to the suspicion of dyssynchrony. In some cases, ambulatory ECG recordings may be warranted. It is important to recognize, however, that a normal ECG does not exclude the diagnosis of a cardiomyopathy or severe valvular heart disease as a cause of CHF.

3.4. Pulmonary function testing

Spirometry is most useful to establish the diagnosis of obstructive lung disease in patients with dyspnea. A normal spirometry virtually excludes fixed restrictive or obstructive lung disease. In patients with suspected reactive airway disease, spirometry may be obtained after methacholine provocation or after exercise. In those patients identified as having obstructive airway disease at baseline, the test may be repeated after inhaling the bronchodilators to determine if reactive airway disease is present. It is important to recognize, however, that spirometry may reveal a pattern of restrictive airway disease in patients with decompensated heart failure and in those who do not perform an adequate effort during the test. In patients with obstructive and restrictive lung disease, both forced vital capacity (FVC) and forced expiratory volume in 1 s (FEV1) are reduced; however, FEV1 is proportionally lower in obstructive lung disease, and a ratio of FEV1/FVC <0.7 is suggestive of COPD. Total lung capacity (TLC), functional residual capacity, and residual volume (RV) may be increased in obstructive lung disease and are typically reduced in restrictive lung conditions. In restrictive lung parenchymal disease, all lung volumes are proportionally reduced, whereas in neuromuscular disorders, obesity, and chest wall restriction, the RV and the RV/TLC ratio are increased.

Measuring the diffusing capacity for carbon monoxide (DLCO) may be useful to differentiate conditions wherein there is a reduction in effective lung parenchymal and/or blood volume (DLCO reduced: Pulmonary embolism, pulmonary fibrosis, and anemia) from those wherein there is an increase in effective pulmonary blood volume (DLCO increased: Asthma, obesity, left-to-right cardiac shunts, and erythrocytosis).

Pulse oximetry obtained at rest or during exercise is a sensitive and easy-to-obtain indicator of gas exchange abnormalities. A reduced O_2 saturation may be indicative of lung disease where there is ventilation–perfusion mismatch, right-to-left circulatory shunting in patients with congenital heart disease, or intrapulmonary fistulas.

3.5. Metabolic stress testing

Metabolic or cardiopulmonary stress testing is a useful test to differentiate cardiac from pulmonary etiology of dyspnea when other tests are equivocal and to evaluate the extent of functional limitations and physical fitness. During this test, continuous monitoring of respiratory gas exchange, namely O_2 consumption and CO_2 production, allows to determine the onset of anaerobic metabolism during graded exercise. Other variables such as pulsed oximetry, blood pressure recordings, cardiac output determination, ECG recordings, and minute volume ventilation are collected during the test and provide additional information about the probable cause of a metabolic impairment. A low cardiac output will be manifested as onset of anaerobic metabolism (increased CO_2 production/O_2 intake ratio) at low physical workloads. A low O_2 intake may also be found in patients with severe physical deconditioning. However, in the latter, heart rate, blood pressure, and cardiac output increase normally during exercise. Patients with respiratory limitation to exercise will reach a plateau in their minute volume ventilation before or shortly after reaching anaerobic threshold.

3.6. Echocardiography

Two-Dimensional echocardiographic and Doppler techniques offer the ability to quantitatively evaluate LV systolic and diastolic function. The noninvasive nature of the test means that changes in therapy and hemodynamic interventions can be assessed by serial evaluation, allowing the clinician to adjust treatment for the individual depending upon responses.

3.6.1. Left ventricular systolic function assessment
Left Ventricular ejection fraction and stroke volume. LV EF may be calculated from end-diastolic volume, generally determined by using the modified Simpson method, and any measure of stroke volume. Stroke volume is most commonly measured by subtracting the end-systolic volume derived by 2-D echocardiography from the value of end-diastolic volume (see Chapter 2). Stroke volume may also be determined by Doppler interrogation of the LVOT. The diameter of LVOT, D, is measured in the parasternal long-axis view and the LVOT area is calculated by the formula, $D^2/4$. Stroke distance is obtained from the VTI obtained by pulsed wave Doppler interrogation of the LVOT and stroke volume is calculated as VTI × $LVOT_{area}$. Despite errors that may be encountered due to the assumption that the LVOT is circular in cross-section and squaring of any error in the measurement of LVOT diameter, this method is more accurate in the setting of poor ventricular function.[58] One possible source of discrepancy between the 2-D and the Doppler-derived stroke volume is the volume that is produced by mitral regurgitation. Significant mitral regurgitation will lead to overestimation of LV stroke volume (forward + regurgitant volume) by 2-D echocardiography. Similarly, LV EF will differ if stroke volume is calculated by 2-D method versus Doppler-derived method in the presence of significant mitral regurgitation. Some experts refer to the EF determined by the latter as "effective ejection fraction."

A frequently encountered problem in measuring LV volume in the setting of ventricular dilatation is that of foreshortening, which leads to underestimation of volume and to errors in calculation of LV EF. In obtaining images of the LV cavity for quantitation of

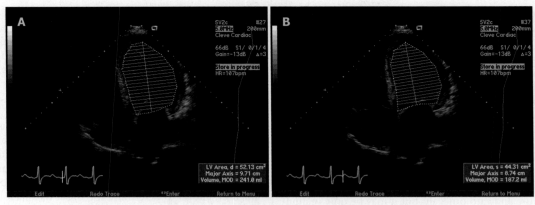

Figure 16.6 (Movie 16.1). Calculation of LV end-diastolic (**A**) and end-systolic (**B**) volumes from 2-dimensional echocardiograhy using the Simpson disc method.

volume, it is vital to ensure that the true apex has been included in the image. This may require the use of lower intercostal spaces or a more lateral transducer position for apical imaging. The use of contrast agents has shown to improve reproducibility in the determination of LV volumes and EF in patients with technically limited examinations. Their use is recommended in patients in whom the endocardial border of two or more myocardial segments cannot be adequately visualized. It has been shown that volumes measured by contrast echocardiography are 10% to 20% larger and correlate better with CMR volumes since endocardial trabeculations are often mistaken as true endocardial borders in noncontrast studies.

Real-time 3-D echocardiography has demonstrated superior accuracy for calculation of volumes, when compared to 2-D echocardiography. More recently, the use of real-time 3-D echocardiography for the measurement of ventricular volumes and EF in patients with heart failure has been shown to be accurate (see Chapter 11), although the method shows systematic underestimation in patients with very large ventricles when compared to CMR imaging.[59] Reason for this includes difficulty in encompassing the entire LV within the pyramidal imaging volume, a problem which may also occur with 2-D echocardiographic methods. Nevertheless, 3-D echocardiography is superior compared to 2-D echocardiography for determination of volumes of irregular shaped ventricles.

The most common indication for performing an echocardiogram is the assessment of LV function. While conventional 2-D echocardiography provides quantitative methods of evaluating LV function, it relies on geometric modeling of the ventricle, with measurements obtained in two orthogonal planes. Using the modified Simpson rule, a calculation of LV volumes can be obtained at end-diastole and systole (Fig. 16.6, movie 16.1). Problems exist, however, with the accuracy and reproducibility of volumes and masses obtained by this method. The extrapolations of geometric models give rise to many of these errors, particularly when the ventricle is asymmetric, as in the case of an LV aneurysm.[10–12] In addition, foreshortened views of the LV also contribute to errors in quantification.[13–15]

To date, numerous studies have proven the accuracy and reproducibility of measurements of LV volumes and EF obtained by 3-D echocardiography.[16–21] Comparisons between measurements made by 3-D echocardiography and both CMR and postmortem measurements have shown excellent correlation. New computer-generated algorithms employing automated frame-by-frame detection of the endocardial surface allow for direct quantification of LV volumes without multiplane or geometrical model assumptions (Figures 16.7 and 16.8, movies 16.2, 16.3, 16.4). In addition to reducing analysis time, these techniques have also shown good accuracy, when compared with CMR.[15]

Given the demonstrated accuracy of the technique for the assessment of global LV indices, use of real-time 3-D echocardiography for the diagnosis of regional wall motion abnormalities represents a natural progression. Studies assessing real-time 3-D echocardiography to assess regional wall motion[19,22–24] have demonstrated good correlation to CMR, even in patients with suboptimal acoustic images. Real-time 3-D echocardiography images can be segmented and analyzed by the standard 17-segment model (Fig. 16.9), and each of these segments can be tracked for changes in regional volume over time, generating graphical analyses of regional wall volumes during systole and diastole.

The multisegmental analysis provided by real-time 3-D echocardiography lends itself to use in stress testing. Capable of scanning the entire LV along with its complex motion in a few cardiac cycles from a single transducer position,[25] 3-D technology applied to stress echocardiography reduces many of the difficulties associated with the conventional 2-D stress echocardiography—imaging from multiple locations on the chest and inaccurate alignment of prestress and poststress images for accurate comparison. Several studies have shown comparable accuracies of 3-D stress echocardiography with 2-D studies for detecting myocardial ischemia and coronary artery stenosis.[26–29] In fact, real-time 3-D echocardiography may identify apical wall motional abnormalities more readily than 2-D studies.[30]

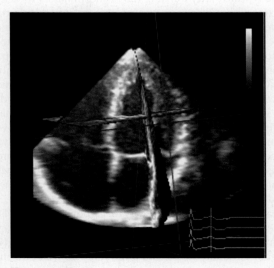

Figure 16.7 (Movie 16.2). Cross-plane 3-dimensional image of the cardiac chambers obtained from the apical window.

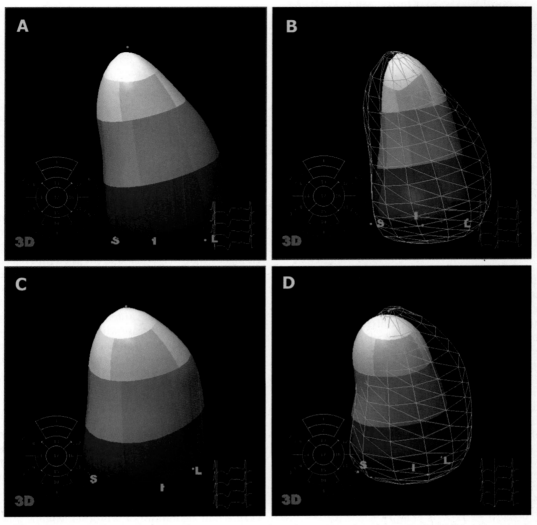

Figure 16.8 (Movies 16.3 and 16.4). End-diastolic (**A,C**) and end-systolic (**B,D**) LV volume casts derived from 3-dimensional echocardiography in a normal patient (top) and a patient with apical dyskinesis (bottom).

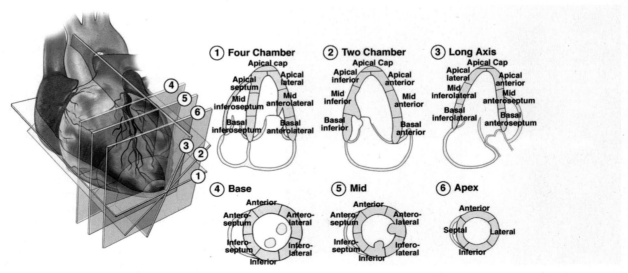

Figure 16.9 Nomenclature for LV segmentation adopted by the American Societies of Nuclear Cardiology, Echocardiography and Cardiac Magnetic Resonance.

Left ventricular (+) dP/dt A simple index of LV systolic function is the rate of change in left ventricular pressure (dP/dt) during early systole. This parameter may be estimated in patients with mitral regurgitation (MR) from a continuous wave Doppler recording of the MR signal. Left atrial pressure remains fairly constant during early systole and the instantaneous velocity derived from the Doppler display reflects the pressure gradient between the LV and the LA.

The slope of the Doppler velocity curve between 1 and 3 m/s is used to measure LV dP/dt (Fig. 16.10). Using the simplified Bernoulli equation, this represents a change in pressure from 4 (4×1^2) to 36 (4×3^2) mm Hg, a difference of 32 mm Hg. Thus, dP/dt (in mm Hg/s) is calculated by 32/(time taken for the velocity to increase from 1 to 3 m/s). Values are normally >1,200 mm Hg/s, and in the setting of ventricular systolic dysfunction, dP/dt is often <1,000 mm Hg/s.[60]

Left ventricular wall stress. Most commonly used noninvasive measures of LV systolic function, such as EF, are highly dependent upon loading conditions and as such cannot differentiate between the effects of changes in preload and afterload and true changes in myocardial contractility. Stress describes force per unit area and LV wall stress, the load opposing ejection, provides an index of LV myocardial systolic function, which is less dependent on preload. This is particularly useful when the effect of hemodynamic manipulations is studied or when the relationship between wall stress and ejection phase indices is examined.[61] Wall stress is, however, quite dependent upon afterload, as can be seen from the equations below, and must be considered in the context of systolic blood pressure.

A number of measures of LV wall stress may be made by echocardiography. Meridional stress describes wall stress parallel to the long axis of the ventricle and is calculated by the following formula:

Meridional end-systolic

$$\text{wall stress} = 0.334 \frac{P \times LVIDs}{PWT\left(1 + \dfrac{PWT}{LVIDs}\right)} \quad \text{(Eq. 16.1)}$$

where P is systolic blood pressure, LVIDs is LV systolic diameter, and PWT is posterior wall thickness, and wall stress is expressed

in dynes/cm². Meridional wall stress is elevated in dilated cardiomyopathy.[62]

Circumferential wall stress is the wall stress in a circular direction around the major axis of the ventricle. The formula for its calculation is given by:

Circumferential end-systolic wall stress =

$$\frac{1.33 \times P\sqrt{Ac}}{\sqrt{Am+Ac}-\sqrt{Ac}} \times \left[\frac{\dfrac{4(Ac)^{3/2}}{\pi L^2}}{\sqrt{Am+Ac}+\sqrt{Ac}}\right] \quad \text{(Eq. 16.2)}$$

where L is left ventricular long-axis dimension, Ac is LV cavity area, and Am is LV myocardial area.

It can be seen from both of the above formulas that LV dilatation, LV thinning, and increases in systolic blood pressure will all result in increased LV wall stress. In normal hearts, circumferential wall stress is higher than meridional wall stress, but this relationship is altered in dilated cardiomyopathy, due to the more spherical ventricular shape, so that the two stress values may be almost equal.[63]

Wall stress calculations assume that the LV endocardium has a constant radius of curvature, which may not be true in the setting of coronary artery disease where ventricular shape can be irregular. In this situation, regional wall stress may be measured, but this requires very complex mathematical formulations. In general, wall stress measurements remain more useful as a research tool than a day-to-day clinical measure.

Elastance. Ees may be calculated using echocardiographically determined LV end-systolic volume measurements[64] and end-systolic pressure measured invasively, using a ventricular catheter, or noninvasively, using carotid pressure tracings obtained at the dicrotic notch.[65] While elastance is sensitive to acute alterations in contractility, its use in CHF is confounded by the fact that Ees is independently affected by LV volume and is therefore less reliable in dilated hearts. Correction algorithms for ventricular volume may be applied, but controversy remains about whether this is clinically useful.[66] In addition, due to the errors involved in accurate measurement of LV end-systolic pressure and the need for hemodynamic manipulation, this useful measure of ventricular contractility is also used largely for research rather than as a day-to-day clinical tool.

Myocardial velocities, strain, and strain rate. In technical terms, TDI differs from standard Doppler by eliminating the high pass filter and using low gain amplification to display the velocities of the myocardium. TDI velocities may be displayed in spectral pulsed mode or in color encoded 2-D maps (Fig. 16.11) superimposed over structural images.[67] The technical principles and limitations of these modalities are similar to those encountered with standard Doppler flow systems. Myocardial velocities may be obtained from multiple locations of the myocardium. In a typical spectral display (Fig. 16.12), the myocardial velocity waveform displays a positive wave representing ventricular systole (S_M) and two waves corresponding to early filling (E_M) and atrial contraction (A_M). From the apical acoustic windows, the diastolic myocardial velocities obtained from any of the LV myocardial segments appear as a mirror image of the mitral inflow early (E) and atrial (A) filling velocities. In normal humans, the peak of E_M precedes the peak of LV filling E velocity suggesting that active relaxation of the myocardium generates negative pressures in the LV cavity that initiate LV filling. TDI velocities are affected not only by regional LV mechanical events but also by global

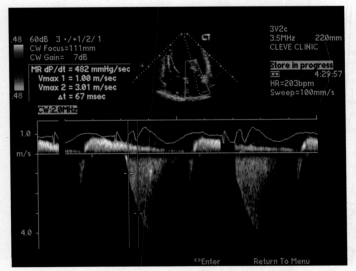

Figure 16.10 Calculation of dP/dt from the mitral regurgitation continuous wave Doppler signal in a patient with dilated cardiomyopathy.

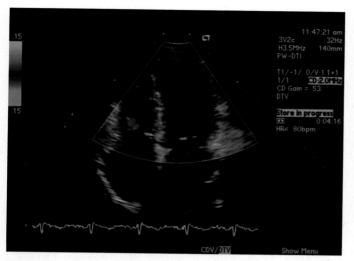

Figure 16.11 Example of color tissue Doppler 2-dimensional velocity map obtained during diastole.

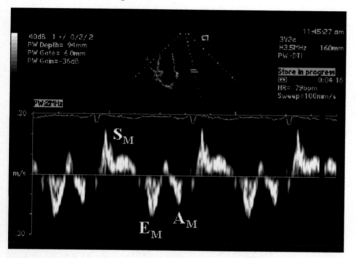

Figure 16.12 Normal tissue Doppler pattern showing the systolic (S_M), early diastolic (E_M), and atrial contraction (A_M) longitudinal velocities recorded at the lateral wall.

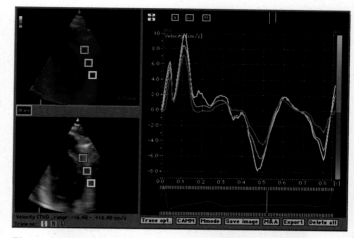

Figure 16.13 Determination of regional myocardial longitudinal velocities by tissue Doppler imaging (TDI) showing the normal apex-to-base velocity gradients (yellow–red).

translation and rotation of the heart. Accordingly, spectral TDI velocities are usually obtained from the apical acoustic window, since LV longitudinal velocities are less affected by translational motion.[68] Alternatively, translational motion may be corrected by off-line analysis from color-encoded TDI velocities. One method plots the velocity of each adjacent scan line from the distance from epicardium to endocardium. From a parasternal color M-mode image, the rates of circumferential fiber shortening and lengthening are proportional to the slope of velocity/distance regression line. The value of this slope has been referred to as myocardial velocity gradient.

Myocardial strain may be quantified noninvasively using cardiac magnetic resonance (CMR), TDI, or high frame rate 2-D echocardiography with speckle tracking. TDI-derived strain quantifies tissue deformation based on Doppler velocity shifts (Fig. 16.13). Unlike tissue Doppler velocities, tissue strain is less affected by segmental tethering and translational motion; therefore, it primarily reflects the intrinsic deformation of the myocardial segment within the sample region. The SR of a segment of a given length (L_0) is given by SR $= (V_1 - V_2)/L_0$, where V_1 and V_2 are the tissue Doppler velocities at each end of the segment (L_0). Strain (ε) represents the

percentage deformation for the given segment over its initial value and is obtained by integrating SR over the systolic (shortening) or diastolic interval (lengthening) of the cardiac cycle. Recent studies have demonstrated a closed correlation between SR and indices of LV contractility and between ε and LV stroke volume. Unfortunately, Doppler-derived strain is limited to interrogating segments aligned in parallel with the Doppler angle of incidence.

More recently, strain analysis derived from 2-D speckle tracking has become available. One of the special characteristics of static B-scan ultrasound imaging is an appearance of speckle patterns within the tissue, which are the result of constructive and destructive interference of ultrasound back-scattered from structures smaller than a wavelength of ultrasound.[69] This speckle pattern is unique for each myocardial region and is relatively stable throughout the cardiac cycle. Myocardial motion can be analyzed by tracking the movement of these speckles by filtering out random speckles and then performing an autocorrelation to estimate the motion of stable structures. This relatively new technique has been well validated with tagged CMR studies. An automated algorithm follows the change in spatial position of the speckles in a specified region in each frame and calculates the displacement, velocity, strain, and SR of a defined myocardial segment. An important advantage of speckle-derived strain is that, unlike Doppler-derived strain, it does not require alignment of the plane of motion with the direction of the ultrasound beam, thus allowing the interrogation of LV from all acoustic windows and in all spatial directions to calculate radial, circumferential, and longitudinal deformation indices. Speckle tracking is ideally suited to quantitatively assess regional LV wall motion and has the ability to demonstrate significantly decreased wall thickening in areas of hypokinetic or akinetic wall motion (Figs. 16.14 and 16.15, movies 16.5, 16.6).[70]

Left ventricular torsion. Torsional deformation may be quantified by magnetic resonance imaging (MRI) or by echocardiography from either TDI velocities or high frame rate 2-D echocardiography with speckle-tracking.[71,72] Using TDI, myocardial velocities are recorded at the septum and lateral wall of basal and apical short-axis images. The difference between septal and lateral velocity at each level represents the twisting velocity. Torsional velocity is calculated as the difference between apical and basal twisting velocities. By speckle tracking, torsion is determined from similar short-axis images, and it is determined as the difference in degrees of angular rotation between both levels.

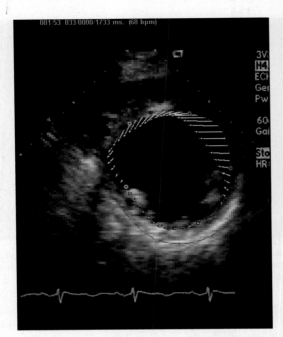

Figure 16.14 (Movie 16.5). Myocardial deformation vectors determined by velocity-vector imaging showing akinesis of the inferoseptal segments in a patient with myocardial infarction.

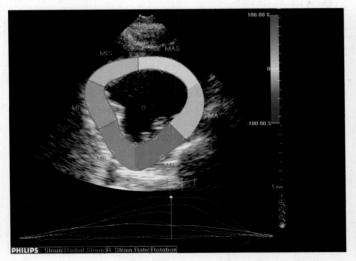

Figure 16.15 (Movie 16.6). Speckle tracking-derived radial strain map indicating reduced strain (*pink*) in the anterior segments of a patient with anterior myocardial infarction.

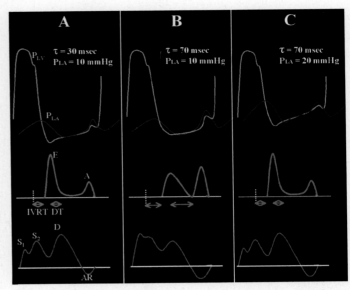

Figure 16.16 Corresponding LV and LA pressure tracings and mitral inflow patterns in patients with normal diastolic function (**A**); impaired LV relaxation (**B**); and pseudonormal diastolic function (**C**). IVRT, isovolumic relaxation time; P_{LA}, mean LA pressure; DT, early LV filling deceleration time; E, early LV filling velocity; A, atrial contraction velocity; S, pulmonary venous systolic velocity; D, pulmonary venous diastolic velocity; AR, pulmonary venous atrial reversal velocity; and τ, time constant of isovolumic relaxation.

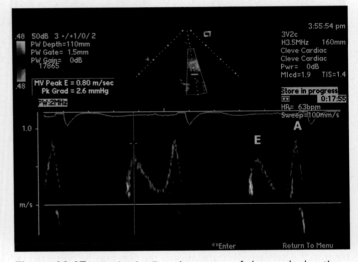

Figure 16.17 Mitral pulse Doppler pattern of abnormal relaxation.

3.6.2. Left ventricular diastolic function

Echocardiography is the most comprehensive technique for establishing the diagnosis and mechanism of diastolic function. 2-D echocardiography allows identification of LA size, LV cavity size and mass, and systolic function, helping to establish the cause and chronicity of diastolic dysfunction.[73] The precision of the measurements obtained by echocardiography has been corroborated by several clinical and pathologic studies.[74] 2-D echocardiography also allows evaluation of the distensibility of the caval and hepatic veins, which is useful for estimating right atrial pressure.[75]

Once the anatomic information has been obtained by 2-D echocardiography, the use of transmitral flow Doppler provides functional information. This study allows precise measurement

of ventricular filling velocity. The simplified Bernoulli equation allows direct relation of this velocity (v) and the pressure gradients of the atrium (P_A) and the left ventricle (P_V): $P_V - P_A \approx 4(v)^2$ (Fig. 16.16). In patients in sinus rhythm, Doppler study of ventricular filling is composed of an early filling wave (E) and an atrial contraction (A) velocity (Fig. 16.17). During early filling, ventricular relaxation causes a reduction in ventricular pressure to less than the atrial pressure, creating a pressure gradient. In accordance with the isovolumetric relaxation hemodynamic formula ($p = p_0 e^{-t/\tau}$), when the atrial pressure (P_A) varies, the decrease in the velocity of intraventricular pressure ($(-) dP/dt$) varies in accordance with p_A/τ, so that E is directly proportional to atrial pressure and the relaxation velocity of the LV ($1/\tau$).[76] At the end of the early filling stage, the decrease in LA pressure and the simultaneous increase in intraventricular pressure reduce the pressure gradient, causing deceleration of early filling flow. The operating stiffness of the left ventricle (S) is the principal determinant of deceleration of the early filling velocity (E_{DT}). In stiff ventricles, the deceleration time is reduced, as the filling volume causes a sudden increase in intraventricular pressure, equalizing this pressure with the LA pressure and causing the rapid cessation of early filling flow: $E_{DT} = 70/S^2$. The physical determinants of the ventricular filling wave during atrial contraction (A) are the same as those that determine the E-wave.[77,78] Muscular contraction of the LA increases atrial pressure and, therefore, the atrioventricular gradient, causing acceleration of the A-wave flow. The relaxation of LA and the simultaneous increase in ventricular pressure cause deceleration of A. The LA function and LV distensibility are the factors that fundamentally contribute to the occurrence of these events. The E/A relationship is the keystone for the interpretation of diastolic function on Doppler echocardiography. Nevertheless, since E and A wave velocity are determined by various confounding variables, its correct interpretation tends to require complementary information.

Several studies have shown that the filling velocities of LV vary depending on spatial location. The maximum velocity E changes as the flow is displaced from the mitral orifice toward the apex. In ventricles functioning normally, E is rapidly displaced and reaches higher amplitude near the apex, probably due to the suction caused by the apical relaxation accelerating the flow.[79] In patients with abnormal relaxation, E is greater near the mitral orifice, decreasing in amplitude and displacing itself more slowly toward the ventricular apex. This information can be easily obtained by means of an M-mode color Doppler imaging study. The propagation velocity (v_p) of the early filling wave on M-mode color Doppler imaging allows qualitative estimation of LV relaxation (Fig. 16.18).[80,81] In contrast with the E wave on pulsed Doppler, v_p is relatively independent of atrial pressure,[82] so the pattern of normal filling can be distinguished from that of pseudonormal filling (increased filling pressures).[83] The digital information obtained on M-mode color Doppler imaging can also be quantitatively analyzed. Using a simplified form of the Euler differential equation, the spatial–temporal distribution of the velocities can be applied to calculate the intraventricular pressure gradients: $\rho\left[\frac{\partial v}{\partial t} + v\frac{\partial v}{\partial e}\right] = -\frac{\partial p}{\partial e}$. These pressure gradients physiologically generate the ventricular filling suction.[84,85] M-mode color Doppler imaging can also be useful to estimate LA pressure in combination with

pulsed Doppler imaging of ventricular filling. The propagation velocity (v_p) from M-mode color Doppler imaging of ventricular filling is inversely related to the isovolumetric relaxation constant (τ) and is relatively independent of atrial pressure. On the other hand, the E wave filling on ventricular Doppler imaging is determined by atrial pressure and relaxation: $\left(E \propto \frac{P_A}{\tau}\right)$.[86,87] Therefore, atrial pressure can be noninvasively estimated as:

$$P_A = k \times \frac{E}{v_p}.$$ [88] (Eq. 16.3)

A Doppler study of PV flow complements the interpretation of ventricular filling flow, particularly in the study of atrial function. PV flow in patients in sinus rhythm has three characteristic waves: (a) the S wave, which represents filling of the atrium during ventricular systole, (b) the D wave, which represents a second filling phase during ventricular diastole, and (c) the AR wave, which represents the reserve flow toward the pulmonary veins during atrial contraction (Fig. 16.19). Since there are no valves that impede retrograde flow from the left atrium to the pulmonary veins, the relation between the amplitude and the duration of the A filling wave of the left ventricle and the AR wave in the pulmonary veins depends on the stiffness of LV: $K \approx AR_{dur} - A_{dur}$.[89]

Applying the same physical principle used to analyze blood flow, TDI Doppler studies can be adapted to obtain the velocity of myocardial movement during diastole.[90] Several studies have shown a direct relationship between ventricular relaxation and TDI E_m, which also appears to be less influenced by atrial pressure. This method has proven to be useful for differentiating restrictive cardiomyopathy from constrictive pericarditis. Similar to the application of M-mode color Doppler imaging, the E_m wave of tissue Doppler can be used in combination with transmitral E wave to estimate LA pressure.[91]

The normal Doppler pattern for ventricular filling is characterized by a prominent E, with rapid acceleration and gradual deceleration. The E wave amplitude is determined by rapid relaxation. The A wave is of lesser proportion due to the low LA volume at the end of the early filling phase and, therefore, E/A > 1. M-mode color Doppler imaging shows a propagation velocity (v_p) > 45 cm/s and TDI shows E_m > 8 cm/s (Fig. 16.20).

In impaired LV relaxation, the E amplitude is reduced. Given that atrial contraction begins before ventricular relaxation is complete,

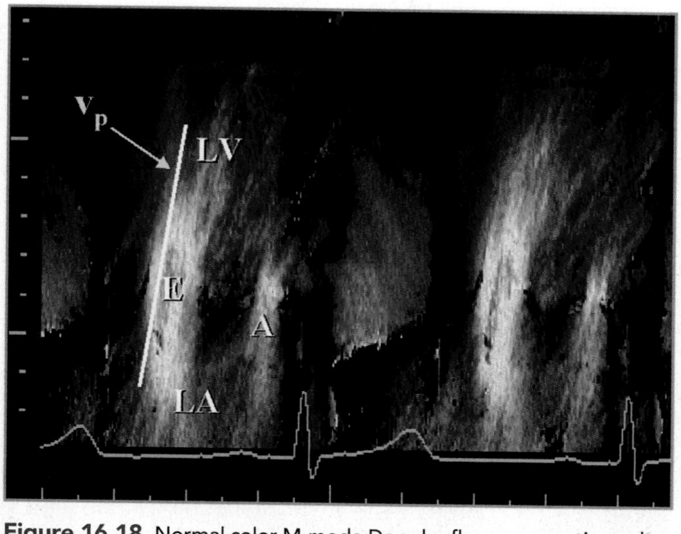

Figure 16.18 Normal color M-mode Doppler flow propagation velocity (v_p), measured as the slope of the first aliasing velocity from the mitral leaflet tips to the LV apex.

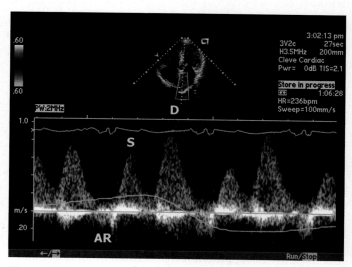

Figure 16.19 Blunted pulmonary venous velocity pattern (S/D < 1).

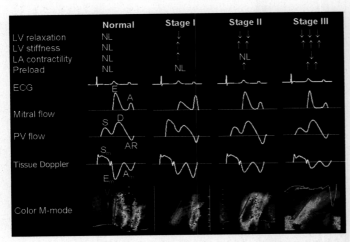

Figure 16.20 Typical changes in mitral inflow, pulmonary venous (PV) flow, and tissue Doppler and color M-mode propagation velocity and corresponding physiologic alterations expected with varying degrees of diastolic dysfunction.

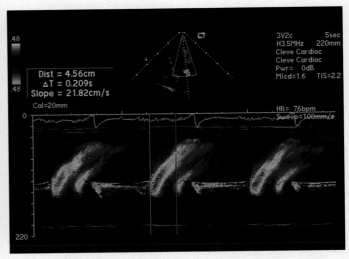

Figure 16.21 Reduced color M-mode Doppler flow propagation velocity obtained from a patient with dilated cardiomyopathy.

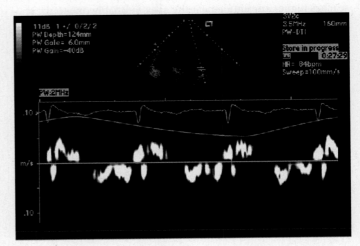

Figure 16.22 Abnormal tissue Doppler velocities obtained from a patient with dilated cardiomyopathy.

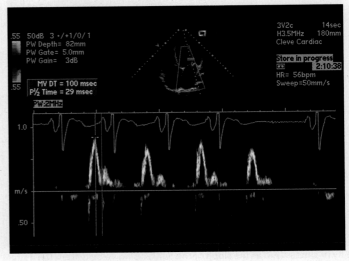

Figure 16.23 Mitral pulse Doppler restrictive pattern.

the volume in the LA at the end of early filling increases, which in turn increases the atrial ejection volume and, therefore, the A amplitude. An impaired LV relaxation pattern is characterized by an $E/A < 1$ and an $E_{DT} > 240$ ms.[92,93] An impaired relaxation pattern is common in individuals of advanced age and in patients with hypertensive,[94] hypertrophic,[95] and ischemic cardiomyopathies.[96] These patients frequently present with few symptoms, but tend to have reduced cardiac output during exercise. The impaired relaxation pattern tends to be associated with the presence on auscultation of an S4 atrial gallop. M-mode color Doppler imaging shows a propagation velocity (v_p) < 45 cm/s and TDI shows $E_m < 8$ cm/s.

As diastolic dysfunction advances, cardiac output diminishes, which in turn causes a reduction in renal excretion of sodium and water and the elevation of LA pressure. This elevated pressure, in turn, produces changes in the mitral flow pattern in the opposite manner to those changes caused by abnormal relaxation (Fig. 16.16). The isovolumetric relaxation time is shortened, as atrial pressure advances the moment of mitral opening. The E amplitude is increased while the A decreases due to the reduction in ventricular distensibility. This pattern is indistinguishable from a normal filling pattern and is frequently observed in patients with dilated, hypertrophic, and restrictive cardiomyopathy. Certain clinical and echocardiographic characteristics help distinguish a pseudonormal filling pattern from a normal filling pattern. These include the presence of systolic dysfunction or other echocardiographic findings suggestive of heart disease, such as dilation of the LA. Pulmonary vein flow tends to demonstrate a blunted S wave, prominent reverse atrial contraction wave (AR) > 35 cm/s, and $AR_{dur} > A_{dur}$. M-mode color Doppler imaging shows a propagation velocity (v_p) < 45 cm/s (Fig. 16.21) and TDI shows $E_m < 8$ cm/s (Fig. 16.22). These allow a normal filling pattern to be distinguished from a pseudonormal filling pattern.

An excessive increase in atrial pressure ultimately causes a marked shortening in isovolumetric relaxation time. In the restrictive filling pattern, the early filling deceleration time (E_{DT}) is shortened due to increased ventricular stiffness (Fig. 16.23). The amplitude and duration of A are reduced significantly. The restrictive filling pattern is typically seen in patients with advanced congestive symptoms, with auscultatory detection of an S3 ventricular gallop,[97] and is associated with increased cardiac mortality rate. The restrictive filling pattern is characterized by an E/A ratio > 2 and an $E_{DT} < 150$ ms. The reverse atrial contraction wave (AR) is prominent, unless atrial function has deteriorated. M-mode color Doppler imaging shows a propagation velocity (v_p) < 45 cm/s and TDI shows E_m < 8 cm/s.

Table 16.4 summarizes the normal values, guidelines for interpretation, and pitfalls of common echocardiographic indices of diastolic function.

3.6.3. Left ventricular myocardial performance index

A novel Doppler method that combines LV systolic and diastolic performance is the Tei index.[98] This index takes into account: (1) the isovolumic contraction time (ICT, interval between the end of mitral valve closure and aortic valve opening), which is inversely proportional to LV (+) dP/dt, thus representing LV contractility; (2) the ejection time (ET, from aortic valve opening to aortic valve closure), which is proportional to stroke volume; and (3) the isovolumic relaxation time (IVRT, from aortic valve closure to mitral valve opening), which is inversely proportional to LV (−) dP/dt, thus expressing diastolic relaxation. The Tei index can be obtained by the following formula: LV Tei index = [(isovolumic contraction time + isovolumic relaxation time)/LV ejection time]. These intervals are measured from separate pulsed Doppler recordings of the mitral inflow and aortic outflow. Since the distance between mitral valve closure to mitral valve opening in the next heart beat (a) = IVC + ET + IVRT, the actual formula is represented as: LV Tei index = (a − ET)/ET. An alternative approach for the measurement of Tei index uses a TDI recording obtained from the four-chamber view at the basal septum level.[99] This method has the advantage of using a single recording since TDI allows measurements of both systolic and diastolic intervals. Studies have shown that the Tei index increases in patients with LV dysfunction, regardless of the etiology, and values >0.6 are typically associated with symptomatic CHF.[100]

3.6.4. Right ventricular function

In the parasternal long-axis and apical four-chamber views, the normal RV has a smaller diameter than the LV. The RV should have a crescent shape in the short-axis view whereas the LV has a circular geometry. Therefore, the RV side of the interventricular septum is normally convex and the LV side concave. In RV volume overload, the interventricular septum may appear flattened or assume a reverse concavity only during diastole, whereas in RV pressure overload, these changes are seen in systole.[101] RV end-systolic and end-diastolic areas and fractional area change can be traced from the apical four-chamber view, with a modest correlation (r = 0.7–0.85) compared to radionuclide ventriculography or CMR.[102,103] The reproducibility of these measurements is, however, limited by foreshortening and changes in angulation. In many patients, visualization of the RV free wall may also be limited by lung interference.

A very useful semiquantitative method to estimate RV function is the measurement of tricuspid annular plane systolic excursion (TAPSE). This is obtained by measuring the level of systolic excursion of the lateral tricuspid valve annulus toward the apex in the four-chamber view. Studies have shown a good correlation between TAPSE and RV EF determined by radionuclide angiography.[104]

Alternative methods to TAPSE that evaluate RV free wall longitudinal motion use pulsed or color TDI. A peak systolic velocity <11 cm/s has been reported to identify RV dysfunction with sensitivity and specificity of 90% and 85%, respectively.[105] TDI velocities have been used to identify RV involvement in patients with inferior wall myocardial infarction.[106] Strain and SR imaging of the RV have been attempted but, by large, these methods do not appear to offer significant advantage over TDI velocities. Obtaining adequate data for strain calculation in the RV is difficult, given the limited thickness of RV free wall and the limited number of acoustic windows available. Nevertheless, studies have

TABLE 16.4
NORMAL VALUES, INTERPRETATION, AND PITFALLS OF INDICES OF DIASTOLIC FUNCTION

	Normal values	Interpretation	Pitfalls
E/A ratio	≥1.0	Low value indicates reduced LV relaxation or low filling pressures	Normal value indicates normal LV relaxation or increased filling pressures
E_{DT}	>150 ms	Low value indicates increased LV stiffness and filling pressures	May be short in young subjects with vigorous LV relaxation or in normal ventricles with volume overload
S/D ratio	≥1.0	Low value indicates elevated LA pressure	May be reduced in young subjects with vigorous relaxation and patients with mitral insufficiency or atrial fibrillation
TDI E_M	>8.0 cm/s	Low value indicates reduced LV relaxation	May exhibit regional variability in ischemic heart disease and hypertrophic cardiomyopathy
Color M-mode v_p	>45 cm/s	Low value indicates reduced LV relaxation	May be "pseudo-normalized" in patients with small LV cavity
E/E_M ratio	<8	High value indicates increased LA pressure	Range 8–15 undetermined
AR_{dur}−A_{dur}	>0 ms	High value indicates elevated LV end-diastolic pressure and LV stiffness	Difficult to measure by transthoracic echocardiography
LA area	<20 cm²	High value suggests chronically elevated LA pressure	Does not reflect acute changes; may be increased in mitral insufficiency and atrial fibrillation

E/A, early-to-atrial contraction pulsed LV filling Doppler velocity; E_{DT}, Early LV filling Doppler deceleration time; S/D, systolic-to-diastolic pulmonary venous pulsed Doppler velocity; E_M, tissue Doppler early diastolic velocity (measured at the basal septum, from the apical four-chamber view); v_p, LV early filling propagation velocity; A_{dur}, LV filling Doppler atrial contraction duration; AR_{dur}, pulmonary venous pulsed Doppler atrial reversal duration; and LA, left atrium.

Figure 16.24 Images obtained by equilibrium radionuclide angiocardiography (ERNA) at end-diastole and end-systole in a patient with normal cardiac function.

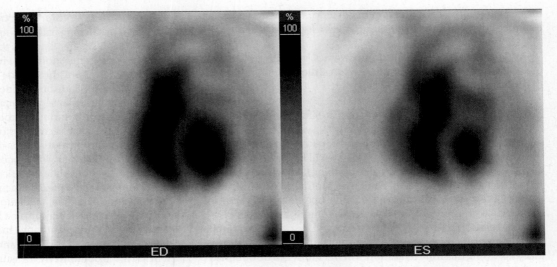

shown good correlation between strain determined invasively by sonomicrometry and TDI-derived strain.[107]

The Doppler index of myocardial performance (Tei index) may be applied and can be used for evaluation of RV performance. It is calculated as RV Tei index = [(isovolumic contraction time + isovolumic relaxation time)/RV ejection time]. An increased RV Tei index predicts poor outcome in patients with primary pulmonary hypertension and in patients with left-sided chronic heart failure.[108]

3.7. Nuclear scintigraphy

Radioactive tracers can be injected as a bolus and tracked during first pass through the vascular system, attached to red blood cells and in equilibrium within the vascular space or as myocardial perfusion tracers that define the endocardial borders of LV. (1) First pass radionuclide angiography (FPRNA) and equilibrium radionuclide angiocardiography (ERNA) have been the most commonly used techniques that are capable of assessing global and regional systolic and diastolic function at rest and following supine or upright exercise. These modalities have the advantages of providing true 3-D measurements that are independent of geometric assumptions, with high accuracy and reproducibility based on measured radioactive counts. ^{99m}Tc pertechnetate is the radioisotope of choice and it is attached to the patient's own red blood cells using different labeling methods that vary in time, expense, and labeling efficiency.

Most ERNA studies are performed using planar techniques with the patient positioned in the left anterior oblique view, which allows the best separation of the LV and RV for independent and accurate volume measurements in each chamber (Fig. 16.24). The labeled red blood cells circulate in the vascular space and the patient's ECG signal is used to set the timing for acquisition of each heart beat at 8 to 32 individual time intervals, which may vary from 10 to 150 ms depending on heart rate. Information from > 400 heartbeats is divided among the time intervals and used to reconstruct a time–activity curve (Fig. 16.25).

First pass techniques require administration of a compact intravenous bolus of radioactivity, using a very high temporal resolution and high count rate camera system to follow the radioactivity as it traverses the LV and RV. Serial gated images at 25 to 50 ms temporal resolution are acquired and the resultant time–activity curve allows systolic and diastolic function analysis of the RV and LV at rest or following exercise or pharmacologic stress. The FPRNA method is less utilized than ERNA method since it requires high-count rate using multicrystal camera systems, which are optimal for the technique.

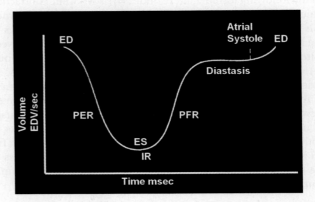

Figure 16.25 Typical parameters measured from the LV volume curve obtained by radionuclide angiocardiography. ED, end-diastole; ES, end-systole; PER, peak ejection rate; PFR, peak filling rate; and IR, isovolumic relaxation.

3.7.1. LV systolic function

Radionuclide approaches for assessing LV systolic function require the generation of a curve plotting the changes in radioactivity, which is proportional to changes in LV volume over time. From this time–activity curve, the first derivative, which measures the change in volume over time, is calculated and used to calculate the most rapid changes in ejection and the time when the maximal rate occurs. For systolic function analysis, changes in heart rate and arrhythmias can be handled by eliminating 10% to 20% of heart beats that significantly deviate from the mean cardiac cycle length. The left side of the time–activity curve prior to end-systole provides information on the systolic function of the ventricle as expressed by the rate of ejection, measured as end diastolic volumes/second (EDV/s), and the time at which this peak ejection occurs, expressed as time to peak ejection rate. This peak ejection rate is decreased in patients with ischemic heart disease or with cardiomyopathies, even before EF is significantly impaired.

Gated single photon emission computed tomography (SPECT) myocardial perfusion imaging can also evaluate LV systolic function. Analysis is usually performed during stress acquisition, and it is usually limited to myocardial perfusion studies using Technetium compounds since they provide higher count rate than Thallium-201. The acquired scintigraphic counts are divided usually in eight separate time intervals to reconstruct a movie. It is important to recognize that acquisition is performed several minutes after peak stress, thus transient changes in LV function may have resolved by the time the data is acquired. In patients with extensive transmural myocardial infarction, the absence of counts may not allow to differentiate akinetic, dyskinetic, or aneurysmal segments. Thus, LV function estimation may be inaccurate in these cases. In patients with LV hypertrophy and/or small LV cavity, LV volumes may be underestimated and EF overestimated due to partial volume effects caused by limited spatial resolution.

3.7.2. Left ventricular diastolic function

From the same time–activity curve previously described, the first derivative, which measures the change in volume over time, is calculated and used to calculate the most rapid changes in filling and the time when the maximal rate occurs. To attain sufficient temporal resolution for assessment of diastolic function, the data should be acquired in at least 16 phases per cardiac cycle. Unlike systolic function analysis where changes in heart rate and arrhythmias have relatively little influence, diastolic parameters are markedly affected by heart rate variability during acquisition and processing. The peak-filling rate represents the most rapid ventricular filling, is normalized to EDV/s, and is normally >2.5. This peak-filling rate declines in subjects with impaired LV relaxation, including apparently healthy elderly.[109] The time to achieve the peak-filling rate is an important measurement of diastolic function and is <180 ms in normal ventricles. The percent of stroke volume filling that occurs during the rapid filling phase may also be derived from the time–activity curve, and it is normally >70% of the stroke volume, decreasing in subjects with impaired LV relaxation. It is important to recognize that factors such as age, heart rate, adrenergic state, and medications will alter all these parameters in the absence of pathology.[110] Elevated LV filling pressure in patients with CHF and restrictive LV filling may increase peak-filling rate, in a manner similar to that described in Doppler LV filling patterns.

3.7.3. Right ventricular function

Nuclear cardiology techniques are ideal for examination of the RV because they rely on a count-based method that is independent of geometry. RV EF and regional wall motion may be assessed by ERNA or FPRNA. A left anterior oblique projection is typically used in ERNA to separate the LV from the RV counts. Studies have shown excellent correlation between RVEF by ERNA and FPRNA.[111,112] However, RV evaluation by ERNA may be limited in many patients in whom it is difficult to adequately separate

the RV from the RA. FPRNA is performed in the right anterior oblique view with ECG gating as the bolus passes through the right side of the heart. With gating, there is a summation of data from several cardiac cycles. Since data are obtained during first pass, overlapping with LV counts is avoided by adding only the data of those cardiac cycles that are occurring before detection of LV counts. Acquisition may be performed with or without ECG gating, although the latter is not commonly done since it requires acquisition with high sensitivity cameras and collimators. Determination of RV EF by FPRNA has been shown to correlate better with CMR than ERNA determinations.[113]

3.8. Computed tomography

For evaluation of LV function, CCT needs to be performed using ECG gating with retrospective reconstruction. The use of tube current modulation to reduce radiation exposure does not interfere with the assessment of LV function. However, LV function assessment cannot be performed in studies acquired using prospective ECG gating. It has been shown that CCT has high accuracy in assessing global LV volumes and EF.[114,115] This accuracy depends on the temporal resolution of the scanner, the number of phases reconstructed, and on the appropriate phase selection. At least 10 cardiac phases should be reconstructed at 10% intervals (Fig. 16.26, movie 16.7). End-diastole corresponds usually to the 0% phase, centered within the first 100 ms after the QRS. End-systole is selected as the minimum volume, usually corresponding to the 30% to 40% phase, according to heart rate. One of the advantages of CCT is its true 3-D submillimeter resolution. A disadvantage is its lower temporal resolution compared to echocardiography and CMR. Thus, it is possible to miss the true end-systolic volume in some cases. Choosing 5% instead of 10% step increments has been shown to decrease the ES volume by 1 ± 0 mL and increase the calculated EF by 0.4 ± 0.1%,[116] but this generates larger datasets requiring longer transmission time and significantly increased storage capacity. CCT, compared with CMR and echocardiography, tends to yield slightly larger volumes and lower EF.[117] These differences may be explained by the effect of the contrast load and/or the common use of β-blockers to perform the test. Several methods may be used to calculate the EF, including area–length, Simpson rule, and the volumetric voxel count using automated edge detection (Fig. 16.27). By this method, the volume of the LV cavity is selected using a Hounsfield unit threshold, with the only input required from the user being the selection of mitral annular and

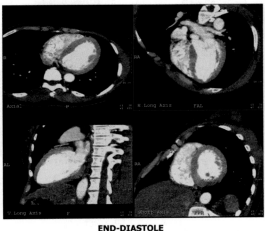
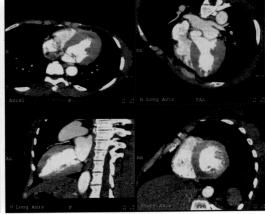

END-DIASTOLE   **END-SYSTOLE**

Figure 16.26 (Movie 16.7). Cardiac CT visualization of end-diastolic and end-systolic volumes in the axial, four-chamber, two-chamber, and sort-axis views.

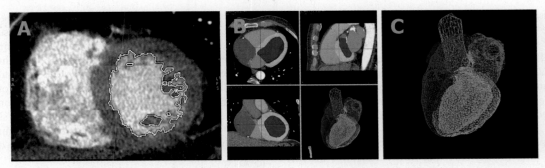

Figure 16.27 Cardiac CT determination of chamber volumes: (**A**) automated threshold-based method to detect the endocardial boundary; (**B**) chamber segmentation; and (**C**) 3-dimensional model.

aortic valve planes. By definition, papillary muscles are excluded from the LV volume. This is an important consideration when comparing with echocardiography and CMR, where the papillary muscles are often included. In patients with small LV cavity and concentric LVH, this volume difference may be significant.

Regional wall thickening may be assessed by CCT. This is particularly important when evaluating patients with acute chest pain and coronary artery disease to recognize possible myocardial injury. Wall thickness and LV mass may be measured from the end-diastolic phase. Temporal derivatives such as the velocity of wall thickening and thinning or the peak ejection or filling rates are, in theory, possible to obtain but their accuracy is limited by the low temporal resolution of CCT.

CCT can be used for assessment of RV performance with the addition of retrospective ECG gating and the use of dedicated cardiac analysis software. Compared with CMR, CCT is an accurate and reliable noninvasive technique for evaluating RV measurements.[118,119] Assessing RV function with CCT requires a specialized contrast injection protocol to opacify the RV. Most investigators propose a biphasic contrast injection. Temporal resolution is limited with CCT. Radiation exposure is comparable, or greater than, with radionuclide ventriculography. Thus, evaluation of RV function by cardiac CT is usually complementary to other information being sought, rather than a primary indication for the test.

High-resolution CT may also be useful to establish the diagnosis and determine the severity of interstitial lung disease, Bronchiectasis, and pulmonary embolism as the cause of dyspnea. About 85% of patients who present honeycombing on CT have idiopathic pulmonary fibrosis.[120]

3.9. Cardiac magnetic resonance

3.9.1. Left ventricular systolic function
Left ventricular stroke volume. CMR is an excellent technique for the determination of flow. The signal measured during MR image acquisition has two components, magnitude and phase. The phase of the signal can provide information about the velocity of moving protons (see Chapter 6). To obtain LV stroke volume, a velocity-encoded phase contrast acquisition is made at the level of the ascending aorta. The LV stroke volume is determined as the product of the cross-sectional area of the aorta, measured from the corresponding cine magnitude image, and the average velocity integrated over the systolic ejection period. In the presence of aortic regurgitation, the diastolic flow is subtracted to obtain the forward stroke volume.

Left ventricular volumes, mass, and ejection fraction. CMR is considered the "gold standard" for quantifying ventricular volumes, EF, and myocardial mass.[121] Although LV volumes may

be measured from four-chamber and two-chamber images, in a similar manner as in echocardiography, the most common method uses short-axis acquisitions (Fig. 16.28). CMR offers two distinct advantages over echocardiography: (1) A precise spatial location and angulation may be obtained from localizer images to plan each image acquisition, and (2) The acquisition planes are not limited to the selected acoustic windows. A series of 10 to 15 contiguous, LV short-axis slices of 5 to 10 mm thickness are acquired using gradient echo, balanced or steady-state free precession cine-"bright-blood" sequences using ECG-gating and breath-holding.

Endocardial and epicardial contours are drawn during off-line postprocessing in a dedicated computer workstation. Volumetric quantification is based on Simpson rule: LV volume = sum of volumes of all slices. Myocardial mass is calculated as the difference of the epicardial and the endocardial volumes multiplied by muscle specific density. Unlike 2-D echocardiography, CMR LV volumes and mass determinations do not rely on any geometrical assumption, making it more accurate for the evaluation of patients with cardiomyopathies.[122] The higher reproducibility of CMR makes it an ideal method for serial evaluation after therapeutic intervention, reducing the sample size required to evaluate efficacy in clinical trials.[123]

Left ventricular strain. Myocardial strain and SR determinations can be made in cine-CMR sequences using tissue tagging.[124] Tags are bands where magnetization is altered and signal is nulled by selectively applying specialized radiofrequency pulses. The tags

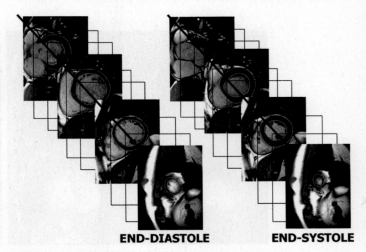

END-DIASTOLE   **END-SYSTOLE**

Figure 16.28 CMR determination of LV and RV mass and function. Tracings are done off-line on 10–15 contiguous slices at end-diastole and end-systole. Volumes are calculated by the Simpson disc method.

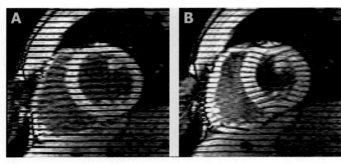

Figure 16.29 (**Movie 16.8**). Cine-tagged CMR images showing the deformation of the nulled bands from end-diastole (**A**) to end-systole (**B**).

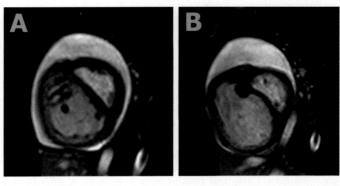
Figure 16.30 Evidence of RV dilatation, hypertrophy, and reversed-systolic septal curvature in a patient with severe pulmonary hypertension. (**A**) end-diastole; (**B**) end-systole.

are typically applied at end-diastole and followed during systolic contraction (Fig. 16.29, movie 16.8). With myocardial contraction, the tag lines deform and the space between tag lines is compressed. Using dedicated postprocessing algorithms, the intersection points of perpendicular tag lines are followed in space to determine strain and SR. Compared to 2-D echo speckle tracking and TDI-derived strain, CMR strain determinations have lower spatial and temporal resolution. However, strain deformation can be measured in any segment and in any direction by CMR.

3.9.2. Left ventricular diastolic function

Velocity-encoded (phase-contrast) cine-CMR is a widely available and established pulse sequence that provides quantitative determination of intraventricular blood flow. Phase-contrast CMR measurements of mitral and PV flow are feasible in most patients with heart failure. Application of three-dimensional mitral valve flow measurements may overcome difficulties related to the motion of the mitral valve plane during the cardiac cycle. In patients with amyloidosis, there is a good correlation between echocardiography and phase-contrast CMR in estimating LV filling E/A, E_{DT}, and PV S/D ratios.[125] CMR tagging and phase-encoding may be applied to measure diastolic myocardial velocities and SR, although these have not been extensively validated.

3.9.3. Right ventricular function

CMR has excellent accuracy and reproducibility for assessment of RV function and RV volumes.[126,127] Anatomical images of the RV may be obtained in the short-axis direction or axial planes. By either method, 10 to 15 contiguous sections are acquired using a cine sequence, as described previously for the RV. RV volumes are determined as the sum of the subvolumes of each slice obtained from computer-aided manual tracings.[128] CMR is superior to echocardiography for the assessment of dilated RV since no geometrical assumptions are made. CMR is the ideal method for serial follow-up of patients with congenital heart disease and for establishing the diagnosis of RV dysplasia, given its ability to visualize all the segments of RV from multiple anatomical planes. In patients with pulmonary hypertension, CMR may accurately quantify RV volumes, EF, and mass and qualitatively quantify the severity of pulmonary hypertension based on pulmonary artery distensibility and the degree of interventricular septal systolic convexity toward the LV (Fig. 16.30).

3.9.4. Myocardial tissue characterization

Probably the most important value of CMR in patients with ventricular dysfunction is myocardial characterization or "virtual histology." By exploiting the different T1 and T2 characteristics of water,

fat, and other tissue components, CMR may identify the extent of myocardial edema after myocardial infarction (Fig. 16.31) or in certain cardiomyopathies such as sarcoidosis. In the latter, detection of myocardial edema correlates with disease activity and may be useful for management decisions. Special sequences such as T2* may be used to characterize infiltrative disorders. This sequence in particular is very useful to establish the diagnosis and severity of iron overload in hemochromatosis and hemosiderosis. But probably the most useful application for tissue characterization by CMR is delayed enhancement after gadolinium administration. Gadolinium chelates are paramagnetic agents that on first pass, enhance the venous and arterial circulation, including the capillary-rich myocardium. After initial assessment of myocardial perfusion, gadolinium gradually disappears from the blood pool and is excreted through the kidneys. In areas where the myocardium is injured, scarred or fibrotic, there is delayed "wash-in" and "wash-out" of gadolinium. After acute myocardial infarction, gadolinium enters the intracellular space of death cells due to their disrupted membrane. In areas of increased fibrosis caused by remote infarction

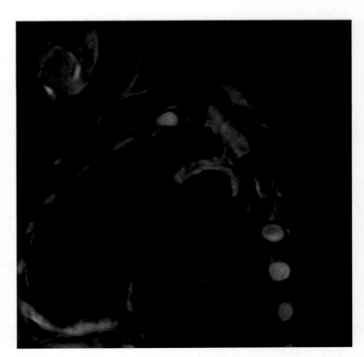
Figure 16.31 Triple-inversion recovery CMR sequence used to demonstrate myocardial edema in the anteroseptal wall after recent myocardial infarction.

or in cardiomyopathies, gadolinium accumulates in the increased interstitial space. These fibrotic or scarred areas show up as bright or "hyperenhanced" areas of myocardium when "delayed" images are taken, typically 10 to 15 min after injection. A special inversion signal given prior to the main pulse sequence is used to "null" signal from the normal myocardium so that it can be more easily distinguished from the abnormal, hyperenhanced myocardium. Specific patterns of delayed hyperenhancement correspond with certain cardiovascular diseases, and can be used to distinguish ischemic from nonischemic cardiomyopathy, as well as differentiate between different forms of infiltrative cardiomyopathies.

Several studies have reported excellent correlation between scar tissue by CMR and postmortem examination of infarcted myocardium.[129] In patients with ischemic cardiomyopathy, CMR allows accurate discrimination between viable and nonviable myocardium (Fig. 16.32). Myocardial scar in ischemic cardiomyopathy, invariably involving the subendocardial regions in the distribution territory of a coronary artery, is demonstrated in patients with MI.[130] The inplane spatial resolution of down to 1 × 1 mm permits to differentiate subendocardial from transmural infarction. Dysfunctional myocardial regions with less than 50% transmural infarct extension are likely to recover following

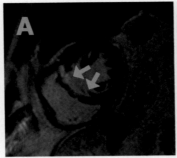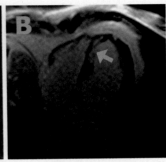

Figure 16.32 Evidence of myocardial gadolinium delayed enhancement in a patient with transmural anteroseptal infarct. (**A**) short-axis; (**B**) four-chamber views.

revascularization.[131] Delayed-enhanced CMR has a sensitivity of 94% and a specificity of 84% when compared with FDG-PET for the detection of viable myocardium in patients with ischemic cardiomyopathy and LV dysfunction.[132]

The relative value and limitations of noninvasive imaging modalities for evaluation of LV systolic and diastolic function indices are summarized in Table 16.5.

TABLE 16.5
RELATIVE VALUE AND LIMITATIONS OF NONINVASIVE IMAGING MODALITIES FOR EVALUATION OF LV FUNCTION INDICES

	Value	Limitations	Preferred indications
Systolic function			
Echocardiography	Portable, inexpensive, complementary valve information	Lower reproducibility, limited by acoustic windows in 5%–10% patients	Initial evaluation, serial assessment, critically ill patients
CMR	High reproducibility, precise quantification, tissue characterization	Costly, limited to hemodynamically stable and cooperative patients	Evaluation of "borderline" patients, viability assessment, determination of specific etiology
Gated MPI	Complementary ejection fraction, regional wall motion assessment during stress MPI	Unreliable in patients with large infarcts, overestimates LV ejection fraction in small LV cavity, increased wall thickness, no valvular assessment	Complementary during stress MPI
RNA	Applicable to most patients, high reproducibility	Radiation exposure, no valvular assessment	Evaluation of "borderline" patients, serial comparisons
CCT	High spatial resolution, reproducibility	Radiation exposure, limited valvular assessment	Complementary to other CCT indications
Diastolic function			
Echocardiography	Most complete hemodynamic assessment	Occasional misinterpretations caused by unknown hemodynamic confounding variables	Essential for the evaluation of patients with dyspnea and CHF
CMR	LV mass evaluation, tissue characterization	Limited hemodynamic assessment	Useful to determine the etiology of CHF
Gated MPI	Not validated	Low temporal resolution	None established
RNA	Reproducible volumetric filling times and rates	Frequent misinterpretations caused by unknown hemodynamic confounding variables	Complementary during evaluation of ejection fraction
CCT	Not validated	Low temporal resolution	None established

CMR, cardiac magnetic resonance; MPI, myocardial perfusion imaging; RNA, radionuclide angiography; and CCT, cardiac computed tomography.

4. PROGNOSIS AND TREATMENT

The LV EF has been shown to be a powerful prognostic index in patients with coronary artery disease, cardiomyopathies, and valvular heart disease. A reduced LV EF is associated with decreased long-term survival after myocardial infarction and in patients with CHF, independent of functional class and other clinical characteristics. The increase of cardiac events is noted once the LV EF falls below 40% and continues to increase as the value is further reduced. Arbitrarily, different clinical trials have defined cutoff values of 30% or 35% to define a "higher risk" substrate. It is important to remember than in most clinical studies, these values have been established based on echocardiographic results. Most experts will accept values from CMR or radionuclide ventriculography as equivalent, but not those obtained from gated SPECT myocardial perfusion studies, given the inherent limitations of this technique previously discussed. The prognostic values of end-diastolic and, most importantly, end-systolic dimensions have also been established in patients with ischemic and nonischemic cardiomyopathies as well as in those with valvular heart disease. In patients with regurgitant valve lesions, end-systolic diameters >4.5 to 5 cm are associated with increased cardiovascular events and are therefore considered as indication for valve repair or replacement, even in asymptomatic patients. In addition to LV systolic function indices, RV function indices are also strong independent predictors of increased adverse event rates in patients with CHF, congenital heart disease, and pulmonary hypertension.[133-135]

Several studies have shown that diastolic dysfunction is associated with increased morbidity and mortality in the community. In the Cardiovascular Health Study,[136] both high (>1.5) and low (<0.7) E/A ratios were predictive of the development of CHF during a mean follow-up of 5.2 years. In the Strong Heart Study,[137] the prognostic value of high and low E/A ratios were investigated in 3,008 American–Indian participants. A high (>1.5) E/A ratio was predictive of all-cause and cardiac mortality (adjusted HRs [95% CI] for all-cause and cardiac death, 1.73 [0.99–3.03] and 2.8 [1.19–6.75], respectively) during a mean follow-up of 3 years. Finally, in the Olmstead county study,[4] the prognostic value of diastolic dysfunction assessed by both pulsed Doppler and TDI was investigated. Both mild and moderate or severe diastolic dysfunction were predictive of all-cause death during a median of 3.5 person-years of follow-up (adjusted HRs [95% CI] of mild and moderate or severe diastolic dysfunction, 8.31 [3.00–23.1] and 10.2 [3.28–31.0], respectively).

The association of systolic and diastolic function with survival has been examined in 102 patients with dilated cardiomyopathy and an EF of 0.23 ± 0.08.[138] In this study, markers of diastolic dysfunction, including a short E_{DT} and an increased E LV inflow velocity, were more strongly associated with symptoms than the reduced EF. An E_{DT} < 130 had incremental prognostic value to a reduced (<0.25) EF. The strong prognostic value of E_{DT} has also been demonstrated in patients with ischemic and restrictive cardiomyopathies. More recently, a reduced (<3 cm/s) TDI E_m was shown to predict 4-year mortality and provided incremental prognostic value to other clinical risk factors and Doppler echocardiographic variables in 182 CHF patients with an EF < 0.50.[139]

The myocardial performance (Tei) index has also shown important prognostic value pathophysiology in relation with cardiac function. In patients with cardiac amyloidosis, an increase in Tei index predicted decreased survival better than EF.[140] The prognostic utility of Tei index has been also demonstrated in dilated cardiomyopathy, myocardial infarction, chronic heart failure, and others.[141-143]

The prognostic significance of LA enlargement in cardiovascular diseases has been demonstrated in many studies. Left atrial size is associated with the outcome of patients with myocardial infarction. An LA volume index > 32 mL/m² measured a median of 1 day after admission was a powerful and independent predictor of mortality in patients with acute myocardial infarction. In the studies of left ventricular dysfunction population, an LA greater than 4.17 cm in diameter was closely associated with increased risk of death and cardiovascular hospitalization.[144]

The presence and extent of CMR delayed enhancement also have important prognostic implications. In patients with ischemic heart disease, dysfunctional myocardial regions with less than 50% transmural infarct extension have a good chance of functional recovery after myocardial infarction[145] or with coronary artery bypass surgery.[146] Even segments with reduced myocardial thickness may recover after revascularization if there is <50% transmural scar extension.[147] The extent of delayed enhancement has also been shown to have important negative prognostic implications for patients with dilated cardiomyopathy, independent of baseline ventricular functional parameters.[148]

5. FUTURE DIRECTIONS

Over the last two decades, noninvasive imaging techniques have emerged as very powerful tools to evaluate global and regional myocardial function. Noninvasive methods have largely replaced invasive hemodynamic assessment in the clinical practice, and today the cardiac catheterization laboratory is no longer a diagnostic but rather a therapeutic environment. In the near-future, noninvasive methods may also gradually replace or reduce the need for invasive hemodynamic monitoring in the intensive care setting.

Noninvasive determination of LV and RV function is an integral part in clinical decision making in patients with known or suspected CHF. Whereas echocardiography remains the most useful method, given its low cost, safety, and adaptability to the critical setting, CMR provides important complementary information with its unique ability to provide "virtual histology." The ability to demonstrate myocardial edema, microvascular obstruction, and the presence or extent of myocardial obstruction makes CMR a powerful tool to establish the etiology and the extent of injury. CMR may potentially prove to be a method to evaluate response to novel therapeutic interventions. Although CCT has been shown to be accurate and reproducible, its role may be limited to provide complementary information in those patients who have been imaged for the evaluation of the coronary anatomy, given the required use of contrast and use of ionizing radiation. Radionuclide methods for the evaluation of LV function are also accurate and reproducible but unlike echocardiography, they cannot provide important information such as myocardial wall thickness, valvular function, and hemodynamic assessment. They may continue to play an important role as an alternative to the patients with limited echocardiographic windows and with contraindications for CMR imaging.

The application of 3-D imaging techniques is likely to replace 2-D imaging techniques for the evaluation of global LV and RV function. Unlike 2-D imaging techniques, 3-D imaging is not limited by geometrical assumptions; therefore, it should prove to be more accurate and reproducible. Quantitative echocardiographic CMR and echocardiographic assessment of regional myocardial function should also provide greater accuracy and reproducibility when compared to the traditional qualitative visual assessment. To gain acceptance, clinical trials will require demonstrating that the adoption of these novel methods leads to improvement in quality and in clinical outcomes. This is an additional challenge that new technologies will face in this new era of cost-containment.

REFERENCES

1. Pratter MR, Curley FJ, Dubois J, et al. Cause and evaluation of chronic dyspnea in a pulmonary disease clinic. *Arch Intern Med.* 1989;149:2277–2282
2. American Thoracic Society. Dyspnea. Mechanisms, assessment, and management: A consensus statement. *Am J Respir Crit Care Med.* 1999;159:321–340.
3. DePaso WJ, Winterbauer RH, Lusk JA, et al. Chronic dyspnea unexplained by history, physical examination, chest roentgenogram, and spirometry. Analysis of a seven-year experience. *Chest.* 1991;100:1293–1299.
4. Redfield MM, Jacobsen SJ, Burnett JC Jr, et al. Burden of systolic and diastolic ventricular dysfunction in the community: Appreciating the scope of the heart failure epidemic. *JAMA.* 2003;289:194–202.
5. Elliott MW, Adams L, Cockcroft A, et al. The language of breathlessness. Use of verbal descriptors by patients with cardiopulmonary disease. *Am Rev Respir Dis.* 1991;144:826–832.
6. Pauwels RA, Buist AS, Ma P, et al. GOLD Scientific Committee. Global strategy for the diagnosis, management and prevention of chronic obstructive pulmonary disease. *Respir Care.* 2001;46:798–825.
7. Baicu CF, Zile MR, Aurigemma GP, et al. Left ventricular systolic performance, function, and contractility in patients with diastolic heart failure. *Circulation.* 2005;111:2306–2312.
8. Suga H, Sagawa K. Instantaneous pressure–volume relationships and their ratio in the excised, supported canine left ventricle. *Circ Res.* 1974;35:117–126.
9. Kawaguchi M, Hay I, Fetics B, et al. Combined ventricular systolic and arterial stiffening in patients with heart failure and preserved ejection fraction: Implications for systolic and diastolic reserve limitations. *Circulation.* 2003;107(5):656–658.
10. Greenberg NL, Firstenberg MS, Castro PL, et al. Doppler-derived myocardial systolic strain rate is a strong index of left ventricular contractility. *Circulation.* 2002;105(1):99–105.
11. Weidemann F, Jamal F, Sutherland GR, et al. Myocardial function defined by strain rate and strain during alterations in inotropic states and heart rate. *Am J Physiol.* 2002;283(2):H792–H799.
12. Streeter DD Jr, Spotnitz HM, Patel DP, et al. Fiber orientation in the canine left ventricle during diastole and systole. *Circ Res.* 1969;24:339–347.
13. Arts T, Reneman RS. Dynamics of left ventricular wall and mitral valve mechanics—a model study. *J Biomech.* 1989;22:261–271.
14. Beyar R, Yin FC, Hausknecht M, et al. Dependence of left ventricular twist-radial shortening relations on cardiac cycle phase. *Am J Physiol.* 1989;257:H1119–H1126.
15. Ingels NB Jr, Hansen DE, Daughters GT II, et al. Relation between longitudinal, circumferential, and oblique shortening and torsional deformation in the left ventricle of the transplanted human heart. *Circ Res.* 1989;64:915–927.
16. Rademakers FE, Buchalter MB, Rogers WJ, et al. Dissociation between left ventricular untwisting and filling. Accentuation by catecholamines. *Circulation.* 1992;85:1572–1581.
17. Stuber M, Scheidegger MB, Fischer SE, et al. Alterations in the local myocardial motion pattern in patients suffering from pressure overload due to aortic stenosis. *Circulation.* 1999;100:361–368.
18. Bell SP, Nyland L, Tischler MD, et al. Alterations in the determinants of diastolic suction during pacing tachycardia. *Circ Res.* 2000;87:235–240.
19. Dong SJ, Hees PS, Siu CO, et al. MRI assessment of LV relaxation by untwisting rate: A new isovolumic phase measure of tau. *Am J Physiol Heart Circ Physiol.* 2001;281:H2002–H2009.
20. Nikolic S, Yellin EL, Tamura K, et al. Passive properties of canine left ventricle: Diastolic stiffness and restoring forces. *Circ Res.* 1988;62:1210–1222.
21. Yellin EL, Hori M, Yoran C, et al. Left ventricular relaxation in the filling and nonfilling intact canine heart. *Am J Physiol.* 1986;250:H620–H629.
22. Yturralde FR, Gaasch WH. Diagnostic criteria for diastolic heart failure. *Prog CV Dis.* 2005;47:314–319.
23. Aurigemma GP, Gaasch WH. Diastolic heart failure. *N Engl J Med.* 2004;351:1097–1105.
24. Katz AM, Zile MR. New molecular mechanism in diastolic heart failure. *Circulation.* 2006;113:1922–1925.
25. Gaasch WH, LeWinter MM. *Left Ventricular Diastolic Dysfunction and Heart Failure.* Philadelphia, PA: Lea & Febiger; 1994:3–140.
26. Katz AM. *Physiology of the Heart.* New York, NY: Raven Press; 1992:151–177.
27. Grossman W. *Diastolic Relaxation of the Heart.* Boston: Martinez Nijhoff; 1988.
28. Morgan JP. Mechanisms of disease: Abnormal intracellular modulation of calcium as a major cause of cardiac contractile dysfunction. *N Engl J Med.* 1991;325:625.
29. Courtois M and Ludbrook PA. Intraventricular pressure transients during relaxation and filling. In: Gaasch WH, LeWinter MM, eds. *Left Ventricular Diastolic Dysfunction and Heart Failure.* Philadelphia: Lea & Febiger; 1994:150–166.
30. Ling D, Rankin JS, Edwards CH, et al. Regional diastolic mechanics of the left ventricle in the conscious dog. *Am J Physiol.* 1979;236:(Heart Circ Physiol 5):H323–H330.
31. Weiss JL, Frederiksen JW, Weisfeldt ML. Hemodynamic determinants of the time-course of fall in canine left ventricular pressure. *J Clin Invest.* 1976;58:751–760.
32. Factor SM, Flomenbaum M, Zhao MJ, et al. The effect of acutely increased ventricular cavity pressure on intrinsic myocardial connective tissue. *J Am Coll Cardiol.* 1988;12:1582.
33. Templeton GH, Donald IT, Mitchell JH, et al. Dynamic stiffness of papillary muscle during contraction and relaxation. *Am J Physiol.* 1973;224:692–698.
34. Janicki JS, Matsubara BB. Myocardial collagen and left ventricular diastolic function. In: Gaasch WH, LeWinter MM, eds. *Left Ventricular Diastolic Dysfunction and Heart Failure.* Philadelphia, PA: Lea & Febiger; 1994:125–140.
35. Robinson TF, Factor SF, Sonnenblick EH. The heart as a suction pump. *Sci Am.* 1986;254:84.
36. Janicki JS, Matsubara BB, Kabour A. Myocardial collagen and its functional role. *Adv Exp Med Biol.* 1993;346:291–298.
37. Nishimura RA, Abel MD, Hatle LK, et al. Relation of pulmonary vein to mitral flow velocities by transesophageal Doppler echocardiography. Effect of different loading conditions. *Circulation.* 1990;81(5):1488.
38. Manning WJ, Leeman DE, Gotch PJ, et al. Pulsed Doppler evaluation of atrial mechanical function after electrical cardioversion of atrial fibrillation. *J Am Coll Cardiol.* 1989;13:617.
39. Polak JF, Holman BL, Wynne J, et al. Right ventricular ejection fraction: An indicator of increased mortality in patients with congestive heart failure associated with coronary artery disease. *J Am Coll Cardiol.* 1983;2:217–224.
40. de Groote P, Millaire A, Foucher-Hossein C, et al. Right ventricular ejection fraction is an independent predictor of survival in patients with moderate heart failure. *J Am Coll Cardiol.* 1998;32:948–954.
41. Mehta SR, Eikelboom JW, Natarajan MK, et al. Impact of right ventricular involvement on mortality and morbidity in patients with inferior myocardial infarction. *J Am Coll Cardiol.* 2001;37:37–43.
42. Grant RP, Downey FM, MacMahon H. The architecture of the right ventricular outflow tract in the normal human heart and in the presence of ventricular septal defects. *Circulation.* 1961;24:223–235.
43. Dell'Italia LJ. The right ventricle: Anatomy, physiology, and clinical importance. *Curr Probl Cardiol.* 1991;16:653–720.
44. Torrent-Guasp F, Buckberg GD, Clemente C, et al. The structure and function of the helical heart and its buttress wrapping. I. The normal macroscopic structure of the heart. *Semin Thorac Cardio vasc Surg.* 2001;13:301–319.
45. Kono T, Sabbah HN, Rosman H, et al. Left atrial contribution to ventricular filling during the course of evolving heart failure. *Circulation.* 1992;86:1317–1322.
46. Tsang TS, Barnes ME, Gersh BJ, et al. Left atrial volume as a morphophysiologic expression of left ventricular diastolic dysfunction and relation to cardiovascular risk burden. *Am J Cardiol.* 2002;90:1284–1289.
47. Benjamin EJ, D'Agostino RB, Belanger AJ, et al. Left atrial size and the risk of stroke and death: The Framingham Heart study. *Circulation.* 1995;92:835–841.
48. Flaker GC, Fletcher KA, Rothbart RM, et al. Clinical and echocardiographic features of intermittent atrial fibrillation that predict recurrent atrial fibrillation (stroke prevention in atrial fibrillation (SPAF) investigators). *Am J Cardiol.* 1995;76:355–358.
49. Møller JE, Hillis GS, Oh JK, et al. Left atrial volume. A powerful predictor of survival after acute myocardial infarction. *Circulation.* 2003;107:2207–2212.
50. Beinart R, Boyko V, Schwammenthal E., et al. Long-term prognostic significance of left atrial volume in acute myocardial infarction. *J Am Coll Cardiol.* 2004;44:327–334.
51. Rossi A, Cicoira M, Zanolla L, et al. Determinants and prognostic value of left atrial volume in patients with dilated cardiomyopathy. *J Am Coll Cardiol.* 2002;40:1425.
52. Sabharwal N, Cemin R, Rajan K, et al. Usefulness of left atrial volume as a predictor of mortality in patients with ischemic cardiomyopathy. *Am J Cardiol.* 2004;94:760–763.
53. Schabelman S, Schiller NB, Silverman NH, et al. Left atrial volume estimation by two-dimensional echocardiography. *Catheter Cardiovasc Diagn.* 1981;7:165–178.
54. Vandenberg BF, Weiss RM, Kinzey J, et al. Comparison of left atrial volume by two-dimensional echocardiography and cine-computed tomography. *Am J Cardiol.* 1995;75:754–757.
55. Rodevan O, Bjornerheim R, Ljosland M, et al. Left atrial volumes assessed by three- and two-dimensional echocardiography compared to MRI estimates. *Int J Card Imaging.* 1999;15:397–410.
56. Wieczorek SJ, Wu AH, Christenson R, et al. A rapid B-natriuretic peptide assay accurately diagnoses left ventricular dysfunction and heart failure: A multicenter evaluation. *Am Heart J.* 2002;144:834–839.
57. ATS/ACCP Statement on cardiopulmonary exercise testing. American Thoracic Society; American College of Chest Physicians. *Am J Respir Crit Care Med.* 2003;167:211–277.
58. Dubin J, Wallerson DC, Cody RJ, et al. Comparative accuracy of Doppler echocardiographic methods for clinical stroke volume determination. *Am Heart J.* 1990;120:116–123.
59. Shiota T, McCarthy PM, White RD, et al. Initial clinical experience of real-time three-dimensional echocardiography in patients with ischemic and idiopathic dilated cardiomyopathy. *Am J Cardiol.* 1999;84:1068–1073.
60. Bargiggia GS, Bertucci C, Recusani F, et al. A new method for estimating left ventricular dp/dt by continuous wave Doppler-echocardiography. Validation studies at cardiac catheterization. *Circulation.* 1989;80:1287–1292.
61. Roman MJ, Devereaux RB, Cody RJ. Ability of left ventricular stress-shortening relations, end-systolic stress/volume ratio and indirect indexes to detect severe contractile failure in ischemic or idiopathic dilated cardiomyopathy. *Am J Cardiol.* 1989;64:1338–1343.
62. Reichek N, Wilson J, St John Sutton M, et al. Noninvasive determination of left ventricular end-systolic stress. Validation of the method and initial application. *Circulation.* 1982;65:99–108.
63. Douglas PS, Reichek N, Hackney K, et al. Contribution of afterload, hypertrophy and geometry to left ventricular ejection fraction in aortic valve stenosis, pure aortic regurgitation and idiopathic dilated cardiomyopathy. *Am J Cardiol.* 1987;59:1398–1404.

64. Gorcsan J, III, Denault A, Mandarino WA, et al. Left ventricular pressure–volume relations with transesophageal echocardiographic automated border detection: Comparison with conductance-catheter technique. *Am Heart J.* 1996;131:544–552.

65. Marsh JD, Green LH, Wynne J, et al. Left ventricular end-systolic pressure-dimension and stress-length relations in normal human subjects. *Am J Cardiol.* 1979;44:1311–1317.

66. Hsia HH, Starling MR. Is standardization of left ventricular chamber elastance necessary? *Circulation.* 1990;81:1826–1836.

67. Miyatake K, Yamagishi M, Tanaka N, et al. New method for evaluating left ventricular wall motion by color-coded tissue Doppler imaging. In vitro and in vivo studies. *J Am Coll Cardiol.* 1995;25:717–724.

68. Garcia MJ, Rodriguez L, Ares MA, et al. Differentiation of constrictive pericarditis from restrictive cardiomyopathy: Assessment of left ventricular diastolic velocities in the longitudinal axis by Tissue Doppler imaging. *J Am Coll Cardiol.* 1996;27:108–114.

69. Smith SW, Wagner RF. Ultrasound speckle size and lesion signal to noise ratio: Verification of theory. *Ultrason Imaging.* 1984 April;6(2):174–180.

70. Ogawa K, Hozumi T, Sugioka K, et al. Usefulness of automated quantitation of regional left ventricular wall motion by a novel method of two-dimensional echocardiographic tracking. *Am J Cardiol.* 2006 Dec 1;98(11):1531–1537.

71. Notomi Y, Lysyansky P, Setser RM, et al. Measurement of ventricular torsion by two-dimensional ultrasound speckle tracking imaging. *J Am Coll Cardiol.* 2005. Jun 21;45(12):2034–2041.

72. Helle-Valle T, Crosby J, Edvardsen T, et al. New noninvasive method for assessment of left ventricular rotation: Speckle tracking echocardiography. *Circulation.* 2005 Nov 15;112(20):3149–3156.

73. Appleton CP, Hatle LK. The natural history of left ventricular filling abnormalities: Assessment by two-dimensional and Doppler echocardiography. *Echocardiography.* 1992;9:437.

74. Larkin H, Johnson DC, Hunyor SN, et al. Anatomical accuracy of echocardiographically assessed left ventricular wall thickness. *Clin Sci.* 57:1979;55S.

75. Himelman RB, Kircher B, Rockey DC, et al. Inferior vena cava plethora with blunted respiratory response: A sensitive echocardiographic sign of cardiac tamponade. *J Am Coll Cardiol.* 1988;12(6):1470.

76. Choong CY, Abascal VA, Thomas JD, et al. The combined effect of ventricular loading and relaxation on the transmitral flow velocity profile in dogs measured by Doppler echocardiography. *Circulation.* 1988;78:672.

77. Hoit BD, Shao Y, Gabel M, et al. In-vivo assessment of left atrial contractile performance in normal and pathological conditions using a time varying elastance model. *Circulation.* 1994;89:1829.

78. Hoit BD, Shao Y, Tsai LM, et al. Altered left atrial compliance after atrial appendectomy: Influence on left atrial and ventricular filling. *Circ Res.* 1993;72:167–175.

79. Thomas JD, Aragam JR, Rodriguez LL, et al. Spatiotemporal distribution of mitral inflow velocity: Use of the color Doppler M-mode echocardiogram to investigate intracardiac pressure gradients (abstract). *Med Biol Eng Comput.* 1991;29:(Suppl I):130.

80. Brun P, Tribouilloy C, Duval AM, et al. Left ventricular flow propagation during early filling is related to wall relaxation: A color M-mode Doppler analysis. *J Am Coll Cardiol.* 1992;20:420.

81. Stuggard M, Smiseth OA, Risoe C, et al. Intraventricular early diastolic filling during acute myocardial ischemia: Assessment by multigated color M-mode Doppler echocardiography. *Circulation.* 1993;88:2705.

82. Garcia MJ, Smedira NG, Greenberg NL, et al. Color M-mode Doppler flow propagation is a preload insensitive index of left ventricular relaxation. Animal and human validation. *J Am Coll Cardiol.* 2000;35:201–208.

83. Takatsuji H, Mikami T, Urasawa K, et al. A new approach for evaluation of left ventricular diastolic function: Spatial and temporal analysis of left ventricular filling flow propagation by color M-mode Doppler echocardiography. *J Am Coll Cardiol.* 1996;27:365.

84. Greenberg NL, Vandervoort PM, Firstenberg MS, et al. Estimation of diastolic intraventricular pressure gradients by Doppler M-mode echocardiography. *Am J Physiol Heart Circ Physiol.* 2001 Jun;280:(6): H2507–H2515.

85. Bermejo J, Antoranz JC, Yotti R, et al. Spatio-temporal mapping of intracardiac pressure gradients. A solution to Euler's equation from digital postprocessing of color Doppler M-mode echocardiograms. *Ultrasound Med Biol.* 2001;27:621–630.

86. Thomas JD, Weyman AE. Echocardiographic Doppler evaluation of left ventricular diastolic function. Physics and physiology. *Circulation.* 1990;84:977.

87. Thomas JD, Choong CY, Flachskampf F, et al. Analysis of the early transmitral Doppler velocity curve: Effect of primary physiologic changes and compensatory preload adjustment. *J Am Coll Cardiol.* 1990;16:644.

88. Garcia MJ, Ares MA, Asher C, et al. Color M-mode flow velocity propagation: An index of early left ventricular filling that combined with pulsed Doppler peak E velocity may predict capillary wedge pressure. *J Am Coll Cardiol.* 1997;29:448.

89. Rossvoll O, Hatle LK. Pulmonary venous flow velocities recorded by transthoracic Doppler ultrasound: Relation to left ventricular diastolic pressures. *J Am Coll Cardiol.* 1993;21(7):1687.

90. McDicken WN, Sutherland GR, Moran CM, et al. Color Doppler velocity imaging of the myocardium. *Ultrasound Med Biol.* 1992;18:651.

91. Nagueh SF, Middleton KJ, Kopelen HA, et al. Tissue Doppler imaging: A noninvasive technique for evaluation of left ventricular relaxation and estimation of filling pressures. *J Am Coll Cardiol.* 1997;30(6):1527–1533.

92. Klein AL, Tajik AJ. Doppler assessment of diastolic function in cardiac amyloidosis. *Echocardiography.* 1991;8:233.

93. Grodecki PV, Klein AL. Pitfalls in the echo-Doppler assessment of diastolic dysfunction. *Echocardiography.* 1993;10:213.

94. Otto CM, Pearlman AS, Amsler LC. Doppler echocardiographic evaluation of left ventricular diastolic filling in isolated valvular aortic stenosis. *Am J Cardiol.* 1989;63:313–316.

95. Takenaka K, Dabestani A, Gardin JM, et al. Left ventricular filling in hypertrophic cardiomyopathy: A pulsed Doppler echocardiographic study. *J Am Coll Cardiol.* 1986;7:1263.

96. Iliceto S, Amico A, Marangelli V, et al. Doppler echocardiographic evaluation of the effect of atrial pacing-induced ischemia on left ventricular filling in patients with coronary artery disease. *J Am Coll Cardiol.* 1988;11:953.

97. Glower DD, Murrah RL, Olsen CO, et al. Mechanical correlates of the third heart sound. *J Am Coll Cardiol.* 1992;19:450.

98. Tei C. New non-invasive index for combined systolic and diastolic ventricular function. *J Cardiol.* 1995;26:135.

99. Harada T, Masamichi M, Toyono K, et al. Assessment of global left ventricular function by tissue Doppler imaging. *Am J Cardiol.* 2001;88:927–932.

100. Tei C, Nishimura RA, Seward JB, et al. Noninvasive Doppler-derived myocardial performance index: Correlation with simultaneous measurements of cardiac catheterization measurements. *J Am Soc Echocardiogr.* 1997;10:169–178.

101. Feigenbaum H. *Echocardiography.* 6th Ed. Philadelphia: Lippincott Williams and Wilkins, 2005.

102. Schenk P, Globits S, Koller J, et al. Accuracy of echocardiographic right ventricular parameters in patients with different end-stage lung diseases prior to lung transplantation. *J Heart Lung Transplant.* 2000;19:145–153.

103. Kovalova S, Necas J, Cerbak R, et al. Echocardiographic volumetry of the right ventricle. *Eur J Echocardiography.* 2005;6:15–23.

104. Kaul S, Tei C, Hopkins JM, et al. Assessment of right ventricular function using two-dimensional echocardiography. *Am Heart J.* 1984;107:526–531.

105. Meluzin J, Spinarova L, Bakala J, et al. Pulsed Doppler tissue imaging of the velocity of tricuspid annular systolic motion. *Eur Heart J.* 2001;22:340–348.

106. Alam M, Wardell J, Andersson E, et al. Right ventricular function in patients with first inferior myocardial infarction: Assessment by tricuspid annular motion and tricuspid annular velocity. *Am Heart J.* 2000;139:710–715.

107. Jamal F, Bergerot C, Argaud L, et al. Longitudinal strain quantitates regional right ventricular contractile function. *Am J Physiol Heart Circ Physiol.* 2003;285:H2842–H2847.

108. Yeo TC, Dujardin KS, Tei C, et al. Value of a Doppler-derived index combining systolic and diastolic time intervals in predicting outcome in primary pulmonary hypertension. *Am J Cardiol.* 1998;81:1157–1161.

109. Johannessen KA, Cerqueira M, Veith RC, et al. The relation between radionuclide angiography and Doppler echocardiography during contractile changes with infusions of epinephrine. *Int J Cardiol.* 1991;33:149–157.

110. Arrighi JA, Soufer R. Left ventricular diastolic function: Physiology, methods of assessment, and clinical significance. *J Nucl Cardiol.* 1995;2:525–543.

111. Maddahi J, Berman DS, Matsuoka DT, et al. A new technique for assessing right ventricular ejection fraction using rapid multiple-gated equilibrium cardiac blood pool scintigraphy. *Circulation.* 1979;60:581–589.

112. Morrison D, Marshall J, Wright A1, et al. An improved method of right ventricular gated equilibrium blood pool radionuclide ventriculography. *Chest.* 1982;82:607–614.

113. Johnson LL, Lawson MA, Blackwell GG, et al. Optimizing the method to calculate right ventricular ejection fraction from first-pass data acquired with a multicrystal camera. *J Nucl Cardiol.* 1995;2:372–379.

114. Hundt W, Siebert K, Wintersperger BJ, et al. Assessment of global left ventricular function: Comparison of cardiac multidetector-row computed tomography with angiocardiography. *J Comput Assist Tomogr.* 2005;29:373–381.

115. Orakzai SH, Orakzai RH, Nasir K, et al. Assessment of cardiac function using multidetector row computed tomography. *J Comput Assist Tomogr.* 2006;30:555–563.

116. Raman SV, Shah M, McCarthy B, et al. Multidetector row cardiac computed tomography accurately quantifies right and left ventricular size and function compared with cardiac magnetic resonance. *Am Heart J.* 2006;151:736–744.

117. Sugeng L, Mor-Avi V, Weinert L, et al. Quantitative assessment of left ventricular size and function: Side-by-side comparison of real-time three-dimensional echocardiography and computed tomography with magnetic resonance reference. *Circulation.* 2006;114:654–661.

118. Lembcke A, Dohmen PM, Dewey M, et al. Multislice computed tomography for preoperative evaluation of right ventricular volumes and function: Comparison with magnetic resonance imaging. *Ann Thorac Surg.* 2005;79:1344–1351.

119. Koch K, Oellig F, Oberholzer K, et al. Assessment of right ventricular function by 16-detector-row CT: Comparison with magnetic resonance imaging. *Eur Radiol.* 2005;15:312–318.

120. Hunninghake GW, Lynch DA, Galvin JR, et al. Radiologic findings are strongly associated with a pathological diagnosis of usual interstitial pneumonia. *Chest.* 2003;124:1215–1223.

121. Pennell DJ, Sechtem UP, Higgins CB, et al. Clinical indications for cardiovascular magnetic resonance (CMR). Consensus Panel report. *Eur Heart J.* 2004;25:1940–1965.

122. Grothues F, Smith GC, Moon JC, et al. Comparison of interstudy reproducibility of cardiovascular magnetic resonance with two-dimensional echocardiography in normal subjects and in patients with heart failure or left ventricular hypertrophy. *Am J Cardiol.* 2002;90:29–34.

123. Bellenger NG, Davies LC, Francis JM, et al. Reduction in sample size for studies of remodeling in heart failure by the use of cardiovascular magnetic resonance. *J Cardiovasc Magn Reson.* 2000;2:271–278.

124. Zerhouni EA, Parish DM, Rogers WJ, et al. Human heart: Tagging with MR imaging—a method for noninvasive assessment of myocardial motion. *Radiology.* 1988;83:862–973.

125. Rubinshtein R, Glockner JF, Feng D, et al. Comparison of magnetic resonance imaging versus Doppler echocardiography for the evaluation of left ventricular diastolic function in patients with cardiac amyloidosis. *Am J Cardiol.* 2009;103(5). 718–723.

126. Mogelvang J, Stubgaard M, Thomsen C, et al. Evaluation of right ventricular volumes measured by magnetic resonance imaging. *Eur Heart J.* 1988;9:529–533.

127. Grothues F, Moon JC, Bellenger NG, et al. Interstudy reproducibility of right ventricular volumes, function, and mass with cardiovascular magnetic resonance. *Am Heart J.* 2004;147:218–223.

128. Alfakih K, Plein S, Bloomer T, et al. Comparison of right ventricular volume measurements between axial and short axis orientation using steady-state free precession magnetic resonance imaging. *J Magn Reson Imaging.* 2003;18:25–32.

129. Kim RJ, Fieno DS, Parrish TB, et al. Relationship of MRI delayed contrast enhancement to irreversible injury, infarct age and contractile function. *Circulation.* 1999;100:1992–2002.

130. Thomson LE, Kim RJ, Judd RM. Magnetic resonance imaging for the assessment of myocardial viability. *J Magn Reson Imaging.* 2004;19:771–788.

131. Selvanayagam JB, Kardos A, Francis JM, et al. Value of delayed-enhancement cardiovascular magnetic resonance imaging in predicting myocardial viability after surgical revascularization. *Circulation.* 2004;110:1535–1541.

132. Kuhl HP, Beek AM, van der Weerdt AP, et al. Myocardial viability in chronic ischemic heart disease: Comparison of contrast-enhanced magnetic resonance imaging with (18)F-fluorodeoxyglucose positron emission tomography. *J Am Coll Cardiol.* 2003;41:1341–1348.

133. Gavazzi A, Berzuini C, Campana C, et al. Value of right ventricular ejection fraction in predicting short-term prognosis of patients with severe chronic heart failure. *J Heart Lung Transplant.* 1997;16:774–785.

134. Graham TP Jr, Bernard YD, Mellen BG, et al. Long-term outcome in congenitally corrected transposition of the great arteries: A multi-institutional study. *J Am Coll Cardiol.* 2000;36:255–261.

135. D'Alonzo GE, Barst RJ, Ayres SM, et al. Survival in patients with primary pulmonary hypertension. Results from a national prospective registry. *Ann Intern Med.* 1991;115:343–349.

136. Aurigemma GP, Gottdiener JS, Shemanski L, et al. Predictive value of systolic and diastolic function for incident congestive heart failure in the elderly. The cardiovascular study. *J Am Coll Cardiol.* 2001;37:1042–1048.

137. Bella JN, Palmieri V, Roman MJ et al. Mitral ratio of peak early to late diastolic filling velocity as a predictor of mortality in middle-aged and elderly adults. The Strong Heart Study. *Circulation.* 2002;105:1928–1933.

138. Rihal CS, Nishimura RA, Hatle LK et al. Systolic and diastolic dysfunction in patients with clinical diagnosis of dilated cardiomyopathy. Relation to symptoms and prognosis. *Circulation.* 1994;90:2772–2779.

139. Wang M, Yip G, Yu CM, et al. Independent and incremental prognostic value of early mitral annulus velocity in patients with impaired left ventricular systolic function. *J Am Coll* Cardiol. 2005;45:272–277.

140. Tei C, Dujardin KS, Hodge DO, et al. Doppler index combining systolic and diastolic myocardial performance: Clinical value in cardiac amyloidosis. *J Am Coll Cardiol.* 1996;28:658–664.

141. Dujardin KS, Tei C, Yeo TC, et al. Prognostic value of a Doppler index combining systolic and diastolic performance in idiopathic-dilated cardiomyopathy. *Am J Cardiol.* 1998;82:1071–1076.

142. Moller JE, Egstrup K, Kober L, et al. Prognostic importance of systolic and diastolic function after acute myocardial infarction. *Am Heart J.* 2003;145:147–153.

143. Harjai KJ, Scott L, Vivekananthan K, et al. The Tei index: A new prognostic index for patients with symptomatic heart failure. *J Am Soc Echocardiogr.* 2002;15:864–868.

144. Quinones MA, Greenberg BH, Kopelen HA, et al. Echocardiographic predictors of clinical outcome in patients with left ventricular dysfunction enrolled in the SOLVD registry and trials: Significance of left ventricular hypertrophy: Studies of left ventricular dysfunction. *J Am Coll Cardiol.* 2000;35:1237–1244.

145. Gerber BL, Garot J, Bluemke DA, et al. Accuracy of contrast-enhanced magnetic resonance imaging in predicting improvement of regional myocardial function in patients after acute myocardial infarction. *Circulation.* 2002;106:1083–1089.

146. Kim R, Wu E, Rafael A, et al. The use of contrast-enhanced magnetic resonance imaging to identify reversible myocardial dysfunction. *N Engl J Med.* 2000;343:1445–1453.

147. Kim RJ, Shah DJ. Fundamental concepts in myocardial viability assessment revisited: When knowing how much is "alive" is not enough. *Heart.* 2004;90:137–140.

148. Assomull RG, Prasad SK, Burman E, et al. Cardiovascular magnetic resonance, fibrosis and prognosis in dilated cardiomyopathy. *J Cardiovasc Magn Reson.* 2006;8:3–4.

Syncope

Fetnat Fouad-Tarazi
Kenneth A. Mayuga
Huijan Wang

17

1. INTRODUCTION

Syncope has become a well-recognized disease entity that affects all ages. It occurs alone or in association with other medical conditions. Syncope is the ultimate most severe form of abnormal cardiovascular responses to decrease blood pressure; it occurs commonly during upright posture. It may be preceded by any of the other components of the overall spectrum of orthostatic intolerance. Symptoms related to upright posture are essentially due to the effect of gravity on the circulation and the autonomic nervous system (ANS). Such symptoms may present as dizziness, light-headedness, palpitations, nausea, excess sweating, or tremulousness. Mild symptoms can generally be stopped and relieved by changing posture to a sitting or supine position; otherwise, symptoms may continue, increase, and result in loss of consciousness.

Although postural hypotension is a major presentation of postural intolerance, sometimes symptoms provoked by upright posture are not associated with a drop of blood pressure. In some situations, an accentuated increase in heart rate during the upright position is the main feature of the postural imbalance; impaired cardiac filling due to encroachment of ventricular diastole under these circumstances may provoke symptoms; and this category has been identified as postural orthostatic tachycardia syndrome or POTS.

In general, the patients are advised to sit down or lie down at the onset of postural symptoms to avoid falls with subsequent injuries. Occasionally patients find that they automatically start walking when postural symptoms start during passive standing and they report improvement of symptoms when walking; this phenomenon is probably related to assistance of circulatory dynamics by the contracting skeletal muscles allowing a better venous flow to counterbalance the effect of gravity.

2. PREVALENCE

Syncope and orthostatic hypotension are not rare. Syncope was found to occur in 1% to 6% of hospital admissions and up to 3% of emergency department visits.[1]

Syncope in the elderly is particularly risky[2,3] due to possible associated bone injuries and possible concurrent cardiovascular etiologies such as conduction abnormalities and serious arrhythmias; moreover, it's frequently observed that orthostatic hypotension in the elderly may reach very low levels of blood pressures before symptoms appear, an event that may be related to changes in the autoregulatory mechanisms of the cerebral circulation.[4] It has been also noted in institutionalized patients in the elderly age group that orthostatic hypotension may be initiated after a meal—postprandial hypotension.[5] Such events sometimes remain unexplained until postural blood pressure is taken into consideration when blood pressure is measured in both the supine and upright positions.

2.1. Risk stratification of syncope

Although syncope is by definition a transient self-limited loss of consciousness, it was demonstrated that the presence of underlying heart disease is accompanied by a poor prognosis.[6,7] It was reported that 70% of patients experiencing recurrent syncope suffer challenges in their quality of life, 6% sustain fractures, 39% change jobs, and 64% have restricted driving abilities.[8,9] Physiological impacts were also reported in relation to recurrent syncopal events.

Recently, risk stratification of syncope received special attention particularly in relation to decision-making in the emergency room setting; the cost benefit ratio of hospital admission after an emergency department visit has been often questioned.[10,11]

The San Francisco syncope rule is an instrument that was recently designed to identify low risk of serious clinical events over a short term (7 days and 30 days) in patients presenting with syncope or near syncope.[12,13] A 2007 report of Emergency Department patients with serious outcomes found the majority to have brain natriuretic peptide (BNP) elevation of >100 pg/mL, and the authors recommended additional studies to evaluate this finding.[14]

3. PATHOPHYSIOLOGY

Syncope is triggered by the interaction between both biological and environmental factors that modify cardiovascular homeostasis.

The circulatory system is regulated by the ANS as well as by humoral and hormonal factors. The ANS is important in the immediate response of blood pressure and heart rate to altered posture. The hormonal and humoral factors are thought to intervene later to assist in the maintenance of the circulatory balance.

The normal hemodynamic response to gravity while in the upright posture is influenced by several factors including the distensibility of the veins below the level of the heart, the reactivity of arterioles to vasoconstrictor stimuli, and the circulating intravascular blood volume. Furthermore, an increased capillary pressure during venous distension provokes ultra filtration with a shift of fluid from the intravascular space to the interstitial space causing a decrease of plasma volume (estimated at 15% reduction within 20 min of standing). The decreased plasma volume is reflected by increased hematocrit in the upright posture.[15]

Pooling of blood in the veins decreases venous return to the heart with subsequent reduction of stroke volume and cardiac output; consequently, the blood pressure will tend to fall unless compensatory mechanisms come into play including activation of sympathetic outflow, increased catecholamine secretion, and activation of the renin angiotensin system and of the arginine vasopressin system. The role of endothelin, nitric oxide (NO), and other factors such as BNP and kidney perfusion have not been studied extensively.

The regulatory function of the ANS is intricate and very well organized.[16,17] The central autonomic network (CAN) regulating the cardiovascular system is located in the brain stem. The nucleus tractus solitarius (NTS) is a major component of the CAN; it integrates and regulates the sympathetic and parasympathetic components of the ANS. The NTS is located in the dorsal medial aspect of the medulla, anterior to the dorsal vagal nucleus.

Several sensors communicate peripheral circulatory and positional changes to the central nervous system. These sensors respond to changes in blood volume, cardiopulmonary volume, tension in the walls of the large arteries, tension in the walls of the cardiac atria and ventricles, distension of pulmonary alveoli, chemical alterations at specific sites (coronaries, carotid body), skeletal muscle contraction, and possibly the vestibular apparatus.

Afferent connections convey information to the central nervous system; afferent pathways originate from various cardiovascular regions including the carotid sinus, the aortic arch, the atria, the ventricles, the coronaries, as well as the cardiopulmonary area. Sensory afferents are activated by mechanical or chemo sensitive specialized receptors. The efferent connections from the NTS supply the dorsal vagal motor nucleus as well as the reticular formation in the ventral-lateral medulla; they also travel to the hypothalamus, the limbic system, and amygdala. It is thought that the cerebellar vermis is a neural substrate for regulation of voluntary upright posture since an orthostatic positron emission tomography (PET) study showed that cerebellar vermis activation was more marked in the standing position than in the sitting or supine positions.[18] It is well recognized that the physiologic regulatory function of the afferent neural pathways are altered in cardiovascular dysfunction such as hypertension, atherosclerosis, myocardial ischemia, and diabetes mellitus.

The NTS has extensive afferent and efferent connections to the higher brain centers as well as to the cardiovascular system and other organs including respiratory, gastrointestinal, and somatic pathways. Both the chronotropic and inotropic cardiac function and the peripheral vascular tone are influenced by the NTS.

Norephinephrine release causes vasoconstriction, venoconstriction, increased cardiac inotropism, and chronotropism.

It is noteworthy that the main mechanism of loss of consciousness during a syncopal event or obtunded consciousness during near syncope is caused by a fall in blood pressure, which then results in decreased cerebral perfusion. A protective physiologic mechanism is made possible by the phenomenon of the cerebral circulation autoregulation. Through this mechanism the brain perfusion can be preserved in the face of significant changes in blood pressure; regional cerebral blood flow is maintained constant over a range of perfusion pressure from 50 to 140 mm Hg. Blood pressures below the lower limit of autoregulation causes brain hypoxia.[4]

3.1. Classification of orthostatic intolerance and syncope

For practical purposes, a causal classification helps a Medical Care Provider categorize pathways for the diagnosis and treatment of syncope and orthostatic intolerance (Table 17.1).

TABLE 17.1
SYNCOPE CLASSIFICATION BY CAUSE

Cardiovascular	Autonomic neural dysfunction
1. Cardiac	1. Autonomic insufficiency
Arrhythmias	Central
Conduction defects	Afferent
Obstructive heart diseases	Efferent preganglionic disturbance
2. Vascular	Efferent postganglionic disturbance
Reduced arteriolar vascular reactivity	2. Autonomic neural imbalances
Impaired large arterial compliance	(i) Neurocardiogenic syncope/ NCG
Impaired venous contractility	Vasovagal
3. Severe hypovolemia	Vasodepressor
	Mixed types
	(ii) Postural tachycardia syndrome (POTS)
	(iii) Specific reflex types
	Cough
	Laughter
	Micturition
	Defecation
	3. Primary (genetic or degenerative)
	Abnormality initiated in the ANS without other causative factors
	4. Secondary
	Provoked by other illnesses or medications

Each of these diagnoses may be caused by more than one homeostatic abnormality. For example, progressive orthostatic hypotension (POH) may be caused by severe postural venous pooling, reduced vascular reactivity to adrenergic reflexes, and/or autonomic insufficiency. "Autonomic insufficiency" encompasses various types known as pure autonomic failure, multisystem atrophy, amyloid autonomic failure, and diabetic autonomic failure. Reduction of large arterial compliance causes isolated progressive systolic orthostatic hypotension.

Neurocardiogenic (NCG) syncope/presyncope may be caused by severe hypovolemia, accentuated postural venous pooling, hyperkinetic heart syndromes, and/or autonomic imbalance.

Postural orthostatic tachycardia syndrome (POTS) may be caused by severe hypovolemia, accentuated postural venous pooling, hyperkinetic heart syndromes, and/or autonomic imbalance. In some situations, POTS may then progress to become NCG. Figure 17.1 summarizes the hemodynamic alterations found in 194 POTS patients evaluated in 2007 at Cleveland Clinic.

It is still unclear how syncope/presyncope is mediated in valvular and cardiomyopathic obstructive heart disease and pheochromocytoma. It may involve both structural and autonomic reflex abnormalities.

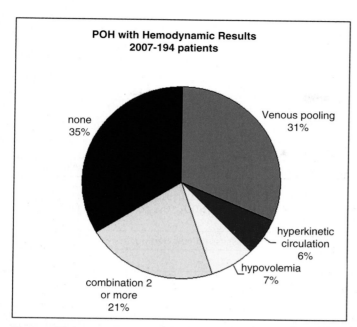

POH with Hemodynamic Results
2007-194 patients

- none 35%
- Venous pooling 31%
- hyperkinetic circulation 6%
- hypovolemia 7%
- combination 2 or more 21%

Figure 17.1 Hemodynamic alterations found in 194 POTS patients evaluated in 2007 at Cleveland Clinic.

It is recognized that patients with migraine, vertigo, sympathetic dystrophy syndrome, and chronic fatigue syndrome may present clinically with homeostatic derangement that operates in parallel to convey new messages to the ANS and subsequently present clinically with cardiovascular manifestations of orthostatic derangement.

4. DIAGNOSTIC TESTS FOR SYNCOPE

A thorough history and physical examination have proven to be the most valuable first steps in obtaining information from the patient, family, and/or bystanders to help differentiate among the various types of syncope and orthostatic intolerance. Further diagnostic workup aims at identification of the underlying biological factors that predispose a person to orthostatic intolerance and/or syncope. Both the cardiovascular/circulatory system and the ANS are major contributors to the individual response to upright posture. Consequently, studies needed for the evaluation of the pathophysiology of orthostatic intolerance/syncope are directed to the cardiovascular system as well as to the ANS. Procedures that help achieve this goal are selected according to the history and physical exam. Normal values for common tests are listed in Table 17.2.

TABLE 17.2
NORMAL VALUES FOR COMMON TESTS

Blood volume test: Results are calculated as excess/deficit in % deviation from ideal (for gender and body surface area)

Plasma volume, total blood volume: Normal deviation 0%–8%, mild deviation 8.1–16, moderate deviation 16.1–24, severe deviation 24.1–32, and extreme deviation >32

Red cell volume: Normal deviation 0%–10%, mild deviation 10.1–20, moderate deviation 20.1–30, severe deviation 30.1–40, and extreme deviation >40

Hematocrit (HCT): 37%–47% in Women; 40%–50% in Men

Cardiac index: 2.9–3.1 L/min/M2

Pulmonary mean transit time: 7–9 s

Vascular resistance: Normal supine 30 Wood units/m², normal response during head-up posture is an increase from baseline.

Hyperkinetic circulation: Cardiac index >3.2 + Pulmonary mean transit time <7 + vascular resistance <28

Hypokinetic circulation: Cardiac index <2.7 + Pulmonary mean transit time >9 + vascular resistance >33

Venous pooling index (Cardiopulmonary volume/Total blood volume):

Supine: normal 14%–18%; supine Venous pooling: <14%; supine venoconstriction: >18%

Postural decrease of cardiopulmonary volume: normal = decrease by 10%–15%, mild postural venous pooling = decrease by 16%–18%, moderate venous pooling = decrease by 18%–24%, marked venous pooling = decrease by 24%–30%, and severe = decrease by >30%

LV ejection fraction: Normal 50%–70%

Valsalva procedure:

Qualitative normal response: BP plateau in late phase II, increased HR in late phase II relative to baseline, Systolic BP Overshoot (rapid increase to above baseline for few cycles) in phase IV associated with slowing of HR in phase IV relative to late phase II and sometimes relative to baseline

Quantitative analysis: [a]Valsalva Ratio [VR] is derived from the maximal heart rate generated by the Valsalva Maneuver divided by the lowest HR occurring within 30 seconds of the peak HR. *Normal VR* varies with age (1.35–1.50 from age 10 to >61yo, VR decreases with advancing age). [a]Vasoconstriction [measured by plethysmography] in phase II and extending to phase IV

VR correlates with the magnitude of SBP overshoot in phase IV due to vagal stimulation via baroreceptor afferent pathway when SBP increases

Abnormal response: Inadequate vasoconstriction in phase II and IV, inability of BP to plateau in late phase II, absence of SBP overshoot in phase IV, inability to increase HR in late phase II, and inability to slow HR in phase IV

(Continued)

TABLE 17.2
NORMAL VALUES FOR COMMON TESTS (Continued)

VR Pitfall: [a]The BP, HR, and extent of arteriolar vasoconstriction in response to the Valsalva procedure are dependent on the extent of fall in venous return during straining. [a]The SBP overshoot in phase IV may be affected by the compliance of the large arteries.

Cold pressor test:

Normal response: increased BP by.10/5 mm Hg and increase of HR by 10 bpm

Plethysmography may show increased flow or increased resistance or bi-phasic response

Abnormal response (Efferent baroreflex arc pathway): no BP rise and chronotropic insufficiency (no increase of HR) during stimulation

Baroreceptor sensitivity:

Normal response: Significant correlation between SBP and next (or next to next) R-R with *r* value >0.70; the corresponding slope varies with age—decreases in advanced age.

Requirement: Decrease or increase in systolic BP by a minimum of 20 mm Hg to be able to assess corresponding change in R-R interval

Head-up Tilt test:

1. *Normal response*

SBP: Decrease within 10–15 mm Hg from baseline

DBP: Increase within 5–10 mm Hg from baseline

HR: Increase within 15–20 bpm from baseline

2. *Abnormal response*

[a]POH

SBP: Decrease >20 mm Hg from baseline

DBP: Decrease >5 mm Hg from baseline

Suggest possible autonomic insufficiency pattern vs. possible postural venous pooling.

If associated chronotropic insufficiency (blunted or no increase of HR) favors Autonomic Insufficiency or Sick Sinus Syndrome or medication effect.

[a]POTS (postural orthostatic tachycardia syndrome); classical definition:

HR: increase >30 bpm from baseline or greater than or equal to 120 bpm within the first 10 min of standing or head-up Tilt.

[a]VVS/VVR (vasovagal syncope/vasovagal response)

SBP: Sudden drop

DBP: Sudden drop

HR: Sudden drop; sometimes, asystole

Symptoms of: Lightheadedness, dizziness, fainting, nausea, diaphoresis, and pallor.

Monitor BP & EKG closely.

[a]VasoDepressor Syncope:

SBP: Sudden drop

DBP: Sudden drop

HR: No drop. <u>NO</u> asystole.

Symptoms of: Lightheadedness, dizziness, fainting, nausea, diaphoresis, and pallor.

Monitor BP & EKG closely.

[a]Possible poor vasoconstriction (decreased vascular reactivity to reflex vasoconstrictor stimuli):

SBP: Decrease within normal limits

DBP: Drop or flat

HRV test (heart rate variability test): In comparison to age and heart rate matched controls, the ratio of high frequency power to low frequency power provides an index of cardiac sympatho–vagal balance. Results are influenced by age and quality of breathing pattern

Ectopic beats, atrial fibrillation, and electronic cardiac pacing interfere with the accuracy of the measurements

The 30:15 R-R ratio measured while standing for one minute indicates the trend of the predominance of sympathetic vs. vagal autonomic cardiac modulation of postural heart rate

QSART test (quantitative sudomotor axon reflex test): It allows noninvasive evaluation of the postganglionic sympathetic sudomotor axon reflex. Latencies and sweat output are assessed at specific sites on the forearm, leg, and foot. Volumes of sweat output are compared to normal for standard sites relative to age and gender

VR, valsalva ratio; SBP, systolic blood pressure; DBP, diastolic blood pressure

A 12-lead ECG with rhythm strip must be obtained in all patients. The ECG is examined for QRS patterns, ECG intervals, ST/T changes, as well as cardiac rhythm. Specialized electrophysiologic evaluation is called upon in special situations such as arrhythmogenic right ventricular dysplasia (ARVD), Brugada syndrome, long QT syndrome, AV block, and pacemaker dysfunction.

An ambulatory cardiac monitoring device is essential in patients with recurrent palpitations, or recurrent presyncope, and syncope with unclear etiology despite standard workup. Continuous ambulatory monitoring plays an important role and has several advantages in diagnosing and evaluating patient symptoms; implantable devices have proven to be effective in detecting some clinically significant arrhythmias that could explain patient symptoms.[19,20] This outpatient monitoring system allows daily dose titration of medications in the outpatient setting while avoiding hospitalization. It is understandable in other types of patients hospitalization with inhospital cardiac telemetry may be necessary for diagnosis and management.[19]

Other electrophysiologic procedures are used under special circumstances such as signal averaging ECG, T-wave alternans, and electrophysiologic testing.

An echocardiogram should be obtained at rest or with stress if history, physical signs, or ECG suggest structural heart disease.

A decision tree for management of syncope/orthostatic intolerance is shown in Figure 17.2.

4.1. The Tilt test

There is no doubt that the Tilt test has proven to be an excellent diagnostic tool for the evaluation of a suspected syncope. The Tilt test not only allows the diagnosis of orthostatic hypotension, POTS, and NCG syncope (vasovagal/vasodepressor) but also provides crucial information about the possible underlying mechanism of the abnormal response to upright posture. Figure 17.3 lists the frequency of diagnosis established by Tilt table test in patients referred to the Cleveland clinic for evaluation of syncope in 2007.

Although there is a consensus about the current definitions of orthostatic hypotension, POTS, and vasovagal response to upright posture,[21,22] a description of the blood pressure and heart rate changes that occurred in the initial part of the test is helpful in understanding and even predicting the underlying biological dysfunction. An initial normal blood pressure response to the Tilt test preceding a gradual orthostatic hypotension suggest a probable circulatory dysfunction rather than autonomic failure. POTS may occur in the first 10 min of the 70 degree tilt (classical definition) although in the standard Tilt test, a rise of heart rate by >30 bpm or above 120 bpm may occur in the late part of the tilt[23]; the underlying mechanism for early versus late POTS may be different, and therefore require different types of treatment.

In this respect, it is essential not only to look at the outcome of the Tilt test, but also the preceding blood pressure, heart rate, and ECG changes that occur before the endpoint of the Tilt test is reached. Even if a patient has a benign cause of syncope such

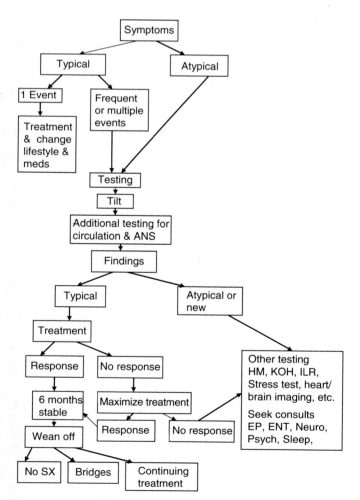

Figure 17.2 Decision tree for management of syncope/orthostatic intolerance.

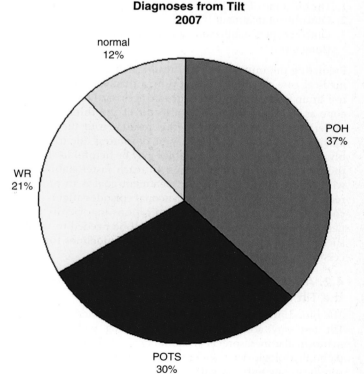

Figure 17.3 Frequency of diagnosis established by Tilt table test in patients referred to the Cleveland clinic for evaluation of syncope in 2007.

as simple NCG response without severe ECG changes, knowledge of the possible underlying mechanism allows triaging of additional testing for a final diagnosis and tailored choice of treatment.[24]

There is no doubt that the Tilt test protocol may influence the outcome of the test. Consequently, the standard Tilt test that was previously recommended by the NASPE/ACC Work Group appears to be the most useful protocol for the diagnosis of the various types of postural intolerance.[25]

Results of the Tilt test may be influenced by current daily medications; they can also be influenced by the administration of a provocative pharmacologic agent or maneuver during the Tilt test.[26,27]

The prognostic importance of the Tilt test needs to be examined in further detail. The "syncope burden" should take into consideration the tolerated duration of the test, the extent of drop of blood pressure, the characteristics of the associated changes in heart rate, PR interval and T-wave, the presence or absence of asystole, the duration of asystole, the presence or absence as well as the extent of sinus arrhythmia, and the presence or absence of premature beats or other dysrhythmia.

Variables that have been used for prediction of the results of the Tilt test differed among groups. Some used data obtained from the data of the Tilt test itself.[28,29] Others reported that variables obtained before the head-up positioning may predict the response to the Tilt test.[30] Others used the "neural networks" computer-based decision-making tool to predict the outcome of the tilt. The panel included 19 variables, and the authors concluded that body composition variables contributed more significantly than cardiovascular variables to the prediction of outcome of the head-up Tilt test.[31]

The question becomes which outcomes the patient will be interested in?

1. The outcome of the Tilt test (diagnostic)?
2. Outcome of treatment (QOL)?
3. Outcome after stabilization and discontinuation of treatment (long-term)?

Predicting the outcome of the head-upTilt test may assist the medical care provider to determine a diagnosis and stop the test at an appropriate time without necessarily reaching syncope as an endpoint. It may also direct the thinking to the underlying factors leading to this result. From the patient's perspective, this knowledge may be of interest due to a possibly shorter test. The same variables may be helpful in selecting the proper choice of medication to reach faster stabilization with treatment. Optimally the treatment goal is to prevent a recurrence of the syncopal/presyncopal episodes after reaching complete stabilization, where medications may be discontinued. However large clinical studies will be needed to validate such an approach and to provide useful guidelines for a successful patient management.[32]

4.2. Additional diagnostic testing after the Tilt test

The blood pressure and heart rate response pattern to head-up Tilt test vary according to the underlying pathophysiologic neurocirculatory disorders. It should be remembered that several pathophysiologic derangements may share the same blood pressure/heart rate response pattern to the Tilt test.

After the head-up Tilt test is completed and the blood pressure and heart rate response pattern is examined, additional testing

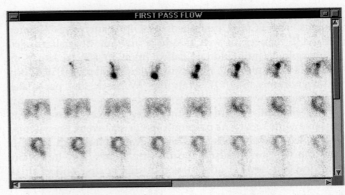

Figure 17.4 Example of radionuclide 99 mTc first-pass ventriculography. Each image (from top left to bottom right) represents the bolus of contrast as it travels from the venous to the systemic circulation in the chest. (**Movie 17.1**)

procedures may be necessary to provide more specific information in regard to the underlying homeostatic problem. These tests are usually done in a tertiary care center.

Laboratory evaluation of ANS function as well as circulatory dynamics provides a means to detect the type of deficit predisposing to postural intolerance and syncope. These tests are used if they appear to be of value in the diagnostic workup of the patient or in the proper selection of therapy. In our hands, measurement of blood volume using radionuclide 131-iodinated serum albumin and hemodynamics (using radionuclide 99 mTc first pass ventriculography) allow noninvasive evaluation of the circulatory parameters.[32-34] (Fig. 17.4, Movie 17.1)

The reasons for additional diagnostic testing are to define the cause of the abnormal response to head-up Tilt test and to target treatment to the specific underlying mechanism of syncope/orthostatic intolerance. Indeed the abnormal response to the Tilt test may be related to low blood volume (hypovolemia), the distribution of the blood volume between the cardiopulmonary and peripheral territories (venous pooling), reduced vascular reactivity (arteriolar vasoconstrictive responses), autonomic dysfunction, hypo adrenergic state, hyperadrenergic state, increased vagal mechanisms, or other modulating factors. Also a specific pattern of blood pressure and heart rate response to the Tilt test may be shared by a number of underlying circulatory abnormalities, each of which will require a different treatment; the differentiation between these various underlying abnormalities requires additional specific tests (Figs. 17.3 and 17.4). Targeting treatment to the specific underlying mechanism of syncope/orthostatic intolerance is the backbone of tailored therapy which is anticipated to improve outcomes.

4.3. Role of imaging in syncope/postural intolerance

4.3.1. Cardiac imaging

Echocardiography is very valuable in the evaluation of anatomical cardiac causes of syncope as well as in the assessment of cardiac systolic and diastolic function prior to initiation of some forms of therapy. Cardiac sympathetic innervation may be evaluated by the use of either 123-I-MIBG or 6-[18-F] fluorodopamine in patients with Parkinson disease.[35-37] The usefulness of cardiac magnetic resonance in the diagnosis of ARVD is well documented.

4.3.2. Imaging of arteries

Carotid ultrasound, carotid wall-lumen ratio, and pulse wave velocity are being used in various centers for both clinical and research purposes to assess large arterial compliance. Arterial plethysmography is being used for determination of vascular reactivity to vasoconstrictor and vasodilator stimuli. Changes in large and small arterial function play an important role in hemodynamic adjustments in response to gravity.

4.3.3. Imaging of veins for venous insufficiency

Using the venous plethysmography technique or radionuclide techniques offers a potential for the determination of the role of preload in syncope/orthostatic hypotension.[34,38,39]

4.3.4. Cerebral imaging

Sympathetic function in the human brain may be evaluated by using quantitative single photon computed tomography (SPECT) and PET scanning.[18,40]

Other cerebral imaging techniques focus on blood flow velocity changes in the large cerebral arteries using ultrasound methods.

5. THERAPY FOR SYNCOPE AND ORTHOSTATIC INTOLERANCE

The treatment goal of syncope/orthostatic intolerance is identification of types that are treatable with devices, ablation techniques, or a surgical approach and prevention of new episodes in those who require medical treatment (Table 17.2).

Another question relates to treatment of syncope/orthostatic intolerance in teenagers/adolescents. Previously, these youngsters were reassured and were told they would outgrow it. In practice, however, adults who present with syncope/orthostatic intolerance often recall having had postural challenges as teenagers. This raises the question as to whether treatment of syncope/orthostatic intolerance in teenagers will prevent future recurrences in adult life. Long-term studies are needed to answer this question.

In general, treatment is based on nonpharmacologic measures as well as pharmacologic agents. In addition, it is necessary to review and adjust current medications and concomitant treatment of the patient's other medical conditions. It is hoped that by achieving a stable medical control of syncope and re-establishment of a balanced ANS as well as a readaptation of the circulatory system, it becomes possible to wean patients off medications. In our experience, weaning patients off medications for the treatment of syncope is often possible after 6 months of clinical stabilization. Clinical experience has shown that after the weaning process, patients would fall into three groups according to their clinical follow-up: (a) Some patients do not require pharmacologic treatment thereafter; (b) Others may need "bridges" of pharmacologic treatment for 2 to 3 weeks when subjected to a flare of postural symptoms triggered by events such as viral illness, stressors, or weight loss; (c) Still others require continuing pharmacologic therapy—patients who have other medical conditions for which they take numerous medications. There has been no formal study to assess this outcome observation.

In addition to long-term treatment goals, managing an acute episode of postural intolerance or syncope is important to the patient as well as the family and bystanders.

5.1. Managing the acute episode

Where physicians and nursing staff in specialized syncope centers have given education, patients have avoided syncope by quick management of premonitory symptoms. Because patients still experience syncope events at home or in public, family members and bystanders should be able to recognize the situation and help the patient recover. The question becomes when should the patient go to a hospital emergency room or facility after a postural event? Suspicion of any serious diagnosis or injury must alert witnesses to call for immediate emergency medical help to transfer the patient safely to a medical emergency facility. At the emergency department, the patient will benefit from determining the seriousness of the acute situation, evaluation of possible other differential diagnoses, and determination of any injury that the patient could have sustained. Emergency departments are equipped to handle such situations and to provide preliminary medical care such as fluid replacement and to advise patients about the next step care. A triaging system at the emergency department is of definite importance to the patient at this time.

Emergency departments must determine both when the patient should be admitted to the hospital and also how much this service impacts the medical system qualitatively and financially.[41,42]

5.2. Prevention of recurrence of postural/syncopal episodes

In our experience, prevention of new attacks has been accomplished by establishing the specific treatment based on identifying the underlying pathophysiology. The development of specialized syncope clinics has allowed the offering of unique services to achieve this purpose.

5.2.1. Nonpharmacologic treatment of postural intolerance/syncope

Nonpharmacologic treatment is the basic treatment that should be offered to all patients with such events. It includes adequate salt intake, adequate hydration using electrolyte-balanced fluids along with water, natural sources of potassium, postural precautions including post meals and post exercise, avoiding decongestants and excess caffeine, avoiding heat exposure, and awareness of the vasodilatory effect of alcohol. Nonpharmacologic treatment also includes the use of support garments (stockings or abdominal binder). Physical therapy and a moderate exercise program geared toward re-establishment of circulatory balance have been useful. Elevation of the head of the bed 6 to 8 in during recumbency is recommended in situations where supine hypertension is an issue. In our experience, physical therapy at home and in a specialized rehabilitation clinics and more specific exercise programs like cardiac rehabilitation phase II programs under supervision have proved valuable in the treatment of postural intolerance/syncope.

5.2.2. Pharmacologic treatment

Pharmacologic treatment of syncope requires special attention. Rather than using general guidelines for a stepwise addition of medications, a tailored approach to treatment helps achieve a quicker re-establishment of clinical improvement. Various classes of medications have been utilized in the treatment of postural intolerance/syncope including (alphabetically)

(1) Anticholinergic agents.
(2) β-blockers (cardioselective, noncardioselective, and sometimes β-blockers with intrinsic sympathomimetic activity).
(3) Calcium channel blockers (Verapamil and Cardizem).
(4) Salt retaining minralocorticoid such as Fludrohydrocortisone (Florinef).
(5) Selective serotonin uptake inhibitors.
(6) Vasoconstrictors.

In the general stepwise treatment approach, it has been customary to start with a β-blocker followed by a fluid/salt retaining agent followed by a vasoconstrictor. Then other medications are added in different sequence according to protocols at different centers.

In the tailored treatment approach, any of the classes of medications can be used as a first line treatment according to the pathophysiology of the condition. Other medications may be added as needed. Alteration of the sequence often is necessary according to the baseline blood pressure and heart rate.

5.2.3. Role of permanent cardiac pacemakers in the treatment of syncope

It was previously thought that the reversal of bradycardia or asystole, which are commonly seen during a vasovagal event, would be ideal to prevent the syncopal episode. However results of multicenter randomized studies did not confirm a consistent beneficial effect of dual chamber pacing (DDD) in the prevention of neurocardiogenic episodes.[43,44]

5.3. Special populations

There is no doubt that tolerability of pharmacologic agents differs in various populations. Dosages need to be adjusted. Special populations include the elderly, children and adolescents, patients with cardiac, renal or hepatic dysfunction, prior history of stroke, and presence of cardiac arrhythmias. Patients who have supine hypertension in association with orthostatic hypotension present a treatment challenge. A fine balance is needed to control both sides of the equation.

6. FUTURE DIRECTIONS

This patient population often has challenging social concerns such as school, work, sports, driving privileges, flying, and vacationing.

Familial types of cardiac syncope are well documented. However not much information is available in syncope/orthostatic intolerance without cardiac disease. Although syncope/orthostatic intolerance may affect more than one member of the same family, genetic information is rare.[45] The question often arises "who to screen"; the answer remains unknown.

REFERENCES

1. Kapoor WN. Current evaluation and management of syncope. *Circulation.* 2002;106:1606–1609.
2. Hood R. Syncope in the elderly. *Clin Geriatr Med.* 2007;351–361.
3. Paul B, Gierob Z, Mangoni AA. Influence of comorbidities and medication use on tilt table test outcome in elderly patients. *PACE.* 2007;30:540–543.
4. Folino AF. Cerebral autoregulation and syncope. *Prog Cardiovasc Dis.* 2007;50:49–80.
5. Maurer MS, Karmally W, Rivadeneira H, et al. Upright posture and postprandial hypotension in elderly persons. *Ann Intern Med.* 2000;133:533–536.
6. Kapoor WN, Hanasu BH. Is syncope a risk factor for poor outcomes? Comparison of patients with and without syncope. *Am J Med.* 1996;100:646–655.
7. Kapoor WN, Karpf M, Wieand S, et al. A prospective evaluation and followup of patients with syncope. *New Eng J Med.* 1983;309:197–204.
8. Linzer M, Pontinan M, Gold DT, et al. Impairment of physical and psychological function in recurrent syncope. *Clin Epidemiol.* 1991;44:1037–1043.
9. Van Dijk N, Sprangers MA, Colman N, et al. Clinical factors associated with quality of life in patients with transient loss of consciousness. *Cardiovasc Electrophysiol.* 2006;17:998–1003.
10. Blanc JJ, L'Her C, Touiza A, et al. Prospective evaluation and outcome of patients admitted for syncope over a one year period. *Eur Heart J.* 2002;23:815–820.
11. Sun BC, Emond JA, Camargo CA, Jr. Direct medical costs of syncope related hospitalizations in the United States. *A J Cardiol.* 2005;95:668–671.
12. Quinn JV, Stiell IG, McDermott DA, et al. Derivation of the San Francisco syncope rule to predict patients with short term serious outcomes. *Ann Emerg Med.* 2004;43:224–232.
13. Quinn JV, Stiell IG, McDermott DA, et al. Prospective validation of the San Francisco syncope rule to predict patients with serious outcomes. *Ann Emerg Med.* 2006;47:448–454.
14. Reed MJ, Newby DE, Coull AJ, et al. *Emerg Med J.* 2007;24:769–773.
15. Yamanouchi Y, Jaalouk S, Shehadeh AA, et al. Venous dysfunction and the change of blood viscosity during head-up tilt. *Pacing Clin Electrophysiol.* 1998;21(3):520–527.
16. Richerson GB. The autonomic nervous system. In: Boron, WF, Boulpaep, EL. eds. *Medical Physiology. A Cellular and Molecular Approach.* Updated Ed. Philadelphia, PA: Elsevier Saunders; 2005:378–398, Chapter 15.
17. Boulpaep EL. Regulation of arterial pressure and cardiac output. In: Boron, WF, Boulpaep, EL. eds. *Medical Physiology. A Cellular and Molecular Approach.* Updated ed. Philadelphia, PA: Elsevier Saunders; 2005:534–557, Chapter 22.
18. Ouchi Y, Okada H, Yoshikawa E, et al. Absolute changes in regional cerebral blood flow in association with upright posture in humans: An orthostatic PET Study. *J Nucl Med.* 2001;42:707–712.
19. Olson JA, Fouts AM, Padanilam BJ, et al. Utility of mobile cardiac outpatient telemetry for the diagnosis of palpitations, presyncope, syncope and the assessment of therapy efficacy. *Cardiovasc Electrophysiol.* 2007;18:473–477.
20. Benezet-Mazuecos J, Ibanez B, Manuel-Rubio J, et al. Utility of in-hospital cardiac remote telemetry in patients with unexplained syncope. *Europace.* 2007;9:1196–1201.
21. Schondorf R, Low PA. Idiopathic postural tachycardia syndromes. Evaluation and management. In: Low, PA. ed. *Clinical Autonomic Disorders.* 1st Ed. Boston, Toronto, London: Little, Brown and Company; 1993:641–652, Chapter 46.
22. Robertson D, Davis TL. Neurological and related causes of syncope: The importance of recognition and treatment. In: Grubb, BP, Olshansky, B. eds. *Syncope: Mechanisms and Management.* Armonk, NY: Futura Publishing Company, Inc.; 1998:223–251, Chapter 8.
23. Mayuga KA, Butters K, Fouad-Tarazi F. Early vs. Late POTS: A re-evaluation of a syndrome. *Clin Auton Res.* 2008;18:155–157.
24. Brignole M, Alboni P, Benditt D, et al. Task force on syncope. European Society of Cardiology. *Eur Heart J.* 2001;22:1256–1306.
25. Benditt D, Fergusson D, Grubb BP, et al. Tilt table testing for assessing syncope: An American College of Cardiology Consensus document. *J Am Coll Cardiol.* 1996;28:263–275.
26. Kapoor WN, Brant N. Evaluation of syncope by upright tilt testing with isoproterenol. A nonspecific test. *Ann Intern Med.* 1992;116(5):358–363.
27. Sankaranarayanan-Prakash E, Pavithran P. A novel tilt testing protocol for investigating patients suspected to have neurally mediated syncope. *Int J Cardiol.* 2007;121:315–316.
28. Mallat Z, Vicaut E, Sangare A, et al. Prediction of head- up tilt test result by analysis of early heart rate variations. *Circulation.* 1997;96:581–584.
29. Pitzalis M, Massari F, Guida P, et al. Shortened head up tilting test guided by systolic pressure reductions in neurocardiogenic syncope. *Circulation.* 2002;105:146–148.
30. Bellard E, Fortrat JO, Schang D, et al. Changes in transthoracic impedance signal predict outcome of 70 degree head up tilt test. *Clin Sci (London).* 2003;104:119–126.
31. Fortrat JO, Schang D, Bellard E, et al. Cardiovascular variables do not predict head-up tilt test outcome better than body composition. *Clin Auton Res.* 2007;17:206–210.
32. Fouad-Tarazi F. Idiopathic hypovolemia. In: Robertson, D, Low, PA, Polinski, RJ. eds. *Primer On the Autonomic Nervous System.* San Diego: Academic Press;1996:286–289.
33. Fouad FM, Tarazi RC, MacIntyre WJ, et al. Venous delay, a major source of error in isotopic cardiac output determination. *Am Heart J.* 1979;97:477–484.
34. Fouad F, MacIntyre WJ, Tarazi RC. Noninvasive measurement of cardiopulmonary blood volume. Evaluation of the centroid method. *J Nucl Med.* 1981;22:205–211.
35. Yoshita M. Differentiation of idiopathic Parkinson's disease from striatonigral degeneration and progressive supranuclear palsy using Iodine-123 meta-iodobenzylguanidine myocardial scintigraphy. *J Neurol Sci.* 1998;155:60–67.
36. Satoh A, Serita T, Seto M, et al. Loss of 123 I-MIBG uptake by the heart in Parkinson's disease: Assessment of cardiac sympathetic denervation and diagnostic value. *J Nucl Med.* 1999;40:371–375.
37. Goldstein D, Holmes C, Li S-T, et al. Cardiac sympathetic denervation in Parkinson disease. *Ann Intern Med.* 2000;133:338–347.

38. Streeten DHP, Anderson GH Jr, Richardson R, et al. Abnormal orthostatic changes in blood pressure and heart rate in subjects with intact sympathetic nervous function: Evidence for excessive venous pooling. *J Lab Clin Med.* 1988;111:326–335.

39. Streeten DH, Scullard TF. Excessive gravitational blood pooling caused by impaired venous tone is the predominant non-cardiac mechanism of orthostatic intolerance. *Clin Sci.* 1996;90:277–285.

40. Arakawa R, Okumura M, Ito H, et al. Quantitative analysis of Norepinephrine transporter in the human brain using PET with (S,S)-18F-FMeNER-D2. *J Nucl Med.* 2008;49:1270–1276.

41. Sun BC, Magione CM, Merchant G, et al. External validation of the San Francisco syncope rule. *Ann Emerg Med.* 2007;49:420–427.

42. Cosgriff TM, Kelly AM, Kerr D. External validation of the San Francisco syncope rule in the Australian context. *Can J Emerg Med.* 2007;9:157–161.

43. Conolly SJ, Sheldon R, Roberts RS, et al. Vasovagal Pacemaker Study investigators. The North American Vasovagal Pacemaker Study [VPS]: A randomized trial of permanent cardiac pacing for the prevention of vasovagal syncope. *J Am Coll Cardiol.* 1999;33:16–20.

44. Conolly SJ, Sheldon R, Thorpe KE, et al. For the VPS II investigators. Pacemaker therapy for prevention of syncope in patients with recurrent severe vasovagal syncope: Second Vasovagal Pacemaker Study [VPS II]. *JAMA.* 2003;289:2224–2229.

45. Garland EM, Black BK, Harris PA, et al. Dopamine-beta-hydroxylase in postural tachycardia syndrome. *Am J Physiol Heart Circ Physiol.* 2007;293:H684–H690.

Hypertension

Rebecca T. Hahn

18

1. INTRODUCTION

1.1. Epidemiology

Hypertension is a major risk factor for significant morbidity and mortality from stroke, cardiovascular, and renal disease. In both developed and developing countries, the prevalence of hypertension in adults exceeds 25% and approaches three quarters of the population beyond the seventh decade.[1] The World Health Organization estimates that hypertension may cause 7.1 million premature deaths and 4.5% of the disease burden worldwide.[2] Because hypertension is a continuous variable, however, we continue to redefine the level at which hypertension should be treated.[3] How to best approach the treatment of hypertension is beyond the scope of this chapter, however, decisions regarding management of hypertension must include an assessment of treatable causes of secondary hypertension as well as an overall assessment of cardiovascular risk and target organ damage.

Hypertensive heart disease is a complex entity involving changes to the cardiac system resulting from arterial hypertension and is the major cause of hypertension-related morbidity and mortality. Many of the disease processes associated with hypertension will be covered in other chapters of this text and include coronary artery disease, congestive heart failure (CHF) (with normal and preserved ejection fraction [EF]), and sudden death. Hypertrophy of the left ventricle secondary to hypertension is a major risk factor for myocardial infarction, stroke, sudden death, and CHF as well as peripheral vascular disease[4–7] and is the primary precursor to hypertensive heart disease. In a recent multicenter, prospective observational study of uncomplicated essential hypertensives[8] for any 39 g increase in left ventricular (LV) mass there was an independent increase in the risk of primary events (37%, 95% confidence interval [CI]: 5 to 80, $p = 0.020$) and total cardiovascular events (40%, 95% CI: 14 to 73, $p = 0.0013$). A twofold to fourfold increase in cardiovascular risk with echocardiographic LV hypertrophy (Echo-LVH) and a sixfold increase in overall morality with ECG–LVH[9] persist after adjustment for the influence of several traditional risk factors.[5,6,9,10] The relationship between the increased LV mass and cardiovascular risk has been shown in diverse patient populations and is not limited to patients with hypertension, but has also been shown in the general population[10,11] and patients with coronary artery disease.[12,13]

Although blood pressure (BP) is a major determinant of LV mass,[14] only 10% to 25% of the variability of LV mass can be attributed to random systolic BP measurements[15] or 24-h mean BP.[16] The development of LVH is thus multifactorial with studies suggesting a role for age, gender, race, body mass index, and neurohormonal stimulation.[17] LV mass increases with age, however, the independent role of age on LV mass is difficult to demonstrate. In an adolescent and young adult population, some studies show an age-related change in LV mass that is independent of body size,[18] however, in a healthy adult population[19] no increase in LV mass could be demonstrated. The Framingham study[20] did document a higher prevalence of LVH in hypertensive women than men (57% vs. 31%) and gender differences in LVH regression have also been shown.[21] The prevalence of LVH is twofold to threefold higher in African Americans than whites, adjusting for differences in BP.[22–24] In addition, diastolic dysfunction is of greater severity in hypertensive patients of African-Caribbean origin than white Europeans even after adjusting for LV mass.[25] Obesity is also a major risk factor for LVH development.[26] The Strong Heart Study[27] evaluated a cohort of unselected adolescents from a specific ethnic group (American Indians) and despite normal BPs, 33.5% of obese adolescents fulfilled criteria for LVH (vs. 3.5% in normal weight adolescents).

Numerous recent studies suggest that regression of hypertensive LVH is associated with improved prognosis. A decrease in cardiovascular events occurs with pharmacologic treatment of BP[28,29,30] as well as nonpharmacologic interventions.[31,32] Regression of LVH also reduces the risk of stroke.[33] A recent meta-analysis of the effect of antihypertensive medications on LV mass[35] included 80 double-blind, randomized trials of BP treatment. The mean LV mass index reduction with active treatment was 9% ± 8%. Among the five classes of antihypertensive drugs used (diuretics, beta-blockers, calcium antagonists, angiotensin converting enzyme inhibitors [ACEI], and angiotensin receptor blockers [ARBs]), beta-blockers reduced LV mass the least (6%, 95% CI: 3 to 8) whereas ARB reduced LV mass the most (13%, 95% CI: 8 to 18). Calcium antagonists (11%, 95% CI: 9 to 13), ACEI (10% 95% CI: 8 to 12), and diuretics (8%, 95% CI: 5 to 10) fell between these two agents. This study mirrors the results of the Losartan Intervention for Endpoint Reduction in Hypertension (LIFE) trial[36] in which 9,193 patients with essential hypertension and ECG–LVH were randomized to treatment with Losartan (and ARB) or atenolol. Losartan-based therapy induced greater reduction in LV mass index than atenolol with adjustment for baseline LV mass index and BP and in-treatment pressure (-21.7 ± 21.8 vs. -17.7 ± 19.6 g/m^2; $p = 0.021$). Subsequent analysis showed that reduction in LV mass reduced the composite endpoint of cardiovascular death, fatal or nonfatal myocardial infarction, and fatal or nonfatal stroke.[36]

In addition to LV mass, LV geometry provides additional prognostic information about patients with hypertension.[5,10] The geometric classification of LV architecture relies on the measurement of LV mass and the relative wall thickness (RWT) defined as

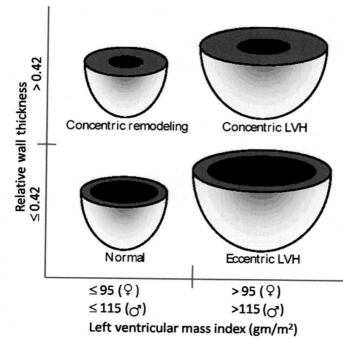

Figure 18.1 LV geometry based on LV mass index and RWT. LVH, left ventricular hypertrophy.

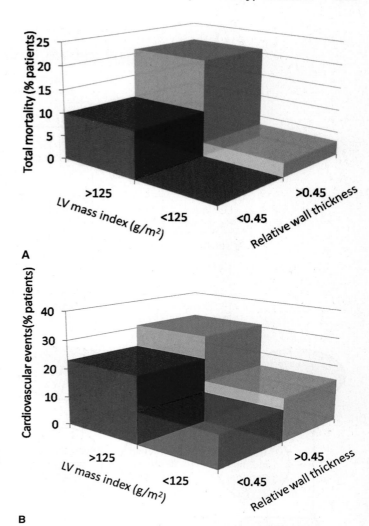

Figure 18.2 Mortality (**A**) and cardiovascular events (**B**) stratified by LV geometry. (Modified from Koren MJ, Devereux RB, Casale PH, et al. Relation of left ventricular mass and geometry to morbidity and mortality in uncomplicated essential hypertension. *Ann Intern Med.* 1991;114:345–352).

two times the posterior wall thickness (PWT) divided by LV internal dimension in diastole. Four types of LV geometry can therefore be described using these two parameters (Fig. 18.1): normal geometry with normal LV mass and RWT, concentric remodeling with normal LV mass and increased RWT, eccentric hypertrophy with increased LV mass and normal RWT, and concentric hypertrophy with increased LV mass and increased RWT. Based on these four categories, Koren et al.[5] showed both total mortality and cardiovascular events could be further stratified by LV geometry (Fig. 18.2). Di Tullio et al.[37] showed that in a population-based case–control study of patients with first ischemic stroke, LV geometry was a strong predictor of stroke risk: concentric hypertrophy carried the greatest stroke risk (adjusted odds ratio [OR], 3.5; 95% CI: 2.0 to 6.2), followed by eccentric hypertrophy (adjusted OR, 2.4; 95% CI: 2.0 to 4.3). LV mass and geometry are strong predictors of morbidity and mortality irrespective of the etiology. Verma et al.[38] found increased baseline LV mass and abnormal geometry increased the risk for morbidity and mortality following high-risk myocardial infarction. Table 18.1 summarizes some of the studies relating risk to cardiac geometry.

Finally, RWT alone carries significant prognostic information. In one study,[39] concentric remodeling (normal LV mass, increased RWT) occurred in 39% of patients with essential hypertension. Adjusting for multiple covariates, the risk of cardiovascular morbid events was higher in the group with concentric remodeling than in the group with normal geometry (relative risk 2.56, 95% CI: 1.20 to 5.45, *p* < 0.01). Increased risk for mortality also exists for this geometry.[40] In this retrospective analysis of a patient referred for echocardiography (*n* = 35,602), concentric remodeling was present in 35% (*n* = 12,362) and LVH in 11% (*n* = 3,958) and each conferred a similar significantly increased risk for all-cause mortality (RR 1.99, 95% CI: 1.88 to 2.18, *p* < 0.0001 and RR 2.13, 95% CI: 1.89 to 2.40, *p* < 0.0001, respectively). Subjects with concentric remodeling who reverted to a normal geometric pattern had improved survival (RR 0.64, 95% CI: 0.42 to 0.97, *p* < 0.03) compared to those who progressed to LV hypertrophy (RR 1.54, 95% CI: 1.01 to 2.47, *p* < 0.05).

2. PATHOPHYSIOLOGY

Hypertension is a heterogeneous disorder with a number of well-defined as well as putative etiologies. Although our understanding of the complexity of the molecular mechanisms of BP control continues to expand,[41] it is difficult to precisely determine the relative contribution of each variable. Despite this limitation, our understanding of the pathophysiology of hypertension has led to the development of targeted antihypertensive medications which may be more effective and thus reduce the economic burden of diagnosing and treating the disease. Only about 5% of people with hypertension have underlying renal, adrenal, or other disorders that can be directly related to an increase in BP, whereas the remaining 95% have essential or primary hypertension.

Elevated BP is an integral component of hypertension and according to Ohm's law, BP is proportional to cardiac output and peripheral vascular resistance. Although seemingly simple, numerous pathways contribute to these two factors (Fig. 18.3). Each

TABLE 18.1
RELATIVE RISKS ACCORDING TO LV GEOMETRY

Patient population	Risk	Concentric remodeling		Eccentric LVH		Concentric LVH	
		HR	95% CI	HR	95% CI	HR	95% CI
HTN/nl LVM[35]	CV Events	2.56	1.2–5.45				
HTN/nl LVM[36]	Mortality	1.54	1.01–2.47				
General Population[40]	Mortality	1.99	1.88–2.18	HR = 2.13 (1.89–2.40)			
Stroke[37]	Stroke			2.4	2.0–4.3	3.5	2.0–6.2
CAD[38]	Mortality/ CV events	3.0	1.9–4.9	3.1	1.9–4.8	5.4	3.4–8.5

HR, hazards ratio: CI, confidence intervals LVH, left ventricular hypertrophy;.
Note: the study by Milani et al. compared concentric remodeling to patients with hypertrophy.

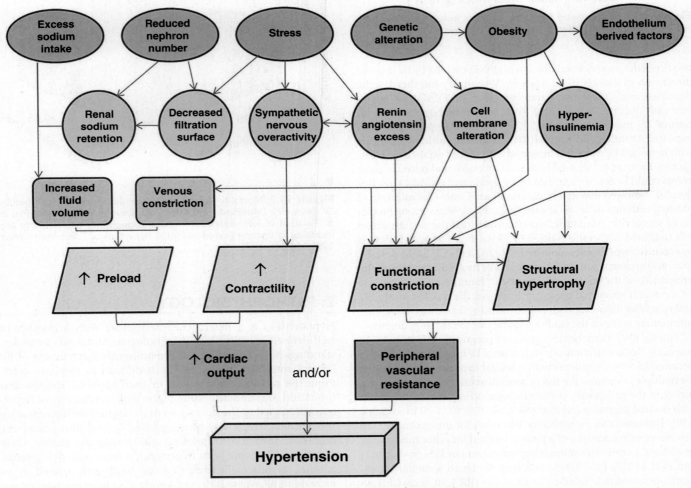

Figure 18.3 Factors contributing to hypertension.

pathway or physiologic system has a wide variety of interactions with BP. The relationship between the pathways, however, has proven to be complex and intertwined. For instance, baroreceptors within the vessel walls sense acute pressure changes and these may trigger release of natriuretic peptides produced in the brain and heart. Vascular tone is controlled not only by the renin–angiotensin–aldosterone system which controls vascular volume homeostasis, but also the kinin–kallikrein system which influences renal salt handling. Factors released by the vessel walls themselves, such as nitric oxide (NO) and endothelin, may alter vascular tone. We are just beginning to understand the impact for example, of insulin resistance which results in hyperinsulinemia and subsequent sodium sensitivity, obesity, and increased sympathetic drive.[42]

The interaction of sodium and fluid balance and vasomotor tone determine BP regulation. There are two major systems that influence BP: the renin–angiotensin–aldosterone system and the autonomic nervous system. The kidneys regulate fluid and electrolytes and are thus the major determinant of BP in essential hypertension.[43-45] The initial stages of hypertension are characterized by reduced sodium membrane exchange/excretion by the kidney, thus requiring a higher than usual BP to maintain extracellular fluid volume. The resulting renal and systemic vasoconstriction causes reduced renal blood flow and stimulates natriuresis. Thus, most patients initially have a lower blood plasma volume and total exchangeable sodium. Reduced renal blood flow and decreased sodium delivery to the distal tubules of the kidney stimulate the renin–angiotensin–aldosterone system (Fig. 18.4), which is the primary regulator of cardiovascular and renal function.

In response to glomerular underperfusion, low sodium delivery, or sympathetic nervous system stimulation, renin is secreted from the juxtaglomerular apparatus of the kidneys. Renin converts angiotensinogen to angiotensin I within the circulation as well within vascular and other tissues. Conversion of angiotensin I to angiotensin II occurs primarily by angiotensin converting enzyme (ACE). Angiotensin II then acts at numerous sites in the body to result in hypertension and end-organ changes (Table 18.2). This active peptide is responsible for a number of physiologic changes: cell growth in the heart and vasculature resulting in cardiac and vascular hypertrophy, systemic vasoconstriction, stimulation of the adrenal gland and aldosterone production, stimulation of the posterior pituitary gland and vasopressin production, as well as stimulation of the thirst reflex in the hypothalamus. All of these effects are regulated by the AT_1 receptor, whereas the AT_2 receptor antagonizes some of the AT_1 effects of vasoconstriction and cell growth. An understanding of this complex relationship has led to the development of hypertension medications such as ACE inhibitors which block the generation of angiotensin II, and ARBs which block AT_1 but stimulate AT_2 receptors. Medications designed to affect this complex cascade such as renin inhibitors continue to be developed.[46] The later stages of hyper-

TABLE 18.2

LIST OF ENDOTHELIAL VASOACTIVE SUBSTANCES AND GROWTH FACTORS

Vasodilating systems	Vasoconstricting systems	Vascular growth factors
Parasympathetic Kallikrein–kinin system Prostaglandins Endothelium-derived relaxing factor (nitric oxide) Atrial natriuretic factor	Sympathetic Calcium Local renin–angiotensin Systems Circulating renin–angiotensin system Endothelin Ouabain Vasopressin Superoxide anion	Insulin like growth factor Growth hormone Parathyroid hormone Tissue oncogenes Angiotensin II

tension are associated with salt sensitivity and the inability of the kidney to excrete a sodium load. Vascular remodeling rapidly ensues resulting in sustained vasoconstriction. Arterial stiffening with age is a separate disease entity manifest by isolated systolic hypertension.

The autonomic nervous system is the second major neurohumoral system that determines BP. The sympathetic nervous system and plasma catecholamines cause arteriolar constriction and dilatation, thus helping to maintain normal BP during daily activity and physical/emotional stress. Like angiotensin II, catecholamine receptors are found in multiple systems throughout the body including the brain, cardiac tissue, the adrenal medulla, kidneys, and blood vessels. The relationship of the sympathetic nervous system to essential hypertension has not been well defined. Prior studies implicating catecholamine excess in essential hypertension[47] showed that an increase in urinary catecholamines was directly related to the severity of hypertension and that catecholamines were the key to understanding low renin hypertension. Although it was an attractive theory, other investigators[48] found no relationship between plasma norepinephrine and epinephrine concentrations in high, normal, and low renin hypertensives in response to postural changes and suggested that renin subgroups had differential responsiveness to adrenergic stimulation. Beta-blockers may thus act on hypertension not by blocking catecholamine effects, but rather by reducing renin release from the kidneys.[49] It appears nonetheless that catecholamines may not have as large a role in chronic BP control compared to the renin–antiogensin–aldosterone system. This is an attractive theory in the setting of the results of the LIFE study. A recent meta-analysis of LV mass response to treatment in patients with essential hypertension confirmed that despite an equivalent BP response, LV mass index decreased the least in response to beta-blockers (6%, 95% CI: 3 to 8) compared to any other class of antihypertensive and angiotensin II receptor antagonist treatment resulted in the greatest reduction (13%, 95% CI: 8 to 18).[34]

Inherited hypertension has long been recognized and more recently been the focus of extensive research. The surge in research stems from two factors: difficulty in defining the exact causes of hypertension and thus targeting therapy, and the recent mechanization of genomics and proteonomics. It is estimated that BP variance may be under a significant degree (35% to 70%) of genetic control.[50] Because of the difficulty in defining the pathophysiology of hypertension, therapies

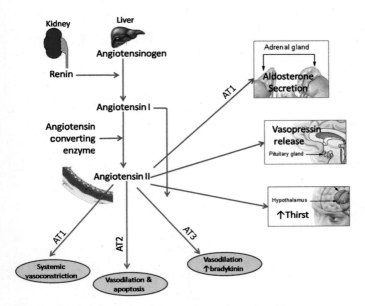

Figure 18.4 Schematic of the renin–angiotensin–aldosterone system. AT_1, angiotensin II receptor 1; AT_2, angiotensin II receptor 2; AT_3, angiotensin (1–7) receptor 3.

for hypertension have been limited to those neurohormonal pathways that have been defined or to the phenotypic treatment of high plasma volume load or high vascular resistance. An understanding of the genetic basis for hypertension would further our understanding of the pathophysiology of the disease and lead to the development of targeted therapy. Complicating the genetic story are the numerous contributing factors including obesity, dyslipidemia, glucose intolerance, alcohol, and salt intake. The interactions between these behavioral and environmental factors with neurohormonal factors may affect the genetic expression of inherited hypertension. Each of these contributing factors may also be under allelic influence, further complicating the genetics of hypertension. Although numerous hypertension genes have been identified, none appear to be the primary BP control gene.

The evaluation of patients with hypertension must include exclusion of the secondary causes of hypertension. Although this population of patients comprises only 2% to 3% of patients with hypertension, these etiologies require specific diagnostic techniques and treatment. Secondary causes of hypertension may include chronic kidney disease, renovascular disease, primary aldosteronism, pheochromocytoma, coarctation of the aorta, thyroid or parathyroid disease, sleep apnea, steroid use or Cushing syndrome, and finally drug-related or drug-induced hypertension.[3] The evaluation of these secondary causes is outlined in Table 18.3.[51] Patients without secondary causes of hypertension have essential hypertension.

TABLE 18.3

CLINICAL PRACTICE GUIDELINE FOR DIAGNOSIS AND MANAGEMENT OF HYPERTENSION IN THE PRIMARY CARE SETTING

Disease	Features	Recommended test/referral
Cushing syndrome and other glucocorticoid excess states including chronic steroid therapy	Amenorrhea Increased dorsal fat Diabetes mellitus Edema Hirsutism Moon facies Purple striae Truncal obesity	History 24-h urine for free cortisol Dexamethasone suppression test
Hyperparathyroidism	Hypercalcemia Polyuria/polydipsia Renal stones	Serum calcium and parathyroid hormone (PTH) level
Hyperthyroidism	Anxiety Brisk reflexes Hyperdefecation Heat intolerance Tachycardia Tremor Weight loss Wide pulse pressure	Thyroid stimulating hormone (TSH) Free T4
Pheochromocytoma	Labile BP Orthostatic hypotension Paroxysms (headaches, palpitations, sweating, pallor) Tachycardia	Plasma metanephrines or 24-h urine for metanephrines and/or catecholamines Consider referral to specialist
Primary hyperaldosteronism	K+ ≤3.5 mEq/L in patients **not** on diuretic therapy; or K+ ≤3 mEq/L in patients **on** diuretic therapy Muscle cramps Polyuria Weakness	Plasma aldosterone and plasma renin activity 24-h urinary aldosterone level on a high sodium diet
Kidney disease	Abnormal urine sediment Elevated serum creatinine Hematuria on two occasions or structural renal abnormality (e.g., abdominal or flank masses) Proteinuria	Urinalysis; estimation of urinary protein excretion and creatinine clearance by using a single random urine test; renal ultrasound may also be considered (See annotation H in original guideline document.) Consider referral to nephrology
Renovascular disease	Abdominal bruits over the renal arteries Abrupt onset of severe HTN Diastolic BP ≥115 mm Hg Initial onset age ≥50 years old	There are a variety of screening tests for renovascular HTN, depending on equipment and expertise in institutions. Magnetic resonance angiography, renal artery Doppler, and postcaptopril renograms are used.

(Continued)

TABLE 18.3

CLINICAL PRACTICE GUIDELINE FOR DIAGNOSIS AND MANAGEMENT OF HYPERTENSION IN THE PRIMARY CARE SETTING (Continued)

Disease	Features	Recommended test/referral
	Worsening BP control when previously stable Evidence of atherosclerotic vascular disease	However, there is no single best test for renovascular HTN, and consultation with experts in your institution is recommended. Intravenous pyelogram is relatively contraindicated in diabetes and no longer recommended as screening test for renovascular disease.
Sleep apnea	Daytime somnolence Snoring or observed apneic episodes	Referral for sleep study
Aortic Coarctation	Weak or delayed femoral pulses	Computerized tomography angiography
Drug or substance induced	Nonsteroidal anti-inflammatory drugs (NSAIDs), including Cox-2 Inhibitors Sympathomimetics (e.g., decongestants, anorectics) Oral contraceptives Adrenal steroids Erythropoietin Cyclosporine, tacrolimus Cocaine, amphetamines Excessive alcohol use Licorice Selected dietary supplements (e.g., ma huang, ephedra, bitter orange)	History Urine toxicology as indicated

Source: Veterans Administration, Department of Defense. VA/DoD clinical practice guideline for diagnosis and management of hypertension in the primary care setting. Washington DC: Veterans Administration, Department of Defense; 2004 Aug.

2.1. Essential hypertension

Essential hypertension is defined by a sustained systolic pressure of >140 mm Hg and a diastolic pressure (DP) of >90 mm Hg with no known cause.[52] Cardiac output may be normal or mildly increased in the early stages of essential hypertension resulting in an increase in total peripheral resistance in order to maintain normal tissue perfusion. Abnormal vascular hyperreactivity is often seen and frequently manifest during stress. High peripheral vascular resistance and associated alteration in renal physiology including reduced renal blood flow and accelerated natriuresis initiate the renin–angiotensin–aldosterone system described earlier.

Essential hypertension is unquestionably a multifactorial disease. Although the renin–angiotensin–aldosterone system is the major cause, there are other factors that contribute to high BP including abnormal endothelial function, salt sensitivity, obesity, and the metabolic syndrome. The endothelium produces a range of vasoactive substances and vascular growth factors (Table 18.2). NO, a potent vasodilator, is scavenged by mitochondrial generated superoxide anion (O_2^-). The resulting reduction in NO as well as O_2^- causes vasoconstriction. Angiotensin II has been shown to stimulate O_2^- production in rats[53,54] however, the results in humans have been inconclusive.[55-57]

Salt sensitivity is still a poorly understood but frequently observed phenomenon. Normal patients will respond to a high-salt diet by decreasing renin levels, therefore decreasing angiotensin II and maintaining mean arterial BP (Fig. 18.5). Conversely, the normal response to a low-salt diet is an increase in renin levels which increases vasoconstriction. BP homeostasis

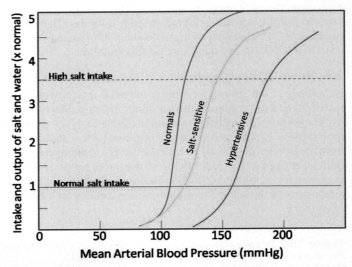

Figure 18.5 Pressure natriuresis in normal and hypertensives and salt-sensitive individuals.

is thus closely related to sodium-stimulated blood volume and renin-induced vasoconstriction. In salt-sensitive individuals, the response to sodium is exaggerated either by enhanced reabsorption of volume and/or a change in the renin responsiveness. Salt sensitivity has dramatic implications in normotensive and hypertensive patients increasing the risk of death significantly (OR = 1.73, CI: 1.02 to 2.94, p = 0.042).[58]

2.2. Aortic coarctation

The evaluation of hypertension in a child or adult should always include the exclusion of coarctation of the aorta which is covered in more depth in Chapter 45. Coarctation of the aorta represents about 6% of congenital heart disease in the adult and presents most commonly a discrete narrowing of aorta at the ligamentum arteriosum particularly in the adult. More diffuse diseases involving the arch or isthmus, as well as diffuse arteriopathy as seen in bicuspid aortic valves also occur. Although coarctation of the aorta can present as an isolated lesion ("simple") when it is associated with other intracardiac or extracardiac effects ("complex"), it is most commonly associated with bicuspid aortic valve.[59]

The examination of an adult with hypertension should include an examination of the symmetry and timing of peripheral pulses which then may lead to measurement of upper and lower extremity BP differential. Normally, the BP in the lower extremity may be 5 to 10 mm Hg higher than that in the upper extremity due to downstream augmentation of the reflected pressure wave. The presence of a delay or decrease in femoral pulse amplitude, or a significant difference in upper extremity to lower extremity BP (>5 to 10 mm Hg),[60] should increase the suspicion of coarctation of the aorta. The measured difference in pressure on examination has correlated with the measured pressure gradient across the coarctation.[61] It is also important to palpate or measure the pressure of both upper extremities given the occasional presence of anomalous great arteries which may cause asymmetry of upper extremity pulses and pressures (Fig. 18.6). A systolic murmur is frequently heard over the precordium or parascapular region. Chest X-ray may reveal significant rib notching and the "3" sign (outline of the outer border of the coarctation). Once the diagnosis of coarctation of the aorta is suspected, further imaging is recommended including echocardiography (Fig. 18.7), computed tomography (CT) angiography, and magnetic resonance imaging (MRI). An echocardiographic Doppler gradient of ≥20 mm Hg resting or provoked (exercise) peak instantaneous gradient may indicate a significant coarctation.[62] CT angiography and MRI aid in the diagnosis of collaterals as well as intracranial vascular abnormalities.

2.3. Renal artery stenosis

Narrowing of the renal artery lumen or renal artery stenosis is increasingly more common and an important treatable cause of hypertension. Although fibromuscular dysplasia is an uncommon cause of hypertension in the young, renal artery obstruction from atherosclerotic disease in older adults is a major concern in our current aging population with increasing prevalence of diabetes and hyperlipidemia. The prevalence of atherosclerotic renal artery stenosis in high-risk populations may be 25% to 50%.[63–66]

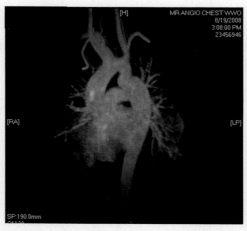

Figure 18.6 MRI of an adult with coarctation of the aorta and abnormal (atretic) left subclavian artery. A 35 mm Hg brachial artery pressure differential between the left and right arms was found.

The renin–angiotensin–aldosterone system plays a primary role in the pathophysiology of hypertension in renal artery stenosis. Narrowing of the renal artery leads to renal hypoperfusion which stimulates production of renin and consequently, angiotensin. Therefore, testing for renal artery stenosis includes physiologic studies to assess the renin–angiotensin–aldosterone system (level of stimulated or unstimulated plasma renin activity or direct renal vein renin measurements), functional studies to assess renal function, perfusion studies to assess relative renal blood flow, and vascular studies to directly image the renal arteries.[66]

Although clinical examination may reveal bruits over major vessels or the renal arteries, clinical suspicion for renal artery stenosis may stem from the presentation of malignant or drug-resistant hypertension in the setting of renal dysfunction. Hypokalemia and hyponatremia may be seen from secondary hyperaldosteronism. Classically, patients with bilateral renal artery stenosis may develop acute renal failure when exposed to ACEI or ARBs. Noninvasive vascular studies to directly image the renal arteries include Doppler ultrasonography,[67,68] spiral CT and MR angiography[69] and are discussed in more detail in Chapters 48 and 49. Perfusion studies to assess relative blood flow include Captopril renography with technetium ^{99m}Tc mercaptoacetyltriglycine (^{99m}Tc MAG$_3$), iodine-labeled orthoiodohippurate (^{131}I OIH), or technetium-labeled diethylenetriamine pentaacetic acid (DTPA) to estimate fractional flow to each kidney.

Captopril renal scan (CRS) is based on the physiology of an ACEI induced fall in filtration pressure in the affected kidney with

Figure 18.7 Doppler/echocardiogram in the suprasternal notch plane. **(A)** Color Doppler of proximal descending aorta turbulent flow across a coarctation. **(B)** Continuous wave Doppler of the peak gradient across the descending aorta with prominent diastolic anterograde flow (*arrows*).

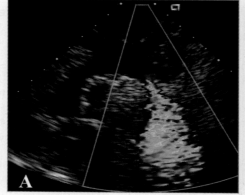

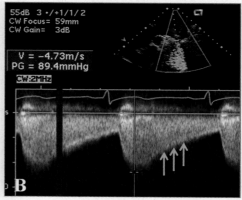

improved function of the contralateral kidney (renin mediated). These changes affect the renal handling of radioactive tracer, amplifying the difference in renal perfusion between the two kidneys. Although a baseline scan can be performed and compared to a postcaptopril scan, the sensitivity and specificity of asymmetric uptake and/or excretion in a single postcaptopril DTPA scan may be as high as 91% to 94% and 93% to 97%, respectively, with high (>93%) negative predictive value.[70] More recent studies suggest, however, that CRS performs differently in populations with high versus low prevalence of disease making it less useful as a screening test.[71] Asymmetric excretion is detected as a delayed (>11 min) time to peak activity or a >1.5-fold difference in glomerular filtration rate between the two kidneys.[72] The study will have limited utility in advanced atherosclerotic disease or significant reduction in renal function.

2.4. Renin–aldosterone disorders

Measurement of renin and total body sodium differentiates between renal and adrenal causes of hypertension.[73] As renin levels increase, there is more vasoconstriction and plasma volume falls leading to lower total body sodium. High renin levels result in increased angiotensin I and subsequently stimulate aldosterone synthesis, angiotensin II, and angiotensin III. In addition, high potassium levels and low sodium levels which increase adrenocorticotropic hormone (ACTH) also stimulate the cortex of the adrenal glands to release aldosterone.

Aldosterone is a mineralocorticoid that acts on distal tubule and collecting duct of the kidneys, resulting in the reabsorbtion of sodium and excretion of potassium. Higher plasma sodium levels lead to water retention and increased circulating blood volume. This in turn increases renal perfusion pressure, resulting in down-regulation of aldosterone secretion in a classic feedback loop.[74] Aldosterone is also produced in extra-adrenal tissues including the brain, cardiac tissue, and blood vessels. Its nonepi-

thelial effects include promotion of inflammation, collagen formation, and fibrosis as well as cellular apoptosis.[74] Excessive LV hypertrophy and reduced myocardial perfusion have also been documented in patients with primary hyperaldosteronism.[75] Aldosterone antagonists reduce collagen synthesis which correlates with the survival benefit seen in patients with clinically significant CHF.[76]

Two forms of hyperaldosteronism therefore exist. PA results in suppression of renin levels, whereas secondary hyperaldosteronism is a result of high renin levels. PA is defined as excessive aldosterone secretion independent of angiotensin II. Because high aldosterone levels suppress renin synthesis, the hallmark of PA is a high aldosterone-to-renin ratio.[77] A high aldosterone-to-renin ratio may also be seen in low renin hypertension, however, using absolute aldosterone concentrations or active renin measurements help to distinguish these two entities as well as saline infusion or fludrocortisone suppression test. The two most common causes of PA are bilateral (rarely unilateral) adrenal hyperplasia accounting for ~68% of cases and aldosterone-producing adenomas which accounts for ~30% of cases. A very small number of cases arise from aldosterone-producing adrenocortical carcinoma, ovarian cancer, or familial hyperaldosteronism. Differential diagnosis of PA requires adrenal gland imaging by CT or MRI, biochemical testing of the aldosterone response to posture, and selective adrenal venous sampling to differentiate unilateral aldosterone-producing adenoma from bilateral hyperplasia.

2.5. Neuroendocrine tumors

Although a rare neuroendocrine tumor, pheochromocytoma as a cause of hypertension is frequently underdiagnosed resulting in catastrophic cardiovascular consequences.[78,79] Familial pheochromocytomas occur in a number of syndromes listed in Table 18.4. Hereditary forms of pheochromocytoma may occur in up to 20% to 30% of patients, often present in younger patients

TABLE 18.4

FAMILIAL PHEOCHROMOCYTOMA SYNDROMES AND THEIR CLINICAL FEATURES

Syndrome	Clinical feature	Gene mutations
Multiple endocrine neoplasia (MEN) type 2a	Medullary thyroid carcinoma Pheochromocytoma Hyperparathyroidism Cutaneous lichen amyloidosis	RET proto-oncogene (chromosome 10q)
Von Hippel–Lindau (VHL) disease type 2	A: Retinal and CNS haemangioblastomas Pheochromocytomas Endolymphatic sac tumors Epididymal cystadenomas B: Renal cell cysts and carcinomas Retinal and CNS haemangioblastomas Pancreatic neoplasms and cysts Pheochromocytomas Endolymphatic sac tumors Epididymal cystadenomas C: Pheochromocytomas only	VHL gene (chromosome 3p)
Neurofibromatosis. type 1	Multiple fibromas on skin and mucosa "Cafè au lait" skin spots Pheochromocytomas	NF1 gene (chromosome 17q)
Familial paragangliomas	Head and neck tumors (carotid-body tumors; vagal, jugular, and tympanic paragangliomas) Pheochromocytomas Abdominal or thoracic paragangliomas (or both)	Germline mutations of B and D subunits of mitochondrial succinate dehydrogenase (SDH B on chromosome 1p and SDH D on chromosome 11q)

(<40 years) and if found in children, are often extra-adrenal (20% to 25%). Numerous gene mutations have been identified for each of the familial syndromes. Adrenal pheochromocytomas usually present in the fourth and fifth decades of life and infrequently (5% to 10%) are metastatic. Extra-adrenal pheochromocytomas have a higher prevalence of malignancy (30% to 40%) which may be genetically determined.

The clinical presentation of pheochromocytomas is protean and thus may be mistaken for any number of other disease processes (Table 18.5). Catecholamine secretion (norepinephrine and epinephrine) is primarily responsible for the major clinical signs including hypertension, tachycardia, pallor, headache, and anxiety. However, centrally acting α_2-agonists that suppress the sympathetic nervous system are very effective in controlling hypertension associated with pheochromocytoma implicating this system in the generation of peripheral vasoconstriction. Patients may have normal BP or sustained hypertension in between episodes of marked increases in BP. Metabolic effects of catecholamines lead to hyperglycemia, lactic acidosis, and weight loss. The presentation may be atypical depending on the associated clinical findings (other tumors) and other secreted peptides or hormones which include dopamine, vasoactive intestinal peptide, ACTH, atrial natriuretic factor, growth hormone-releasing factor, somatostatin, parathyroid hormone-related peptide, calcitonin, serotonin, and others. Dopamine paragangliomas may not present with hypertension, and epinephrine-secreting pheochromocytomas may present with severe hypotension. Numerous triggers of hypertensive paroxysms have been reported including anesthesia, tumor manipulation, postural changes, exertion, anxiety, trauma, pain, drugs/foods with tyramine, and other drugs (histamine, glucagon, phenothiazine, metoclopramide, ACTH). The location of the extra-adrenal tumor may influence the trigger (i.e., micturition with bladder pheochromocytoma).

The majority of pheochromocytomas arise from the chromaffin cells of the adrenal medulla, whereas 15% to 20% arise from extra-adrenal paraganglia. Catecholamine-producing extra-adrenal pheochromocytomas are most frequently found in the abdomen (paraaortic region or around the renal hilum) or pelvis, however, up to 8% may be found in the chest or neck.[80]

Biochemical testing continues to form the cornerstone of diagnosis in suspected pheochromocytomas. Plasma or urine metanephrine and normetanephrine levels have high sensitivity (97% to 99%)[23] however, advances in imaging and genetic testing have led to the diagnosis of familial pheochromocytoma in asymptomatic or normotensive patients. Imaging of adrenal pheochromocytomas can be accomplished with ultrasound, CT, or MRI. Ultrasound for detection of adrenal tumors has a relatively low sensitivity and specificity (83% to 89% and 60%, respectively).[81,82] CT can detect 95% of primary adrenal pheochromocytomas 0.5 to 1.0 cm or larger, and 90% of extra-adrenal pheochromocytomas of at least 1.0 to 2.0 cm in size[83] with a high sensitivity of 85% to 94%, however, the specificity is low (29% to 50%).[84] MRI with T_2-weighted images (high vascularity of pheochromocytoma) has higher sensitivity and specificity compared to CT imaging (93% to 100% and 50% to 100%, respectively).

Adrenal masses are very common[85] and the prediction of malignant or metastatic pheochromocytomas imprecise at best. Thus, function imaging modalities that are specific to pheochromocytomas have a particular utility in this disease. Fortunately, pheochromocytoma cells express specific catecholamine plasma membrane and vesicular transporter systems that allow uptake of metaiodobenzylguanidine (MIBG) and positron-emitting agents. Functional imaging studies include [^{123}I] or [^{131}I] MIBG scintigraphy, 6-[18F]fluorodopamine ([18F] DA), [18F] dihydroxyphenyl-lalanine ([18F] DOPA), [11C] hydroxyephedrine, and [11C] epinephrine positron emission tomography.[84,86] MIBG scintigraphy has a sensitivity of 77% to 90% with a specificity of 95% to 100% for pheochromocytoma.[87,88] These studies play a complementary role in CT or MRI; the combination of an adrenal mass seen on a CT or MRI and uptake on MIBG scanning is definitive in the diagnosis of pheochromocytoma. Functional studies also are useful in localizing metastatic disease with the caveat that dedifferentiated or necrotic tumors may not take up the isotopes. Some would advocate using MIBG scintigraphy prior to surgery in all cases of suspected pheochromocytoma.[84]

2.6. Cushing syndrome

Cushing syndrome is an endocrine disease caused by high levels of cortisol. Normally, ACTH is released by the pituitary gland and acts on the adrenal gland to stimulate release of cortisol. Causes for high cortisol levels include pituitary adenoma (Cushing disease), adrenal hyperplasia or neoplasia and ectopic ACTH production. Cortisol causes hypertension by enhancing the vasoconstrictive effect of epinephrine, or by direct mineralocorticoid activity which is associated with hypokalemia. In addition, other factors may increase the incidence of hypertension including sleep apnea and insulin resistance syndromes. Hypertension is present in 70% to 90% of patients with Cushing syndrome, but resistance hypertension is seen in up to 17% of them. The overall cardiovascular risk is compounded by the associated high-risk

TABLE 18.5
CLINICAL PRESENTATION OF PHEOCHROMOCYTOMA

Cardiac	Hypertension (sustained or paroxysmal) Tachycardia Palpitations Orthostatic hypotension Transient electrocardiographic changes Hypotension and shock Myocardial infarction Arrhythmias Aortic dissection Sudden death
Neurologic	Headaches Tremulousness Encephalopathy Visual disturbances Paresthesias Seizures Stroke Neurogenic pulmonary edema
Endocrine	Hyperglycemia
Gastrointestinal	Abdominal pain Nausea and vomiting Constipation
Psychological	Anxiety Panic
Miscellaneous	Pallor Flushing Heat intolerance Excess sweating Weight loss

factors of diabetes mellitus, the metabolic syndrome, obesity, and dyslipidemia. Consequently, target organ damage is more severe than in patients with essential hypertension.

After screening patients with a dexamethasone suppression test or 24-h urinary measurement of cortisol, those suspected of having Cushing syndrome should have noninvasive imaging of the pituitary sella and the adrenal gland with MRI and CT scanning. Iodocholesterol scintigraphy has also been used to detect adrenal gland hyperactivity.

2.7. Sleep apnea

Obstructive sleep apnea (OSA) is present in 30% to 80% of hypertensive patients[89,90] and may contribute significantly to disease severity and progression.[91,92] High-risk predictors of OSA include obesity, male gender, and age. In OSA, collapse of the pharyngeal airway causes repetitive cessation of ventilation for ≥10 s during ventilatory effort. Hypopnea is a decrease (not complete cessation) of ventilation. The diagnosis is made when patients have ≥5 apneic or hypopneic episodes per hour, with daytime sleepiness. However, in moderate or severe OSA patients can have ≥15 episodes per hour.[93] The cause of disturbed ventilation is pharyngeal collapse posterior to the nasal septum and above the epiglottis. Although the diagnosis can be suspected by history (disruptive snoring, witnessed apnea, obesity, and hypersomnolence), polysomnography is the diagnostic test of choice.

OSA is listed as an identifiable cause of essential hypertension by the Joint National Committee on the Detection and Management of Hypertension.[3] This causal relationship was identified by three lines of research: studies identifying OSA as an independent risk factor for hypertension, a dose-related effect (the worse the OSA, the higher the BP), and finally a treatment-response effect.[89] Treatment of OSA by continuous, positive airway pressure will acutely decrease the BP, however, the chronic effect of BP has been variable. Some studies report modest changes in both daytime and sleep BPs, and others just in sleep BP. The extent of these changes may also be related to the severity of OSA.

The American Heart Association and American College of Cardiology Foundation Scientific Statement on sleep apnea and cardiovascular disease[94] summarizes the magnitude of the problem: "...>85% of patients with clinically significant and treatable OSA have never been diagnosed...." Screening patients for OSA is relatively simple. A clinician evaluating a hypertensive patient, particularly if that patient is older, male, or obese (twofold to fourfold increase risk of OSA), should consider OSA in the diagnosis of secondary causes of hypertension. Because almost all patients with OSA snore (although not all snorers have OSA) and OSA results in disturbed sleep and thus daylong somnolence, physicians can easily screen for OSA by asking the patient or family member three questions: (a) Do you snore a lot? (b) Do you experience excessive daytime sleepiness (i.e., fall asleep during passive activities such as reading an interesting book, watching an interesting program, or driving a car)? (c) Does your partner say you stop breathing or gasp a lot during sleep? The last question fulfills the criteria of "witnessed apnea/hypopnea." Patients who answer in the affirmative may have OSA and should then be sent for polysomnography.

3. DIAGNOSTIC EVALUATION OF THE PATIENT WITH HYPERTENSION

The cardiovascular effects of hypertension are varied in part because of various comorbidities associated with this disease entity, such as age, diabetes, obesity, and coronary artery disease. The earliest presentation may be limited to an abnormal vascular response to stress. Advanced disease will result in heart failure symptoms with diastolic or systolic dysfunction. Between these two presentations is a broad spectrum of diseases with a unifying feature: LV hypertrophy. Numerous studies have shown increased myocardial fibrosis associated with hypertension related LVH.[95-97] This increase in the support structures for the myocytes has been postulated as the etiology for a "stiff heart" and reduced diastolic function in diastolic heart failure (DHF). Recent studies have also shown that the myocytes of patients with DHF actually differ in morphology compared to patients with systolic heart failure (SHF).[98] Cardiomyocyte diameter was higher in DHF and exhibited higher passive force, whereas myofibrillar density was lower in SHF. These cellular alterations help explain changes in cardiac function seen in the hypertensive population with LVH.

LVH is the result of increased afterload and high peripheral vascular resistance. In addition, the prevalence of hypertrophy is influenced by sodium intake and high plasma angiotensin II levels. Remodeling of the ventricle however, is multifactorial, and numerous reports suggest a strong relationship between LV mass and age, obesity, and diabetes[14-21] as well as genetic factors.[99] As discussed previously, LV mass is a strong predictor of adverse cardiovascular events[4-13] and regression of LVH predicts improved outcomes.[19,23-30] The accurate measurement of LV mass is thus an integral part of the evaluation of a patient with hypertension.

Although indirect measures of LV mass by ECG have also predicted adverse outcomes in epidemiologic studies,[100,101] this modality has reasonable specificity (90% to 95%) but poor sensitivity.[102-104] A recent study evaluating the accuracy of ECG criteria for LVH using MRI–LV mass determination[105] showed a sensitivity of only 23% to 26% using various ECG criteria. Thus, ECG should not be used to exclude the diagnosis of LVH. However, given the low cost, ease of acquisition and interpretation, as well as numerous studies on cardiovascular prognosis based on ECG–LVH measurements, this remains a useful tool for the clinician.

Other noninvasive methods of assessing LV mass should improve on the advantages and disadvantages inherent to ECG measurements. Although cost and equipment considerations are important particularly for following medical therapy, accuracy and reproducibility of measurements are the major determinants of clinical utility. The primary tools for measuring LV mass include two-dimensional (2D) and three-dimensional (3D) echocardiography, MRI, and CT. LVH and structural changes to the myocardium and vasculature create the substrate for systolic (both global and regional) and diastolic dysfunction. Although covered elsewhere, the role of noninvasive imaging in assessing these abnormalities will be briefly discussed.

3.1. Echocardiography

3.1.1. M-mode and two-dimensional echocardiographies

Left ventricular mass and left ventricular hypertrophy. M-mode and 2D echocardiographies developed in ~1957 and ~1974, respectively, were the first noninvasive tools to directly measure LV mass. To calculate LV mass from linear dimensions, models of LV geometry were developed. Geiser and Bove[106] made linear measurements on 51 ex-vivo hearts and provided anatomic validation for the truncated ellipsoidal model (95% CI: ±2) and a simpler ellipsoidal model (95% CI: ±22). The latter geometry approximates the D³ formula using M-mode measurements. LV mass is determined by subtracting the LV cavity volume from the volume encompassed by the LV epicardium and multiplying the resultant volume by myocardial density. This method has been validated by LV mass at necropsy in numerous studies.[107-109]

Because of the significantly higher pulse rates with M-mode echocardiography, temporal resolution of this technique exceeds that of 2D imaging. Border delineation is an important aspect of measurement and accuracy in M-mode calculations of LV volume and mass. Investigators at the University of Pennsylvania developed modifications referred to as the Penn convention in which all edges are not included in the parietal thickness measurements (Fig. 18.8).[107] Using the Penn convention as the border definition criteria, LV mass could be calculated using the formula

$$LV\,mass\,(Penn) = 1.04([LVIDd + PWTd + IVSTD]^3 - [LVIDd]^3) - 13.6\,g \qquad \text{(Eq. 18.1)}$$

where LVIDd is the internal LV linear measurements in diastole, PWT and SWT are the PWT diastole and interventricular septal thickness at end diastole, respectively. The American Society of Echocardiography (ASE) subsequently published their recommendations for border measurement[110] calling for use of the leading edge technique. LV mass using the cube formula and this border definition, however, consistently overestimated the anatomic LV mass by about 15% to 20%. Devereux et al.[111] derived a regression equation correcting this overestimation:

$$LV\,Mass\,(ASE) = 0.8\,(1.04\,([LVIDd + PWTd + IVSTD]^3 - [LVIDd]^3)) + 0.6\,g \qquad \text{(Eq. 18.2)}$$

2D imaging can be used to make linear and area measurements.[112,113] These may be taken from multiple imaging planes (apical, or parasternal short- or long-axis views) at the tips of papillary muscles. A current ASE recommendation for chamber quantification[114] is that 2D or 2D-guided M-mode measurements and more recently 2D linear measurements[115] be taken from the minor axis of the LV in the parasternal long-axis view, "approximately at the level of the mitral leaflet tips."

A variation of this method taking linear measurements from the base of the ventricle was validated in a population of patients with LV aneurysms, but yielded significantly smaller internal dimensions and mass.[116] This measurement is performed at the base of LV and can be used to assess basal wall motion in asymmetric ventricle, but is not the accepted standard.

The second recommended method for calculating LV mass utilizes 2D planimetered areas and ventricular long-axis linear measurements in either the area–length (A–L) formula or the truncated ellipsoid (T-E) model.[114] For this calculation, the area of ventricle is measured at the midpapillary muscle level. For endocardial tracing, the papillary muscles are excluded as are prominent trabeculations. For the epicardial area, the visceral pericardium and right ventricular trabeculations are excluded. A long-axis measurement from apical views is also required. Obtaining an accurate long-axis measurement from the level of the mitral annulus to the apex of the LV cavity is essential for the A–L method. The semimajor axis and truncated semimajor axis are used in the T-E formula (Fig. 18.9).

The final 2D method for calculating LV mass is the biplane method of discs using the modified Simpson's rule (Fig. 18.10). In this method, two orthogonal apical views are traced, excluding the papillary muscles. Areas of discs of equal height (the number of discs set by predetermined algorithms) are calculated using the diameters in each plane and the resulting volumes summed. This method is particular useful for asymmetric ventricles but still assumes an ellipsoid area for each disc. To calculate the mass, the volume of the endocardial volume is subtracted from the epicardial volume and multiplied by myocardial density. Validation for this method has been limited however, because complete endocardial and epicardial borders are difficult to image. Takeuchi et al.[117] recently calculated LV mass on 205 patients using M-mode, 2D, 3D, and CMR imaging. After correlating 3D echocardiography to cardiac MRI in one group of patients, they then compared M-mode and 2D biplane Simpson's rule methods using 3D echo as the gold standard. Correlation with 3D was excellent for both methods.

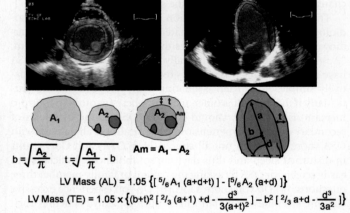

$$b = \sqrt{\frac{A_2}{\pi}} \qquad t = \sqrt{\frac{A_1}{\pi}} - b \qquad A_m = A_1 - A_2$$

$$LV\,Mass\,(AL) = 1.05\left\{[\tfrac{5}{6}A_1\,(a+d+t)] - [\tfrac{5}{6}A_2\,(a+d)]\right\}$$

$$LV\,Mass\,(TE) = 1.05 \times \left\{(b+t)^2\left[\tfrac{2}{3}(a+1)+d-\frac{d^3}{3(a+t)^2}\right] - b^2\left[\tfrac{2}{3}a+d-\frac{d^3}{3a^2}\right]\right\}$$

Figure 18.9 Two methods for estimating LV mass based on A–L formula and the truncated ellipsoid (T-E) formula, from short-axis (**left**) and apical four-chamber (**right**) 2D echo views. Where A_1, total LV area; A_2, LV cavity area; A_m, myocardial area, a is the long or semimajor axis from widest minor axis radius to apex, b is the short-axis radius (back calculated from the short-axis cavity area), and d is the truncated semimajor axis from widest short-axis diameter to mitral annulus plane. Assuming a circular area, the radius (b) is computed and mean wall thickness (t) is derived from the short-axis epicardial and cavity areas. (Adapted from Lang R, Bierig M, Devereux R, et al. Recommendations for chamber quantification: A report from the American Society of Echocardiography's Guidelines and Standards Committee and the Chamber Quantification Writing Group, developed in conjunction with the European Association of Echocardiography, a Branch of the European Society of Cardiology. *J Am Soc Echocardiogr.* 2005;18:1440–1463.).

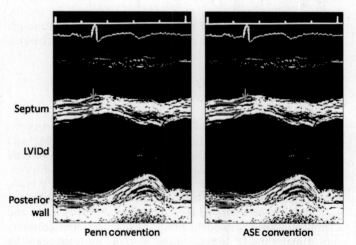

Figure 18.8 Border measurement techniques: Penn convention and ASE convention. *Red arrows* indicate location measurement. *Green arrow* shows the right ventricular echoes from the moderator band that is excluded from LV measurements. ASE, American Society of Echocardiography; LVIDd, Lv internal dimensional in a diastole.

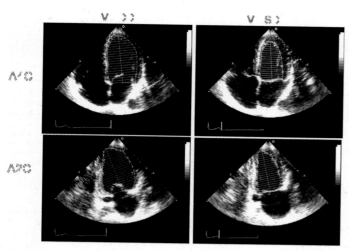

Figure 18.10 2D measurements for volume calculations using biplane method of discs (modified Simpson's rule) in apical 4-chamber (*4Ch*) and apical 2-chamber (*2Ch*) views at end diastole and at end systole. Papillary muscles should be excluded from the cavity in the tracing.

Multiple limitations to M-mode and 2D calculations of LV mass must be recognized. First, validation studies by necropsy are limited in sample size with some studies showing poor correlation.[107,108,111,118–120] In addition, asymmetric ventricles may not only be accurately measured using linear measurements but also be inaccurately characterized by two orthogonal planes. The accuracy of echocardiographically determined LV mass measurements is summarized in Table 18.6. Finally, the variability of measurements is not trivial. In one study,[121] these difference were as much as 28 to 29 g for paired measurements for an individual. The long-term variability of LV mass (average follow-up of 5 years) in a normal population was associated with changes in body weight, BP, and sodium intake. When these variables were adjusted for, the change in LV mass in an individual was <6 g (95% CI of <23 g) and the intra-patient difference did not exceed 10%.[122] In a population of hypertensives[123] using the ASE recommendations, the between-study standard deviation of LV mass was only 6 g/m². LV mass estimates have been shown to be stable despite acute changes in LV geometry caused by acute hypertension[124] or relief of volume load.[125]

The prevalence of LVH in hypertension varies significantly based on the study population, measurement method, and cut-point criteria for LVH. In addition, because body size and habitus are associated with LV size, normalizing LV mass for some index of body size is an accepted practice. Although the most common index has been body surface area (BSA) with reduced variability due to body size and gender,[126] this index significantly underestimates LV mass in obese patients.[127] Using height to index LV mass would more accurately estimate LV mass and cardiovascular risk associated with LVH. Numerous groups have shown that indexing to height to the power of 2.7 (height$^{2.7}$) more accurately estimates LVH and risk.[34,128] In one of the largest studies comparing various LV mass indexes, Liao et al.[129] evaluated 988 patients with LV mass determination by M-mode ASE convention and followed them for 7 years. Unindexed LV mass and indexing for four different heights and two different BSA methods of body size predicted all-cause death and cardiac deaths with no significant difference among them. Importantly, those patients who fulfilled both BSA and height indexed criteria for LVH had the greatest average LV masses. The ASE has thus listed partition values for LV mass based on BSA, height, and height$^{2.7}$ in their quantitation guidelines. It is reasonable to use BSA in most clinical cases, realizing that this index will incorporate some of the risks for obesity into the LVH determination. The ASE recommendations for LV quantification[108] has determine partition values for LV mass, mass index (to BSA, height, and height$^{2.7}$) and is reproduced in Table 18.7.

TABLE 18.6
LV MASS VALIDATION STUDIES USING THE 2D OR M-MODE ECHOCARDIOGRAPHIC CALCULATIONS

Geometric model	Reference	Number of subjects	Reference standard	Cross-sectional views	Convention	LV mass R	LV mass SEE(g)
Prolate Ellipsoid	Devereux[107]	34	Postmortem	M-mode MV tips	Penn	0.96	29
	Devereux[111]	52	Postmortem	M-mode MV tips	ASEM-mode	0.9	47
	Devereux[111]	52	Postmortem	M-mode MV tips	Penn	0.86	59
	Woythaler[108]	48	Postmortem	M-mode MV tips	ASE M-mode	0.81	51
	Park[118]	34	Postmortem	M-mode MV tips	ASE M-mode	0.78	20
	Qin[195]	27	MRI	M-mode	ASE M-mode	0.38	124
	Takeuchi[150]	150	MRI	M-mode	ASE M-mode	0.76	21
Area length	Park[118]	34	Postmortem	SAX-Pap; 4Ch		0.66	34
	Qin[195]	27	MRI	SAX-Pap; 4Ch		0.83	45
Truncated ellipsoid	Devereux[111]	9	Postmortem	SAX-Pap; 4Ch		0.82	
	Park[118]	34	Postmortem	SAX-Pap; 4Ch		0.66	34
Modified Simpson's rule	Helak[120]	13 in vitro	Direct	6-11 SAX	Wyatt	0.93	89.5
	Takeuchi[117]	150	RT3D	4Ch, 2Ch		0.91	5
		150	RT3D	3D-guided 2D 4Ch, 2Ch		0.95	11

TABLE 18.7
ASE REFERENCE LIMITS AND PARTITION VALUES OF LEFT VENTRICULAR MASS AND GEOMETRY

	Women				Men			
	Reference Range	Mildly abnormal	Moderately abnormal	Severely abnormal	Reference Range	Mildly abnormal	Moderately abnormal	Severely abnormal
Linear Method								
LV Mass (g)	67–162	163–186	187–210	≥211	88–224	225–258	259–292	≥293
LV Mass/ BSA (g/ m²)	43–95	96–108	109–121	≥122	49–115	116–131	132–148	≥149
LV Mass/ Height (g/ m)	41–99	100–115	116–128	≥129	52–126	127–144	145–162	≥163
LV Mass/ Height$^{2.7}$ (g/ m$^{2.7}$)	18–44	45–51	52–58	≥59	20–48	49–55	56–63	≥64
RWT	0.22–0.42	0.43–0.47	0.48–0.52	≥0.53	0.24–0.42	0.43–0.46	0.47–0.51	≥0.52
SWT (cm)	0.6–0.9	1.0–1.2	1.3–1.5	≥1.6	0.6–0.9	1.0–1.3	1.4–1.6	≥1.7
PWT (cm)	0.6–0.9	1.0–1.2	1.3–1.5	≥1.6	0.6–0.9	1.0–1.3	1.4–1.6	≥1.7
2D Method								
LV Mass (g)	66–150	151–171	172–182	≥193	96–200	201–227	228–254	≥255
LV Mass/ BSA (g/ m²)	44–88	89–100	101–112	≥113	56–102	102–116	117–130	≥131

LV, left ventricle; BSA, body surface area; RWT, relative wall thickness; SWT, septal wall thickness; PWT, posterior wall thickness.
Source: Modified from Lang R, Bierig M, Devereux R, et al. Recommendation for chamber Quantification: A report from the American Society of Echocardiography's Guidelines and Standards Committee and the Chamber Quantification Writing Group, developed in conjuction with the European Association of Echocardiography, a Branch of the European Society of Cardiology. *J Am Soc Echocardiogr.* 2005; 18:1440–1463.

As noted previously, LV geometry further stratifies risk based on the measurement of LV mass and RWT (Figs. 18.1 and 18.2). RWT is defined as

$$(PWT \times 2) / LVIDd \qquad (Eq. 18.3)$$

where PWT, posterior wall thickness in diastole and LVIDd, LV internal dimensions in diastole. RWT provides additional prognostic information independent of LV mass. In a population-based case–control study of patients with first ischemic stroke,[34] an increased LVRWT was independently associated with stroke after adjustment for LV mass (OR, 1.6; 95% CI: 1.1 to 2.3). RWT, end-systolic stress, and systolic BP were independently associated with midwall fractional shortening (MWFS) (a measure of systolic function) and RWT and age were independently associated with isovolumic relaxation time (a surrogate for diastolic dysfunction).[130]

Left ventricular systolic function. The assessment of LV function is another important aspect of hypertensive heart disease. Numerous studies have shown that LVH can predict the development of CHF.[5-10] Reduced systolic function may occur due to subendocardial ischemia or decreased coronary blood reserve or flow however, the development of LVH is not just determined by the pressure load and wall stress. The traditional way of measuring systolic function has been EF. Although numerous formulas using linear dimensions have been proposed for calculating LV volumes, the ASE recommends using the biplane Simpson's method of discs (Fig. 18.10).

Studies of hypertensives early in the disease process have shown normal to increased EF even in the setting of LVH. Endocardial shortening, which plays a major role in the determination of volume and EF however, does not account for the different fiber orientations throughout the thickness of the LV wall. Because end-systolic stress at the endocardium is not transmitted transmurally, and transmural thickening is not uniform with the endocardial portion of the wall thickening more than the epicardial portion, it would make sense that the midwall shortening during systole might be an afterload independent measure of ventricular function. The midwall fibers of the ventricle are oriented more circumferentially, making perpendicular measurements (shortening) of this set of fibers ideal. Numerous studies show that MWFS, which can be measured easily by parasternal short-axis M-modes or 2D images, may be a better measure of systolic function than endocardial fraction shortening[131] particularly when indexed for end-systolic stress.[132,133] In patient with LVH and normal LVEF, MWFS is abnormal in the setting of high BP[134] and acute DHF,[135] is reduced in patients with diastolic dysfunction,[136] can predict LV diastolic abnormalities,[137] can predict the development of CHF,[138] and can precede diastolic dysfunction.[139]

MWFS is calculated as formula (Eq. 18.4)[140,141]:

$$MWFS = \frac{([LVIDd \pm MWd]-[LVIDs \pm MWs]}{LVIDd+MWd} \times 100 \qquad (Eq. 18.4)$$

where LVIDd, LV internal dimension in diastole; MWd, midwall diastolic thickness; LVIDs, LV internal dimension in systole; MWs, midwall systolic thickness.

In this formula, MWd is half of the end-diastolic wall thickness and is defined as formula (Eq. 18.5):

$$MWd = SWTd / 2 + PWTd / 2 \qquad (Eq. 18.5)$$

where SWTd, septal wall thickness in diastole; PWTd, posterior wall thickness in diastole.

MWs however, cannot be calculated the same way, since the mid wall migrates toward the epicardium in systole. Instead, MWs is calculated using the diastolic LV mass. Because of conservation of mass, the diastolic LV mass must equal the systolic LV mass (formula 3):

$$(LVIDd + MWd)^3 - LVIDd^3 = (LVIDs + MWs)^3 - LVIDs \quad (Eq. 18.6)$$

Solving for MWs thus yields

$$MWs = [(LVIDd + SWTd/2 + PWTd/2)^3 - LVIDd^3 + LVIDs^3]^{1/3} - LVIDs \quad (Eq. 18.7)$$

The final formula for MWFS thus becomes

$$MWFS = \frac{([LVIDd + SWTd/2 + PWTd/2] - [LVIDs + MWs])}{(LVIDd + SWTd/2 + PWTd/2)} \times 100 \quad (Eq. 18.8)$$

An example of the calculation is shown in Figure 18.11 with reference limits[111] in Table 18.8.

3D echocardiography has recently been used to assess 3D midwall EF ($3DEF_{mw}$). MWFS and $3DEF_{mw}$ correlated significantly with LV mass and were better discriminators of LVH and normal LV mass compared to endocardial indices.[142]

Tissue Doppler for evaluation of systolic function[143,144] is another useful tool in patients with hypertension.[145,146] Multiple studies have shown that in patients with hypertension and normal EF, there is a significant reduction in systolic tissue velocities (from multiple positions at the level of the mitral annulus as well as mid septal region) which parallel the prevalence of LVH and diastolic dysfunction.[145] Longitudinal systolic tissue Doppler velocities were linearly related to worsening global diastolic dysfunction but not to global EF.[146]

Hypertension is a major risk factor for the development of CHF.[147-149] According to the Framingham study,[147] the hazard for developing heart failure in hypertensive compared with normotensive subjects was about twofold in men and threefold in women. Multivariable analyses revealed that hypertension had a high population-attributable risk for CHF, accounting for 39% of cases in men and 59% in women. Coronary artery disease

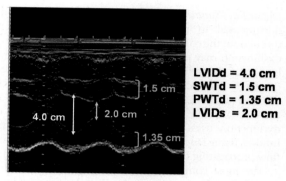

LVIDd = 4.0 cm
SWTd = 1.5 cm
PWTd = 1.35 cm
LVIDs = 2.0 cm

Calculation of midwall fractional shortening:
MWS = [(LVIDd + SWTd/2 + PWTd/2)³ - LVIDd³ + LVIDs³]¹⁄³ - LVIDs
MWFS = ([LVIDd + SWTd/2 + PWTd/2] - [LVIDs + MWs]) x 100 / (LVIDd + SWTd/2 + PWTd/2)

MWs = (157 - 64 + 8)^(1/3) - 2.0 = 2.65 cm
MWFS = (5.43 - (2 + 2.65) x 100 / 5.425
     = 14%

Figure 18.11 Sample calculation of M-mode derived mid wall fractional shortening (MWFS) in a hypertensive patient with normal EF. Although the EF is 80%, the MWFS is reduced (14%). MWs, midwall systolic thickness; LVIDd, LV internal dimensions in diastole; LVIDs, LV internal dimensions in systole; SWTd, septal wall thickness in diastole; PWTd, posterior wall thickness in diastole.

preceded the development of CHF in 60% of cases. Treatment of hypertension reduces the risk for developing CHF by up to 50%.[150-152] LVH is an independent risk factor for CHF, and LVH regression also confers a reduced risk.[147]

The prevalence of asymptomatic LV systolic dysfunction in the general population is ~2%,[153,154] but may occur in 4% to 14% of hypertensive patients.[155,156] Patients with essential hypertension and EFs of <50% at initial evaluation, had a nearly 10-fold risk of hospitalization for CHF compared to patients with normal EF.[149] This finding on echocardiography should prompt aggressive pharmacologic and nonpharmacologic treatment of hypertension.

TABLE 18.8
REFERENCE LIMITS FOR MIDWALL FRACTION SHORTENING

	Women				Men			
	Reference range	Mildly abnormal	Moderately abnormal	Severely abnormal	Reference range	Mildly abnormal	Moderately abnormal	Severely abnormal
Linear method								
Endocardial fractional shortening (%)	27–45	22–27	17–21	≤16	25–43	20–24	15–19	≤14
Midwall fractional shortening (%)	15–23	13–14	11–12	≤10	14–22	12–13	10–11	≤10
2D method								
Ejection fraction (%)	≥55	45–54	30–44	<30	≥55	45–54	30–44	<30

Source: Modified from Lang R, Bierig M, Devereux R, et al. Recommendation for chamber Quantification: A report from the American Society of Echocardiography's Guidelines and Standards Committee and the Chamber Quantification Writing Group, developed in conjuction with the European Association of Echocardiography, a Branch of the European Society of Cardiology. *J Am Soc Echocardiogr.* 2005; 18:1440–1463.

Diastolic function. Abnormal diastolic function is well documented in patients with hypertension and may occur throughout the course of the disease. The development of diastolic dysfunction may precede the development of LVH and thus may be one of the earliest changes associated with hypertensive heart disease.[157–159] Structural changes in the myocardium such as altered collagen and myocardial cell architecture have been postulated as the mechanism.[160] The echocardiographic evaluation of diastolic dysfunction uses Doppler of the mitral and pulmonary vein inflows, tissue Doppler of the mitral annulus, color M-mode of the flow propagating into the ventricle, and left atrial (LA) volume.

The most common echocardiographic tool used for assessing LV diastolic function is the Doppler flow profile across the LV inflow tract and pulmonary veins. Both diastolic function and preload affect the *E:A* ratio[161] however, various estimates of LV filling pressure using mitral inflow and pulmonary venous inflow allowed differentiation of normal *E:A* ratio, from pseudonormal *E:A* ratio (high filling pressures in the setting of impaired relaxation).[162] Tissue Doppler of the mitral annulus and color M-mode for flow propagation velocities are less preload-independent measures of diastolic function. Combining either of these two parameters with the mitral E wave has allowed for the assessment of ventricular preload and estimates of pulmonary capillary wedge pressure. Echocardiographic estimates of LV end-DP and pulmonary capillary wedge pressure have correlated well with invasive hemodynamics.

Does echocardiography measure the actual diastolic function of the ventricle, or the surrogate of diastolic dysfunction filling pressures? Numerous studies have correlated echocardiographic parameters of diastolic dysfunction with direct measurements of the relaxation constant tau. Oki et al.[163] showed a strong correlation between tau and basal posterior wall myocardial early diastolic velocity ($r = -0.81$, $p < 0.0001$) in 40 patients with normal and abnormal diastolic functions. There was no significant relationship between tau and transmitral E or E deceleration time. Kasner et al.[164] studied diastolic function in "heart failure with normal ejection fraction" patients by directly measuring the indexes for diastolic relaxation (tau, dP/dt[min]), LV end-diastolic pressure, and LV end-diastolic pressure–volume relationship (stiffness, b [dP/dV], and stiffness constant, beta), correlated these with mitral inflows, *E'/A'* and *E/E'* (lateral). These parameters detected diastolic function in 70%, 81%, and 86% of patients, respectively. In this study, the single best index to detect diastolic dysfunction was *E/E'* (lateral) >8. A complete discussion of the usage of imaging techniques to measure diastolic function can be found in Chapter 16.

Left atrial volume. LA size has been shown to be a predictor of atrial fibrillation, stroke, CHF, and overall cardiovascular risk.[165–168] LA volume has been evaluated in numerous epidemiological studies across diverse populations[169] and shown to be linearly related to filling pressures, LV mass, and BP. LA volume predicts all-cause mortality and cardiovascular events. Because LA size reflects LV diastolic dysfunction and increased LV filling pressures, it is closely related to both hypertension[170,171] and LV mass.[172] In fact, the ability of LA size to predict mortality is attenuated when LV mass,[128] LV hypertrophy,[173] or diastolic function[174] are considered.

The thin-walled left atrium is sensitive to filling pressures and remodels in response to chronic pressure and volume overload. Chronic pressure overload of the LA may occur secondary to increased LA afterload (mitral valve disease[175] and LV diastolic dysfunction[176]) as well as fibrosis of the left atrium with reduced LA compliance.[177] Chronic volume overload occurs with valvular regurgitation and high output states (i.e., arteriovenous fistulas,

chronic anemia, or athletic heart). In the absence of primary atrial pathology, mitral valve disease, or atrial fibrillation, increased LA volume is a measure of chronically increased ventricular pressures. In response to high LV filling pressure, the LA pressure increases to maintain cardiac output[178] with LA remodeling occurring after chronic pressure overload. Thus, LA volume adds incremental information to instantaneous diastolic grade assessment by reflecting the chronicity of LA pressure overload.[179,180]

LA volume and LA anteroposterior dimension are not linearly related. LA volume is a more accurate and reproducible estimate of LA size compared to 3D reference standards such as MRI[181] and CT.[182] LA volume is also superior to LA dimension in predicting outcomes.[183] MRI can not only measure LA volume, but by creating a volume–time curve it may also determine LA volume change, reservoir function, EF, and mean filling and emptying rates.[184] Methods for measuring LA volume by 2D echocardiography include the biplane A–L method and the biplane Simpson's rule.[102,185] Both measurements require imaging of the entire left atrium from two orthogonal views. Gender difference in LA dimensions is primarily due to differences in body size and thus, indexing for BSA is an accepted method for adjusting for these differences.[186] Published reference values for maximum and minimum LA volumes are 22 ± 6 and $9 \pm 4 \, \text{mL/m}^2$, respectively.[187,188] The same limitations of LV volume and mass measurements apply to measuring the LA including failure to image the entire LA wall and off-axis image orientation.

3.1.2. Three-dimensional echocardiography

The discussions above about geometric assumptions for calculation of LV mass could not highlight more appropriately the need for a 3D solution to the measurements of LV size and function. 3D echocardiography offers multiple advantages over 2D echocardiography. Historically, 3D echocardiograms were reconstructed from 2D data sets. Some of the earliest 3D reconstructions utilized freehand 2D scanning while tracking the transducer position and orientation with an acoustic locator or spark gap. LV mass measurements using this system showed high correlation ($r = 0.9$) with MRI with a standard error of the estimate of only 11 g but an interobserver variability of 13%.[189] Gated sequential scanning methods acquired 2D images sequentially in a rotational, fanlike or parallel manner, from a single acoustic window, gated to ECG and respirations. Correlation of LV volumes with MRI was very high (0.9 to 0.95).

The development of matrix array transducers of more than 3,000 elements has made real-time 3D echocardiography a clinical reality. These probes allow acquisition of volumes of data with acceptable volume rates, thus allowing for wide-angle acquisitions by splicing subvolumes or real-time volume acquisitions. Because there are multiple display options for 3D volume sets, LV mass can be calculated by numerous methods using off-line analysis software. The earliest methods of calculating LV mass reconstructed the LV chamber in multiple 2D short-axis views. This allows for a direct application of the Simpson's rule, where planimetry of the epicardial area and endocardial area of each slice can generate a volume and mass. Although time-consuming, this method has been validated against postmortem LV weights and MRI. LV mass measurements can now be calculated using semiautomated endocardial border detection of the entire volume set with an assumed wall thickness but with manual adjustments if needed (Fig. 18.12). A significant reduction in standard error of the estimate is seen in most studies (Table 18.9).[117,190–196] Takeuchi et al.[117] also showed, however, that using real-time 3D to guide acquisition of two orthogonal planes LV mass could be measured using the modified biplane Simpson's rule. They found excellent correlation

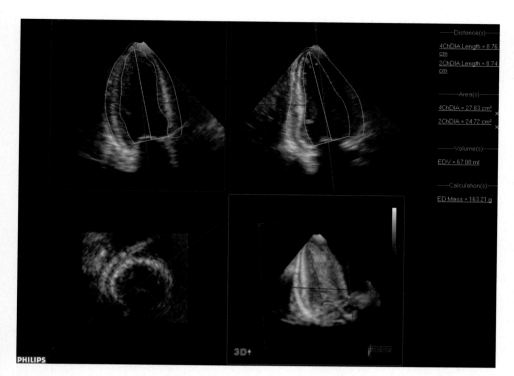

Figure 18.12 The 3D LV mass measurement of the same patient in Figure 18.11, using semiautomated mass measurements (=162 g). LV mass calculation by M-mode measurements overestimates the 3D LV mass calculation by 44 g.

TABLE 18.9
LV MASS VALIDATION STUDIES USING THE THREE-DIMENSIONAL ECHOCARDIOGRAPHIC MEASUREMENTS

Author	3D technique	Subjects	Reference standard	R	SEE (gm)	Mean difference ± 1 SD	Interobserver variability (%)
Gopal et al.[189]	Free hand, spark gap locator	15	MRI	EDV, 0.90	11		13
Gopal et al.[190]	Free hand, spark gap locator	20 (pre-transplant)	Explanted hearts	0.99	11.9	−4.9	23.3
Lee et al.[191]	RT3D	25	MRI	0.95	6	5±26	
Mor-Avi et al.[192]	RT3D	21	MRI	0.90		4±14	0.23
Takeuchi et al.[117]	Rt3D	21 (LVH)	MRI	0.95	20	−14±29	11
Ven den Bosch et al.[193]	RT3D	20 (CHD)	MRI	0.94	19	10±19	
Jenkins et al.[194]	RT3D	50	MRI			0±38	
Qin et al.[195]	RT3D	27 (COM,AR)	MRI	0.92	29	−9±33	
Caiani et al.[196]	RT3D automated	21	MRI	0.96	11	−2±12	12
Takeuchi et al.[197]	RT3D	55	MRI	0.95		−2±19.9	

between 3D guided 2D LV mass calculations compared to real-time 3D LV mass ($r = 0.95$, bias = −4.6 ± 12.5 g).

3.2. Cardiac magnetic resonance and multidetector computed tomography

Advantages of cardiac magnetic resonance (CMR) include its high spatial and reasonable temporal resolution (≥20 per s). Obtaining a combination of T_1- and T_2-weighted images allows for morphology and tissue characterization. Contrast agents (gadolinium DTPA) allow assessment of perfusion (first pass) and late enhancement (viability or other pathologies). Finally, morphologic and functional assessment is improved by the ability to acquire images in any cardiac plane. Thus, although 2D echocardiography remains the primary modality for assessment

of LV volumes and mass, CMR (Fig. 18.13) has been the noninvasive gold standard given its superior accuracy and reproducibility.[198–202] Interstudy reproducibility of CMR versus 2D echo was performed by Grothues et al.,[203] by conducting two sequential MR and echocardiographic studies on a heterogeneous group of 60 subjects; 20 normals, 20 with LVH, and 20 with CHF. Interstudy reproducibility was higher for CMR measurements of LV size and function ($r = 0.94$ to 0.99) and more variable for echocardiographic measurements ($r = 0.65$ to 0.98). In patients with LVH, the coefficient of variability for LV mass measurements (defined as the standard deviation of the mean difference between two measures divided by the mean value of the LV mass) was 13.5% for Echo LV mass versus 3.6% for CMR LV mass. Because MRI images are gated acquisitions, temporal resolution is lower when com-

Figure 18.13 Multiple short-axis imaging planes using CMR for Simpson's method of volume and mass calculations: endocardial tracing (*red*) and epicardial tracing (*green*).

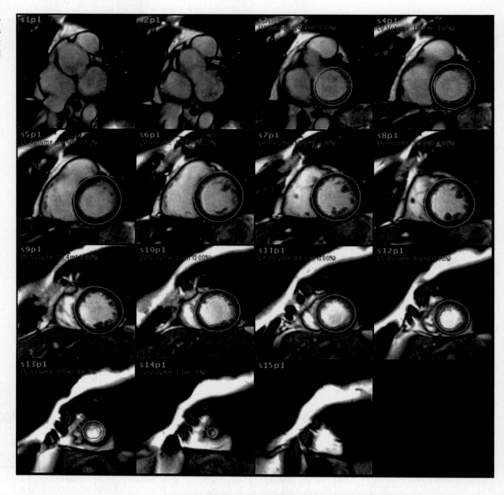

pared to 2D echocardiography. Arrhythmias will further reduce spatial resolution and significantly increase acquisition time.

CT has theoretically similar advantages to CMR with regard to multiplane reconstruction however, there are significant disadvantages. CT temporal resolution does not compare to CMR, and a second significant disadvantage is the need to use nonionic contrast agents and significant radiation dose for imaging. Because of the limited temporal resolution, patients with high heart rates frequently require beta-blockers prior to imaging. Studies comparing LV quantification by CT and CMR have been conflicting. Schlosser et al.[204] found that CT significantly overestimated the volumes and underestimated LV mass calculations, although EF did not differ significantly. The mean difference between CT and CMR was 11.7 ± 15.9 g ($p < 0.05$). However, other studies[205] have shown a closer correlation ($r = 0.95$) with mean difference between CT and CMR of 6.5 ± 7.5 g. Using 64-slice CT compared to echo and CMR, Wu et al.[206] showed excellent correlation between CT and CMR for LV volumes ($r = 0.98$ to 0.99) and EF ($r = 0.97$) however, there were significantly larger end-diastolic volumes on CT in patients with low HR (<70 bpm) than high HR (≥70 bpm) compared to CMR. Using CMR as the gold standard, CT measured volume by modified biplane Simpson's rule (Fig. 18.14) and EF have a higher correlation than 2D measures of volume.[207] These differences may be attributed to the contrast load and the hemodynamic effect of β-blockers.

3.3. Echocardiographic and nuclear stress testing

There are multiple reasons for which stress testing may be useful in the hypertensive population; evaluation of appropriate

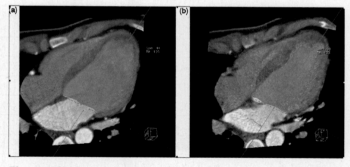

Figure 18.14 The four-chamber view of the 64-slice CT at end diastolic (**a**) and end systolic (**b**) phase. (Reproduced with permission from Annuar BR, Liew CK, Chin SP, et al. Assessment of global and regional left ventricular function using 64-slice multi-slice computed tomography and 2D echocardiography: A comparison with cardiac magnetic resonance. *Eur J Rad.* 2008;65:112–119.).

exercise vasoreactivity, evaluation of stress-induced systolic dysfunction, the evaluation of obstructive coronary disease, and the evaluation of exercise-induced/exacerbated diastolic dysfunction. In the setting of LVH, however, ST segment depressions are unreliable markers for ischemia, reducing diagnostic accuracy to 59%.[208]

Sympathetic nervous system stimulation with stress causes an increase in cardiac output driven initially by predominant increase in stroke volume from increased inotropy and increased venous return. At higher levels of stress, the increase in cardiac output is driven by the increase in heart rate. The mean arterial BP is stable. In resting normotensives, an exaggerated BP response (defined as +2 standard deviations of systolic pressure) has been shown to predict the development of sustained hypertension[209-211] portending a twofold to threefold risk of future hypertension. These patients are also characterized by a greater prevalence of LVH,[212] resting diastolic dysfunction,[213] endothelial dysfunction, and inflammatory markers.[214] Recent investigators[215] measured the neurohormonal levels following exercise in patients with exaggerated stress-induced BP response and compared them to controls. They showed that renin, aldosterone, and catecholamines were increased equally in both groups, however, the level of angiotensin II was significantly increased in the study group. The most recent practice guidelines published by the American College of Cardiology/American Heart Association recognizes that there is no absolute definition of a hypertensive response to exercise but recommends considering a systolic BP of >250 mm Hg and a diastolic BP of >115 mm Hg as relative indications for test termination.[216]

Exaggerated BP response may also be seen in patients with DHF which may in part explain the symptoms of dyspnea on exertion seen in these patients. Compared to a hypertensive-only group, patients with DHF (previously hospitalized for pulmonary congestion and symptoms and signs of heart failure but normal LV EF >50%) had significantly higher resting angiotensin II and brain natriuretic protein (BNP) levels and higher in BP response to exercise.[217] In addition, resting angiotensin II and BNP were higher in the patients with DHF than the control hypertensive group. Administration of an ARB significantly lowered the BNP levels in the DHF group and increased exercise tolerance.

Doppler estimates of LV filling pressures are accurate even in sinus tachycardia[218] thus, estimations of LV filling pressures can be performed during stress. Multiple studies have evaluated the feasibility of measuring diastolic parameters during treadmill[219] and supine bicycle testing.[220] Two studies looked at the feasibility and accuracy of measuring E/E' during stress compared to invasive hemodynamics. Burgess et al.[221] studied two groups of patients; 37 unselected patients presenting for left heart catheterization were referred for supine bicycle exercise and 166 consecutive patients referred for treadmill exercise testing. Mitral inflow pulsed Doppler (apical 4ch) and tissue Doppler of the medial (septal) mitral annulus could be made in all patients at rest and with exercise with the caveat that, if the mitral inflow profile was fused due to tachycardia, repeat measures were performed at lower heart rates. The correlation between E/E'(septal) and mean LVDP at rest was good ($r = 0.67$, $p < 0.01$) but less strong during exercise ($r = 0.59$, $p < 0.01$), with an exercise E/E'(septal) of >13 having a sensitivity and specificity of 73% and 96%, respectively, for detecting a LVDP of >15 mm Hg. This cutoff, when applied to the noninvasive group, had a sensitivity and specificity of 48% and 90%, respectively, for predicting reduced exercise capacity. A cutoff of E/E' >10 however, had a sensitivity and specificity of 71% and 69% respectively, for predicting patients who could not complete eight metabolic equivalents (METS) of exercise.

The second study compared echocardiographic and invasive hemodynamic measures of LV filling during stress in patients with dyspnea with normal EF.[222] Simultaneous Doppler and invasive measurements revealed that noninvasive Doppler of the mitral annulus at rest and with exercise was a reliable estimate of PCWP. An E/E' (septal) ratio of <15 during exercise had a sensitivity of 89% for predicting a normal PCWP, and all patients with a ratio of >15 during exercise had a PCWP >20 mm Hg.

In patients with essential hypertension and normal resting EF, stress may uncover underlying systolic myocardial dysfunction unrelated to coronary artery disease.[223,224] This may be a manifestation of impaired function reserved in hypertensive patients[225] and has been correlated with LV mass.[226] Numerous studies have shown that myocardial perfusion defects may occur in the setting of LVH in the absence of significant coronary artery disease.[227-229] Thus, despite studies suggesting a high specificity of ECG changes in the setting of LVH for myocardial perfusion defect,[230] these defects are not specific for coronary artery disease. Nonetheless, perfusion defects on nuclear stress tests have prognostic importance. Elhendy et al.[231] showed that in patients with ECG–LVH, the annual mortality rate was significantly higher for patients with single vessel distribution abnormalities or multivessel abnormalities (3.2% vs. 8%, respectively) versus a normal scan (1.4%).

4. FUTURE DIRECTIONS

In 1628, William Harvey described the potential functional significance of fiber orientation of the ventricular mass.[232] Anatomic studies have produced two theories of myocardial fiber arrangement; the ventricular wall is a series of stacked sheets of different orientation[233] or the myocardium is a continuous helical band of muscle.[234,235] Both theories of myocardial fiber array have been called into question with data supporting a 3D network of fibers with angulated connections of myocytes.[236] There is agreement however, that fiber arrangement dictates how the heart functions to eject blood and "Models based on uniform myocardial fiber structure cannot explain wall movement in normal subjects and are likely to have significant limitations if used to investigate LV function in disease."[237] Despite decades of prognostic information gathered in incredibly diverse populations for the simplistic EF, it seems likely that we will rely on the newer methods of assessing myocardial function in the future. Measuring tissue deformation or strain seems a likely candidate for improving our assessment of cardiac function however, myocyte shortening, typically ~15% of its length, cannot entirely explain about the >50% volume ejected from the left ventricle in normal individuals. The initial descriptions of ventricular contraction as "the wringing of a linen cloth to squeeze out the water"[238] seem plausible from descriptions of the helical angle of fiber array.[239] Then McDonald,[240] using radio-opaque markers attached to the epicardium, directly appreciated the counterclockwise rotation of the left ventricle when observed from the apex. With the development of MRI, a better understanding of muscle mechanics has led to an understanding of strain, strain rate (SR), and torsion. A new technology has been developed to measure these indices with echocardiography, thus bringing these tools out of the research and into the clinical sphere.

4.1. Strain and strain rate

Myocardial strain is defined as the deformation of the myocardium and can be expressed as the change in length normalized to the original length. Strain is thus a dimensionless ratio which can be expressed in percent. Positive strain is stretching, whereas negative strain is shortening or compression in relation to the original length. Peak negative strain is thus one of the most common strain measurements to describe myocardial strain. A more complete description of strain and SR is discussed in Chapter 16.

Initial MRI studies[241,242] measured 2D strain by tagged MR images. From these images, SR can be measured. The first echocardiographic method for measuring SR was the use of tissue velocity, since the longitudinal tissue velocity gradient is related to the change in length by the formula:

$$VG = \frac{(v_2 - v_1)}{L} = \frac{dL/dt}{L} \qquad \text{(Eq. 18.9)}$$

and thus the velocity gradient equals the rate of natural strain and the natural strain equals the time integral of the velocity gradient:

$$d\varepsilon_N = \frac{dL}{L} = VG\,dt \quad \text{and} \quad VG = \frac{d\varepsilon_N}{dt} \quad \text{and} \quad \varepsilon_N = \int VG\,dt \qquad \text{(Eq. 18.10)}$$

Tissue velocity can be measured by tissue Doppler, M-mode Doppler, or 2D color Doppler. There are inherent problems with measuring SR and deriving strain from Doppler. We know that velocities measured by Doppler are dependent on the angle of insonation and this measure of strain is highly angle dependent. The angle of insonation thus changes not only by image position, but also by the inherent curvature of the ventricular wall. In addition, given the dependence on a parallel insonation beam, only longitudinal strain can be measured reproducibly. Finally, tissue Doppler signals are of high amplitude but low velocity and the signal-to-noise ratio is low.

Strain can also be determined by echocardiographic speckle tracking. A small region of the 2D image exhibits a defined speckle pattern. By tracking this pattern from frame to frame, the change in position (distance) can be determined over time. This is a versatile method of measuring the change in length over time, since it could potentially measure change in any direction (longitudinal, circumferential, or radial). Speckle strain method is dependent on high enough frame rates to distinguish speckles moving over time.

Strain and SR have been studied in the hypertensive population and provide insight into the phenomenon of "heart failure with normal EF." Given the changes in myocyte and extracellular matrix composition stimulated by hypertension, measuring of strain may be a more accurate and sensitive method of assessing myocardial systolic function in this population compared to EF. Poulsen et al.[243] studied Doppler tissue tracking strain measurements in 40 patients with essential hypertension and compared them to controls. They found that global abnormalities in longitudinal systolic SR were seen in patients with abnormal diastolic filling patterns and global and regional abnormalities in strain were significantly related to systolic BP and LV mass.[187] Other studies have confirmed the correlation of systolic strain and LV mass and BP.[244] Abnormal longitudinal strain has also been shown to occur even in the absence of diastolic dysfunction[245,246] and may be related to markers of collagen deposition.[246]

Abnormal segmental relaxation has also been documented with strain imaging. Pavlopoulos and Nihoyannopoulos[247] showed that in a population of essential hypertensives, the number of segments with abnormal diastolic SR varied with the severity of diastolic dysfunction, worsening with progression from hypertension alone, to hypertension with asymptomatic diastolic dysfunction, to hypertension with symptomatic diastolic dysfunction. The number of segments with abnormal diastolic SR was also related to the severity of LVH and SBP, and negatively correlated systolic strain and SR. After the development of LVH, regional abnormalities in strain continue to be seen.[248]

4.2. Torsion

The arrangement of myocardial fibers has been described as subendocardial right-handed helix, and subepicardial left-handed helix.[249] In theory, this twisting motion may reduce intramyo-

cardial strain and energy expenditure. Torsion is variably been defined as the net twist (in degree of rotation) alone, or twist divided by the length over which the twist occurs. Torsion initially was described on cineradiography, but subsequently was observed by tagged MRI[250] and more recently by tissue Doppler imaging[251] and speckle tracking.[252] Torsion has been studied in the hypertensive population. When compared to normal controls, patients with DHF frequently have normal to increased systolic torsion.[253] Untwisting however, may be reduced and delayed[254] which may to be related to markers of collagen deposition.[246]

With the development of real-time 3D technology, assessing 3D strain (Figs. 18.15 and 18.16)[255] and torsion have now

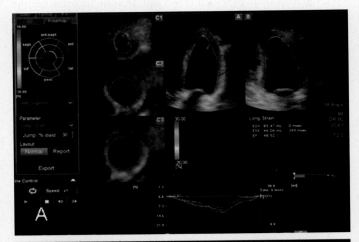

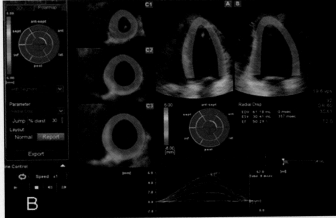

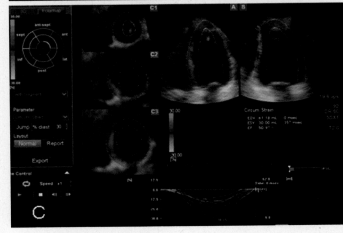

Figure 18.15 Speckle tracking from a singe 3D data set. (**A**) Longitudinal strain, (**B**) Radial strain, and (**C**) Circumferential strain.

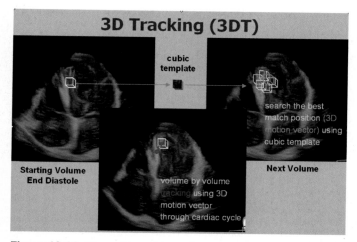

Figure 18.16 3D speckle tracking technique using cubic pattern matching for 3D myocardial data set by a numerical modeling study. (Reproduced from Abe Y, Kawagishi1 T, Ohuchi H, et al. Accurate detection of regional contraction using novel 3-dimensional speckle tracking technique. *J Am Coll Cardiol.* 2008;51 (Suppl A; A116.), with permission).

become a reality. The inherent benefit of assessing strain in three dimensions hardly needs mentioning. Given the complex nature of myocardial structure and function and the clear regionality of both systolic and diastolic dysfunction in hypertension, not to mention other cardiac disease processes such as coronary artery disease, rapid assessment of myocardial deformation may add to our understanding of these diseases as well as provide a more accurate prognostic measure of cardiovascular risk.

REFERENCES

1. Staessen JA, Wang J, Bianchi G, et al. Essential hypertension. *Lancet.* 2003;361:1629–1641.
2. World Health Organization, International Society of Hypertension Writing Group. 2003. World Health organization (WHO)/International Society of Hypertension (ISH) statement on management of hypertension. *J Hypertens.* 2003;21(11):1983–1992.
3. Chobonian AV, Bakris GL, Black HR, et al. Seventh report of the joint national committee on prevention, detection, evaluation and treatment of high blood pressure. *Hypertension.* 2003;42:1206–1252.
4. Casale PN, Devereux RB, Milner M, et al. Value of echocardiographic measurement of left ventricular mass in predicting cardiovascular morbid events in hypertensive men. *Ann Intern Med.* 1986;105:173–178.
5. Koren MJ, Devereux RB, Casale PH, et al. Relation of left ventricular mass and geometry to morbidity and mortality in uncomplicated essential hypertension. *Ann Intern Med.* 1991;114:345–352.
6. Ghali JK, Liao Y, Simmons B, et al. The prognostic role of left ventricular hypertrophy in patients with or without coronary artery disease. *Ann Intern Med.* 1992;117:831–836.
7. Verdecchia P, Porcellati C, Schillaci G, et al. Ambulatory blood pressure: An independent predictor of prognosis in essential hypertension. *Hypertension.* 1994;24:793–801.
8. Verdecchia P, Carini G, Circo A, et al. Left ventricular mass and cardiovascular morbidity in essential hypertension: the MAVI study. *J Am Coll Cardiol.* 2001;38:1829–1835.
9. Levy D, Salomon M, D'Agostino RB, et al. Prognostic implications of baseline electrocardiographic features and their serial changes in subjects with left ventricular hypertrophy. *Circulation.* 1994;90:1786–1793.
10. Levy D, Garrison RJ, Savage DD, et al. Prognostic implications of echocardiographically determined left ventricular mass in the Framingham Heart Study. *N Engl J Med.* 1990;322:1561–1566.
11. Bikkina M, Levy D, Evans JC, et al. Left ventricular mass and the risk of stroke in an elderly cohort. The Framingham Heart Study. *J Am Med Assoc.* 1994; 272:33–36.
12. Bolognese L, Dellavese P, Rossi L, et al. Prognostic value of left ventricular mass in uncomplicated acute myocardial infarction and one–vessel coronary artery disease. *Am J Cardiol.* 1994;73:1–5.
13. Liao Y, Cooper RS, McGee DL, et al. The relative effects of left ventricular hypertrophy, coronary artery disease, and ventricular dysfunction on survival among black adults. *J Am Med Assoc.* 1995;273:1592–1597.
14. Baker B, O'Kelly B, Szalai JP, et al. Determinants of left ventricular mass in early hypertension. *Am J Hypertens.* 1998;11:1248–1251.
15. Devereux RB, Pickering TG, Harshfield BA, et al. Left ventricular hypertrophy in patients with hypertension: Importance of blood pressure response to regulatory recurring stress. *Circulation.* 1983;68:470–476.
16. Gosse P, Ansoborio P, Jullien V, et al. Ambulatory blood pressure and left ventricular hypertrophy. *Blood Press Monit.* 1997;2:70–74.
17. Celentano A, Mancini FP, Crivaro M, et al. Cardiovascular risk factors, angiotensin-converting enzyme gene I/D polymorphism, and left ventricular mass in systemic hypertension. *Am J Cardiol.* 1999;83(8):1196–1200.
18. Cain PA, Ahl R, Hedstrom E, et al. Physiological determinants of the variation in left ventricular mass from early adolescence to late adulthood in healthy subjects. *Clin Physiol Funct Imaging.* 2005;25:332–339.
19. Dannenberg AL, Levy D, Garrison RJ. Impact of age on echocardiographic left ventricular mass in a healthy population (the Framingham Study). *Am J Cardiol.* 1989;64:1066–1068.
20. Levy D, Anderson, KM, Savage DD, et al. Echocardiographically detected left ventricular hypertrophy: Prevalence and risk factors. The Framingham Heart Study. *Ann Intern Med.* 1988;108:7–13.
21. Gerdts E, Okin PM, de Simone G, et al. Gender differences in left ventricular structure and function during antihypertensive treatment: The Losartan Intervention for Endpoint Reduction in Hypertension Study. *Hypertension.* 2008;51:1109–1114.
22. Dunn FG, Oigman W, Sungaard-Riise K, et al. Racial differences in cardiac adaptation to essential hypertension determined by echocardiographic indexes. *J Am Coll Cardiol.* 1983;1:1348–1351.
23. Kizer JR, Arnett DK, Bella JN, et al. Differences in left ventricular structure between black and white hypertensive adults: The Hypertension Genetic Epidemiology Network study. *Hypertension.* 2004;43:1182–1188.
24. Drazner MH, Dries DL, Peshock RM, et al. Left ventricular hypertrophy is more prevalent in blacks than whites in the general population: The Dallas Heart Study. *Hypertension.* 2005;46:124–129.
25. Sharp A, Tapp R, Francis DP, et al. Ethnicity and left ventricular diastolic function in hypertension: An ASCOT (Anglo-Scandinavian Cardiac Outcomes Trial) Substudy. *J Am Coll Cardiol.* 2008;52:1015–1021.
26. Chinali M, de Simone G, Roman MJ, et al. Impact of obesity on cardiac geometry and function in a population of adolescents: The Strong Heart Study. *J Am Coll Cardiol.* 2006;4:2267–2273.
27. Kuperstein R, Hanly P, Niroumand M, et al. The importance of age and obesity on the relation between diabetes and left ventricular mass. *J Am Coll Cardiol.* 2001;37(7):1957–1962.
28. Muiesan ML, Salvetti M, Rizzoni D, et al. Association of change in left ventricular mass with prognosis during long-term antihypertensive treatment. *J Hypertens.* 1995;13:1091–1095.
29. Verdecchia P, Schillaci G, Borgioni C, et al. Prognostic significance of serial changes in left ventricular mass in essential hypertension. *Circulation.* 1998;97:48–54.
30. Devereux RB, Wachtell K, Gerdts E, et al. Prognostic significance of left ventricular mass change during treatment of hypertension. *J Am Med Assoc.* 2004;292:2350–2356.
31. MacMahon SW, Wilcken DEL, McDonald GJ. The effect of weight reduction on left ventricular mass: a randomized controlled trial in young, overweight hypertensive patients. *N Engl J Med.* 1986;314:334–339.
32. Jula AM, Karanko HM. Effects on left ventricular hypertrophy of long-term non- pharmacological treatment with sodium restriction in mild to moderate essential hypertension. *Circulation.* 1994;89:1023–1031.
33. Verdecchia P, Angeli F, Gattobigio R, et al. Regression of left ventricular hypertrophy and prevention of stroke in hypertensive subjects. *Am J Hypertens.* 2006;19:493–499.
34. Klingbeil AU, Schneider M, Martus P, et al. A meta-analysis of the effects of treatment on left ventricular mass in essential hypertension. *Am J Med.* 2003;115:41–45.
35. Okin PM, Devereux RB, Jern S, et al. Regression of electrocardiographic left ventricular hypertrophy during antihypertensive treatment and the prediction of major cardiovascular events. *J Am Med Assoc.* 2004;292:2343–2349.
36. Devereux RB, Dahlöf B, Gerdts E, et al. Regression of hypertensive left ventricular hypertrophy by Losartan compared with Atenolol. *Circulation.* 2004;110:1456–1462.
37. Di Tullio MR, Zwas DR, Sacco RL, et al. Left ventricular mass and geometry and the risk of ischemic stroke. *Stroke.* 2003;Oct 34(10):2380–2384.
38. Verma A, Meris A, Skali H, et al. Prognostic implications of left ventricular mass and geometry following myocardial infarction: The VALIANT (VALsartan In Acute myocardial iNfarcTion) Echocardiographic Study. *J Am Coll Cardiol Img.* 2008;1(5):582–591.
39. Verdecchia P, Schillaci G, Borgioni C, et al. Adverse prognostic significance of concentric remodeling of the left ventricle in hypertensive patients with normal left ventricular mass. *J Am Coll Cardiol.* 1995;25:871–878.
40. Milani RV, Lavie CJ, Mehra MR, et al. Left ventricular geometry and survival in patients with normal left ventricular ejection fraction *Am J Cardiol.* 2006;97:959–963.
41. Lifton RP, Gharavi AG, Geller DS. Molecular mechanisms of human hypertension. *Cell.* 2001;104:545–556.
42. Reaven GM, Lithell H, Landsberg L. Hypertension and associated metabolic abnormalities – the role of insulin resistance and the sympathoadrenal system. *N Engl J Med.* 1996;334:374–381.
43. Cowley AW Jr. Long-term control of blood pressure. *Physiol Rev.* 1992;72:231–300.
44. Guyton AC. Blood pressure control-special role of the kidneys and body fluids. *Science.* 1991;252:1813–1816.
45. Keller G, Zimmer G, Mall G, et al. Nephron number in patients with primary hypertension. *N Engl J Med.* 2003;348:101–108.

46. Sealey JE, Laragh JH. Aliskiren, the first renin inhibitor for treating hypertension: Reactive renin secretion may limit its effectiveness. *Am J Hypertens.* 2007;20:587–597.

47. Esler MD, Nestel PJ. High catecholamine essential hypertension: Clinical and physiological characteristics. *Aust NZJ Med.* 1973;3:117–123.

48. Morganti A, Pickering TG, Lopez-Ovejero JA, et al. High and low renin subgroups of essential hypertension: Differences and similarities in their renin and sympathetic responses to neural and nonneural stimuli. *Am J Cardiol.* 1980;46(2):306–312.

49. Bühler FR, Laragh JH, Vaughan ED Jr, et al. Antihypertensive action of propranolol: Specific anti-renin responses in high and normal renin forms of essential, renal, renovascular and malignant hypertension. *Am J Cardiol.* 1973;32:511–522.

50. Beevers DG, Lip GYH, O'Brien E, eds. *ABC of Hypertension.* 5th Ed. Massachusetts, MA: Blackwell Publishing Inc.; 2007.

51. Veterans Administration, Department of Defense. VA/DoD clinical practice guideline for diagnosis and management of hypertension in the primary care setting. Washington, DC: Veterans Administration, Department of Defense; 2004 Aug.

52. Laragh JH, Blumenfeld JB. *Essential hypertension. In Brenner and Rector's The Kidney, Vol. II.* 6th Ed. Philadelphia: WB Saunders; 2000:1967–2000.

53. Laursen JB, Rajagopalan S, Galis Z, et al. Role of superoxide in angiotensin II–induced but not catecholamine-induced hypertension. *Circulation.* 1997;95:588–593.

54. Kerr S, Brosnan MJ, McIntyre M, et al. Superoxide anion production is increased in a model of genetic hypertension: Role of the endothelium. *Hypertension.* 1999;33:1353–1358.

55. Mehta JL, Lopez LM, Chen L, et al. Alterations in nitric oxide synthase activity, superoxide anion generation, and platelet aggregation in systemic hypertension, and effects of celiprolol. *Am J Cardiol.* 1994;74:901–905

56. Cracowski JL, Baguet JP, Ormezzano O, et al. Lipid peroxidation is not increased in patients with untreated mild-moderate hypertension. *Hypertension.* 2003;41:286–288.

57. Ward NC, Hodgson JM, Puddey IB, et al. Oxidative stress in human hypertension: Association with antihypertensive treatment, gender, nutrition and lifestyle. *Free Radic Biol Med.* 2004;36:226–232.

58. Weinberger MH, Fineberg NS, Fineberg SE, et al. Salt sensitivity, pulse pressure, and death in normal and hypertensive humans. *Hypertension.* 2001;37:429–432.

59. Braverman AC, Guven H, Beardslee MA, et al. The bicuspid aortic valve. *Curr Probl Cardiol.* 2005;30:470–522.

60. Rahiala E, Tikanoja T. Suspicion of aortic coarctation in an outpatient clinic: How should blood pressure measurements be performed? *Clin Physiol.* 2001;21(1):100–104.

61. Park MK, Lee D, Johnson GA. Oscillometric blood pressures in the arm, thigh, and ankle in healthy children and those with aortic coarctation. *Pediatrics.* 1993;91:761–765.

62. Aboulhosn J, Child JS. Left ventricular outflow obstruction: Subaortic stenosis, bicuspid aortic valve, supravalvar aortic stenosis, and coarctation of the aorta. *Circulation.* 2006;114:2412–2422.

63. Harding MB, Smith LR, Himmelstein SI, et al. Renal artery stenosis: Prevalence and associated risk factors in patients undergoing routine cardiac catheterization. *J Am Soc Nephrol.* 1992;2:1608–1616.

64. Missouris CG, Buckenham T, Cappuccio FP, et al. Renal artery stenosis: A common and important problem in patients with peripheral vascular disease. *Am J Med.* 1994;96:10–14.

65. McLaughlin K, Jardin AG, Moss, JG. ABC of arterial and venous disease: Renal artery stenosis. *Br Med J.* 2000;320:1124–1127.

66. Safian RD, Textor SC. Renal artery stenosis. *N Eng J Med.* 2001;344:431–442.

67. Williams GJ, Macaskill P, Chan SF, et al. Comparative accuracy of renal duplex sonographic parameters in the diagnosis of renal artery stenosis: Paired and unpaired analysis. *AJR Am J Roentgenol.* 2007;188:798–811.

68. Radermacher J, Chavan A, Bleck J, et al. Use of Doppler ultrasonography to predict the outcome of therapy for renal-artery stenosis. *New Eng J Med.* 2001;344:410–417.

69. Boudewijn GBC, Nelemans PJ, Kessels AGH, et al. Accuracy of computed tomographic angiography and magnetic resonance angiography for diagnosing renal artery stenosis. *Ann Intern Med.* 2004;141:674–682.

70. Mann SJ, Pickering TG. Detection of renovascular hypertension. *Ann Intern Med.* 1992;117:845.

71. Huot SJ, Hansson JH, Dey H, et al. Utility of captopril renal scans for detecting renal artery stenosis. *Arch Intern Med.* 2002;162:1981–1984.

72. Chen CC, Hoffer PB, Vahjen G, et al. Patients at high risk for renal artery stenosis: A simple method of renal scintigraphic analysis with Tc-99 m DTPA and Captopril. *Radiology.* 1990;176:365–370.

73. Laragh JH, Sealey JE. Renin system under standard for analysis and treatment of hypertensive patients: A means to quantify the vasoconstrictor elements, diagnose curable renal and adrenal causes, assess risk of cardiovascular morbidity, and find the best fit drug regimen. In: Laragh JH, Brenner BM, eds. *Hypertension: Pathophysiology, Diagnosis and Management.* 2nd Ed. New York, NY: Raven Press;1995;18:13–36.

74. Williams JS, Williams GH. 50th Anniversary of aldosterone. *J Clin Endo Metab.* 2003;88:2364–2372.

75. Napoli C, DiGregorio F, Leccese M, et al. Evidence of exercise-induced myocardial ischemia in patients with primary aldosteronism: The Cross-sectional Primary Aldosteronism and Heart Italian Multicenter Study. *J Invest Med.* 1999;47:212–221.

76. Pitt B, Zannad F, Remme WJ. The effect of spironolactone on morbidity and mortality in patients with severe heart failure. *N Engl J Med.* 1999;341:709–717.

77. Rayner B. Primary aldosteronism and aldosterone-associated hypertension. *J Clin Pathol.* 2008;61:825–831.

78. Manger WM. An overview of phaeochromocytoma: History, current concepts, vagaries, and diagnostic challenges. *Ann NY Acad Sci.* 2006;1073:1–20.

79. Lenders JWM, Eisenhofer G, Mannelli M, et al. Phaeochormocytoma. *Lancet* 2005;366:665–675.

80. Atiyeh BA, Barakat AJ, Abumrad NN, et al. Extra-adrenal pheochromocytoma. *J Nephrol.* 1997;10(1):25–29.

81. Lucon AM, Pereira MA, Mendonca BB, et al. Pheochromocytoma: Study of 50 cases. *J Urol.* 1997;157:1208–1212.

82. Abrams HL, Siegelman SS, Adams DF, et al. Computed tomography versus ultrasound of the adrenal gland: A prospective study. *Radiology.* 1982;143:121–128.

83. Pacak K, Linehan WM, Eisenhofer G, et al. Recent advances in genetics, diagnosis, localization and treatment of pheochromocytoma. *Ann Intern Med.* 2001;134:315–329.

84. Ilias I, Pacak K. Current approaches and recommended algorithm for the diagnostic localization of pheochromocytoma. *J Clin Endocrinol Metab.* 2004;89:479–491.

85. Grumbach MM, Biller BM, Braunstein GD, et al. Management of the clinically inapparent adrenal mass ("incidentaloma"). *Ann Intern Med.* 2003;138:424–429.

86. Quint LE, Glazer GM, Francis IR, et al. Pheochromocytoma and paraganglioma: Comparison of MR imaging with CT and I-131 MIBG scintigraphy. *Radiology.* 1987;165:89–93.

87. Fujita A, Hyodoh H, Kawamura Y, et al. Use of fusion images of I-131 metaiodobenzylguanidine, SPECT and magnetic resonance studies to identify a malignant pheochromocytoma. *Clin Nucl Med.* 2000;25:440–442.

88. Bravo EL. Evolving concepts in the pathophysiology, diagnosis and treatment of pheochromocytoma. *Endocr Rev.* 1994;15:356–358.

89. Silverberg DS, Oksenberg A, Iaina A. Sleep-related breathing disorders as a major cause of essential hypertension: Fact or fiction? *Curr Opin Nephrol Hypertens.* 1998;7:353–357.

90. Fletcher EC, DeBehnke RD, Lovoi MS, et al. Undiagnosed sleep apnea in patients with essential hypertension. *Ann Intern Med.* 1985;103:190–195.

91. Nieto FJ, Young TB, Lind BK, et al. Association of sleep-disordered breathing, sleep apnea, and hypertension in a large community-based study. Sleep Heart Health Study. *JAMA.* 2000;283:1829–1836.

92. Peppard PE, Young T, Palta M, et al. Prospective study of the association between sleep-disordered breathing and hypertension. *N Engl J Med.* 2000;342:1378–1384.

93. American Academy of Sleep Medicine Task Force. Sleep-related breathing disorders in adults: Recommendations for syndrome definition and measurement techniques in clinical research. *Sleep.* 1999;22:667–689.

94. Somers VK, White CP, Amin R, et al. Sleep Apnea and Cardiovascular Disease: An American Heart Association/American College of Cardiology Foundation Scientific Statement From the American Heart Association Council for High Blood Pressure Research Professional Education Committee, Council on Clinical Cardiology, Stroke Council, and Council on Cardiovascular Nursing Council. *Circulation.* 2008;118:1080–1111.

95. Weber KT, Brilla CG. Pathological hypertrophy and cardiac interstitium: Fibrosis and renin–angiotensin–aldosterone system. *Circulation.* 1991;83:1849–1865.

96. Querejeta R, Varo N, Lopez B, et al. Serum carboxy-terminal propeptide of procollagen type I is a marker of myocardial fibrosis in hypertensive heart disease. *Circulation.* 2000;101:1729–1735.

97. Alla F, Kearney-Schwartz A, Radauceanu A, et al. Early changes in serum markers of cardiac extra-cellular matrix turnover in patients with uncomplicated hypertension and type II diabetes. *Eur J Heart Fail.* 2006;8:147–153.

98. van Heerebeek L, Borbely A, Niessen HW, et al. Myocardial structure and function differ in systolic and diastolic heart failure. *Circulation.* 2006;113:1966–1973.

99. Post WS, Larson MG, Myers RH, et al. Heritability of left ventricular mass: The Framingham Heart Study. *Hypertension.* 1997;30:1025–1028.

100. Levy D, Salomon M, D'Agostino RB, et al. Prognostic implications of baseline electrocardiographic features and their serial changes in subjects with left ventricular hypertrophy. *Circulation.* 1994;90:1786–1793.

101. Verdecchia P, Angeli F, Reboldi G, et al. Improved cardiovascular risk stratification by a simple ECG index in hypertension. *Am J Hypertens.* 2003;16:646–652.

102. Levy D, Labib SB, Anderson KM, et al. Determinants of sensitivity and specificity of electrocardiographic criteria for left ventricular hypertrophy. *Circulation.* 1990;81:815–820.

103. Casale PN, Devereux RB, Kligfield P, et al. Electrocardiographic detection of left ventricular hypertrophy: Development and prospective validation of improved criteria. *J Am Coll Cardiol.* 1985;6:572–580.

104. Pewsner D, Juni P, Egger M, et al. Accuracy of electrocardiography in diagnosis of left ventricular hypertrophy in arterial hypertension: Systematic review. *Br Med J.* 2007;335:711.

105. Alfakih K, Walters K, Jones T, et al. New gender-specific partition values for ECG criteria of left ventricular hypertrophy: Recalibration against cardiac MRI hypertension. 2004;4:175–179.

106. Geiser EA, Bove KE. Calculation of the left ventricular mass and relative wall thickness. *Arch Pathol.* 1974;97:13–21.

107. Devereux RB, Reichek N. Echocardiographic determination of left ventricular mass in man: Anatomic validation of the method. *Circulation.* 1977;55:613–618.

108. Woythaler N, Singer SL, Kwan OL, et al. Accuracy of echocardiography versus electrocardiography in detecting left ventricular hypertrophy: Comparisons with postmortem mass measurements. *J Am Coll Cardiol.* 1983;2:305–311.

109. Daniels SR, Meyer RA, Liang Y, et al. Echocardiographically determined left ventricular mass index in normal children, adolescents and young adults. *J Am Coll Cardiol.* 1988;12:703–708.

110. Schiller NB, Shah PM, Crawford M, et al. Recommendations for quantitation of the left ventricle by twodimensional echocardiography. American Society of Echocardiography Committee on Standards, Subcommittee on Quantitation of Two-Dimensional Echocardiograms. *J Am Soc Echocardiogr.* 1989;2: 358–367.

111. Devereux RB, Alonso DR, Lutas EM, et al. Echocardiographic assessment of left ventricular hypertrophy: Comparison to necropsy findings. *Am J Cardiol.* 1986;57:450–458.

112. Schnittger I, Gordon EP, Fitzgerald PJ, et al. Standardized intracardiac measurements of two-dimensional echocardiography. *J Am Coll Cardiol.* 1983;2: 934–938.

113. Triulzi M, Gillam LD, Gentile F, et al. Normal adult cross-sectional echocardiographic values: Linear dimensions and chambers area. *Echocardiography.* 1984;1:403–426.

114. Lang R, Bierig M, Devereux R, et al. Recommendations for chamber quantification: A report from the American Society of Echocardiography's Guidelines and Standards Committee and the Chamber Quantification Writing Group, developed in conjunction with the European Association of Echocardiography, a Branch of the European Society of Cardiology. *J Am Soc Echocardiogr.* 2005;18:1440–1463.

115. Ilercil A, O'Grady MJ, Roman MJ, et al. Reference values for echocardiographic measurements in urban and rural populations of differing ethnicity: The strong heart study. *J Am Soc Echocardiogr.* 2001;14:601–611.

116. Ryan T, Petrovic O, Armstrong WF, et al. Quantitative two-dimensional echocardiographic assessment of patients undergoing left ventricular aneurysmectomy. *Am Heart J.* 1986;111:714–720.

117. Takeuchi M, Nishikage T, Mor-Avi V, et al. Measurement of left ventricular mass by real-time three-dimensional echocardiography: Validation against magnetic resonance and comparison with two-dimensional and M-mode measurements. *J Am Soc Echocardiogr.* 2008;21:1001–1005.

118. Park S, Shub C, Nobrega T, et al. Two-dimensional echocardiographic calculation of left ventricular mass as recommended by the American Society of Echocardiography: Correlation with autopsy and M-mode echocardiography. *J Am Soc Echocardiogr.* 1996;9:119–128.

119. Bachenberg TC, Shub C, Hauck AJ, et al. Can anatomical left ventricular mass be estimated reliably by M-mode echocardiography? A clinicopathological study of ninety-three patients. *Echocardiography.* 1991;8:9–15.

120. Helak JW, Reichert NP. Quantitation of human left ventricular mass and volume by two-dimensional echocardiography: In vitro anatomic validation. *Circulation.* 1981;63;1398–1407.

121. Wallerson DC, Devereux RB. Reproducibility of echocardiographic left ventricular measurements. *Hypertension.* 1987;9(suppl 2):6–18.

122. de Simone G, Ganau A, Verdecchia P, et al. Echocardiography in arterial hypertension: When, why and how? *J Hypertens.* 1994;12:1129–1136.

123. Devereux RB, Dahlöf B, Levy D, et al. Comparison of enalapril vs nifedipine to decrease left ventricular hypertrophy in systemic hypertension (The PRESERVE Trial). *Am J Cardiol.* 1996;78:61–65.

124. Matsubara BB, Bregagnollo EA, Tucci PJ. Left ventricular mass estimated by M-mode echocardiogram is not altered by changes in cardiac shape and dimensions due to acute arterial hypertension. *Braz J Med Biol Res.* 1993;26:173–176.

125. Ditchey RV, Schuler G, Peterson KL. Reliability of echocardiographic and electrocardiographic parameters in assessing serial changes in left ventricular mass. *Am J Med.* 1981;70:1042–1050.

126. Devereux RB, Lutas EM, Casale PN, et al. Standardization of M-mode echocardiographic left ventricular anatomic measurements. *J Am Coll Cardiol.* 1984;4:1222–1230.

127. De Simone G, Daniels SR, Devereux RB, et al. Left ventricular mass and body size in normotensive children and adults: Assessment of allometric relations and impact of overweight. *J Am Coll Cardiol.* 1992;20:1251–1260.

128. Zoccali C, Benedetto FA, Mallamaci F, et al. Prognostic impact of the indexation of left ventricular mass in patients undergoing dialysis. *J Am Soc Nephrol.* 2001;12:2768–2774.

129. Liao Y, Cooper RS, Durazo-Arvizu R, et al. Prediction of mortality risk by different methods of indexation for left ventricular mass. *J Am Coll Cardiol.* 1997;29:641–647.

130. Li L, Shigematsu Y, Hamada M, et al. Relative wall thickness is an independent predictor of left ventricular systolic and diastolic dysfunctions in essential hypertension. *Hypertens Res.* 2001;24:493–499.

131. Aurigemma GP, Silver KH, Priest MA, et al. Geometric changes allow normal ejection fraction despite depressed myocardial shortening in hypertensive left ventricular hypertrophy. *J Am Coll Cardiol.* 1995;26:195–202.

132. DeSimone G, Devereux RB, Roman MJ, et al. Assessment of left ventricular function by the midwall fractional shortening/end-systolic stress relation in human hypertension. *J Am Coll Cardiol.* 1994;23:1444–1451.

133. Ballo P, Mondillo S, Guerrini F, et al. Midwall mechanics in physiologic and hypertensive concentric hypertrophy. *J Am Soc Echocardiogr.* 2004;17:418–427.

134. Devereux RB, Roman MJ, Palmieri V, et al. Left ventricular wall stresses and wall stress-mass-heart rate products in hypertensive patients with electrocardiographic left ventricular hypertrophy: The LIFE study. Losartan Intervention for Endpoint Reduction in Hypertension. *J Hypertens.* 2000;18:1129–1138.

135. Vinch CS, Aurigemma GP, Simon HU, et al. Analysis of left ventricular systolic function using midwall mechanics in patients >60 years of age with hypertensive heart disease and heart failure. *Am J Cardiol.* 2005;96:1299–1303.

136. Wachtell K, Papademetrious V, Smith G, et al. Relation of impaired left ventricular filling to systolic midwall mechanics in hypertensive patients with normal left ventricular systolic chamber function: The Losartan Intervention of Endpoint Reduction in Hypertension (LIFE) study. *Am Heart J.* 2004;148:538–544.

137. Schussheim AE, Diamond JA, Jhang JS, et al. Midwall fractional shortening is an independent predictor of left ventricular diastolic dysfunction in asymptomatic patients with systemic hypertension. *Am J Cardiol.* 1998;82:1056–1059.

138. Shimizu G, Hirota Y, Kawamura K. Empiric determination of the transition from concentric hypertrophy to congestive heart failure in essential hypertension. *J Am Coll Cardiol.* 1995;25:888–894.

139. Palmiero P, Maiello M, Nanda N. Is echo-determined left ventricular geometry associated with ventricular filling and midwall shortening in hypertensive ventricular hypertrophy? *Echocardiography.* 2008;25:20–26.

140. Shimizu G, Hirota Y, Kita Y, et al. Left ventricular midwall mechanics in systemic arterial hypertension: Myocardial function is depressed in pressure overload hypertrophy. *Circulation.* 1991;83:1676–1684.

141. Devereux RB, de Simone G, Pickering TG, et al. Relation of left ventricular midwall function to cardiovascular risk factors and arterial structure and function. *Hypertension.* 1998;31:929–936.

142. Jung HO, Sheehan FH, Bolson EL, et al. Evaluation of midwall systolic function in left ventricular hypertrophy: a comparison of 3-dimensional versus 2-dimensional echocardiographic indices. *J Am Soc Echocardiogr.* 2006;19:802–810.

143. Oki T, Tabata T, Mishiro Y, et al. Pulsed tissue Doppler imaging of left ventricular systolic and diastolic wall motion velocities to evaluate differences between long and short axes in healthy subjects. *J Am Soc Echocardiogr.* 1999;12: 308–313.

144. Waggoner AD, Bierig SM. Tissue Doppler imaging: A useful echocardiographic method for the cardiac sonographers to assess systolic and diastolic ventricular function. *J Am Soc Echocardiogr.* 2001;14:1143–1152.

145. Bountioukos M, Schinkel AFL, Bax JJ, et al. The impact of hypertension on systolic and diastolic left ventricular function: A tissue Doppler echocardiographic study. *Am Heart J.* 2006;151:1323.e7–1323.312.

146. Vinereanu D, Nicolaides E, Tweddel AC, et al. "Pure" diastolic dysfunction is associated with long-axis systolic dysfunction. Implications for the diagnosis and classification of heart failure. *Eur J Heart Fail.* 2005;7:820–828.

147. Levy D, Larson MG, Vasan RS, et al. The progression from hypertension to congestive heart failure. *J Am Med Assoc.* 1996;275:1557–1562.

148. Gottdiener JS, Arnold AM, Aurigemma GP, et al. Predictors of congestive heart failure in the elderly: The Cardiovascular Health Study. *J Am Coll Cardiol.* 2000;35:1628–1637.

149. He J, Ogden LG, Bazzano LA, et al. Risk factors for congestive heart failure in US men and women: NHANES I epidemiologic follow-up study. *Arch Intern Med.* 2001;161:996–1002.

150. Kostis JB, Davis BR, Cutler J, et al. SHEP Cooperative Research Group. Prevention of heart failure by antihypertensive drug treatment in older persons with isolated systolic hypertension. *J Am Med Assoc.* 1997;278:212–216.

151. Turnbull F, Blood Pressure Lowering Treatment Trialists' Collaboration. Effects of different blood-pressure-lowering regimens on major cardiovascular events: Results of prospectively-designed overviews of randomised trials. *Lancet.* 2003;362:1527–1535.

152. Schocken DD, Benjamin EJ, Fonarow GC, et al. Prevention of heart failure: A scientific statement from the American Heart Association Councils on Epidemiology and Prevention, Clinical Cardiology, Cardiovascular Nursing, and High Blood Pressure Research; Quality of Care and Outcomes Research Interdisciplinary Working Group; and Functional Genomics and Translational Biology Interdisciplinary Working Group. *Circulation.* 2008;117:2544–2565.

153. Redfield MM, Jacobsen SJ, Burnett JC Jr, et al. Burden of systolic and diastolic ventricular dysfunction in the community: Appreciating the scope of the heart failure epidemic. *J Am Med Assoc.* 2003;289:194–202.

154. Wang TJ, Evans JC, Benjamin EJ, et al. Natural history of asymptomatic left ventricular systolic dysfunction in the community. *Circulation.* 2003;108: 977–982.

155. Verdecchia P, Angeli F, Gattobigio R, et al. Asymptomatic left ventricular systolic dysfunction in essential hypertension: Prevalence, determinants, and prognostic value. *Hypertension.* 2005;45:412–418.

156. Devereux RB, Bella JN, Palmieri V, et al. Hypertension Genetic Epidemiology Network Study Group. Left ventricular systolic dysfunction in a biracial sample of hypertensive adults: The Hypertension Genetic Epidemiology Network (HyperGEN) Study. *Hypertension.* 2001;38:417–423.

157. Kitzman DW, Sheikh KH, Beere PA, et al. Age-related alterations of Doppler left ventricular filling indexes in normal subjects are independent of left ventricular mass, heart rate, contractility and loading conditions. *J Am Coll Cardiol.* 1991;18:1243–1250.

158. Graettinger WF, Neutel JM, Smith DHG, et al. Left ventricular diastolic filling alterations in normotensive young adults with a family history of systemic hypertension. *Am J Cardiol.* 1991;68:51–56.

159. Cuocolo A, Sax FL, Brush JE, et al. Left ventricular hypertrophy and impaired diastolic filling in essential hypertension. *Circulation,* 1990;81:978–986.

160. Mo R, Nordrehaug JE, Omvik P, et al. The Bergen Blood Pressure Study: Prehypertensive changes in cardiac structure and function in offspring of hypertensive families. *Blood Press.* 1995;4:16–22.

161. Garcia MJ, Thomas JD, Klein A. New Doppler echocardiographic application for the study of diastolic function. *J Am Coll Cardiol.* 1998;32:865–875.

162. Rossvoll O, Hatle LK. Pulmonary venous flow velocities recorded by transthoracic Doppler ultrasound: Relation to left ventricular diastolic pressures. *J Am Coll Cardiol*. 21:1687–1696.
163. Oki T, Tabata T, Yamada H, et al. Clinical application of pulsed Doppler tissue imaging for assessing abnormal left ventricular relaxation. *Am J Cardiol*. 1997;79:921–928.
164. Kasner M, Westermann D, Steendijk P, et al. Utility of Doppler echocardiography and tissue Doppler imaging in the estimation of diastolic function in heart failure with normal ejection fraction: A comparative Doppler-conductance catheterization study. *Circulation*. 2007;116:637–647.
165. Benjamin EJ, D'Agostino RB, Belanger AJ, et al. Left atrial size and the risk of stroke and death. The Framingham Heart Study. *Circulation*. 1995;92:835–841.
166. Tsang TS, Gersh BJ, Appleton CP, et al. Left ventricular diastolic dysfunction as a predictor of the first diagnosed nonvalvular atrial fibrillation in 840 elderly men and women. *J Am Coll Cardiol*. 2002;40:1636–1644.
167. Takemoto Y, Barnes ME, Seward JB, et al. Usefulness of left atrial volume in predicting first congestive heart failure in patients ≥65 years of age with well-preserved left ventricular systolic function. *Am J Cardiol*. 2005;96:832–836.
168. Tsang TS, Barnes ME, Gersh BJ, et al. Left atrial volume as a morphophysiologic expression of left ventricular diastolic dysfunction and relation to cardiovascular risk burden. *Am J Cardiol*. 2002;90:1284–1289.
169. Tsang TS, Barnes ME, Gersh BJ, et al. Prediction of risk for first age-related cardiovascular events in an elderly population: The incremental value of echocardiography. *J Am Coll Cardiol*. 2003;42:1199–1205.
170. Vaziri SM, Larson MG, Lauer MS, et al. Influence of blood pressure on left atrial size: The Framingham Heart Study. *Hypertension*. 1995;25:1155–1160.
171. Tedesco MA, DiSalvo G, Ratti G, et al. Left atrial size in 164 hypertensive patients: and echocardiographic and ambulatory blood pressure study. *Clin Cardiol*. 2001;24:603–607.
172. Pearson AC, Gudipati, C, Nagelhout D, et al. Echocardiographic evaluation of cardiac structure and function in elderly subjects with isolated systolic hypertension. *J Am Coll Cardiol*. 1991;17:422–430.
173. Laukkanen JA, Kurl S, Eranen J, et al. Left atrium size and the risk of cardiovascular death in middle-aged men. *Arch Intern Med*. 2005;165:1788–1793.
174. Pritchett AM, Mahoney DW, Jacobsen SJ, et al. Diastolic dysfunction and left atrial volume: A population-based study. *J Am Coll Cardiol*. 2005;45:87–92.
175. Pape LA, Price JM, Alpert JS, et al. Relation of left atrial size to pulmonary capillary wedge pressure in severe mitral regurgitation. *Cardiology*. 1991;78:297–303.
176. Simek CL, Feldman MD, Haber HL, et al. Relationship between left ventricular wall thickness and left atrial size: Comparison with other measures of diastolic function. *J Am Soc Echocardiogr*. 1995;8:37–47.
177. Mehta S, Charbonneau F, Fitchett DH, et al. The clinical consequences of a stiff left atrium. *Am Heart J*. 1991;122:1184–1191.
178. Greenberg B, Chatterjee K, Parmley WW, et al. The influence of left ventricular filling pressure on atrial contribution to cardiac output. *Am Heart J*. 1979;98:742–751.
179. Appleton CP, Galloway, JM, Gonzalez, MS, et al. Estimation of left ventricular filling pressures using two-dimensional and Doppler echocardiography in adult patients with cardiac disease. Additional value of analyzing left atrial size, left atrial ejection fraction and the difference in duration of pulmonary venous and mitral flow velocity at atrial contraction. *J Am Coll Cardiol*. 1993;22:1972–1982.
180. Douglas PS. The left atrium: A biomarker of chronic diastolic dysfunction and cardiovascular disease risk. *J Am Coll Cardiol*. 2003;42:1206–1207.
181. Rodevan O, Bjornerheim R, Ljosland M, et al. Left atrial volumes assessed by three- and two-dimensional echocardiography compared to MRI estimates. *Int J Card Imaging*. 1999;15:397–410.
182. Kircher B, Abbott JA, Pau S, et al. Left atrial volume determination by biplane two-dimensional echocardiography: Validation by cine computed tomography. *Am Heart J*. 1991;121:864–871.
183. Tsang TS, Barnes ME, Bailey KR, et al. Left atrial volume: Important risk marker of incident atrial fibrillation in 1,655 older men and women. *Mayo Clin Proc*. 2001;76:467–475.
184. Jarvinen VM, Kupari MM, Poutanen VP et al. A simplified method for the determination of left atrial size and function using cine magnetic resonance imaging. *Magn Reson Imaging*. 1996;14:215–226.
185. Lester SJ, Ryan EW, Schiller NB, et al. Best method in clinical practice and in research studies to determine left atrial size. *Am J Cardiol*. 1999;84:829–832.
186. Vasan RS, Larson MG, Levy D, et al. Distribution and categorization of echocardiographic measurements in relation to reference limits: The Framingham Heart Study: formulation of a height- and sex-specific classification and its prospective validation. *Circulation*. 1997;96:1863–1873.
187. Schiller N, Foster E. Analysis of left ventricular systolic function. *Heart*. 1996;75(Suppl 2):17–26.
188. Triposkiadis F, Tentolouris K, Androulakis A, et al. Left atrial mechanical function in the healthy elderly: New insights from a combined assessment of changes in atrial volume and transmitral flow velocity. *J Am Soc Echocardiogr*. 1995;8: 801–809.
189. Gopal AS, Keller AM, Shen Z, et al. Three-dimensional echocardiography: In vitro and in vivo validation of left ventricular mass and comparison with conventional echocardiographic methods. *J Am Coll Cardiol*. 1994;24:504–513.
190. Gopal AS, Schnellbaecher MJ, Shen Z, et al. Freehand three-dimensional echocardiography for measurement of left ventricular mass: In vivo anatomic validation using explanted human hearts. *J Am Coll Cardiol*. 1997;30:802–810.
191. Lee, D, Fuisz AR, Fan PH, et al. Real-time 3-dimensional echocardiographic evaluation of left ventricular volume: Correlation with magnetic resonance imaging—A validation study. *J Am Soc Echocardiogr* 2001;14:1001–1009.
192. Mor-Avi V, Sugeng L, Weinert L, et al. Fast measurement of left ventricular mass with real-time three-dimensional echocardiography: Comparison with magnetic resonance imaging. *Circulation*. 2004;110:1814–1818.
193. van den Bosch AE, Robbers-Visser D, Krenning BJ, et al. Comparison of tealtime three-dimensional echocardiography to magnetic resonance imaging for assessment of left ventricular mass. *Am J Cardiol*. 2006;97:113–117.
194. Jenkins C, Bricknell K, Hanekom L, et al. Reproducibility and accuracy of echocardiographic measurements of left ventricular parameters using real-time three-dimensional echocardiography. *J Am Coll Cardiol*. 2004;44:878–886.
195. Qin JX, Jones M, Travaglini A, et al. The accuracy of left ventricular mass determined by real-time three-dimensional echocardiography in chronic animal and clinical studies: A comparison with postmortem examination and magnetic resonance imaging. *J Am Soc Echocardiogr*. 2005;18:1037–1043.
196. Caiani EG, Corsi C, Sugeng L, et al. Improved quantification of left ventricular mass echocardiography detection with real time three dimensional based on endocardial and epicardial surface. *Heart*. 2006;92:213–219.
197. Oe H, Hozumi T, Arai K, et al. Comparison of accurate measurement of left ventricular mass in patients with hypertrophied hearts by real-time three-dimensional echocardiography versus magnetic resonance imaging. *Am J Cardiol*. 2005;95:1263–1267.
198. Higgins CB. Which standard has the gold? *J Am Coll Cardiol*. 1992;19:1608–1609.
199. Semelka RC, Tomei E, Wagner S, et al. Normal left ventricular dimensions and function: Interstudy reproducibility of measurements with cine MR imaging. *Radiology*. 1990;174:763–768.
200. Pattynama PM, Lamb HJ, van der Velde EA, et al. Left ventricular measurements with cine and spin-echo MR imaging: A study of reproducibility with variance component analysis. *Radiology*. 1993;187:261–268.
201. Shapiro EP, Rogers WJ, Beyar R, et al. Determination of left ventricular mass by MRI in hearts deformed by acute infarction. *Circulation*. 1989;79:706–711.
202. Lorenz CH, Walker ES, Morgan VL, et al. Normal human right and left ventricular mass, systolic function and gender differences by cine magnetic resonance imaging. *J Cardiovasc Magn Reson*. 1999;1:7–21.
203. Grothues F, Smith GC, Moon JCC, et al. Comparison of interstudy reproducibility of cardiovascular magnetic resonance with two-dimensional echocardiography in normal subjects and in patients with heart failure or left ventricular hypertrophy. *Am J Cardiol*. 2002;90:29–34.
204. Schlosser T, Pagonidis K, Herborn CU, et al. Assessment of left ventricular parameters using 16-MDCT and new software for endocardial and epicardial border delineation. *Am J Roentgenol*. 2005;184(3):765–773.
205. Raman SV, Shah M, McCarthy B, et al. Multi-detector row cardiac computed tomography accurately quantifies right and left ventricular size and function compared with cardiac magnetic resonance. *Am Heart J*. 2006;151:736–744.
206. Wu YW, Tadamur E, Yamamuro M, et al. Estimation of global and regional cardiac function using 64-slice computed tomography; a comparison study with echocardiography, gated-SPECT and cardiovascular magnetic resonance. *Int J Cardiol*. 2008;128:69–76.
207. Annuar BR, Liew CK, Chin SP, et al. Assessment of global and regional left ventricular function using 64-slice multi-slice computed tomography and 2D echocardiography: A comparison with cardiac magnetic resonance. *Eur J Rad*. 2008;65:112–119.
208. Meyers DG, Bendon KA, Hankins JH, et al. The effect of baseline electrocardiographic abnormalities on the diagnostic accuracy of exercise-induced ST segment changes. *Am Heart J*. 1900;119:272–276.
209. Jette M, Landry F, Sidney K, et al. Exaggerated blood pressure response to exercise in the detection of hypertension. *J Cardiopulm Rehabil*. 1988;8:171–177.
210. Allison TG, Cordeiro MA, Miller TD, et al. Prognostic significance of exercise-induced systemic hypertension in healthy subjects. *Am J Cardiol*. 1999;83:371–375.
211. Majahalme S, Turjanmaa V, Tuomisto M, et al. Blood pressure responses to exercise as predictors of blood pressure level after 5 years. *Am J Hypertens*. 1997;10:106–116.
212. Polonia J, Martins L, Bravo-Faria F, et al. Higher left ventricle mass in normotensive with exaggerated blood pressure responses to exercise associated with higher ambulatory blood pressure load and sympathetic activity. *Eur Heart J*. 1992;13(Suppl A):30–36.
213. Takamura T, Onishi K, Sugimoto T, et al. Patients with a hypertensive response to exercise have impaired left ventricular diastolic function. *Hypertens Res*. 2008;31:257–263.
214. Jae SY, Fernhall B, Lee M, et al. Exaggerated blood pressure response to exercise is associated with inflammatory markers. *J Cardiopulm Rehabil*. 2006;26:145–149.
215. Shim CY, Ha JW, Park S, et al. Exaggerated blood pressure response to exercise is associated with augmented rise of angiotensin II during exercise. *J Am Coll Cardiol*. 2008;52:287–92.
216. Gibbons RJ, Balady BJ, Bricker JT et al. ACC/AHA 2002 Guideline Update for Exercise Testing A Report of the American College of Cardiology/American Heart Association Task Force on Practice Guidelines (Committee on Exercise Testing). Accessed online at http://www.acc.org/qualityandscience/clinical/guidelines/exercise/exercise_clean.pdf
217. Kato S, Onishi K, Yamanaka T, et al. Exaggerated hypertensive response to exercise in patients with diastolic heart failure. *Hypertens Res*. 2008;31:679–684.
218. Nagueh SF, Mikati I, Kopelen HA, et al. Doppler estimation of left ventricular filling pressure in sinus tachycardia: A new application of tissue Doppler imaging. *Circulation*. 1998;98:1644–1650.
219. Ha JW, Lulic F, Bailey KR, et al. Effects of treadmill exercise on mitral inflow and annular velocities in healthy adults. *Am J Cardiol*. 2003;91:114–115.

220. Ha JW, Oh JK, Pellikka PA, et al. Diastolic stress echocardiography: A novel noninvasive diagnostic test for diastolic dysfunction using supine bicycle exercise Doppler echocardiography. *J Am Soc Echocardiogr.* 2005;18:63–68.

221. Burgess MI, Jenkins C, Sharman JE, et al. Diastolic stress echocardiography: hemodynamic validation and clinical significance of estimation of ventricular filling pressures with exercise. *J Am Coll Cardiol.* 2006;47:1891–1900.

222. Talreja DR, Nishimura RA, Oh JK. Estimation of left ventricular filling pressure with exercise by Doppler echocardiography in patients with normal systolic function: A Simultaneous echocardiographic–cardiac catheterization study. *J Am Soc Echocardiogr* 2007;20:477–479.

223. Wasserman AG, Katz RJ, Varghese PJ, et al. Exercise radionuclide ventriculographic responses in hypertensive patients with chest pain. *N Engl J Med.* 1984;311:1276–1280.

224. Miller DD, Ruddy TD, Zusman RM, et al. Left ventricular ejection fraction response during exercise in asymptomatic systemic hypertension. *Am J Cardiol.* 1987;59:409–413.

225. Tubau JF, Szlachicic J, Braun S, et al. Impaired left ventricular functional reserve in hypertensive patients with left ventricular hypertrophy. *Hypertension.* 1989;14:1–8.

226. Drazner MH, Rame JE, Marino ED, et al. Increased left ventricular mass is a risk factor for the development of a depressed left ventricular ejection fraction within five years: The Cardiovascular Health Study. *J Am Coll Cardiol.* 2004;43:2207–2215.

227. Houghton JL, Frank MJ, Carr AA, et al. Relations among impaired coronary flow reserve, left ventricular hypertrophy and thallium perfusion defects in hypertensive patients. *J Am Coll Cardiol.* 1990;15:43–51.

228. Aguirre JM, Rodriguez E, Ruiz De Azua E, et al. Segmentary coronary reserve in hypertensive patients with echocardiographic left ventricular hypertrophy, gammagraphic ischemia and normal coronary angiography. *Eur Heart J.* 1993;2(Suppl J):25–31.

229. Fragasso G, Lu C, Dabrowski P, et al. Comparison of stress/rest myocardial perfusion tomography, dipyridamole and dobutamine stress echocardiography for the detection of coronary disease in hypertensive patients with chest pain and positive exercise test. *J Am Coll Cardiol.* 1999;34:441–447.

230. Vashist A, Victoria A, Blum S, et al. Do electrocardiographic changes with adenosine myocardial perfusion imaging predict ischemia in patients with left ventricular hypertrophy? *Nuc Med Commun.* 2004;25(6):553–556.

231. Elhendy A, Schinkel AF, van Domburg RT, et al. Prognostic implications of stress Tc-99m tetrofosmin myocardial perfusion imaging in patients with left ventricular hypertrophy. *J Nucl Cardiol.* 2007;14(4):550–554.

232. Harvey W. An anatomical disquisition on the motion of the heart and blood in animals (1628). In: Willis FA, Keys TE, eds. *Cardiac Classics.* London: Henry Kimpton; 1941:19–79.

233. Pettigrew JB. On the arrangement of the muscular fibres in the ventricles of the vertebrate heart, with physiological remarks. *Philos Trans.* 1864;154:445–500.

234. Torrent-Gausp F. *Anatomia Functional del Corazon.* Madrid: Paz Montalvo; 1957:62–68.

235. Buckberg GD, Clemente C, Cox JL, et al. The structure and function of the helical heart and its buttress wrapping. IV. Concepts of dynamic function from the normal macroscopic helical structure. *Semin Thorac Cardiovas Surg.* 2001;13:342–357.

236. Anderson RH, Sanchez-Quintana D, Niederer P, et al. Structural–functional correlates of the 3-dimensional arrangement of the myocytes making up the ventricular walls. *J Thorac Cardiovasc Surg.* 2008;136:10–18.

237. Greenbaum RA, Ho SY, Gibson DG, et al. Left ventricular fibre architecture in man. *Br Heart J.* 1981;45:248–253.

238. Lower R. Tractus de Corde. In: Gunther RT, ed. *Early Science in Oxford, Vol. 9.* Oxford, UK: Sawsons; 1968:1669.

239. Streeter DD Jr, Bassett DL. An engineering analysis of myocardial fiber orientation in pig's left ventricle in systole. *Anat Rec.* 1966; 155:503–511.

240. McDonald IG. The shape and movements of the human left ventricle during systole. A study by cineangiography and by cineradigrgaphy of epicardial markers. *Am J Cardiol.* 1970;26:221–230.

241. Young AA, Axel L. Three-dimensional motion and deformation of the heart wall: Estimation with spatial modulation of magnetization: a model-based approach. *Radiology.* 1992;185:241–247.

242. O'Dell WG, Moore CC, Hunter WC, et al. Three-dimensional myocardial deformations calculation with displacement field fitting to tagged MR images. *Radiology.* 1995;195:829–835.

243. Poulsen SH, Andersen NH, Ivarsen PI, et al. Doppler tissue imaging reveals systolic dysfunction in patients with hypertension and apparent "isolated" diastolic dysfunction. *J Am Soc Echocardiogr.* 2003;16:724–731.

244. Sironi AM, Pingitore A, Ghione S, et al. Early hypertension is associated with reduced regional cardiac function, insulin resistance, epicardial, and visceral fat. *Hypertension.* 2008;51:282–288.

245. Takemoto Y, Pellikka PA, Wang J, et al. Analysis of the interaction between segmental relaxation patterns and global diastolic function by strain echocardiography. *J Am Soc Echocardiogr.* 2005;18:901–906.

246. Kang, SJ, Lim HS, Choi BJ, et al. Longitudinal strain and torsion assessed by two-dimensional speckle tracking correlate with the serum level of tissue inhibitor of matrix metalloproteinase-1, a marker of myocardial fibrosis, in patients with hypertension. *J Am Soc Echocardiogr.* 2008;21:907–911.

247. Pavlopoulos, H, Nihoyannopoulos P. Abnormal segmental relaxation patterns in hypertensive disease and symptomatic diastolic dysfunction detected by strain echocardiography. *J Am Soc Echocardiogr.* 2008;21: 899–906.

248. Biederman RW, Doyle M, Young AA, et al. Marked regional left ventricular heterogeneity in hypertensive left ventricular hypertrophy patients: A Losartan Intervention For Endpoint Reduction In Hypertension (LIFE) cardiovascular magnetic resonance and echocardiographic substudy. *Hypertension.* 2008;52:279–286.

249. Wu MT, Tseng WY, Su MY, et al. Diffusion tensor magnetic resonance imaging mapping the fiber architecture remodeling in human myocardium after infarction: Correlation with viability and wall motion. *Circulation.* 2006;114: 1036–1045.

250. Buchalter MB, Weiss JL, Rogers WJ, et al. Noninvasive quantification of left ventricular rotational deformation in normal humans using magnetic resonance imaging myocardial tagging. *Circulation.* 1990;81:1236–1244.

251. Notomi Y, Setser RM, Shiota T, et al. Assessment of left ventricular torsional deformation by Doppler tissue imaging: Validation study with tagged magnetic resonance imaging. *Circulation.* 2005;111:1141–1147.

252. Helle-Valle T, Crosby J, Edvardsen T, et al. New noninvasive method for assessment of left ventricular rotation: speckle tracking echocardiography. *Circulation.* 2005;112:3149–3156.

253. Wang J, Khoury DS, Yue Y, et al. Preserved left ventricular twist and circumferential deformation, but depressed longitudinal and radial deformation in patients with diastolic heart failure. *Eur Heart J.* 2008;29:1283–1289.

254. Takeuchi M, Borden WB, Nakai H, et al. Reduced and delayed untwisting of the left ventricle in patients with hypertension and left ventricular hypertrophy: A study using two-dimensional speckle tracking imaging. *Eur Heart J.* 2007;28:2756–2762.

255. Abe Y, Kawagishi1 T, Ohuchi H, et al. Accurate detection of regional contraction using novel 3-dimensional speckle tracking technique. *J Am Coll Cardiol.* 2008;51(Suppl A); A116.

Claudication

Jeffrey W. Olin

19

1. INTRODUCTION

Claudication is the primary symptom that occurs in patients with peripheral arterial disease (PAD). The ACC/AHA Practice Guidelines[1] on the Management of Patients with PAD define PAD as "a diverse group of disorders that lead to progressive stenosis or occlusion, or aneurysmal dilatation, of the aorta and its noncoronary branch arteries, including the carotid, upper extremity, visceral, and lower extremity arterial branches." However, for purposes of this chapter, we will use the term PAD to denote vascular diseases caused by atherosclerosis of the aorta and lower extremity arteries leading to stenosis or occlusion of an artery.

2. EPIDEMIOLOGY OF PERIPHERAL ARTERIAL DISEASE

PAD is a marker of systemic atherosclerosis. The prevalence of PAD is approximately 12% in the adult population and there appears to be an equal prevalence in men and women.[2,3] However, this percentage is dependent on the age of the cohort studied (Table 19.1). Almost 20% of adults over the age of 70 years have PAD.[4] In an elderly hypertensive population from the Systolic Hypertension in the Elderly Program (SHEP), the prevalence of PAD was 38% in black men, 25% in white men, 41% in black women, and 23% in white women.[5] Findings from a national cross-sectional survey of PAD awareness, risk, and treatment: new resources for survival (PARTNERS) found that PAD afflicts 29% of patients who are either ≥70 years old or 50 to 69 years old who have a 10-pack year history of smoking or have diabetes.[6] Despite the strikingly high prevalence of this disease, especially in the elderly, this disease is underdiagnosed since it often presents with atypical symptoms or no lower extremity symptoms at all. The PARTNERS study demonstrated that more than 70% of primary care providers whose patients were screened in this study were unaware of the presence of PAD.[6]

The clinical presentation of PAD may vary from intermittent claudication, atypical leg pain, rest pain, ischemic ulcers to gangrene or no symptoms at all. Claudication is the typical symptomatic expression of PAD. However, the prevalence of asymptomatic disease is thought to be higher than symptomatic PAD with an estimated ratio of 0.9 to 7.7:1.[7] The Walking and Leg Circulation Study evaluated the symptoms in patients with PAD. Of the 460 patients with PAD, 19.8% had no exertional leg pain, 28.5% had atypical leg pain, 32.6% had classic intermittent claudication, and 19.1% had pain at rest.[8] Results from large epidemiologic studies suggest that only 2% to 6% of patients ≥60 years of age are symptomatic with intermittent claudication, despite the high prevalence

of PAD in that population studied.[9] The Rotterdam Study identified a 19.1% prevalence of PAD in its cohort population; however, intermittent claudication was reported in only 6.3% in the PAD group.[10] Similarly, the Edinburgh Artery Study surveyed 1,592 subjects aged 55 to 74 years and identified a 4.5% prevalence of intermittent claudication while the prevalence of asymptomatic PAD was 8.0%.[11] The results of these studies make it readily apparent that more patients with PAD are asymptomatic or have atypical leg symptoms than classic intermittent claudication.

2.1. Risk factors associated with peripheral arterial disease

2.1.1. Age

The most common risk factors associated with PAD are increasing age, diabetes, and smoking (Fig. 19.1).[12] PAD increases with age and there is a 1.5- to 2-fold increase in prevalence of PAD for every 10-year increase in age. Individuals 65 years of age or older in the Framingham Heart Study and persons 70 years of age and over in the National Health and Nutrition Examination Study (NHANES) were at increased risk for the development of PAD.[1] There was a strong association between age and the prevalence of PAD in the NHANES study (Table 19.1). The prevalence was 4.3% in subjects >40 years of age compared to 14.5% for those over 70 years of age.[3] Others have reported similar findings; there is a 2% to 3% prevalence of PAD [defined by an abnormal ankle-brachial index (ABI)] in individuals 50 years of age or under, but 20% in individuals greater than 75 years of age.[1,13] Higher prevalence rates were also observed in cardiovascular heart study (CHS), which recruited older, Medicare-eligible adults (25% for individuals 80 to 84 years of age and 30% for those 85 years of age and up) and the PARTNERS program (prevalence of 29%) in patients over 70 or 50 to 69 years of age with a history of smoking or diabetes.[14] PAD may be present in younger individuals (50 years of age or under), although this represents a very small percentage of cases.

2.1.2. Smoking

Smoking is the single most important modifiable risk factor for the development of PAD and its complications (intermittent claudication and critical limb ischemia). Smoking increases the risk of PAD by approximately fourfold compared to that of nonsmokers and results in earlier onset of symptoms by almost a decade with an apparent dose-response relationship between the pack/year history and PAD risk.[14-16] Smokers are more likely to have poorer survival rates (death attributed to increased cardiovascular events), progression to critical limb ischemia, amputation, and decreased arterial bypass graft patency rates when compared to nonsmokers. Both former and current smokers are at increased risk for PAD.

TABLE 19.1
PREVALENCE OF PAD

	Subjects (no.)	Age	ABI	Prevalence (%)	Claudication (%)
PARTNERS(6)	6,417	≥70 or >50 with Diabetes Mellitus (DM) or tobacco history	≤0.9	29	11
Rotterdam(10)	7,715	≥55	<0.9	19	6
Edinburgh(11)	1,592	55–74	<0.9	18	5
CHS(38)	5,714	≥65	<0.9	13	1
ARIC(41)	15,106	45–64	≤0.9	3	1

Risk factors for PAD (TASC II)

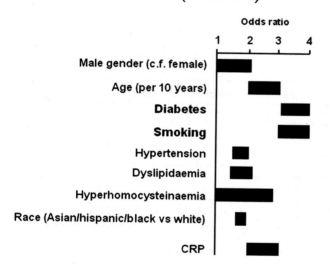

TASC II Inter-society consensus for the management of PAD. 2006

Figure 19.1 Risk factors for PAD. (Reproduced from Smith SC, Jr., Milani RV, Arnett DK, et al. Atherosclerotic vascular disease conference: Writing group II: Risk factors. *Circulation.* 2004;109(21):2613–2616, with permission.).

However, patients who are able to stop smoking are less likely to develop critical limb ischemia and have improved survival rates.[17] It is unclear why the association between smoking and PAD is about twice as strong as that for coronary artery disease (CAD).[15]

2.1.3. Diabetes mellitus

Diabetes increases the risk of developing symptomatic and asymptomatic PAD by 1.5- to 4-fold compared to nondiabetic individuals and leads to an increased risk for cardiovascular events and early mortality.[18–20] In the Framingham Heart Study, 20% of symptomatic patients with PAD had diabetes. In all likelihood, this is an underestimation because the diagnosis was from symptoms of intermittent claudication rather than objective testing.[21] In the NHANES survey[14] using the ABI, 26% of individuals with PAD were identified with diabetes while in the Edinburgh Artery Study, the prevalence of

PAD was greater in individuals with diabetes or an impaired glucose tolerance test (20.6%) compared to individuals with normal glucose tolerance (12.5%).[22] More recently, the Atherosclerosis Risk in Communities (ARIC) Study reported that a prior history of diabetes with insulin treatment was independently associated with a greater incidence of PAD while the Multi-Ethnic Study of Atherosclerosis (MESA) study reported that 26% of women and 27.5% of men with an ABI <0.9 had PAD.[19,23]

In patients with diabetes, the prevalence and extent of PAD also appear to correlate with the age of the individual and the duration and severity of their disease.[20] Diabetes mellitus is a stronger risk factor for PAD in women than men and the prevalence of PAD is higher in African Americans and Hispanics with diabetes when compared to non-Hispanic whites.[13,18,23,24] Patients with diabetes develop occlusive disease in the infrapopliteal arteries more than nondiabetics and are also more likely to develop microangiopathy, neuropathy, and impaired wound healing.[18] Diabetics may also present later in life with PAD that is more severe and progresses more rapidly. They have a higher risk for ischemic ulceration and gangrene and diabetes is the most common cause for amputation in the United States.[18]

2.1.4. Hyperlipidemia

In the Framingham Heart Study, an elevated level of cholesterol was associated with a twofold increased risk for intermittent claudication.[24] In NHANES survey, more than 60% of individuals with PAD had hypercholesterolemia while in the PARTNERS program, the prevalence of hyperlipidemia in patients with known PAD was 77%.[14,6] Hyperlipidemia increases the adjusted likelihood of developing PAD by 10% for every 10 mg/dL rise in total cholesterol.[25] The 2001 National Cholesterol Education Program Adult Treatment Panel (NCEP) III considered PAD a CAD risk equivalent.[26]

2.1.5. Hypertension

Almost every study has shown a strong association between hypertension and PAD and as many as 50% to 92% of patients with PAD have hypertension.[27] In the NHANES survey and the PARTNERS program, PAD and hypertension were encountered together in about 74% and 92% of enrolled subjects, respectively.[6,14] In the Cardiovascular Health Study, 52% of patients with an ABI < 0.9 had high blood pressure[28] and data from the Framingham Study demonstrated a 2.5- to 4-fold increased risk of developing intermittent claudication in both men and women with hypertension.[24] In the SHEP trial, 25.5% of the participants had an ABI under 0.9.[29] Taken together, these studies underscore the high prevalence of PAD in patients with hypertension.

The Seventh Report of the Joint National Committee on Prevention, Detection, Evaluation and Treatment of High Blood Pressure (JNC 7) acknowledged that PAD is equivalent in risk to ischemic heart disease.[30] Patients with hypertension and PAD are at greatly increased risk for the development of stroke and myocardial infarction (MI) independently of other risk factors.[27] In SHEP, there was a two to threefold increase in total and cardiovascular mortality in older adults with systolic hypertension while in the ARIC study, men with hypertension and PAD were four to five times more likely to have a stroke or transient ischemic attack (TIA), although this association was not significant in women.[29]

Other risk factors that are associated with an increased prevalence of PAD include race and ethnicity, inflammation, chronic kidney disease, genetics, hypercoagulable states, β_2 microglobulin, homocysteine, and the metabolic syndrome.[31-33] A full discussion of these nontraditional risk factors is beyond the scope of the chapter.

3. CLINICAL PRESENTATION

PAD causes two major consequences: there is a decrease in overall well-being and quality of life due to claudication and atypical leg pain and there is a markedly increased morbidity and all-cause

and cardiovascular mortality. Treatment should be directed at each of these facets. The clinical presentation, natural history, and outcomes in patients with PAD are summarized in Figure 19.2.

3.1. Symptoms

While claudication is the most common symptom that is associated with PAD, a majority of patients are either asymptomatic or have atypical symptoms. In a cross-sectional survey of 1,592 subjects aged 55 to 74 years old, the prevalence of PAD was 21.5% but only 4.5% of the subjects had symptoms.[11] In the PARTNERS program, classic symptoms of intermittent claudication only occurred in 11% of patients.[6]

Classic claudication as described in the Rose questionnaire describes muscular leg pain that occurs with exercise (usually walking). This "pain" can be described as an aching, heaviness, tiredness, cramping, pain, burning, or tightness and has three notable characteristics: (i) it is reproducible with a similar level of exercise from day to day; (ii) it disappears after 2- to 5 min of standing; and (iii) it occurs at the same distance once walking has been resumed.

When patients are asked if they have "pain," many will say no. It is helpful to ask the patients if they have *discomfort* when they walk. Patients who predominately have aortoiliac disease may experience exercise induced hip, buttock, or thigh discomfort or merely a sense of *power failure*. If patients walk until the symp-

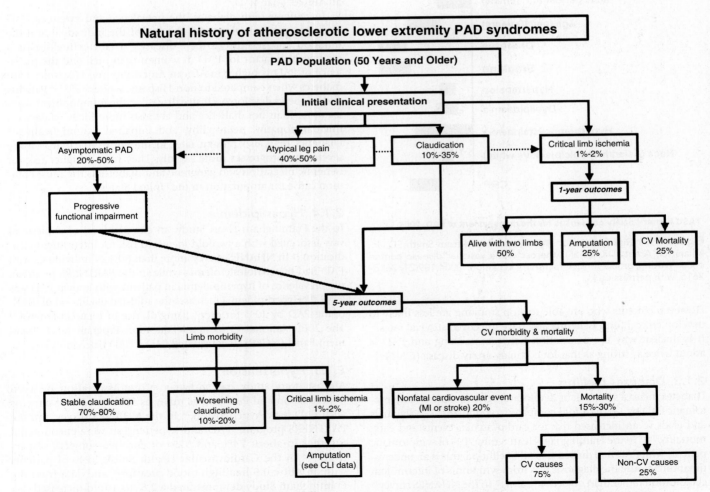

Figure 19.2 Clinical presentation, natural history, and outcomes in patients with atherosclerotic PAD. (Reproduced from Weitz JI, Byrne J, Clagett GP, et al. Diagnosis and treatment of chronic arterial insufficiency of the lower extremities: A critical review. *Circulation.* 1996;94(11):3026–3049, with permission.).

toms become so severe that they can no longer walk, it may take 15 or 20 min to get relief and they may have to sit down. This is because they have built up so much lactic acid in their muscle that it takes time to return to normal.

The discomfort is usually experienced one level distal to the level of obstruction (i.e., superficial femoral artery or popliteal obstruction causes calf claudication). When multilevel disease exists, the symptoms occur in the most distal segment. It is helpful to try and quantify the degree of disability by recording the distance when the discomfort first starts (initial claudicating distance) and the distance when the patient must stop walking (absolute or maximal claudication distance).

Patients with claudication have significant functional disability similar to patients with New York Heart Association Class III heart failure and severe chronic obstructive lung disease.[34] From the standpoint of the limb, the prognosis of PAD is favorable in that the symptom of claudication remains stable in 75% of subjects over a 10-year period of time (Fig. 19.2). The remainder of patients may progress to either disabling claudication or critical limb ischemia requiring revascularization or, less commonly, amputation.[8]

When patients progress to critical limb ischemia, they develop pain at rest, ischemic ulcerations, or gangrene. These patients are at a much greater risk of limb loss and also have a higher likelihood of suffering from a MI, stroke, or cardiovascular death.[1,9] The pain is often severe and starts distally in the toes and foot. The pain is worse with the leg elevated (e.g., at night when the patient is in bed) and relieved with dependency (hanging the leg over the side of the bed or getting up and standing or sitting in a chair). As the degree of ischemia worsens, patients may experience parasthesias, coldness of the extremity, muscular weakness, and stiffness of the foot and ankle joints. The two most commonly used classifications of severity are shown in Tables 19.2 and 19.3.

3.1.1. Differential diagnosis of claudication

There are a large number of conditions that should be considered in patients who present with exercise induced leg discomfort. There are several vascular conditions that may cause claudication other than PAD caused by atherosclerosis. These include: popliteal artery entrapment syndrome, cystic adventitial disease, fibromuscular dysplasia of the iliac or lower extremity arteries, endofibrosis of the iliac artery associated with cycling, external compression on the artery, and, less commonly, atheromatous embolization or vasculitis. Rarely, arthritis, myositis, and compartment syndrome may be mistaken for vascular claudication. Patients with venous obstruction (especially of the iliac veins) may develop venous claudication. In this condition, patients experience the feeling that the leg is "bursting" when walking and they must stop.

However, the most common conditions associated with symptoms that may commonly be confused with claudication are spinal stenosis and lumbar radiculopathy. In fact, it is not uncommon for elderly patients to have both PAD from atherosclerosis and spinal stenosis (pseudoclaudication). It is only by a detailed history that one can distinguish which of these two common conditions is causing the symptoms in an individual patient (Table 19.4).

3.2. Physical examination

A carefully performed cardiovascular physical examination is imperative. Specifically related to patients with PAD, the blood pressure should be obtained from each arm since associated subclavian artery disease is not uncommon in patients with atherosclerosis in other locations. A blood pressure difference of 20 mm Hg or more may indicate innominate, subclavian, or axillary artery disease. In addition, one should listen for bruits over the carotid and subclavian arteries and if present, they are described as systolic or diastolic, or both.[35] The abdominal aorta should be palpated in all individuals and if enlarged, the patient should undergo an abdominal ultrasound. The femoral, popliteal,

TABLE 19.2
FONTAINE CLASSIFICATION

Stage	Description
I	Asymptomatic and ankle brachial index <0.9
II	Intermittent claudication
III	Daily rest pain
IV	Focal tissue necrosis

TABLE 19.3
RUTHERFORD CLASSIFICATION

Grade	Category	Description
0	0	Asymptomatic
I	1	Mild claudication
I	2	Moderate claudication
I	3	Severe claudication
II	4	Ischemic rest pain
III	5	Minor tissue loss
IV	6	Major tissue loss

TABLE 19.4
DIFFERENTIATING PAD FROM SPINAL STENOSIS

Description of symptom	Intermittent claudication	Pseudoclaudication
Character of discomfort	Pain, tightness, cramping, heaviness, tiredness, burning	Same plus tingling, weakness, clumsiness
Location of discomfort	Buttock, hip, thigh, calf, foot	Same
Exercise induced	Yes	Yes or No
Distance to claudication	Same each time	Usually variable
Occurs with standing	No	Yes
Relief	Stop walking and stand	Often, must sit down or change body position

Source: Modified from Krajewski LP, Olin JW. Atherosclerosis of the aorta and lower extremity arteries. In: Young JR, Olin JW, Bartholomew JR, eds. *Peripheral Vascular Diseases.* 2nd Ed. C.V. Mosby Co; 1996.

dorsalis pedis, and posterior tibial arteries should be palpated and described as normal (2+), diminished (1+), or absent (0). Since popliteal and femoral arteries may become aneurysmal, this should also be noted on the physical examination. The dorsalis pedis pulse may be absent in up to 12% of individuals and thus is not considered an abnormal finding. However, it is never normal to have an absent posterior tibial pulse and the inability to detect the posterior tibial pulse usually indicates that the patient has PAD. Careful inspection of the feet should be undertaken to look for pallor, cyanosis or rubor, ulcerations, trophic changes, muscular atrophy, and tinea infection.

4. CLINICAL OUTCOMES

PAD is most often diagnosed by an ABI ≤ 0.9. The ABI is the ratio of the ankle systolic pressure to the arm systolic pressure. Using a hand-held continuous wave Doppler ultrasound device, the higher systolic pressure measured from either the posterior tibial or dorsalis pedis artery (in each leg) is compared with the highest brachial artery pressure taken from either arm (Fig. 19.3). A low ABI has been shown to be an independent predictor of increased mortality.[29,36-40] Patients with an ABI < 0.9 have approximately a 25% mortality within 5 years.[38] The incidence of TIA/stroke and cardiac events is proportional to a decrease in the ABI.[28,41] Patients with an ABI < 0.9 are twice as likely to have a history of MI, angina, and congestive heart failure than patients with an ABI of 1.0 to 1.5.[28,41] The mortality in patients with intermittent claudication is two to three times higher than in age- and sex-matched controls, with 75% of PAD patients dying from cardiovascular events.[24] In a 10-year prospective study by Criqui et al.,[42] both PAD patients with and without a history of cardiovascular disease had significantly increased risk of dying from any cause, cardiovascular, and coronary heart disease than age-matched controls.[42] The 10-year mortality increased as the severity of PAD increased (Fig. 19.4A). The all-cause mortality was 3.1 times greater and cardiovascular disease mortality 5.9 times greater in those patients with PAD compared to patients without PAD (Fig. 19.4B). The risk of cardiovascular events is similar between PAD patients with claudication and those without symptoms.[43] In a study of 2,023 middle-aged asymptomatic men without CAD, an ABI less than 0.9 was independently associated with higher coronary and cardiovascular mortality than in subjects with a normal ABI.[44] The extremely high morbidity and mortality in the PAD population is due to MI and stroke.[45,46] Both the ARIC and Edinburgh Artery Studies correlated an

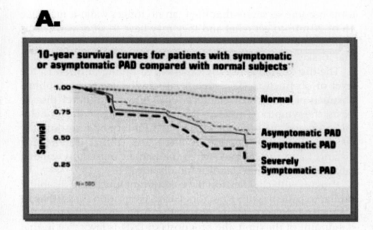

A.

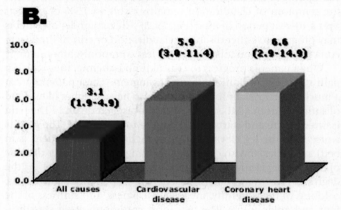

B.

Figure 19.4 A: Kaplan Meier survival demonstrating that as the severity of PAD worsens, mortality increases over a 10-year period of time. Note that even those subjects with asymptomatic PAD have a marked decrease in survival. **B:** The relative risk of dying from any cause is 3.1 times greater in those with PAD compared to those without and there is a 5.9 times greater risk of dying from a cardiovascular death in subjects with PAD compared to subjects without PAD.

increased risk of stroke and TIA with increased PAD severity.[41,43] The combination of known coronary or cerebrovascular disease with PAD has been shown to increase mortality risk. The Bypass Angioplasty Revascularization Investigation (BARI) trial demonstrated that patients with multivessel CAD and PAD had a 4.9 times greater relative risk of death compared to those individuals without PAD.[47] In a pooled analysis of mortality in eight large randomized percutaneous coronary intervention (PCI) trials involving 19,867 patients, Saw and colleagues demonstrated that the 7 day, 30 day, 6 month, and 1 year death or MI rates were significantly higher in those patients with PAD who underwent PCI compared to those without PAD who underwent PCI (Fig. 19.5).[48]

5. PATHOPHYSIOLOGY OF INTERMITTENT CLAUDICATION

The classic symptom of PAD is claudication, a word derived from the Latin word *claudicato*, meaning to limp. The discomfort is from reversible muscle ischemia. The pathophysiologic abnormalities (Table 19.5) that have been observed in patients with PAD are complex and the details are beyond the scope of this chapter. However, some basic principles are worthy of brief discussion.

Calculation of the ankle brachial index

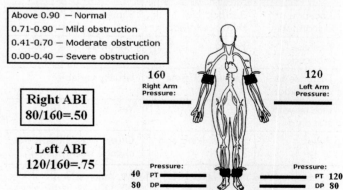

Above 0.90	— Normal
0.71-0.90	— Mild obstruction
0.41-0.70	— Moderate obstruction
0.00-0.40	— Severe obstruction

Right ABI
80/160=.50

Left ABI
120/160=.75

160
Right Arm Pressure:

120
Left Arm Pressure:

Pressure:
40 PT
80 DP

Pressure:
PT 120
DP 80

Figure 19.3 Method for the calculation of the ankle-brachial index.

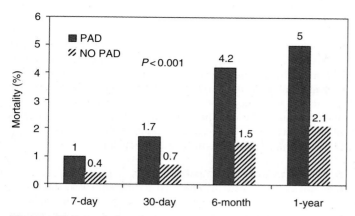

Figure 19.5 Pooled analysis of eight large randomized trials in 19,867 patients who underwent PCI demonstrating that the mortality was higher in patients with PAD who underwent PCI compared to patients without PAD who underwent PCI.

Blood flow is determined by the systemic blood pressure and the resistance to flow as represented by the formula (flow = pressure ÷ resistance). In normal subjects, exercise causes vasodilatation and thus a decrease in peripheral vascular resistance. Therefore, flow will increase with exercise and because resistance also decreases, there is no decrease in pressure distally in the normal individual. However, in PAD, two physiological mechanisms occur: (i) exercise causes increased demand for oxygen, yet only a fixed amount of blood can be delivered distally because of an obstruction to blood flow and (ii) there is vasodilatation to decrease outflow resistance. Thus, a fixed amount of blood is delivered to a dilated arterial segment causing a decrease in ankle pressure with exercise. This is expressed more completely in Poiseuille's equation that defines the relationship between resistance, pressure, and flow: Pressure drop across stenosis = flow $[8\,L\eta]$ ÷ πr^4 where L is the length of stenosis, r is the internal radius, and η is the viscosity.[49]

In addition to the hemodynamic abnormalities that occur in patients with PAD, there are abnormalities of muscle structure and function. Muscle biopsies of patients with PAD have shown a decrease in the type II fast twitch fiber area. These findings have been associated with muscle weakness.[50] It has also been demonstrated that patients with claudication develop progressive denervation over time.[51] These abnormalities have important clinical implications since patients with claudication have slow walking speed, decreased step length, and cadence and impaired gait stability.[49] Hiatt and others have suggested that the reduced exercise capacity in patients with PAD cannot be explained by alterations in limb blood flow alone since there are so many other abnormalities in muscle and nerve structure, function, and metabolism.[49]

6. DIAGNOSTIC EVALUATION IN PATIENTS WITH PERIPHERAL ARTERIAL DISEASE AND CLAUDICATION

6.1. Nonimaging methods

Of all the noninvasive methods for the diagnosis of PAD, ABI, segmental blood pressure, and pulse volume waveform analysis are the only techniques that provide physiologic information about perfusion in the limb. All other techniques provide excellent anatomic information but little, if any, physiologic information.

TABLE 19.5
ABNORMALITIES OBSERVED IN PAD

Changes in PAD	Possible consequences
Hemodynamic Arterial stenosis/occlusion Collateral formation Increased blood viscosity Endothelial dysfunction Muscle capillary proliferation	Pressure drop across stenosis Inability to increase flow relative to demand Partial compensation for arterial stenosis Reduced flow Altered arteriolar regulation of flow Increased oxygen diffusion capacity
Oxidant Stress Free radical generation White cell activation Mitochondrial DNA deletions	Endothelial and muscle injury Contributes to oxidant injury Reflection of mitochondrial oxidant stress/injury
Structural Distal axonal denervation Reinnervation Type II fiber loss	Muscle weakness Partial compensation Decreased muscle mass/strength
Metabolic Increased oxidative enzymes Short chain acylcarnitine Decreased activity of complexes I and III of electron transport chain	Partial compensation for flow and metabolic abnormalities Reflects altered oxidative metabolism Muscle accumulation related to performance Reduced potential for generation of ATP; increased production of reactive oxygen species and altered metabolic intermediate accumulation

PAD, Peripheral arterial disease
Source: Regensteiner JG, Wolfel EE, Brass EP, et al. Chronic changes in skeletal muscle histology and function in peripheral arterial disease. *Circulation*. 1993;87(2):413–421.

It is important to recognize that the systolic pressure in the arterial system *increases* from the central aorta to the peripheral arteries. This is caused by reflection waves from the arterioles, bifurcation points and branches, which amplify the systolic pressure wave in the peripheral artery. In addition, the distensibility of the central aorta tends to dampen the peak of the systolic wave centrally, contributing to the same phenomenon. Conditions that increase stiffness in the peripheral arteries, most commonly calcification, will result in an exaggerated increase in the difference between peripheral and central systolic pressure.

A continuous wave Doppler device is used to detect flow distal to a pneumatic cuff. The cuff is inflated to occlusive pressure and then gradually deflated, with the Doppler device positioned over the downstream artery. The systolic pressure is the point at which the flow signal is restored during cuff deflation. Traditionally, systolic pressures are measured in both arms and ankles. Other locations for pressure measurement include the upper and lower thigh, calf, ankle, transmetatarsal region, and the digits.[52] The cuff width should be proportional to the circumference of the limb segment under investigation, otherwise spuriously elevated or reduced values can be obtained. The measurement of segmental blood pressures is useful in not only determining if the disease is present but it can also help in localizing the arterial segments involved as well.

6.1.1. Ankle-brachial Index

Using a hand-held continuous wave Doppler ultrasound device, the ratio between the systolic pressure measured over the posterior tibial or dorsalis pedis arteries is compared to the systolic blood pressure in the arms. The higher of the two arm blood pressures is used and the higher of the dorsalis pedis or posterior tibial artery in each leg is used for the calculation (Fig. 19.3). A normal ABI is 0.9 to 1.40. A value over 1.40 indicates that the blood vessels are calcified, and not compressible. Under these circumstances, the ABI is not an accurate representation of the circulatory status and pulse volume waveforms or toe pressures should be used instead. Any reduction in the ABI value indicates reduced arterial flow to the lower extremity.[53,54] Measurement of the ABI does not define the level of obstructive disease, but it is accurate, simple to obtain, and correlates with severity of the disease. A value ≤0.9 and >0.4 reflects mild to moderate disease and is consistent with patients experiencing claudication, whereas an ABI ≤ 0.4 denotes severe disease and is consistent with short distance claudication or rest pain. Patients exhibiting critical limb ischemia almost always have an ABI < 0.40 and have multilevel disease. ABI is the method most commonly used to define lower extremity PAD in large population-based studies. Moreover, it has been correlated with clinical outcomes of different patient populations with vascular risk factors and CAD.[40,42]

The diagnostic value of the ABI is limited in disease states that lead to noncompressibility of blood vessels, e.g., patients with diabetes or renal failure. In these circumstances, the ABI is artifactually increased (>1.40) or may be falsely read as normal, thus underestimating the disease severity. It has been shown in the Strong Heart Study that an ABI > 1.40 is associated with increased all-cause and cardiovascular mortality.[40] In cases of arterial calcification, the toe brachial index (TBI) (the ratio of the systolic pressure of the toe to that of the arm) should be utilized.

It should be noted that the ABI can be normal in the face of a hemodynamically significant stenosis. This most commonly occurs in patients with aortoiliac occlusive disease. For example, if there is a 50% iliac stenosis, the pulse and the systolic pressure at rest may be normal. If the patients give a history of claudication, they should undergo a treadmill test to reproduce their symptoms and the ankle systolic pressures should be measured before and after exercise. As discussed later, if the ankle pressure (and ABI) decreases, the diagnosis of PAD is secure. The decreased pressure is due to a fixed amount of blood being delivered to the dilated vascular bed distally.

6.1.2. Segmental limb pressures

Limb pressures are usually measured at different levels: upper and lower thighs, calf, ankle, metatarsal, and digits. After the ABI is calculated, the cuffs are sequentially inflated to occlusive pressures and then are gradually deflated. The Doppler device is placed on a pedal artery and the systolic pressure at each level is recorded. Normally, the difference between systolic pressure at two consecutive levels should be <20 mm Hg. A larger difference indicates obstructive disease in the artery proximal to the cuff. The difference between the two limbs at the same level should be <20 mm Hg. A larger difference indicates obstructive disease proximal to the cuff on the side with the lower pressure (Fig. 19.6).[52] In addition to comparing pressures at different levels, the absolute levels of pressure may be of value: an ankle pressure < 40 mm Hg and/or a toe pressure < 30 mm Hg are considered to be signs of very poor perfusion and unfavorable predictors of ulcer healing.

It is important to understand that pressures measured using this technique may be artifactually high. Using cuff measurement, the proximal thigh pressure is expected to be 20 to 30 mm Hg higher than the brachial pressure. In addition to the increasing systolic pressure in the peripheral arteries, it is also possible that the pressure inside the cuff may not be fully transmitted to the artery embedded deep in the thigh. This may result in overestimation of the systolic pressure in the proximal thigh and underestimation of possible aortoiliac obstruction. Therefore, if the systolic pressure in the thigh is equal to or lower than the brachial pressure, this should raise the possibility of aortoiliac disease.

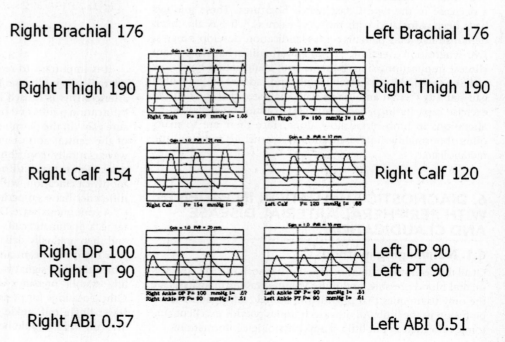

Figure 19.6 Segmental blood pressures and pulse volume waveform analysis. Note that the ABI is reduced bilaterally (0.57 on the right and 0.51 on the left). The degree of reduction in the ABI should lead to the suspicion that there is multilevel disease. There is a pressure drop from the thigh to the calf bilaterally, which indicates superficial femoral or popliteal artery disease, and from the calf to the ankle bilaterally, which indicates tibial peroneal disease. Also of note, the calf pulse volume waveforms should be 1.5 times the amplitude of the thigh waveforms. The lack of augmentation is also suggestive of superficial femoral or popliteal artery disease.

Right Brachial 176

Left Brachial 176

Right Thigh 190

Right Thigh 190

Right Calf 154

Right Calf 120

Right DP 100
Right PT 90

Left DP 90
Left PT 90

Right ABI 0.57

Left ABI 0.51

Under these circumstances, a Doppler waveform at the common femoral artery (Fig. 19.7) provides additional useful information. If it is normal (triphasic), it is very unlikely that the patient has iliac disease.

6.1.3. Doppler velocity patterns

One of the valuable diagnostic clues that can be provided by a vascular laboratory is analysis of the velocity waveforms of arterial flow. These waveforms are obtained using a Doppler device placed over the different segments of the arterial tree. The changes in the direction and velocity of arterial flow can be displayed on a screen and printed for documentation.

The normal Doppler tracing is described as "triphasic": a main forward-flow systolic phase, a reverse-flow phase coinciding with late systole, and a secondary smaller forward-flow phase seen in diastole.[55] The tracing is unlikely to be abnormal unless the obstructive lesion exceeds 50% diameter stenosis. With early disease, the reverse-flow phase is lost leading to a "biphasic" wave (Fig. 19.7). The amplitude of the forward systolic wave diminishes and the wave becomes "monophasic" with more advanced disease. Although only qualitative, the presence of a triphasic wave distally virtually excludes significant proximal obstruction. By obtaining waveforms at different levels, the location of the obstructive lesion can be identified.

6.1.4. Pulse volume recordings (PVR)

During the cardiac cycle, there are pulsatile volume changes in the limb. Since the volume of tissue and venous blood is relatively constant, the change in volume is directly related to the arterial flow. Using the same pneumatic cuffs that were utilized to measure segmental blood pressure, these volume changes can be measured using a pulse volume recorder (Fig. 19.6). The cuff is inflated to a set pressure ~60 mm Hg (in the presence of severe ischemia, especially in the foot and toe, the pressure in the cuff should be reduced). With each heartbeat, the limb expands leading to a change in the cuff pressure. That change can be presented on a spectral display and printed on a graduated chart, producing a plethysmographic tracing. Generally, every 1 mm Hg change in the cuff pressure produces 20 mm of deflection on the spectral display. The PVR tracings are similar to arterial pulse wave tracings: rapid systolic upstroke followed by a rapid downstroke, interrupted by a prominent dicrotic notch. With mild disease, the dicrotic notch is blunted. As the disease progresses, the change in volume (and hence the amplitude of the tracing) is diminished. In very severe obstructive lesions, the wave is almost flat, indicat-

ing no significant change in limb volume during systole.[56] PVR provides a qualitative assessment of flow-mediated changes and when combined with segmental blood pressures, it is a very useful tool to assess the lower extremity circulation.[57]

6.1.5. Exercise testing

Similar to cardiac stress testing, the purpose of exercise testing in the evaluation of PAD is to reproduce the physiologic conditions that result in intermittent claudication. The treadmill exercise protocol can be either constant-grade (speed of 2 miles per h and 12% incline for 5 min) or variable-grade (2 miles per h and 0% incline increasing by 2% every 2 min). Performance parameters that are monitored include (i) development of symptoms, (ii) duration of exercise, and (iii) change in ankle systolic pressure with exercise.

A normal individual should be able to perform this level of exercise for the 5-min duration without developing claudication and with no or little drop in the ankle pressure.[58]. A small drop in pressure (<20 mm Hg) may be noted, but it is expected to return to pre-exercise levels within 2 to 3 min. A patient who stops exercise within the first minute due to leg symptoms usually has severe disease that is very limiting or a nonvascular cause of leg pain. If symptoms develop after 3 to 5 min, the disease is milder in severity and the patient's lifestyle should be factored in the decision to proceed with revascularization. A drop in ankle pressure >20 mm Hg (or a significant reduction in pulse amplitude by PVR) at the end of the exercise is considered positive for obstructive disease.[52] The time for recovery of systolic pressure at the ankle to pre-exercise levels is also proportional to the severity of obstruction.[59] Development of leg pain without a drop in ankle pressure is almost always due to causes other than ischemia.[60]

Exercise testing has several advantages; it establishes the diagnosis of PAD in patients with normal or mildly reduced resting ABI, but with significant symptoms (Fig. 19.8). In our vascular laboratory, we routinely perform an exercise study in all patients with a normal ABI in whom the indication for the study was claudication. Exercise is also a valuable objective measure of the functional impairment the patient is experiencing. The comparison of the patient's performance before and after the treatment (medical, endovascular, or surgical) is a good measure of treatment success and can be used as an objective follow-up test.

6.1.6. Duplex ultrasonography

Duplex imaging involves several modalities: brightness or B-mode imaging, color Doppler ultrasonography, and pulsed wave Doppler. B-mode or gray-scale imaging displays a two-dimensional (2D) image of the arterial wall and lumen within the surrounding tissue using transducers of variable frequencies (2 to 3 MHz for aorta, iliac, renal, and mesenteric arteries and 5.0 to 7.5 MHz for femoral and more distal arteries). Due to the difference in acoustic properties of the arterial wall layers and components of atherosclerotic plaques, the ultrasound reflections can be reconstructed into different shades of gray-scale. Pulsed-wave Doppler ultrasound complements the 2D imaging by providing a Doppler waveform of the flow velocity within the lumen. The angle of insonation must be ≤60 degree (Chapter 3). This allows the analysis of direction, velocity, and pattern of arterial flow. Color-coding the Doppler signal facilitates the examination of specific arterial segment.

The resolution of the gray-scale image permits a rough evaluation of the lesion and atheroma characteristics, but does not allow accurate assessment of stenosis severity. The addition of color Doppler and pulsed-wave Doppler ultrasound results in a dramatic improvement of the sensitivity and specificity of the technique.[61]

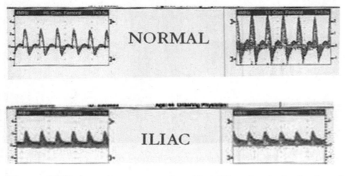

Figure 19.7 A continuous wave hand-held Doppler device is placed over the common femoral artery. A normal exam shows a triphasic waveform **(top)** indicating no proximal obstruction. When the Doppler waveform shows a biphasic or monophasic waveform **(bottom)**, there is common femoral or iliac artery occlusive disease.

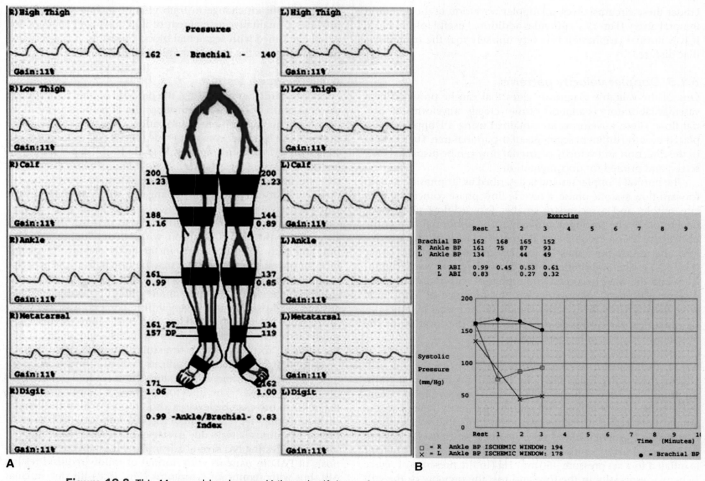

Figure 19.8 This 44-year-old male noted bilateral calf discomfort when walking two blocks. The pulse examination was normal bilaterally. **A:** The ABI was normal on the right (0.99) and only mildly reduced on the left (0.83). **B:** He exercised at 2MPH and a 12% incline and developed claudication at 1 min and 22 s and had to stop walking because of severe pain at 2 min and 29 s. The right ankle pressure decreased from 161 to 87 mm Hg and the left ankle pressure decreased from 134 to 34 mm Hg confirming the presence of PAD.

Because color-coding allows interrogation of specific segments surveyed by B-mode imaging, spectral waveforms from the segment of interest are obtained and compared to spectral waveforms from adjacent segments. At a stenotic segment, flow velocity increases proportionally to the severity of the stenosis (Fig. 19.9). Diagnostic criteria have been developed that allow an estimation of the stenosis severity based on the Doppler waveforms obtained at the segment of interest and comparing it with waveforms obtained in a more proximal, apparently normal segment.[62] More recently, a simpler, but more reliable, classification has been adopted in which arteries are classified into patent with mild disease, patent with ≥50% stenosis, and occluded. The main criterion for diagnosis of a hemodynamically significant lesion (angiographic diameter stenosis as ≥50%) is doubling of the peak systolic velocity (PSV) at the lesion site compared to the "normal" proximal segment and a PSV >200 cm/s with turbulence demonstrated on color Doppler.[63,64] With less significant stenoses, the increase in PSV is less pronounced, the reverse-flow component of the triphasic wave is preserved, and spectral broadening is less apparent.

Compared to digital subtraction angiography (DSA), duplex imaging is an accurate tool in detection of significant stenoses (>50% diameter reduction) and totally occluded vessels. The sensitivity and specificity of duplex imaging in detection of significant lesions are 92% and 97%, respectively. For total occlusions, the sensitivity and specificity are 95% and 99%, respectively.[63,65,66]

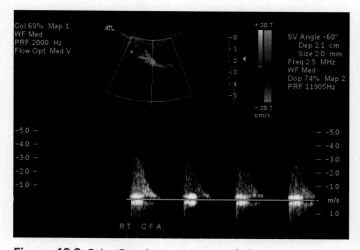

Figure 19.9 Color Doppler examination of the common femoral artery demonstrating a severe stenosis. The color Doppler shows marked turbulence to flow (mosaic color pattern). The pulsed wave spectral Doppler demonstrates a markedly increased PSV (350 cm/s). In addition, there is a visual bruit (dense white area at the baseline of each beat) thought to be due to vibration of the blood vessel wall and suggests that the stenosis is severe.

In general, >95% of the lower extremity arterial segments can be adequately visualized, with the exception of the peroneal artery, which can be examined in about 82% of patients.[63]

Duplex ultrasound is also valuable in identifying the exact site of obstruction in patients with disease (Fig. 19.10A). This in turn is critical in planning endovascular or surgical therapy. Moreover, it is useful in the follow-up of patients who had undergone endovascular [percutaneous transluminal angioplasty [(PTA)/stent] or surgical revascularization (Fig. 19.11). In those situations, the segments of interest are well defined and there are baseline studies performed before and after the procedure for reference. Every patient who has undergone either endovascular or surgical revascularization should be placed into a surveillance program to detect restenosis before the artery occludes. The surveillance should consist of an ABI and duplex ultrasound of the bypass graft or angioplasty/stent site. If a problem is identified, an angiogram should be performed. Surveil-

lance should be done soon after the procedure to have a baseline at 3 months, 6 months, and every 6 months thereafter.[67]

Gray-scale imaging is also important in identifying and measuring aortic and peripheral aneurysm dimensions, hematomas, and pseudoaneurysms. With the latter, it is of great value in guiding and following percutaneous ultrasound guided thrombin injection.[68,69]

6.2. Imaging methods

6.2.1. Magnetic resonance angiography

Magnetic resonance angiography (MRA) of the aorta and peripheral vasculature can be performed rapidly with excellent image quality. MRA has two fundamental advantages: contrast agents for MRA lack renal toxicity and images are obtained without the use of ionizing radiation.

Noncontrast MRA can be performed using "time of flight" methods (Chapter 10). In this method, background tissue is suppressed

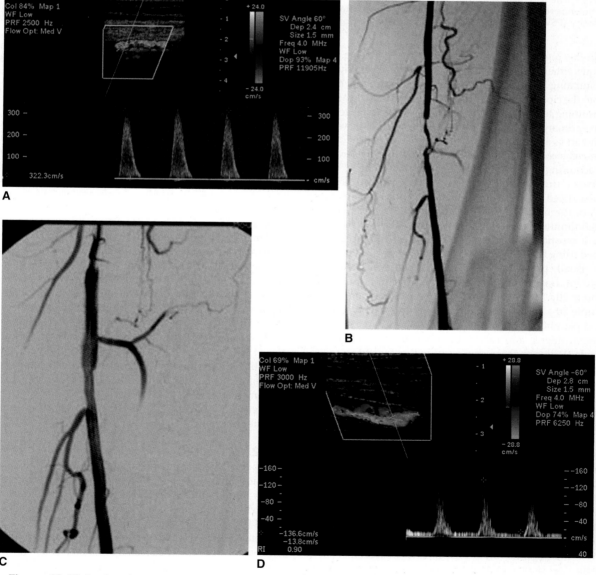

Figure 19.10 Duplex ultrasound showing marked turbulence to flow (mosaic color pattern in the mid portion of the superficial femoral artery) (**A**). This is a focal area of stenosis and is confirmed by the increase in the peak systolic velocity (PSV) (322 cm/s) and a monophasic waveform. This type of focal lesion usually does very well with an endovascular approach. This digital subtraction angiogram demonstrates focal superficial femoral artery (SFA) stenosis before (**B**) and after (**C**) stent implantation. Surveillance duplex ultrasound of the stented segment 3 months following stent implantation (**D**). There is good color filling of the stented superficial femoral artery and there is normalization of the velocity of blood flow (peak systolic velocity (PSV) 137 cm/s).

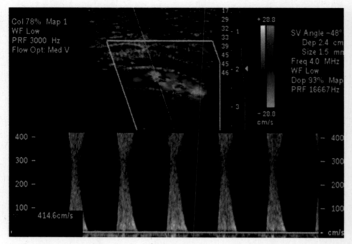

Figure 19.11 There is severe instent restenosis present. There is marked turbulence to flow (color aliasing) and an increase in the peak systolic velocity (PSV) and aliasing within the below knee popliteal stent.

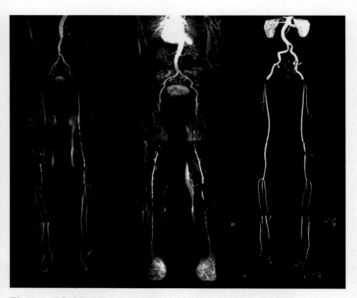

Figure 19.12 Multistation three-dimensional magnetic resonance angiogram (MRA) in several patients with claudication, which demonstrates superficial femoral artery disease (**left and middle panel**). Note that calcification is not visualized on MRA and the patent vessel lumen is well visualized. The panel on the right shows a normal MRA from the renal arteries to the ankles.

while the in-flowing blood signal is bright on MRA imaging. With this technique, either arterial or venous signal can be selectively visualized by saturating blood in the unwanted vascular territory before it moves into the cross-sectional imaging slice. Time of flight MRA is a time-consuming technique that is susceptible to flow-related signal loss. The primary applications of time-of-flight MRA are venous imaging and act as a supplement to other arterial sequences.

Contrast-enhanced 3-dimensional (3D) MRA is a newer technique for acquiring noninvasive angiographiclike images.[70–73] In many practices, this method has become the standard because of improved speed of acquisition, excellent image quality, and robustness of the method. Contrast-enhanced 3D MRA uses an injected gadolinium-based contrast medium followed by rapid 3D magnetic resonance imaging (MRI). Contrast-enhanced MRA is performed using fast 3D spoiled gradient echo pulse sequences. Imaging is usually performed in the coronal plane with a field of view of ≈40 cm. Images are obtained during breath-holding and require about 20 s. When multiple areas of the body are examined, multiple 20-s acquisitions are used. For example, for an aortogram and peripheral runoff, three MRA volumes are obtained: the abdomen, thighs, and calves. Because hundreds of images are acquired, 3D image processing is subsequently performed to project vessels in views of high diagnostic interest (Fig. 19.12).

Advanced MR methods use techniques such as partial k-space sampling, rectangular field of view, and real-time fluoroscopic imaging to further improve image quality. Additional slices can be acquired in the slice select direction by interpolating between adjacent acquired slices to improve the "smoothness" of the reconstructed 3D images.

For the aorta, contrast-enhanced MRA images are readily reformatted to provide information about the cross-sectional size of aortic aneurysms, extent and origin of aortic dissection, and branch vessel involvement. Abdominal MRA is increasingly being used to evaluate the abdominal aorta and its branches, particularly the renal arteries. The quality of MRA is so good that it (or CT angiography) has virtually replaced diagnostic angiography when evaluating patients with PAD to determine what type of intervention is most appropriate. The success of MRA in identifying small runoff vessels meets or exceeds that of traditional catheter-based angiography.[74]

MRA of the thigh and iliac vessels is commonly performed with the 3D contrast-enhanced method. A "bolus chase" technique is used, which substantially reduces examination times relative to

time-of-flight methods.[75] Bolus chase MRA involves manual or automated translation of the patient after a moderate, sustained infusion of gadolinium contrast agent via peripheral vein. Using current technology, CE 3D MRA has a sensitivity of ~90% and specificity of ~97% in detection of hemodynamically significant stenoses in any of the lower extremity arteries as compared to DSA.[67]

By acquiring volumetric or 3D data sets, it is possible to postprocess on independent workstations and enable reformations of the images in multiple views.[76–78]

In addition to detecting stenosis or occlusion of an artery, MRI can be used to assess the vessel wall directly for early atherosclerotic changes. In vivo studies have shown that MRI can distinguish among a variety of lipid mixtures typically found in human plaque.[79,80] T2-weighted MRI sequences offer good contrast for distinguishing plaque components and interrogating the vessel wall. Shinnar et al.[81] reported very high sensitivities and specificities of MRI in detecting various plaque components.

While MR angiography is a useful diagnostic modality for diagnosing significant PAD, it is not useful for following patients after placement of endovascular stents. Duplex ultrasound remains the diagnostic test of choice for detecting restenosis after angioplasty and stenting.[67]

6.2.2. Computed tomographic angiography

Computed tomographic angiography (CTA) is a vascular imaging technique that can be performed rapidly and safely for assessment of many vascular diseases. With the advent of multidetector-row CTA, excellent image quality is now possible with higher resolution than could be obtained previously with single-detector-row technology. Current multidetector-row scanners acquire up to 64 simultaneous interweaving helices. CTA has several advantages over conventional angiography, including volumetric acquisition, which permits visualization of the anatomy from multiple angles and in multiple planes after a single acquisition; improved visualization of soft tissues and other adjacent anatomic structures; less invasiveness; and thus fewer complications.[67,82,83] CTA has several advantages over MRA, including wider availability of scanners, higher spatial resolution, absence of flow-related phenomena that may distort MRA images, and capability to visualize calcification and metallic implants such as endovascular stents or stent grafts (Fig. 19.13). The main disadvantage of CTA compared with MRA is exposure to ionizing radiation.

Rapid CTA acquisition of images is critical because the images are obtained during the arterial phase of an intravenous (IV) contrast injection. The multidetector-row CTA has an increased speed of acquisition by increasing table feed, thus reducing exposure times.[84] These features allow for greater longitudinal coverage for a given scan duration and greater spatial resolution (i.e., imaging the thoracoabdominal, aortoiliac, and lower extremities), which may require up to 1,400 mm of coverage. More rapid acquisition also allows for a reduction in the amount of iodinated contrast material needed without significantly affecting the degree of arterial enhancement. Moreover, rapid acquisition permits more uniform vascular enhancement, thin section scans of large anatomic territories during a single breath-hold, improved visualization of small branch vessels and calcified plaque, and decreased pulsation-related artifacts.[67,84]

The initial image output from all CT scans consists of sets of contiguous or overlapping transverse cross-sections. These are always formally interpreted in the same manner as any CT scan, with full attention to all nonvascular structures, including bones, bowel, visceral organs, and lungs. To create angiographic representations, post processing of the volumetric data is necessary. The best postprocessed images are created from overlapping images, usually 50% to 80%. In the absence of overlap, the angiographic images may have a marked stair-step appearance.

For visualization and analysis, four postprocessing techniques may be used at the workstation: multiplanar reformation, maximum intensity projection (MIP), shaded surface display, and volumetric rendering. Each of these techniques has advantages and disadvantages depending on clinical application, anatomic area of interest, and image acquisition technique used.[85] These techniques allow manipulation of raw data to optimize visualization of relevant lesions or disease processes. An important common pitfall is the selective visualization of the maximally opacified vascular lumen. Both automated and manual creation of postprocessed images risk inadvertent rejection of critical vascular and nonvascular information. Postprocessed images alone should not be used for interpretation of CTAs. It is important to base the diagnosis on the source data available (axial images).

PAD is frequently multifocal; thus, lower-extremity arterial inflow and runoff should be imaged in its entirety. Before the advent of multidetector-row CT, limitations in scanning speed with single-detector-row CT yielded insufficient spatial resolution of the lower-extremity inflow and runoff to adequately characterize occlusive and aneurysmal disease in arteries that may be only 2 to 3 mm in diameter and span a distance of >1 m.[82] Recently, however, the greater longitudinal coverage of multidetector-row CT has been successfully used in imaging the entirety of the lower-extremity inflow and runoff.[86] For arterial segments identified with conventional angiography, Rubin et al. found 100% concordance with CT angiography.[82] Moreover, CT depicted 26 additional segments that could not be analyzed with conventional angiography because of improved arterial opacification distal to the occluded segments. The overall accuracy of multidetector CT angiography in patients with PAD is excellent (Table 19.6).

6.2.3. Digital subtraction angiography

Vascular imaging with ultrasound, CTA, and MRA has replaced catheter-based techniques in the initial diagnostic evaluation of patients in most circumstances. Angiography for diagnosis is reserved primarily for clarification of inadequate or conflicting results from physiological testing and cross-sectional vascular imaging. Despite a paradigm shift away from conventional angiography as a purely diagnostic technique, its importance in intervention has increased dramatically. DSA is a cornerstone technology in peripheral vascular intervention and will likely remain so for the foreseeable future.

In most institutions, DSA has replaced screen-film angiography for vascular applications. The resolution of DSA is less than that of screen film but can approach three to four line pairs per millimeter with current equipment. The standard imaging matrix is now 1,024 × 1,024, with image intensifiers that range up to 16 in. in diameter.

A number of major developments in DSA hardware and software contribute to greater diagnostic accuracy, faster procedures, and improved outcomes of interventions. Bolus chasing, rapid image acquisition, vessel diameter analysis, regional pixel shifting, image-stacking, 3D reconstructions from rotational angiograms, and even angioscopic representations of DSA data are now routinely available. The smaller diameter of catheters and devices, use of alternative access sites such as the radial artery, and access site management with closure devices and hemostatic agents have contributed greatly to the improved overall safety of angiographic procedures.[67]

The major attributes of DSA that contribute to its importance in vascular imaging are the ability to selectively evaluate individual vessels, access to direct physiologic information

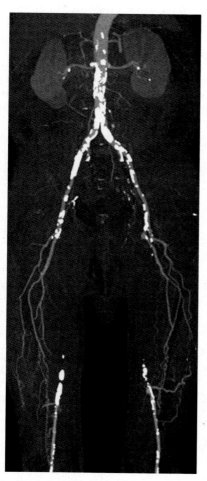

Figure 19.13 Multidetector CT angiogram [maximum intensity projection (MIP)] of the aorta and lower extremity arteries in a patient with calf claudication. There is extensive calcification of the aortoiliac segments and bilateral superficial femoral artery occlusions, which reconstitute (via collaterals from the profunda femoral artery) the above knee popliteal artery.

TABLE 19.6

RESULTS OF RECENT STUDIES COMPARING MULTIDETECTOR CT WITH DIGITAL SUBTRACTION ANGIOGRAPHY

Author, Year (Ref)	No. of Patients	MDCT rows	Section thickness (mm)	Sensitivity (%)	Specificity (%)
Willmann, 2005[93]	39	16	0.75	96–97	96–97
Edwards, 2005[94]	44	4	3.2	72–79	93
Romano, 2004[95]	42	4	3.2	93	95
Catalano, 2004[96]	50	4	3	96	93
Ota, 2004[97]	24	4	2	99	99
Martin, 2003[98]	41	4	5	92	97
Ofer, 2003[99]	18	4	3.2	91	92

NOTE: All sensitivities and specificities are reported for detection of ≥50% stenosis with the exception of the report by Martin et al. which is ≥75%. MDCT, multidetector CT.
Source: Modified from Hiatt MD, Fleischmann D, Hellinger JC, et al. Angiographic imaging of the lower extremities with multidetector CT. *Radiol Clin North Am.* 2005;43(6):1119–1127, ix.

such as pressure gradients, the ability to perform intravascular ultrasound, and its use as a platform for intervention. Exposure to ionizing radiation, use of iodinated contrast agents, and risks related to vascular access and catheterization are limitations of this technique. Nevertheless, until an alternative platform for intervention is developed or devices that are completely MRI-compatible become available, DSA will continue to have a central role in the management of patients with vascular disease.

Tables 19.7 and 19.8 summarize the benefits and limitations and differences of the various tests used to diagnose and follow patients with PAD.

7. FUTURE DIRECTIONS

Therapeutic angiogenesis is the concept of growing new blood vessels from existing vessels. Numerous studies have attempted to use this strategy of administering growth factors, to stimu-

TABLE 19.7

NONINVASIVE AND INVASIVE VASCULAR DIAGNOSTIC TOOLS: BENEFITS AND LIMITATIONS

Diagnostic tool*	Benefits	Limitations
Ankle-brachial indices (ABI)	A quick cost-effective way to establish or refute the diagnosis of PAD (see text) Useful to monitor the efficacy of therapeutic interventions	May not be accurate when systolic blood pressure cannot be abolished by inflation of an air-filled blood pressure cuff (noncompressible vessels at the level of the ankle), as occurs in some diabetic, elderly, or renal failure individuals
Toe-brachial indices	A quick cost-effective way to establish or refute the diagnosis of PAD (see text) Can measure digital perfusion when small-vessel arterial disease is present Useful in individuals with noncompressible vessels at the level of the ankle	Requires small cuffs and careful technique to preserve accuracy
Segmental pressure examination	Useful to establish or refute the diagnosis of PAD (see text) Useful to provide anatomic localization of lower extremity disease Can provide data to predict limb survival and wound healing Useful to monitor the efficacy of therapeutic interventions	May not be accurate when systolic blood pressure cannot be abolished by inflation of an air-filled blood pressure cuff (noncompressible vessels at the level of the ankle), as occurs in some diabetic, elderly, or renal failure individuals
Pulse volume recording	Useful to establish the diagnosis of PAD Helpful in predicting outcome in CLI and risk of amputation Can be used to monitor limb perfusion after revascularization procedures	Usefulness maintained in patients with noncompressible vessels (ABI >1.3–1.4) Qualitative, not quantitative measure of perfusion May not be accurate in more distal segments Less accurate than other noninvasive tests in providing arterial anatomic localization of PAD May be abnormal in patients with low cardiac output

(Continued)

TABLE 19.7

NONINVASIVE AND INVASIVE VASCULAR DIAGNOSTIC TOOLS: BENEFITS AND LIMITATIONS (Continued)

Diagnostic tool*	Benefits	Limitations
Duplex ultrasound	Can establish the diagnosis of PAD, establish anatomic localization, and define severity of lower extremity arterial stenosis Can be useful to select candidates for endovascular or surgical revascularization Can be useful to follow patients after endovascular or surgical revascularization for restenosis	Accuracy is diminished in aortoiliac arterial segments in some individuals (obesity or bowel gas) Dense arterial calcification can limit diagnostic accuracy Sensitivity is diminished for detection of stenosis downstream from a proximal stenosis
Toe-up exercise testing with pre-exercise and postexercise ABIs	Useful to diagnose PAD when resting ABI values are normal Can be performed in the absence of a treadmill with increased convenience and low cost	Provides qualitative (rather than quantitative) exercise diagnostic results Lower workload may not elicit symptoms in all individuals with claudication
Treadmill exercise testing, with and without pre-exercise and postexercise ABIs	Helps to differentiate claudication from pseudoclaudication in individuals with exertional leg symptoms Useful to diagnose PAD when resting ABI values are normal Objectively documents the magnitude of the symptom limitation in patients with claudication, especially when used with a standardized treadmill protocol Demonstrates the safety of exercise and provides data to individualize exercise prescriptions in individuals with claudication before initiation of a formal program of therapeutic exercise training Useful to measure the objective functional response to claudication therapeutic interventions	Requires the use of a motorized treadmill, with or without continuous electrocardiographic monitoring as well as staff familiar with exercise testing protocols
Magnetic resonance angiography (MRA)	Useful to assess PAD anatomy and presence of significant stenosis Useful to help select patients who are candidates for endovascular or surgical revascularization Helpful to provide associated soft tissue diagnostic information that may be associated with PAD (e.g. aneurysms, popliteal entrapment, and cystic adventitial disease	May overestimate the degree of stenosis Not useful in patients who have metallic stents in place Cannot be used in patients with contraindications to magnetic resonance techniques (pacemakers, defibrillators, intracranial metallic stents, clips, coils, and other devices) Gadolinium needs to be avoided in individuals with an eGFR <30 mL/min/1.73^2
Multidetector computed tomographic angiography (CTA)	Useful to assess PAD anatomy and presence of significant stenosis Useful to help select patients who are candidates for endovascular or surgical revascularization Helpful to provide associated soft tissue diagnostic information that may be associated with PAD (e.g., aneurysms, popliteal entrapment, and cystic adventitial disease Metal clips, stents, and metallic prostheses do not cause significant CTA artifacts Scan times are faster than for MRA	Requires iodinated contrast and ionizing radiation Use may be limited in patients with significant renal insufficiency
Catheter-based angiography	In the past, angiography was the definitive method for anatomic evaluation of PAD when revascularization is planned However, with multidetector CTA and Gd enhanced MRA, the need for catheter-based angiography is now rarely needed for diagnostic purposes alone Contrast angiography is used during the performance of endovascular procedures	Invasive evaluation is associated with a small risk of bleeding, infection, vascular access complications (e.g., dissection, pseudoaneurysm, AV fistula, closure device injury, or hematoma), atheroembolism, contrast allergy, and contrast nephropathy

*Tools are listed in order from least invasive to most invasive, from the least to most costly.
CLI, critical limb ischemia; PAD, peripheral arterial disease.
Source: Modified from Hirsch AT, Haskal ZJ, Hertzer NR, et al. ACC/AHA 2005 Practice Guidelines for the management of patients with peripheral arterial disease (lower extremity, renal, mesenteric, and abdominal aortic): A collaborative report from the American Association for Vascular Surgery/Society for Vascular Surgery, Society for Cardiovascular Angiography and Interventions, Society for Vascular Medicine and Biology, Society of Interventional Radiology, and the ACC/AHA Task Force on Practice Guidelines (Writing Committee to Develop Guidelines for the Management of Patients With Peripheral Arterial Disease): Endorsed by the American Association of Cardiovascular and Pulmonary Rehabilitation; National Heart, Lung, and Blood Institute; Society for Vascular Nursing; TransAtlantic Inter-Society Consensus; and Vascular Disease Foundation. *Circulation.* 2006;113(11):e463–e654.

TABLE 19.8
COMPARISON OF DUPLEX ULTRASOUND, MRA, AND CTA

	Duplex ultrasound	MRA	CTA
Accurate in diagnosis of disease severity and location	++++	++++	++++
Identify calcification	++++	–	++++
Provide roadmap for intervention	++	++++	++++
Useful for follow-up after surgical revascularization	++++	+	+++
Useful for follow-up after stent implantation	++++	–	+++
Cost effective	++++	+	+

MRA, Magnetic resonance angiography; CTA, Computed tomographic angiography.

late angiogenesis, and to bypass obstructions in the coronary and peripheral circulation. The Therapeutic Angiogenesis with Recombinant Fibroblast Growth Factor-2 for Intermittent Claudication (TRAFFIC) trial used a single intra-arterial infusion of recombinant fibroblast growth factor-2 (rFGF-2) in patients with intermittent claudication.[87] At 90 days, patients who received one dose of rFGF-2 had significantly improved peak walking time compared to those who received placebo. A repeat infusion at 30 days had no additional effects. Despite these promising results, the Regional Angiogenesis with Vascular Endothelial growth factor (RAVE) trial showed no difference in peak walking time between PAD patients who received a single intramuscular administration of vascular endothelial growth factor (VEGF) in an adenovirus vector versus patients who received placebo.[88] Disparity in these randomized trials could be explained by differences in the angiogenic growth factors, the vehicle used, or the mode of delivery. Recently, a randomized pilot trial examined the efficacy and safety of intramuscular injections of bone marrow-mononuclear cells into the legs of patients with chronic limb ischemia.[89] The hypothesis of this study was that injected marrow cells would supply endothelial progenitor cells, angiogenic growth factors, and cytokines to enhance angiogenesis. Twenty-four weeks after implantation, PAD patients who received bone marrow cells had significantly improved ABI, transcutaneous oximetry, and peak walking time compared to controls. Data will be available soon on the use of hypoxia-inducible factor 1 α as a potential treatment for patients with claudication.[90] The future of therapeutic angiogenesis is certainly challenging, but with continued research it may find utility in treating PAD patients refractory to medical and surgical interventions. Better resolution with MRA and CTA will allow visualization of the new blood vessel growth that occurs with therapeutic angiogenesis.

Imaging has made dramatic advances over the last decade. The quality of the images from ultrasound, MRA, CTA, and DSA has continued to improve and will do so in the immediate future. MR compatible stents are on the horizon, and there has been early work on MR guided interventional therapy.[91,92]

REFERENCES

1. Hirsch AT, Haskal ZJ, Hertzer NR, et al. ACC/AHA 2005 Practice Guidelines for the management of patients with peripheral arterial disease (lower extremity, renal, mesenteric, and abdominal aortic): A collaborative report from the American Association for Vascular Surgery/Society for Vascular Surgery, Society for Cardiovascular Angiography and Interventions, Society for Vascular Medicine and Biology, Society of Interventional Radiology, and the ACC/AHA Task Force on Practice Guidelines (Writing Committee to Develop Guidelines for the Management of Patients With Peripheral Arterial Disease): Endorsed by the American Association of Cardiovascular and Pulmonary Rehabilitation; National Heart, Lung, and Blood Institute; Society for Vascular Nursing; Trans-Atlantic Inter-Society Consensus; and Vascular Disease Foundation. *Circulation.* 2006;113(11):e463–e654.
2. Criqui MH, Fronek A, Barrett-Connor E, et al. The prevalence of peripheral arterial disease in a defined population. *Circulation.* 1985;71(3):510–515.
3. Regensteiner JG, Hiatt WR. Current medical therapies for patients with peripheral arterial disease: A critical review. *Am J Med.* 2002;112(1):49–57.
4. Newman AB, Sutton-Tyrrell K, Kuller LH. Lower-extremity arterial disease in older hypertensive adults. *Arterioscler Thromb.* 1993;13(4):555–562.
5. Hirsch AT, Criqui MH, Treat-Jacobson D, et al. Peripheral arterial disease detection, awareness, and treatment in primary care. *JAMA.* 2001;286(11):1317–1324.
6. Dormandy J, Heeck L, Vig S. Intermittent claudication: A condition with underrated risks. *Semin Vasc Surg.* 1999;12(2):96–108.
7. McDermott MM, Greenland P, Liu K, et al. The ankle brachial index is associated with leg function and physical activity: The Walking and Leg Circulation Study. *Ann Intern Med.* 2002;136(12):873–883.
8. Dormandy JA, Rutherford RB. Management of peripheral arterial disease (PAD). TASC Working Group. TransAtlantic Inter-Society Consensus (TASC). *J Vasc Surg.* 2000;31(1 Pt 2):S1–S296.
9. Meijer WT, Hoes AW, Rutgers D, et al. Peripheral arterial disease in the elderly: The Rotterdam Study. *Arterioscler Thromb Vasc Biol.* 1998;18(2):185–192.
10. Fowkes FG, Housley E, Cawood EH, et al. Edinburgh Artery Study: Prevalence of asymptomatic and symptomatic peripheral arterial disease in the general population. *Int J Epidemiol.* 1991;20(2):384–392.
11. Norgren L, Hiatt WR, Dormandy JA, et al. Inter-Society Consensus for the Management of Peripheral Arterial Disease (TASC II). *Eur J Vasc Endovasc Surg.* 2007;33(suppl 1):S1–75.
12. Smith SC, Jr., Milani RV, Arnett DK, et al. Atherosclerotic Vascular Disease Conference: Writing group II: Risk factors. *Circulation.* 2004;109(21):2613–2616.
13. Selvin E, Erlinger TP. Prevalence of and risk factors for peripheral arterial disease in the United States: Results from the National Health and Nutrition Examination Survey, 1999–2000. *Circulation.* 2004;110(6):738–743.
14. Kannel WB, Shurtleff D. The Framingham study. Cigarettes and the development of intermittent claudication. *Geriatrics.* 1973;28(2):61–68.
15. Powell JT, Edwards RJ, Worrell PC, et al. Risk factors associated with the development of peripheral arterial disease in smokers: A case-control study. *Atherosclerosis.* 1997;129(1):41–48.
16. Jonason T, Bergstrom R. Cessation of smoking in patients with intermittent claudication. Effects on the risk of peripheral vascular complications, myocardial infarction and mortality. *Acta Med Scand.* 1987;221(3):253–260.
17. Peripheral arterial disease in people with diabetes. *Diabetes Care.* 2003;26(12):3333–3341.
18. McDermott MM, Liu K, Criqui MH, et al. Ankle-brachial index and subclinical cardiac and carotid disease: The multi-ethnic study of atherosclerosis. *Am J Epidemiol.* 2005;162(1):33–41.
19. Selvin E, Marinopoulos S, Berkenblit G, et al. Meta-analysis: Glycosylated hemoglobin and cardiovascular disease in diabetes mellitus. *Ann Intern Med.* 2004;141(6):421–431.
20. Muntner P, Wildman RP, Reynolds K, et al. Relationship between HbA1c level and peripheral arterial disease. *Diabetes Care.* 2005;28(8):1981–1987.
21. MacGregor AS, Price JF, Hau CM, et al. Role of systolic blood pressure and plasma triglycerides in diabetic peripheral arterial disease. The Edinburgh artery study. *Diabetes Care.* 1999;22(3):453–458.
22. Wattanakit K, Folsom AR, Selvin E, et al. Risk factors for peripheral arterial disease incidence in persons with diabetes: The Atherosclerosis Risk in Communities (ARIC) study. *Atherosclerosis.* 2005;180(2):389–397.
23. Kannel WB, McGee DL. Update on some epidemiologic features of intermittent claudication: The Framingham study. *J Am Geriatr Soc.* 1985;33(1):13–18.
24. Hiatt WR, Hoag S, Hamman RF. Effect of diagnostic criteria on the prevalence of peripheral arterial disease. The San Luis Valley Diabetes study. *Circulation.* 1995;91(5):1472–1479.
25. Executive Summary of the Third Report of The National Cholesterol Education Program (NCEP) Expert Panel on Detection, Evaluation, And Treatment of High Blood Cholesterol In Adults (Adult Treatment Panel III). *JAMA.* 2001;285(19):2486–2497.
26. Olin JW. Hypertension and peripheral arterial disease. *Vasc Med.* 2005;10(3):241–246.
27. Newman AB, Siscovick DS, Manolio TA, et al. Ankle-arm index as a marker of atherosclerosis in the Cardiovascular Health Study. Cardiovascular Heart Study (CHS) Collaborative Research Group. *Circulation.* 1993;88(3):837–845.
28. Newman AB, Tyrrell KS, Kuller LH. Mortality over four years in SHEP participants with a low ankle-arm index. *J Am Geriatr Soc.* 1997;45(12):1472–1478.
29. Chobanian AV, Bakris GL, Black HR, et al. The Seventh Report of the Joint National Committee on Prevention, Detection, Evaluation, and Treatment of High Blood Pressure: The JNC 7 report. *JAMA.* 2003;289(19):2560–2572.

30. Bartholomew JR, Olin JW. Pathophysiology of peripheral arterial disease and risk factors for its development. *Cleve Clin J Med.* 2006;73(suppl 4):S8–S14.
31. Fung ET, Wilson AM, Zhang F, et al. A biomarker panel for peripheral arterial disease. *Vasc Med.* 2008;13(3):217–224.
32. Wilson AM, Kimura E, Harada RK, et al. Beta2-microglobulin as a biomarker in peripheral arterial disease: Proteomic profiling and clinical studies. *Circulation.* 2007;116(12):1396–1403.
33. Ware JE, Jr. The status of health assessment 1994. *Annu Rev Public Health.* 1995;16:327–354.
34. Olin JW. Evaluation of the peripheral circulation. In: Izzo JL, Black HR, eds. *Hypertension Primer.* Dallas: American Heart Association; 2007.
35. Vogt MT, Cauley JA, Newman AB, et al. Decreased ankle/arm blood pressure index and mortality in elderly women. *JAMA.* 1993;270(4):465–469.
36. McKenna M, Wolfson S, Kuller L. The ratio of ankle and arm arterial pressure as an independent predictor of mortality. *Atherosclerosis.* 1991;87(2–3):119–128.
37. Newman AB, Shemanski L, Manolio TA, et al. Ankle-arm index as a predictor of cardiovascular disease and mortality in the Cardiovascular Health Study. The Cardiovascular Health Study Group. *Arterioscler Thromb Vasc Biol.* 1999;19(3):538–545.
38. Criqui MH, Coughlin SS, Fronek A. Noninvasively diagnosed peripheral arterial disease as a predictor of mortality: Results from a prospective study. *Circulation.* 1985;72(4):768–773.
39. Resnick HE, Lindsay RS, McDermott MM, et al. Relationship of high and low ankle brachial index to all-cause and cardiovascular disease mortality: The Strong Heart study. *Circulation.* 2004;109(6):733–739.
40. Zheng ZJ, Sharrett AR, Chambless LE, et al. Associations of ankle-brachial index with clinical coronary heart disease, stroke and preclinical carotid and popliteal atherosclerosis: The Atherosclerosis Risk in Communities (ARIC) study. *Atherosclerosis.* 1997;131(1):115–125.
41. Criqui MH, Langer RD, Fronek A, et al. Mortality over a period of 10 years in patients with peripheral arterial disease. *N Engl J Med.* 1992;326(6):381–386.
42. Leng GC, Lee AJ, Fowkes FG, et al. Incidence, natural history and cardiovascular events in symptomatic and asymptomatic peripheral arterial disease in the general population. *Int J Epidemiol.* 1996;25(6):1172–1181.
43. Kornitzer M, Dramaix M, Sobolski J, et al. Ankle/arm pressure index in asymptomatic middle-aged males: An independent predictor of ten-year coronary heart disease mortality. *Angiology.* 1995; 46(3):211–219.
44. Criqui MH, Denenberg JO, Langer RD, et al. The epidemiology of peripheral arterial disease: Importance of identifying the population at risk. *Vasc Med.* 1997;2(3):221–226.
45. Ness J, Aronow WS. Prevalence of coexistence of coronary artery disease, ischemic stroke, and peripheral arterial disease in older persons, mean age 80 years, in an academic hospital-based geriatrics practice. *J Am Geriatr Soc.* 1999;47(10):1255–1256.
46. Burek KA, Sutton-Tyrrell K, Brooks MM, et al. Prognostic importance of lower extremity arterial disease in patients undergoing coronary revascularization in the Bypass Angioplasty Revascularization Investigation (BARI). *J Am Coll Cardiol.* 1999;34(3):716–721.
47. Saw J, Bhatt DL, Moliterno DJ, et al. The influence of peripheral arterial disease on outcomes: A pooled analysis of mortality in eight large randomized percutaneous coronary intervention trials. *J Am Coll Cardiol.* 2006;48(8):1567–1572.
48. Hiatt WR, Brass EP. Pathophysiology of Intermittent Claudication. In: Creager MA, Dzau VJ, Loscalzo J, eds. *Vascular Medicine, a Companion to Braunwald's Heart Disease.* Philadelphia, Pa: Saunders, Elsevier; 2006: 239–247.
49. Regensteiner JG, Wolfel EE, Brass EP, et al. Chronic changes in skeletal muscle histology and function in peripheral arterial disease. *Circulation.* 1993;87(2):413–421.
50. England JD, Ferguson MA, Hiatt WR, et al. Progression of neuropathy in peripheral arterial disease. *Muscle Nerve.* 1995;18(4):380–387.
51. Strandness DE, Jr. Noninvasive vascular laboratory and vascular imaging. In: Young J.R. OJWBJR, ed. *Peripheral Vascular Diseases.* St. Louis: Mosby Publishing Company; 1996: 33–64.
52. Carter SA. Clinical measurement of systolic pressures in limbs with arterial occlusive disease. *JAMA.* 1969;207(10):1869–1874.
53. Carter SA. Indirect systolic pressures and pulse waves in arterial occlusive diseases of the lower extremities. *Circulation.* 1968;37(4):624–637.
54. Hirsch AT, Criqui MH, Treat-Jacobson D, et al. Peripheral arterial disease detection, awareness, and treatment in primary care. *JAMA.* 2001;286(11):1317–1324.
55. Strandness DE, Jr., Schultz RD, Sumner DS, et al. Ultrasonic flow detection. A useful technic in the evaluation of peripheral vascular disease. *Am J Surg.* 1967;113(3):311–320.
56. Darling RC, Raines JK, Brener BJ, et al. Quantitative segmental pulse volume recorder: A clinical tool. *Surgery.* 1972;72(6):873–877.
57. Raines JK. Use of pulse volume recorder in peripheral arterial disease. In: Bernstein EF, ed. *Noninvasive Diagnostic Techniques in Vascular Disease.* St Louis: The CV Mosby Co.; 1985.
58. King LT, Strandness DE, Jr., Bell JW. The hemodynamic response of the lower extremities to exercise. *J Surg Res.* 1965;148:167–171.
59. Sumner DS, Strandness DE, Jr. The relationship between calf blood flow and ankle blood pressure in patients with intermittent claudication. *Surgery.* 1969;65(5):763–771.
60. Strandness DE, Jr., Zierler RE. Exercise ankle pressure measurements in arterial disease. In: Bernstein EF, ed. *Noninvasive Diagnostic Techniques in Vascular Disease.* St Louis: The CV Mosby Co.; 1985.
61. Hatsukami TS, Primozich JF, Zierler RE, et al. Color Doppler imaging of infrainguinal arterial occlusive disease. *J Vasc Surg.* 1992;16(4):527–531.
62. Jager KA, Ricketts HJ, Strandness DE, Jr. Duplex scanning for the evaluation of lower limb arterial disease. In: Bernstein EF, ed. *Noninvasive Diagnostic Techniques in Vascular Disease.* St. Louis: The CV Mosby Co.; 1985.
63. Moneta GL, Yeager RA, Antonovic R, et al. Accuracy of lower extremity arterial duplex mapping. *J Vasc Surg.* 1992;15(2):275–283.
64. Ligush J, Jr., Reavis SW, Preisser JS, et al. Duplex ultrasound scanning defines operative strategies for patients with limb-threatening ischemia. *J Vasc Surg.* 1998;28(3):482–490.
65. Kohler TR, Nance DR, Cramer MM, et al. Duplex scanning for diagnosis of aortoiliac and femoropopliteal disease: A prospective study. *Circulation.* 1987;76(5):1074–1080.
66. Whelan JF, Barry MH, Moir JD. Color flow Doppler ultrasonography: Comparison with peripheral arteriography for the investigation of peripheral vascular disease. *J Clin Ultrasound.* 1992;20(6):369–374.
67. Olin JW, Kaufman JA, Bluemke DA, et al. Atherosclerotic Vascular Disease Conference: Writing Group IV: Imaging. *Circulation.* 2004;109(21):2626–2633.
68. La Perna L, Olin JW, Goines D, et al. Ultrasound-guided thrombin injection for the treatment of postcatheterization pseudoaneurysms. *Circulation.* 2000;102(19):2391–2395.
69. Webber GW, Jang J, Gustavson S, et al. Contemporary management of postcatheterization pseudoaneurysms. *Circulation.* 2007;115(20):2666–2674.
70. Prince MR, Meaney JF. Expanding role of MR angiography in clinical practice. *Eur Radiol.* 2006;16(suppl 2):B3–B8.
71. Ersoy H, Zhang H, Prince MR. Peripheral MR angiography. *J Cardiovasc Magn Reson.* 2006;8(3):517–528.
72. Prince MR. Peripheral vascular MR angiography: The time has come. *Radiology.* 1998;206(3):592–593.
73. Prince MR, Narasimham DL, Stanley JC, et al. Breath-hold gadolinium-enhanced MR angiography of the abdominal aorta and its major branches. *Radiology.* 1995;197(3):785–792.
74. Grist TM. MRA of the abdominal aorta and lower extremities. *J Magn Reson Imaging.* 2000;11(1):32–43.
75. Rofsky NM, Johnson G, Adelman MA, et al. Peripheral vascular disease evaluated with reduced-dose gadolinium-enhanced MR angiography. *Radiology.* 1997;205(1):163–169.
76. Rofsky NM, Adelman MA. MR angiography in the evaluation of atherosclerotic peripheral vascular disease. *Radiology.* 2000;214(2):325–338.
77. Goyen M, Ruehm SG, Debatin JF. MR angiography for assessment of peripheral vascular disease. *Radiol Clin North Am.* 2002;40(4):835–846.
78. Ho VB, Corse WR. MR angiography of the abdominal aorta and peripheral vessels. *Radiol Clin North Am.* 2003;41(1):115–144.
79. Choudhury RP, Fuster V, Badimon JJ, et al. MRI and characterization of atherosclerotic plaque: Emerging applications and molecular imaging. *Arterioscler Thromb Vasc Biol.* 2002;22(7):1065–1074.
80. Helft G, Worthley SG, Fuster V, et al. Atherosclerotic aortic component quantification by noninvasive magnetic resonance imaging: An in vivo study in rabbits. *J Am Coll Cardiol.* 2001;38(5):1149–1154.
81. Shinnar M, Fallon JT, Wehrli S, et al. The diagnostic accuracy of ex vivo MRI for human atherosclerotic plaque characterization. *Arterioscler Thromb Vasc Biol.* 1999;19(11):2756–2761.
82. Rubin GD, Schmidt AJ, Logan LJ, et al. Multi-detector row CT angiography of lower extremity arterial inflow and runoff: Initial experience. *Radiology.* 2001;221(1):146–158.
83. Rubin GD, Shiau MC, Leung AN, et al. Aorta and iliac arteries: Single versus multiple detector-row helical CT angiography. *Radiology.* 2000;215(3):670–676.
84. Rubin GD. Techniques for performing multidetector-row computed tomographic angiography. *Tech Vasc Interv Radiol.* 2001;4(1):2–14.
85. Addis KA, Hopper KD, Iyriboz TA, et al. CT angiography: In vitro comparison of five reconstruction methods. *Am J Roentgenol.* 2001;177(5):1171–1176.
86. Katz DS, Hon M. CT angiography of the lower extremities and aortoiliac system with a multi-detector row helical CT scanner: Promise of new opportunities fulfilled. *Radiology.* 2001;221(1):7–10.
87. Lederman RJ, Mendelsohn FO, Anderson RD, et al. Therapeutic angiogenesis with recombinant fibroblast growth factor-2 for intermittent claudication (the TRAFFIC study): A randomised trial. *Lancet.* 2002;359(9323):2053–2058.
88. Rajagopalan S, Mohler ER, III, Lederman RJ, et al. Regional angiogenesis with vascular endothelial growth factor in peripheral arterial disease: A phase II randomized, double-blind, controlled study of adenoviral delivery of vascular endothelial growth factor 121 in patients with disabling intermittent claudication. *Circulation.* 2003;108(16):1933–1938.
89. Tateishi-Yuyama E, Matsubara H, Murohara T, et al. Therapeutic angiogenesis for patients with limb ischaemia by autologous transplantation of bone-marrow cells: A pilot study and a randomised controlled trial. *Lancet.* 2002;360(9331):427–435.
90. Kelly BD, Hackett SF, Hirota K, et al. Cell type-specific regulation of angiogenic growth factor gene expression and induction of angiogenesis in nonischemic tissue by a constitutively active form of hypoxia-inducible factor 1. *Circ Res.* 2003;93(11):1074–1081.
91. Lederman RJ, Guttman MA, Peters DC, et al. Catheter-based endomyocardial injection with real-time magnetic resonance imaging. *Circulation.* 2002;105(11):1282–1284.
92. Lederman RJ. Cardiovascular interventional magnetic resonance imaging. *Circulation.* 2005;112(19):3009–3017.

93. Willmann JK, Baumert B, Schertler T, et al. Aortoiliac and lower extremity arteries assessed with 16-detector row CT angiography: Prospective comparison with digital subtraction angiography. *Radiology*. 2005;236(3):1083–1093.

94. Edwards AJ, Wells IP, Roobottom CA. Multidetector row CT angiography of the lower limb arteries: A prospective comparison of volume-rendered techniques and intra-arterial digital subtraction angiography. *Clin Radiol*. 2005;60(1):85–95.

95. Romano M, Mainenti PP, Imbriaco M, et al. Multidetector row CT angiography of the abdominal aorta and lower extremities in patients with peripheral arterial occlusive disease: Diagnostic accuracy and interobserver agreement. *Eur J Radiol*. 2004;50(3):303–308.

96. Catalano C, Fraioli F, Laghi A, et al. Infrarenal aortic and lower-extremity arterial disease: Diagnostic performance of multi-detector row CT angiography. *Radiology*. 2004;231(2):555–563.

97. Ota H, Takase K, Igarashi K, et al. MDCT compared with digital subtraction angiography for assessment of lower extremity arterial occlusive disease: Importance of reviewing cross-sectional images. *Am J Roentgenol*. 2004;182(1):201–209.

98. Martin ML, Tay KH, Flak B, et al. Multidetector CT angiography of the aortoiliac system and lower extremities: A prospective comparison with digital subtraction angiography. *Am J Roentgenol*. 2003;180(4):1085–1091.

99. Ofer A, Nitecki SS, Linn S, et al. Multidetector CT angiography of peripheral vascular disease: A prospective comparison with intraarterial digital subtraction angiography. *Am J Roentgenol*. 2003;180(3):719–724.

100. Hiatt MD, Fleischmann D, Hellinger JC, et al. Angiographic imaging of the lower extremities with multidetector CT. *Radiol Clin North Am*. 2005;43(6):1119–1127.

101. Weitz JI, Byrne J, Clagett GP, et al. Diagnosis and treatment of chronic arterial insufficiency of the lower extremities: A critical review. *Circulation*. 1996;94(11):3026–3049.

Acute Neurological Deficits

20

Ennis J. Duffis
Majaz Moonis
Dennis A. Tighe

1. INTRODUCTION

Stroke and transient ischemic attack (TIA) represent neurological emergencies. The effective treatment and prognosis of these conditions rely heavily on prompt evaluation. In addition, management decisions are dependent on fully understanding the mechanism of stroke as secondary prevention strategies vary according to presumed etiology of stroke. Since most causes of stroke are related to disorders of the cardiovascular system, it is important for the cardiologist to become familiar with the diagnosis and treatment of these conditions. Several noninvasive methods are widely available to aid in the diagnosis of acute stroke and the evaluation of the causes of stroke. Here we review the incidence, classification, and diagnostic modalities for the evaluation of acute stroke and selected causes of ischemic stroke including stroke of cardio-embolic origin.

2. EPIDEMIOLOGY

Stroke is the third leading cause of death in the United States. Each year, ~700,000 strokes occur, of which 500,000 are new strokes and 200,000 are recurrent.[1] The vast majority of strokes are ischemic in origin with a minority attributable to intracerebral hemorrhage.[2] Cardio-embolic stroke accounts for ~15% to 20% of all ischemic strokes. TIA has been estimated to occur in 240,000 persons per year.[3] In developed countries, the most important risk factors for stroke and TIA remain hypertension, cigarette smoking, and hyperlipidemia.

TIA has been classically defined as a transient neurological deficit lasting less than 24 h. The neurological symptoms must be referable to vascular distribution within the brain, and thus caused by presumed relative ischemia of that area without infarction. The classical definition is in most cases inadequate as magnetic resonance imaging (MRI) evidence suggests that tissue ischemia leads to infarction in the vast majority of cases after only 60 min.[4] Consequently, a new tissue-based definition of TIA has been proposed that relies on the evidence of infarction. This definition is based on a reversible neurological deficit within 60 min and absence of demonstrable imaging abnormalities.[5]

3. CLASSIFICATION AND PATHOPHYSIOLOGY OF STROKE

Stroke can be classified into ischemic stroke and hemorrhagic stroke. Ischemic stroke denotes a condition in which the brain parenchyma receives an inadequate supply of blood typically as a result of arterial vascular occlusion. Hemorrhagic stroke refers to bleeding within the brain parenchyma. About 85% to 90% of all strokes are ischemic in origin.[5] Ischemic strokes can be further subdivided according to presumed etiology into thrombotic, cardio-embolic, undetermined, or small vessel. Some strokes may occur because of global hypoperfusion.

Thrombotic stroke is usually the result of a local disease process within the arterial wall. In most industrialized nations, hypertension, diabetes, cigarette smoking, and hyperlipidemia are the most common risk factors for the development of atherosclerosis. Atherosclerotic plaque in turn narrows the vessel lumen. This process leads to hypoperfusion of brain tissue supplied by the artery. With longstanding atherosclerosis, collateral circulation may develop from nearby arteries as a compensatory mechanism. Ischemic stroke typically develops through a thrombotic cascade beginning with local endothelial damage leading to plaque rupture with platelet and fibrin aggregation, which further narrows the blood vessel lumen causing occlusion. Other less common causes of thrombosis include arteritis, vascular dissection, and hypercoagulable states.

Embolic stroke refers to occlusion of vessels by material from a distant source. Embolism from nearby artery (artery to artery embolism) can occur as a result of thrombotic or atheromatous debris dislodging from a large artery downstream, such as seen in embolism from the internal carotid artery to the ophthalmic artery causing amaurosis fugax. The embolic material may also be of cardiac origin as seen in a variety of conditions including atrial fibrillation (AF), patent foramen ovale (PFO), and valvular vegetations.

Stroke due to hypoperfusion may first affect vulnerable areas of the brain such as those supplied by watershed from major arterial territories. The gray matter in the brain is exquisitely sensitive to ischemia. Compared to other vital organs, the brain does not tolerate a lack of perfusion well for more than a few minutes. Prolonged periods of cerebral hypoperfusion can cause generalized infarction in multiple vascular territories leading to generalized cytotoxic edema within the cerebrum.

3.1. Clinical presentation of ischemic stroke

The clinical presentation of stroke varies according to the arterial territory involved. Table 20.1 summarizes the common stroke syndromes by arterial territory. It may be difficult to determine the pathophysiology of stroke based on presentation alone. However, thrombotic stroke may be preceded by recurring or "stuttering" symptoms attributable to the same vascular distribution. As an example, recurrent transient aphasia can be seen with high grade stenotic lesions of the left middle cerebral artery (MCA) prior to the onset of full blown left MCA syndrome, including right

269

TABLE 20.1
SELECTED STROKE SYNDROMES BY VASCULAR DISTRIBUTION

Vascular distribution	Signs and symptoms (variable according to the extent of territory involved)
Middle cerebral artery (MCA)	Contralateral hemiparesis and sensory impairment, homonymous hemianopia, aphasia (dominant hemisphere), contralateral neglect (nondominant hemisphere)
Anterior cerebral artery	Weakness and sensory impairment of contralateral lower extremity, urinary incontinence
Posterior cerebral artery	Contralateral sensory loss (thalamic involvement), occulomotor nerve palsy and contralateral hemiplegia (midbrain involvement, Weber syndrome), contralateral homonymous hemianopia with central sparing (involvement of occipital cortex)
Vertebral artery/ Posterior inferior cerebellar artery (PICA)	Ipsilateral deviation of tongue with contralateral hemiparesis and sensory impairment (medial medullary syndrome) vertigo, nausea, vomiting, ipsilateral Horner syndrome and contralateral loss of pain and temperature sensation (lateral medullary syndrome, Vertebral or PICA)
Basilar artery	Somnolence or coma (as part of "top of the basilar syndrome"), bilateral quadriplegia, and mutism (locked in syndrome)

TABLE 20.2
WELL-DEFINED CLINICAL AND RADIOLOGIC LACUNAR SYNDROMES

Lacunar syndrome	Signs and symptoms	Localization
Clumsy-hand dysarthria	Dysarthria, dysphagia; facial weakness and ipsilateral weakness, primarily affecting distal upper extremity (hand)	Basal pons or corona radiata
Pure motor hemiparesis	Weakness of entire hemibody (face, arm, and leg)	Contralateral internal capsule
Pure sensory stroke	Numbness of entire hemibody	Contralateral thalamus or corona radiata
Pure sensory motor stroke	Weakness and numbness of entire hemibody	Contralateral thalamo-capsular region
Ataxic hemiparesis	Weakness and ataxia (i.e., out of proportion to the degree of weakness) of hemibody	Basal pons or internal capsule

hemiplegia, aphasia, and left gaze deviation. In contrast, embolic strokes are typically maximal at onset and a patient may have no symptoms prior to the development of a stroke syndrome.

Lacunar syndromes represent a distinct group of stroke syndromes that have been often well defined with respect to localization. They are caused by occlusions of small penetrating arteries. The classical lacunar syndromes include pure motor, pure sensory, ataxic-hemiparesis, and clumsy-hand dysarthria. The localization and clinical presentation of these syndromes are summarized in Table 20.2.

The presentation of hemorrhagic stroke may be similar to that of ischemic stroke. In fact, it is often difficult to distinguish hemorrhagic from ischemic strokes based solely on clinical grounds. Neurological findings as in ischemic stroke are also determined by the location of the hemorrhage. Often, noncontrast head computed tomography (NCCT) scanning is necessary to distinguish between the two.

3.2. Cardiogenic embolism

Among patients with acute ischemic strokes, ~15% to 20% suffer events that may be classified as definitely originating from a cardiac source.[6] In another 30% of patients, while the cause of ischemic strokes may not be known firmly, so-called cryptogenic strokes, certain characteristic may suggest a cardio-embolic mechanism. Intracardiac thrombus is the most common source of embolic material; however, tumor fragments, vegetations, air, fat, and atherosclerotic debris may also travel to the cerebral circulation causing acute ischemia and neurological deficits. With the existence of a number of possible "cardiac sources" for acute cerebral ischemia, consideration of the radiological pattern of the stroke (multiple vascular territories involved or involvement of a single large vessel with normal or near normal arterial imaging), the patient's age, the commonality of conditions in the general population, and the medical history of the patient may allow for a more focused differential diagnosis and imaging evaluation. Some patients, especially the elderly, may exhibit evidence for multiple potential cardio-embolic lesions. Potential cardio-embolic sources can be classified (Table 20.3) based on their potential for embolism,[7] on the prevalence of these lesions in the general population, or on their potential embolic mechanism.[8] The following discussion will focus on the first classification scheme.

3.2.1. Conditions associated with high embolic potential

Atrial fibrillation. AF is a common disorder estimated to affect ~2.3 million people in the Untied States.[9] The prevalence is higher among men and doubles with each decade of life. While being uncommon prior to age 60, almost 9% of individuals aged 80 to 89 years have AF.[9] The most common risk factors for development of AF include systemic hypertension (most important), diabetes mellitus, and obesity.[9] Patients with heart failure (HF), coronary heart disease, and valvular heart disease are also at increased risk for development of AF. Whether permanent or paroxysmal, AF is a potent risk factor for embolic stroke; about 45% of all embolic strokes can be attributed to AF and the estimated hazard ratio of nonvalvular AF is 4 to 5 (up to 15 for those with mitral stenosis) compared to those in sinus rhythm.[9,10] The increased risk of stroke is largely attributable to

TABLE 20.3

RISK POTENTIAL FOR LESIONS ASSOCIATED WITH CARDIOEMBOLISM

Major risk established	Minor or uncertain risk

Atrial Dysrhythmias
  Atrial fibrillation (AF)
  Atrial flutter
	Complex aortic atheromata

Left ventricular thrombus
  Recent myocardial infarction
  Dilated cardiomyopathy
  LV aneurysm
	Interatrial septal abnormalities
	  Patent foramen ovale (PFO)
	  Atrial septal aneurysm (ASA)

Valvular vegetations
  Infective
  Noninfective
	Spontaneous echocardiographic contrast (SEC)

Prosthetic heart valves
  Mechanical
  Biological
	Native heart valve disorders
	  Mitral valve prolapse
	  Mitral annular calcification
	  Valvular excrescences
	  Calcific aortic stenosis

Cardiac tumors
  Atrial myxoma
  Papillary fibroelastoma	

Mitral stenosis	

exceed 10% when multiple risk factors are present.[12,19,20] For low-risk patients, aspirin appears to be sufficient to reduce stroke risk.[10,20,21] When the estimated risk for thromboembolism is higher, antiplatelet therapy is insufficient to prevent stroke and therapy with warfarin is documented to significantly reduce the risk of thromboembolism.[10,20,21] Although left atrial thrombosis can occur among patients with sinus rhythm, the incidence is very low [0.1% of transesophageal echocardiography (TEE) examinations] unless coexisting cardiac pathology such as mitral valve (MV) disease (especially mitral stenosis), SEC material, or severe left ventricular (LV) dysfunction is present.[22,23]

Atrial flutter. Atrial flutter is a relatively common arrhythmia that accounts for about 10% of all supraventricular tachycardias. The risk of thromboembolism for this arrhythmia is not as clearly established as that for AF.[10,24] Early studies suggested that the risk for thromboembolism was low. More recently, several retrospective studies have shown a rather substantial thromboembolic risk (about 1.6% per year) to be associated with the presence of chronic atrial flutter.[24,25] Based on this more recent data, it is recommended that a strategy of risk stratification similar to that used for AF be employed to guide antithrombotic therapy for these patients.[10,21]

Left ventricular thrombus. Formation of thrombus within the LV cavity occurs most often in the settings of myocardial infarction and dilated cardiomyopathy. Approximately 2% of patients with acute myocardial infarctions will suffer a stroke within the first 30 days and half of these events will occur within the first 5 days.[26,27] For those with large, primarily anterior myocardial infarctions that involve the apex (Fig. 20.3), the risk for formation of LV thrombus is much higher; the estimated incidence is 12% versus 2% for infarctions involving other sites.[28] A Class I recommendation for use of echocardiography is given for assessment of possible mural thrombus in this situation.[29] The risk for embolism is highest in the first 2 weeks after infarction and when the thrombus protrudes into the LV cavity or is mobile.[26,30,31] In contrast, systemic embolization is believed to occur infrequently when the infarction is >4 months old. In the presence of chronic myocardial infarction with formation of an LV aneurysm, thrombus, often layered and nonmobile, may be present in up to 50% of patients.[26] Observational data[32,33] suggest that the incidence of thromboembolism in this situation is low unless a protruding and/or mobile thrombus is observed.

Among patients with HF and low LV ejection fractions (LVEF), the reported incidence of stroke ranges from 1.3% to 3.5% per year.[27,34] The risk of thromboembolism increases with increasing

stasis of blood and thrombus formation within the left atrium (LA) with subsequent distal embolization.[11] Approximately 90% of the thrombi forming in the LA can be localized to the left atrial appendage (LAA) (Fig. 20.1 and **Movie 20.1**). Left atrial thrombi are found in 20% to 40% of patients with recent thromboembolism.[11] Risk factors for ischemic stroke due to systemic embolization in AF include prior stroke or TIA, a history of hypertension, diabetes mellitus, HF, and advancing age.[12] The presence of spontaneous echocardiographic contrast (SEC) (Fig. 20.2 and **Movie 20.2**) and low LAA filling velocities has also been associated with increased risk of thrombus formation and systemic embolization.[13–16] It should be noted that only about two-thirds of strokes in patients with AF can be directly attributed to embolism of left atrial thrombus, other mechanisms may be operative in the remaining one-third.[11,17,18] With "lone" AF, the annual risk for thromboembolism is low, being <1% per year. This annual risk (Tables 20.4 and 20.5) may

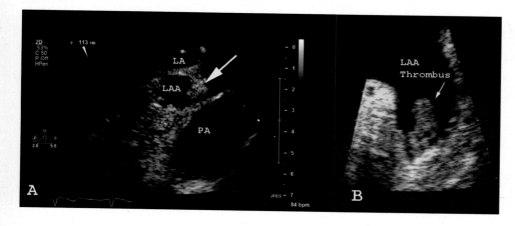

Figure 20.1 Examples of LAA thrombi as seen on transesophageal echocardiography (TEE). In both panels, the LAA mass *(arrow)* protrudes into the cavity and exhibits an echotexture distinct from the surrounding tissue. In real time, the characteristics of the mass shown in (**A**) are better appreciated (**Movie 20.1**). Care must be taken to distinguish LAA thrombus from pectinate muscles, normal thin protruding structures found in the vast majority of patients. LA, left atrium; PA, pulmonary artery.

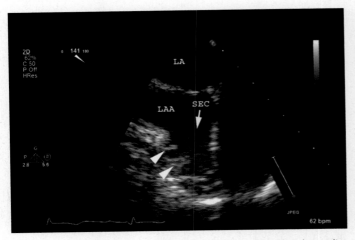

 Figure 20.2 This magnified transesophageal echocardiogram image demonstrates increased echodensity within the LAA consistent with the presence of spontaneous echocardiographic contrast (SEC) material. In real time (**Movie 20.2**), a characteristic swirling appearance is noted. Pectinate muscles are also noted (*arrow heads*). LA, left atrium.

TABLE 20.5
THROMBOEMBOLIC EVENT RATES IN ATRIAL FIBRILLATION BY BASELINE CHADS2 SCORE AND ANTICOAGULATION THERAPY STATUS

CHADS2 score	Warfarin-treated	No warfarin
0	0.25 (0.11–0.55)	0.49 (0.30–0.78)
1	0.72 (0.50–1.03)	1.52 (1.19–1.94)
2	1.27 (0.94–1.72)	2.50 (1.98–3.15)
3	2.20 (1.61–3.01)	5.27 (4.15–6.70)
4	2.35 (1.44–3.83)	6.02 (3.90–9.29)
5 or 6	4.60 (2.72–7.76)	6.88 (3.42–13.84)

Note: Event rates per 100-person years (95% confidence interval). *Source*: Adapted from Go AS, Hylek EM, Chang Y et al. Anticoagulation therapy for stroke prevention in atrial fibrillation. How well do randomized trials translate into clinical practice? *JAMA*. 2003;290:2685–2692.

TABLE 20.4
CHADS2 SCORE: CLINICAL PARAMETERS AND POINT VALUES

Clinical parameter	Points assigned
CHF (recent)	1
Hypertension	1
Age ≥75 years	1
Diabetes mellitus	1
Stroke or transient ischemic attack (TIA) (history of)	2

The total score is determined by summing the point values assigned to the clinical parameters present. A score of 0 to 6 is possible.

New York Heart Association (NYHA) classification, lower LVEF,[35] and concomitant occurrence of other risk factors for thromboembolism, such as AF or the presence of prosthetic heart valves. The risk of thromboembolism does not appear to depend upon the etiology of HF; those with ischemic and nonischemic cardiomyopathies appear to suffer embolic events at similar rates. A recent report[34] showed that the absolute risk of stroke among patients with NYHA

Class II or III HF and LVEF ≤35% in sinus rhythm appears to be about 1% per year; the risk appears to increase as the LVEF declines. At present, randomized trials among HF patients with low LVEF are lacking to appropriately guide primary preventive therapy. Anticoagulation is recommended for patients with AF or a prior embolic event.[36] While echocardiography remains the primary modality to visualize intracavitary thrombus, recent data suggest that cardiac magnetic resonance (CMR)[37] may be a more sensitive and specific technique for identification of LV mural thrombus.

Valvular vegetations. Endocarditis, infectious or sterile, involving the left-sided heart valves often exhibits a great potential for systemic embolization. The lesion of endocarditis, the vegetation composed of platelets and fibrin, may be quite friable and prone to embolization of fragments (Fig. 20.4 and **Movie 20.3**). Among patients with active infective endocarditis (IE), systemic embolization is estimated to occur in 22% to 50% of cases.[38,39] The central nervous system is involved in about 65% of the embolic events and more than 90% of those emboli are recognized to travel to the distribution of the MCA.[38] The embolic risk of infective material is recognized to be greater with vegetations involving the MV compared to the aortic valve (incidence 25% vs. 10%, respectively), with size or length of the vegetations exceeding 10 mm, and with enhanced vegetation mobility.[38,40,41] A greater propensity for systemic embolization is also recognized in the presence of certain pathogens such as fungi, *Staphylococcus aureus*, *Streptococcus bovis*, HACEK microorganisms, and Abiotrophia

Figure 20.3 A layered echodensity at the left ventricular (LV) apex consistent with thrombus is shown (**A**). With injection of a transpulmonary echo contrast agent (**B**), no penetration of the contrast material to the LV apex is observed. LA, left atrium; RA, right atrium; RV, right ventricle.

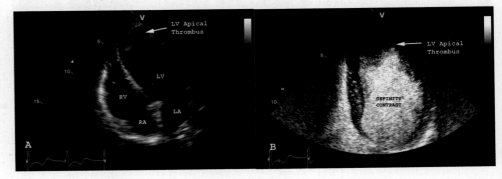

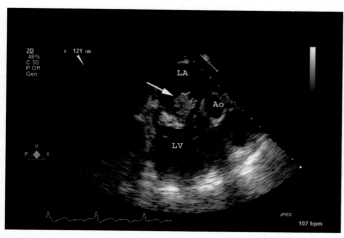

Figure 20.4 A transesophageal echocardiographic view in a vertical plane shows an inhomogeneous echodenisty *(arrow)* diffusely involving the mitral leaflet and prolapsing into the LA. In this patient with *S. aureus* bacteremia, such a finding is highly consistent with an infectious etiology for the vegetation. In real time **(Movie 20.3)**, the vegetation is demonstrated to be highly mobile with friable elements.

organisms.[38,39] The risk of embolization is greatest in the period prior to initiation of appropriate antimicrobial therapy and shortly after initiation of therapy.[42] This risk drops significantly when appropriate therapy has been delivered for at least 2 weeks.[38,42]

Aseptic vegetations (also known as nonbacterial thrombotic endocarditis), due to focal injury to the valvular endothelium and also composed of platelets and fibrin, may be observed in 19% to 63% of patients with disease processes characterized by hypercoagulability such as with various malignancies and certain autoimmune disorders.[43] While the true incidence and embolic potential of these lesions are difficult to estimate as other risk factors for stroke may be present, recent reports testify to the commonality of this condition among patients with predisposing conditions and their apparent high embolic potential.[43–45]

Prosthetic heart valves. Artificial heart valves are associated with a significant potential for systemic embolization.[46–49] The majority of these events involves the cerebral circulation. Prevalence estimates range from 1% to 4% per year depending upon anticoagulation status.[46–49] Even with adequate levels of anticoagulation, the risk of embolization among patients with mechanical prostheses approaches 1% to 2% per year.[46,48,49] While the long-term risk of embolization from biological valves is less, averaging about 0.7% per year for patients in sinus rhythm, an increased risk is observed in the first 3 months following implantation.[50] Factors associated with increased

risk for embolization include inadequate anticoagulation status, mitral location, type of prosthesis (caged-ball vs. tilting disk), presence of multiple valve prostheses, prior systemic embolization, reduced LVEF, age over 70 years, and AF.[46,48,49]

Primary cardiac tumors. Primary cardiac tumors are rare, being found in about 0.02% of autopsies. The most common primary tumors involving the left heart are atrial myxomas and papillary fibroelastomas. Atrial myxomas are considered to have high embolic potential[51] while the embolic potential of papillary fibroelastomas appears to be moderate. The mechanisms underlying cerebral embolism can include detachment of tumor fragments or dislodgement of superimposed thrombus. Atrial myxoma, often a benign tumor of endocardial origin, is the most common primary cardiac tumor (Chapters 10 and 51). While any endocardial surface can be involved, about 75% of these tumors arise from a stalk within the LA in the region of the fossa ovalis.[51] Macroscopically, myxomas may appear polyploid, pedunculated, or rounded and can possess a smooth or lobulated surface. Many are discovered incidentally by echocardiography performed for other indications, but systemic embolism, often to the retinal or cerebral circulation, can occur in up to 30% to 40% of cases.[51] Atrial myxoma is estimated to account for about 1% of strokes in young patients.[26] In rare instances, bacteria may infect a myxoma leading to vegetation formation and systemic embolization. The recommended treatment of choice is surgical excision.

Papillary fibroelastomas (Fig. 20.5 and **Movie 20.4**), benign avascular papillomas derived from the endocardium, are the second most commonly encountered primary cardiac tumor.[52] These tumors, which account for 75% of all tumors involving the cardiac valves, are more commonly found to affect the left-sided valves, with aortic valve involvement being more frequent than mitral involvement.[52,53] The size of these tumors can vary significantly; however, most have a diameter <10 mm.[52,53] Grossly, fibroelastomas exhibit multiple papillary fronds and attach to the endocardium, sometimes via a stalk.[52,53] On echocardiography, these tumors may exhibit mobility and present a fronded appearance. They rarely interfere with valve function.[53] Similar to the myxomas, fibroelastomas may be discovered incidentally; however, a common clinical presentation is cerebral ischemia due to presumed embolism.[52] Predictors of clinical events include tumor mobility, size >10 mm, and location on the aortic valve.[52] While treatment of incidentally found fibroelastomas remains controversial, surgical excision is recommended if an embolic event has occurred or when high-risk characteristics are identified.

3.2.2. Lesions associated with lesser or uncertain embolic potential

Complex aortic atherosclerosis. Autopsy data[54] have shown that ulcerated atherosclerotic plaques in the aortic arch are more

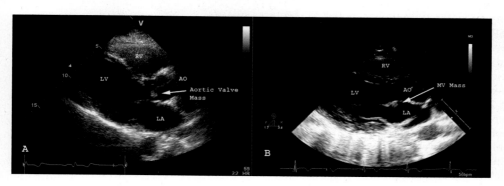

Figure 20.5 Two examples of mass lesions involving the cardiac valves *(arrows)* are shown. The mass lesions are rounded and move synchronously with the excursions of the valve leaflets **(Movie 20.4)**. In each case, the mass does not interfere with valve function. The appearances and locations of these valvular masses are typical of papillary fibroelastomas. AO, aorta; LA, left atrium; LV, left ventricle; MV, mitral valve; RV, right ventricle.

Figure 20.6 Examples showing complex aortic atheromatous disease. In (**A**), a protruding, and in real time (**Movie 20.5**), highly mobile plaque is observed in the aortic arch. In (**B**), a protruding, ulcerated plaque with mobile elements (**Movie 20.6**) is demonstrated.

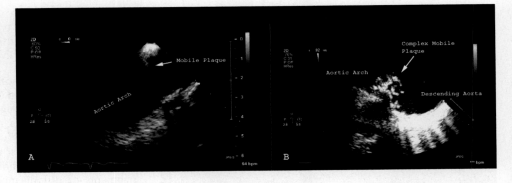

commonly present among patients with ischemic strokes than among those with other neurological conditions. With the advent of routine TEE in the 1980s, several investigators further established a link between the presence of atherosclerosis involving the ascending aorta (AO) and aortic arch and ischemic neurological events.[55–57] The prevalence of severe aortic plaque among stroke patients is estimated to be 14% to 21%, a range similar in magnitude to that of AF and carotid artery disease.[58] Several studies have identified specific characteristics of atherosclerotic plaques, such as thickness ≥4 mm, presence of ulcerations, mobile protruding elements, and lack of calcifications as being associated with higher risk of recurrent brain infarctions.[55–59] The presence of these "complex" or "severe" plaques (Fig. 20.6 and **Movies 20.5 and 20.6**) may impart a risk of brain embolism as high as 10% to 12% per year.[58] The presence of aortic atherosclerosis has also been reported to be a significant independent predictor of stroke among patients with AF.[18]

Emboli originating from these plaques may be of three distinct types: cholesterol emboli, atheromatous emboli, and emboli due to mural thrombus. Aortic manipulation at the time of surgery or during percutaneous catheter-based procedures has also been associated with brain infarctions presumed due to atheroembolic events.[60] Off-pump surgery and a brachial approach may reduce embolic events in these situations. However, as most patients with cerebral embolizations have not undergone a prior procedure that can be linked to the event, and since most patients have multiple lesions as well as other potential causes of stroke, interest has focused on medical therapies designed to reduce the risk of recurrent events. At present, no randomized controlled trial is available to guide therapeutic decision making. Observational data suggest that administration of HMG-CoA reductase inhibitors reduces the risk of recurrent events, while no such data are available to support the use of warfarin or antiplatelet agents for this indication.[61]

The studies described previously included symptomatic patients referred for diagnostic evaluations. Recent data have called into question the role of aortic atherosclerosis as an independent risk factor for cerebral embolism. Data from the Stroke Prevention: Assessment of Risk in a Community (SPARC) trial,[62] a prospective population-based TEE study, showed that while the prevalence of aortic atherosclerosis increased with age, it most commonly involved the descending thoracic AO; the prevalence of complex aortic atherosclerosis in the proximal portions of the AO was low (0.2% in the ascending AO and 2.2% in the aortic arch). A follow-up publication from this group showed that after controlling for comorbidities, the presence of complex aortic plaques did not predict the occurrence of cerebrovascular events.[63] In a more recently published case-control study, Petty et al.[64] found similar results; aortic atherosclerotic debris was not associated with cerebrovascular ischemic events but appeared to be a marker of more generalized atherosclerosis. Based on these findings, it appears that complex aortic atherosclerosis, while capable of causing cerebral embolization in selected patients,[58] may not be as prevalent a source of stroke as reported previously.

Abnormalities of the atrial septum: Patent foramen ovale and atrial septal aneurysm. A PFO is an obligate component of the fetal circulation that closes spontaneously after birth in the majority of subjects. In ~25% to 30% of the general population, this tunnellike connection between the septum primum and septum secundum does not fuse, leading to a potentially open channel for passage of material from the venous to the arterial circulation when the pressures in the right atrium (RA) exceed those in the LA.[62,65] With aging, the percentage of patients with a PFO declines; however, the size of a PFO tends to be greater.[65] The prevalence of PFO among patients with cryptogenic stroke is higher than that found in the general population.[66] The primary mechanism for cerebral events is believed to be paradoxical embolization of material (thrombus greater than air or fat) via the PFO from right to left. In support of this mechanism, thrombus transiting a PFO can be documented (Fig. 20.7). However, in clinical practice, this finding is rare. While increased incidences of proximal and pelvic vein thromboses are reported among patients with PFO and cryptogenic stroke,[67,68] such pathology is often not found clinically.[69] In addition, most patients with cerebral events do not report having performed activities or maneuvers that would

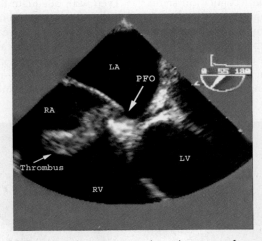

Figure 20.7 A thrombus transiting through a patent foramen ovale (PFO) is demonstrated. This patient suffered both pulmonary and arterial embolisms. LA, left atrium; LV, left ventricle; RA, right atrium; RV, right ventricle.

tend to increase right atrial pressure transiently just prior to the occurrence of acute cerebral events. Other mechanisms postulated for cerebral events in the setting of a PFO include the local formation of thrombus within the PFO tunnel due to stagnant blood flow and possibly a susceptibility to atrial arrhythmia with formation of atrial thrombus.[70] Though these mechanisms seem plausible, imaging studies of patients with PFOs and stroke rarely identify such pathology. Nonetheless, a strong association has been reported between the presence of PFO and cryptogenic strokes, primarily among individuals ≤55 years old.[66,70,71] Contrary to previously held beliefs, recent data suggest that paradoxical embolization via a PFO may also be an important cause of cerebral ischemia among older patients.[72] Given the prevalence of PFO in the general population and that about 30% of all ischemic strokes are cryptogenic in nature, it has been estimated that ~70,000 cerebral events per annum in the United States may be attributable to paradoxical embolizations via a PFO.[73] Factors purported to increase the risk for paradoxical embolization (Fig. 20.8 and Movies 20.7 and 20.8) include size of the PFO (separation ≥ 4 mm), the extent to which microbubbles appear in the LA, the presence of an atrial septal aneurysm (ASA), septal hypermobility, the presence of a prominent Eustachian valve or a Chiari complex, and right-to-left shunting at rest. However, the data regarding the importance of these risk factors are somewhat clouded. The frequency of ASA is documented to be greater among those with cerebral ischemic events than among control subjects (7.9% vs. 2.2%, respectively; OR 3.65).[74] In addition, among patients with a prior ischemic stroke treated with aspirin,[75] recurrent events were much more common among the subgroup with PFO and ASA as compared to PFO or ASA in isolation (15.2% vs. ≤4.0%, respectively; p = 0.04) at 4 years. In this same study, however, the degree of inducible right-to-left shunting, as measured by the number of microbubbles appearing in the LA, was not found to be a significant predictor of recurrent events. Results from the Patent Foramen Ovale in Cryptogenic Stroke Study (PICSS)[76] further showed that recurrent stroke was not more common with larger size PFOs, defined as a separation ≥2 mm or ≥10 microbubbles appearing in the LA. In contrast to the results of the study of Mas et al.,[75] the presence of an ASA in PICSS did not confer an increased risk of recurrent stroke in this older population treated with aspirin or warfarin. Among patients with a PFO and prior stroke or TIA, the risk of recurrent cerebral ischemia is reported to be 3% to 16% per year.[73] Medical therapy with antiplatelet agents or warfarin and interventional therapies, such as surgical or percutaneous PFO closures, has been shown to reduce the risk of recurrent events.[70,77] In the absence of randomized controlled clinical trials, however, the optimal therapeutic strategy remains unknown.

All the data described previously on the risk of cerebral events associated with PFO and ASA were obtained in populations presenting after clinical events for diagnostic evaluations. Little was known previously about the risk associated with these conditions in the general population. Several recent population-based studies[78–80] have raised doubts about the independent role of PFO and ASA as risk factors for ischemic strokes. These studies uniformly concluded that no association could be established between the presence of a PFO and subsequent risk of ischemic stroke. Due to its relatively low prevalence in the general population, the role of ASA in ischemic stroke could not be supported or refuted by these studies; this cohort will require further investigation.

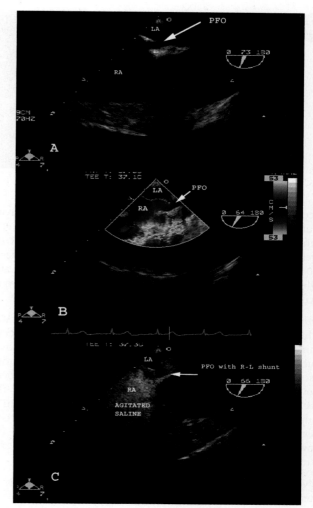

 Figure 20.8 Transesophageal echocardiographic views demonstrating a patent foramen ovale (PFO). In (**A**) (**Movie 20.7**), a tunnellike separation between the septum primum and septum secundum (arrow) is demonstrated. In (**B**), a still frame using color-flow Doppler demonstrates the dynamic nature of the separation of this tunnellike defect; in this case, a separation of up to 5 mm is shown. With injection of agitated saline and opacification of the right atrium (RA) (**C**), a large right-to-left shunt across the PFO is demonstrated (**Movie 20.8**). LA, left atrium.

Spontaneous echocardiographic contrast. SEC, also known as "smoke," is commonly observed in the LA or LAA among patients with AF, in the presence of low LAA flow velocities, when MV disease is present, and with LV dysfunction; conditions all known to cause stasis of blood flow.[81] Characterized by its swirling appearance on TEE, SEC is considered a prothrombotic condition.[81] In particular, the presence of "dense" SEC has been associated with an increased prevalence of left atrial thrombus[13] and a high risk of cerebral thromboembolism among patients with nonvalvular AF.[14–16] Since SEC occurs primarily in association with other conditions causing stasis of blood flow, it may simply represent a marker of increased thromboembolic risk rather than an independent risk factor for stroke.

Conditions affecting the heart valves. Mitral valve prolapse Early studies indicated that mitral valve prolapse (MVP) was a putative risk factor for stroke in young patients (<45 years old).[82]

Figure 20.9 Zoom-magnified apical four-chamber transthoracic views (**A, B**) with posterior tilt demonstrating extensive MAC ("toothpaste" tumor). A mobile echodensity (arrows) involving the left ventricular (LV) aspect of the annular calcification is shown (**Movie 20.9**). This elderly patient suffered several embolic strokes. LA, left atrium; RA, right atrium.

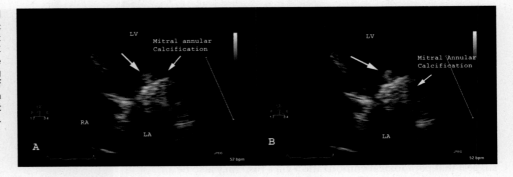

Recent case-control[83] and population-based[84] studies have refuted this association by demonstrating that young patients with uncomplicated MVP do not exhibit an increased risk for cerebral ischemic events. However, among a subgroup of patients >50 years old or with thickened mitral leaflets, Avierinos and colleagues[84] found that an excess of ischemic neurological events occurred.

Mitral annular calcification   Mitral annular calcification (MAC), a chronic degenerative process characterized by deposition of calcium and lipid in the fibrous support of the MV, is commonly found with aging and has been associated with atherosclerotic vascular disease. In population-based studies, MAC has been shown to be a strong, independent risk factor for stroke.[85,86] The mechanism of stroke in MAC most likely relates to its association with risk factors for vascular disease and the presence of complex aortic atheromata;[87,88] however, in some cases (Fig. 20.9 and **Movie 20.9**), it may serve as a direct source of thrombotic, calcific, or infectious embolic material.[89,90]

Valve excrescences   Excrescences, thin filamentous structures often attached at the valve closure lines, are common findings at autopsy or during TEE performed in unselected subjects.[62] With increased use of TEE to examine patients with suspected cardiac sources of embolism, valve excrescences were found to be present in excess compared to controls.[91] The presumed mechanisms for embolic events include embolization of strand fragments or superimposed thrombi. However, among the patients examined in these early studies, alternative cardiac sources of embolism were frequently identified. Recent longitudinal studies[92,93] have shown valve excrescences to be commonly present on the left-sided heart valves (prevalence 38% to 47%) of normal subjects. In addition, they were not more prevalent among those suffering cardioembolism and, when medical therapy was used, were not associated with an increased risk of recurrent cerebral embolic events or death. Given the strength of this data, an independent association between valve excrescences and cardioembolism seems unlikely.

3.2.3. Other conditions

Several conditions can mimic stroke or TIA and should be considered when evaluating patients with acute neurological deficits including those with focal deficits. Typically, routine laboratory testing and a thorough history can serve to differentiate stroke from other conditions. Hypoglycemia and other metabolic derangements should always be considered, particularly in patients presenting with change in mental status. Focal seizure may present with rhythmic contraction of one limb or hemibody followed by paralysis, so-called Todd palsy. Complex migraine may likewise present with focal deficits including hemiplegia.

More commonly, visual scotomata associated with migraine may be confused with amaurosis fugax. A history of migraine or headache at presentation can be easily obtained from the history and can serve to differentiate the two. However, caution should be taken as migraine may produce stroke in some patients. Other conditions to consider in the differential include arterial dissection, syncope or presyncope, brain tumor, dural sinus thrombosis, head trauma, multiple sclerosis or other demyelinating disorders, peripheral vertigo, systemic infection, and functional deficits (conversion reactions).

4. DIAGNOSTIC EVALUATION

4.1. Neuroimaging in acute stroke

After careful history and physical exam, the first step in evaluation of acute stroke is the exclusion of hemorrhagic infarction. The presence of intracerebral hemorrhage is an absolute contraindication to treatment with thrombolytic agents and is therefore important to recognize. The imaging modality of choice to exclude hemorrhage is noncontrast CT. Acute blood should appear as an area of increased density relative to the normal brain parenchyma (Flow diagram, **Figs. 20.10 and 20.11**). Density on CT scanning is typically reported in Hounsfield units (HU). Blood typically corresponds to 50 to 80 HU. MRI has also been shown to have a good sensitivity for identification of acute hemorrhage; however, its utility in the acute setting is limited by the fact that compared to CT, it is a relatively time consuming modality.

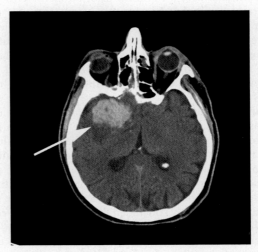

Figure 20.10 Noncontrast head computed tomography (NCCT) showing hyperdensity (arrow) in the area of the right temporal lobe corresponding to the presence of intracerebral hemorrhage.

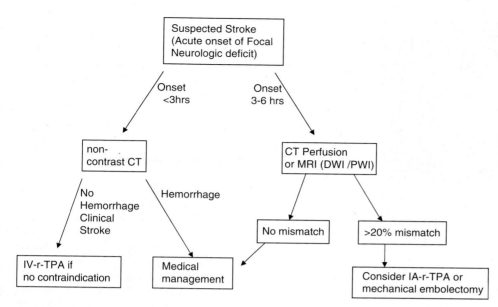

Figure 20.11 Flow diagram: Early evaluation of suspected stroke. DWI, diffusion weighted imaging; PWI, perfusion weighted imaging.

Once hemorrhage has been excluded and the diagnosis of ischemic stroke is confirmed clinically within 3 h of stroke onset, treatment with intravenous (IV) recombinant tissue plasminogen activator (r-TPA) should be initiated unless a contraindication exists. It should be recognized that patients with large clot burdens (internal carotid artery, proximal MCA stem, and basilar artery occlusions) may not do well with IV thrombolysis. Imaging modalities available may be helpful in deciding whether patients should receive IV or intra-arterial (IA) interventions.

4.1.1. Computed tomography (CT) and CT perfusion

Relative to MRI, CT scanning is far less sensitive for identification of infarction in the acute phase of stroke. In fact, CT may be entirely normal in appearance within the first 24 h of onset of stroke. If present, the early CT findings of stroke may include obscuration of the lentiform nucleus, hyperdense MCA sign (representing blood clot within the vessel lumen), as well as loss of gray–white distinction within the insular cortex. The radiographic evolution of infarction proceeds with the appearance of a more clearly defined area of hypodensity (typically within 24 h), which corresponds to the area of infarction (Fig. 20.12). The main advantage of CT scanning over other modalities is that it allows for a rather timely evaluation and is available at most hospitals. The addition of CT angiography (CTA) allows for rapid visualization of the cervical and intracranial vasculature. This added information may help in some situations to guide therapy as more proximal vascular occlusion may not respond favorably to IV thrombolysis.[94] In this situation, other therapies such as administration of IA thrombolytic agents may be necessary. Finally, CT is the imaging modality of choice to exclude hemorrhage.

The relatively new technique of CT perfusion can be employed in the early phase of stroke to improve the detection of areas of infarction (core) as well as tissue around it which is ischemic but not yet infarcted, the so-called penumbra. The technique utilizes the acquisition of sequential images through a selected location (e.g., just above the orbits) during a timed IV contrast bolus. The parameters of cerebral blood flow (CBF), cerebral blood volume (CBV), and mean transit time (MTT) of the bolus can then be calculated. Different combinations of these parameters have been used to identify the infarct core and the ischemic penumbra. Data

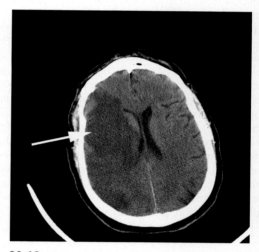

Figure 20.12 Noncontrast head computed tomographic scan obtained at 48 h after symptom onset showing evolution of right middle cerebral artery (MCA) territory infarct corresponding to the area of hypodensity (arrow). There is evidence of surrounding edema and mild right-to-left shift of midline structures.

obtained from CT perfusion should be viewed with caution as currently no uniform agreement exists as to what parameters most accurately predict final infarct or penumbra size.

4.1.2. Magnetic resonance imaging and MR perfusion

MRI is extremely sensitive in identifying infarction even in the very early stages of evolving ischemic stroke. The addition of diffusion weighted imaging (DWI) sequences can further increase the sensitivity of MRI, making it possible to identify ischemic changes as early as 30 min from symptom onset. This technique relies on the detection of restricted diffusion of water molecules between two radiofrequency pulses. The resulting images obtained display areas of restricted diffusion as increased intensity (brightness), which correspond to areas of infarction. Both acute (hours) and subacute (days) infarction may appear bright on DWI sequences as there is component of T2 "built into" DWI. Differentiating between the two is easily accomplished with the use of apparent diffusion coef-

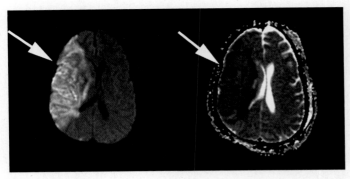

Figure 20.13 On DWI, left panel, hyperintensity in the distribution of the right middle cerebral artery (MCA) *(arrow)* is shown. ADC, right panel, shows corresponding hypointensity *(arrow)*, which signifies an acute stroke.

ficient (ADC) map. Areas of acute infarction should appear hyperintense (bright) on DWI and hypointense (dark) on ADC map (Fig. 20.13). Subacute infarction should appear hyperintense on both sequences. The phenomenon of restricted diffusion typically lasts anywhere from 10 to 14 days; therefore, chronic (months to years) infarctions should not appear bright on DWI.

The technique of MR perfusion, much like CT perfusion, allows for identification of infarct core and penumbra. The most widely used technique, dynamic susceptibility contrast, involves the administration of an IV contrast agent (gadolinium), which is then tracked using fast gradient echo techniques. Contrast agent at the level of the capillaries produces decreased signal intensity. Common parameter measurements obtained include CBF, CBV, time to peak (TTP), and MTT. Areas with relatively prolonged MTT and low CBV represent the most vulnerable tissue. As with CT perfusion, the optimal parameters to define the ischemic penumbra are still disputed. The data processing involved in perfusion measurement is time consuming, a limiting factor in its utility.

The major advantage of MR in acute stroke is its high sensitivity in identifying infarction, particularly with DWI sequence early on

in the evolution of stroke even when CT scan may appear entirely normal. It is also highly sensitive in detecting acute blood. The main reason MR has not yet completely replaced CT scanning in acute evaluation of stroke is its relatively limited availability. Not all hospitals are equipped with MR scanners and even those that are equipped, such as academic medical centers, experience a substantial delay in "Emergency room (ER) to scan time" relative to CT scanning. In addition, longer scan times compared to CT limit its utility in the acute emergency setting where time literally equals brain.

4.2. Evaluation of specific causes of stroke
4.2.1. Carotid artery stenosis
Clinical trials have demonstrated a clear benefit with respect to secondary stroke prevention favoring carotid endarterectomy over medical management in selected patients.[95,96] The accurate diagnosis and quantification of carotid stenosis is thus paramount to the management of patients presenting with TIA or ischemic stroke. Several diagnostic modalities for the evaluation of carotid stenosis are currently available, including Duplex ultrasound, CTA, magnetic resonance angiography (MRA), and conventional angiography. The advantages and limitations of each method are summarized in Table 20.6 and discussed below.

Calculating the degree of stenosis. Three methods are used commonly for estimating the degree of carotid stenosis. Two of these methods were derived from clinical trials comparing endarterectomy and medical management, the North American Symptomatic Endarterectomy Trial (NASCET)[95] and the European Carotid Surgery Trial (ECST).[96] Using the NASCET method,[95] the diameter of the most stenotic part of the vessel (B) is subtracted from the diameter of the normal internal carotid lumen (A) and expressed as a fraction of that diameter or (A–B)/A. The ECST method[96] subtracts the most stenotic portion of the vessel (C) from the estimated original diameter of the vessel (D) and expresses it as a fraction of the original vessel diameter (D–C)/D. The final method, common carotid method, compares the residual lumen at the most stenotic portion (E) to the lumen of the common carotid artery (F) [(F–E)/F]. When comparing the same stenotic

TABLE 20.6
IMAGING OF THE CAROTID ARTERIES

Imaging study	Main advantages	Limitations
Carotid Doppler	Noninvasive, relatively accurate, widely available	Accuracy dependent on operator experience, unreliable in distinguishing complete occlusion from severe stenosis
MRA	Noninvasive, extremely sensitive (particularly with contrast enhancement), allows for visualization of major cervical and intracranial vasculature, allows identification of potential "tandem lesions"	Longer image acquisition times prevent utility in unstable patients, contraindicated in patients with pacemakers and other metallic implants, gadolinium contrast has potential for nephrotoxicity
CTA	Noninvasive, rapid image acquisition, relatively sensitive, allows for visualization of major cervical and intracranial vessels to identify "tandem lesions"	Potential for contrast induced nephropathy, limits use in patients with renal insufficiency, potential for anaphylactic reaction to contrast
Conventional angiography	Considered the "gold standard" for evaluation of carotid stenosis, allows for visualization of major cervical and intracranial vessels	Limited to selected centers, potential for procedure related complications including stroke, contrast reaction, and hemorrhage

CTA, computed tomographic angiography; MRA, magnetic resonance angiography.

vessel, the ECST and common carotid methods tend to give higher degrees of stenosis compared to the NASCET method. A 50% stenosis reported using the NASCET method is roughly equivalent to a 75% stenosis using the other two methods. Current guidelines for the management of symptomatic carotid stenosis are based on combined analysis of the data from both NASCET and ECST trials utilizing the NASCET method of stenosis measurement. All three methods were devised for use with digital subtraction angiography (DSA); however, they may be applied to any of the diagnostic modalities discussed below.

Cerebral angiography. This modality is considered the gold standard in the evaluation of carotid artery stenosis. The major clinical trials comparing medical and surgical management of symptomatic carotid artery stenosis used cerebral angiography as the diagnostic imaging technique to define carotid artery stenosis. DSA techniques allow for shorter procedure durations and smaller quantities of contrast material administration. The procedure involves using fluoroscopy to guide a catheter into the aortic arch and then into the carotid arteries. Iodinated contrast material is then injected to opacify the vessels. Two to three projections of the carotids are then obtained; however, up to 32 projections can be obtained using rotational angiography.

The prime advantage of angiography is that it allows for visualization of the major cervical and intracranial vessels allowing for identification of tandem lesions, which may impact management. The major disadvantage of angiography is that it is invasive when compared to the other imaging modalities. Major complications of the procedure may include retroperitoneal hemorrhage, contrast reactions including anaphylaxis to iodinated contrast, stroke, and TIA. However, the incidence of major complications is extremely rare, on the order of 1%.[97] Lastly, angiography is only available at specialized centers, which limits its utility as the initial diagnostic modality of choice.

Duplex ultrasound. Carotid duplex ultrasound uses Doppler measurements of systolic velocity to estimate the degree of stenosis within the vessel wall. Higher peak systolic velocities correspond to higher degree of stenosis. Other common measurements of stenosis include the carotid index (peak internal carotid velocity to common carotid velocity). The NASCET investigators[98] used a carotid index (peak internal carotid velocity to common carotid velocity) of 4 or greater to obtain sensitivities and specificities of 91% and 87%, respectively.

The main advantages of carotid duplex ultrasound are its wide availability and noninvasive nature. In addition, it is a relatively accurate diagnostic modality. The overall sensitivity of carotid duplex ultrasound ranges from 81% to 89% in identifying patients with high-grade stenosis of 70% to 99%.[99,100]

The main limitation of carotid duplex ultrasound is the inherent operator-related variability. The accuracy of the test varies widely with operator experience. In addition, carotid ultrasound is notoriously inadequate in distinguishing patients with near occlusion from complete carotid occlusion.[101] Finally, carotid ultrasound may be less accurate in the evaluation of 50% to 69% stenoses when compared with higher (>70%) grade stenoses.[102] Thus, this technique may potentially miss patients with symptomatic stenoses of 60% to 70% severity who have also been shown to benefit from endarterectomy.[103]

CT angiography. CTA is becoming increasingly widespread in its use. Blood vessels are opacified on CT scan after the administration of IV contrast material. The technique thus allows

for a three-dimensional reconstruction of the cervical and/or intracranial vasculature (Fig. 20.14). The sensitivity of CTA for the evaluation of carotid artery stenosis compared to the gold standard angiography is reported to be in the range of 76% to 85% with a specificity of 94%.[100,104] CTA may be comparable to angiography in detecting complete occlusion of the carotid with sensitivities of 97% and specificities of 98% being reported.[104]

The main advantage of CTA is its wide availability. Images can be obtained quickly (within 15 to 20 min). This is particularly advantageous in the ER with respect to evaluation of acute stroke where visualization of the major vessels can help to guide treatment. The major disadvantage of CTA is that it requires the administration of contrast material, exposing the patient to the potential of allergic reactions and contrast-induced nephropathy.

MR angiography. Intensity differences between flowing blood and surrounding tissue can be detected using MR allowing for suppression of tissue and reconstruction of images depicting the vasculature. One MR sequence used in angiography is time of flight (TOF), which relies on the phenomenon of flow related enhancement (flowing blood appears bright). Processing of the source images using maximal intensity pixel postprocessing (MIP) projects only the brightest pixels in the final image, thus only vascular structures are displayed. Three-dimensional images can then be easily reconstructed (Fig. 20.15). Another common technique, contrast enhanced MRA, uses administration of gadolinium contrast, typically through an injector, to improve the detection of slow flow and to eliminate flow-related artifact.

The main advantage of MRA is that it is an extremely sensitive diagnostic modality yet remains noninvasive. Contrast enhanced MRA is more sensitive than TOF approaching sensitivities of 95% to 100% compared to DSA.[100,105,106] Similar to CTA, the major cervical and intracranial vessels can be visualized in tandem with MRA. A major disadvantage of MRA is that this technique tends to overestimate the degree of stenosis when compared to angiography. In addition, MRA is somewhat limited in its availability when compared to CT/CTA or carotid Doppler. MRA is contraindicated in patients with pacemakers, older cerebral aneurysm clips, or other metallic implants. Finally, nephrogenic systemic fibrosis has been associated with gadolinium exposure in patients with severely impaired renal function.[107]

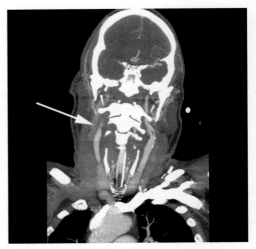

Figure 20.14 Computed tomographic angiogram of the head and neck showing complete occlusion of the right internal carotid artery in the neck approximately at its bifurcation from the common carotid artery (*arrow*).

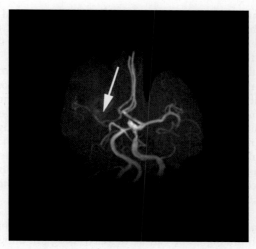

Figure 20.15 Magnetic resonance angiogram of the head showing occlusion of the right middle cerebral artery (MCA) *(arrow)*. Reconstitution in the supraclinoid segment through collateral circulation is present. The right anterior cerebral artery and MCA are also shown with diminished flow related signal being fed through collaterals.

4.2.2. Evaluation of intracranial arterial stenosis

Intracranial arterial stenosis accounts for ~10% of all ischemic strokes. Blacks, Hispanics, and Asians are more commonly affected than Caucasians. The rate of recurrent stroke in intracranial stenosis is high, with a clear increase in risk for stenoses greater than 70% and recently symptomatic.[108] These patients may be considered for treatment with emerging therapies such as intracranial stenting and angioplasty given the high rate of medical treatment failure. Correctly identifying intracranial stenosis is thus important in secondary prevention strategies. The most widely available modalities to evaluate the intracranial circulation include transcranial Doppler (TCD), CTA, MRA, and conventional angiography.

Transcranial Doppler ultrasonography. TCD allows for noninvasive evaluation of the major intracranial arteries through the skull. For example, insonation of the MCA is achievable through a temporal window. Similarly, the ophthalmic artery can be insonated through an orbital window. Information about the velocity of blood flow as well as direction can be obtained. Overall interpretation of a TCD study can yield important information regarding both the presence of stenotic narrowed vessels as well as presence of any collateral blood flow.

There has been limited evaluation of the accuracy of TCD in detection of intracranial stenosis compared with conventional angiography. A recent review[109] comparing TCD with angiography in the diagnosis of >50% MCA stenosis reported a sensitivity and specificity of 92% for mean flow velocity of >80 cm/s. Increasing the cutoff velocity to 100 cm/s yielded a sensitivity and specificity of 100% and 97%, respectively, with a positive predictive value (PPV) of 88% and negative predictive value (NPV) of 100%. TCD may be less reliable in evaluation of vertebrobasilar stenosis.[110] A recent multicenter prospective trial, The Stroke Outcomes and Neuroimaging of Intracranial Atherosclerosis (SONIA) trial,[111] demonstrated a PPV of 36% and NPV of 86% for TCD in identification of large proximal artery intracranial stenosis. The relatively higher NPV of TCD suggests that its utility in evaluation of intracranial stenosis is greatest for excluding the diagnosis. However, positive findings should be confirmed with another method.

MR angiography. This technique has been described previously with respect to evaluation of carotid stenosis. Sensitivities of MR angiography for the evaluation of intracranial stenosis have been reported to range from 86% to 95%.[112,113] Investigators from the SONIA trial reported a PPV of 59% and NPV of 91% for MRA in detection of intracranial stenosis.[111] Here, again the utility of MR angiography is likely in excluding intracranial disease.

CT angiography. CTA shows great promise as an accurate method for the noninvasive diagnosis of intracranial stenosis (Fig. 20.16). The sensitivity of CTA compared to conventional angiography has been reported to be as high as 97.1% with specificity of 99.5% for detection of intracranial stenosis ≥50%.[114] The same study reported a sensitivity and specificity of 100% for complete occlusion. Preliminary evidence also suggests that CTA may be more sensitive than MRA in detection of intracranial stenosis.[115]

Conventional angiography. This procedure has been described previously in relationship to evaluation of carotid artery stenosis. Angiography is also considered the gold standard technique in evaluation of intracranial stenosis (Fig. 20.17). The Warfarin Aspirin Symptomatic Intracranial Disease (WASID) study[116]

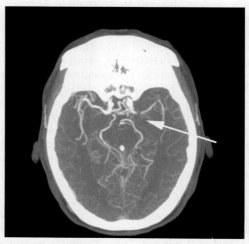

Figure 20.16 Computed tomographic angiogram of the head showing severe intracranial stenosis of the proximal (M1) portion of the left middle cerebral artery (MCA) *(arrow)*. Distal flow is still present within the vessel.

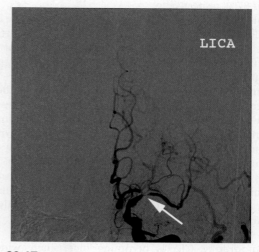

Figure 20.17 Anterior–posterior view of a conventional cerebral angiogram from the left internal carotid artery (LICA) injection. Note narrowing of the proximal (M1) portion of the left middle cerebral artery (MCA) *(arrow)* as seen in the CT angiogram (Fig. 20.16).

utilized the following equation to quantify the degree of stenosis of intracranial vessels:

$$[1-(Ds/Dn)] \times 100 \qquad \text{(Eq. 20.1)}$$

where Ds represents the diameter of the most stenotic portion of the vessel and Dn is the diameter of the normal vessel distal to the lesion. This method has been proposed as a standard measure of intracranial stenosis.

4.2.3. Evaluation of cardio-embolic stroke

Echocardiography. A potential cardiac source of embolism should be highly suspected among patients lacking standard risk factors for stroke, in young patients, and when suggestive signs on neuroimaging are present. The history, physical examination, and results of the ECG and rhythm monitoring may point to causes such as a recent myocardial infarction, HF due to low ejection fraction, a murmur suggestive of valvular heart disease, peripheral signs of IE, or atrial arrhythmia.

Echocardiography is often used to confirm suspected findings and is indicated when a definite cause for stroke is not found or when therapeutic decisions will depend on its results[29] (Table 20.7). In clinical practice, the first cardiac imaging test often selected is transthoracic echocardiography (TTE), particularly among patients over 45 years of age with clinically overt heart disease. TTE is particularly well suited to identify pathology such as poor LV function, focal wall motion abnormalities, LV intracavitary thrombus, LV aneurysm, and MAC. While other potential cardiac sources of embolism such as valvular vegetations, interatrial shunts, and aortic atheromata can be identified using the transthoracic approach, the sensitivity of TTE for detecting these lesions is lower than TEE, even when newer techniques such as harmonic imaging are employed.[117-119] In contrast to TTE, TEE provides superior anatomical detail for structures such as the LA, interatrial septum, MV, and aortic arch. TCD ultrasonography performed during IV agitated saline injection has been demonstrated to exhibit similar diagnostic accuracy to TEE for identifying right-to-left shunts; however, it cannot provide specific information about the level of the shunt (atrial vs. transpulmonic) and anatomical detail about the interatrial septum.[120]

The use and sequence of echocardiography in acute ischemic neurological events remain an area of controversy. Little controversy exists about the ability of echocardiography to identify potential cardio-embolic sources among patients with otherwise unexplained large vessel or multiple foci strokes. TEE has been consistently shown to offer higher sensitivity than TTE.[8,121,122] Emerging data[123] also suggest that lacunar strokes can be attributed to cardioembolism in some cases[123]; however, the use of echocardiography to identify potential cardiac sources of embolism in this group is less well studied. The controversy regarding the routine use of echocardiography for identifying potential cardio-embolic sources in all patients with acute neurological deficits stems from uncertainty in its added value over known clinical information. Echocardiography is costly and, when TEE is performed, may be associated with significant procedure-related morbidities. Some findings may be of uncertain significance. In addition, many embolic strokes can be linked to conditions, for example AF, for which anticoagulation is required regardless of identifying the embolic source. Lastly, for certain lesions, such as SEC or aortic atheromata, it is unclear what specific therapy is best for the lesion identified and how therapy would be modified in relation to that recommended based on existing clinical information.

Efforts to determine the cost-effectiveness of echocardiography as applied to patients with acute neurological deficits have

TABLE 20.7
ACC/AHA/ASE RECOMMENDATIONS FOR ECHOCARDIOGRAPHY IN PATIENTS WITH NEUROLOGICAL EVENTS

Class I
1. Younger patients (typically <45 years old)
2. Older patients (typically >45 years old) with neurological events without evidence of cerebrovascular disease or other obvious cause
3. Patients for whom a clinical therapeutic decision (e.g., anticoagulation) will depend on the results of echocardiography

Class IIa
Patients with suspicion of embolic disease and with cerebrovascular disease of questionable significance

Class IIb
Patients with a neurological event and intrinsic cerebrovascular disease of a sufficient nature to cause the clinical event

Class III
Patients for whom the results of echocardiography will not impact a decision to institute anticoagulant therapy or otherwise alter the approach to diagnosis or treatment

Source: From Cheitlin MD, Armstrong WF, Aurigemma GP, et al. ACC/AHA/ASE 2003 Guideline Update for the Clinical Application of Echocardiography. A report of the American College of Cardiology/American Heart Association Task Force on Practice Guidelines (ACC/AHA/ASE Committee to Update the 1997 Guidelines for the Clinical Application of Echocardiography). 2003, American College of Cardiology Web Site available at: www.acc.org/clinical/guidelines/echo/index.pdf.

yielded conflicting results based upon the assumptions used to conduct the analyses.[124,125] McNamara et al.[124] concluded that TEE was a cost-effective procedure among all patients in normal sinus rhythm with new-onset stroke. In contrast, Meenan et al.[125] found that TEE was a cost-effective procedure only when performed among the subset of patients in normal sinus rhythm with a pretest probability of intracardiac thrombus $\geq5\%$. In all other cases, these investigators concluded that performing a TEE was not a cost-effective strategy. Differences in the assumptions of prevalence of disease and the patient populations and conditions studied may explain the contrasting conclusions about the use of TEE for this indication.

The types of analyses described above are limited because they evaluate cost-effectiveness from a societal perspective and not that of the individual patient. In addition, these analyses are limited by the quality of data available, heterogeneity of diagnostic criteria, and effectiveness of prevalent medical therapies. At present, firm recommendations regarding the application of echocardiography in the individual patient cannot be given. Some argue that echocardiography should be used in all patients with ischemic neurological deficits to clarify the mechanism of stroke[122,126,127] while the results of the available cost analyses[124,125] and recent clinical studies[128-130] argue in favor of a more restrained approach. At present, given this conflicting data, it seems prudent when evaluating the individual patient to use echocardiography selectively based upon the history and physical examination and likelihood of the presence of a cardio-embolic source and when treatment plans would be modified based on the results of echocardiography. In general, echocardiography, especially TEE, is more likely to yield important results among younger patients (usually considered to be <45 to 50 years old) than in older individuals and among patients with otherwise unexplained strokes.[8,130]

5. FUTURE DIRECTIONS

r-TPA is the only FDA-approved treatment for ischemic stroke within 3 h of onset. National estimates of the use of r-TPA suggest that a mere 2% of all stroke patients receive this treatment.[131] This is likely in part due to the rather narrow 3-h therapeutic window. Much of the focus of stroke neurologists has been in identifying ways to extend the time window for treatment. Selection of patients for thrombolysis beyond 3 h may be aided by the detection of salvageable brain tissue (penumbra) as seen on perfusion scanning with either perfusion CT or MR perfusion. Indeed, some reports have suggested that implementing MR perfusion in selection of patients may help to identify patients that may benefit from r-TPA even after 3 h.[132,133] As a result, efforts are underway to attempt to improve the reliability of detecting ischemic penumbra.[134] Other modalities besides MR and CT perfusion may also be of use. As an example, single positron emission CT (SPECT) imaging is widely available and with relatively fast data acquisition, it shows promise in identifying patients at high risk for bleeding after thrombolysis.[135]

In terms of cardio-embolic sources, the results of trials that define the optimal therapeutic strategy for patients with PFO and ASAs are awaited. Research is also being focused on the relative impact of newer noninvasive imaging modalities, such as cardiac MR and multidetector CT as compared to TEE, in the evaluation of patients with presumed cardio-embolic strokes.

REFERENCES

1. Rosamond W, Flegal K, Furie K, et al. Heart disease and stroke statistics—2008 update: A report from the American Heart Association Statistics Committee and Stroke Statistics Subcommittee. *Circulation.* 2008;117:e25–e146.
2. Thom T, Haase N, Rosamond W, et al. Heart disease and stroke statistics—2006 update: A report from the American Heart Association Statistics Committee and Stroke Statistics Subcommittee. *Circulation.* 2006;113:e85.
3. Kleindorfer D, Panagos P, Pancioli A, et al. Incidence and short-term prognosis of transient ischemic attack in a population-based study. *Stroke.* 2005;36:720–723.
4. Crisostomo RA, Garcia MM, Tong DC, et al. Detection of diffusion-weighted MRI abnormalities in patients with transient ischemic attack: Correlation with clinical characteristics. *Stroke.* 2003;34:932–937.
5. Albers GW, Caplan LR, Easton JD, et al. Transient ischemic attack—proposal for a new definition. *N Engl J Med.* 2002;347:1713–1716.
6. Cardiogenic brain embolism. The second report of the Cerebral Embolism Task Force. *Arch Neurol.* 1989;46:727–743.
7. Hart RG. Cardiogenic embolism to the brain. *Lancet.* 1992;339:589–594.
8. Manning WJ. Role of transesophageal echocardiography in the management of thromboembolic stroke. *Am J Cardiol.* 1997;80:19D–28D.
9. Kannel WB, Benjamin EJ. Status of the epidemiology of atrial fibrillation. *Med Clin North Am.* 2008;92:17–40.
10. Fuster V, Rydén LE, Cannom DS, et al. ACC/AHA/ESC 2006 guidelines for the management of patients with atrial fibrillation: A report of the American College of Cardiology/American Heart Association Task Force on Practice Guidelines and the European Society of Cardiology Committee for Practice Guidelines (Writing Committee to Revise the 2001 Guidelines for the Management of Patients With Atrial Fibrillation). *J Am Coll Cardiol.* 2006;48:e149–e246.
11. Hart RG, Halperin JL. Atrial fibrillation and stroke. Concepts and controversies. *Stroke.* 2001;32:803–808.
12. Gage BF, Waterman AD, Shannon W, et al. Validation of clinical classification schemes for predicting stroke. Results from the National registry of Atrial Fibrillation. *JAMA.* 2001;285:2864–2870.
13. Fatkin D, Feneley M. Stratification of thromboembolic risk of atrial fibrillation by transthoracic echocardiography and transesophageal echocardiography: The relative role of left atrial appendage function, mitral valve disease, and spontaneous echocardiographic contrast. *Prog Cardiovasc Dis.* 1996;39:57–68.
14. Zabalgoitta M, Halperin JL, Pearce LA, et al. Transesophageal echocardiographic correlates of clinical risk of thromboembolism in nonvalvular atrial fibrillation. *J Am Coll Cardiol.* 1998;31:1622–1626.
15. Kamp O, Verhorst PMJ, Welling RC, et al. Importance of left atrial appendage flow as a predictor of thromboembolic events in patient with atrial fibrillation. *Eur Heart J.* 1999;20:979–985.
16. Bernhardt P, Schmidt H, Hammerstingl C, et al. Patients with atrial fibrillation and dense spontaneous echo contrast at high risk. *J Am Coll Cardiol.* 2005;45:1807–1812.
17. Stollberger C, Chnupa P, Kronik G, et al. Transesophageal echocardiography to assess embolic risk in patients with atrial fibrillation. *Ann Intern Med.* 1998;128:630–638.
18. The Stroke Prevention in Atrial Fibrillation Investigators Committee on Echocardiography. Transesophageal echocardiographic correlates of thromboembolism in high-risk patients with nonvalvular atrial fibrillation. *Ann Intern Med.* 1998;128:639–647.
19. Lip GYH, Lim HS. Atrial fibrillation and stroke prevention. *Lancet Neurol.* 2007;6:981–993.
20. Go AS, Hylek EM, Chang Y et al. Anticoagulation therapy for stroke prevention in atrial fibrillation. How well do randomized trials translate into clinical practice? *JAMA.* 2003;290:2685–2692.
21. Scholten MF, Thornton AS, Mekel JM, et al. Anticoagulation in atrial fibrillation and flutter. *Europace.* 2005;7:492–499.
22. Omran H, Rang B, Schmidt H, et al. Incidence of left atrial thrombi in patients in sinus rhythm and a recent neurological deficit. *Am Heart J.* 2000;140:658–662.
23. Agmon Y, Khandheria BK, Gentile F, et al. Clinical and echocardiographic characteristics of patients with left atrial thrombus and sinus rhythm. Experience in 20643 consecutive transesophageal echocardiographic examinations. *Circulation.* 2002;105:27–31.
24. Lanzarotti CJ, Olshansky B. Thromboembolism in chronic atrial flutter: Is the risk underestimated? *J Am Coll Cardiol.* 1997;30:1506–1511.
25. Wood KA, Eisenberg SJ, Kalman JM, et al. Risk of thromboembolism in chronic atrial flutter. *Am J Cardiol.* 1997;79:1043–1047.
26. Weir NU. An update on cardioembolic stroke. *Postgrad Med J.* 2008;84:133–142.
27. Doufekias E, Segal AZ, Kizer JR. Cardiogenic and aortogenic brain embolism. *J Am Coll Cardiol.* 2008;51:1049–1059.
28. Chiarella F, Santoro E, Domenicucci S, et al. Predischarge two-dimensional echocardiographic evaluation of left ventricular thrombosis after acute myocardial infarction in the GISSI-3 study. *Am J Cardiol.* 1998;81:822–827.
29. Cheitlin MD, Armstrong WF, Aurigemma GP, et al. ACC/AHA/ASE 2003 Guideline Update for the Clinical Application of Echocardiography. A report of the American College of Cardiology/American Heart Association Task Force on Practice Guidelines (ACC/AHA/ASE Committee to Update the 1997 Guidelines for the Clinical Application of Echocardiography). 2003, American College of Cardiology Web Site available at: www.acc.org/clinical/guidelines/echo/index.pdf.
30. Visser CA, Kan G, Meltzer RS, et al. Embolic potential of left ventricular thrombus after myocardial infarction: A two-dimensional echocardiographic study of 119 patients. *J Am Coll Cardiol.* 1985;5:1276–1280.
31. Keren A, Goldberg S, Gottlieb S, et al. Natural history of left ventricular thrombi: Their appearance and resolution in the posthospitalization period of acute myocardial infarction. *J Am Coll Cardiol.* 1990;15:790–800.
32. Lapeyre AC, Steele PM, Kazimer FJ, et al. Systemic embolism in chronic left ventricular aneurysm: Incidence and the role of anticoagulation. *J Am Coll Cardiol.* 1985;6:534–538.
33. Cabin HS, Roberts WC. Left ventricular aneurysm, intra-aneurysmal thrombus and systemic embolus in coronary heart disease. *Chest.* 1980;77:586–589.
34. Freudenberger RS, Hellkamp AS, Halperin JL, et al. Risk of thromboembolism in heart failure. An analysis from the Sudden Cardiac Death in Heart Failure Trial (SCD-HeFT). *Circulation.* 2007;115:2637–2641.
35. Loh E, St. John Sutton M, Wun CC, et al. Ventricular dysfunction and the risk of stroke after myocardial infarction. *N Engl J Med.* 1997;336:251–257.
36. Hunt SA, Abraham WT, Chin MH, et al. ACC/AHA 2005 Guideline Update for the Diagnosis and Management of Chronic Heart Failure in the Adult: A Report of the American College of Cardiology/American Heart Association Task Force on Practice Guidelines (Writing Committee to Update the 2001 Guidelines for the Evaluation and Management of Heart Failure). American College of Cardiology Web Site. Available at: http://www.acc.org/clinical/guidelines/failure//index.pdf.
37. Srichai MB, Junor C, Rodriguez LL, et al. Clinical, imaging, and pathological characteristics of left ventricular thrombus: A comparison of contrast-enhanced magnetic resonance imaging, transthoracic echocardiography, and transesophageal echocardiography with surgical or pathological validation. *Am Heart J.* 2006;152:75–84.
38. Bayer AS, Bolger AF, Taubert KA, et al. Diagnosis and management of infective endocarditis and its complications. *Circulation.* 1998;98:2936–2948.
39. Baddour LM, Wilson WR, Bayer AS, et al. Infective endocarditis: Diagnosis, antimicrobial therapy, and management of complications: A statement for healthcare professionals from the Committee on Rheumatic Fever, Endocarditis, and Kawasaki Disease, Council on Cardiovascular Disease in the Young, and the Councils on Clinical Cardiology, Stroke, and Cardiovascular Surgery and Anesthesia, American Heart Association: Endorsed by the Infectious Disease Society of America. *Circulation.* 2005;111:e394–e434.
40. DiSalvo G, Habib G, Pergola V, et al. Echocardiography predicts embolic events in infective endocarditis. *J Am Coll Cardiol.* 2001;37:1069–1076.
41. Thuny F, DiSalvo G, Belliard O, et al. Risk of embolism and death in infective endocarditis: Prognostic value of echocardiography. A prospective multicenter study. *Circulation.* 2005;112:69–75.
42. Vilacosta I Graupner C, San Roman JA, et al. Risk of embolization after initiation of antibiotic therapy for infective endocarditis. *J Am Coll Cardiol.* 2002;39:1489–1495.
43. Reisner SA, Brenner B, Haim N, et al. Echocardiography in nonbacterial thrombotic endocarditis: From autopsy to clinical entity. *J Am Soc Echocardiogr.* 2000;13:876–881.
44. Dutta T, Karas MG, Segal AZ, et al. Yield of transesophageal echocardiography for nonbacterial thrombotic endocarditis and other cardiac sources of embolism in cancer patients with cerebral ischemia. *Am J Cardiol.* 2006;97:894–898.

45. Edoute Y, Haim N, Rinkevich D, et al. Cardiac valvular vegetations in cancer patients: A prospective echocardiographic study of 200 patients. *Am J Med.* 1997;102:252–258.

46. Bonow RO, Carabello BA, Chatterjee K, et al. ACC/AHA 2006 Guidelines for the Management of Patients with Valvular Heart Disease: A Report of the American College of Cardiology/American Heart Association Task Force on Practice Guidelines (Writing Committee to Develop Guidelines for the Management of Patients With Valvular Heart Disease). American College of Cardiology Web Site. Available at: http://www.acc.org/clinical/guidelines/valvular/index.pdf.

47. Hammermeister K, Sethi GK, Henderson WG, et al. Outcomes 15 years after valve replacement with a mechanical versus a bioprosthetic valve: Final report of the Veterans Affairs Randomized Trial. *J Am Coll Cardiol.* 2000;36:1152–1158.

48. Vongpatanasin W, Hillis LD, Lange RA. Prosthetic heart valves. *N Engl J Med.* 1996;335:407–416.

49. Salem D, Stein PD, Al-Ahmad A, et al. Antithrombotic therapy in valvular heart disease—native and prosthetic. *Chest.* 2004;126:457S–482S.

50. Heras M, Chesebro JH, Fuster V, et al. High risk of thromboemboli early after bioprosthetic cardiac valve replacement. *J Am Coll Cardiol.* 1995;25:1111–1119.

51. Reyen K. Cardiac myxomas. *N Engl J Med.* 1995;333:1610–1617.

52. Gowda RM, Khan IA, Nair CK, et al. Cardiac papillary fibroelastoma: A comprehensive analysis of 725 cases. *Am Heart J.* 2003;146:404–410.

53. Sun JP, Asher CR, Yang XS, et al. Clinical and echocardiographic characteristics of papillary fibroelastomas. A retrospective and prospective study in 162 patients. *Circulation.* 2001;103:2687–2693.

54. Amarenco P, Duyckaerts C, Tzourio C, et al. The prevalence of ulcerated plaques in the aortic arch in patients with stroke. *N Engl J Med.* 1992;326:221–225.

55. Amarenco P, Cohen A, Tzourio C, et al. Atherosclerotic disease of the aortic arch and the risk of ischemic stroke. *N Engl J Med.* 1994;331:1474–1479.

56. The French Study of Aortic Plaques in Stroke Group. Atherosclerotic disease of the aortic arch as a risk factor for recurrent ischemic stroke. *N Engl J Med.* 1996;334:1216–1221.

57. Tunick PA, Perez JL, Kronzon I. Protruding atheromas in the thoracic aorta and systemic embolization. *Ann Intern Med.* 1991;115:423–427.

58. Kronzon I, Tunick PA. Aortic atherosclerotic disease and stroke. *Circulation.* 2006;114:63–75.

59. Cohen A, Tzourio C, Bertrand B, et al. Aortic plaque morphology and vascular events. A follow-up study in patients with ischemic stroke. *Circulation.* 1997;96:3838–3841.

60. Blauth CI, Cosgrove DM, Webb BW, et al. Atheroembolism from the ascending aorta. *J Thorac Cardiovasc Surg.* 1992;103:1104–1112.

61. Tunick PA, Nayar AC, Goodkin GM, et al. Effect of treatment on the incidence of stroke and other emboli in 519 patients with severe thoracic aortic plaque. *Am J Cardiol.* 2002;90:1320–1325.

62. Meissner I, Whisnant JP, Khandheria BK, et al. Prevalence of potential risk factors for stroke assessed by transesophageal echocardiography and carotid ultrasonography: The SPARC study. *Mayo Clin Proc.* 1999;74:862–869.

63. Meissner I, Khandheria BK, Sheps SG, et al. Atherosclerosis of the aorta: Risk factor, risk marker, or innocent bystander? A prospective population-based transesophageal echocardiography study. *J Am Coll Cardiol.* 2004;44:1018–1024.

64. Petty GW, Khandheria BK, Meissner I, et al. Population-based study of the relationship between atherosclerotic debris and cerebrovascular ischemic events. *Mayo Clin Proc.* 2006;81:609–614.

65. Hagen PT, Scholz DG, Edwards WD. Incidence and size of patent foramen ovale during the first 10 decades of life: An autopsy study of 965 normal hearts. *Mayo Clin Proc.* 1984;59:17–20.

66. Lechat P, Mas JL, Lascault G, et al. Prevalence of patent foramen ovale in patients with stroke. *N Engl J Med.* 1998;318:1148–1152.

67. Stollberger C, Slany J, Schuster I, et al. The prevalence of deep venous thrombosis in patients with suspected paradoxical embolism. *Ann Intern Med.* 1993;119:461–465.

68. Cramer SC, Rordorf G, Maki JH, et al. Increased pelvic vein thrombi in cryptogenic stroke. Results of the Paradoxical Emboli from Large Veins in Ischemic Stroke (PELVIS) Study. *Stroke.* 2004;35:46–50.

69. Stollberger C, Finsterer J, Slany J. Why is venous thrombosis only rarely detected in patients with suspected paradoxical embolism? *Thromb Res.* 2002;105:189–191.

70. Homma S, Sacco RL. Patent foramen ovale and stroke. *Circulation.* 2005;112:1063–1072.

71. Overell JR, Bone I, Lees KR. Interatrial septal abnormalities and stroke: A meta-analysis of case-control studies. *Neurology.* 2000;55:1172–1179.

72. Handke M, Harloff A, Olschewski M, et al. Patent foramen ovale and cryptogenic stroke in older patients. *N Engl J Med.* 2007;357:2262–2268.

73. Meier B, Lock JE. Contemporary management of patent foramen ovale. *Circulation.* 2003;107:5–9.

74. Agmon Y, Khandheria BK, Meisner I, et al. Frequency of atrial septal aneurysms in patients with cerebral ischemic events. *Circulation.* 1999;99:1942–1944.

75. Mas JL, Arquizan C, Lamy C, et al. Recurrent cerebrovascular events associated with patent foramen ovale, atrial septal aneurysm, or both. *N Engl J Med.* 2001;345:1740–1746.

76. Homma S, Sacco RL, Di Tullio MR, et al. Effect of medical treatment in stroke patients with patent foramen ovale. Patent foramen ovale in Cryptogenic Stroke Study. *Circulation.* 2002;105:2625–2631.

77. Windecker S, Wahl A, Nedeltchev K, et al. Comparison of medical treatment with percutaneous closure of patent foramen ovale in patients with cryptogenic stroke. *J Am Coll Cardiol.* 2004;44:750–758.

78. Meissner I, Khandheria BK, Heit JA, et al. Patent foramen ovale: Innocent or guilty? Evidence from a prospective population-based study. *J Am Coll Cardiol.* 2006;47:440–445.

79. Petty GW, Khandheria BK, Meissner I, et al. Population-based study of the relationship between patent foramen ovale and cerebrovascular ischemic events. *Mayo Clin Proc.* 2006;81:602–608.

80. Di Tullio MR, Sacco RL, Sciacca RR, et al. Patent foramen ovale and the risk of ischemic stroke in a multiethnic population. *J Am Coll Cardiol.* 2007;49:797–802.

81. Patel SV, Flaker G. Is early cardioversion for atrial fibrillation safe in patients with spontaneous echocardiographic contrast? *Clin Cardiol.* 2008;31:148–152.

82. Barnett HJ, Boughner DR, Taylor DW, et al. Further evidence relating mitral-valve prolapse to cerebral ischemic events. *N Engl J Med.* 1980;302:139–144.

83. Gilon D, Buonanno FS, Joffe MM, et al. Lack of evidence of an association between mitral-valve prolapse and stroke in young patients. *N Engl J Med.* 1999;341:3–13.

84. Avierinos JF, Brown RD, Foley DA, et al. Cerebral ischemic events after diagnosis of mitral valve prolapse. A community-based study of incidence and predictive factors. *Stroke.* 2003;34:1339–1345.

85. Benjamin EJ, Plehn JF, D'Agostino RB, et al. Mitral annular calcification and the risk of stroke in an elderly cohort. *N Engl J Med.* 1992;327:374–379.

86. Kizer JR, Wiebers DO, Whisnant JP, et al. Mitral annular calcification, aortic valve sclerosis, and incident stroke in adults free of clinical cardiovascular disease. The Strong Heart Study. *Stroke.* 2005;36:2533–2537.

87. Karas MG, Francescone S, Segal AZ, et al. Relation between mitral annular calcium and complex aortic atheroma in patients with cerebral ischemia referred for transesophageal echocardiography. *Am J Cardiol.* 2007;99:1306–1311.

88. Pujadas R, Abroix A, Anguera N, et al. Mitral annular calcification as a marker of complex aortic atheroma in patients with stroke of uncertain etiology. *Echocardiography.* 2008;25:124–132.

89. Stein JH, Soble JS. Thrombus associated with mitral valve calcification. A possible mechanism for embolic stroke. *Stroke.* 1995;26:1697–1699.

90. Lin CS, Schwartz I, Chapman I. Calcification of the mitral annulus fibrosis with systemic embolization. A clinicopathological study of 16 cases. *Arch Pathol Lab Med.* 1987;111:411–414.

91. Freedberg RS, Goodkin GM, Perez JL, et al. Valve strands are strongly associated with systemic embolization: A transesophageal echocardiographic study. *J Am Coll Cardiol.* 1995;26:1709–1712.

92. Roldan CA, Shively BK, Crawford MH. Valve excrescences: Prevalence, evolution and risk for cardioembolism. *J Am Coll Cardiol.* 1997;30:1308–1314.

93. Homma S, Di Tullio MR, Sciacca RR, et al. Effect of aspirin and warfarin therapy in stroke patients with valvular strands. *Stroke.* 2004;35:1436–1442.

94. Linfante I, Llinas RH, Selim M, et al. Clinical and vascular outcomes in internal carotid versus middle cerebral artery occlusions after intravenous tissue plasminogen activator. *Stroke.* 2002;33:2066–2071.

95. North American Symptomatic Carotid Endarterectomy Trial Collaborators. Beneficial effect of carotid endarterectomy in symptomatic patients with high-grade carotid stenosis. *N Engl J Med.* 1991;325:445–453.

96. European Carotid Surgery Trialists' Collaborative Group. MRC European carotid surgery trial: Interim results for symptomatic patients with severe (70%–99%) or with mild (0%–29%) carotid stenosis. *Lancet.* 1991;337:1235–1243.

97. Willinsky RA, Taylor SM, TerBrugge K, et al. Neurologic complications of cerebral angiography: Prospective analysis of 2,899 procedures and review of the literature. *Radiology.* 2003;227:522–528.

98. Moneta GL, Edwards JM, Chitwood RW, et al. Correlation of North American Symptomatic Carotid Endarterectomy Trial (NASCET) angiographic definition of 70% to 99% internal carotid artery stenosis with duplex scanning. *J Vasc Surg.* 1993;17:152–157.

99. Mittl RL Jr, Broderick M, Carpenter JP, et al. Blinded-reader comparison of magnetic resonance angiography and duplex ultrasonography for carotid artery bifurcation stenosis. *Stroke.* 1994;25:4–10.

100. Wardlaw JM, Chappell FM, Best JJ, et al. Non-invasive imaging compared with intra-arterial angiography in the diagnosis of symptomatic carotid stenosis: A meta-analysis. *Lancet.* 2006;367:1503–1512.

101. Furst G, Saleh A, Wenserski F, et al. Reliability and validity of noninvasive imaging of internal carotid artery pseudo-occlusion. *Stroke.* 1999;30:1444–1449.

102. Sabeti S, Schillinger M, Mlekusch W, et al. Quantification of internal carotid artery stenosis with duplex US: Comparative analysis of different flow velocity criteria. *Radiology.* 2004;232:431–439.

103. Barnett HJ, Taylor DW, Eliasziw M, et al. Benefit of carotid endarterectomy in patients with symptomatic moderate or severe stenosis. North American Symptomatic Carotid Endarterectomy Trial Collaborators. *N Engl J Med.* 1998;339:1415–1425.

104. Koelemay MJ, Nederkoorn PJ, Reitsma JB, et al. Systematic review of computed tomographic angiography for assessment of carotid artery disease. *Stroke.* 2004;35:2306–2312.

105. Borisch I, Horn M, Butz B, et al. Preoperative evaluation of carotid artery stenosis: Comparison of contrast-enhanced MR angiography and duplex sonography with digital subtraction angiography. *Am J Neuroradiol.* 2003;24:1117–1122.

106. Scarabino T, Carriero A, Giannatempo GM, et al. Contrast-enhanced MR angiography (CE MRA) in the study of the carotid stenosis: Comparison with digital subtraction angiography (DSA). *J Neuroradiol.* 1999;26:87–91.

107. Thomsen HS, Marckmann P, Logager VB. Nephrogenic systemic fibrosis (NSF): A late adverse reaction to some of the gadolinium based contrast agents. *Cancer Imaging.* 2007;7:130–137.

108. Kasner SE, Chimowitz MI, Lynn MJ, et al. Predictors of ischemic stroke in the territory of a symptomatic intracranial arterial stenosis. *Circulation.* 2006;113;555–563.

109. Navarro JC, Lao AY, Sharma VK, et al. The accuracy of transcranial Doppler in the diagnosis of middle cerebral artery stenosis. *Cerebrovasc Dis.* 2007;23(5–6):325–30.

110. Rorick MB, Nichols FT, Adams RJ. Transcranial Doppler correlation with angiography in detection of intracranial stenosis. *Stroke.* 1994;25:1931–1934.

111. Feldmann E, Wilterdink JL, Kosinski A, et al. The Stroke Outcomes and Neuroimaging of Intracranial Atherosclerosis (SONIA) trial. *Neurology.* 2007;68:2099–2106.

112. Stock KW, Radue EW, Jacob AL, et al. Intracranial arteries: Prospective blinded comparative study of MR angiography and DSA in 50 patients. *Radiology.* 1995;195:451–456.

113. Sadikin C, Teng MM, Chen TY. The current role of 1.5T non-contrast 3D time-of-flight magnetic resonance angiography to detect intracranial steno-occlusive disease. *J Formos Med Assoc.* 2007;106:691–699.

114. Nguyen-Huynh MN, Wintermark M, English J, et al. How accurate is CT angiography in evaluating intracranial atherosclerotic disease? *Stroke.* 2008;39:1184–1188.

115. Bash S, Villablanca JP, Jahan R, et al. Intracranial vascular stenosis and occlusive disease: Evaluation with CT angiography, MR angiography, and digital subtraction angiography. *Am J Neuroradiol.* 2005;26:1012–1021.

116. Samuels OB, Joseph GJ, Lynn MJ, et al. A standardized method for measuring intracranial arterial stenosis. *Am J Neuroradiol.* 2000;21:643–646.

117. Reynolds HR, Jagen MA, Tunick PA, et al. Sensitivity of transthoracic versus transesophageal echocardiography for the detection of native valve vegetations in the modern era. *J Am Soc Echocardiogr.* 2003;16:67–70.

118. Ha JW, Shin MS, Kang S, et al. Enhanced detection of right-to-left shunt through patent foramen ovale by transthoracic contrast echocardiography using harmonic imaging. *Am J Cardiol.* 2001;87:669–671.

119. Schwammenthal E, Schwammenthal Y, Tanne D, et al. Transcutaneous detection of aortic arch atheromas by suprasternal harmonic imaging. *J Am Coll Cardiol.* 2002;39:1127–1132.

120. Droste DW, Silling K, Stypmann J, et al. Contrast transcranial Doppler ultrasound in the detection of right-to-left shunts: Time window and threshold in microbubble numbers. *Stroke.* 2000;31:1640–1645.

121. Pearson AC, Labovitz AJ, Tatineni S, et al. Superiority of transesophageal echocardiography in detecting cardiac source of embolism in patients with cerebral ischemia of uncertain etiology. *J Am Coll Cardiol.* 1991;17:66–72.

122. De Bruijn SFTM, Agema WRP, Lammers GJ, et al. Transesophageal echocardiography is superior to transthoracic echocardiography in management of patients of any age with transient ischemic attack or stroke. *Stroke.* 2006;37:2531–2534.

123. Ulrich JN, Hesse B, Schuele S, et al. Single-vessel versus multivessel territory acute ischemic stroke: Value of transesophageal echocardiography in the differentiation of embolic stroke. *J Am Soc Echocardiogr.* 2006;19:1165–1169.

124. McNamara RL, Lima JAC, Whelton PK, et al. Echocardiographic identification of cardiovascular sources of emboli to guide clinical management of stroke: A cost-effectiveness analysis. *Ann Intern Med.* 1997;127:775–787.

125. Meenan RT, Saha S, Chou R, et al. Cost-effectiveness of echocardiography to identify intracardiac thrombus among patients with first stroke or transient ischemic attack. *Med Decis Making.* 2007;27:161–177.

126. De Abreu TT, Mateus S, Correia J. Therapy implications of transthoracic echocardiography in acute ischemic stroke patients. *Stroke.* 2005;36:1565–1566.

127. Strandberg M, Marttila RJ, Helenius H, et al. Transoesophageal echocardiography in selecting patients for anticoagulation after ischemic stroke or transient ischemic attack. *J Neurol Neurosurg Psychiatry.* 2002;73:29–33.

128. Leung DY, Black IW, Cranney GB, et al. Selection of patients for transesophageal echocardiography after stroke and systemic embolic events. Role of transthoracic echocardiography. *Stroke.* 1995;26:1820–1824.

129. Warner MF, Momah KI. Routine transesophageal echocardiography for cerebral ischemia. Is it really necessary? *Arch Intern Med.* 1996;156:1719–1723.

130. Wolber T, Maeder M, Atefy R, et al. Should routine echocardiography be performed in all patients with stroke? *J Stroke Cerebrovasc Dis.* 2007;16:1–7.

131. Kleindorfer D, Lindsell J, Brass L, et al. National US estimates of recombinant tissue plasminogen activator use: ICD-9 codes substantially underestimate. *Stroke.* 2008;39:924–928.

132. Thomalla G, Schwark C, Sobesky J, et al. Outcome and symptomatic bleeding complications of intravenous thrombolysis within 6 hours in MRI-selected stroke patients: Comparison of a German multicenter study with the pooled data of ATLANTIS, ECASS, and NINDS tPA trials. *Stroke.* 2006;37:852–858.

133. Albers GW, Thijs VN, Wechsler L, et al. Magnetic resonance imaging profiles predict clinical response to early reperfusion: The diffusion and perfusion imaging evaluation for understanding stroke evolution (DEFUSE) study. *Ann Neurol.* 2006;60:508–517.

134. Wintermark M, Albers GW, Alexandrov AV, et al. Acute stroke imaging research roadmap. *Stroke.* 2008;39:1621–1628.

135. Alexandrov AV, Masdeu JC, Devous MD Sr, et al. Brain single-photon emission CT with HMPAO and safety of thrombolytic therapy in acute ischemic stroke. Proceedings of the meeting of the SPECT Safe Thrombolysis Study Collaborators and the members of the Brain Imaging Council of the Society of Nuclear Medicine. *Stroke.* 1997;28:1830–1834.

Molecular Imaging in Heart Failure

21

Hina Chaudhry
Randolph Hutter

1. INTRODUCTION

Medical diagnosis and treatment have become increasingly dependent on interdisciplinary efforts which are rapidly advancing clinical practice and biomedical research. There has been a remarkable growth in cardiovascular imaging techniques and applications in recent years. The traditional imaging methods were based on structural and physiological assessments. However, the ongoing revolution in molecular medicine dictates a need to develop accurate imaging techniques to precisely monitor the effects of molecular therapies. In this chapter, we will review the current approaches being utilized for molecular imaging in heart failure (HF), gene therapy, stem cell transplantation, atherosclerosis, and apoptosis.

2. PATHOPHYSIOLOGY

Approximately 5 million patients have HF in the United States at any given time, and an estimated 500,000 new cases are diagnosed yearly.[1] HF is the leading cause of hospitalization, morbidity, and mortality in patients >60 years of age.[2] Despite recent advances in the past decade in surgical and medical treatment of HF, nearly 300,000 patients die of HF as a primary or secondary cause every year.[3] Therefore, HF imposes a major epidemiological burden on society as well as healthcare costs estimated at $35 billion in 2008.[4] Given that the only definitive treatment for HF is cardiac transplantation, it is disconcerting to note that the number of available donors in the United States peaked at 2,525 in 1994 and has steadily declined since.[5] Due to this staggering mismatch in the numbers of HF patients and heart donors, the need to find alternative treatments is a critical imperative. Other approaches being explored include cardiac gene therapy and cardiac stem cell transplantation. These two topics are discussed in subsequent sections of this chapter.

HF is initiated by direct damage to cardiomyocytes, which is due to a combination of genetic and environmental factors. The disease then continues or progresses due to the activation of signaling pathways involving neurohormones and cytokines that further destabilize functions of both myocyte and nonmyocyte cells. "Remodeling" is the term used to describe the cellular and structural changes accompanying this process.

The principal intracellular alterations within cardiomyocytes that are representative of left ventricular (LV) remodeling include loss of contractile proteins, impaired excitation contraction coupling, a decreased responsiveness to β-adrenergic stimulation, and an attempted return to the fetal gene program characterized by decreased expression of the α-myosin heavy chain gene with

increased expression of the β-myosin heavy chain. There is also evidence of increased DNA synthesis after acute injury characterizing efforts to re-enter the cell cycle.[6] Failing cardiomyocytes also have reduced phosphocreatine content and display altered metabolic activity with a downregulation of fatty acid oxidation, increased glycolysis and glucose oxidation, reduced respiratory chain activity, and impaired reserve for mitochondrial oxidative flux.[7] These metabolic adaptations prolong cell viability by ensuring more efficient oxygen consumption and energy production. However, despite these processes, muscle cell loss progresses in LV remodeling through both necrosis and apoptosis.[7] The components and volume of the extracellular matrix also undergo significant changes in HF, as evidenced by increased interstitial, perivascular, and replacement fibrosis. Further, impairment of LV diastolic relaxation, compliance, and contractile function ensues with a decline in coronary flow reserve. Myocardial fibrosis in chronic HF is regulated by a balance between collagen synthesis, its degradation by matrix metalloproteinases (MMPs), and the regulation of MMPs by tissue inhibitors of metalloproteinases (TIMPs) that bind and inactivate MMPs. The dynamic nature of this process is manifested by the potential for reversibility in response to therapeutic interventions such as coronary revascularization, administration of drugs that inhibit the renin-angiotensin-aldosterone or β-adrenergic systems, or biventricular pacing.[8]

Given the pace of advances in understanding the molecular biology and genetic make-up of HF, enhanced by the development of numerous genetically altered small animal models, there is a clear need for early serial evaluation of molecular and cellular alterations that culminate in LV dysfunction. Therefore, cardiac noninvasive imaging in HF has evolved in two parallel directions to fulfill these requirements. Firstly, existing imaging modalities have been modified such that they can be utilized for the imaging of small animal models. Secondly, a number of imaging probes are now available that can target macromolecules and biologic processes in intact organisms. In this section, the current status of a select group of imaging probes with the potential to target macromolecules and biologic pathways involved in LV remodeling is summarized.

3. IMAGING

3.1. Molecular imaging in left ventricular remodeling

Rapid developments are underway in the field of molecular imaging with the goals of providing patient-specific, noninvasive molecular and anatomic information within the context of a systemic or organ-based disease. Such studies may potentiate better diagnostic information, allow a more intelligent choice of therapeutic interventions, and permit improved monitoring of treatment response.[9] Nuclear imaging techniques such as single-photon emission tomography (SPECT) and positron emission tomography (PET) are well suited for cardiac molecular imaging owing to the large number of potentially available molecular targets, high intrinsic sensitivity, and excellent depth of penetration.[9] PET is especially advantageous, given its quantitative nature and high spatial resolution. A combination of PET and computed tomography (PET-CT) can allow for high-resolution anatomic information to be superimposed on molecular imaging data. Quantitative PET can be used to evaluate several metabolic and hemodynamic parameters, including glucose uptake and phosphorylation, glucose oxidation, fatty acid uptake and oxidation, blood flow, and mitochondrial membrane potential.[8] Cardiac magnetic resonance (CMR) imaging is also a rapidly evolving molecular imaging modality with the introduction of an increasing number of high-affinity molecular probes imaged at exceptionally high spatial resolution.[10]

Within the field of HF, molecular imaging is evolving to include imaging and monitoring of myocardial metabolic substrate utilization, apoptosis, collagen matrix turnover, expression of various components of the renin-angiotensin system (RAS), and autonomic innervation, and to track stem cells used for myocardial regeneration (discussed in section 3.3).

3.1.1. Imaging metabolic substrate utilization

LV remodeling in both ischemic and nonischemic cardiomyopathy involves altered myocardial substrate utilization.[11,12] In ischemic cardiomyopathy, viable myocardium remains metabolically active with a shift from free fatty acid (aerobic) to glucose (anaerobic) utilization. The suppression of fatty acid oxidation is seemingly an adaptive process aimed at more efficient oxygen consumption and energy production. This, in turn, is associated with downregulation of peroxisome proliferator-activated receptor α (PPARα), a transcription factor controlling the expression of key enzymes for fatty acid oxidation. Indirect evidence for the favorable effect of this metabolic adaptation comes from the observation that chronic partial inhibition of myocardial free fatty acid oxidation by a selective inhibitor of long-chain 3-ketoacyl thiolase results in improved exercise tolerance, LV systolic and diastolic function, and contractile reserve, and retards LV remodeling in HF.[11] It also appears that the beneficial effects of long-term β-adrenergic receptor and RAS antagonists in HF are, at least in part, due to a switch in cardiomyocyte metabolism from fatty acid to glucose uptake and oxidation.[13] Favorable redistribution in absolute blood flow and associated increases in regional and global LV function have also been shown with β-adrenergic receptor blockers[14] (Fig. 21.1).

A number of nuclear molecular probes have been used to assess myocardial substrate[15] utilization in HF. Using quantitative PET, myocardial glucose and fatty acid metabolism can be analyzed by the use of ^{18}F-2-fluoro-2-glucose (FDG) and ^{11}C-palmitate.[7] FDG is a glucose analog that is phosphorylated by hexokinase to FDG-6-phosphate, but is not metabolized further in the glycolytic pathway, and becomes trapped in the myocardium. Increased utilization of FDG by ischemic myocardium results from molecular signals, in response to ischemic ATP depletion, which aim to maintain cellular viability.[16] ^{11}C-palmitate is a labeled long-chain fatty acid that is esterified by thiokinase to ^{11}C-acyl-CoA and is trapped in the myocyte. ^{11}C-acyl-CoA then enters the intracellular lipid pool as ^{11}C-glyceride and ^{11}C-phospholipid or enters the mitochondria via the

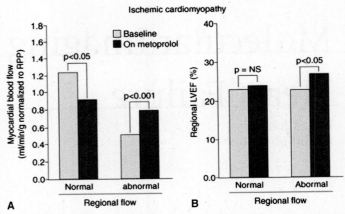

Figure 21.1 A,B: Quantitative PET flow measurements can be used to study the effects of 6 months of medical treatment with the β-blocker metoprolol on absolute myocardial blood flow and function in patients with ischemic cardiomyopathy. **A:** There is a favorable redistribution of absolute blood flow from normally perfused myocardium to abnormally perfused myocardium following metoprolol therapy. **B:** Increased myocardial blood flow is associated with an improvement in the regional left ventricular ejection fraction (LVEF) in the abnormally perfused regions of myocardium; myocardial regions with normal baseline perfusion show no change in regional LVEF. The reduction in blood flow in nonischemic regions by β blockade most probably reflects the reduction in myocardial oxygen demands induced by the reduction in myocardial contractility and work. On the other hand, the decrease in myocardial oxygen demand of the ischemic area by β blockade could restore vascular autoregulation and allow the ischemic vasculature to regulate its blood flow. By decreasing myocardial oxygen demand (decrease in heart rate) and increasing myocardial oxygen supply (increased subendocardial blood flow in ischemic myocardium), treatment with metoprolol results in an improvement in oxygen balance of the ischemic myocardium. (Adapted from Bennett SK, et al. Effect of metoprolol on absolute myocardial blood flow in patients with heart failure secondary to ischemic or nonischemic cardiomyopathy. *Am J Cardiol.* 2002;89(12):1431–1434.)

carnitine shuttle, where it is degraded by β-oxidation. Other PET tracers being assessed for comprehensive evaluation of myocardial metabolic activity include ^{11}C-glucose for assessment of glucose uptake and oxidation in the citric acid cycle and ^{11}C-acetate for determination of oxidative metabolism and oxygen consumption.[7]

Another interesting development in this area is the use of the radioiodine-labeled branched-chain fatty acid, β-methyl-p-[^{123}I]-iodophenyl-pentadecanoic acid (BMIPP), which enables assessment of fatty acid metabolism using SPECT technology. BMIPP is taken up by the myocyte and undergoes ATP-dependent thioesterification, but does not undergo significant mitochondrial β-oxidation.[15] As a result, BMIPP is trapped in the intracellular lipid pool. After a transient ischemic event, persistent and prolonged metabolic disturbances in fatty acid metabolism can occur for up to 30 h, termed "ischemic memory."[15] This metabolic stunning can be assessed by BMIPP and has been observed both among patients undergoing clinically indicated myocardial perfusion SPECT studies as well as in patients presenting with acute coronary syndrome.[12,15]

3.1.2. Imaging the renin-angiotensin system

The RAS is a proficient regulator of human physiology and is frequently activated early in HF. It is associated with LV remodeling and myocardial fibrosis through its primary effector peptide angiotensin II. An increase in angiotensin-converting enzyme

(ACE) has been seen in association with myocardial fibrosis and inhibition of RAS modulates LV remodeling in HF. It is now known that the various components of RAS are locally produced in the heart and that knowledge of the tissue expression of these enzymes and peptides could have important implications for the proper management of patients with HF.[8,17] The discovery of the tissue RAS and its ability for local production of effector hormones (autocrine effects) has encouraged the development of PET tracers targeting ACE.[18]

Two [18F]-radiolabeled ACE inhibitors have been reported thus far: [18F]-captopril (FCAP) and [18F]-fluorobenzoyl-lisinopril (FBL).[19] FBL is superior to FCAP for imaging tissue-bound ACE, owing to its higher affinity for tissue rather than plasma ACE. In an ex vivo study of explanted hearts of patients with ischemic cardiomyopathy, FBL was shown to specifically bind to tissue ACE with the highest activity in regions adjacent to infarcted myocardium (Fig. 21.2).[18] If reproduced in vivo, this imaging technique has the potential to enable tissue ACE activity to be monitored in HF.

The angiotensin II type 1 receptor (AT$_1$R) has also been shown to be an effective molecular target for labeling. A fluorescent-labeled and a [99mTc]-labeled AT$_1$R ligand peptide were studied in a murine model of acute myocardial infarction (MI).[20] Fluorescent AT$_1$R ligand was administered intravenously in mice with recent MI, followed by in vivo optical imaging by real-time fluorescence microscopy of the beating heart. Distinct dense uptake was observed in the infarct area at 1 to 6 weeks after infarction. The uptake was markedly reduced at 12 weeks in the infarct zone, but not in border zone regions adjacent to the infarct. Histological, immunohistochemical, and two-photon microscopy confirmed localization of the tracer within the myofibroblasts. Nuclear imaging, using microSPECT-CT, showed increased uptake of AT$_1$R ligand in the peri-infarct border zone as compared to remote regions.

3.1.3. Imaging myocardial autonomic innervation

HF is a hyperadrenergic state characterized by elevated plasma norepinephrine levels that, in turn, result in downregulation and uncoupling of cardiac β-adrenergic receptors. This leads to progressive impairment of LV systolic function by altering postsynaptic signal transduction. The altered sympathetic tone in HF is also directly linked to worsening of the disease and prognosis, with elevated risk of sudden death. Thus, noninvasive methods to determine the state of cardiac autonomic regulation are of great clinical interest.

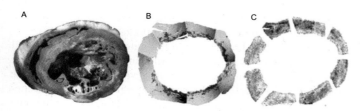

Figure 21.2 A–C: The presence and distribution of ACE activity in relation to collagen replacement in human heart tissue removed from a cardiac transplant recipient with ischemic cardiomyopathy. **A:** Gross pathology of a midventricular slice with corresponding contiguous midventricular slices **(B)** stained with Picrosirius red stain to assess collagen replacement and **(C)** autoradiographic images of the slice after labeling with [18F]fluorobenzyl-linsinopril (FBL). FBL binding to ACE is nonuniform in infarct, peri-infarct, remote, and noninfarct segments. Increased FBL binding can be seen in the segments adjacent to the collagen replacement. (Adapted from Dilsizian V, et al. Evidence for tissue angiotensin-converting enzyme in explanted hearts of ischemic cardiomyopathy using targeted radiotracer technique. *J Nucl Med.* 2007;48(2):182–187.)

Investigators in several studies have demonstrated that [123I]-metaiodobenzylguanidine (MIBG) imaging can provide powerful diagnostic and prognostic information in patients with HF. MIBG competes with norepinephrine for reuptake in presynaptic vesicles (Fig. 21.3A) and has been successfully used to study cardiac presynaptic sympathetic innervations. In patients with HF, MIBG scans typically show a reduced heart-mediastinum uptake ratio, heterogeneous distribution within the myocardium, and increased MIBG washout from the heart[21-23] (Fig. 21.3B and C). For example, Arimoto et al.[24] demonstrated that patients with abnormally rapid washout levels had a significantly higher cardiac event rate than did those with normal washout levels (57% vs. 12%, $p < 0.0001$) during a follow-up period of 6 to 30 months. Kyuma et al.[25] showed incremental prognostic levels when the plasma brain natriuretic peptide level and the heart-mediastinum uptake ratio were used together. More importantly, in a pilot study, Arora et al.[26] demonstrated that patients with implantable cardioverter defibrillator (ICD) discharge had a substantially lower MIBG heart-mediastinum tracer uptake ratio, higher MIBG defect scores, and more extensive sympathetic denervation. Clearly, larger studies are needed in the future. Development of this modality to assess the cardiac autonomic state may help identify patients who would most significantly benefit from an ICD by identifying those at increased risk for potentially fatal arrhythmias thus allowing a more cost-effective implementation of ICDs.

3.2. Imaging in cardiac gene therapy

Gene transfer is one of the most promising aspects of molecular medicine in the 21st century. It is characterized by the transfer to and expression of DNA in somatic cells in an individual with resultant therapeutic effects. In cardiovascular disease, gene therapy can enable the expression of therapeutic factors in the myocardium.[27] Successful application of gene therapy is composed of at least three elements: (a) the proper vector for gene delivery, (b) delivery method of the vector to the target tissue, and (c) a gene with therapeutic efficacy being expressed in a specific patient population.

The ideal vector should be able to efficiently deliver a specific gene to a target tissue while minimizing local and systemic toxicity, delivering a sufficient concentration with the proper duration to induce a therapeutic change, and avoiding germ line transmission to offspring. No single vector has all of these attributes as yet, and thus the type of vector chosen needs to be tailored to the specific clinical application. Vectors can either be viral or nonviral vectors. The common viral vectors include adenovirus, adeno-associated virus, gutless adenovirus, and lentivirus. Nonviral vectors can be liposomes, plasmids, and naked DNA.[28] Techniques of vector delivery to the myocardium include (a) direct epicardial injection, (b) endocardial injection, (c) intracoronary infusion, (d) retrograde coronary sinus infusion, and (e) pericardial injection.[29]

A variety of therapeutic genes have been utilized for expression in the heart depending on the intended application. In animal trials, successful gene therapy has been demonstrated for the following: (a) treatment of CAD by using angiogenic factors such as vascular endothelial growth factor (VEGF),[30] fibroblast growth factor (FGF),[31] and hypoxia-inducible factor 1α[32]; (b) reduction of restenosis postangioplasty through inhibition of smooth muscle cell proliferation with suicide gene therapy using thymidine kinase[33]; (c) improvement of congestive HF with gene transfer of a calcium adenosine triphosphatase pump (SERCA2a)[34]; (d) inhibition of atherosclerosis with overexpression of a high-density lipoprotein receptor[35]; (e) reduction of hypoxia-induced apoptosis of cardiomyocytes[36]; and (f) reactivation of the cardiomyocyte

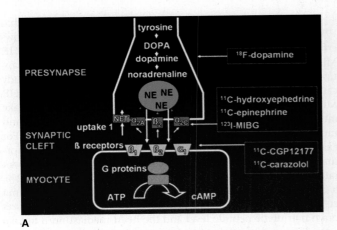

A

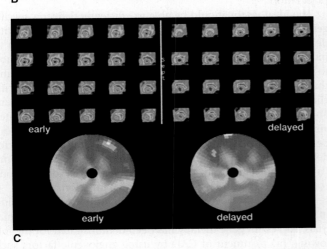

B

C

Figure 21.3 A–C: ^{123}I-MIBG imaging in patients with HF. **A:** Schematic shows most commonly used radioligands for assessment of cardiac presynaptic and postsynaptic processes. **B:** SPECT MIBG study in healthy volunteer. Short-axis tomograms and reconstructed polar maps show normal MIBG distribution and washout. **C:** SPECT MIBG study in patient with dilated cardiomyopathy. Short-axis tomograms and reconstructed polar maps show decreased and heterogeneous myocardial MIBG activity. ATP, adenosine triphosphate; DOPA, dihydroxyphenylalanine; cAMP, cyclic adenosine monophosphate; NE, norepinephrine. (Reproduced from Carrio I. Cardiac neurotransmission imaging. *J Nucl Med.* 2001;42(7):1062–1076, with permission.)

cell cycle utilizing cyclin A2 with subsequent restoration of cardiac function following MI.[37]

These initial encouraging results in animals have led to the initiation of several clinical trials. There are ~500 ongoing gene therapy trials in the United States and at least 46 of these have cardiovascular applications.[38] The bulk of these studies are aimed at testing safety and efficacy of angiogenic agents and, to a lesser extent, factors that prevent restenosis. During the 1990s, several phase 1 open-label trials that involved small numbers of patients with myocardial ischemia and peripheral arterial disease yielded positive results.[39–41] However, phase 2 randomized, double-blind, placebo-controlled trials have yielded conflicting and sometimes disappointing results. Gene therapy trials utilizing either VEGF or FGF have failed to show any consistent improvement in various parameters, such as symptoms, ejection fraction, wall motion scores, myocardial perfusion, and restenosis rate.[42–46]

There are, however, important lessons to be learned from these trials. They have shown that angiogenesis is a complex process regulated by the intersection of various growth factors and may be difficult to be induced by using a single protein or gene. The ideal injection method, delivery vector, and patient population remain to be defined. There is a continued need to determine the pharmacokinetics and pharmacodynamics of therapeutic gene expression so that gene therapy can proceed further to widespread clinical use, and this process is similar to that of the research and development of experimental drugs.

An ongoing human clinical trial investigating gene therapy to target the dysfunctional cardiomyocyte in HF is yielding promising initial results.[47] The Calcium Up-Regulation by Percutaneous Administration of Gene Therapy in Cardiac Disease (CUPID) study utilizes gene transfer of SERCA2a, a major cardiac calcium cycling protein, via an adeno-associated viral (AAV) vector. AAV is derived from a nonpathogenic virus with long-term transgene expression as well as clinically established favorable safety profile. Thus far, even though each cohort is too small to conduct statistical analyses, clinically significant meaningful improvements in functional status and/or cardiac function were observed in most subjects receiving AAV1/SERCA2a.

Recent developments in the field of gene therapy such as directed evolution[48] to produce vectors that can transduce specific cell types offer much greater specificity in targeting approaches, therefore significantly lowering toxicity and other unwanted side effects.

In all gene therapy trials thus far, as there is no accurate method of assessing gene expression in vivo, investigators are unable to determine whether the lack of symptomatic improvement is due to poor injection technique, insufficient gene expression, the host inflammatory response, or an inappropriate candidate gene.[49]

Most molecular imaging studies to date have been conducted in the field of cancer biology.[50,51] Imaging of cardiac transgene expression has been established in several proof-of-principle studies that involved the injection of various reporter genes into the myocardium with assessment of kinetics of transgene expression over time through the use of optical bioluminescence, micro-PET, and clinical PET imaging.[52–56] The concept of imaging reporter-gene expression (Fig. 21.4) involves a reporter gene that is introduced into the target tissue through either viral or nonviral vectors. The promoter region that regulates the transcription of the reporter gene can be constitutive (always on), inducible (able to be turned on or off), or tissue specific (expressed only in target tissue). Once the reporter gene is transcribed and the mRNA has been translated into a reporter protein product, this reporter protein can interact with the reporter probe. This interaction may be mediated by an enzyme (i.e., phosphorylation

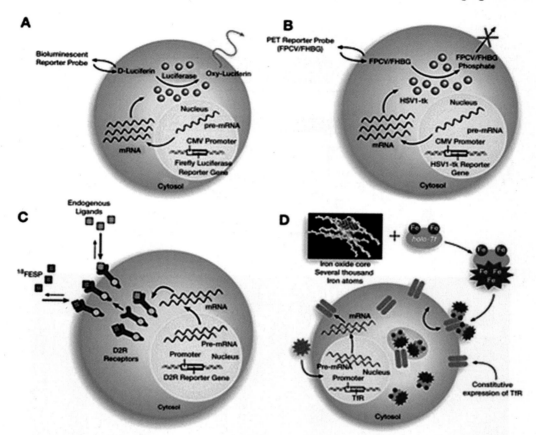

Figure 21.4 A–D: Four strategies of imaging reporter gene and reporter probe. **A:** Enzyme-based bioluminescence imaging. Expression of the firefly luciferase reporter gene leads to the firefly luciferase reporter enzyme, which catalyzes the reporter probe (D-luciferin) that results in a photochemical reaction. This yields low levels of photons that can be detected and quantified by a charge-coupled device camera. **B:** Enzyme-based PET imaging. Expression of the herpes simplex virus type 1 thymidine kinase (HSV1-tk) reporter gene leads to the thymidine kinase reporter enzyme, HSV1-TK, which phosphorylates and traps the PET reporter probe 9-(4-[^{18}F]fluoro-3-hydroxymethylbutyl)guanine (FHBG) intracellularly. Radioactive decay of ^{18}F isotopes can be detected with PET. **C:** Receptor-based PET imaging. 3-(2-[^{18}F]fluoroethyl) spiperone (^{18}FESP) is a reporter probe that interacts with the dopamine 2 receptor (D2R) to result in probe trapping on or in cells expressing the D2R gene. **D:** Receptor-based MRI. Overexpression of engineered transferrin receptor (TfR) results in increased cell uptake of the transferrin-monocrystalline iron oxide nanoparticles. These changes result in a detectable contrast change on MR image. FPCV, 8-[^{18}F]fluoropenciclovir, holo-Tf, holo-transferrin. (Reproduced from Wu JC, Tseng JR, Gambhir SS. Molecular imaging of cardiovascular gene products. *J Nucl Cardiol.* 2004;11(4):491–505, with permission.)

of a reporter probe with intracellular trapping of metabolites) or a receptor (i.e., binding of a radio-labeled ligand to cell surface receptors).[28] There is quite a degree of flexibility within these systems. By altering various components, the reporter gene can provide information about efficiency of gene transfer into cells, regulation of DNA by promoters, and the patterns of intracellular protein trafficking. Additionally, the reporter probe itself need not be altered if one wishes to study a different biological process altogether, and this may save valuable time in synthesizing and validating new radiotracer agents.

Two studies have demonstrated the feasibility of linking a PET reporter gene to a therapeutic gene.[57,58] In this approach, an adenovirus with two constitutive cytomegalovirus (CMV) promoters driving a $VEGF_{121}$ therapeutic gene and an $HSV1$-$sr39tk$ PET reporter gene separated by polyadenine sequences was constructed (Ad-CMV-VEGF$_{121}$-CMV-HSV1-sr39tk) (Fig. 21.5A). Wu et al.[53] injected the construct into the rat myocardium in an MI model. Reporter gene expression, which indirectly reflects the $VEGF_{121}$ therapeutic gene expression, persisted for only ~2 weeks because of host immune response against the adenovirus. At 2 months, there was no substantial improvement in myocardial contractility, perfusion,

or metabolism as measured using echocardiography, ^{13}N ammonia perfusion, and FDG imaging between study and control groups (Fig. 21.5B). Thus, this study underscores the importance of monitoring the pharmacokinetics of gene expression. It also demonstrates the proof of principle that any other cardiac therapeutic genes of interest (i.e., hypoxia-inducible factor 1α, SERCA2a, heat shock protein, or endothelial nitric oxide synthase) can likewise be coupled to a PET reporter gene for noninvasive monitoring.

In future studies, the following features would be helpful additions to the arsenal of cardiac gene therapy: (a) less immunogenic vectors such as adeno-associated virus that can prolong gene expression in the heart; (b) vectors that are specifically able to transduce a given cell type; (c) cardiac tissue-specific promoters (i.e., troponin or myosin light chain kinase) to diminish unwanted extracardiac expression; (d) joint delivery of proangiogenic genes with stem cells to enhance revascularization; (e) delivery of myogenic genes with or without stem cells to induce therapeutic myogenesis; and (f) multimodality molecular imaging approaches that can monitor the location, magnitude, and duration of transgene expression, along with their downstream functional effects.[28,49]

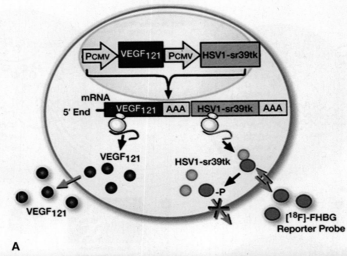

A

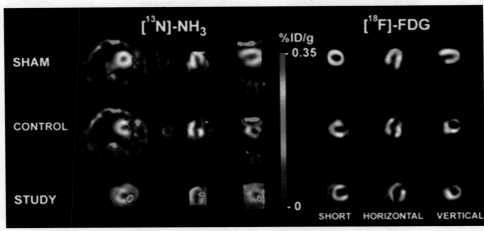

B

Figure 21.5 A,B: Molecular imaging of cardiac perfusion, metabolism, and gene expression. **A:** Schematic of Ad-CMV-VEGF$_{121}$-CMV-HSV1-sr39tk mediated gene expression. The translated product of *VEGF$_{121}$* is soluble and excreted extracellularly, whereas the translated product of *HSV1-sr39tk* (HSV1-sr39TK) traps FHBG intracellularly by phosphorylation. P$_{CMV}$, CMV promoter. **B:** At day 2, representative images showing normal perfusion ([^{13}N]–NH$_3$) and metabolism (FDG) in a sham rat, anterolateral infarction in a control rat, and anterolateral infarction in a study rat (Ad-CMV-VEGF$_{121}$-CMV-HSV1-sr39tk) in short, vertical, and horizontal axes (gray scale). The color scale is expressed as percentage injected dose per gram (%ID/g) for FHBG uptake. Only the study rat showed robust *HSV1-sr39tk* reporter gene activity near the site of injection. (Reproduced from Wu JC, et al. Molecular imaging of the kinetics of vascular endothelial growth factor gene expression in ischemic myocardium. *Circulation*. 2004;110(6):685–691, with permission.)

3.3. Imaging in stem cell transplantation

It is widely agreed that the regenerative capacity of the human heart is clinically inadequate to compensate for the severe loss of myocardial mass that is noted in catastrophic MI or other myocardial diseases. Laboratory experiments and some recent clinical trials suggest that cell-based therapies can improve cardiac function, and the implications of these studies are causing great excitement with regard to cardiac regeneration. Bone marrow-derived progenitor cells and other progenitor cells can differentiate into vascular cell types, restoring blood flow. More recently, endogenous cardiac stem cells have been shown to differentiate into multiple cell types present in the heart, including cardiomyocytes. These findings are generating optimism that the progression to HF can potentially be prevented or even reversed with cell-based therapy (CBT). The current constituents of the stem and progenitor cell (SPCs) pool are quite diverse: bone marrow, peripheral blood, fat, skeletal and cardiac muscle, embryonic tissue, and more recently, induced pluripotent cells which are adult cells that have been subjected to molecular "reprogramming" back to a pluripotent cell.[59,60]

Clinical trials in cardiac CBT have exploited the underlying assumption that repopulation of infarcted myocardium can be achieved with stem cells. Studies have thus far focused on chronic HF or acute MI (Table 21.1). The bulk of incoming clinical evidence has indicated that CBT shows promise for myocardial repair in terms of improving structure and function.[61] Nonetheless, ongoing debate regarding specifics in regard to CBT has highlighted important unresolved questions: whether different cell types are required according to type of injury and time since injury; clarification of the underlying mechanisms in trans-differentiation, angiogenesis, paracrine effects, and resident cardiac stem cell activation; how to achieve functional engraftment (including electromechanical coupling with surrounding myocardium and

TABLE 21.1
RANDOMIZED CLINICAL TRIALS IN CARDIAC CBT

Trial	No of patients	Main cardiovascular characteristic	Cell types and numbers	Duration of follow-up (months)	Reported effects
Congestive heart failure					
TOPCARE-CHD; Assmus et al. (2006)[91]	75	EF < 35%	Unfractionated BMMNCs and CPCs: 2.2×10^8	3	↑Global LVEF, BMMNCs > CPCs = control
MAGIC; Menasché et al. (2006)[92]	97	EF < 35%	Skeletal myoblasts: high dose 8×10^8; low dose 4×10^8	6	No change in global LVEF, ↓LV remodeling, no proarrhythmia (all had ICDs)
Acute MI					
BOOST; Wallert et al. (2004)[93]	60	5 days after STEMI	Unfractionated BMMNCs: 2.5×10^9	18	↑Global LVEF at 6 months, no difference at 18 months
Janssens et al. (2006)[94]	67	1 day after STEMI	Unfractionated BMMNCs: 3.0×10^8	4	↓Infarct size, no change in global LVEF
ASTAMI; Lunde et al. (2006)[95]	100	6 days after STEMI	Unfractionated BMMNCs: 7.0×10^7	6	No change in global LVEF
REPAIR-AMI; Schachinger et al. (2006)[96]	204	5 days after STEMI	Unfractionated BMMNCs: 2.4×10^8	12	↑Global LVEF

Menashé P, Alfieri O, Janssens S, et al. The myoblast autologous grafting in ischemic cardiomyopathy (MAGIC) trial: first randomized placebo-controlled study of myoblast transplantation. *Circulation.* 2008;117(9):1189–1200.
BMMNC, bone-marrow-derived mononuclear cell; CPC, circulating progenitor cell; EF, ejection fraction; ICD, implantable cardioverter-defibrillator; LV, left ventricular; LVEF, left ventricular ejection fraction; STEMI, ST-segment elevation myocardial infarction.
Source: Adapted from Ly HQ, Frangioni JV, Hajjar RJ. Imaging in cardiac cell-based therapy: In vivo tracking of the biological fate of therapeutic cells. *Nat Clin Pract Cardiovasc Med.* 2008;5(Suppl. 2):S96–S102.

SPC retention and survival); and the need to fully understand the adverse effects of the therapy such as immunogenicity, arrhythmogenesis, and tumorigenicity. While the route of delivery for SPCs might affect cell distribution during administration, other phenomena such as cell recirculation, homing, or cell death will ultimately affect stem cell spread and engraftment. The ability to detect signal from appropriately labeled SPCs will also be affected, thus influencing the ability to track outcomes.

It is becoming clear to physicians and scientists that parallel developments in cell-based therapies and in vivo imaging modalities will reinforce the clinical gains to be made in this exciting field. In this section, we discuss the advantages and inherent shortcomings of various imaging techniques.

3.3.1. In vivo molecular and cellular imaging of CBT
In order to make CBT more feasible, the fate of SPCs needs to be closely examined. A more rigorous understanding of the scientific and mechanistic underpinnings will likely lead to more consistent results in clinical trials.[62,63] There is a definitive need for noninvasive in vivo imaging modalities that allow accurate and serial assessment of CBT. The ideal modality would utilize high-affinity probes that can safely interact with biologic tissues (i.e., vascular and cellular membranes) and exhibit a high degree of sensitivity for the detection of cell fate in terms of survival, apoptosis, proliferation, differentiation, or fusion. Conventional imaging modalities allow objective assessment of structural (chamber size and area of scar) and functional (flow, perfusion, and contractility) parameters. In vivo

imaging can track the biological fate of SPCs by targeting fundamental cellular processes within specific microenvironments.

Imaging reporter genes. As described above, reporter gene insertion achieves stable transfection of target tissues with the gene product (enzymes, receptors, or transporters), which can be activated by exposure of an imaging probe. Activation catalyzes an enzymatic reaction that results in emission of an intracellular imaging signal. Reporter genes are minimally affected by physiological processes. As described in the section on cardiac gene therapy above, adenovirus has been utilized to target the expression of herpes simplex virus type 1 mutant thymidine kinase (*HSV1-sr39tk*) in pioneering studies that highlight the usefulness of this kind of molecular imaging.[52] High numbers of cells can be visualized on optical imaging (5×10^5 transfected cells).[64]

Serial visualization of transgene expression would reliably track cell viability (constitutive expression of the reporter gene product would occur only in viable cells), proliferation (reporter genes undergo chromosomal integration and are passed on with each cellular division), and differentiation (restrictive promoters sensitive to endogenous molecules only active in mature cells can provide information on differentiation pathways). Additional advantages are cardiac specificity through the use of cardiac promoter sequences such as myosin light chain kinase 2, troponin T, or a myosin heavy chain which would render posttranscriptional gene expression limited to cardiac cells.[65,66] Newer generation viral vectors derived through directed evolution[48] allow the transduction of specific cell types, thus greatly enhancing control over the targeting of gene expression.

The use of reporter genes in SPC tracking has notable limitations as well. Adenoviral vectors only provide transient transgene expression. Other vector systems such as lentivirus or retrovirus provide sustained transfection but are associated with the risk of insertional mutagenesis. There remain questions regarding the robustness of the signal as the detected signal could reflect the magnitude of transgene expression instead of cell survival. Additionally, concerns remain about host immune reactions or disturbances of cellular homeostasis.

3.3.2. Optical imaging

Optical imaging relies on two complementary imaging methods: bioluminescence and fluorescence. The former detects light at wavelengths of 400 to 700 nm generated by the enzymatic reaction catalyzed by firefly luciferase. However, the need to inject nonhuman, immunogenic substrates (D-luciferin and coelenterazine) and the high absorption and scatter of emitted light in living tissue preclude the use of bioluminescence in clinical applications. Conversely, fluorescence optical imaging uses organic (green fluorescence protein, polymethamines) or organic/hybrid (quantum dots) contrast agents. Two promising fluorescence modalities are near-infrared fluorescence and quantum dot optical imaging.

Near-infrared fluorophores are visible at wavelengths 700 to 1000 nm, have low absorption, and scatter photons at visible wavelengths.[67] This technique offers high sensitivity tomographic imaging and versatility; it is well-suited for single-cell-level detection by conventional microscopy[68] and large animal disease models.[69,70] Two major limitations are: tissue penetration is only 4 to 10 cm, although "stealth" near-infrared fluorescent probes might allow deep-tissue visualization[71]; and fluorophore dilution, which arises from cell division and following cell death, from uptake by non-SPCs such as macrophages.

Quantum dots comprise nanometer-sized fluorescent particles coupled to cellular or molecular probes and possess several characteristics rendering them ideal tracers relative to other organic fluorescent probes. These include resistance to photo-bleaching, a broad excitation spectrum (greater sensitivity), good signal stability, and suitability for longitudinal assessment, because they are not susceptible to chemical degradation within the cell.[72] This method of optical imaging is feasible in vivo as efforts to conjugate quantum dots to endothelial progenitor cells[73] and embryonic stem cells[74] have been successful without compromise of cellular survival and proliferation.

3.3.3. Radionuclide imaging

Although radionuclide imaging is routinely used for the assessment of myocardial viability and metabolism, nuclear imaging agents are well suited to track SPCs. Their use can be extended to biological processes such as cell homing, engraftment, and extracellular matrix activation because of their high sensitivity (10^{-11} to 10^{-12} pmol/l).[75]

In single-photon emission CT (SPECT), a rotating collimated γ camera is used to detect high-energy γ-ray emission. PET detects γ rays emitted after positron annihilation. Overall, PET is more sensitive than SPECT because of the use of higher-energy photons, coincident detection, and greater detector efficiency. Tracers used for direct labeling of cells in radionuclide imaging include ^{111}In-labeled oxine, [99m]Te-labeled hexamethylprophylene amine oxine (HMPAO), and ^{18}F-labeled fluorodeoxyglucose (FDG). Cell labeling can be achieved in the following ways: direct loading with the radioactive agent; enzymatic conversation and retention of a radioactive substrate; or receptor-mediated binding. With ^{111}In oxine cell labeling, up to ~10,000 cells could be detectable.[76] Use of radiolabeled probes offers high labeling efficiency, high signal-to-noise ratio, accurate cell quantification, correlation with cell viability, monitoring of cell differentiation, and more sensitive tracking of progenitor stem cell number.[77]

Despite advances such as hybrid systems that combine CT and PET/SPECT, tracking of radioisotope-labeled SPCs has limitations (radiation exposure notwithstanding). Nonspecific tracer uptake by normal tissue, as well as photon attenuation by tissue, can reduce sensitivity and, more importantly, limit quantification of cells. Detection at the single-cell level remains a significant technical challenge as it is still difficult to concentrate radioactive agents in SPCs.[78] Alterations in cell function and proliferation of transplanted cells have not been fully elucidated and need to be carefully ascertained. Finally, long-term tracking remains a challenge due to the short half-life of currently available radioisotopes, leading to loss of signal.

3.3.4. Magnetic resonance imaging

In vivo MRI tracking is feasible due to unparalleled three-dimensional, whole-body capabilities and innovative direct labeling techniques that provide near cellular level resolution (25 to 50 μm). Novel agents such as gadolinium-based or superparamagnetic-iron-oxide (SPIO)-based agents can be internalized and provide signal amplification detectable by T1 (longitudinal relaxation rate) or T2/T2* (transverse relaxation rate) contrast.

Labeling is achieved via endogenous membrane mechanisms (endocytosis or pinocytosis) or by use of transfection agents (poly-L-lysine, protamine sulfate, lipofectamine), facilitating internalization for cells lacking such mechanisms.[79] The ratio of particle size to uptake for internalization of the contrast agent is a determining stem for signal emission from labeled cells. The emission level will ultimately influence the lower threshold of detectability.[80] According to preclinical data, with the use of MRI, the minimum detectable numbers of SPCs implanted are 10^5 with MPIO[81] and 10^8 with superparamagnetic iron oxide (USPIO).[82]

Direct labeling of stem cells with gadolinium-based agents creates an inherently high detection threshold as well as requirement of bulky scaffolds to increase the T1 effect. T2/T2* contrast agents are more widely used. In preclinical studies, in vivo detection and localization of MRI signal from labeled stem cells (i.e., embryonic stem cells[83] and mesenchymal stem cells[84]) have correlated with histopathological assessment. Current formulations of the superparamagnetic agents are biocompatible, safe, and nontoxic. Newer magnetic nanoparticles could offer important advantages for MRI analysis in studies of cardiac CBT. Conjugating a cross-linked iron oxide to the Tat protein (involved in membrane translocation signal of HIV) generates a contrast agent that has good magnetic and fluorescence labeling capacity and efficiency, strong signal emission or relaxivity, and lack of immunogenicity.[85,86] From a clinical perspective, MRI has a clear advantage over other modalities as it is able to obtain serial assessments of cardiac structure, function and perfusion with real-time MRI-guided delivery devices, and to enable monitoring of labeled SPCs.[87]

While high spatial resolution remains one of its strengths, MRI also has limitations.[88] It is the least sensitive imaging modality regarding detection of tracers as compared to radionuclide and optical imaging.[89] This low sensitivity is in part due to contrast agent transfer to non-SPCs (such as macrophages) following cell death. Concerns have been expressed over effects of iron oxide compounds on SPC differentiation.

Antibody nanoparticles of iron dextran beads show promise as imaging probes, having both ease of labeling (through cell surface interaction) and no reported untoward effects on cellular activity, although persistence of the probe following cell death remains problematic.[90] There are a number of issues of quantitation that need to be resolved. These include signal dilution from cell division, problematic correlation between signal intensity and cell number due to variable intracellular iron oxide uptake, and detection at the single-cell level being hindered by cardiac motion.

4. FUTURE DIRECTIONS

Currently, most of the imaging techniques discussed in this chapter have been used as research tools. Several trials, however, are being conducted to study their applications in the clinical setting. Preliminary results suggest that MIBG may be a useful clinical tool to identify HF patients at risk for cardiac events. The results of these studies could lead to the use of this test to identify patients who may benefit from automated implantable cardioverter defibrillator (AICD) implantation.

As gene therapy and cell transplantation become accepted therapeutic strategies, imaging will be needed to direct therapy and to monitor response. Advances in both hardware and molecular imaging probes will help to advance this promising field in the future.

REFERENCES

1. Hunt SA, Baker DW, Chin MH, et al. ACC/AHA guidelines for the evaluation and management of chronic heart failure in the adult: Executive summary. A report of the American College of Cardiology/American Heart Association Task Force on Practice Guidelines (Committee to revise the 1995 Guidelines for the Evaluation and Management of Heart Failure). *J Am Coll Cardiol.* 2001;38(7):2101–2113.
2. Massie BM, Shah NB. Evolving trends in the epidemiologic factors of heart failure: Rationale for preventive strategies and comprehensive disease management. *Am Heart J.* 1997;133(6):703–712.
3. Haldeman GA, Croft JB, Giles WH, et al. Hospitalization of patients with heart failure: National Hospital Discharge Survey, 1985 to 1995. *Am Heart J.* 1999;137(2):352–360.
4. American Heart News. Available at: www.americanheart.org.
5. Rose EA. A new continuous-flow LV assist device for patients with end-stage heart failure. *Nat Clin Pract Cardiovasc Med.* 2008;5(2):80–81.
6. Buja LM, Vela D. Cardiomyocyte death and renewal in the normal and diseased heart. *Cardiovasc Pathol.* 2008;17(6):349–374.
7. Shirani J, Narula J, Eckelman WC, et al. Early imaging in heart failure: Exploring novel molecular targets. *J Nucl Cardiol.* 2007;14(1):100–110.
8. Shirani J, Narula J, Eckelman WC, et al. Novel imaging strategies for predicting remodeling and evolution of heart failure: Targeting the Renin-Angiotensin system. *Heart Fail Clin.* 2006;2(2):231–247.
9. Jaffer FA, Weissleder R. Seeing within: Molecular imaging of the cardiovascular system. *Circ Res.* 2004;94(4):433–445.
10. Jaffer FA, Libby P, Weissleder R. Molecular imaging of cardiovascular disease. *Circulation.* 2007;116(9):1052–1061.
11. Bertomeu-Gonzalez V, Bouzas-Mosquera A, Kaski JC. Role of trimetazidine in management of ischemic cardiomyopathy. *Am J Cardiol.* 2006;98(5A):19J–24J.
12. Kawai Y, Tsukamoto E, Nozaki Y, et al. Significance of reduced uptake of iodinated fatty acid analogue for the evaluation of patients with acute chest pain. *J Am Coll Cardiol.* 2001;38(7):1888–1894.
13. Stanley WC, Recchia FA, Lopaschuk GD. Myocardial substrate metabolism in the normal and failing heart. *Physiol Rev.* 2005;85(3):1093–1129.
14. Bennett SK, Smith MF, Gottlieb SS, et al. Effect of metoprolol on absolute myocardial blood flow in patients with heart failure secondary to ischemic or nonischemic cardiomyopathy. *Am J Cardiol.* 2002;89(12):1431–1434.
15. Dilsizian V, Bateman TM, Bergmann SR, et al. Metabolic imaging with β-methyl-p-[^{123}I]-iodophenyl-pentadecanoic acid identifies ischemic memory after demand ischemia. *Circulation.* 2005;112(14):2169–2174.
16. Young LH, Li J, Baron SJ, et al. AMP-activated protein kinase: A key stress signaling pathway in the heart. *Trends Cardiovasc Med.* 2005;15(3):110–118.
17. Paul M, Poyan Mehr A, Kreutz R. Physiology of local renin-angiotensin systems. *Physiol Rev.* 2006;86(3):747–803.
18. Dilsizian V, Eckelman WC, Loredo ML, et al. Evidence for tissue angiotensin-converting enzyme in explanted hearts of ischemic cardiomyopathy using targeted radiotracer technique. *J Nucl Cardiol.* 2007;48(2):182–187.
19. Hwang DR, Eckelman WC, Mathias CJ, et al. Positron-labeled angiotensin-converting enzyme (ACE) inhibitor: Fluorine-18-fluorocaptopril. Probing the ACE activity in vivo by positron emission tomography. *J Nucl Med.* 1991;32(9):1730–1737.
20. van den Borne SW, Isobe S, Verjans JW, et al. Molecular imaging of interstitial alterations in remodeling myocardium after myocardial infarction. *J Am Coll Cardiol.* 2008;52(24):2017–2028.
21. Carrio I. Cardiac neurotransmission imaging. *J Nucl Med.* 2001;42(7):1062–1076.
22. Henderson EB, Kahn JK, Corbett JR, et al. Abnormal I-123 metaiodobenzylguanidine myocardial washout and distribution may reflect myocardial adrenergic derangement in patients with congestive cardiomyopathy. *Circulation.* 1988;78(5 Pt 1):1192–1199.
23. Schofer J, Spielmann R, Schuchert A, et al. Iodine-123 meta-iodobenzylguanidine scintigraphy: A noninvasive method to demonstrate myocardial adrenergic nervous system disintegrity in patients with idiopathic dilated cardiomyopathy. *J Am Coll Cardiol.* 1988;12(5):1252–1258.
24. Arimoto T, Takeishi Y, Fukui A, et al. Dynamic 123I-MIBG SPECT reflects sympathetic nervous integrity and predicts clinical outcome in patients with chronic heart failure. *Ann Nucl Med.* 2004;18(2):145–150.
25. Kyuma M, Nakata T, Hashimoto A, et al. Incremental prognostic implications of brain natriuretic peptide, cardiac sympathetic nerve innervation, and noncardiac disorders in patients with heart failure. *J Nucl Med.* 2004;45(2):155–163.
26. Arora R, Ferrick KJ, Nakata T, et al. I-123 MIBG imaging and heart rate variability analysis to predict the need for an implantable cardioverter defibrillator. *J Nucl Cardiol.* 2003;10(2):121–131.
27. Wu JC, Yla-Herttuala S. Human gene therapy and imaging: Cardiology. *Eur J Nucl Med Mol Imaging.* 2005;32(Suppl. 2):S346–S357.
28. Wu JC, Tseng JR, Gambhir SS. Molecular imaging of cardiovascular gene products. *J Nucl Cardiol.* 2004;11(4):491–505.
29. Yla-Herttuala S, Alitalo K. Gene transfer as a tool to induce therapeutic vascular growth. *Nat Med.* 2003;9(6):694–701.
30. Takeshita S, Pu LQ, Stein LA, et al. Intramuscular administration of vascular endothelial growth factor induces dose-dependent collateral artery augmentation in a rabbit model of chronic limb ischemia. *Circulation.* 1994;90(5 Pt 2):II228–II234.
31. Brogi E, Wu T, Namiki A, et al. Indirect angiogenic cytokines upregulate VEGF and bFGF gene expression in vascular smooth muscle cells, whereas hypoxia upregulates VEGF expression only. *Circulation.* 1994;90(2):649–652.
32. Shyu KG, Wang MT, Wang BW, et al. Intramyocardial injection of naked DNA encoding HIF-1alpha/VP16 hybrid to enhance angiogenesis in an acute myocardial infarction model in the rat. *Cardiovasc Res.* 2002;54(3):576–583.
33. Steg PG, Tahlil O, Aubailly N, et al. Reduction of restenosis after angioplasty in an atheromatous rabbit model by suicide gene therapy. *Circulation.* 1997;96(2):408–411.
34. Miyamoto MI, del Monte F, Schmidt U, et al. Adenoviral gene transfer of SERCA2a improves left-ventricular function in aortic-banded rats in transition to heart failure. *Proc Natl Acad Sci USA.* 2000;97(2):793–798.
35. Kozarsky KF, Donahee MH, Glick JM, et al. Gene transfer and hepatic overexpression of the HDL receptor SR-BI reduces atherosclerosis in the cholesterol-fed LDL receptor-deficient mouse. *Arterioscler Thromb Vasc Biol.* 2000;20(3):721–727.
36. Matsui T, Li L, del Monte F, et al. Adenoviral gene transfer of activated phosphatidylinositol 3′-kinase and Akt inhibits apoptosis of hypoxic cardiomyocytes in vitro. *Circulation.* 1999;100(23):2373–2379.
37. Woo YJ, Panlilio CM, Cheng RK, et al. Therapeutic delivery of cyclin A2 induces myocardial regeneration and enhances cardiac function in ischemic heart failure. *Circulation.* 2006;114(Suppl. 1):I206–I213.
38. National Institutes of Health Office of Biotechnology Advances. Clinical trials in human gene transfer: Query of clinical trials. Available at: http://www4.od.nih.gov/oba/rac/trialquery/index.asp.
39. Rosengart TK, Lee LY, Patel SR, et al. Angiogenesis gene therapy: Phase I assessment of direct intramyocardial administration of an adenovirus vector expressing VEGF121 cDNA to individuals with clinically significant severe coronary artery disease. *Circulation.* 1999;100(5):468–474.
40. Symes JF, Losordo DW, Vale PR, et al. Gene therapy with vascular endothelial growth factor for inoperable coronary artery disease. *Ann Thorac Surg.* 1999;68(3):830–836, discussion 836–837.
41. Vale PR, Losordo DW, Milliken CE, et al. Left ventricular electromechanical mapping to assess efficacy of phVEGF(165) gene transfer for therapeutic angiogenesis in chronic myocardial ischemia. *Circulation.* 2000;102(9):965–974.
42. Henry TD, Annex BH, McKendall GR, et al. The VIVA trial: Vascular endothelial growth factor in ischemia for vascular angiogenesis. *Circulation.* 2003;107(10):1359–1365.
43. Simons M, Annex BH, Laham RJ, et al. Pharmacological treatment of coronary artery disease with recombinant fibroblast growth factor-2: Double-blind, randomized, controlled clinical trial. *Circulation.* 2002;105(7):788–793.
44. Grines CL, Watkins MW, Mahmarian JJ, et al. A randomized, double-blind, placebo-controlled trial of Ad5FGF-4 gene therapy and its effect on myocardial perfusion in patients with stable angina. *J Am Coll Cardiol.* 2003;42(8):1339–1347.
45. Grines CL, Watkins MW, Helmer G, et al. Angiogenic Gene Therapy (AGENT) trial in patients with stable angina pectoris. *Circulation.* 2002;105(11):1291–1297.
46. Hedman M, Hartikainen J, Syvanne M, et al. Safety and feasibility of catheter-based local intracoronary vascular endothelial growth factor gene transfer in the prevention of postangioplasty and in-stent restenosis and in the treatment of chronic myocardial ischemia: Phase II results of the Kuopio Angiogenesis Trial (KAT). *Circulation.* 2003;107(21):2677–2683.
47. Jaski BE, Jessup ML, Mancini DM, et al. Calcium upregulation by percutaneous administration of gene therapy in cardiac disease (CUPID Trial), a first-in-human phase 1/2 clinical trial. *J Card Fail.* 2009;15(3):171–181.

48. Li W, Asokan A, Wu Z, et al. Engineering and selection of shuffled AAV genomes: A new strategy for producing targeted biological nanoparticles. *Mol Ther*. 2008;16(7): 1252–1260.

49. Pislaru S, Janssens SP, Gersh BJ, et al. Defining gene transfer before expecting gene therapy: Putting the horse before the cart. *Circulation*. 2002;106(5): 631–636.

50. Tjuvajev JG, Finn R, Watanabe K, et al. Noninvasive imaging of herpes virus thymidine kinase gene transfer and expression: A potential method for monitoring clinical gene therapy. *Cancer Res*. 1996;56(18):4087–4095.

51. Gambhir SS, Barrio JR, Wu L, et al. Imaging of adenoviral-directed herpes simplex virus type 1 thymidine kinase reporter gene expression in mice with radiolabeled ganciclovir. *J Nucl Med*. 1998;39(11):2003–2011.

52. Wu JC, Inubushi M, Sundaresan G, et al. Positron emission tomography imaging of cardiac reporter gene expression in living rats. *Circulation*. 2002;106(2): 180–183.

53. Wu JC, Inubushi M, Sundaresan G, et al. Optical imaging of cardiac reporter gene expression in living rats. *Circulation*. 2002;105(14):1631–1634.

54. Inubushi M, Wu JC, Gambhir SS, et al. Positron-emission tomography reporter gene expression imaging in rat myocardium. *Circulation*. 2003;107(2): 326–332.

55. Bengel FM, Anton M, Richter T, et al. Noninvasive imaging of transgene expression by use of positron emission tomography in a pig model of myocardial gene transfer. *Circulation*. 2003;108(17):2127–2133.

56. Chen IY, Wu JC, Min JJ, et al. Micro-positron emission tomography imaging of cardiac gene expression in rats using bicistronic adenoviral vector-mediated gene delivery. *Circulation*. 2004;109(11):1415–1420.

57. Wu JC, Chen IY, Wang Y, et al. Molecular imaging of the kinetics of vascular endothelial growth factor gene expression in ischemic myocardium. *Circulation*. 2004;110(6):685–691.

58. Anton M, Wittermann C, Haubner R, et al. Coexpression of herpesviral thymidine kinase reporter gene and VEGF gene for noninvasive monitoring of therapeutic gene transfer: An in vitro evaluation. *J Nucl Med*. 2004;45(10): 1743–1746.

59. Ly HQ, Frangioni JV, Hajjar RJ. Imaging in cardiac cell-based therapy: In vivo tracking of the biological fate of therapeutic cells. *Nat Clin Pract Cardiovasc Med*. 2008;5(Suppl. 2):S96–S102.

60. Daley GQ, Lensch MW, Jaenisch R, et al. Broader implications of defining standards for the pluripotency of iPSCs. *Cell Stem Cell*. 2009;4(3):200–201, author reply 202.

61. Boyle AJ, Schulman SP, Hare JM, et al. Is stem cell therapy ready for patients? Stem cell therapy for cardiac repair. Ready for the next step. *Circulation*. 2006;114(4):339–352.

62. Fuster V, Sanz J. Gene therapy and stem cell therapy for cardiovascular diseases today: A model for translational research. *Nat Clin Pract Cardiovasc Med*. 2007;4(Suppl. 1):S1–S8.

63. Rosenzweig A. Cardiac cell therapy—mixed results from mixed cells. *N Engl J Med*. 2006;355(12):1274–1277.

64. Wu JC, Chen IY, Sundaresan G, et al. Molecular imaging of cardiac cell transplantation in living animals using optical bioluminescence and positron emission tomography. *Circulation*. 2003;108(11):1302–1305.

65. Franz WM, Rothmann T, Frey N, et al. Analysis of tissue-specific gene delivery by recombinant adenoviruses containing cardiac-specific promoters. *Cardiovasc Res*. 1997;35(3):560–566.

66. Meyer N, Jaconi M, Landopoulou A, et al. A fluorescent reporter gene as a marker for ventricular specification in ES-derived cardiac cells. *FEBS Lett*. 2000;478(1–2): 151–158.

67. Frangioni JV. In vivo near-infrared fluorescence imaging. *Curr Opin Chem Biol*. 2003;7(5):626–634.

68. Nakayama A, Bianco AC, Zhang CY, et al. Quantitation of brown adipose tissue perfusion in transgenic mice using near-infrared fluorescence imaging. *Mol Imaging*. 2003;2(1):37–49.

69. De Grand AM, Frangioni JV. An operational near-infrared fluorescence imaging system prototype for large animal surgery. *Technol Cancer Res Treat*. 2003;2(6):553–562.

70. Hoshino K, Kimura T, De Grand AM, et al. Three catheter-based strategies for cardiac delivery of therapeutic gelatin microspheres. *Gene Ther*. 2006;13(18): 1320–1327.

71. Chen J, Tung CH, Mahmood U, et al. In vivo imaging of proteolytic activity in atherosclerosis. *Circulation*. 2002;105(23):2766–2771.

72. Gao X, Yang L, Petros JA, et al. In vivo molecular and cellular imaging with quantum dots. *Curr Opin Biotechnol*. 2005;16(1):63–72.

73. Murasawa S, Kawamoto A, Horii M, et al. Niche-dependent translineage commitment of endothelial progenitor cells, not cell fusion in general, into myocardial lineage cells. *Arterioscler Thromb Vasc Biol*. 2005;25(7):1388–1394.

74. Chang GY, Xie X, Wu JC. Overview of stem cells and imaging modalities for cardiovascular diseases. *J Nucl Cardiol*. 2006;13(4):554–569.

75. Blankenberg FG, Strauss HW. Nuclear medicine applications in molecular imaging. *J Magn Reson Imaging*. 2002;16(4):352–361.

76. Jin Y, Kong H, Stodilka RZ, et al. Determining the minimum number of detectable cardiac-transplanted ^{111}In-tropolone-labelled bone-marrow-derived mesenchymal stem cells by SPECT. *Phys Med Biol*. 2005;50(19):4445–4455.

77. Bengel FM. Nuclear imaging in cardiac cell therapy. *Heart Fail Rev*. 2006;11(4):325–332.

78. Frangioni J, Hajjar R. In vivo tracking of stem cells for clinical trials in cardiovascular disease. *Circulation*. 2004;110(21):3378–3383.

79. Montet-Abou K, Montet X, Weissleder R, et al. Transfection agent induced nanoparticle cell loading. *Mol Imaging*. 2005;4(3):165–171.

80. Metz S, Bonaterra G, Rudelius M, et al. Capacity of human monocytes to phagocytose approved iron oxide MR contrast agents in vitro. *Eur Radiol*. 2004;14(10):1851–1858.

81. Hill JM, Dick AJ, Raman VK, et al. Serial cardiac magnetic resonance imaging of injected mesenchymal stem cells. *Circulation*. 2003;108(7):1009–1014.

82. Frank J, Miller B, Arbab A, et al. Clinically applicable labeling of mammalian and stem cells by combining superparamagnetic iron oxides and transfection agents. *Radiology*. 2003;(2):480–487.

83. Arai T, Kofidis T, Bulte JW, et al. Dual in vivo magnetic resonance evaluation of magnetically labeled mouse embryonic stem cells and cardiac function at 1.5 t. *Magn Reson Med*. 2006;55(1):203–209.

84. Amado LC, Saliaris AP, Schuleri KH, et al. Cardiac repair with intramyocardial injection of allogeneic mesenchymal stem cells after myocardial infarction. *Proc Natl Acad Sci USA*. 2005;102(32):11474–11479.

85. Lewin M, Carlesso N, Tung CH, et al. Tat peptide-derivatized magnetic nanoparticles allow in vivo tracking and recovery of progenitor cells. *Nat Biotechnol*. 2000;18(4):410–414.

86. Bulte JW, Douglas T, Witwer B, et al. Magnetodendrimers allow endosomal magnetic labeling and in vivo tracking of stem cells. *Nat Biotechnol*. 2001;19(12):1141–1147.

87. Graham JJ, Lederman RJ, Dick AJ. Magnetic resonance imaging and its role in myocardial regenerative therapy. *Regen Med*. 2006;1(3):347–355.

88. Arbab AS, Liu W, Frank JA. Cellular magnetic resonance imaging: Current status and future prospects. *Expert Rev Med Devices*. 2006;3(4):427–439.

89. Zhou R, Acton PD, Ferrari VA. Imaging stem cells implanted in infarcted myocardium. *J Am Coll Cardiol*. 2006;48(10):2094–2106.

90. Bara C, Ghodsizad A, Niehaus M, et al. In vivo echocardiographic imaging of transplanted human adult stem cells in the myocardium labeled with clinically applicable CliniMACS nanoparticles. *J Am Soc Echocardiogr*. 2006;19(5): 563–568.

91. Assmus B, Honold J, Schächinger V, et al. Transcoronary transplantation of progenitor cells after myocardial infarction. *N Engl J Med*. 2006;355(12):1222–1232.

92. Menasché P, Alfieri O, Janssens S, et al. The Myoblast Autologous Grafting in Ischemic Cardiomyopathy (MAGIC) trial: first randomized placebo-controlled study of myoblast transplantation. *Circulation*. 2008;117(9):1189–1200.

93. Wollert KC, Meyer GP, Lotz J, et al. Intracoronary autologous bone-marrow cell transfer after myocardial infarction: the BOOST randomised controlled clinical trial. *Lancet*. 2004;364(9429):141–148.

94. Janssens S, Dubois C, Bogaert J, et al. Autologous bone marrow-derived stem-cell transfer in patients with ST-segment elevation myocardial infarction: double-blind, randomised controlled trial. *Lancet*. 2006;367(9505):113–121.

95. Lunde K, Solheim S, Aakhus S, et al. Intracoronary injection of mononuclear bone marrow cells in acute myocardial infarction. *N Engl J Med*. 2006;355(12): 1199–1209.

96. Schächinger V, Erbs S, Elsässer A. REPAIR-AMI Investigators. Intracoronary bone marrow-derived progenitor cells in acute myocardial infarction. *N Engl J Med*. 2006;355(12):1210–1221.

Assessment of Risk in the Asymptomatic Patient

22

Paolo Raggi
Nikolaos Alexopoulos
Dalton McLean
Stamatios Lerakis

1. INTRODUCTION

The field of atherosclerosis research has witnessed extraordinary advances in the last few decades. Along with an exceptional amount of research on the pathophysiology and biology of atherosclerosis, came the discovery of numerous serological markers of risk as well as a rapid development of techniques to image atherosclerosis or to assess its indirect effects on the cardiovascular system. In this chapter, we attempt to summarize the large amount of evidence collected in the past two decades surrounding the diagnostic and prognostic utility of these tools.

2. EPIDEMIOLOGY

Cardiovascular disease (CVD) is a global health problem and it is quickly becoming a priority issue even in developing countries. Gender, race, age, genetic, ethnic, and regional variations of risk factors are responsible for the different rates of CVD noted around the world. According to the statistics of the American Heart Association,[1] two in every three US men and in excess of one in every two US women at the age of 40 have a lifetime chance of developing CVD. This simple piece of information clearly underlines the seriousness of this condition for our western societies. A look at the published statistics reveals a very large disease burden and an associated massive cost. In 2005 the prevalence of CVD in the United States was nearing 81 million people and the associated annual total mortality was almost 870,000 lives. The two most frequent causes of death from CVD were coronary heart disease (CHD) (50%) and stroke (16%) (Fig. 22.1). Over eight million people had suffered a myocardial infarction as of 2005 and about 900,000 new myocardial infarctions were recorded yearly. Among these, 157,000 died each year. There is a 10-year lag between women and men for development of CHD and about a 20 year lag for serious clinical events such as myocardial infarction and sudden cardiac death. Estimates reveal that every 26 seconds an American suffers a coronary event and about one every minute dies from such an event.

The prevalence of stroke in 2005 was 5.8 million; it is estimated that every 40 seconds someone in the United States suffers a stroke with a yearly incidence reported at about 780,000 and 151,000 deaths per year. The male to female incidence ratio for stroke decreases with increasing age with higher rates of stroke in women older than 80 years of age. Blacks show almost twice the risk of stroke compared with Whites. Men have a higher mortality from stroke across all ethnic groups compared to women, with black men and women showing about 20% to 25% higher overall death rate from stroke compared to all other ethnic groups. Despite the greater mortality from each incidental stroke demonstrated by men, as a consequence of their longer lives, more men die of stroke each year.

Peripheral arterial disease (PAD) affected approximately eight million people in 2005 in the United States; PAD increases with age and disproportionately affects Blacks more than other racial groups. Interestingly, there is no greater incidence and prevalence of PAD in men than women. PAD is associated with a fivefold to sixfold increased risk of cardiovascular morbidity and death. Amputation, the most devastating complication of PAD, is performed in about 5% to 7% of patients with mild to moderate intermittent claudication. The overall ten-year survival of patients requiring amputation is 50% or less compared with 90% survival for age-matched control subjects.

In the last 30 years there has been a slowing of incident CVD among Americans of all races, although about 40% of the people who experience an acute coronary event in a given year will die. Furthermore, despite significant improvement in prevention, early detection and treatment of stroke, 8% to 12% of ischemic strokes and about 40% of hemorrhagic strokes still result in death within 30 days from the occurrence of the event. Despite the general trend toward reduction of cardiovascular events, CVD death rates have not declined as much in women of diverse racial subsets as in men. Interestingly, despite the fact that CVD is the leading killer of women of all ages, the prevalence of obstructive coronary artery disease (CAD) in women is low with black and Hispanic women having a lower prevalence of obstructive CAD compared to their white nonhispanic counterparts when referred for evaluation of stable and unstable chest pain syndromes.[2]

As a result of the burden of CVD the number of hospital admissions and office and emergency department visits burgeoned to several tens of millions a year with an associated expansion of diagnostic and interventional procedures. Ultimately, the 2008 estimated cost of CHD alone in the United States (not including cerebrovascular disease and PAD but including the cost of long-term complications such as congestive heart failure) is estimated near $160 billion.

CVD is a complex health problem with multiple variations depending on numerous risk factors affecting all ethnicities in every corner of the world.[3] Because the magnitude of the effect on every society can be severe, preventive strategies, early detection methods, and cost effective treatments are necessary.

3. PATHOPHYSIOLOGY OF ATHEROSCLEROSIS

The precise causative factors of the atherosclerotic process have been the focus of intense research and debate for a long time.

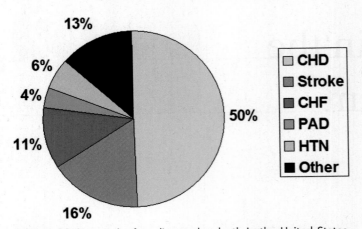

Figure 22.1 Causes of cardiovascular death in the United States. (Modified from AHA statistics at http://www.americanheart.org/downloadable/heart/1200082005246HS_Stats%202008.final.pdf.)

The predominant theory, presently, is one that revolves around the primary role of cholesterol as the necessary stimulus for the initiation of a cascade of events that eventually brings to the formation of advanced atherosclerotic plaques and their rupture with or without repair. The most relevant discovery of the 20th century in the field of atherosclerosis research may have been the elucidation of the role played by inflammation in the initiation and perpetuation of the cascade alluded to above. Virchow wrote in 1860: "*I have no hesitation....in admitting an inflammation of the inner arterial coat to be the starting point of the so-called atheromatous degeneration....*"[4] So if inflammation is responsible for this type of vascular disease, how does the process begin? What makes cholesterol particles penetrate between endothelial cells and accumulate in the subendothelial space? How does inflammation come into play? It would appear that no matter what noxious stimuli one applies, induction of experimental diabetes, balloon injury of the endothelium, and others, the animal model will not develop advanced atherosclerotic plaques unless serum cholesterol levels are elevated or the animal is unable to

handle cholesterol particles such as in the low density lipoprotein (LDL) receptor deficient (LDL R −/−) or the *apoE*-knockout (*apoE* −/−) mouse.[5] In the next few paragraphs we will succinctly review the suggested stages of plaque development and expansion as viewed today.[6,7]

Prior to the formation of true atheromas, raised lesions known as fatty streaks appear in the aorta of most humans at a very young age. These lesions, which consist of the accumulation of lipid-laden macrophages in the subendothelial space along with rare lymphocytes, may or may not progress to full-blown atherosclerotic lesions. In the presence of high serum cholesterol levels, LDL particles penetrate and are retained in the subendothelial space where they undergo oxidation and generate several phospholipids that activate the endothelial cells (Fig. 22.2). Endothelial cells appear to be particularly sensitive to activating stimuli in areas of low shear stress, and they begin to express adhesion molecules such as vascular–cell adhesion molecule-1 (VCAM-1). Circulating monocytes become "sticky" and adhere to activated endothelial cells via receptors expressed on their surface interacting with adhesion molecules. The adhesiveness of monocytes to the endothelium appears to be increased by the arrival of platelets in the area of growing vascular damage. Indeed, the contact of platelet surface glycoproteins IIb/IIIa with receptors on the endothelial cells contributes to the further activation of the latter.

Chemoatractant factors (known as *chemokines*) released from the subendothelial space are then responsible for stimulating the migration of the adherent monocytes and lymphocytes to the intimal space beneath the endothelium. After penetrating in the intima, monocytes differentiate into macrophages that express several surface receptors of vital importance for innate immunity. Some of these, known as *toll-like receptors*, can be activated by the interaction with several noxious stimuli such as oxidized LDL (oxLDL), endotoxins, and heat-shock proteins with the resultant release of mediators of inflammation such as cytokines, tissue factor, chemokines, oxygen radical species, proteases (collagenases, matrix metalloproteinases-*MMP*, and myeloperoxidase-*MPO*), and others. The progressive accumulation of oxidized lipids in macrophages eventually engulfs these cells turning them into the

Figure 22.2 Simplified schema of the pathophysiology of atherosclerosis. (Courtesy of Eric Jablonowski, Department of Radiology, Emory Universtiy, Atlanta, GA.)

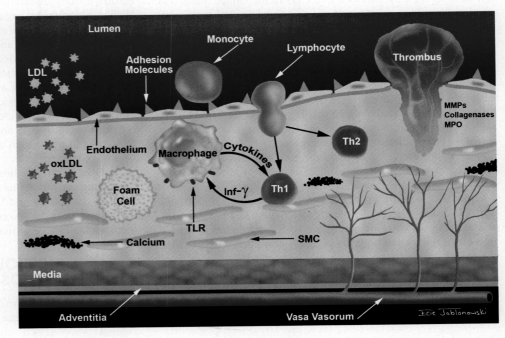

pathognomonic cell type of atherosclerosis, the *foam cell*. Several other types of inflammatory cells are found in the context of the growing atherosclerotic plaque like lymphocytes, mast cells, and dendritic cells. CD4+ T-lymphocytes are the most numerous although some natural-killer and CD8+ T-lymphocytes are also present. Cytokine stimulation may turn the T-helper lymphocyte into an effector cell capable of producing *interferon-γ*. This cytokine improves the efficiency of antigen presentation from the activated macrophage to the T-lymphocyte (mostly of the T-helper 1 type) and promotes further release of inflammatory mediators such as tumor necrosis factor (TNF)-α, interleukin-1 (IL-1), and interleukin-6 (IL-6). The release of large quantities of cytokines, not only from the vessel wall but from fat tissue as well, induces the production of acute phase reactants from the liver (serum amyloid A and C-reactive protein) that can be measured in the peripheral blood. The knowledge that some of the phases described above play a pivotal role in the development of atherosclerosis is provided by animal models such as the *toll-like receptor* knockout or the *interferon-γ* knockout mouse models where atherosclerosis is strongly inhibited or the demonstration that systemic infusion of *interferon-γ* in *apoE* –/– mice causes an intense acceleration of atherosclerosis.

There are also several mechanisms predisposed to act as inhibitors of the growing atherosclerotic process. Investigators have identified a few anti-inflammatory cytokines such as interleukin-10 and transforming growth factor-β (TGF-β) apparently responsible for an inhibitory function on the activated T-lymphocyte. The accumulation of *MMP1* and *MMP-9* is accompanied by the intralesional collection of tissue inhibitors of metalloproteinases (*TIMP*). Both vascular and splenic B-lymphocytes produce antibodies that link to oxLDL and apoptotic cell membranes, thereby contributing to the elimination of these promoters of inflammation and atherosclerosis. Finally, the adipose tissue appears to have a very important role in the control of the atherosclerotic plaque development both as a promoter, via the secretion of cytokines such as interleukin-1, resistin, and tumor necrosis factor, and as an inhibitor via adipokines such as adiponectin and possibly leptin.

The histology of a plaque prone to rupture has been inferred from postmortem studies of patients that succumbed to acute coronary syndromes or sudden cardiac death. It has become common knowledge that a plaque with a relatively large lipid core covered by a thin fibrous cap and demonstrating active inflammatory changes, particularly in the vicinity of the plaque hinges, may be the type of plaque more likely to cause an acute thrombotic event (*the vulnerable plaque*). These plaques usually demonstrate strong positive staining for *MMP* and *MPO* near the fracture point of the fibrous cap, suggesting that the digesting activity of proteases released by inflammatory cells may play a causative role in the acute disruption of the plaque. Besides sudden fissuring of the plaque cap, superficial erosion of the same has been shown in patients who succumbed to sudden cardiac death. The sudden exposure of plaque contents that follows plaque fissuring and erosion causes the creation and propagation of an intravascular thrombus that often manifest with dramatic clinical syndromes such as acute myocardial infarction, stroke, and sudden death.

Nonetheless, other pathological changes that occur in the vessel wall can have important effects on plaque formation and destabilization. Namely, the proliferation of vasa vasorum that occurs in several models of atherosclerosis has stimulated the interest of investigators for many years.[8] Exposure to noxious stimuli induces neovascularization of the growing atherosclerotic plaque; oxidative stress, nicotine, and hypertension have been shown to modulate the expression of growth factors capable of inducing vasa vasorum proliferation, likely via induction of relative vessel wall hypoxia. As a result, numerous vessels appear on the adventitial surface of the artery and penetrate the vessel wall to reach the subintimal space. Interestingly, neovascularization is more intense in lipid-rich and inflamed plaques with a thin cap. Furthermore, vasa vasorum proliferation appears to be more prominent toward the shoulders of a rupture-prone plaque. These vessels contain a very limited number of smooth muscle cells and pericytes and are therefore particularly permeable and fragile. The latter factors allow leaking of intravascular substances in the plaque, such as reactive oxygen species (ROS), oxLDL, and inflammatory cells. Therefore, although not yet conclusively proven, it is conceivable that vessel wall neovascularization may provide enough inciting momentum for plaque development with a radical reversal of the "intra-luminal" hypothesis of atherosclerosis. Vasa vasorum can contribute to destabilization of atherosclerotic plaques not only by means of transporting toxic mediators but also by causing sudden intralesional hemorrhage, with noticeable increase in intraplaque pressure and subsequent disruption of the fibrous cap. Furthermore, intralesional hemorrhage has been demonstrated even in the absence of cap disruption.

One final component of the atherosclerotic plaque that deserves mentioning is calcium. Calcification of the atherosclerotic plaque has been known to occur for centuries. For a long time this process was believed to be secondary to passive accumulation of calcium in the plaque, possibly as a consequence of sequential intralesional hemorrhagic episodes. However in 1860 Virchow wrote: "*For here we have really to do with an ossification, and not merely, as has recently been maintained, with a mere calcification; the plates which pervade the inner wall of the vessel are real plates of bone,*" a luminary ahead of his times![4] It is now known that calcification occurs via an active process resembling bone formation under the control of complex enzymatic and cellular pathways.[9,10] A large number of in vitro studies have highlighted the involvement in the process of vascular calcification of osteoblastlike cells, cytokines, transcription factors, and bone morphogenic proteins found in normal bone. Calcification of the intima is characterized by cellular apoptosis,[11] inflammation, lipoprotein and phospholipid accumulation and finally hydroxyapatite deposition. Calcification is first noted in the lipid core of the atheroma, juxtaposed to inflammatory cells that infiltrate the fibrocalcific plaque.[12-14] Endothelial cells in healthy arteries exert a vaso-protective effect against calcification by expressing matrix GLA protein (MGP), a potent vitamin K dependent inhibitor of vascular calcification.[15] Its deficiency in MGP-knockout mice results in disseminated soft tissue and vascular calcification with premature demise of the experimental animal.[16] Cola et al.[15] incubated coronary artery endothelial cells with oxLDL and TNF-α and monitored the ensuing gene expression. They observed that some bone morphogenic proteins, such as MGP or BMP-2, constituently expressed at very low levels, were strongly expressed after exposure to atherogenic stimuli. Macrophages also exert an important role in the synthesis and deposition of collagenous proteins that work as a template for hydroxyapatite deposition. Tyson et al.[17] identified a subset of macrophages that can differentiate in vitro into osteoclastlike cells and express a number of bone specific proteins such as osteopontin, bone sialoprotein, alkaline phosphatase, and bone-GLA protein. The authors hypothesized that the lack of inhibiting factors such as osteoprotegerin, as shown in prior studies,[18,19] could trigger the osteoblastic differentiation of macrophages. Finally, some investigators hypothesized that pericytes (the endothelial cells of vasa vasorum) could potentially express osteoblasticlike phenotypic characteristics and contribute to the calcification of the growing plaque. The basic mechanism initiating the process of calcification is unknown but it appears to require apoptosis of intralesional cells,[11] likely smooth muscle cells; the apoptotic bodies would then work as nucleating foci of calcification. The teleological aim of plaque calcification is also unknown with some researchers suggesting that it may have a reparative, stabilizing effect on the plaque[20,21] and others noting a greater fragility of calcified vessels.[22-24] The latter hypothesis is supported by in vitro experiments showing a greater propensity to fracture in plaques with calcification near the shoulders as compared to plaques containing large plates of calcification at the border between the intima and the media.[25] The uncertainty regarding the role of arterial calcification sparked a very lively debate that revolved around the opposite view that calcification of the atherosclerotic plaque is a benign versus an ominous finding. Neither position may be entirely correct, in that some calcification may be a marker of a stable plaque while the other may identify unstable milieus as explained above. Furthermore, it is now recognized that despite the fact that intraluminal thrombosis occurs frequently, simultaneously, and/or sequentially at several sites in the same coronary tree or carotid artery, most occurrences are not followed by an acute event due to the ability of the vessel wall to repair itself and the powerful anticoagulant activity of the intravascular milieu. It would appear, therefore, that rather than pursuing the single vulnerable or high-risk atherosclerotic plaque our preventive efforts should focus on the identification of the *"vulnerable, high-risk individual,"* who may possess a complement of factors (proinflammatory, procoagulant, proarrhythmic, etc.) that predispose him/her to the occurrence of sudden events.[26]

The above brief synopsis of the pathogenesis of atherosclerosis provides a list of the potential targets of investigation to assess risk in asymptomatic patients: serum lipoproteins, serum markers of inflammation and several other proteins, imaging of the lipid core, the fibrous cap, calcium, vasa vasorum, iron from intraplaque hemorrhaging, etc. In the following paragraphs, we will review the current literature on several of these noninvasive techniques to assess risk in the population.

4. DIAGNOSTIC EVALUATION

4.1. Serum biomarkers

4.1.1. Low density lipoprotein cholesterol

Numerous epidemiological studies and prospective clinical trials have demonstrated that elevated total and LDL cholesterol are strong and modifiable risk factors for CHD.[27] Patients with homozygous familial hypercholesterolemia with very high LDL cholesterol levels experience myocardial infarction and cardiac death in the first few decades of life.[28] Conversely, when cholesterol is low, CHD risk is low despite the existence of other risk factors.[29,30] Since the early experiments of Anitschkow in 1913,[31] it became very clear that atherosclerotic lesions could be induced in animals with high cholesterol diets without the need for other risk factors (for example diabetes mellitus). The genetically manipulated LDL receptor −/− rabbit or *apoE* −/− mouse develops atherosclerosis rapidly as a consequence of very elevated levels of LDL cholesterol. In post to World War II Japan. the average cholesterol level was 160 mg/dL, and heart disease rates were extremely low despite a high prevalence of smoking and hypertension in the population.[32] All of these observations and others suggest that cholesterol and cholesterol fractions elevation are necessary factors for induction of atherosclerosis that may, nonetheless, be accelerated by other contributing factors such as diabetes and smoking.

The main results of the Lipid Research Clinic—Coronary Primary Prevention Trial—were published in 1984 and for the first time they provided demonstration of the fact that LDL reduction affords a significant decrease in cardiovascular events.[33] This study was followed by extensive research on cholesterol and LDL lowering, especially with statins but other treatments as well. A metaanalysis published in 2005 of 14 controlled, randomized studies of 90,056 subjects treated with statins (46% without known CVD) showed an overall 12% reduction in all-cause mortality and 19% reduction in cardiovascular mortality per mmol/L (40 mg/dL) LDL reduction.[34] The mortality reduction was significant both for patients with and without CVD at baseline. LDL cholesterol has been found to have a log-linear relationship with CHD, so that for a given mg/dL LDL change, the corresponding change in relative risk of CHD is the same for any starting level of LDL cholesterol.[35] This relationship holds even at very low LDL levels.

Other facts support the notion that lifetime low LDL is protective of risk of CVD. Cohen et al.[30] analyzed 3,363 black and 9,524 white subjects for mutations in the gene encoding proprotein convertase subtilisin/kexin type 9 (PCSK9). Mutations that lead to reduced expression of this gene confer lifelong low LDL cholesterol. A mutation in PCSK9 was found in 2.6% of black subjects and was associated with a 28% lower LDL and an 88% lower risk of CHD. In white subjects, the mutation was found in 3.2% of the population and was associated with a 15% reduction in LDL and a 47% reduction in CHD risk.

Although large scale statin trials have consistently shown an approximate 30% reduction in CHD events compared to placebo, patients still experience a residual large burden of events.[34,36,37] Several factors could be invoked to explain this apparent paradox: (a) beyond LDL, part of the residual risk must be secondary to nonlipid factors such as smoking, hypertension, and diabetes mellitus; (b) we may not be targeting low enough LDL levels; and (c) there could be significant residual lipid-related CHD risk that is not addressed by LDL-lowering alone. Targeting an even lower LDL compared to the goal levels set by The National Cholesterol Education Program Adult Treatment Panel III (NCEP ATP III) in 2001 has shown clinical benefit in further studies.[38-43] Indeed, current recommendations recognize that in patients at high risk LDL <70 mg/dL confers greater protection from CHD events than LDL <100 mg/dL.[35] Interestingly, Leeper et al.[44] have shown that statin therapy for 2 years reduces all-cause mortality even among patients with baseline LDL <40 mg/dL. Finally, a number of lipid particles, other than mere LDL cholesterol, have been extensively investigated for better risk stratification and as targets for therapeutic intervention.

4.1.2. Small, dense LDL

Measurement of LDL particle size (large, buoyant versus small, dense) has been proposed as a method to better stratify CHD risk beyond that total LDL level. LDL particles differ in metabolic behavior based on size, with small, dense LDL being more atherogenic than large, buoyant LDL. Small, dense LDL particles are more easily oxidized and transported to the subendothelium, allowing for a quicker contribution to the development of atherosclerotic plaque than large, buoyant LDL.[45] Studies have shown that the presence of small, dense LDL, found in 30% to 35% of Caucasian males, is associated with a threefold increase in CAD risk.[45-47] However, it is unclear whether the measurement of small, dense LDL adds additional information beyond measurement of triglycerides, as in most of the studies, small, dense LDL was not an independent risk factor due to its strong association with increased triglyceride levels.

4.1.3. Oxidized LDL

OxLDL is formed when LDL is exposed to oxidizing substances such as hydrogen peroxide and superoxide anion from inflammatory cells in the vessel wall and to oxidizing products of MPO. OxLDL is avidly taken up by scavenger receptors on macrophages in the vessel wall, leading to the formation of foam cells—a fundamental element in the development of the atherosclerotic plaque.[48,49] Given its apparent role in the development of atherosclerotic plaque, oxLDL has been investigated as a marker of CHD risk. Elevated oxLDL has been linked to increased carotid intima-media thickness (IMT) in asymptomatic patients,[50–53] and baseline oxLDL level predicted progression of IMT independently of other risk factors.[54] Tsimikas et al.[55] measured oxLDL in 504 patients undergoing coronary angiography. Higher oxLDL correlated with more extensive CAD. In the overall cohort, elevated oxLDL was predictive of CAD independently of all tested risk factors except lipoprotein(a) (Lp(a)). However, in patients below 60 years of age, oxLDL was predictive of coronary disease independently of Lp(a). Toshima et al.,[56] similarly, showed that oxLDL was higher in patients with angiographic CAD compared to those without CAD. In the multiethnic study of atherosclerosis (MESA) study oxLDL was associated with subclinical atherosclerosis assessed as presence of plaque on carotid imaging, presence of coronary artery calcium (CAC), or an ankle brachial index <0.9.[57]

Paradoxically, in the REVERSAL trial prolonged exposure to statin therapy with either pravastatin or atorvastatin resulted in 17% to 48% increase in serum oxidized phospholipids despite an effect of these drugs on plaque volume as assessed by intravascular ultrasound (IVUS).[58] There is currently no reproducible and standardized method to measure oxLDL; as a consequence this marker is not recommended as a target for testing or therapy. Nonetheless, the available evidence suggests a potential role of oxLDL as a marker of CAD risk, especially in patients under 60 years of age.

4.1.4. High-density lipoprotein cholesterol

High-density lipoprotein (HDL) cholesterol plays a complex role in atherosclerosis. The purported most important anti-atherogenic function of HDL is to reverse cholesterol transport from atherosclerotic plaques to the liver for further processing and excretion into the bile.[59] Additional potential effects include inhibition of expression of adhesion molecules on the endothelial surface (Fig. 22.2) that favor the adhesion and penetration of monocytes into the subintimal space[60] and reduction of LDL oxidation, rendering it less atherogenic.[61] Although HDL is generally thought of as "good" cholesterol, certain conditions such as chronic inflammation can induce the production of HDL particles depleted of their antiatherogenic characteristics.[62] Low HDL levels are common among the American population; as much as 26.4% of subjects over 20 years of age have HDL <40 mg/dL.[63]

There is a strong relationship between low HDL cholesterol and increased CHD risk. An analysis of four large prospective trials showed a 2% CHD risk decrease in men and 3% decrease in women for each 1% higher level of HDL.[64] The Framingham Heart Study showed an inverse relationship between HDL cholesterol levels and CAD incidence.[65] The Munster Heart Study showed that HDL <35 mg/dL (compared to HDL ≥35 mg/dL) conferred three times greater CAD risk,[66] and the Physicians' Health Study similarly demonstrated that low HDL is an independent risk factor for CAD.[67] Despite the rather strong evidence that low HDL cholesterol is an independent risk factor for CHD, trials aiming at raising HDL to lower CHD risk have given mixed results and are so far unconvincing. The only positive result was obtained in the Veterans Administration—HDL Intervention Trial (VA-HIT) where a small (6%) increase in HDL was associated with an absolute risk reduction of 4.4% for nonfatal myocardial infarction or death from coronary causes.[68] A later trial, the bezafibrate infarct prevention study, showed that bezafibrate raised HDL cholesterol by 18%, but over a mean of 6.2 years, there was only a nonsignificant trend toward lower fatal or nonfatal myocardial infarctions or sudden death in the bezafibrate group compared to placebo.[69]

4.1.5. Triglycerides

Triglycerides have also received in depth attention as possible biomarkers of elevated CHD risk. Triglycerides are produced endogenously in the liver and carried in very-low-density lipoproteins (VLDL) or are absorbed from dietary fat and carried in chylomicrons. It has been difficult to separate the independent contribution of triglycerides to CHD risk since hypertriglyceridemia is often associated with other cardiovascular risk factors, such as low HDL levels, hyperinsulinemia, type 2 diabetes mellitus, obesity, and increased levels of small dense LDL.[70,71] However, there is now strong evidence that hypertriglyceridemia is an independent risk factor for CHD, especially in women. A metaanalysis of prospective trials including 57,277 patients showed a significant correlation between hypertriglyceridemia and increasing CHD risk independently of HDL level and other risk factors.[70] The Munster heart study showed an increasing CHD risk independent of other risk factors as triglycerides rose from 2.3 to 9.0 mmol/L.[66] Interestingly, triglyceride levels do not appear in most risk calculation equations except for the PROCAM, underlying the greater weight attributed to LDL compared to other lipid markers.

4.1.6. Non-HDL cholesterol

Non-HDL cholesterol, calculated by subtracting HDL from total cholesterol, takes into account all unmeasured particles in the standard lipid profile such as LDL, VLDL, intermediate-density lipoproteins (IDL), chylomicron remnants, lipoprotein(a), and potentially others. Unlike LDL, non-HDL measurement accounts for all types of atherogenic lipid particles. The National Cholesterol Education Program-ATP III identified non-HDL cholesterol as a secondary treatment target after the LDL target is reached for patients with triglycerides >200 mg/dL.[72] The goal for non-HDL cholesterol was set at 30 mg/dL higher than the goal for LDL cholesterol.[72] Though non-HDL cholesterol is highly correlated with LDL when triglycerides are <150 mg/dL, the correlation weakens substantially when triglycerides are >150 mg/dL.[73] Consequently, non-HDL cholesterol appears to be a better predictor of CHD events than LDL in patients with hypertriglyceridemia. Liu et al.[74] reported on a group of 5,794 subjects from the Framingham heart study initially free from CHD for whom LDL cholesterol was measured and non-HDL cholesterol was calculated. In this population, non-HDL cholesterol was predictive of CHD events at all triglyceride levels while LDL cholesterol was only predictive of CHD events in patients with triglycerides <200 mg/dL. Within each non-HDL category (<160 mg/dL, 160 to 189 mg/dL, and ≥190 mg/dL), LDL was not predictive of CHD events. However, within each LDL category, non-HDL was predictive of CHD events. In the women's health study, non-HDL cholesterol was found to be the strongest marker of CHD risk in 15,632 females without baseline CVD.[75] In a study of 1,611 asymptomatic subjects submitted to computed tomography (CT) screening for CAC, non-HDL cholesterol showed a much closer association with this marker of atherosclerosis than any other lipid particle serum value.[76] As non-HDL cholesterol appears to be a better predictor of CHD risk than LDL, it may become the primary lipid index in the future. It is an especially relevant measurement for the 16% of American population and the 37% of diabetic subjects with severe hyper-triglyceridemia,[77] in whom LDL may be less predictive. Finally, it appears that triglycerides add prognostic information beyond LDL cholesterol measurement but not beyond non-HDL cholesterol measurement.[78]

4.1.7. Lipoprotein(a)

Lp(a) is an extension to apolipoprotein B-100 and its physiological function is unknown.[79] Lp(a) binds and transports oxidized phospholipids, a function that may partly explain its proatherogenic nature.[80]

It appears to be a marker of cardiovascular risk, especially for young patients with premature atherosclerosis.[81,82] The cardiovascular health study (3,942 without known CVD) showed a threefold increase in risk of death from cardiovascular causes for patients in the highest quintile versus the lowest quintile of Lp(a) during a follow-up period of 7.4 years. The association, however, was seen only in males.[83] The link of Lp(a) with CHD appears to be the strongest for very high levels of Lp(a) (>30 mg/dL); in fact, Lp(a) >30 mg/dL is an independent predictor of angiographic CAD.[84,85] Based on the available data, Lp(a) may be most useful for risk assessment in younger patients, especially males, with a family history of premature CAD or multiple risk factors.

4.1.8. Homocysteine

Homocysteine is an amino acid derived from the catabolism of another amino acid, methionine. The B vitamins, B_2, B_6, and B_{12}, are involved in the metabolic break-down pathways for homocysteine.[86] Therefore, hyperhomocysteinemia can be caused by B vitamin deficiencies.

The first suggestion of an interaction between elevated homocysteine and atherosclerosis was suggested by McCully in 1969.[87] He noted that children with certain inborn errors of metabolism leading to extreme hyperhomocysteinemia developed early atherosclerotic disease.[87] Early observational studies linked elevated homocysteine to risk of CAD and stroke in the general population. Boushey et al.[88] conducted a meta analysis of predominantly retrospective studies and showed a link between reduction in homocysteine levels and decrease in CVD. More recent prospective studies continue to show an association, albeit less marked than earlier retrospective studies, between hyperhomocysteinemia and CVD, especially stroke. The homocysteine studies collaboration analyzed data from 9,025 patients in 12 prospective cohort studies showing that a 25% lower homocysteine level was associated with a significant 19% lower stroke risk and 11% lower risk of ischemic heart disease after adjusting for other cardiovascular risk factors.[89] Additionally, low dietary folate intake, leading to hyperhomocysteinemia, has been correlated to stroke and ischemic heart disease in prospective observational studies.[90]

Homozygosity for a variant allele of methylene tetrahydrofolate reductase, an enzyme playing a role in homocysteine metabolism, results in approximately 25% higher homocysteine levels compared to the wild type. Two metaanalyses assessed the risk of CVD among subjects homozygous for this variant allele. Casas et al.[91] reviewed data on 6,324 cases and 7,604 controls and showed an odds ratio for stroke of 1.26 (95% CI 1.14 to 1.40) for homozygous patients compared to controls. A second metaanalysis involving 26,000 cases and 31,183 controls showed only a weak association between homozygosity for the variant allele and ischemic heart disease with an odds ratio of 1.14 (95% CI 1.05 to 1.24).[92] The authors of the latter metaanalysis noted a strong heterogeneity among studies. Overall, there appears to be a stronger

association between hyperhomocysteinemia and stroke and a weaker association between hyperhomocysteinemia and ischemic heart disease. According to a metaanalysis including 25 randomized controlled trials, treatment with folic acid can reduce homocysteine levels by about 23%, and vitamin B_{12} added to folate can reduce homocysteine by an additional 7%.[93] Despite the efficacy of these treatments for lowering homocysteine, data from four large randomized clinical trials of homocysteine-lowering have been disappointing.[94-97] None showed significant benefit for prevention of major cardiovascular events by lowering homocysteine using folic acid and B vitamins. The Heart Outcomes Prevention Evaluation-2 (HOPE-2) trial did show a 25% reduction in risk of stroke for patients receiving folic acid and vitamins B_6 and B_{12} though this was a secondary endpoint in the study.[96]

4.1.9. Uric acid

Uric acid is generated by xanthine oxidase as the final breakdown product of purine metabolism.[98] About two-thirds of uric acid is excreted in the urine. Thus, hyperuricemia is most often the result of inadequate renal uric acid clearance.[99] Hyperuricemia has been frequently associated with essential hypertension.[100,101] In this context, elevated uric acid has been considered a direct hypertension inducer,[102] although it may also be a marker of renal dysfunction, which can lead to both hyperuricemia and hypertension.

There is a significant body of epidemiological evidence identifying elevated uric acid as a risk marker of CVD. Analysis of the National Health and Nutrition Examination Study (NHANES I), including data from 5,926 subjects whose uric acid levels were measured at baseline, showed that hyperuricemia was significantly associated with all-cause and ischemic heart disease mortality.[103] This relationship remained significant after adjustment for traditional CHD risk factors and was stronger for women than for men. Not all epidemiologic studies have supported the association of CHD and uric acid. An analysis from the Framingham heart study did not show a significant association.[103] Among patients with angiographic CAD, those in the highest quartile of uric acid were five times more likely to die than those in the lowest quartile.[104] A 26% increase in mortality was associated with a 1 mg/dL rise in uric acid level.

As said earlier, elevated uric acid is common among hypertensive patients and may be related to problems with renal uric acid clearance. Verdecchia et al.[105] showed that serum uric acid level was a strong predictor of CHD and all-cause mortality among 1,720 patients with hypertension after adjustment for multiple traditional risk factors. In the Systolic Hypertension in the Elderly Trial (SHEP), 4,327 patients with hypertension were treated with chlorthalidone or placebo.[106] The baseline uric acid level was an independent predictor of CHD, and the benefit of chlorthalidone as far as the reduction in CHD events was limited to patients whose uric acid levels did not rise.

4.1.10. B-type natriuretic peptide and N-terminal pro-B-type natriuretic peptide

Pro-BNP is released by the cardiac ventricles mainly in response to elevated wall stress leading to myocyte stretch. However, other factors, including ischemia and inflammation, may trigger pro-BNP release independently of elevated wall stress.[107] Pro-BNP is cleaved to yield active B-type Natriuretic Peptide (BNP) and the inactive N-Terminal pro-B-type Natriuretic Peptide (NT-pro-BNP). The main utility for measurement of serum BNP or NT-pro-BNP level lies in assessment of patients with suspected or known congestive heart failure. Some data, however, are available regarding a role for BNP in cardiovascular risk assessment. BNP and NT-pro-BNP levels have been shown to be predictive of the extent of CAD[108,109] and the risk of events among patients with stable known CAD.[110-112] Blankenberg et al.[113] assessed NT-pro-BNP, nine inflammatory markers, and microalbuminuria in the Heart Outcomes Prevention Evaluation (HOPE) study for risk stratification of recurrent cardiovascular events. NT-pro-BNP was the only marker showing incremental risk stratification beyond traditional risk factors. Marz et al.[114] showed that increasing NT-pro-BNP was predictive of all-cause and cardiovascular mortality in stable patients undergoing coronary angiography. Of these patients, 31% had no detectable coronary disease, but NT-pro-BNP remained predictive of mortality. NT-pro-BNP was also predictive of mortality independent of the presence of clinical heart failure or left ventricular systolic dysfunction. BNP and NT-pro-BNP appears to be prognostic markers among asymptomatic patients as well.[115-117] In an analysis of 3,346 patients from the Framingham heart study without heart failure at baseline who were followed for a mean of 5.2 years, higher BNP levels were found to correlate with increasing risk of all-cause mortality, first cardiovascular event, heart failure, and stroke.[116] Increasing BNP level was not, however, significantly associated with CHD events when defined as recognized or unrecognized myocardial infarction, coronary insufficiency, or angina pectoris. Currently, there is no clear role established for measurement of BNP or NT-pro-BNP in the risk assessment of asymptomatic patients without known CHD. However, one could envision a future role for BNP or NT-pro-BNP in a multimarker risk assessment strategy.

Inflammation and atherosclerosis. Vessel wall inflammation plays a central role in the development of atherosclerotic plaque as discussed in a prior section of this chapter. The initial noxious stimulus leads to endothelial dysfunction with expression of cellular adhesion molecules on the endothelial surface. As discussed earlier, circulating leukocytes interact with endothelial cellular adhesion molecules, leading to diapedesis and collection in the vessel intima.[118] The accumulation of these cells in the sub-intimal space leads to a complex cascade of events and—among others—the release of proinflammatory cytokines such as interleukin-1β, tumor necrosis factor-α, interleukin-6, and monocyte chemoattractant protein-1.[119] Macrophages and lymphocytes in the intima secrete further inflammatory cytokines, triggering a spiral of inflammation and oxidation. Given the central role for inflammation and oxidative stress in atherogenesis, it is not surprising that markers of inflammation and oxidative stress have been studied as markers of risk of cardiovascular events and several have been associated with an increased risk. The white blood cell count, the most basic measure of systemic inflammation, has been correlated with the risk of CHD and cardiac death independently of other risk factors in populations without known vascular disease.[120,121]

4.1.11. C-Reactive protein
C-reactive protein (CRP) is an acute phase reactant produced primarily in the liver but, apparently, in atherosclerotic plaque by smooth muscle cells and/or endothelial cells as well.[122] It remains unclear whether also CRP plays a direct causal atherogenic role or is simply a marker of developing inflammatory disease.[123] This molecule has been extensively studied in the setting of primary prevention of CVD. Large observational, prospective studies in patients without known CVD with follow-up periods of up to 10 years have shown baseline CRP to correlate with future cardiovascular death, myocardial infarction, stroke, and PAD. These studies have shown that the predictive ability of CRP is independent of

diabetes, triglycerides, body mass index, and other covariates considered in the Framingham risk score (FRS).[124-133] In the women's health study, the investigators measured CRP and LDL at baseline in a cohort of 27,939 women and followed them for a mean of 8 years.[128] After adjusting for diabetes, blood pressure, smoking status, age, and hormone replacement status, increasing quintiles of CRP showed a strong correlation with an increasing risk of a first cardiovascular event. This correlation remained significant after adjustment for LDL levels and FRS.[128] Interestingly, cardiovascular risk was higher in patients with low LDL and high CRP than patients with high LDL and low CRP. This study suggested that CRP may be a stronger predictor of cardiovascular events than LDL. In 2002, the Centers for Disease Control and the American Heart Association endorsed CRP use in the intermediate risk population for further risk stratification.[134] For patients with elevated CRP, statins have been shown to lower the level independently of LDL reduction.[135,136] An ongoing randomized controlled trial, *The Justification for the Use of statins in Primary prevention: an Intervention Trial Evaluating Rosuvastatin* (JUPITER), has been recently prematurely terminated and at the time of this writing the official results have not been published although a preliminary report has been released on the internet (http://www.astrazeneca.com/pressrelease/5385.aspx). This trial sought to define the role of CRP as a target of therapy in patients without known CVD and average to low LDL (<130 mg/dL).[137] Patients with elevated CRP (≥2 mg/L) but LDL <130 mg/dL were randomized to rosuvastatin 20 mg versus placebo. This study should provide important information on the utility of CRP in the primary prevention setting.

4.1.12. Interleukin-6
IL-6 is a proinflammatory cytokine involved in the acute-phase response and also found in the context of the atherosclerotic plaque. Hepatic release of CRP is promoted by IL-6 and IL-1β.[138] Ridker et al.[139] examined the relationship between future myocardial infarction and IL-6 level among a population of apparently healthy men. IL-6 was found to be predictive of future myocardial infarction independently of other risk factors, including CRP. At this time, there is no IL-6 assay available for general clinical use.

4.1.13. Myeloperoxidase
MPO is a heme peroxidase secreted by neutrophils, monocytes, and macrophages at sites of inflammation. Its primary biological role is in host defense against pathogens. However, the products of MPO, hypochlorous acid, tyrosyl radical, and nitrogen dioxide can cause oxidative damage and contribute to atherosclerosis.[140] Oxidative stress from MPO is involved in LDL oxidation,[141] foam cell formation,[142] plaque vulnerability,[143,144] and HDL oxidation (rendering HDL dysfunctional).[145]

There is evidence for MPO use as a marker of CHD risk. Increased levels of MPO correlate with endothelial dysfunction as measured by brachial artery reactivity.[146] Zhang et al.[147] conducted a case-control study involving 158 patients with documented CAD and 175 without angiographic CAD (controls). After adjustment for traditional risk factors, white blood cell count and FRS, an odds ratio of 11.9 (CI 5.5 to 25.5), was found for CAD for the highest versus lowest quartiles of leukocyte-MPO and an odds ratio of 20.4 (CI 8.9 to 47.2) was found for CAD for the highest versus lowest quartiles of blood-MPO. Brennan et al.[148] assessed 604 patients presenting to the emergency department with chest pain but without evidence for myocardial infarction on initial testing. Higher MPO predicted increased risk of myocardial infarction within 16 h of presentation as well as major adverse cardiac events at 30 days and 6 months. Since most of the data on the association between MPO and CHD have been obtained in the setting of acute coronary syndromes or known CVD, the ability of MPO to risk stratify patients in a primary prevention remains unknown.

4.1.14. Lipoprotein-associated phospholipase A2

Lipoprotein-associated phospholipase A_2 (Lp-PLA$_2$) is an enzyme that hydrolyzes oxLDL, generating proatherogenic lysophosphatidylcholine and oxidized fatty acids.[149] Lp-PLA$_2$ is produced in atherosclerotic plaque by foam cells. After production, it has a high affinity for and travels with LDL particles, though small amounts are also found attached on HDL. Given its localization in the atherosclerotic plaque and production by foam cells, Lp-PLA$_2$ has been investigated as a risk marker for CHD.[150] In addition, as some animal studies have shown that inhibition of the enzyme slows the atherosclerotic progress, it may be not only a marker but also a factor influencing the very atherosclerotic process.[151] However, this concept is controversial as other studies suggested that increased expression of Lp-PLA$_2$ decreases atherosclerosis progression.[152-155] For example, hereditary deficiency of Lp-PLA$_2$ in Japanese subjects is linked with an increased risk of CVD.[152]

Clinical studies have investigated the potential link of Lp-PLA$_2$ and CHD in primary prevention populations. The link was first investigated in the West of Scotland Coronary Prevention Study (WOSCOPS).[156] Lp-PLA$_2$ levels were divided into quintiles, with a statistically significant CHD risk increase for the 3rd to the 5th quintile compared to the lower quintiles. The correlation of Lp-PLA$_2$ with CHD risk was independent of traditional risk factors and appeared to be a stronger risk marker than CRP in this population.[156] In the MONitoring of Trends and Determinants in Cardiovascular Disease (MONICA) study, Lp-PLA$_2$ level predicted coronary events in males over a 14-year follow-up but LDL was not measured, and the independence of Lp-PLA$_2$ from LDL could not be assessed.[157] The Atherosclerosis Risk in Communities (ARIC) study showed that Lp-PLA$_2$ predicted the development of CAD independent of LDL only in patients with LDL <130 mg/dL.[127] A case-control study from the women's health study failed to show Lp-PLA$_2$ as an independent predictor of CHD after adjustment for LDL.[158] Hence, further research appears necessary to determine whether this biomarker modifies CHD risk beyond LDL serum levels. Based on current evidence, its best use could be in further risk stratification of intermediate risk patients with LDL levels <130 mg/dL. An immunoassay for Lp-PLA$_2$ mass concentration has received US Food and Drug Administration clearance (PLAC test, diaDexus, San Francisco, CA).

4.1.15. Isoprostanes

Isoprostanes are nonenzymatic molecules derived from the free-radical catalyzed peroxidation of arachidonic acid that circulate in the plasma and are excreted in the urine.[159,160] Isoprostane levels can be measured and are a sensitive marker for oxidative stress. High levels of isoprostanes have been found in atherosclerotic plaque removed from carotid arteries.[161] Urinary isoprostane levels correlate with plasma LDL and elevated isoprostane levels have been noted in patients with diabetes, smoking, and hyperhomocysteinemia.[159,160] Both in unstable angina and during acute myocardial infarction, elevated isoprostanes have been measured in the urine and coronary sinuses of patients undergoing percutaneous coronary intervention or thrombolysis.[159,160] Finally, CAC and isoprostane levels were assayed in a cohort of 2,850 subjects.[162] After adjustment for CRP and traditional risk factors, a high versus low isoprostane level was associated with a 24% higher likelihood of having CAC. Based on available data,

isoprostanes are a promising marker, but there is no prognostic data for CHD risk available at this time.

4.1.16. Fibrinogen

Fibrinogen is a major factor in the common pathway of the coagulation cascade and also acts as an acute-phase reactant. As such, it has been investigated as a marker of CHD risk. A metaanalysis involving 4,018 patients yielded a combined relative risk of 1.8 (95% CI 1.6 to 2.0) for CHD when comparing the highest tertile to the lowest tertile of fibrinogen.[163]

4.1.17. Neopterin

Neopterin, a pyrazolopyridine derivative of the guanosine triphosphate-biopterin pathway, elevates in chronic inflammatory processes. Elevated neopterin has been correlated with an increased risk of CHD events. Avanzas et al.[164] followed patients with chronic stable angina for 1 year and showed that elevated neopterin levels predicted adverse cardiac events. Neopterin has also been investigated as a marker for risk stratification of patients suffering from acute coronary syndromes.[165] Neopterin levels were shown to correlate closely with the thrombolysis in myocardial infarction (TIMI) risk score: as TIMI risk score increased, neopterin level increased. Ray et al. analyzed data from the Pravastatin or Atorvastatin Evaluation Infection-TIMI 22 (PROVE IT TIMI-22) trial and showed that a neopterin level ≥12.11 mmol/L measured 7 days and 4 months after an acute coronary syndrome was associated with an increased risk of death or recurrent events.[166] Further research is needed to assess the role of neopterin as an independent risk factor for CHD in primary prevention populations.

4.1.18. Bilirubin

Bilirubin is a heme degradation end product, but its role now seems more complex with the emergence of data showing antioxidant and anti-inflammatory properties. These properties suggest that bilirubin may be an inhibitor of atherosclerosis. Bilirubin has been shown to act at all steps in the development of atherosclerotic plaque. It inhibits endothelial dysfunction, and low bilirubin is correlated with impaired endothelial function.[167,168] It inhibits endothelial expression of vascular cell adhesion molecule-1 and monocyte transmigration into the vascular intima.[169,170] Bilirubin additionally inhibits the formation of oxLDL, intimal smooth muscle proliferation, and thrombus formation.[171-173] Heme oxygenase is the enzyme catalyzing the rate-limiting step in heme metabolism to bilirubin. Increased heme oxygenase activity has been shown to decrease experimental atherosclerosis.[174] The antiatherogenic effect of heme oxygenase may be due primarily to bilirubin, as administration of bilirubin reproduces the protective effect of heme oxygenase induction.[168]

Based upon its physiological role, higher bilirubin levels would be expected to be protective against CVD. In patients without known CHD, low bilirubin has been associated with increased carotid intimal thickness.[175] Patients with Gilbert syndrome, who have hereditary unconjugated hyperbilirubinemia, have a very low prevalence of CAD.[176] Early case-control and cross-sectional studies suggested an inverse relationship between CAD and bilirubin level in men and women. Schwertner et al.[177] showed that a 50% lower total bilirubin among male Air Force pilots was associated with a 47% higher risk of CAD. Data from the Framingham offspring study have been analyzed to assess the effect of bilirubin levels on CHD events.[178,179] In this cohort study, 4,276 subjects without known CHD at baseline were followed for a mean 21.9 years. Higher bilirubin was associated with lower risk for development of myocardial infarction, CAD, or any cardiovascular event during follow-up among men, but the association was not strong among women. Analysis of data from NHANES 1999 to 2004, a cross-sectional examination of the United States population, showed that a 0.1 mg/dL increment in serum bilirubin was associated with a 9% lower odds (OR 0.9, 95% CI 0.86 to 0.96) of stroke and 6% lower odds (OR 0.94, 95% CI 0.90 to 0.98) of PAD as defined by either leg ankle-brachial index ≤0.9.[180,181] The available data suggest that bilirubin has vascular protective effects; therefore, low bilirubin may be helpful in identifying patients, especially men, at risk for vascular disease.

4.2. Imaging biomarkers

4.2.1. Coronary artery calcium

The tenet of atherosclerosis imaging is that identification of subclinical disease allows early aggressive modification of risk in those at highest risk of future events with potentially optimal gain. CAC is a sensitive indicator of atherosclerosis and it has been extensively studied for risk stratification of asymptomatic individuals first with electron beam computed tomography (EBCT) and more recently with multi detector computed tomography (MDCT) scanners (Fig. 22.3). The most recent generations MDCT scanners, however, have made it possible to obtain consistently good angiographic images of the coronary arteries that clearly demonstrate the presence of luminal stenoses as well as noncalcified plaques. It is therefore natural to question whether in the era of noninvasive CT coronary angiography (CTA) there is still a role for CAC scoring. In the following paragraphs we will address both the utility of CAC and that of CTA for risk stratification.

Quantitative measurement of CAC can be performed with three different scores: the Agatston score, the volume score, and more recently the mass scoring method.[182] While the Agatston method was developed for the EBCT scanners, acquiring axial images at 3 mm intervals, and was based on the assumption that CAC has a minimum attenuation of 130 Hounsfield units,[183] it has been extensively applied to MDCT imaging, and several publications have shown a fair to good numerical correlation between the Agatston score measured by EBCT and MDCT.[184,185] Despite the fact that the volume and mass scores may be more reproducible, especially with MDCT,[186] most publications have reported the Agatston score that has become the universally accepted reporting method.

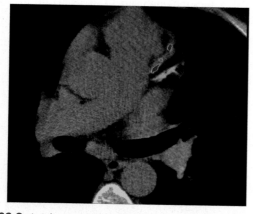

Figure 22.3 Axial computed tomography images of the chest; coronary artery calcium in an asymptomatic patient with hypertension and family history of premature coronary artery disease. The software uses color coding to differentiate plaques seen along the left anterior descending coronary artery and its branch according to the calcium concentration in the plaque (the darker the color the greater the plaque attenuation).

Histopathologic and autopsy studies have demonstrated that CAC amounts to about 20% of the total plaque volume. Although the presence of CAC is pathognomonic of the presence of atherosclerosis, its absence on chest CT imaging cannot be taken as absolute proof of absence of atherosclerotic disease. In fact, multiple correlative studies employing either invasive or noninvasive angiographic techniques have shown that about 5% to 8% of patients without CAC may have a critical coronary artery lesion (>50% luminal stenosis).[187,188] This, however, appears to be true particularly in symptomatic patients[189] and may not apply to the majority of asymptomatic subjects screened for atherosclerosis.

Prognostic role of coronary artery calcium. Several publications have demonstrated the independent and incremental prognostic value of CAC over traditional risk factors both for the prediction of all cause mortality and cardiovascular events. Shaw et al.[190] reported that the adjusted relative risk for all-cause death was 1.64, 1.74, 2.54, and 4.03 for CAC scores of 11 to 100, 101 to 400, 401 to 1,000, and greater than 1,000 compared to a CAC of 1 to 10 in a cohort of 10,377 asymptomatic patients followed for a mean of 5 years. The area under the receiver operating characteristic curve (AUC) to predict death was greater for CAC than for traditional risk factors (0.72 to 0.78, p <0.001).

Greenland et al.[191] followed 1,312 subjects for a median of 7 years after CAC screening. All patients had at least one risk factor for atherosclerosis and the primary endpoint was either nonfatal myocardial infarction or cardiovascular death. A CAC score >300 was associated with a hazard ratio of 3.9 for the occurrence of a primary event during follow-up. The addition of CAC to traditional risk factors provided incremental prognostic value for the prediction of a cardiac event, although this was true only in patients with a baseline FRS >10% at 10 years.

In the St. Francis heart study,[192] 4,613 asymptomatic subjects 50 to 70 years old were followed for 4.3 years after CAC screening. The baseline CAC score was higher in the 119 patients who suffered cardiovascular events than those without events [median score (interquartile range): 384 (127, 800) versus 10 (0, 86); p <0.0001]. For subjects with a CAC score ≥ 100 versus <100, the relative risk (95% confidence interval) of nonfatal myocardial infarction and death was 9.2 (4.9 to 17.3). The CAC score predicted cardiovascular events independently of standard risk factors and CRP (p = 0.004) and was superior to the FRS (AUC 0.79 ± 0.03 vs. 0.69 ± 0.03, p = 0.0006). Similarly, LaMonte et al.,[193] Taylor et al.,[194] and Kondos et al.[195] added further evidence that CAC works well in intermediate risk patients to improve risk prediction.

The utility of CAC screening has also been investigated in special subsets of the populations such as women, diabetic patients, and the elderly. Two original investigations and one metaanalysis supported the utility of CAC for risk stratification in women. Raggi et al.[196] compared the occurrence of all-cause death in approximately 4,000 women and 6,000 men referred for CAC screening by primary care physicians. CAC scores were lower in women than men (p <0.0001), but death rates were higher among older, diabetic, hypertensive, and smoking patients of both sexes. In risk-adjusted models, women had a greater probability of death than men for any CAC score. Importantly, CAC added incremental prognostic value to the FRS (p <0.0001) in both sexes.

Lakoski et al.[197] conducted gender analyses of the MESA data and noted that a CAC score >0 was a strong predictor of coronary heart and CVD events in 2,684 women considered at low-risk by Framingham categories compared to patients without CAC (hazard ratio 6.5 and 5.2, respectively). Finally in a metaanalysis of three prospective and two observational registries, Bellasi et al.[198]

concluded that CAC screening is equally accurate in stratifying risk for all-cause death and CVD events in women and men.

Several clinical studies have shown that glucose intolerance and insulin resistance are associated with increased prevalence of CAC[199,200]; similarly frank diabetes mellitus is associated with a greater extent of CAC compared to the nondiabetic population.[201] Both Wong et al.[202] and Anand et al.[203] demonstrated an increasing incidence of inducible ischemia on stress myocardial perfusion imaging in diabetic patients with greater amounts of CAC. Type-2 diabetic patients with a CAC score of ≤10, 11 to 100, 101 to 400, 401 to 1,000, and >1,000, had an incidence of myocardial ischemia of 0%, 18%, 23%, 48%, and 71%, respectively,[203] and morbidity and mortality increased proportionally with the CAC score and ischemic burden.[203] In an observational registry, Raggi et al.[204] showed a higher all-cause mortality rate for any extent of CAC in diabetic than nondiabetic subjects ($p > 0.001$). Of interest, the 5-year mortality of diabetic patients with little or no CAC (approximately 30% of a cohort of 903 diabetic patients) was as low as that of nondiabetic subjects without CAC (about 1% at the end of follow-up).

CAC maintains its utility as a tool for risk stratification in the elderly. In the prospective Rotterdam study, 2,013 participants (men 71 ± 5.7 years of age) were submitted to CAC screening as well as measurement of traditional cardiovascular risk factors.[205] Men and women in the highest CAC score category showed an adjusted odds ratio for myocardial infarction of 7.7 (95% CI 4.1 to 14.5) and 6.7 (95% CI 2.4 to 19.1), respectively compared to the lowest score category (0 to 100).[205] The predictive power of CAC was independent of the FRS category (low, intermediate, or high). Raggi et al.[206] followed 35,388 patients with 3,570 subjects ≥ 70 years old at screening for an average period of 5.8 ± 3 years. They reported an expected increase in all-cause mortality with increasing age (relative hazard per age decile increase: 1.09; CI: 1.08 to 1.10, $p < 0.0001$) and with higher death rates among men than women (hazard ratio: 1.53; 1.32 to 1.77, $p < 0.0001$). Nonetheless, increasing CAC scores were associated with decreasing survival rates across all age deciles ($p < 0.0001$), suggesting that CAC is predictive even in older age. Finally, using CAC score categories, over 40% of elderly patients were reclassified to either lower or higher risk categories compared to their original FRS group.[206] This was likely due to a reduction in risk attributed to age, the variable carrying most weight in the Framingham equations, in the absence of subclinical atherosclerosis.

Finally, a very important question that needed to be addressed is whether CAC has the same predictive value in subjects of different races. Until recently, most of the published data on CAC had been collected in Caucasians. Data from the MESA study as well as other series[207,208] demonstrated that Caucasians have a higher prevalence of CAC and larger CAC scores than other races and this raised the question of the validity of CAC in nonCaucasians. Two recent publications addressed the value of CAC as a marker of risk in four different races (Caucasian, African-American, Chinese, and Hispanic) in the United States. Nasir et al.[208] evaluated the use of CAC to predict all-cause mortality (505 deaths during 10 years of follow-up) in 14,812 patients. The prevalence of CAC was highest in Whites, although Blacks and Hispanics had a greater clustering of risk factors for CAD. Despite a lower prevalence of CAC and lower scores compared to other races, black patients demonstrated the highest mortality rates even after multivariable adjustment for clinical risk factors and baseline CAC scores ($p < 0.0001$). Compared with Whites, the relative risk of death was 2.97 (CI:1.87 to 4.72) in Blacks, 1.58 (CI: 0.92 to 2.71) in Hispanics, and 0.85 (CI: 0.47 to 1.54) in Chinese patients. Detrano et al.[209] showed

that CAC is a strong predictor of cardiovascular death, nonfatal myocardial infarction, angina, and revascularization (total events = 162) independent of race in 6,722 MESA patients (the risk increased 7.7-fold in patients with a CAC score between 101 and 300 compared to 0- and 9.7-fold in patients with a score >300). Furthermore, CAC added incremental prognostic value beyond traditional risk factors for the prediction of events in all races.[209] Hence, CAC appears to be an excellent marker of risk in all races so far investigated, although the prognostic significance of score categories may vary between racial groups.

The evidence surrounding CAC was recently reviewed in two statements of the American Heart Association[210] and the American College of Cardiology,[211] who recognized the potential utility of CAC screening for refinement of risk assessment in intermediate risk patients.

4.2.2. Contrast-enhanced coronary computed tomographic angiography

In view of the recent technological advances in cardiac CT, it may be logical to question whether the risk discriminating ability of CAC may not be surpassed by the information obtained with coronary CT angiography. The latter has demonstrated excellent accuracy in excluding (negative predictive value: 95% to 98%) and less optimal accuracy in confirming the presence of luminal stenoses (positive predictive value ~70%) compared to invasive angiography.[212,213] However, this technology allows the acquisition of additional information of great potential utility such as the presence of noncalcified obstructive and noncalcified and nonobstructive plaque (Fig. 22.4) and ventricular functional data. Indeed, in two recent studies the presence of nonobstructive disease has been linked with a more unfavorable outcome than the complete absence of luminal encroachment by atherosclerotic plaques.[214,215]

Numerous investigators have attempted to separate lipid-rich from fibrotic plaques by assessing the mean attenuation (density) of areas apparently containing noncalcified plaques and performed comparative studies of CT and IVUS. MDCT appears to underestimate plaque volume compared to IVUS and shows modest (53%) to good sensitivity (83%) for the identification of noncalcified plaques compared to IVUS. The mean CT attenuation of lipid rich plaques, that appear hypo-echogenic on IVUS, is significantly lower than that of hyper-echogenic (i.e., fibrotic) plaques with values ranging from 14 to 58 HU for the former to

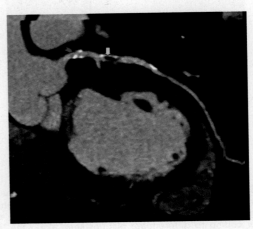

Figure 22.4 Computed tomography coronary angiography showing mixed atherosclerotic plaques with noncalcified (*red arrow head*) and calcified areas (*yellow arrow*).

90 to 120 HU for the latter.[216–218] Computed tomography angiography performed in patients with acute coronary syndromes show less coronary artery calcification, larger and more numerous low attenuation plaques,[219,220] and positive remodeling[221] compared to patients with stable angina. Motoyama et al.[221] reported that the simultaneous presence of positive remodeling, areas of low attenuation, and spotty calcification on CT angiography identifies with 95% accuracy the culprit plaque associated with an acute coronary syndrome. Although attractive, the use of mean attenuation to identify the lipid-rich, fracture prone plaque suffers from a fundamental flaw; most investigators reported a substantial overlap between CT attenuation values of lipid-rich and fibrotic plaques, indicating that relying exclusively on measurement of mean plaque attenuation may not be sufficient to define its vulnerability. Furthermore, there are several other considerations to be made that may temper the enthusiasm for performing CTA in asymptomatic subjects. The presence and degree of luminal stenosis on invasive angiography has not been shown to be predictive of severity and time to events.[222] Furthermore, correction of luminal stenoses has not been shown to improve survival or reduce the occurrence of myocardial infarction.[223] There is currently no proven and reproducible method to quantify noncalcified plaque burden. A recent study suggested that the incremental value of detecting noncalcified plaque over the simpler calcium score is minimal in asymptomatic patients. In this study the investigators found coronary atherosclerotic plaques in 215 of 1,000 Korean subjects, but only 40 (4%) had noncalcified plaques (calcium score = 0).[224]

Finally, the radiation exposure provided by CT angiography is high (close to that of a stress nuclear test and larger than that of an uncomplicated diagnostic invasive coronary angiogram). It is therefore logical to conclude that CT angiography should not be considered a screening tool for refinement of risk prediction in asymptomatic subjects, at this time. The American College of Cardiology recently endorsed a list of appropriate uses of CT angiography and screening for asymptomatic CAD was excluded.[225]

4.2.3. Epicardial adipose tissue

Growing evidence suggests that regional fat distribution, rather than just total body fat, plays an important role in cardiovascular risk. Excess visceral adipose tissue, especially around the abdominal viscerae, holds a stronger association with the metabolic syndrome and with CVD than overall obesity or subcutaneous adipose tissue.[226–230] Epicardial adipose tissue (EAT) is a type of visceral fat that shares a common embryonic origin with abdominal visceral adipose tissue.[231] EAT is most plentiful in the interventricular and atrioventricular grooves. As it increases, it covers the right ventricular free wall and then the left ventricular wall.[232]

The adipose tissue has a variety of functions besides fat storage. It produces adipokines, i.e., cytokines and chemokines secreted by adipocytes and the inflammatory cells located within adipose tissue. Adipokine production may have a central role in the association between obesity and CVD.[233] Adipokines, such as IL-1β, IL-6, IL-8, IL-10, TNF-α, adiponectin, leptin, monocyte chemoattractive protein-1 (MCP-1), plasminogen activator inhibitor-1 (PAI-1), and resistin, have paracrine and endocrine functions that may influence vascular inflammation and atherosclerosis.

EAT is ideally situated to have a paracrine effect on the epicardial coronary arteries since there is no fascia separating them from EAT. Adipokines from EAT may diffuse directly to the vascular intima from the perivascular fat, leading to the initiation of inflammation, atherosclerosis development, and plaque instability.[234,235] Mazurek et al.[236] showed that inflammatory adipokines

were elevated in EAT from patients with CAD undergoing coronary artery bypass grafting but not from subcutaneous adipose tissue, suggesting a unique role for EAT in CAD development. Biopsy samples of EAT and subcutaneous adipose tissue were obtained from 42 patients undergoing coronary artery bypass. Higher levels of MCP-1, IL-1β, IL-6, and TNF-α were found in EAT than in subcutaneous tissue, and EAT inflammation was independent of the presence or absence of whole-body obesity. Support for a paracrine effect of EAT on the development of CAD also has come from studies of intramyocardial segments of coronary arteries, such as myocardial bridge segments. These segments, naturally free of any fat wrapping, tend to be free of atherosclerotic lesions.[237–240]

Given the above postulated connection between EAT and coronary atherosclerosis, there is considerable interest in EAT as a CAD risk marker. EAT has been measured by several means including echocardiography, magnetic resonance imaging (MRI), and noncontrast computed tomography (CT). By echocardiogram, EAT appears as a hypo-echoic free space between the visceral pericardium and the epicardium. The thickness of this free space is measured on the right ventricular free wall in the parasternal long and short axis views. The thickest EAT is usually found on the surface of the right ventricular free wall.[241] Since EAT is distributed nonuniformly over the epicardial surface and there is significant interindividual variation in EAT distribution, doubt remains about the correlation of echocardiographic EAT thickness measurement at a single point with total EAT volume. Additionally, echocardiographic EAT assessment is dependent on the acoustic window and may be less accurate in obese patients. CT has also been used to measure EAT (Fig. 22.5). Gorter et al.[242] compared several CT methods to measure EAT. Measurement of total EAT volume was found to be the most reproducible, although this method is time consuming. Ding et al.[243] shortened the analysis time by measuring EAT volume only around the proximal coronary arteries; this reduced the analysis time to 10 min, or approximately 50% less than the traditional method. Interestingly, this new method was highly reproducible and correlated well with CT measurement of the entire EAT volume.

Current research suggests that elevated EAT is linked to increased CAD risk. Two recent studies correlated an increasing CAC score on cardiac CT with increasing EAT.[243,244] This association was independent of visceral abdominal fat and traditional cardiac

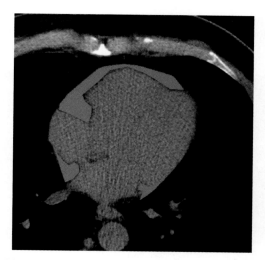

Figure 22.5 Axial image of the heart showing an example of epicardial adipose tissue measurement (*pink area*); the area can be drawn manually or by means of a semi-automatic tool.

risk factors. Several other investigators sought a link between EAT and coronary disease on coronary angiography. Taguchi et al.[245] submitted a population of 251 Japanese males, of which 70 were obese, to CT imaging to measure EAT, visceral abdominal fat, and subcutaneous fat. The presence of CAD was established by coronary angiography. The presence of CAD was closely associated with increased EAT, more so than visceral abdominal fat or subcutaneous fat. Four studies correlated EAT thickness measured on the right ventricular free wall by echocardiography with coronary angiography findings. Three of the studies[246-248] showed that EAT thickness was greater in patients with CAD and that increasing severity of CAD correlated with increasing EAT thickness. The fourth study[249] found no significant correlation between EAT thickness and CAD.

Hence, EAT volume has the potential to emerge as a screening test for subclinical coronary atherosclerosis and as a marker to help risk stratify subjects carrying risk factors for atherosclerosis. CT seems to be the winning imaging technique at this time because of its use of execution and reproducibility. The next necessary step will be to establish a correlation between EAT volume and risk of CHD events in prospective studies.

4.2.4. Carotid intima media thickness

The presence of extracardiac atherosclerosis has long been recognized as a marker of coronary atherosclerosis and has been clearly linked with an adverse cardiovascular outcome. Specifically, the association of carotid atherosclerosis with coronary atherosclerosis is high.[250] The presence of obstructive carotid artery stenosis diagnosed by Duplex ultrasonography, however, is an indicator of advanced atherosclerotic disease. On the contrary, the assessment of carotid IMT has established itself as a surrogate marker of preclinical atherosclerosis.[251] Indeed, although IMT is a measure of the composite thickness of both the tunica intima and the tunica media, and it can be increased in diseases that mainly affect the media, it correlates with atherosclerotic vascular disease in several arterial beds including the coronary arteries.

Intimal media thickness measurement. Carotid IMT is usually measured using ultrasound equipment with high frequency transducers (preferably 6 to 12 MHz linear array transducers) and dedicated software (Fig. 22.6). IMT is usually measured using B-mode imaging, although some investigators have used M-mode because of its greater temporal resolution.[252] The common carotid artery, the bulb, and the internal and external carotid arteries are meticulously scanned using different angles to better detect the

thickest wall area and the presence of a plaque. With B-mode ultrasound it is possible to visualize a double-line pattern on both near and far carotid artery walls on longitudinal plane images. The double-line pattern represents the leading edges of the lumen-intima and media-adventitia interfaces and ensures that the sonographer is imaging the vessel at its truest diameter.[253] Typically IMT is measured in end-diastole in the far wall of the common or internal carotid artery; in fact the far wall usually shows the double-line pattern in greater detail than in near wall. The measurement can be made manually by trained readers or by means of automated edge detection calipers. Inter-adventitial and lumen diameter measurements must also be obtained as IMT is significantly correlated with the arterial diameter.

The site of measurement of IMT is a matter of great debate and it can be performed in the common carotid artery, the carotid bulb, and the internal carotid artery. Measurement of IMT in the common carotid artery is easier and can be achieved in most cases, whereas the bulb and the internal carotid artery may not be accessible in all subjects, especially those with a short neck. Furthermore, the common carotid usually shows a thicker IMT and this renders the measurement more reproducible. However, measurement of IMT at multiple sites may provide additional information in terms of prognosis.[254] A multiple measurement protocol that includes several measurements at all three sites is usually applied and the mean of the maximum wall thickness at all sites is used.[255]

Most authorities prefer not to include plaques in the measurement of IMT and report the presence of plaques separately. Atherosclerotic plaque is defined as a focal structure encroaching into the arterial lumen that measures at least 0.5 mm in thickness, or 50% of the surrounding IMT value, or demonstrates a thickness of 1.5 mm when measured from the media-adventitia interface to the lumen-intima interface (Fig. 22.7).[253] The presence of carotid plaques is a strong predictor of cardiovascular events. In fact, their presence is associated with increased risk of stroke and myocardial infarction.[256,257] Attempts at characterizing the *"vulnerability"* of carotid plaques by ultrasound, has brought to the identification of echolucent plaques as being a marker of high risk. In the study by Honda et al.,[258] the presence of echolucent carotid plaques in patients with stable CAD was associated with an increased risk of future acute coronary events independent of other risk factors.

Clinical significance of intimal media thickness. Carotid wall thickness varies with age, race, and sex, on average being thicker in men than in women.[259] On average, IMT increases by almost 0.03 mm/year in patients with CAD, but only by 0.01 mm/year in subjects without coronary CAD.[260,261] Data from large population studies indicate that IMT in black subjects exceeds IMT in white patients in both genders.[262] Furthermore, the Bogalusa study showed that the relationship between childhood risk factors and IMT in adulthood differs among different races.[263] It is therefore preferable to use age, race, and gender-specific reference values of IMT rather than an absolute threshold; however, in middle aged subjects an IMT of 1 mm or more is considered abnormal, because IMT above this value has been clearly associated with a poor outcome.[264] Recently in a British population, the upper limits of IMT of the common carotid artery for participants of age 35 to 39, 40 to 49, 50 to 59, and 60 years or older were 0.60, 0.64, 0.71, and 0.81 mm, respectively, whereas at the bifurcation they were 0.83, 0.77, 0.85, and 1.05 mm, respectively.[265]

Age, cardiovascular risk factors, and genetic background are important determinants of IMT. Furthermore, a significant part

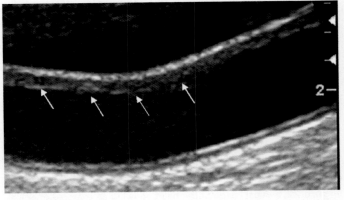

Figure 22.6 Example of a segment of the proximal left common carotid artery showing a thick intima-media layer (*white arrows*).

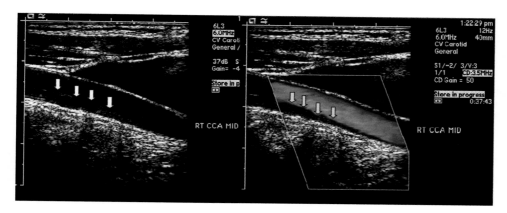

Figure 22.7 A: Smooth, homogeneous plaque along the mid portion of the right common carotid artery of a 53-year-old smoker (*white arrows*). **B:** Color Doppler filling of the lumen of the carotid artery highlights better the presence of the plaque, confirming that it is not an artifact (*yellow arrows* point at the atherosclerotic plaque).

of the variation of IMT depends on lifestyle characteristics. For example, it has been shown that Japanese Americans have a thicker IMT than native Japanese subjects probably due to the adoption of western lifestyle and a higher prevalence of metabolic disorders.[266] Body mass index, abdominal adiposity, and physical inactivity are also associated with an increased carotid IMT.[267,268] Interestingly, data from the ARIC study showed that a higher rate of IMT progression is associated with low income in white patients but with high income in black patients, indicating differential associations of socioeconomic status with atherosclerosis among races.[269]

IMT is increased in the presence of many cardiovascular risk factors, such as smoking, hypertension, diabetes mellitus, and hypercholesterolemia.[268,270] The combination of multiple risk factors is associated with even higher IMT values, as is the presence of the metabolic syndrome.[271] Furthermore, IMT in adulthood is related to the presence of cardiovascular risk factors during childhood, denoting that IMT reflects the impact of risk factors on atherosclerosis development.[272]

IMT is a strong predictor of cardiovascular events, such as myocardial infarction and stroke, although one study found no association in men.[256] In the ARIC study, a 0.2 mm thicker IMT was associated with a 28% higher relative risk of stroke and 33% higher relative risk of myocardial infarction.[264] In the Rotterdam Study IMT predicted an increased risk of stroke and myocardial infarction.[273] Similar results were also obtained from the Cardiovascular Health Study.[254] In most, yet not all studies, IMT was associated with cardiovascular events independently of the presence of traditional cardiovascular risk factors. Although there is evidence that the predictive value of IMT is higher in high-risk populations,[257] the CAPS Study showed that IMT also predicts cardiovascular mortality in low-risk asymptomatic subjects.[274] It is often assumed that the relationship between carotid IMT and cardiovascular risk is linear; however, a recent metaanalysis demonstrated that it is nonlinear in most populations, especially for myocardial infarction.[275] The risk associated with a specific increase in IMT is age-dependent, the risk being higher in younger individuals (<50 years) with an increased IMT.[275]

The prognostic value of IMT has also been evaluated along with that of ankle-brachial index (ABI). The two indices appear equivalent, but, when taken together, they have higher prognostic value than each taken alone.[276] Of note, IMT is a better predictor of stroke than CAC, at least in the elderly,[277] whereas in the MESA study CAC was a stronger predictor of future cardiovascular events than IMT.[278] Finally, IMT predicts myocardial infarction independently of the presence of atherosclerosis in the aorta or the lower extremities.[279]

Carotid IMT has been used as a surrogate end-point in intervention studies of various antiatherogenic treatments, including statins, antihypertensive agents, such as calcium antagonists, β-blockers and angiotensin converting enzyme inhibitors, and recently insulin sensitizing agents.[280–284] In the ARBITER study, atorvastatin 80 mg/daily lowered LDL cholesterol by 49%, to 76 ± 23 mg/dL, and pravastatin 40 mg/daily lowered LDL cholesterol by 27%, to 110 ± 30 mg/dL. In the pravastatin group, IMT stabilized, whereas in the atorvastatin group the IMT decreased ($p = 0.03$ for the difference between treatment arms) during a 12 month follow–up period.[280] In ARBITER-2, the addition of niacin to statins induced a further reduction in IMT.[282] Interestingly, in the ENHANCE trial,[283] a combination of ezetimibe 10 mg/daily and simvastatin 80 mg/dL to lower LDL cholesterol in familiar hypercholesterolemia patients to a lower level than simvastatin 80 mg/daily failed to demonstrate a benefit in terms of IMT regression. Finally, in the CHICAGO trial[284] the thiazolidinedione agent pioglitazone (15 to 45 mg/daily) halted the progression of IMT while sulfonylurea glimepiride (1 to 4 mg/daily) did not in 462 diabetes type-2 adult patients treated for 18 months. Numerous other studies have employed IMT as an endpoint of therapy as shown in the limited list displayed in Table 22.1.

As carotid IMT reflects the effects of several determinants of atherosclerosis on vascular structure, the American Heart Association and the European Society of Hypertension/European Society of Cardiology suggest that the measurement of carotid IMT may add to the overall risk prediction, especially in individuals at intermediate pretest risk.[251,285] The European Society of Hypertension and the European Society of Cardiology further recommend that IMT be measured as an assessment of target-organ damage in all patients with arterial hypertension.[285]

4.2.3. Cardiovascular magnetic resonance imaging

Cardiovascular magnetic resonance (CMR) can be employed to image atherosclerotic plaques of large vessels and characterize plaque composition.[286] CMR differentiates plaque components on the basis of biochemical and biophysical parameters such as physical state, water content, and molecular motion and diffusion.[287] Given its ability to differentiate plaque components, CMR has the potential to distinguish unstable atherosclerotic from stable plaques (see Chapter 23), potentially providing important prognostic information. An unstable plaque is more likely to cause clinical events, even if it is nonobstructive.[288] Histological characteristics that identify vulnerable plaque include a large necrotic lipid core, a thin fibrous cap overlying the plaque, intraplaque hemorrhage, and inflammation with activated macrophages in close proximity to the fibrous cap.[289,290]

TABLE 22.1

STUDIES OF ATHEROSCLEROSIS REGRESSION USING IMT AS ENDPOINT

Study acronym	Study type	Number of patients	Type of treatment	Carotid IMT change/Year (mm)	Carotid IMT change/Year (mm)	p-value
CLAS	Prospective and randomized 2 and 4 year follow-ups	78	Colestipol-Niacin vs. Placebo	Colestipol-Niacin 2 year: −0.005 4 year: −0.05	Placebo 2 year: 0.004 ± 0.06 4 year: 0.005 ± 0.08	0.0001 0.0004
ACAPS	Prospective and randomized 3 year follow-up	919	Placebo + Placebo Lovastatin + Placebo Lovastatin + Warfarin	0.006 ± 0.003 −0.009 ± 0.003 −0.03 ± 0.003		NS 0.01 0.06 (all values compared to baseline)
ASAP	Prospective and randomized 2 year follow-up	325 patients with familiar hyper-cholesterolemia	Atorvastatin 80 mg/d vs. Simvastatin 40 mg/d	Atorvastatin −0.031	Simvastatin 0.036	0.0001
ARBITER-1	Prospective and randomized 1 year follow-up	161	Atorvastatin 80 mg/d vs. Pravastatin 40 mg/d	Atorvastatin −0.034 ± 0.021	Pravastatin 0.025 ± 0.017	0.03
ARBITER-2	Prospective and randomized 1 year follow-up	167 with low HDL	Niacin + Statins vs. Placebo + Statins	Niacin + Statins 0.044 ± 0.1 (p < 0.001 compared to baseline)	Placebo + Statins 0.014 ± 0.1 (p = NS compared to baseline)	0.08
ENHANCE	Prospective and randomized 2 year follow-up	720 patients with familial hyper-cholesterolemia	Simvastatin 80 mg/d + ezetimibe 10 mg/d vs. Simvastatin 80 mg/d + Placebo	Ezetimibe 0.0111 ± 0.0038	Placebo 0.0058 ± 0.0037	0.29
CHICAGO	Prospective and randomized 72 week follow-up	462 patients with type 2 diabetes mellitus	Pioglitazone (15–45 mg/d) vs. Glimepiride (1–4 mg/d)	Pioglitazone −0.001	Glimepiride + 0.012	0.02

Most CMR plaque imaging is being performed currently on whole-body 1.5-Tesla MR systems though there has been some investigation of 3.0-Tesla MR systems. The use of 3.0-Tesla CMR has been shown to improve signal-to-noise ratio 1.4- to 2.4-fold over 1.5-Tesla CMR for carotid plaque imaging,[291-293] and recent work by Maroules et al.[294] showed that 3.0-Tesla CMR allows shorter scan time than 1.5-Tesla CMR. In vivo CMR plaque imaging and characterization have been performed utilizing a multi-contrast approach with high-resolution black blood spin echo, fast spin echo-based MR, and bright blood sequences. The most effective black blood sequence is double inversion recovery. Using this method, the signal from the flowing blood is suppressed and turned black for optimal characterization of the vessel wall.[295-297] Identification of plaque characteristics such as size of lipid core, calcified nodules, intraplaque hemorrhage, and thickness of the fibrous cap requires the use of contrast weighting (T_1, T_2, and proton density) with black blood imaging.[298] Calcium is hypointense on T_1, T_2, and proton density weighting; the lipid core is hyperintense with proton density and T1 weighting but hypointense with T2 weighting, and fibrous plaque components are hyperintense on T_1, T_2, and proton density weighting.[299] Bright blood imaging (3D time-of-flight [TOF]) can be employed to assess the thickness of the fibrous cap and the morphological integrity of

atherosclerotic plaques.[300] Finally, contrast-enhanced MRI (CE-MRI) using gadolinium for evaluation of atherosclerotic plaque has been investigated. Fibrous tissue has been found to enhance with contrast, so CE-MRI may be useful for the assessment of fibrous cap thickness.[301,302] Plaque contrast enhancement has also been associated with elevated serum inflammatory markers, suggesting that a contrast-enhancing plaque may be more inflamed and thus a higher-risk plaque.[303,304]

Saam et al.[305] used both CMR and histological examination of carotid endarterectomy specimens from 40 patients to assess CMR identification of plaque composition. MRI measurements of lipid core, dense fibrous tissue, and loose fibrous matrix were statistically equivalent to histological measurements. Calcification, however, was underestimated by CMR. A similar recent study assessed 12 carotid endarterectomy specimens by both CMR and histological examination.[306] Compared to histological examination, CMR demonstrated a sensitivity and specificity of 92% and 74% for lipid core, 82% and 94% for fibrous tissue, and 72% and 87% for loose connective tissue. In contrast to the study by Saam et al., in this study CMR had a sensitivity and specificity of 98% and 99% for plaque calcification. CMR has also been shown to detect intraplaque hemorrhage with 90% sensitivity and 74% specificity, and CMR and histological examination showed moderate to high agreement for the classification of different stages of intraplaque hemorrhage.[307] Using in vivo multi-contrast CMR, Yuan et al. detected the presence of a lipid core and acute intraplaque hemorrhage in human carotid arteries with a sensitivity of 85% and a specificity of 92%.[308]

Direct MR thrombus imaging (MRDTI, a technique sensitive to methemoglobin in the plaque) has been used to detect complex carotid disease with intraplaque hemorrhage.[309-311] Moody et al.[310] compared MRDTI findings with endarterectomy specimens and showed a sensitivity and specificity of 84% for the detection of complex plaque in the carotid artery ipsilateral to an old TIA or stroke. Murphy et al.[312] described a high prevalence of complex carotid plaques with MRDTI ipsilateral to a recent TIA or stroke, but a significantly lower prevalence in the contralateral carotid and complete absence of complex plaque in healthy controls. Finally, elevated serum levels of inflammatory markers such as fibrinogen and CRP[313] or IL-6 and intercellular adhesion molecule-1 and vascular cell adhesion molecule-1[304] have been shown to be associated with increased wall thickness of the aorta and carotid arteries on CMR.

A number of small studies have investigated the clinical use of CMR for the detection of atherosclerotic plaques at high risk of rupture, to track plaque progression and to assess the effect of lipid-lowering treatment on plaque volume and composition. Yuan et al.[309] studied 53 consecutive patients (mean age 71, in 49 men) scheduled for carotid endarterectomy who were submitted to CMR of the carotid arteries prior to surgery. Twenty-eight patients had a recent history of TIA or stroke ipsilateral to the index carotid lesion, and 25 were asymptomatic. The fibrous cap was categorized as intact-thick, intact-thin, or ruptured on CMR images. Ruptured caps were significantly more frequent than thick-intact caps in symptomatic patients (70% vs. 9%, $p = 0.001$). Takaya et al.[314] showed that patients with carotid intraplaque hemorrhage had accelerated plaque progression over 18 months. Therefore, intraplaque hemorrhage may be a stimulus for atherosclerosis progression. In a study of 154 patients with asymptomatic 50% to 79% stenosis by carotid Doppler, high risk plaque characteristics (intraplaque hemorrhage, thin or ruptured fibrous cap, and large necrotic lipid cores) were highly associated with future cerebrovascular events.[315] Similarly, U-King-Im et al.[316] in a case control study involving 18 symptomatic and 19 asymptomatic patients with >50% carotid stenosis by Doppler showed that patients with symptomatic stenosis had more complex atherosclerotic lesions, with a greater risk of ruptured fibrous cap, intraplaque hemorrhage, and large necrotic lipid core. A study of 192 patients undergoing CMR after carotid Doppler showed that a significant percentage of patients with <50% carotid stenosis by ultrasound have complex atherosclerotic lesions (surface disruption, calcified nodule, and intraplaque hemorrhage) and are thus presumably at higher risk of clinical events than would be predicted by degree of stenosis alone.[317]

Finally, in an investigation from the MESA, Wasserman et al.[318] showed that high serum total cholesterol, but no other CHD risk factor, is strongly associated with the presence of a large lipid core in carotid artery atherosclerotic plaques by CMR.

CMR is as accurate for aortic plaque detection as it is for carotid plaque. Furthermore, several studies have shown a good correlation between CMR findings and histological examination of aortic plaques.[319-322] In asymptomatic Framingham Study subjects, the prevalence of aortic atherosclerosis by CMR increased significantly with patients' age and was higher in the abdominal aorta than in the thoracic aorta.[323] Similarly, in 102 symptomatic patients undergoing coronary angiography,[313] plaques were noted by CMR more frequently in the abdominal (90%) than in the thoracic aorta (61%) and were more prevalent in patients with established CAD. In a study of 146 patients undergoing coronary angiography and thoracic and abdominal aortic imaging by CMR, not only were aortic plaques more common in patients with CAD but complex aortic plaques were also associated with myocardial infarction and with complex coronary lesions (vulnerable plaques). These findings suggest that complex aortic plaques found by CMR may be a marker of coronary plaque instability and may identify high risk patients.

Another interesting application of CMR is the study of plaque regression in the carotid arteries as well as the aorta. In a case-control study, Zhao et al.[324] observed that the carotid arteries of patients treated with long-term, aggressive lipid-lowering therapy contained plaques with smaller lipid cores on CMR and more calcification than untreated subjects. Corti et al.[325] followed prospectively the progression of carotid and aortic plaques in 51 asymptomatic hypercholesterolemic subjects treated with statins. Treatment effect was assessed as change in lumen area (LA), vessel wall thickness (VWT), and vessel wall area (VWA) from baseline. Significant ($p = 0.01$) reductions in maximal VWT and VWA (10% and 11% for aortic and 8% and 11% for carotid plaques, respectively), without changes in LA, were reported at 12 months. Further decreases in VWT and VWA ranging from 12% to 20% were observed at 18 and 24 months along with a slight but significant increase (ranging from 4% to 6%) in LA.[326]

The effect of moderate versus aggressive lipid lowering on plaque regression was addressed in a prospective study by Lima et al.[327] The investigators used a combination of surface and transesophageal CMR to enhance detection of thoracic aorta plaque regression in 27 asymptomatic subjects treated with either a moderate dose (20 mg/day) or a high dose (80 mg/day) of simvastatin. Both plaque volume and plaque area regressed significantly ($p < 0.02$ for both measurements) during a follow-up period of 6 months, while the vessel LA did not change. The degree of plaque regression over this period was directly related to the degree of LDL lowering. Similarly, in 43 patients randomized for 2 years to low dose (5 mg) or high dose (20 mg) rosuvastatin, aggressive LDL reduction was associated with halting of progression of carotid artery disease and reduction in lipid core size.[328] Yonemura et al.[329] showed the same effect on aortic plaque using a randomization of atorvastatin 5 mg daily versus 20 mg daily. Bezafibrate treatment in 22 hypertriglyceridemic patients induced atherosclerotic plaque regression in both the thoracic and abdominal aorta as measured by baseline and follow-up CMR.[330] Finally, in an experimental rabbit model, Corti et al.[331] used CMR to demonstrate that PPAR-gamma agonists enhance the effect of statins on atherosclerotic plaque regression and composition.

Very little data are available regarding use of CMR for plaque characterization in the coronary arteries that are obviously very mobile and smaller than the aorta and carotid arteries. Attempts at identifying coronary artery plaque have been made using both breath-holding black-blood techniques[332] and a real-time navigator for respiratory gating.[333] Kim et al.[334] investigated 136 patients with type 1 diabetes without known CVD. Coronary plaque burden, expressed as mean right coronary artery wall thickness, was greater in patients with diabetic nephropathy than in those without. In a small sample of the MESA population, Macedo et al.[335] demonstrated a greater coronary artery wall thickness in patients with two or more risk factors. Interestingly, this held true even in the few patients without CAC but with more than two risk factors for atherosclerosis, suggesting that a 0 calcium score may not completely exclude the presence of atherosclerosis in the vessel wall. Despite these initial encouraging results it is obvious that the future of coronary MR imaging is still far from coming.

4.3. Endothelial function

The vascular endothelium is composed of a single layer of cells representing the border between the blood pool and the vascular wall. Contrary to older views that interpreted the endothelium as a simple barrier, it is now known that it has multiple functions that may play a key role in the homeostasis of the cardiovascular system. The endothelium serves as a paracrine organ, and it produces a large number of substances that affect vascular tone, smooth muscle cell proliferation, the thrombotic/thrombolytic state, cellular adhesion, and vessel wall inflammation.[336] Table 22.2 is a comprehensive yet not exhaustive summary of the substances secreted by endothelium and their role.

One of the first observations of the pivotal role played by the endothelium in the regulation of vascular tone was published by Furchgott and Zawadzki,[337] who showed that the vasodilatory effect of acetylcholine was strictly dependent on the presence of intact endothelium. They attributed this effect to an unknown signal molecule they named EDRF, i.e., endothelium-derived relaxing factor. Six years later and after extensive research, Louis J Ignarro together with and independently of Robert Furchgott, demonstrated that EDRF is actually nitric oxide (NO). This is produced from L-arginine by the action of the enzyme endothelial NO synthase (eNOS) and diffuses to the vascular smooth muscle cells, where it produces relaxation. One of the physiological activators of eNOS is shear stress; this represents an adaptive mechanism to an increased cardiac output. NO, along with other substances with vasorelaxing, such as prostacyclin, or vasoconstricting, such as endothelin-1 properties (Table 22.1), regulates vascular tone and tissue perfusion.

While in normal state endothelium regulates vascular homeostasis in a well-controlled manner, various conditions, including all risk factors for atherosclerosis, induce endothelial dysfunction. In the presence of noxious stimuli fact the *endothelium is activated*, and the endothelial function changes from the previous "silent mode" to an activated state that aims, amongst others, at the initiation of a host defense response. A central role in the initiation of this response is played by ROS, which are produced normally during an infection and pathophysiologically in the presence of cardiovascular risk factors. The activated endothelium responds by increasing production of substances that promote vasoconstriction, cellular adhesion, smooth muscle proliferation, thrombosis, and vascular wall inflammation. The result is the deregulation of physiological vascular homeostasis with significant pathophysiological and clinical consequences.[119]

4.3.1. Assessment of endothelial function

Several methods can be utilized to assess endothelial function, each of them focusing on a different aspect (Fig. 22.8). These methods may generally be identified as (i) those that measure the concentration of a biomarker in the serum or plasma and (ii) those that assess the endothelium-dependent vasomotion of an artery.

The biomarkers are both molecules and circulating cells. The molecules that can be measured include adhesion molecules, such as the intercellular adhesion molecule-1 (ICAM-1), the vascular cell adhesion molecule-1 (VCAM-1), E-selectin, P-selectin,

TABLE 22.2

BIOLOGICALLY ACTIVE SUBSTANCES SECRETED BY THE ENDOTHELIUM, CATEGORIZED ACCORDING TO THEIR ACTIONS

Regulation of vascular tone

Vasodilating substances
– Nitric oxide (NO)
– Prostacycline (PGI_2)
– Hyperpolarizing endothelial factor (EDHF)
– Bradykinin
– Adenosine
– C-natriuretic peptide

Vasoconstricting subtances
– Endothelin-1 (ET-1)
– Vasoconstricting prostanoids
   Prostaglandin H_2 (PGH_2)
   Thromboxane (TXA_2)
– Angiotensin-II

Regulation of coagulation

Antithrombotic substances
– Nitric oxide (NO)
– Prostacycline-I_2 (PGI_2)
– Tissue plasminogen activator (t-PA)
– Heparin
– Thrombomodulin

Substances that promote thrombosis
– Endothelin-1 (ET-1)
– Thromboxane (TXA_2)
– Angiotensin-II
– Tissue plasminogen activator inhibitors (PAI)
– von Willebrand factor (vWF)
– Tissue factor (TF)

Regulation of inflammation

Anti-inflammatory substances
– Interleukin-10 (IL-10)
– Adiponectin

Substances that promote inflammation
– Cytokines
   Interleukins (IL-1β, IL-6)
   Tissue necrosis factor-α (TNF-α)
– Adhesion molecules

Vascular cell adhesion molecule-1 (VCAM-1)

Intercellular adhesion molecule-1 (ICAM-1)

P-Selectin, E-Selectin

Soluble CD40 ligand

and the soluble CD40 ligand, and cytokines, such as interleukins 6 and 18, TNF-α, and endothelin-1. These methods rely on the assumption that the increase in the circulating levels of these inflammatory and vasoconstricting substances is a sign of endothelial activation. The circulating cells that can be measured are of two different types: the circulating endothelial cells and the circulating endothelial progenitor cells. While circulating endothelial cells arise from damaged endothelium and they are a

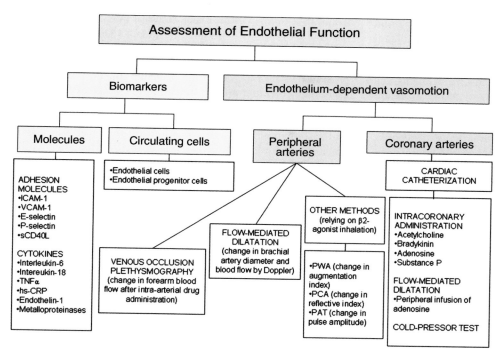

Figure 22.8 Methods to assess endothelial function. Endothelial function can be assessed either by measuring the circulating level of a biomarker or by measuring the endothelium-dependent vasomotion of a coronary or a peripheral artery.

sign of endothelial injury, circulating progenitor endothelial cells are probably a sign of regeneration and attempted repair of the damaged endothelium.[338]

The methods that measure the endothelium-dependent vasodilation of an artery use a stimulus, to which a normally functioning endothelium responds with production of vasodilating substances, mainly NO, and produce subsequent arterial dilation. On the contrary, arteries with dysfunctional endothelium do not dilate to the same degree or may even constrict. The most typical type of stimulus used for this purpose is the intra-arterial administration of acetylcholine or bradykinin. A similar effect, however, can be attained with artificial creation of local shear stress that can also increase NO production from the endothelium. It should be noted that while the methods relying on biomarkers likely assess the endothelial function of the whole body, those measuring vasodilation in response to a stimulus measure the endothelial function of the specific arterial segment under study, i.e., the coronary arteries or a peripheral artery. There are several noninvasive and invasive methods for the assessment of endothelium-dependent vasomotion of the coronary or the peripheral arteries; the most commonly used are forearm plethysmography, flow-mediated dilatation (FMD) of the brachial artery, and quantitative coronary angiography after intracoronary administration of acetylcholine.

Assessment of endothelial function of the coronary arteries. The assessment of the endothelial function of the coronary arteries can be performed with quantitative coronary angiography before and after intracoronary administration of a vasoactive drug, such as acetylcholine. As it was initially observed, normal coronary arteries respond to acetylcholine with dilatation. On the contrary, coronary arteries containing atherosclerotic plaques and/or dysfunctional endothelium either dilate minimally or constrict after intracoronary acetylcholine infusion.[339,340] The vasoconstrictor response has been attributed to a direct effect of acetylcholine on muscarinic smooth muscle

receptors. The response of the coronary arteries is not identical in all coronary segments for a given patient[341,342]; however, the response is generally in the same direction in all coronaries of the same patient, both the coronary arteries with plaques and those that appear normal. This finding denotes that endothelial dysfunction is not confined to the specific arterial segment that has "macroscopic" disease, but it is generalized.[343] Several evolutions of this method have been applied; the response to a wide range of endothelial agonists, such as substance P, adenosine, and bradykinin, has also been measured, as well as physiological responses to cold-pressor testing and dilation of the proximal segment of a coronary artery after distal infusion of adenosine.[344]

Assessment of endothelial function of the peripheral arteries. The invasive nature of the assessment of coronary endothelial function inhibits its use for population studies and for repeated testing. Furthermore, the finding that endothelial dysfunction is generalized and not confined to the diseased coronary vessels led to the investigation of methods to assess peripheral endothelial function. The first method used for this purpose was actually a fairly invasive one that used occlusion venous plethysmography with intra-arterial infusion of endothelium-dependent vasoactive substances, such as acetylcholine. The results of these measurements correlated closely with those of coronary endothelial function, but the intra-arterial infusion of drugs was an obvious drawback of the method. The first noninvasive method used to assess endothelial function, and that of the largest dissemination today, is the ultrasound-based method of measuring FMD of the brachial artery, which will be further described in the following paragraphs. Other less established methods for evaluation of peripheral endothelial function rely on the ability of the β_2-agonist salbutamol to reduce arterial stiffness in a NO-dependent manner without significant reduction in arterial pressure, when inhaled.[345] The assessment of arterial stiffness can be done with pulse wave analysis using radial arterial tonometry, pulse contour analysis by digital photoplethysmography, or digital pulse amplitude tonometry.[345,346]

Flow-mediated dilatation of the brachial artery. This method was originally described in 1992 by Celermajer et al.[347] in a landmark study of children and adults at risk of developing atherosclerosis. The method has since been used in numerous clinical studies and has been the topic of consensus documents that addressed its characteristics both in terms of technical details and performance. This method is based on the measurement of the diameter of the brachial artery by 2D-ultrasound before and after an increase in shear stress induced by reactive hyperemia. The hyperemia occurs in response to prolonged ischemia of the upper limb produced with a blood pressure cuff inflated at suprasystolic pressure. During the ischemic period the vessels of the ischemic region are dilated as a result of hypoxia. After the release of the blood pressure cuff, flow increases sharply as a result of the decreased peripheral vascular resistance. The sudden increase in flow increases shear stress that acts as a stimulus for the endothelium to release NO.[348]

The method is operator dependent and should be performed by adequately trained personnel. Since there are multiple factors affecting arterial vasomotion, several precautions should be taken to avoid possible confounding factors. In particular, the subject should ideally be in a fasting state or have had only a low fat meal, and he/she should have abstained from exercise, smoking, and caffeine for at least 4 to 6 h prior to testing. All vasoactive medications should be withheld for at least four half-lives, if possible. Cardiovascular risk factors, medications, recent/current infections, and the stage of menstrual cycle in women should be recorded. The measurements are made in a quiet, temperature-controlled room, with the subject resting in the supine position for at least 10 min before the measurements are made. The brachial artery is imaged in the longitudinal view, just below the antecubital fossa. Fine adjustments of the probe are made to obtain the clearest B-mode image through the center of the vessel with optimal contrast between the anterior and posterior vessel walls and the lumen of the vessel. A B-mode recording is then obtained followed by a spectral Doppler recording of blood flow signal from the center of the vessel prior to inflation and after the deflation of a sphygmomanometer cuff. The cuff is typically inflated about 50 mm Hg above the subject's systolic blood pressure for 5 min. The site where the sphygmomanometric cuff should be placed, either proximal to the probe (above the antecubital fossa) or distally (on the forearm), is still a matter of debate, although most authorities prefer the forearm positioning. Brachial artery FMD is calculated as the maximum change in vessel diameter from baseline, expressed as a percentage. On cuff deflation the resultant reactive hyperemia is measured by flow Doppler and the change in flow from baseline is expressed as a percentage change in time velocity integral between baseline and postdeflation Doppler recordings (Fig. 22.9). After at least 10 min from releasing the cuff—enough time for the artery to return to baseline conditions—endothelium-independent dilatation of the brachial artery can be evaluated 3 to 5 min after sublingual administration of nitroglycerin. An adequate response to nitroglycerin denotes integrity of the muscular function of the artery examined. FMD may also be studied in the radial, axillary, femoral, and posterior tibial arteries. It should be noted, however, that arteries smaller than 2.5 mm in diameter are difficult to measure, and vasodilation is generally less difficult to perceive in vessels larger than 5 mm in diameter. FMD of the brachial artery is the most commonly performed and best validated technique for the noninvasive assessment of peripheral endothelial function.

FMD of the brachial artery is closely related to coronary endothelial function. This has been clearly demonstrated in the landmark study of Anderson et al.[343] in which patients with normal or atherosclerotic coronary arteries were submitted both to coronary and brachial artery reactivity testing. It has therefore been suggested that FMD measurement of the brachial artery could be regarded as an indirect noninvasive assessment of coronary endothelial function.[336]

Prognostic value of endothelial function assessment. Endothelial function is impaired in the presence of various risk factors for CAD, i.e., hypertension, diabetes mellitus, dyslipidemia, smoking, obesity, and in various disease states, i.e., CAD, heart failure, and erectile dysfunction.[349–351] Endothelial dysfunction is correlated with the cardiovascular risk, as estimated by the FRS, especially in low-risk populations.[352]

The association of endothelial dysfunction with various disease states is complex. Not only endothelial dysfunction is encountered in these diseases, but it also plays a significant role in their pathogenesis. Although the characteristics of this cause-effect relationship are still debated,[349] there is evidence that, through alterations in vascular homeostasis, endothelial dysfunction is implicated in the pathogenesis of hypertension, and it is considered the main pathophysiological pathway for erectile dysfunction[351] and a key event in the progression of atherosclerosis.[119, 336]

The prognostic significance of endothelial function assessment has been evaluated in different population subsets. In patients with CAD endothelial dysfunction is an independent predictor of poor outcome. This has been demonstrated for the assessment of both coronary and peripheral endothelial function.[353–356] The independent predictive value of endothelial function has also been demonstrated in patients with PAD.[357] Furthermore, brachial FMD is a strong and independent predictor of in-stent restenosis in patients undergoing coronary revascularization[358,359] and of cardiovascular events in patients undergoing vascular surgery.[360]

The independent predictive value of endothelial function assessment is not as well-documented in patients without

Figure 22.9 Doppler recording of blood flow at baseline (**left panel**) and postcuff inflation (**right panel**) in the radial artery. Note the large increase in arterial flow measured as area under the curve of the spectral Doppler signal (*yellow areas*).

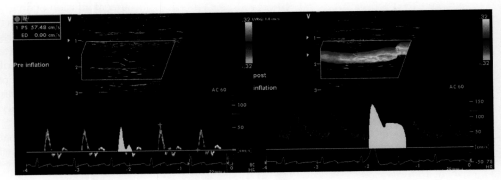

established CVD. Findings supporting its independent predictive value were obtained in hypertensive patients[361] and from an unselected population of elderly subjects.[362] In the latter population, Yeboah et al.[362] measured brachial FMD in 2,792 individuals between 72 and 98 years old, most of them free of known atherosclerotic disease, and found that FMD provided incremental prognostic information beyond other factors such as age, gender, diabetes mellitus, cigarette smoking, systolic and diastolic blood pressure, baseline CVD status, and total cholesterol.

In contrast, in a mixed population of patients at risk for CVD, brachial FMD was not found to be an independent predictor of cardiovascular events, beyond a univariate association.[363] However in the same population, cardiovascular events were independently predicted by markers of cardiac and arterial structure such as carotid IMT and left ventricular mass. Furthermore, in a general population of middle-aged subjects without history of myocardial infarction of stroke, although brachial FMD predicted future cardiovascular events, when entered in the multivariate analysis, this association lost its statistical significance.[364] While most studies have shown that the assessment of endothelial function provides independent prognostic information in populations with established CVD, in the asymptomatic population with risk factors such evidence is lacking. The latter, however, is the population that would benefit most from interventions aiming at reversing endothelial dysfunction early in the course of atherosclerosis.

Flow mediated vasodilation to assess effects of therapy. Several studies have evaluated the reversibility of endothelial dysfunction by means of pharmacological and nonpharmacological interventions. Improvement of several nutritional and behavioral aspects of patients' lifestyle may partly reverse endothelial dysfunction. Examples are the reversal of endothelial dysfunction after smoking cessation[365,366] and the beneficial effects of the consumption of flavonoid-rich beverages and ascorbic acid and the addition of dietary L-arginine supplementation.[367,368] Drugs that have a favorable effect on endothelial function are several lipid-lowering and antihypertensive drugs, such as statins, angiotensin converting enzyme inhibitors, calcium antagonists, and some β-adrenergic blockers.[369] Although it is not clear if reversal of endothelial function is per se associated with reduced cardiovascular risk, the drugs that reverse endothelial dysfunction also reduce cardiovascular risk; this may at least in part be mediated by the amelioration of endothelial function, with stabilization or slowing of the atherosclerotic process.

4.4. Arterial elastic properties and wave reflections

4.4.1. Physiology of the arterial system

The arterial system has two main functions, a conduit function and a cushioning function. As a conduit system, it provides the peripheral tissues with blood, which is essential for their nutrition. During a lifetime, 200,000,000 liters of blood is transferred through the aorta at a speed of 0.5 to 1 m/s under normal conditions. As a cushioning system, the arterial system converts the pulsatile flow of the ejecting ventricles to a continuous flow at the level of the capillaries, thus preventing damage of arterioles and capillaries. Under normal circumstances, these two functions are fulfilled with great efficiency. The result is that the mean pressure along the whole arterial system up to the level of arterioles is rather uniform and the mean pressure during the whole cardiac cycle is only 5 mm Hg lower than the mean pressure during the systolic (i.e., ejecting) phase alone.[370]

4.4.2. Factors determining the elastic properties of arteries

The elastic properties of the arteries are responsible for the cushioning function of the arterial system. The elastic performance of an artery depends on intra-arterial pressure and the intrinsic elastic properties of the artery. The level of arterial pressure determines wall stress and changes in blood pressure produce passive changes in arterial elastic properties. On the other hand, the intrinsic elastic properties of an artery depend on its geometrical characteristics and the structure, composition, and nutritional status of its wall. Changes in the intrinsic elastic properties produce active changes in arterial elastic properties.[371] The main parameter that determines the intrinsic elastic properties of an artery is the composition of the arterial wall, and especially of the tunica media. The elements of the tunica media playing the largest role are elastin and collagen, although the intercellular matrix is obviously also involved. Although the adventitia influences in part wall stress, it does directly affect arterial elasticity since it does not contain any component with significant elastic properties.[370]

Elastin and collagen have different elastic properties. The elastic/collagen ratio in the arterial wall largely determines its elastic properties. This ratio decreases gradually toward the periphery, while the number of smooth muscle cells increases gradually. This fact, along with different geometrical characteristics between the center and the periphery, is mainly responsible for the change in arterial elastic properties along the arterial tree. The most distensible segment of the arterial tree is the ascending aorta, whereas toward the periphery, there is a continuous gradual increase in arterial stiffness.[372]

4.4.3. Pulse wave velocity

Each ventricular contraction produces a sequence of arterial distension and recoils that quickly radiates as a wave (pulse wave) toward the periphery. The speed at which this wave travels (pulse wave velocity: PWV) should be kept distinct from the speed at which blood travels in the arterial system, as these are very different concepts. PWV is the analog of the speed of any wave, such as sound or light. As the speed of sound is determined by the properties of the space in which it travels (i.e., greater in a solid material, slower in water, and even lower in air), PWV is influenced by the viscoelastic properties of the conduits in which it travels, i.e., the arteries.[370] In fact, in distensible arteries, PWV is reduced, whereas in stiff arteries it is increased. In accordance with the previously mentioned gradual decrease in arterial distensibility from the center to the periphery, PWV is increased gradually in the same direction. In humans, PWV increases from 4 to 5 m/s in the ascending aorta to 5 to 6 m/s in the abdominal aorta then to 8 to 9 m/s in the iliac and femoral arteries.[372] The clinical appraisal of the travel of the pulse wave in the arterial system is the synchronous palpation of the carotid and femoral artery pulse. In the carotid artery the pulse is palpated before that in the femoral artery.

4.4.4. Wave reflections

The pulse wave generated by the ejection of blood from the left ventricle travels toward the periphery, but at certain switch sites it is reflected and a portion of it returns toward the center.[373] These reflection sites are mainly constituted by major arterial bifurcations and at the level of arterioles. Each reflected wave travels at the same speed as the forward (i.e., native) wave in the same arterial segment, but in the opposite direction. PWV is high relative to the length of the arterial tree, therefore the reflected wave typically returns early enough to merge with the incident wave before the end of each cardiac cycle. In the periphery, (i.e., brachial artery) the travel time for the reflected waves is shorter than that at the level of the ascending aorta, both because of a shorter distance to cover and higher traveling velocity. As a consequence, at the periphery the reflected waves merge with the forward wave early in systole, thus augmenting peripheral, i.e., brachial systolic pressure, whereas in the ascending aorta, the waves merge at a much later point, with less or absent augmentation of the aortic systolic pressure. This gradual increase in systolic blood pressure from the center (i.e., ascending aorta) to the periphery (i.e., brachial artery) is called pressure amplification.[372,373] Wave reflections do not solely depend on arterial stiffness, but they are affected by other parameters of arterial function, such as vascular tone and microcirculation.[372]

4.4.5. Ventricular–Vascular coupling

In subjects with compliant arteries and low PWV, the reflected waves merge with the forward wave in diastole at the level of ascending aorta. This augmented diastolic pressure facilitates coronary perfusion. In cases with less distensible (stiff) arteries, the reflected waves merge with the forward wave at the level of ascending aorta early in the cardiac cycle, mainly in systole. This augments the systolic portion of the pressure waveform with subsequent increase in left ventricular afterload. The decrease in coronary perfusion, due to loss of diastolic augmentation along with the increase in left ventricular afterload may predispose to subendocardial ischemia.[370,372,373]

4.4.6. Assessment of arterial elastic properties and wave reflections

As previously explained, the elastic properties of the arterial tree are not uniform. Hence, the assessment of elastic properties can be made in various arterial segments with different results. Local determination of arterial stiffness is confined to a specific site of the arterial tree, where one or more parameters of arterial elastic properties, i.e., distensibility can be measured. Regional determination of arterial stiffness assesses the elastic properties of a much larger segment of the arterial tree, i.e., aorta, where parameters like PWV can be measured. Determination of systemic arterial stiffness assesses the elastic properties of the whole arterial tree. Finally, there are methods that specifically evaluate wave reflections and assess central hemodynamics, i.e., ascending aortic pressures.[374]

The determination of arterial stiffness in various vascular beds provides different information, and the results from one level cannot be extrapolated to all vascular beds. Since the aorta is the part of the arterial system with the greatest distensibility and the one that plays the major role in the cushioning function of the arterial system, it has been the primary site of measurement, and it probably represents the site where the measurements have the most pathophysiological and clinical significance. However, other sites, such as the carotid arteries, or the assessment of wave reflections are also pathophysiologically important and provide clinically important data.[372]

4.4.7. Local level assessment of arterial elastic properties

When assessing arterial elastic properties at the local level, one or more parameters are calculated from measurements of the arterial area (or diameter) and pressure. Such parameters are (i) *distensibility*, which represents the relative change in LA (or diameter) during systole for a given pressure change.

$$\text{Distensibility} = \Delta A / A \times \Delta P, \qquad \text{(Eq. 22.1)}$$

where A is the diastolic area (or diameter); ΔA is the change in area (or diameter) from diastole to systole; and ΔP is the pulse pressure at the site of measurement; (ii) *compliance*, which represents the absolute change in LA during systole for a given pressure change.

$$\text{Compliance} = \Delta A / \Delta P \qquad \text{(Eq. 22.2)}$$

(iii) the *Peterson elastic modulus*, which is the inverse of distensibility: the pressure change driving an increase in relative LA (or diameter),

$$\text{Peterson} = A \times \Delta P / \Delta A \qquad \text{(Eq. 22.3)}$$

Several noninvasive methods can be used to evaluate local arterial stiffness. These methods rely on measurement of the systo-diastolic arterial diameter using an imaging modality. The imaging modality most commonly used is ultrasound. Specific echo-tracking devices, such as WallTrack®, NIUS®, and Artlab®, have been developed to accurately measure arterial diameters.[374] The arterial sites that can be examined with ultrasound include the ascending aorta,[375] the aortic arch, the descending aorta (using transesophageal echocardiography),[376] the abdominal aorta,[377] and the carotid,[377] femoral,[377,378] brachial,[378] and radial[377,379,380] arteries. Magnetic resonance imaging may also be used to assess local arterial stiffness in various arterial sites, although it is most frequently used for the aorta.[381]

The indexes of arterial stiffness mentioned above require measurement of blood pressure. To avoid the error introduced by peripheral pressure amplification, the pressure used should be local pressure. Local pressure can be derived by applanation tonometry of the vessel in question and calibration of the waveform to brachial mean and diastolic pressures or automatic calculation using transfer function processing with the SphygmoCor® device (see wave reflections measurement).

4.4.8. Regional level assessment of arterial elastic properties

The most commonly used index of regional arterial stiffness is PWV. PWV is calculated as the distance between two arterial sites divided by the relative time delay between the R-wave on the surface ECG and the onset of the arterial pulse at these two sites (transit time, Fig. 22.10). PWV has an inverse relationship with distensibility. As an artery stiffens, i.e., it becomes less distensible, PWV increases. As it has been previously stated, the most pathophysiologically significant region for the assessment of PWV is the aorta, i.e., carotid–femoral PWV. Although other arterial segments can also be used, such as the carotid–radial or the femoral–tibial, they do not have the same pathophysiologic and prognostic significance as carotid–femoral PWV.[372] PWV is usually measured using the foot-to-foot velocity method (foot of the carotid pulse waveform to foot of femoral pulse waveform) from various waveforms, including pressure,[382] distension,[383] and spectral Doppler.[384] The distance covered by the waves is usually assimilated to the surface distance between the two recording sites. This is a source of inaccuracy in the calculation of PWV that also leads to discrepancy among the results of various laboratories. For carotid–femoral PWV, some investigators recommend either (i) using the total distance between the carotid and femoral artery or (ii) subtracting the distance from the carotid location to the sternal notch from the total distance or (iii) subtracting the distance from the carotid location to the sternal notch from the distance between the sternal notch and the femoral site of measurement.[372] For intervention studies with repeated measurements the distance used is not usually a problem, because it is always kept the same by the same investigators; however, to be able to

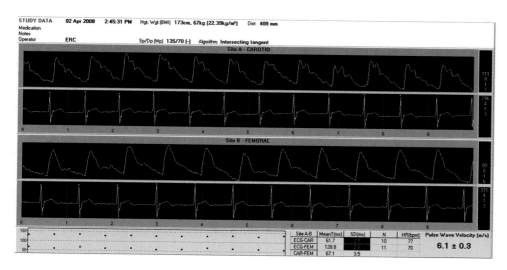

Figure 22.10 Pulse wave velocity: The time delay between the R-wave (green dot at the tip of the R-wave on the ECG) and the foot of the pressure wave (green dot on the pressure curve upstroke) in the carotid and the femoral artery is measured in several cardiac cycles by the device. The mean electrical–mechanical delay in the carotid artery is substracted from that in the femoral artery to calculate the transit time. The carotid–femoral distance is measured on the body surface and the aortic (i.e., carotid–femoral) pulse wave velocity is then calculated by dividing the distance by the transit time.

compare results obtained in different populations obtained in different laboratories and to calculate normative values, the distance used should be standardized.

The Doppler-based method for measuring PWV requires acquiring signals from the right common carotid and the femoral artery. The Doppler signals are not acquired simultaneously and to measure PWV the operator calculates the time delay between the onset of each Doppler signal from the R wave of simultaneously recorded ECGs. Then, the time delay of the femoral signal is subtracted from the time delay of the carotid signal, to calculate the transit time.[385] The two most commonly used methods employ specific devices equipped with pressure sensors. The SphygmoCor® device (AtCor Medical, Sydney, Australia) uses a tonometer to acquire the pressure waveform from the carotid and the femoral artery. The transit delay is measured again in relation to the R wave of the surface ECG. The Complior® (Artech Medical, Pantin, France) device uses two mechano-transducers to simultaneously acquire the pressure waveform from the carotid and the femoral artery and the transit time is measured during the same cardiac beat.[385] Simultaneous recording of the carotid and the femoral signals can also be performed using two Doppler probes.[384] Finally, although rarely used, cardiovascular MRI can be used to measure aortic PWV and the results obtained with this method are very similar to that of the pressure-based methods described above.[386]

4.4.9. Assessment of systemic arterial elastic properties
There are several methods of evaluating systemic stiffness, either by considering the circulatory system as an electrical circuit and analyzing the diastolic decay of the pressure waveform or by measuring aortic flow and calculating aortic pressure.[372,385] Though attractive, due to the potential ability to measure the stiffness of the entire arterial system, there is a lack of prognostic information with these techniques, and they are presently not recommended for clinical applications.

4.4.10. Wave reflections—central pressures
Wave reflections can be evaluated with applanation tonometry and dedicated software for noninvasive recording and analysis of the arterial pulse (SphygmoCor®, AtCor Medical, Sydney, Australia). The central (aortic) pressure waveform can be derived from radial artery recordings, with the use of a generalized transfer function,

which has been shown to give an accurate estimate of the central arterial pressure waveform and its characteristics.[370,387] The aortic pressure waveform may also be derived from carotid recordings, without the use of a transfer function.[388] Carotid waveforms, however, are not always easy to obtain in obese subjects and may pose a minor risk for patients with carotid atherosclerosis.[372]

As described earlier, the arterial pressure waveform is a composite of the forward pressure wave and the reflected waves. In elastic vessels, reflected waves tend to return to the aortic root during diastole. In the case of stiff arteries, PWV rises and the reflected waves return earlier, adding to the forward wave and augmenting the systolic pressure.[373] This phenomenon can be quantified through the augmentation index (AIx)—defined as the difference between the second and first systolic peaks expressed as a percentage of the pulse pressure (Fig. 22.11). Higher values of AIx indicate increased wave reflections from the periphery and vice versa. The AIx may be expressed as a negative number if the reflected waves return in diastole and do not augment the systolic portion of the pressure waveform.[374] AIx is an index of wave reflections and does not depend on the absolute pressure.

Applanation tonometry can also be used to calculate central pressures based on the assumption that mean pressure is constant

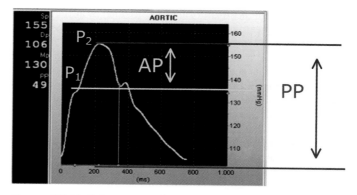

Figure 22.11 Pulse wave analysis: Ascending aorta pressure waveform derived via a mathematical transform from the pressure waveform of the radial artery (not shown). The inflection point in the ascending portion of the pressure waveform identifies the merging point of the incident and the reflected waves. The augmentation index is calculated as the ratio of AP/PP. AP, augmented pressure; PP, pulse pressure.

throughout the arterial tree. Although diastolic pressure does not significantly change along the arterial tree, aortic systolic pressure, which represents left ventricular afterload, and aortic pulse pressure are much lower than at the periphery (i.e., brachial artery), especially in young patients with elastic arteries.[372,373] One of the difficulties in central pressure estimation is that, contrary to the measurement of AIx, the central pressures should be calibrated to the peripheral pressures, which are usually measured at the brachial artery with a sphygmomanometer. This is a potential source of error, which cannot be avoided; however, it is the same error imported in every blood pressure measurement traditionally used for the estimation of cardiovascular risk and for hypertension management.

4.4.11. Clinical significance of arterial stiffness

Arterial stiffness increases with advancing age. This increase is due to alterations in the wall, especially in the tunica media, including elastin fragmentation, collagen accumulation, inflammation, calcification, and medial smooth muscle necrosis.[370] The effect of age on aortic stiffness and wave reflections was evaluated in the normal population in the Anglo Cardiff Collaborative Study, where for the first time the investigators tried to define normal AIx and aortic PWV values across a wide range of ages.[389] According to the findings of this study, the influence of age before the age of 50 is higher on the AIx than on aortic PWV; on the contrary, beyond the age of 50, the influence of age is higher on PWV.[389]

Arterial stiffness and wave reflections are increased in the presence of all cardiovascular risk factors, including smoking, hypertension, dyslipidemia, diabetes mellitus, and obesity; in many CVDs, including CAD, congestive heart failure, and stroke; and in many nonprimary CVDs, including chronic renal disease, rheumatoid arthritis, vasculitis, and other connective tissue disorders.[372,375,377,379,380,384,390,391] The increase in arterial stiffness and wave reflections observed in the presence of cardiovascular risk factors and CVD states establish them as markers of cardiovascular risk.

Indeed, arterial stiffness and wave reflections have been associated with an increased risk of cardiovascular events. This has been demonstrated for both aortic stiffness and wave reflections in patients with CAD.[392,393] In patients without overt CVD or in asymptomatic patients, data are available on aortic PWV. Aortic PWV is an independent predictor of cardiovascular events, as it has been shown in various population subsets, including patients with hypertension,[394,395] type 2 diabetes,[384] end-stage renal disease,[396] in elderly subjects,[397,398] and also in the general population.[399-401] The prognostic information provided by aortic stiffness in patients with cardiovascular risk factors and/or in asymptomatic patients is independent of and incremental over the information provided by traditional risk factors or risk scores such as the Framingham score.[394] Several less robust data exist for the prognostic information of carotid artery stiffness[402] and wave reflections,[403] but research is still ongoing. In contrast, the independent predictive value of other measures of arterial stiffness, such as limb PWV, is questionable.[372]

Arterial stiffness and wave reflections can be reduced with various pharmacological and nonpharmacological means. The former include various antihypertensive agents and statins, while the latter include exercise training and dietary changes, such as weight loss, moderate alcohol and cocoa consumption, and low-salt diet.[372,403-405] The decrease in arterial stiffness and wave reflections is associated with a decrease in cardiovascular risk.[372] There is evidence that the decrease in cardiovascular risk associated with a decrease in arterial stiffness and wave reflections is independent of changes in other markers of cardiovascular risk, even brachial

blood pressure.[406] This has clearly been demonstrated in the CAFÉ study[403] in which, despite a similar reduction in brachial artery systolic pressure, the drug combination that induced a greater reduction in central aortic pressure was the one that also resulted in a greater reduction in cardiovascular events.

The important prognostic information provided by the study of arterial stiffness and wave reflections is highlighted in the guidelines of the European Society of Hypertension.[285] In the 2007 guidelines for management of arterial hypertension, the European Society recommended that aortic PWV be measured as a marker of end-organ damage in all hypertensive patients.[285]

4.4.12. Ankle brachial index

The presence of PAD is often overlooked and this is particularly problematic in patients with atherosclerosis in other vascular beds. Nonetheless, the importance of this condition is underlined by the results of prospective and randomized trials such as the Heart Protection Study; in this study PAD in the absence of known CAD was a better predictor of cardiovascular events than did CAD in the absence of PAD.[407] Additionally, in CAD patients, PAD has been found to be a stronger risk factor for cardiac and cerebrovascular death and overall mortality than prior MI.[408]

The ABI is a simple, noninvasive, and inexpensive test that can be performed in the office or clinical setting. The ABI is used in the diagnosis of PAD in symptomatic patients and in the assessment of vascular risk in asymptomatic patients; it is calculated as the ratio of the ankle to brachial systolic blood pressure, and a value of <0.9 indicates the presence of flow-limiting arterial stenoses along the course of the arterial beds investigated. An ABI between 0.9 and 0.4 is interpreted as mild to moderate PAD and an ABI <0.4 is an indication of severe PAD.[409] ABI <0.9 is 95% sensitive and 99% specific for angiographically documented PAD.[410,411] Overall, the test has a sensitivity of 90% and a specificity of 98% for detecting >50% stenosis in the arteries of the lower extremities.[412,413] The intra-observer variability of ABI among trained observers is about 7%.[414,415]

In a systematic review of the literature, the sensitivity and specificity of ABI <0.8 to 0.9 to predict incident CHD were 16.5% and 92.7%, for incident stroke were 16% and 92.2%, and for cardiovascular mortality were 41% and 87.9%, respectively.[416] Hence, it would appear that a negative test is highly predictive of low adverse cardiovascular risk and may therefore be useful as a screening test.

Several studies have demonstrated that after adjusting for conventional risk factors a low ABI is an independent predictor of cardiovascular risk[251,417,418] and may actually improve the prognostic value of the FRS.[419] The ABI could therefore be used as an adjunct to a global risk assessment based on traditional cardiovascular risk factors.

In this light, the American Heart Association defines ABI as a strong and independent risk factor for cardiovascular mortality and it suggests that it could be used to detect subclinical disease in the prevention of CAD mortality and stroke.[251] The AHA recognizes that ABI may be a useful addition to the assessment of CHD risk in selected populations, especially among people >50 years of age or among those who appear to be at intermediate or higher risk for CVD on the basis of traditional risk factors. According to the current guidelines of the AHA, ABI is defined as the ratio of the highest of the systolic blood pressures measured at the level of the ankle in two different arteries (either the anterior dorsalis pedis or the posterior tibial) and the highest of the two systolic blood pressures measured in the upper limbs.[409,420]

Studies have evaluated the prognostic value of different methods to calculate ABI. When the higher of two ankle pressures is used for ABI calculation, a group of patients at high-risk for cardiovascular events may be overlooked; with a simple modification of the formula (use of the lower instead of the higher of two ankle pressures) more patients at risk may be identified. In fact, in the AtheroGene Study of patients with known atherosclerosis, the prevalence of PAD was 25% when the higher of two ankle pressures was used[421] and 36% when the lower of the two ankle pressures was used[421] and the long-term event rate (death, myocardial infarction, and stroke after 6.6 year median follow-up) was significantly higher in those diagnosed with PAD than those without (28.4% vs. 14.8%). The probable explanation for these findings is that by using the lower rather than the higher of two pressures from the same leg, the investigators maximized their potential to identify stenotic disease in the lower extremity under analysis, therefore increasing the overall estimation of risk. In another study, McDermott et al.[422] used the average of two pressures from the same foot to calculate the ABI and found that this method was more predictive than the highest or lowest foot pressure to predict walking distance and walking velocity.

A supranormal ABI (i.e., >1.4) is found in patients with generalized stiffening of blood vessels and advanced medial calcification. This condition is most commonly seen in diabetic patients and patients with chronic kidney disease. Interestingly, there is a U-shaped association between ABI and mortality, with a significantly increased risk in both low (<0.9) and high (>1.4) ABI groups. However, the U-shaped relationship between ABI and mortality could not be explained by a higher prevalence of diabetes mellitus, hypertension, and chronic kidney disease among patients with either low or high ABI in the Strong Heart Study. Patients at both extremes appeared to be at a higher risk of cardiovascular events.[423]

5. FUTURE DIRECTIONS

The preceding pages detailed the state of the art of numerous serological tests and noninvasive imaging modalities developed in the past several decades to enhance our ability to detect atherosclerosis and predict the risk of events inherent with its presence. These advances have been embraced by many clinicians practicing preventive medicine and have without a doubt improved the overall approach to the *"patient at risk."* Implementation of several of these techniques has demonstrated that risk is often more closely related to the vascular status (*vascular age*) of the individual than to his/her anagraphical age and conventional risk factors. Several questions remain unanswered, however. Large prospective studies are still needed to ascertain the predictive value of markers such as noncalcified plaque on CT and plaque composition assessed by cardiac MRI. Endothelial dysfunction has not been clearly established as a marker of risk in asymptomatic subjects with significant risk factors for CAD. The optimal combination of serological and imaging markers is not clear; at the same time it is not entirely clear which patient is the most appropriate for screening. In this light, if we limit our scope to the intermediate risk patients, are we going to underestimate risk in a large portion of patients considered to be at low risk by clinical markers? At the same time, if we only focus on the intermediate risk patients are we going to neglect that several high risk patients may actually be at lower risk? Despite all the obstacles, this remains a very viable research venue as one may envision a reduction in large-scale randomized morbidity and mortality trials and an increase in the number of trails based on surrogate outcome measures.

Nonetheless, future studies will obviously need to concentrate on establishing a correlation between imaging of plaque progression and future cardiovascular events, and clinicians should not forget two other immensely important principles as we approach a new era: *"primum non nocere"* (__first do no harm__) and be considered of the ___cost of practice___ for the entire society.

REFERENCES

1. American heart association statistics. Available from: http://www.american-heart.org/downloadable/heart/1200082005246HS_Stats%202008.final.pdf.
2. Shaw LJ, Shaw RE, Merz CN, et al. Impact of ethnicity and gender differences on angiographic coronary artery disease prevalence and in-hospital mortality in the American College of Cardiology-National Cardiovascular Data Registry. *Circulation.* 2008;117(14):1787–1801.
3. Yusuf S, Reddy S, Ounpuu S, et al. Global burden of cardiovascular diseases: Part II: Variations in cardiovascular disease by specific ethnic groups and geographic regions and prevention strategies. *Circulation.* 2001;104(23):2855–2864.
4. Virchow R. *Cellular Pathology as Based upon Physiological and Pathological Histology.* London: John Churchill; 1860.
5. Steinberg D. Hypercholesterolemia and inflammation in atherogenesis: Two sides of the same coin. *Mol Nutr Food Res.* 2005;49(11):995–998.
6. Hansson GK. Inflammation, atherosclerosis, and coronary artery disease. *N Engl J Med.* 2005;352(16):1685–1695.
7. Stoll G, Bendszus M. Inflammation and atherosclerosis: Novel insights into plaque formation and destabilization. *Stroke.* 2006;37(7):1923–1932.
8. Doyle B, Caplice N. Plaque neovascularization and antiangiogenic therapy for atherosclerosis. *J Am Coll Cardiol.* 2007;49(21):2073–2080.
9. Johnson RC, Leopold JA, Loscalzo J. Vascular calcification: Pathobiological mechanisms and clinical implications. *Circ Res.* 2006;99(10):1044–1059.
10. Doherty TM, Fitzpatrick LA, Inoue D, et al. Molecular, endocrine, and genetic mechanisms of arterial calcification. *Endocr Rev.* 2004;25(4):629–672.
11. Proudfoot D, Skepper JN, Hegyi L, et al. Apoptosis regulates human vascular calcification in vitro: Evidence for initiation of vascular calcification by apoptotic bodies. *Circ Res.* 2000;87(11):1055–1062.
12. Doherty TM, Asotra K, Fitzpatrick LA, et al. Calcification in atherosclerosis: Bone biology and chronic inflammation at the arterial crossroads. *Proc Natl Acad Sci USA.* 2003;100(20):11201–11206.
13. Aikawa E, Nahrendorf M, Figueiredo JL, et al. Osteogenesis associates with inflammation in early-stage atherosclerosis evaluated by molecular imaging in vivo. *Circulation.* 2007;116(24):2841–2850.
14. Qin X, Corriere MA, Matrisian LM, et al. Matrix metalloproteinase inhibition attenuates aortic calcification. *Arterioscler Thromb Vasc Biol.* 2006;26(7):1510–1516.
15. Cola C, Almeida M, Li D, et al. Regulatory role of endothelium in the expression of genes affecting arterial calcification. *Biochem Biophys Res Commun.* 2004;320(2):424–427.
16. Luo G, Ducy P, McKee MD, et al. Spontaneous calcification of arteries and cartilage in mice lacking matrix GLA protein. *Nature.* 1997;386(6620):78–81.
17. Tyson KL, Reynolds JL, McNair R, et al. Osteo/chondrocytic transcription factors and their target genes exhibit distinct patterns of expression in human arterial calcification. *Arterioscler Thromb Vasc Biol.* 2003;23(3):489–494.
18. Dhore CR, Cleutjens JP, Lutgens E, et al. Differential expression of bone matrix regulatory proteins in human atherosclerotic plaques. *Arterioscler Thromb Vasc Biol.* 2001;21(12):1998–2003.
19. Bucay N, Sarosi I, Dunstan CR, et al. Osteoprotegerin-deficient mice develop early onset osteoporosis and arterial calcification. *Genes Dev.* 1998;12(9):1260–1268.
20. Beckman JA, Ganz J, Creager MA, et al. Relationship of clinical presentation and calcification of culprit coronary artery stenoses. *Arterioscler Thromb Vasc Biol.* 2001;21(10):1618–1622.
21. Huang H, Virmani R, Younis H, et al. The impact of calcification on the biomechanical stability of atherosclerotic plaques. *Circulation.* 2001;103(8):1051–1056.
22. Fitzgerald PJ, Ports TA, Yock PG. Contribution of localized calcium deposits to dissection after angioplasty. An observational study using intravascular ultrasound. *Circulation.* 1992;86(1):64–70.
23. Schmermund A, Erbel R. Unstable coronary plaque and its relation to coronary calcium. *Circulation.* 2001;104(14):1682–1687.
24. Mosseri M, Satler LF, Pichard AD, et al. Impact of vessel calcification on outcomes after coronary stenting. *Cardiovasc Revasc Med.* 2005;6(4):147–153.
25. Veress AI, Cornhill JF, Herderick EE, et al. Age-related development of atherosclerotic plaque stress: A population-based finite-element analysis. *Coron Artery Dis.* 1998;9(1):13–19.
26. Naghavi M, Libby P, Falk E, et al. From vulnerable plaque to vulnerable patient: A call for new definitions and risk assessment strategies: Part II. *Circulation.* 2003;108(15):1772–1778.
27. Law MR, Wald NJ, Thompson SG. By how much and how quickly does reduction in serum cholesterol concentration lower risk of ischaemic heart disease? *BMJ.* 1994;308(6925):367–372.
28. Tsimikas S, Mooser V. Molecular biology of lipoproteins and dyslipidemias. In: Chien KR, ed. *Molecular Basis of Cardiovascular Disease: A Companion to Braunwald's Heart Disease.* Philadelphia, PA: WB Saunders Co.; 2004:365–384.

29. Grundy SM, Wilhelmsen L, Rose G, et al. Coronary heart disease in high-risk populations: Lessons from Finland. *Eur Heart J.* 1990;11(5):462–471.

30. Cohen JC, Boerwinkle E, Mosley TH, Jr, et al. Sequence variations in PCSK9, low LDL, and protection against coronary heart disease. *N Engl J Med.* 2006;354(12):1264–1272.

31. Steinberg D. Thematic review series: The pathogenesis of atherosclerosis. An interpretive history of the cholesterol controversy: Part I. *J Lipid Res.* 2004;45(9):1583–1593.

32. Gore I, Nakashima T, Imai T, et al. Coronary atherosclerosis and myocardial infarction in Kyushu, Japan, and Boston, Massachusetts. *Am J Cardiol.* 1962;10:400–406.

33. The Lipid Research Clinics Coronary Primary Prevention Trial results. I. Reduction in incidence of coronary heart disease. *JAMA.* 1984;251(3):351–364.

34. Baigent C, Keech A, Kearney PM, et al. Efficacy and safety of cholesterol-lowering treatment: Prospective meta-analysis of data from 90,056 participants in 14 randomised trials of statins. *Lancet.* 2005;366(9493):1267–1278.

35. Grundy SM, Cleeman JI, Merz CN, et al. Implications of recent clinical trials for the National Cholesterol Education Program Adult Treatment Panel III guidelines. *Circulation.* 2004;110(2):227–239.

36. Superko HR. Beyond LDL cholesterol reduction. *Circulation.* 1996;94(10):2351–2354.

37. Libby P. The forgotten majority: Unfinished business in cardiovascular risk reduction. *J Am Coll Cardiol.* 2005;46(7):1225–1228.

38. O'Keefe JH, Jr, Cordain L, Harris WH, et al. Optimal low-density lipoprotein is 50 to 70 mg/dl: Lower is better and physiologically normal. *J Am Coll Cardiol.* 2004;43(11):2142–2146.

39. Cannon CP, Braunwald E, McCabe CH, et al. Intensive versus moderate lipid lowering with statins after acute coronary syndromes. *N Engl J Med.* 2004;350(15):1495–1504.

40. LaRosa JC, Grundy SM, Waters DD, et al. Intensive lipid lowering with atorvastatin in patients with stable coronary disease. *N Engl J Med.* 2005;352(14):1425–1435.

41. Shepherd J, Barter P, Carmena R, et al. Effect of lowering LDL cholesterol substantially below currently recommended levels in patients with coronary heart disease and diabetes: The Treating to New Targets (TNT) study. *Diabetes Care.* 2006;29(6):1220–1226.

42. Nissen SE, Tuzcu EM, Schoenhagen P, et al. Effect of intensive compared with moderate lipid-lowering therapy on progression of coronary atherosclerosis: A randomized controlled trial. *JAMA.* 2004;291(9):1071–1080.

43. Wiviott SD, Cannon CP, Morrow DA, et al. Can low-density lipoprotein be too low? The safety and efficacy of achieving very low low-density lipoprotein with intensive statin therapy: A PROVE IT-TIMI 22 substudy. *J Am Coll Cardiol.* 2005;46(8):1411–1416.

44. Leeper NJ, Ardehali R, deGoma EM, et al. Statin use in patients with extremely low low-density lipoprotein levels is associated with improved survival. *Circulation.* 2007;116(6):613–618.

45. Berneis KK, Krauss RM. Metabolic origins and clinical significance of LDL heterogeneity. *J Lipid Res.* 2002;43(9):1363–1679.

46. Rizzo M, Barbagallo CM, Severino M, et al. Low-density-lipoprotein peak particle size in a Mediterranean population. *Eur J Clin Invest.* 2003;33(2):126–133.

47. St-Pierre AC, Cantin B, Dagenais GR, et al. Low-density lipoprotein subfractions and the long-term risk of ischemic heart disease in men: 13-year follow-up data from the Quebec Cardiovascular Study. *Arterioscler Thromb Vasc Biol.* 2005;25(3):553–559.

48. Navab M, Ananthramaiah GM, Reddy ST, et al. The oxidation hypothesis of atherogenesis: The role of oxidized phospholipids and HDL. *J Lipid Res.* 2004;45(6):993–1007.

49. Parthasarathy S, Santanam N, Ramachandran S, et al. Oxidants and antioxidants in atherogenesis. An appraisal. *J Lipid Res.* 1999;40(12):2143–2157.

50. Hulthe J, Fagerberg B. Circulating oxidized LDL is associated with subclinical atherosclerosis development and inflammatory cytokines (AIR Study). *Arterioscler Thromb Vasc Biol.* 2002;22(7):1162–1167.

51. Jarvisalo MJ, Lehtimaki T, Raitakari OT. Determinants of arterial nitrate-mediated dilatation in children: Role of oxidized low-density lipoprotein, endothelial function, and carotid intima-media thickness. *Circulation.* 2004;109(23):2885–2889.

52. Liu ML, Ylitalo K, Salonen R, et al. Circulating oxidized low-density lipoprotein and its association with carotid intima-media thickness in asymptomatic members of familial combined hyperlipidemia families. *Arterioscler Thromb Vasc Biol.* 2004;24(8):1492–1497.

53. Zhang B, Bai H, Liu R, et al. Serum high-density lipoprotein-cholesterol levels modify the association between plasma levels of oxidatively modified low-density lipoprotein and coronary artery disease in men. *Metabolism.* 2004;53(4):423–429.

54. Wallenfeldt K, Fagerberg B, Wikstrand J, et al. Oxidized low-density lipoprotein in plasma is a prognostic marker of subclinical atherosclerosis development in clinically healthy men. *J Intern Med.* 2004;256(5):413–420.

55. Tsimikas S, Brilakis ES, Miller ER, et al. Oxidized phospholipids, Lp(a) lipoprotein, and coronary artery disease. *N Engl J Med.* 2005;353(1):46–57.

56. Toshima S, Hasegawa A, Kurabayashi M, et al. Circulating oxidized low density lipoprotein levels. A biochemical risk marker for coronary heart disease. *Arterioscler Thromb Vasc Biol.* 2000;20(10):2243–2247.

57. Holvoet P, Jenny NS, Schreiner PJ, et al. The relationship between oxidized LDL and other cardiovascular risk factors and subclinical CVD in different ethnic groups: The Multi-Ethnic Study of Atherosclerosis (MESA). *Atherosclerosis.* 2007;194(1):245–252.

58. Choi SH, Chae A, Miller E, et al. Relationship between biomarkers of oxidized low-density lipoprotein, statin therapy, quantitative coronary angiography, and atheroma: Volume observations from the REVERSAL (Reversal of Atherosclerosis with Aggressive Lipid Lowering) study. *J Am Coll Cardiol.* 2008;52(1):24–32.

59. Toth PP. Reverse cholesterol transport: High-density lipoprotein's magnificent mile. *Curr Atheroscler Rep.* 2003;5(5):386–393.

60. Toth PP. Reducing cardiovascular risk by targeting high-density lipoprotein cholesterol. *Curr Atheroscler Rep.* 2007;9(1):81–88.

61. Aviram M, Hardak E, Vaya J, et al. Human serum paraoxonases (PON1) Q and R selectively decrease lipid peroxides in human coronary and carotid atherosclerotic lesions: PON1 esterase and peroxidase-like activities. *Circulation.* 2000;101(21):2510–2517.

62. Ansell BJ. The two faces of the 'good' cholesterol. *Cleve Clin J Med.* 2007;74(10):697–700, 3–5.

63. CRUSADE Quarter 3, 2004 Results.; 2004 [updated 2004; cited]; Available from: http://www.crusad-equ.com/Main/Ecab/Slides/CRUSADEResults_2004Q3.ppt.

64. Gordon DJ, Probstfield JL, Garrison RJ, et al. High-density lipoprotein cholesterol and cardiovascular disease. Four prospective American studies. *Circulation.* 1989;79(1):8–15.

65. Castelli WP, Garrison RJ, Wilson PW, et al. Incidence of coronary heart disease and lipoprotein cholesterol levels. The Framingham Study. *JAMA.* 1986;256(20):2835–2838.

66. Assmann G, Cullen P, Schulte H. The Munster Heart Study (PROCAM). Results of follow-up at 8 years. *Eur Heart J.* 1998;19(Suppl A):A2–A11.

67. Stampfer MJ, Sacks FM, Salvini S, et al. Prospective study of cholesterol, apolipoproteins, and the risk of myocardial infarction. *N Engl J Med.* 1991;325(6):373–381.

68. Rubins HB, Robins SJ, Collins D, et al. Gemfibrozil for the secondary prevention of coronary heart disease in men with low levels of high-density lipoprotein cholesterol. Veterans Affairs High-Density Lipoprotein Cholesterol Intervention Trial Study Group. *N Engl J Med.* 1999;341(6):410–418.

69. Secondary prevention by raising HDL cholesterol and reducing triglycerides in patients with coronary artery disease: The Bezafibrate Infarction Prevention (BIP) study. *Circulation.* 2000;102(1):21–27.

70. Hokanson JE, Austin MA. Plasma triglyceride level is a risk factor for cardiovascular disease independent of high-density lipoprotein cholesterol level: A meta-analysis of population-based prospective studies. *J Cardiovasc Risk.* 1996;3(2):213–219.

71. Criqui MH, Heiss G, Cohn R, et al. Plasma triglyceride level and mortality from coronary heart disease. *N Engl J Med.* 1993;328(17):1220–1225.

72. Executive Summary of The Third Report of The National Cholesterol Education Program (NCEP) expert panel on detection, evaluation, and treatment of high blood cholesterol in adults (Adult Treatment Panel III). *JAMA.* 2001;285(19):2486–2497.

73. Abate N, Vega GL, Grundy SM. Variability in cholesterol content and physical properties of lipoproteins containing apolipoprotein B-100. *Atherosclerosis.* 1993;104(1–2):159–171.

74. Liu J, Sempos CT, Donahue RP, et al. Non-high-density lipoprotein and very-low-density lipoprotein cholesterol and their risk predictive values in coronary heart disease. *Am J Cardiol.* 2006;98(10):1363–1368.

75. Ridker PM, Rifai N, Cook NR, et al. Non-HDL cholesterol, apolipoproteins A-I and B100, standard lipid measures, lipid ratios, and CRP as risk factors for cardiovascular disease in women. *JAMA.* 2005;294(3):326–333.

76. Orakzai SH, Nasir K, Blaha M, et al. Non-HDL cholesterol is strongly associated with coronary artery calcification in asymptomatic individuals. *Atherosclerosis.* 2009;202(1):289–295. Epub 2008 Mar25.

77. Shepherd J. Does statin monotherapy address the multiple lipid abnormalities in type 2 diabetes? *Atheroscler Suppl.* 2005;6(3):15–19.

78. Pischon T, Girman CJ, Sacks FM, et al. Non-high-density lipoprotein cholesterol and apolipoprotein B in the prediction of coronary heart disease in men. *Circulation.* 2005;112(22):3375–3383.

79. Utermann G. Genetic architecture and evolution of the lipoprotein(a) trait. *Curr Opin Lipidol.* 1999;10(2):133–141.

80. Edelstein C, Pfaffinger D, Hinman J, et al. Lysine-phosphatidylcholine adducts in kringle V impart unique immunological and potential pro-inflammatory properties to human apolipoprotein(a). *J Biol Chem.* 2003;278(52):52841–52847.

81. Sandkamp M, Funke H, Schulte H, et al. Lipoprotein(a) is an independent risk factor for myocardial infarction at a young age. *Clin Chem.* 1990;36(1):20–23.

82. Foody JM, Milberg JA, Robinson K, et al. Homocysteine and lipoprotein(a) interact to increase CAD risk in young men and women. *Arterioscler Thromb Vasc Biol.* 2000;20(2):493–499.

83. Ariyo AA, Thach C, Tracy R. Lp(a) lipoprotein, vascular disease, and mortality in the elderly. *N Engl J Med.* 2003;349(22):2108–2115.

84. Danesh J, Collins R, Peto R. Lipoprotein(a) and coronary heart disease. Meta-analysis of prospective studies. *Circulation.* 2000;102(10):1082–1085.

85. Armstrong VW, Cremer P, Eberle E, et al. The association between serum Lp(a) concentrations and angiographically assessed coronary atherosclerosis. Dependence on serum LDL levels. *Atherosclerosis.* 1986;62(3):249–257.

86. Finkelstein JD. Methionine metabolism in mammals. *J Nutr Biochem.* 1990;1(5):228–237.

87. McCully KS. Vascular pathology of homocysteinemia: Implications for the pathogenesis of arteriosclerosis. *Am J Pathol.* 1969;56(1):111–128.

88. Boushey CJ, Beresford SA, Omenn GS, et al. A quantitative assessment of plasma homocysteine as a risk factor for vascular disease. Probable benefits of increasing folic acid intakes. *JAMA.* 1995;274(13):1049–1057.

89. Homocysteine and risk of ischemic heart disease and stroke: A meta-analysis. Homocysteine Studies Collaboration. *JAMA.* 2002;288(16):2015–2022.

90. Kaul S, Zadeh AA, Shah PK. Homocysteine hypothesis for atherothrombotic cardiovascular disease: Not validated. *J Am Coll Cardiol.* 2006;48(5):914–923.

91. Casas JP, Bautista LE, Smeeth L, et al.. Homocysteine and stroke: Evidence on a causal link from mendelian randomisation. *Lancet.* 2005;365(9455): 224–232.

92. Lewis SJ, Ebrahim S, Davey Smith G. Meta-analysis of MTHFR 677C- >T polymorphism and coronary heart disease: Does totality of evidence support causal role for homocysteine and preventive potential of folate? *BMJ.* 2005;331(7524):1053.

93. Dose-dependent effects of folic acid on blood concentrations of homocysteine: A meta-analysis of the randomized trials. *Am J Clin Nutr.* 2005;82(4): 806–812.

94. Toole JF, Malinow MR, Chambless LE, et al. Lowering homocysteine in patients with ischemic stroke to prevent recurrent stroke, myocardial infarction, and death: The Vitamin Intervention for Stroke Prevention (VISP) randomized controlled trial. *JAMA.* 2004;291(5):565–575.

95. Bonaa KH, Njolstad I, Ueland PM, et al. Homocysteine lowering and cardiovascular events after acute myocardial infarction. *N Engl J Med.* 2006;354(15):1578–1588.

96. Lonn E, Yusuf S, Arnold MJ, et al. Homocysteine lowering with folic acid and B vitamins in vascular disease. *N Engl J Med.* 2006;354(15):1567–1577.

97. Albert CM, Cook NR, Gaziano JM, et al. Effect of folic acid and B vitamins on risk of cardiovascular events and total mortality among women at high risk for cardiovascular disease: A randomized trial. *JAMA.* 2008;299(17):2027–2036.

98. Sica DA, Schoolwerth AC. Part 1. Uric acid and losartan. *Curr Opin Nephrol Hypertens.* 2002;11(5):475–482.

99. Johnson RJ, Kivlighn SD, Kim YG, et al. Reappraisal of the pathogenesis and consequences of hyperuricemia in hypertension, cardiovascular disease, and renal disease. *Am J Kidney Dis.* 1999;33(2):225–234.

100. Breckenridge A. Hypertension and hyperuricaemia. *Lancet.* 1966;1(7427): 15–18.

101. Tykarski A. Evaluation of renal handling of uric acid in essential hypertension: Hyperuricemia related to decreased urate secretion. *Nephron.* 1991;59(3): 364–368.

102. Selby JV, Friedman GD, Quesenberry CP, Jr. Precursors of essential hypertension: Pulmonary function, heart rate, uric acid, serum cholesterol, and other serum chemistries. *Am J Epidemiol.* 1990;131(6):1017–1027.

103. Fang J, Alderman MH. Serum uric acid and cardiovascular mortality the NHANES I epidemiologic follow-up study, 1971–1992. National Health and Nutrition Examination Survey. *JAMA.* 2000;283(18):2404–2010.

104. Bickel C, Rupprecht HJ, Blankenberg S, et al. Serum uric acid as an independent predictor of mortality in patients with angiographically proven coronary artery disease. *Am J Cardiol.* 2002;89(1):12–17.

105. Verdecchia P, Schillaci G, Reboldi G, et al. Relation between serum uric acid and risk of cardiovascular disease in essential hypertension. The PIUMA study. *Hypertension.* 2000;36(6):1072–1078.

106. Franse LV, Pahor M, Di Bari M, et al. Serum uric acid, diuretic treatment and risk of cardiovascular events in the Systolic Hypertension in the Elderly Program (SHEP). *J Hypertens.* 2000;18(8):1149–1154.

107. Goetze JP, Christoffersen C, Perko M, et al. Increased cardiac BNP expression associated with myocardial ischemia. *FASEB J.* 2003;17(9):1105–1107.

108. Ndrepepa G, Braun S, Niemoller K, et al. Prognostic value of N-terminal probrain natriuretic peptide in patients with chronic stable angina. *Circulation.* 2005;112(14):2102–2107.

109. Kragelund C, Gronning B, Kober L, et al. N-terminal pro-B-type natriuretic peptide and long-term mortality in stable coronary heart disease. *N Engl J Med.* 2005;352(7):666–675.

110. Weber M, Dill T, Arnold R, et al. N-terminal B-type natriuretic peptide predicts extent of coronary artery disease and ischemia in patients with stable angina pectoris. *Am Heart J.* 2004;148(4):612–620.

111. Ndrepepa G, Braun S, Mehilli J, et al. Plasma levels of N-terminal pro-brain natriuretic peptide in patients with coronary artery disease and relation to clinical presentation, angiographic severity, and left ventricular ejection fraction. *Am J Cardiol.* 2005;95(5):553–557.

112. Sahinarslan A, Cengel A, Okyay K, et al. B-type natriuretic peptide and extent of lesion on coronary angiography in stable coronary artery disease. *Coron Artery Dis.* 2005;16(4):225–229.

113. Blankenberg S, McQueen MJ, Smieja M, et al. Comparative impact of multiple biomarkers and N-Terminal pro-brain natriuretic peptide in the context of conventional risk factors for the prediction of recurrent cardiovascular events in the Heart Outcomes Prevention Evaluation (HOPE) Study. *Circulation.* 2006;114(3):201–208.

114. Marz W, Tiran B, Seelhorst U, et al. N-terminal pro-B-type natriuretic peptide predicts total and cardiovascular mortality in individuals with or without stable coronary artery disease: The Ludwigshafen Risk and Cardiovascular Health Study. *Clin Chem.* 2007;53(6):1075–1083.

115. Kistorp C, Raymond I, Pedersen F, et al. N-terminal pro-brain natriuretic peptide, C-reactive protein, and urinary albumin levels as predictors of mortality and cardiovascular events in older adults. *JAMA.* 2005;293(13):1609–1616.

116. Wang TJ, Larson MG, Levy D, et al. Plasma natriuretic peptide levels and the risk of cardiovascular events and death. *N Engl J Med.* 2004;350(7):655–663.

117. De Sutter J, De Bacquer D, Cuypers S, et al. Plasma N-terminal pro-brain natriuretic peptide concentration predicts coronary events in men at work: A report from the BELSTRESS study. *Eur Heart J.* 2005;26(24):2644–2649.

118. Luster AD. Chemokines–chemotactic cytokines that mediate inflammation. *N Engl J Med.* 1998;338(7):436–445.

119. Ross R. Atherosclerosis–An inflammatory disease. *N Engl J Med.* 1999;340(2): 115–126.

120. Shankar A, Mitchell P, Rochtchina E, et al. The association between circulating white blood cell count, triglyceride level and cardiovascular and all-cause mortality: Population-based cohort study. *Atherosclerosis.* 2007;192(1):177–183.

121. Margolis KL, Manson JE, Greenland P, et al. Leukocyte count as a predictor of cardiovascular events and mortality in postmenopausal women: The Women's Health Initiative Observational Study. *Arch Intern Med.* 2005;165(5):500–508.

122. Calabro P, Willerson JT, Yeh ET. Inflammatory cytokines stimulated C-reactive protein production by human coronary artery smooth muscle cells. *Circulation.* 2003;108(16):1930–1932.

123. Hirschfield GM, Gallimore JR, Kahan MC, et al. Transgenic human C-reactive protein is not proatherogenic in apolipoprotein E-deficient mice. *Proc Natl Acad Sci USA.* 2005;102(23):8309–8314.

124. Ridker PM, Stampfer MJ, Rifai N. Novel risk factors for systemic atherosclerosis: A comparison of C-reactive protein, fibrinogen, homocysteine, lipoprotein(a), and standard cholesterol screening as predictors of peripheral arterial disease. *JAMA.* 2001;285(19):2481–2485.

125. Ridker PM. Clinical application of C-reactive protein for cardiovascular disease detection and prevention. *Circulation.* 2003;107(3):363–369.

126. Cushman M, Arnold AM, Psaty BM, et al. C-reactive protein and the 10-year incidence of coronary heart disease in older men and women: The cardiovascular health study. *Circulation.* 2005;112(1):25–31.

127. Ballantyne CM, Hoogeveen RC, Bang H, et al. Lipoprotein-associated phospholipase A2, high-sensitivity C-reactive protein, and risk for incident coronary heart disease in middle-aged men and women in the Atherosclerosis Risk in Communities (ARIC) study. *Circulation.* 2004;109(7):837–842.

128. Ridker PM, Rifai N, Rose L, et al. Comparison of C-reactive protein and low-density lipoprotein cholesterol levels in the prediction of first cardiovascular events. *N Engl J Med.* 2002;347(20):1557–1565.

129. Pai JK, Pischon T, Ma J, et al. Inflammatory markers and the risk of coronary heart disease in men and women. *N Engl J Med.* 2004;351(25):2599–2610.

130. Danesh J, Wheeler JG, Hirschfield GM, et al. C-reactive protein and other circulating markers of inflammation in the prediction of coronary heart disease. *N Engl J Med.* 2004;350(14):1387–1397.

131. Ridker PM, Cushman M, Stampfer MJ, et al. Inflammation, aspirin, and the risk of cardiovascular disease in apparently healthy men. *N Engl J Med.* 1997;336(14):973–979.

132. Ridker PM, Buring JE, Cook NR, et al. C-reactive protein, the metabolic syndrome, and risk of incident cardiovascular events: An 8-year follow-up of 14 719 initially healthy American women. *Circulation.* 2003;107(3):391–397.

133. Ridker PM, Cook N. Clinical usefulness of very high and very low levels of C-reactive protein across the full range of Framingham Risk Scores. *Circulation.* 2004;109(16):1955–1959.

134. Pearson TA, Mensah GA, Alexander RW, et al. Markers of inflammation and cardiovascular disease: Application to clinical and public health practice: A statement for healthcare professionals from the Centers for Disease Control and Prevention and the American Heart Association. *Circulation.* 2003;107(3): 499–511.

135. Jialal I, Stein D, Balis D, et al. Effect of hydroxymethyl glutaryl coenzyme a reductase inhibitor therapy on high sensitive C-reactive protein levels. *Circulation.* 2001;103(15):1933–1935.

136. Albert MA, Danielson E, Rifai N, et al. Effect of statin therapy on C-reactive protein levels: The pravastatin inflammation/CRP evaluation (PRINCE): A randomized trial and cohort study. *JAMA.* 2001;286(1):64–70.

137. Ridker PM, Fonseca FA, Genest J, et al. Baseline characteristics of participants in the JUPITER trial, a randomized placebo-controlled primary prevention trial of statin therapy among individuals with low low-density lipoprotein cholesterol and elevated high-sensitivity C-reactive protein. *Am J Cardiol.* 2007;100(11):1659–1664.

138. Ikonomidis I, Andreotti F, Economou E, et al. Increased proinflammatory cytokines in patients with chronic stable angina and their reduction by aspirin. *Circulation.* 1999;100(8):793–798.

139. Ridker PM, Rifai N, Stampfer MJ, et al. Plasma concentration of interleukin-6 and the risk of future myocardial infarction among apparently healthy men. *Circulation.* 2000;101(15):1767–1772.

140. Shishehbor MH, Brennan ML, Aviles RJ, et al. Statins promote potent systemic antioxidant effects through specific inflammatory pathways. *Circulation.* 2003;108(4):426–431.

141. Hazen SL, Heinecke JW. 3-Chlorotyrosine, a specific marker of myeloperoxidase-catalyzed oxidation is markedly elevated in low density lipoprotein isolated from human atherosclerotic intima. *J Clin Invest.* 1997;99(9):2075–2081.

142. Podrez EA, Febbraio M, Sheibani N, et al. Macrophage scavenger receptor CD36 is the major receptor for LDL modified by monocyte-generated reactive nitrogen species. *J Clin Invest.* 2000;105(8):1095–1108.

143. Hazen SL. Myeloperoxidase and plaque vulnerability. *Arterioscler Thromb Vasc Biol.* 2004;24(7):1143–1146.

144. Sugiyama S, Okada Y, Sukhova GK, et al. Macrophage myeloperoxidase regulation by granulocyte macrophage colony-stimulating factor in human atherosclerosis and implications in acute coronary syndromes. *Am J Pathol.* 2001;158(3):879–891.

145. Bergt C, Pennathur S, Fu X, et al. The myeloperoxidase product hypochlorous acid oxidizes HDL in the human artery wall and impairs ABCA1-dependent cholesterol transport. *Proc Natl Acad Sci USA.* 2004;101(35):13032–13037.

146. Vita JA, Brennan ML, Gokce N, et al. Serum myeloperoxidase levels independently predict endothelial dysfunction in humans. *Circulation.* 2004;110(9):1134–1139.
147. Zhang R, Brennan ML, Fu X, et al. Association between myeloperoxidase levels and risk of coronary artery disease. *JAMA.* 2001;286(17):2136–2142.
148. Brennan ML, Penn MS, Van Lente F, et al. Prognostic value of myeloperoxidase in patients with chest pain. *N Engl J Med.* 2003;349(17):1595–1604.
149. Macphee CH. Lipoprotein-associated phospholipase A2: A potential new risk factor for coronary artery disease and a therapeutic target. *Curr Opin Pharmacol.* 2001;1(2):121–125.
150. Mcconnell JP, Hoefner DM. Lipoprotein-associated phospholipase A2. *Clin Lab Med.* 2006;26(3):679–697.
151. Blackie JA, Bloomer JC, Brown MJ, et al. The identification of clinical candidate SB-480848: A potent inhibitor of lipoprotein-associated phospholipase A2. *Bioorg Med Chem Lett.* 2003;13(6):1067–1070.
152. Yamada Y, Ichihara S, Fujimura T, et al. Identification of the G994->T missense in exon 9 of the plasma platelet-activating factor acetylhydrolase gene as an independent risk factor for coronary artery disease in Japanese men. *Metabolism.* 1998;47(2):177–181.
153. Noto H, Hara M, Karasawa K, et al. Human plasma platelet-activating factor acetylhydrolase binds to all the murine lipoproteins, conferring protection against oxidative stress. *Arterioscler Thromb Vasc Biol.* 2003;23(5):829–835.
154. Hase M, Tanaka M, Yokota M, et al. Reduction in the extent of atherosclerosis in apolipoprotein E-deficient mice induced by electroporation-mediated transfer of the human plasma platelet-activating factor acetylhydrolase gene into skeletal muscle. *Prostaglandins Other Lipid Mediat.* 2002;70(1–2):107–118.
155. Quarck R, De Geest B, Stengel D, et al. Adenovirus-mediated gene transfer of human platelet-activating factor-acetylhydrolase prevents injury-induced neointima formation and reduces spontaneous atherosclerosis in apolipoprotein E-deficient mice. *Circulation.* 2001;103(20):2495–2500.
156. Packard CJ, O'Reilly DS, Caslake MJ, et al. Lipoprotein-associated phospholipase A2 as an independent predictor of coronary heart disease. West of Scotland Coronary Prevention Study Group. *N Engl J Med.* 2000;343(16):1148–1155.
157. Koenig W, Khuseyinova N, Lowel H, et al. Lipoprotein-associated phospholipase A2 adds to risk prediction of incident coronary events by C-reactive protein in apparently healthy middle-aged men from the general population: Results from the 14-year follow-up of a large cohort from southern Germany. *Circulation.* 2004;110(14):1903–1908.
158. Blake GJ, Dada N, Fox JC, et al. Prospective evaluation of lipoprotein-associated phospholipase A(2) levels and the risk of future cardiovascular events in women. *J Am Coll Cardiol.* 2001;38(5):1302–1306.
159. Pratico D, Rokach J, Lawson J, et al. F2-isoprostanes as indices of lipid peroxidation in inflammatory diseases. *Chem Phys Lipids.* 2004;128(1–2):165–171.
160. Morrow JD. Quantification of isoprostanes as indices of oxidant stress and the risk of atherosclerosis in humans. *Arterioscler Thromb Vasc Biol.* 2005;25(2):279–286.
161. Waters DD, Alderman EL, Hsia J, et al. Effects of hormone replacement therapy and antioxidant vitamin supplements on coronary atherosclerosis in postmenopausal women: A randomized controlled trial. *JAMA.* 2002;288(19):2432–2440.
162. Gross M, Steffes M, Jacobs DR, Jr, et al. Plasma F2-isoprostanes and coronary artery calcification: The CARDIA Study. *Clin Chem.* 2005;51(1):125–131.
163. Danesh J, Collins R, Appleby P, et al. Association of fibrinogen, C-reactive protein, albumin, or leukocyte count with coronary heart disease: Meta-analyses of prospective studies. *JAMA.* 1998;279(18):1477–1482.
164. Avanzas P, Arroyo-Espliguero R, Quiles J, et al. Elevated serum neopterin predicts future adverse cardiac events in patients with chronic stable angina pectoris. *Eur Heart J.* 2005;26(5):457–463.
165. Johnston DT, Gagos M, Raio N, et al. Alterations in serum neopterin correlate with thrombolysis in myocardial infarction risk scores in acute coronary syndromes. *Coron Artery Dis.* 2006;17(6):511–516.
166. Ray KK, Morrow DA, Sabatine MS, et al. Long-term prognostic value of neopterin: A novel marker of monocyte activation in patients with acute coronary syndrome. *Circulation.* 2007;115(24):3071–3078.
167. Gullu H, Erdogan D, Tok D, et al. High serum bilirubin concentrations preserve coronary flow reserve and coronary microvascular functions. *Arterioscler Thromb Vasc Biol.* 2005;25(11):2289–2294.
168. Kawamura K, Ishikawa K, Wada Y, et al. Bilirubin from heme oxygenase-1 attenuates vascular endothelial activation and dysfunction. *Arterioscler Thromb Vasc Biol.* 2005;25(1):155–160.
169. Pae HO, Oh GS, Lee BS, et al. 3-Hydroxyanthranilic acid, one of L-tryptophan metabolites, inhibits monocyte chemoattractant protein-1 secretion and vascular cell adhesion molecule-1 expression via heme oxygenase-1 induction in human umbilical vein endothelial cells. *Atherosclerosis.* 2006;187(2):274–284.
170. Ishikawa K, Navab M, Leitinger N, et al. Induction of heme oxygenase-1 inhibits the monocyte transmigration induced by mildly oxidized LDL. *J Clin Invest.* 1997;100(5):1209–1216.
171. Ollinger R, Bilban M, Erat A, et al. Bilirubin: A natural inhibitor of vascular smooth muscle cell proliferation. *Circulation.* 2005;112(7):1030–1039.
172. Neuzil J, Stocker R. Free and albumin-bound bilirubin are efficient co-antioxidants for alpha-tocopherol, inhibiting plasma and low density lipoprotein lipid peroxidation. *J Biol Chem.* 1994;269(24):16712–16719.
173. Lindenblatt N, Bordel R, Schareck W, et al. Vascular heme oxygenase-1 induction suppresses microvascular thrombus formation in vivo. *Arterioscler Thromb Vasc Biol.* 2004;24(3):601–606.
174. Ishikawa K, Sugawara D, Goto J, et al. Heme oxygenase-1 inhibits atherogenesis in Watanabe heritable hyperlipidemic rabbits. *Circulation.* 2001;104(15):1831–1836.
175. Erdogan D, Gullu H, Yildirim E, et al. Low serum bilirubin levels are independently and inversely related to impaired flow-mediated vasodilation and increased carotid intima-media thickness in both men and women. *Atherosclerosis.* 2006;184(2):431–437.
176. Vitek L, Jirsa M, Brodanova M, et al. Gilbert syndrome and ischemic heart disease: A protective effect of elevated bilirubin levels. *Atherosclerosis.* 2002;160(2):449–456.
177. Schwertner HA, Jackson WG, Tolan G. Association of low serum concentration of bilirubin with increased risk of coronary artery disease. *Clin Chem.* 1994;40(1):18–23.
178. Djousse L, Rothman KJ, Cupples LA, et al. Effect of serum albumin and bilirubin on the risk of myocardial infarction (the Framingham Offspring Study). *Am J Cardiol.* 2003;91(4):485–488.
179. Djousse L, Levy D, Cupples LA, et al. Total serum bilirubin and risk of cardiovascular disease in the Framingham offspring study. *Am J Cardiol.* 2001;87(10):1196–1200, A4, 7.
180. Perlstein TS, Pande RL, Beckman JA, et al. Serum total bilirubin level and prevalent lower-extremity peripheral arterial disease: National Health and Nutrition Examination Survey (NHANES) 1999 to 2004. *Arterioscler Thromb Vasc Biol.* 2008;28(1):166–172.
181. Perlstein TS, Pande RL, Creager MA, et al. Serum total bilirubin level, prevalent stroke, and stroke outcomes: NHANES 1999–2004. *Am J Med.* 2008;121(9):781e1–788e1.
182. Rumberger JA, Kaufman L. A rosetta stone for coronary calcium risk stratification: Agatston, volume, and mass scores in 11,490 individuals. *AJR Am J Roentgenol.* 2003;181(3):743–748.
183. Agatston AS, Janowitz WR, Hildner FJ, et al. Quantification of coronary artery calcium using ultrafast computed tomography. *J Am Coll Cardiol.* 1990;15(4):827–832.
184. Becker CR, Kleffel T, Crispin A, et al. Coronary artery calcium measurement: Agreement of multirow detector and electron beam CT. *AJR Am J Roentgenol.* 2001;176(5):1295–1298.
185. Knez A, Becker C, Becker A, et al. Determination of coronary calcium with multi-slice spiral computed tomography: A comparative study with electron-beam CT. *Int J Cardiovasc Imaging.* 2002;18(4):295–303.
186. McCollough CH, Ulzheimer S, Halliburton SS, et al. Coronary artery calcium: A multi-institutional, multimanufacturer international standard for quantification at cardiac CT. *Radiology.* 2007;243(2):527–538.
187. Becker A, Leber A, White CW, et al. Multislice computed tomography for determination of coronary artery disease in a symptomatic patient population. *Int J Cardiovasc Imaging.* 2007;23(3):361–367.
188. Cheng VY, Lepor NE, Madyoon H, et al. Presence and severity of noncalcified coronary plaque on 64-slice computed tomographic coronary angiography in patients with zero and low coronary artery calcium. *Am J Cardiol.* 2007;99(9):1183–1186.
189. Henneman MM, Schuijf JD, Pundziute G, et al. Noninvasive evaluation with multislice computed tomography in suspected acute coronary syndrome: Plaque morphology on multislice computed tomography versus coronary calcium score. *J Am Coll Cardiol.* 2008;52(3):216–222.
190. Shaw LJ, Raggi P, Schisterman E, et al. Prognostic value of cardiac risk factors and coronary artery calcium screening for all-cause mortality. *Radiology.* 2003;228(3):826–833.
191. Greenland P, LaBree L, Azen SP, et al. Coronary artery calcium score combined with Framingham score for risk prediction in asymptomatic individuals. *JAMA.* 2004;291(2):210–215.
192. Arad Y, Goodman KJ, Roth M, et al. Coronary calcification, coronary disease risk factors, C-reactive protein, and atherosclerotic cardiovascular disease events: The St. Francis Heart Study. *J Am Coll Cardiol.* 2005;46(1):158–165.
193. LaMonte MJ, FitzGerald SJ, Church TS, et al. Coronary artery calcium score and coronary heart disease events in a large cohort of asymptomatic men and women. *Am J Epidemiol.* 2005;162(5):421–429.
194. Taylor AJ, Bindeman J, Feuerstein I, et al. Coronary calcium independently predicts incident premature coronary heart disease over measured cardiovascular risk factors: Mean three-year outcomes in the Prospective Army Coronary Calcium (PACC) project. *J Am Coll Cardiol.* 2005;46(5):807–814.
195. Kondos GT, Hoff JA, Sevrukov A, et al. Electron-beam tomography coronary artery calcium and cardiac events: A 37-month follow-up of 5635 initially asymptomatic low- to intermediate-risk adults. *Circulation.* 2003;107(20):2571–2476.
196. Raggi P, Shaw LJ, Berman DS, et al. Gender-based differences in the prognostic value of coronary calcification. *J Womens Health (Larchmt).* 2004;13(3):273–283.
197. Lakoski SG, Greenland P, Wong ND, et al. Coronary artery calcium scores and risk for cardiovascular events in women classified as "low risk" based on Framingham risk score: The multi-ethnic study of atherosclerosis (MESA). *Arch Intern Med.* [Comparative Study Journal Article Multicenter Study Research Support N I H Extramural]. 2007;167(22):2437–2442.
198. Bellasi A, Lacey C, Taylor AJ, et al. Comparison of prognostic usefulness of coronary artery calcium in men versus women (results from a meta- and pooled analysis estimating all-cause mortality and coronary heart disease death or myocardial infarction). *Am J Cardiol.* [Comparative Study Journal Article]. 2007;100(3):409–414.
199. Dabelea D, Kinney G, Snell-Bergeon JK, et al. Effect of type 1 diabetes on the gender difference in coronary artery calcification: A role for insulin resistance? The Coronary Artery Calcification in Type 1 Diabetes (CACTI) Study. *Diabetes.* [Comparative Study Journal Article Multicenter Study Research Support U S Gov't P H S]. 2003;52(11):2833–2839.
200. Meigs JB, Larson MG, D'Agostino RB, et al. Coronary artery calcification in type 2 diabetes and insulin resistance: The framingham offspring study. *Diabetes*

Care. [Journal Article Research Support Non-U S Gov't Research Support U S Gov't P H S]. 2002;25(8):1313–1319.

201. Wong ND, Sciammarella MG, Polk D, et al. The metabolic syndrome, diabetes, and subclinical atherosclerosis assessed by coronary calcium. *J Am Coll Cardiol.* 2003;41(9):1547–1553.

202. Wong ND, Rozanski A, Gransar H, et al. Metabolic syndrome and diabetes are associated with an increased likelihood of inducible myocardial ischemia among patients with subclinical atherosclerosis. *Diabetes Care.* 2005;28(6):1445–1450.

203. Anand DV, Lim E, Hopkins D, et al. Risk stratification in uncomplicated type 2 diabetes: Prospective evaluation of the combined use of coronary artery calcium imaging and selective myocardial perfusion scintigraphy. *Eur Heart J.* 2006;27(6):713–721.

204. Raggi P, Shaw LJ, Berman DS, et al. Prognostic value of coronary artery calcium screening in subjects with and without diabetes. *J Am Coll Cardiol.* 2004;43(9):1663–1669.

205. Vliegenthart R, Oudkerk M, Hofman A, et al. Coronary calcification improves cardiovascular risk prediction in the elderly. *Circulation.* 2005;112(4):572–577.

206. Raggi P, Gongora MC, Gopal A, et al. Coronary artery calcium to predict all-cause mortality in elderly men and women. *J Am Coll Cardiol.* 2008;52(1):17–23.

207. Bild DE, Detrano R, Peterson D, et al. Ethnic differences in coronary calcification: The Multi-Ethnic Study of Atherosclerosis (MESA). *Circulation.* 2005;111(10):1313–1320.

208. Nasir K, Shaw LJ, Liu ST, et al. Ethnic differences in the prognostic value of coronary artery calcification for all-cause mortality. *J Am Coll Cardiol.* 2007;50(10):953–960.

209. Detrano R, Guerci AD, Carr JJ, et al. Coronary calcium as a predictor of coronary events in four racial or ethnic groups. *N Engl J Med. [Journal Article Research Support NIH Extramural].* 2008;358(13):1336–1345.

210. Budoff MJ, Achenbach S, Blumenthal RS, et al. Assessment of coronary artery disease by cardiac computed tomography: A scientific statement from the American Heart Association Committee on Cardiovascular Imaging and Intervention, Council on Cardiovascular Radiology and Intervention, and Committee on Cardiac Imaging, Council on Clinical Cardiology. *Circulation.* 2006;114(16):1761–1791.

211. Greenland P, Bonow RO, Brundage BH, et al. ACCF/AHA 2007 clinical expert consensus document on coronary artery calcium scoring by computed tomography in global cardiovascular risk assessment and in evaluation of patients with chest pain: A report of the American College of Cardiology Foundation Clinical Expert Consensus Task Force (ACCF/AHA Writing Committee to Update the 2000 Expert Consensus Document on Electron Beam Computed Tomography) developed in collaboration with the Society of Atherosclerosis Imaging and Prevention and the Society of Cardiovascular Computed Tomography. *J Am Coll Cardiol.* 2007;49(3):378–402.

212. Hamon M, Biondi-Zoccai GG, Malagutti P, et al. Diagnostic performance of multislice spiral computed tomography of coronary arteries as compared with conventional invasive coronary angiography: A meta-analysis. *J Am Coll Cardiol. [Comparative Study Journal Article Meta-Analysis Review].* 2006;48(9):1896–1910.

213. Hamon M, Morello R, Riddell JW, et al. Coronary arteries: Diagnostic performance of 16- versus 64-section spiral CT compared with invasive coronary angiography—meta-analysis. *Radiology. [Comparative Study Journal Article Meta-Analysis].* 2007;245(3):720–731.

214. Pundziute G, Schuijf JD, Jukema JW, et al. Prognostic value of multislice computed tomography coronary angiography in patients with known or suspected coronary artery disease. *J Am Coll Cardiol.* 2007;49(1):62–70.

215. Min JK, Shaw LJ, Devereux RB, et al. Prognostic value of multidetector coronary computed tomographic angiography for prediction of all-cause mortality. *J Am Coll Cardiol.* 2007;50(12):1161–1170.

216. Leber AW, Knez A, Becker A, et al. Accuracy of multidetector spiral computed tomography in identifying and differentiating the composition of coronary atherosclerotic plaques: A comparative study with intracoronary ultrasound. *J Am Coll Cardiol. [Comparative Study Evaluation Studies Journal Article Research Support Non-US Gov't].* 2004;43(7):1241–1247.

217. Schroeder S, Kopp AF, Baumbach A, et al. Noninvasive detection and evaluation of atherosclerotic coronary plaques with multislice computed tomography. *J Am Coll Cardiol.* 2001;37(5):1430–1435.

218. Pohle K, Achenbach S, Macneill B, et al. Characterization of non-calcified coronary atherosclerotic plaque by multi-detector row CT: Comparison to IVUS. *Atherosclerosis.* 2007;190(1):174–180.

219. Leber AW, Knez A, White CW, et al. Composition of coronary atherosclerotic plaques in patients with acute myocardial infarction and stable angina pectoris determined by contrast-enhanced multislice computed tomography. *Am J Cardiol.* 2003;91(6):714–718.

220. Schuijf JD, Beck T, Burgstahler C, et al. Differences in plaque composition and distribution in stable coronary artery disease versus acute coronary syndromes; non-invasive evaluation with multi-slice computed tomography. *Acute Card Care.* 2007;9(1):48–53.

221. Motoyama S, Kondo T, Sarai M, et al. Multislice computed tomographic characteristics of coronary lesions in acute coronary syndromes. *J Am Coll Cardiol.* 2007;50(4):319–326.

222. Ambrose JA, Tannenbaum MA, Alexopoulos D, et al. Angiographic progression of coronary artery disease and the development of myocardial infarction. *J Am Coll Cardiol.* 1988;12(1):56–62.

223. Boden WE, O'Rourke RA, Teo KK, et al. Optimal medical therapy with or without PCI for stable coronary disease. *N Engl J Med.* 2007;356(15):1503–1516.

224. Choi EK, Choi SI, Rivera JJ, et al. Coronary computed tomography angiography as a screening tool for the detection of occult coronary artery disease in asymptomatic individuals. *J Am Coll Cardiol.* 2008;52:357–365.

225. Hendel RC, Patel MR, Kramer CM, et al. ACCF/ACR/SCCT/SCMR/ASNC/NASCI/SCAI/SIR 2006 appropriateness criteria for cardiac computed tomography and cardiac magnetic resonance imaging: A report of the American College of Cardiology Foundation Quality Strategic Directions Committee Appropriateness Criteria Working Group, American College of Radiology, Society of Cardiovascular Computed Tomography, Society for Cardiovascular Magnetic Resonance, American Society of Nuclear Cardiology, North American Society for Cardiac Imaging, Society for Cardiovascular Angiography and Interventions, and Society of Interventional Radiology. *J Am Coll Cardiol.* 2006;48(7):1475–1497.

226. Bjorntorp P. Abdominal obesity and the development of noninsulin-dependent diabetes mellitus. *Diabetes Metab Rev.* 1988;4(6):615–622.

227. Despres JP. Is visceral obesity the cause of the metabolic syndrome? *Ann Med.* 2006;38(1):52–63.

228. Folsom AR, Prineas RJ, Kaye SA, et al. Incidence of hypertension and stroke in relation to body fat distribution and other risk factors in older women. *Stroke.* 1990;21(5):701–706.

229. Lebovitz HE, Banerji MA. Point: Visceral adiposity is causally related to insulin resistance. *Diabetes Care.* 2005;28(9):2322–2325.

230. Zamboni M, Armellini F, Sheiban I, et al. Relation of body fat distribution in men and degree of coronary narrowings in coronary artery disease. *Am J Cardiol.* 1992;70(13):1135–1138.

231. Ho E, Shimada Y. Formation of the epicardium studied with the scanning electron microscope. *Dev Biol.* 1978;66(2):579–585.

232. Iacobellis G, Corradi D, Sharma AM. Epicardial adipose tissue: Anatomic, biomolecular and clinical relationships with the heart. *Nat Clin Pract Cardiovasc Med.* 2005;2(10):536–543.

233. Fain JN. Release of interleukins and other inflammatory cytokines by human adipose tissue is enhanced in obesity and primarily due to the nonfat cells. *Vitam Horm.* 2006;74:443–477.

234. Weisberg SP, McCann D, Desai M, et al. Obesity is associated with macrophage accumulation in adipose tissue. *J Clin Invest.* 2003;112(12):1796–1808.

235. Moreno PR, Purushothaman KR, Fuster V, et al. Intimomedial interface damage and adventitial inflammation is increased beneath disrupted atherosclerosis in the aorta: Implications for plaque vulnerability. *Circulation.* 2002;105(21):2504–2511.

236. Mazurek T, Zhang L, Zalewski A, et al. Human epicardial adipose tissue is a source of inflammatory mediators. *Circulation.* 2003;108(20):2460–2466.

237. Robicsek F, Thubrikar MJ. The freedom from atherosclerosis of intramyocardial coronary arteries: Reduction of mural stress–a key factor. *Eur J Cardiothorac Surg.* 1994;8(5):228–235.

238. Kawawa Y, Ishikawa Y, Gomi T, et al. Detection of myocardial bridge and evaluation of its anatomical properties by coronary multislice spiral computed tomography. *Eur J Radiol.* 2007;61(1):130–138.

239. Ishii T, Asuwa N, Masuda S, et al. The effects of a myocardial bridge on coronary atherosclerosis and ischaemia. *J Pathol.* 1998;185(1):4–9.

240. Ishii T, Asuwa N, Masuda S, et al. Atherosclerosis suppression in the left anterior descending coronary artery by the presence of a myocardial bridge: An ultrastructural study. *Mod Pathol.* 1991;4(4):424–431.

241. Schejbal V. Ventricle–morphology [Epicardialfattytissueoftheright. Morphometry and functional significance]. *Pneumologie.* 1989;43(9):490–499.

242. Gorter PM, van Lindert AS, de Vos AM, et al. Quantification of epicardial and peri-coronary fat using cardiac computed tomography; reproducibility and relation with obesity and metabolic syndrome in patients suspected of coronary artery disease. *Atherosclerosis.* 2008;197(2):896–903.

243. Ding J, Kritchevsky SB, Harris TB, et al. The association of pericardial fat with calcified coronary plaque. *Obesity (Silver Spring).* 2008;16(8):1914–1919.

244. de Vos AM, Prokop M, Roos CJ, et al. Peri-coronary epicardial adipose tissue is related to cardiovascular risk factors and coronary artery calcification in postmenopausal women. *Eur Heart J.* 2008;29(6):777–783.

245. Taguchi R, Takasu J, Itani Y, et al. Pericardial fat accumulation in men as a risk factor for coronary artery disease. *Atherosclerosis.* 2001;157(1):203–209.

246. Jeong JW, Jeong MH, Yun KH, et al. Echocardiographic epicardial fat thickness and coronary artery disease. *Circ J.* 2007;71(4):536–539.

247. Eroglu S, Sade LE, Yildirir A, et al. Epicardial adipose tissue thickness by echocardiography is a marker for the presence and severity of coronary artery disease. *Nutr Metab Cardiovasc Dis.* 2009;19(3):211–217.

248. Ahn SG, Lim HS, Joe DY, et al. Relationship of epicardial adipose tissue by echocardiography to coronary artery disease. *Heart.* 2008;94(3):e7.

249. Chaowalit N, Somers VK, Pellikka PA, et al. Subepicardial adipose tissue and the presence and severity of coronary artery disease. *Atherosclerosis.* 2006;186(2):354–359.

250. Gofman JW, Malamud N, Simon A, et al. The interrelationship between cerebral and coronary atherosclerosis; a preliminary report. *Geriatrics.* 1956;11(9):413–418.

251. Smith SC, Jr., Greenland P, Grundy SM. AHA conference proceedings. Prevention conference V: Beyond secondary prevention: Identifying the high-risk patient for primary prevention: Executive summary. *Circulation.* 2000;101(1):111–116.

252. Roman MJ, Naqvi TZ, Gardin JM, et al. Clinical application of noninvasive vascular ultrasound in cardiovascular risk stratification: A report from the American Society of Echocardiography and the Society of Vascular Medicine and Biology. *J Am Soc Echocardiogr.* 2006;19(8):943–954.

253. Mitchell CK, Aeschlimann SE, Korcarz CE. Carotid intima-media thickness testing: Technical considerations. *J Am Soc Echocardiogr.* 2004;17(6):690–692.

254. O'Leary DH, Polak JF, Kronmal RA, et al. Carotid-artery intima and media thickness as a risk factor for myocardial infarction and stroke in older adults. Cardiovascular Health Study Collaborative Research Group. *N Engl J Med.* 1999;340(1):14–22.

255. Bots ML, Evans GW, Riley WA, et al. Carotid intima-media thickness measurements in intervention studies: Design options, progression rates, and sample size considerations: A point of view. *Stroke.* 2003;34(12):2985–2994.

256. Johnsen SH, Mathiesen EB, Joakimsen O, et al. Carotid atherosclerosis is a stronger predictor of myocardial infarction in women than in men: A 6-year follow-up study of 6226 persons: The Tromso Study. *Stroke.* 2007;38(11):2873–2880.

257. Prati P, Tosetto A, Vanuzzo D, et al. Carotid intima media thickness and plaques can predict the occurrence of ischemic cerebrovascular events. *Stroke.* 2008;39(9):2470–2476.

258. Honda O, Sugiyama S, Kugiyama K, et al. Echolucent carotid plaques predict future coronary events in patients with coronary artery disease. *J Am Coll Cardiol.* 2004;43(7):1177–1184.

259. Ebrahim S, Papacosta O, Whincup P, et al. Carotid plaque, intima media thickness, cardiovascular risk factors, and prevalent cardiovascular disease in men and women: The British Regional Heart Study. *Stroke.* 1999;30(4):841–850.

260. Li S, Chen W, Srinivasan SR, et al. Race (black-white) and gender divergences in the relationship of childhood cardiovascular risk factors to carotid artery intima-media thickness in adulthood: The Bogalusa Heart Study. *Atherosclerosis.* 2007;194(2):421–425.

261. Crouse JR, III, Tang R, Espeland MA, et al. Associations of extracranial carotid atherosclerosis progression with coronary status and risk factors in patients with and without coronary artery disease. *Circulation.* 2002;106(16):2061–2066.

262. Ranjit N, Diez-Roux AV, Chambless L, et al. Socioeconomic differences in progression of carotid intima-media thickness in the Atherosclerosis Risk in Communities study. *Arterioscler Thromb Vasc Biol.* 2006;26(2):411–416.

263. Belcaro G, Nicolaides AN, Ramaswami G, et al. Carotid and femoral ultrasound morphology screening and cardiovascular events in low risk subjects: A 10-year follow-up study (the CAFES-CAVE study(1)). *Atherosclerosis.* 2001;156(2):379–387.

264. Chambless LE, Heiss G, Folsom AR, et al. Association of coronary heart disease incidence with carotid arterial wall thickness and major risk factors: The Atherosclerosis Risk in Communities (ARIC) Study, 1987–1993. *Am J Epidemiol.* 1997;146(6):483–494.

265. Lim TK, Lim E, Dwivedi G, et al. Normal value of carotid intima-media thickness–A surrogate marker of atherosclerosis: Quantitative assessment by B-mode carotid ultrasound. *J Am Soc Echocardiogr.* 2008;21(2):112–116.

266. Watanabe H, Yamane K, Egusa G, et al. Influence of westernization of lifestyle on the progression of IMT in Japanese. *J Atheroscler Thromb.* 2004;11(6):330–334.

267. Folsom AR, Eckfeldt JH, Weitzman S, et al. Relation of carotid artery wall thickness to diabetes mellitus, fasting glucose and insulin, body size, and physical activity. Atherosclerosis Risk in Communities (ARIC) Study Investigators. *Stroke.* 1994;25(1):66–73.

268. Gnasso A, Irace C, Mattioli PL, et al. Carotid intima-media thickness and coronary heart disease risk factors. *Atherosclerosis.* 1996;119(1):7–15.

269. Denarie N, Simon A, Chironi G, et al. Difference in carotid artery wall structure between Swedish and French men at low and high coronary risk. *Stroke.* 2001;32(8):1775–1779.

270. Kuller L, Borhani N, Furberg C, et al. Prevalence of subclinical atherosclerosis and cardiovascular disease and association with risk factors in the Cardiovascular Health Study. *Am J Epidemiol.* 1994;139(12):1164–1179.

271. Sipila K, Moilanen L, Nieminen T, et al. Metabolic syndrome and carotid intima media thickness in the health 2000 survey. *Atherosclerosis.* 2009;204(1):276–281.

272. Raitakari OT, Juonala M, Kahonen M, et al. Cardiovascular risk factors in childhood and carotid artery intima-media thickness in adulthood: The cardiovascular risk in young finns study. *JAMA.* 2003;290(17):2277–2283.

273. Bots ML, Hoes AW, Koudstaal PJ, et al. Common carotid intima-media thickness and risk of stroke and myocardial infarction: The Rotterdam Study. *Circulation.* 1997;96(5):1432–1437.

274. Lorenz MW, von Kegler S, Steinmetz H, et al. Carotid intima-media thickening indicates a higher vascular risk across a wide age range: Prospective data from the Carotid Atherosclerosis Progression Study (CAPS). *Stroke.* 2006;37(1):87–92.

275. Lorenz MW, Markus HS, Bots ML, et al. Prediction of clinical cardiovascular events with carotid intima-media thickness: A systematic review and meta-analysis. *Circulation.* 2007;115(4):459–467.

276. Price JF, Tzoulaki I, Lee AJ, et al. Ankle brachial index and intima media thickness predict cardiovascular events similarly and increased prediction when combined. *J Clin Epidemiol.* 2007;60(10):1067–1075.

277. Newman AB, Naydeck BL, Ives DG, et al. Coronary artery calcium, carotid artery wall thickness, and cardiovascular disease outcomes in adults 70 to 99 years old. *Am J Cardiol.* 2008;101(2):186–192.

278. Folsom AR, Kronmal RA, Detrano RC, et al. Coronary artery calcification compared with carotid intima-media thickness in the prediction of cardiovascular disease incidence: The Multi-Ethnic Study of Atherosclerosis (MESA). *Arch Intern Med.* 2008;168(12):1333–1339.

279. van der Meer IM, Bots ML, Hofman A, et al. Predictive value of noninvasive measures of atherosclerosis for incident myocardial infarction: The Rotterdam Study. *Circulation.* 2004;109(9):1089–1094.

280. Taylor AJ, Kent SM, Flaherty PJ, et al. ARBITER: Arterial Biology for the Investigation of the Treatment Effects of Reducing Cholesterol: A randomized trial comparing the effects of atorvastatin and pravastatin on carotid intima medial thickness. *Circulation.* 2002;106(16):2055–2060.

281. Terpstra WF, May JF, Smit AJ, et al. Effects of amlodipine and lisinopril on intima-media thickness in previously untreated, elderly hypertensive patients (the ELVERA trial). *J Hypertens.* 2004;22(7):1309–1316.

282. Taylor AJ, Sullenberger LE, Lee HJ, et al. Arterial Biology for the Investigation of the Treatment Effects of Reducing Cholesterol (ARBITER) 2: A double-blind, placebo-controlled study of extended-release niacin on atherosclerosis progression in secondary prevention patients treated with statins. *Circulation.* 2004;110(23):3512–3517.

283. Kastelein JJ, Akdim F, Stroes ES, et al. Simvastatin with or without ezetimibe in familial hypercholesterolemia. *N Engl J Med.* 2008;358(14):1431–1443.

284. Mazzone T, Meyer PM, Feinstein SB, et al. Effect of pioglitazone compared with glimepiride on carotid intima-media thickness in type 2 diabetes: A randomized trial. *JAMA.* 2006;296(21):2572–2581.

285. Mancia G, De Backer G, Dominiczak A, et al 2007 Guidelines for the management of arterial hypertension: The Task Force for the Management of Arterial Hypertension of the European Society of Hypertension (ESH) and of the European Society of Cardiology (ESC). *Eur Heart J.* 2007;28(12):1462–1536.

286. Fayad ZA, Fuster V, Nikolaou K, et al. Computed tomography and magnetic resonance imaging for noninvasive coronary angiography and plaque imaging: Current and potential future concepts. *Circulation.* 2002;106(15):2026–2034.

287. Toussaint JF, LaMuraglia GM, Southern JF, et al. Magnetic resonance images lipid, fibrous, calcified, hemorrhagic, and thrombotic components of human atherosclerosis in vivo. *Circulation.* 1996;94(5):932–938.

288. Levin DC, Fallon JT. Significance of the angiographic morphology of localized coronary stenoses: Histopathologic correlations. *Circulation.* 1982;66(2):316–320.

289. Falk E. Plaque rupture with severe pre-existing stenosis precipitating coronary thrombosis. Characteristics of coronary atherosclerotic plaques underlying fatal occlusive thrombi. *Br Heart J.* 1983;50(2):127–134.

290. Fuster V, Moreno PR, Fayad ZA, et al. Atherothrombosis and high-risk plaque: Part I: Evolving concepts. *J Am Coll Cardiol.* 2005;46(6):937–954.

291. Anumula S, Song HK, Wright AC, et al. High-resolution black-blood MRI of the carotid vessel wall using phased-array coils at 1.5 and 3 Tesla. *Acad Radiol.* 2005;12(12):1521–1526.

292. Koktzoglou I, Chung YC, Mani V, et al. Multislice dark-blood carotid artery wall imaging: A 1.5T and 3.0T comparison. *J Magn Reson Imaging.* 2006;23(5):699–705.

293. Yarnykh VL, Terashima M, Hayes CE, et al. Multicontrast black-blood MRI of carotid arteries: Comparison between 1.5 and 3 tesla magnetic field strengths. *J Magn Reson Imaging.* 2006;23(5):691–698.

294. Maroules CD, McColl R, Khera A, et al. Assessment and reproducibility of aortic atherosclerosis magnetic resonance imaging: Impact of 3-Tesla field strength and parallel imaging. *Invest Radiol.* 2008;43(9):656–662.

295. Edelman RR, Chien D, Kim D. Fast selective black blood MR imaging. *Radiology.* 1991;181(3):655–660.

296. Simonetti OP, Finn JP, White RD, et al. "Black blood" T2-weighted inversion-recovery MR imaging of the heart. *Radiology.* 1996;199(1):49–57.

297. Itskovich VV, Mani V, Mizsei G, et al. Parallel and nonparallel simultaneous multislice black-blood double inversion recovery techniques for vessel wall imaging. *J Magn Reson Imaging.* 2004;19(4):459–467.

298. Yuan C, Kerwin WS, Yarnykh VL, et al. MRI of atherosclerosis in clinical trials. *NMR Biomed.* 2006;19(6):636–654.

299. Momiyama Y, Fayad ZA. Aortic plaque imaging and monitoring atherosclerotic plaque interventions. *Top Magn Reson Imaging.* 2007;18(5):349–355.

300. Hatsukami TS, Ross R, Polissar NL, et al. Visualization of fibrous cap thickness and rupture in human atherosclerotic carotid plaque in vivo with high-resolution magnetic resonance imaging. *Circulation.* 2000;102(9):959–964.

301. Wasserman BA, Smith WI, Trout HH, III, et al. Carotid artery atherosclerosis: In vivo morphologic characterization with gadolinium-enhanced double-oblique MR imaging initial results. *Radiology.* 2002;223(2):566–573.

302. Yuan C, Kerwin WS, Ferguson MS, et al. Contrast-enhanced high resolution MRI for atherosclerotic carotid artery tissue characterization. *J Magn Reson Imaging.* 2002;15(1):62–67.

303. Kerwin W, Hooker A, Spilker M, et al. Quantitative magnetic resonance imaging analysis of neovasculature volume in carotid atherosclerotic plaque. *Circulation.* 2003;107(6):851–856.

304. Weiss CR, Arai AE, Bui MN, et al. Arterial wall MRI characteristics are associated with elevated serum markers of inflammation in humans. *J Magn Reson Imaging.* 2001;14(6):698–704.

305. Saam T, Ferguson MS, Yarnykh VL, et al. Quantitative evaluation of carotid plaque composition by in vivo MRI. *Arterioscler Thromb Vasc Biol.* 2005;25(1):234–239.

306. Fabiano S, Mancino S, Stefanini M, et al. High-resolution multicontrast-weighted MR imaging from human carotid endarterectomy specimens to assess carotid plaque components. *Eur Radiol.* 2008;18(12):2912–2921. Epub 2008 Aug 27.

307. Chu B, Kampschulte A, Ferguson MS, et al. Hemorrhage in the atherosclerotic carotid plaque: A high-resolution MRI study. *Stroke.* 2004;35(5):1079–1084.

308. Yuan C, Mitsumori LM, Ferguson MS, et al. In vivo accuracy of multispectral magnetic resonance imaging for identifying lipid-rich necrotic cores and intraplaque hemorrhage in advanced human carotid plaques. *Circulation.* 2001;104(17):2051–2056.

309. Yuan C, Zhang SX, Polissar NL, et al. Identification of fibrous cap rupture with magnetic resonance imaging is highly associated with recent transient ischemic attack or stroke. *Circulation.* 2002;105(2):181–185.

310. Moody AR, Allder S, Lennox G, et al. Direct magnetic resonance imaging of carotid artery thrombus in acute stroke. *Lancet.* 1999;353(9147):122–123.

311. Moody AR, Murphy RE, Morgan PS, et al. Characterization of complicated carotid plaque with magnetic resonance direct thrombus imaging in patients with cerebral ischemia. *Circulation.* 2003;107(24):3047–3052.

312. Murphy RE, Moody AR, Morgan PS, et al. Prevalence of complicated carotid atheroma as detected by magnetic resonance direct thrombus imaging in patients with suspected carotid artery stenosis and previous acute cerebral ischemia. *Circulation*. 2003;107(24):3053–3058.
313. Taniguchi H, Momiyama Y, Fayad ZA, et al. In vivo magnetic resonance evaluation of associations between aortic atherosclerosis and both risk factors and coronary artery disease in patients referred for coronary angiography. *Am Heart J*. 2004;148(1):137–143.
314. Takaya N, Yuan C, Chu B, et al. Presence of intraplaque hemorrhage stimulates progression of carotid atherosclerotic plaques: A high-resolution magnetic resonance imaging study. *Circulation*. 2005;111(21):2768–2775.
315. Takaya N, Yuan C, Chu B, et al. Association between carotid plaque characteristics and subsequent ischemic cerebrovascular events: A prospective assessment with MRI–initial results. *Stroke*. 2006;37(3):818–823.
316. U-King-Im JM, Tang TY, Patterson A, et al. Characterisation of carotid atheroma in symptomatic and asymptomatic patients using high resolution MRI. *J Neurol Neurosurg Psychiatry*. 2008;79(8):905–912.
317. Saam T, Underhill HR, Chu B, et al. Prevalence of American Heart Association type VI carotid atherosclerotic lesions identified by magnetic resonance imaging for different levels of stenosis as measured by duplex ultrasound. *J Am Coll Cardiol*. 2008;51(10):1014–1021.
318. Wasserman BA, Sharrett AR, Lai S, et al. Risk factor associations with the presence of a lipid core in carotid plaque of asymptomatic individuals using high-resolution MRI: The multi-ethnic study of atherosclerosis (MESA). *Stroke*. 2008;39(2):329–335.
319. Shinnar M, Fallon JT, Wehrli S, et al. The diagnostic accuracy of ex vivo MRI for human atherosclerotic plaque characterization. *Arterioscler Thromb Vasc Biol*. 1999;19(11):2756–2761.
320. Helft G, Worthley SG, Fuster V, et al. Atherosclerotic aortic component quantification by noninvasive magnetic resonance imaging: An in vivo study in rabbits. *J Am Coll Cardiol*. 2001;37(4):1149–1154.
321. Skinner MP, Yuan C, Mitsumori L, et al. Serial magnetic resonance imaging of experimental atherosclerosis detects lesion fine structure, progression and complications in vivo. *Nat Med*. 1995;1(1):69–73.
322. Worthley SG, Helft G, Fuster V, et al. High resolution ex vivo magnetic resonance imaging of in situ coronary and aortic atherosclerotic plaque in a porcine model. *Atherosclerosis*. 2000;150(2):321–329.
323. Jaffer FA, O'Donnell CJ, Larson MG, et al. Age and sex distribution of subclinical aortic atherosclerosis: A magnetic resonance imaging examination of the Framingham Heart Study. *Arterioscler Thromb Vasc Biol*. 2002;22(5):849–854.
324. Zhao XQ, Yuan C, Hatsukami TS, et al. Effects of prolonged intensive lipid-lowering therapy on the characteristics of carotid atherosclerotic plaques in vivo by MRI: A case-control study. *Arterioscler Thromb Vasc Biol*. 2001;21(10):1623–1629.
325. Corti R, Fayad ZA, Fuster V, et al. Effects of lipid-lowering by simvastatin on human atherosclerotic lesions: A longitudinal study by high-resolution, noninvasive magnetic resonance imaging. *Circulation*. 2001;104(3):249–252.
326. Corti R, Fuster V, Fayad ZA, et al. Lipid lowering by simvastatin induces regression of human atherosclerotic lesions: Two years' follow-up by high-resolution noninvasive magnetic resonance imaging. *Circulation*. 2002;106(23):2884–2887.
327. Lima JA, Desai MY, Steen H, et al. Statin-induced cholesterol lowering and plaque regression after 6 months of magnetic resonance imaging-monitored therapy. *Circulation*. 2004;110(16):2336–2341.
328. Underhill HR, Yuan C, Zhao XQ, et al. Effect of rosuvastatin therapy on carotid plaque morphology and composition in moderately hypercholesterolemic patients: A high-resolution magnetic resonance imaging trial. *Am Heart J*. 2008;155(3):584e1–584e8.
329. Yonemura A, Momiyama Y, Fayad ZA, et al. Effect of lipid-lowering therapy with atorvastatin on atherosclerotic aortic plaques detected by noninvasive magnetic resonance imaging. *J Am Coll Cardiol*. 2005;45(5):733–742.
330. Ayaori M, Momiyama Y, Fayad ZA, et al. Effect of bezafibrate therapy on atherosclerotic aortic plaques detected by MRI in dyslipidemic patients with hypertriglyceridemia. *Atherosclerosis*. 2008;196(1):425–433.
331. Corti R, Osende JI, Fallon JT, et al. The selective peroxisomal proliferator-activated receptor-gamma agonist has an additive effect on plaque regression in combination with simvastatin in experimental atherosclerosis: In vivo study by high-resolution magnetic resonance imaging. *J Am Coll Cardiol*. 2004;43(3):464–473.
332. Fayad ZA, Fuster V, Fallon JT, et al. Noninvasive in vivo human coronary artery lumen and wall imaging using black-blood magnetic resonance imaging. *Circulation*. 2000;102(5):506–510.
333. Botnar RM, Stuber M, Kissinger KV, et al. Noninvasive coronary vessel wall and plaque imaging with magnetic resonance imaging. *Circulation*. 2000;102(21):2582–2587.
334. Kim WY, Astrup AS, Stuber M, et al. Subclinical coronary and aortic atherosclerosis detected by magnetic resonance imaging in type 1 diabetes with and without diabetic nephropathy. *Circulation*. 2007;115(2):228–235.
335. Macedo R, Chen S, Lai S, et al. MRI detects increased coronary wall thickness in asymptomatic individuals: The multi-ethnic study of atherosclerosis (MESA). *J Magn Reson Imaging*. 2008;28(5):1108–1115.
336. Deanfield J, Donald A, Ferri C, et al. Endothelial function and dysfunction. Part I: Methodological issues for assessment in the different vascular beds: A statement by the Working Group on Endothelin and Endothelial Factors of the European Society of Hypertension. *J Hypertens*. 2005;23(1):7–17.
337. Furchgott RF, Zawadzki JV. The obligatory role of endothelial cells in the relaxation of arterial smooth muscle by acetylcholine. *Nature*. 1980;288(5789):373–376.
338. Werner N, Kosiol S, Schiegl T, et al. Circulating endothelial progenitor cells and cardiovascular outcomes. *N Engl J Med*. 2005;353(10):999–1007.
339. Ludmer PL, Selwyn AP, Shook TL, et al. Paradoxical vasoconstriction induced by acetylcholine in atherosclerotic coronary arteries. *N Engl J Med*. 1986;315(17):1046–1051.
340. Cox DA, Vita JA, Treasure CB, et al. Atherosclerosis impairs flow-mediated dilation of coronary arteries in humans. *Circulation*. 1989;80(3):458–465.
341. el-Tamimi H, Mansour M, Wargovich TJ, et al. Constrictor and dilator responses to intracoronary acetylcholine in adjacent segments of the same coronary artery in patients with coronary artery disease. Endothelial function revisited. *Circulation*. 1994;89(1):45–51.
342. Penny WF, Rockman H, Long J, et al. Heterogeneity of vasomotor response to acetylcholine along the human coronary artery. *J Am Coll Cardiol. [Journal Article Research Support Non-US Gov't Research Support US Gov't PHS]*. 1995;25(5):1046–1055.
343. Anderson TJ, Uehata A, Gerhard MD, et al. Close relation of endothelial function in the human coronary and peripheral circulations. *J Am Coll Cardiol*. 1995;26(5):1235–1241.
344. Nabel EG, Selwyn AP, Ganz P. Large coronary arteries in humans are responsive to changing blood flow: An endothelium-dependent mechanism that fails in patients with atherosclerosis. *J Am Coll Cardiol*. 1990;16(2):349–356.
345. Wilkinson IB, Hall IR, MacCallum H, et al. Pulse-wave analysis: Clinical evaluation of a noninvasive, widely applicable method for assessing endothelial function. *Arterioscler Thromb Vasc Biol*. 2002;22(1):147–152.
346. Hayward CS, Kraidly M, Webb CM, et al. Assessment of endothelial function using peripheral waveform analysis: A clinical application. *J Am Coll Cardiol*. 2002;40(3):521–528.
347. Celermajer DS, Sorensen KE, Gooch VM, et al. Non-invasive detection of endothelial dysfunction in children and adults at risk of atherosclerosis. *Lancet*. 1992;340(8828):1111–1115.
348. Corretti MC, Anderson TJ, Benjamin EJ, et al. Guidelines for the ultrasound assessment of endothelial-dependent flow-mediated vasodilation of the brachial artery: A report of the International Brachial Artery Reactivity Task Force. *J Am Coll Cardiol*. 2002;39(2):257–265.
349. Brunner H, Cockcroft JR, Deanfield J, et al. Endothelial function and dysfunction. Part II: Association with cardiovascular risk factors and diseases. A statement by the Working Group on Endothelins and Endothelial Factors of the European Society of Hypertension. *J Hypertens*. 2005;23(2):233–246.
350. Cai H, Harrison DG. Endothelial dysfunction in cardiovascular diseases: The role of oxidant stress. *Circ Res*. 2000;87(10):840–844.
351. Vlachopoulos C, Aznaouridis K, Ioakeimidis N, et al. Unfavourable endothelial and inflammatory state in erectile dysfunction patients with or without coronary artery disease. *Eur Heart J*. 2006;27(22):2640–2648.
352. Witte DR, Westerink J, de Koning EJ, et al. Is the association between flow-mediated dilation and cardiovascular risk limited to low-risk populations? *J Am Coll Cardiol*. 2005;45(12):1987–1993.
353. Schachinger V, Britten MB, Zeiher AM. Prognostic impact of coronary vasodilator dysfunction on adverse long-term outcome of coronary heart disease. *Circulation*. 2000;101(16):1899–1906.
354. Halcox JP, Schenke WH, Zalos G, et al. Prognostic value of coronary vascular endothelial dysfunction. *Circulation*. 2002;106(6):653–658.
355. Heitzer T, Schlinzig T, Krohn K, et al. Endothelial dysfunction, oxidative stress, and risk of cardiovascular events in patients with coronary artery disease. *Circulation*. 2001;104(22):2673–2678.
356. Neunteufl T, Heher S, Katzenschlager R, et al. Late prognostic value of flow-mediated dilation in the brachial artery of patients with chest pain. *Am J Cardiol*. 2000;86(2):207–210.
357. Gokce N, Keaney JF, Jr, Hunter LM, et al. Predictive value of noninvasively determined endothelial dysfunction for long-term cardiovascular events in patients with peripheral vascular disease. *J Am Coll Cardiol. [Journal Article Research Support Non-US Gov't Research Support US Gov't Non-PHS Research Support US Gov't PHS]*. 2003;41(10):1769–1775.
358. Patti G, Pasceri V, Melfi R, et al. Impaired flow-mediated dilation and risk of restenosis in patients undergoing coronary stent implantation. *Circulation*. 2005;111(1):70–75.
359. Kitta Y, Nakamura T, Kodama Y, et al. Endothelial vasomotor dysfunction in the brachial artery is associated with late in-stent coronary restenosis. *J Am Coll Cardiol*. 2005;46(4):648–655.
360. Gokce N, Keaney JF, Jr, Hunter LM, et al. Risk stratification for postoperative cardiovascular events via noninvasive assessment of endothelial function: A prospective study. *Circulation*. 2002;105(13):1567–1572.
361. Perticone F, Ceravolo R, Pujia A, et al. Prognostic significance of endothelial dysfunction in hypertensive patients. *Circulation*. 2001;104(2):191–196.
362. Yeboah J, Crouse JR, Hsu FC, et al. Brachial flow-mediated dilation predicts incident cardiovascular events in older adults: The Cardiovascular Health Study. *Circulation*. 2007;115(18):2390–2397.
363. Fathi R, Haluska B, Isbel N, et al. The relative importance of vascular structure and function in predicting cardiovascular events. *J Am Coll Cardiol*. 2004;43(4):616–623.
364. Shimbo D, Grahame-Clarke C, Miyake Y, et al. The association between endothelial dysfunction and cardiovascular outcomes in a population-based multi-ethnic cohort. *Atherosclerosis*. 2007;192(1):197–203.
365. Celermajer DS, Sorensen KE, Georgakopoulos D, et al. Cigarette smoking is associated with dose-related and potentially reversible impairment of endothelium-dependent dilation in healthy young adults. *Circulation*. 1993;88(5 Pt 1):2149–2155.
366. Raitakari OT, Adams MR, McCredie RJ, et al. Arterial endothelial dysfunction related to passive smoking is potentially reversible in healthy young adults. *Ann Intern Med*. 1999;130(7):578–581.

367. Alexopoulos N, Vlachopoulos C, Aznaouridis K, et al. The acute effect of green tea consumption on endothelial function in healthy individuals. *Eur J Cardiovasc Prev Rehabil.* 2008;15(3):300–305.

368. Treasure CB, Klein JL, Weintraub WS, et al. Beneficial effects of cholesterol-lowering therapy on the coronary endothelium in patients with coronary artery disease. *N Engl J Med.* 1995;332(8):481–487.

369. Clarkson P, Adams MR, Powe AJ, et al. Oral L-arginine improves endothelium-dependent dilation in hypercholesterolemic young adults. *J Clin Invest.* 1996;97(8):1989–1994.

370. Nichols WW, O'Rourke MF. *McDonald's Blood Flow in Arteries.* 4th Ed. London: Edward Arnold; 1998.

371. Stefanadis C, Stratos C, Vlachopoulos C, et al. Pressure-diameter relation of the human aorta. A new method of determination by the application of a special ultrasonic dimension catheter. *Circulation.* 1995;92(8):2210–2219.

372. Laurent S, Cockcroft J, Van Bortel L, et al. Expert consensus document on arterial stiffness: Methodological issues and clinical applications. *Eur Heart J.* 2006;27(21):2588–2605.

373. Vlachopoulos C, O'Rourke M. Genesis of the normal and abnormal arterial pulse. *Curr Probl Cardiol.* 2000;25(5):303–367.

374. O'Rourke MF, Staessen JA, Vlachopoulos C, et al. Clinical applications of arterial stiffness; definitions and reference values. *Am J Hypertens. [Journal Article Review].* 2002;15(5):426–444.

375. Sassalos K, Vlachopoulos C, Alexopoulos N, et al. The acute and chronic effect of cigarette smoking on the elastic properties of the ascending aorta in healthy male subjects. *Hellenic J Cardiol.* 2006;47(5):263–268.

376. Lang RM, Cholley BP, Korcarz C, et al. Measurement of regional elastic properties of the human aorta. A new application of transesophageal echocardiography with automated border detection and calibrated subclavian pulse tracings. *Circulation.* 1994;90(4):1875–1882.

377. Jondeau G, Boutouyrie P, Lacolley P, et al. Central pulse pressure is a major determinant of ascending aorta dilation in Marfan syndrome. *Circulation.* 1999;99(20):2677–2681.

378. Kool MJ, van Merode T, Reneman RS, et al. Evaluation of reproducibility of a vessel wall movement detector system for assessment of large artery properties. *Cardiovasc Res.* 1994;28(5):610–614.

379. Laurent S, Hayoz D, Trazzi S, et al. Isobaric compliance of the radial artery is increased in patients with essential hypertension. *J Hypertens.* 1993;11(1):89–98.

380. Giannattasio C, Failla M, Stella ML, et al. Alterations of radial artery compliance in patients with congestive heart failure. *Am J Cardiol.* 1995;76(5):381–385.

381. Resnick LM, Militianu D, Cunnings AJ, et al. Direct magnetic resonance determination of aortic distensibility in essential hypertension: Relation to age, abdominal visceral fat, and in situ intracellular free magnesium. *Hypertension.* 1997;30(3 Pt 2):654–659.

382. Asmar R, Benetos A, Topouchian J, et al. Assessment of arterial distensibility by automatic pulse wave velocity measurement. Validation and clinical application studies. *Hypertension.* 1995;26(3):485–490.

383. van der Heijden-Spek JJ, Staessen JA, Fagard RH, et al. Effect of age on brachial artery wall properties differs from the aorta and is gender dependent: A population study. *Hypertension.* 2000;35(2):637–642.

384. Cruickshank K, Riste L, Anderson SG, et al. Aortic pulse-wave velocity and its relationship to mortality in diabetes and glucose intolerance: An integrated index of vascular function? *Circulation.* 2002;106(16):2085–2090.

385. Pannier BM, Avolio AP, Hoeks A, et al. Methods and devices for measuring arterial compliance in humans. *Am J Hypertens.* 2002;15(8):743–753.

386. Rogers WJ, Hu YL, Coast D, et al. Age-associated changes in regional aortic pulse wave velocity. *J Am Coll Cardiol.* 2001;38(4):1123–1129.

387. Pauca AL, O'Rourke MF, Kon ND. Prospective evaluation of a method for estimating ascending aortic pressure from the radial artery pressure waveform. *Hypertension.* 2001;38(4):932–937.

388. Chen CH, Ting CT, Nussbacher A, et al. Validation of carotid artery tonometry as a means of estimating augmentation index of ascending aortic pressure. *Hypertension.* 1996;27(2):168–175.

389. McEniery CM, Yasmin, Hall IR, Qasem A, et al. Normal vascular aging: Differential effects on wave reflection and aortic pulse wave velocity: The Anglo-Cardiff Collaborative Trial (ACCT). *J Am Coll Cardiol.* 2005;46(9):1753–1760.

390. Avalos I, Chung CP, Oeser A, et al. Increased augmentation index in rheumatoid arthritis and its relationship to coronary artery atherosclerosis. *J Rheumatol.* 2007;34(12):2388–2394.

391. Raggi P, Bellasi A, Ferramosca E, et al. Association of pulse wave velocity with vascular and valvular calcification in hemodialysis patients. *Kidney Int.* 2007;71(8):802–807.

392. Weber T, Auer J, O'Rourke MF, et al. Increased arterial wave reflections predict severe cardiovascular events in patients undergoing percutaneous coronary interventions. *Eur Heart J.* 2005;26(24):2657–2663.

393. Stefanadis C, Dernellis J, Tsiamis E, et al. Aortic stiffness as a risk factor for recurrent acute coronary events in patients with ischaemic heart disease. *Eur Heart J.* 2000;21(5):390–396.

394. Boutouyrie P, Tropeano AI, Asmar R, et al. Aortic stiffness is an independent predictor of primary coronary events in hypertensive patients: A longitudinal study. *Hypertension.* 2002;39(1):10–15.

395. Laurent S, Boutouyrie P, Asmar R, et al. Aortic stiffness is an independent predictor of all-cause and cardiovascular mortality in hypertensive patients. *Hypertension.* 2001;37(5):1236–1241.

396. Blacher J, Guerin AP, Pannier B, et al. Impact of aortic stiffness on survival in end-stage renal disease. *Circulation.* 1999;99(18):2434–2439.

397. Meaume S, Benetos A, Henry OF, et al. Aortic pulse wave velocity predicts cardiovascular mortality in subjects >70 years of age. *Arterioscler Thromb Vasc Biol.* 2001;21(12):2046–2050.

398. Sutton-Tyrrell K, Najjar SS, Boudreau RM, et al. Elevated aortic pulse wave velocity, a marker of arterial stiffness, predicts cardiovascular events in well-functioning older adults. *Circulation.* 2005;111(25):3384–3390.

399. Mattace-Raso FU, van der Cammen TJ, Hofman A, et al. Arterial stiffness and risk of coronary heart disease and stroke: The Rotterdam Study. *Circulation.* 2006;113(5):657–663.

400. Shokawa T, Imazu M, Yamamoto H, et al. Pulse wave velocity predicts cardiovascular mortality: Findings from the Hawaii-Los Angeles-Hiroshima study. *Circ J.* 2005;69(3):259–264.

401. Willum-Hansen T, Staessen JA, Torp-Pedersen C, et al. Prognostic value of aortic pulse wave velocity as index of arterial stiffness in the general population. *Circulation.* 2006;113(5):664–670.

402. Blacher J, Pannier B, Guerin AP, et al. Carotid arterial stiffness as a predictor of cardiovascular and all-cause mortality in end-stage renal disease. *Hypertension.* 1998;32(3):570–574.

403. Williams B, Lacy PS, Thom SM, et al. Differential impact of blood pressure-lowering drugs on central aortic pressure and clinical outcomes: Principal results of the Conduit Artery Function Evaluation (CAFE) study. *Circulation.* 2006;113(9):1213–1225.

404. Vlachopoulos C, Aznaouridis K, Alexopoulos N, et al. Effect of dark chocolate on arterial function in healthy individuals. *Am J Hypertens.* 2005;18(6):785–791.

405. Balkestein EJ, van Aggel-Leijssen DP, van Baak MA, et al. The effect of weight loss with or without exercise training on large artery compliance in healthy obese men. *J Hypertens.* 1999;17(12 Pt 2):1831–1835.

406. Guerin AP, Blacher J, Pannier B, et al. Impact of aortic stiffness attenuation on survival of patients in end-stage renal failure. *Circulation.* 2001;103(7):987–992.

407. MRC/BHF Heart Protection Study of cholesterol lowering with simvastatin in 20,536 high-risk individuals: A randomised placebo-controlled trial. *Lancet.* 2002;360(9326):7–22.

408. Eagle KA, Rihal CS, Foster ED, et al. Long-term survival in patients with coronary artery disease: Importance of peripheral vascular disease. The Coronary Artery Surgery Study (CASS) Investigators. *J Am Coll Cardiol.* 1994;23(5):1091–1095.

409. Hirsch AT, Haskal ZJ, Hertzer NR, et al. ACC/AHA 2005 Practice Guidelines for the management of patients with peripheral arterial disease (lower extremity, renal, mesenteric, and abdominal aortic): A collaborative report from the American Association for Vascular Surgery/Society for Vascular Surgery, Society for Cardiovascular Angiography and Interventions, Society for Vascular Medicine and Biology, Society of Interventional Radiology, and the ACC/AHA Task Force on Practice Guidelines (Writing Committee to Develop Guidelines for the Management of Patients With Peripheral Arterial Disease): Endorsed by the American Association of Cardiovascular and Pulmonary Rehabilitation; National Heart, Lung, and Blood Institute; Society for Vascular Nursing; transatlantic Inter-Society Consensus; and Vascular Disease Foundation. *Circulation.* 2006;113(11):e463–e654.

410. Hiatt WR, Marshall JA, Baxter J, et al. Diagnostic methods for peripheral arterial disease in the San Luis Valley Diabetes Study. *J Clin Epidemiol.* 1990;43(6):597–606.

411. Newman AB, Sutton-Tyrrell K, Rutan GH, et al. Lower extremity arterial disease in elderly subjects with systolic hypertension. *J Clin Epidemiol.* 1991;44(1):15–20.

412. Yao ST, Hobbs JT, Irvine WT. Ankle systolic pressure measurements in arterial disease affecting the lower extremities. *Br J Surg.* 1969;56(9):676–679.

413. Ouriel K, McDonnell AE, Metz CE, et al. Critical evaluation of stress testing in the diagnosis of peripheral vascular disease. *Surgery.* 1982;91(6):686–693.

414. Matzke S, Franckena M, Alback A, et al. Ankle brachial index measurements in critical leg ischaemia–the influence of experience on reproducibility. *Scand J Surg.* 2003;92(2):144–147.

415. Kaiser V, Kester AD, Stoffers HE, et al. The influence of experience on the reproducibility of the ankle-brachial systolic pressure ratio in peripheral arterial occlusive disease. *Eur J Vasc Endovasc Surg.* 1999;18(1):25–29.

416. Doobay AV, Anand SS. Sensitivity and specificity of the ankle-brachial index to predict future cardiovascular outcomes: A systematic review. *Arterioscler Thromb Vasc Biol.* 2005;25(7):1463–1469.

417. Criqui MH, Langer RD, Fronek A, et al. Mortality over a period of 10 years in patients with peripheral arterial disease. *N Engl J Med.* 1992;326(6):381–386.

418. Kuller LH, Shemanski L, Psaty BM, et al. Subclinical disease as an independent risk factor for cardiovascular disease. *Circulation.* 1995;92(4):720–726.

419. Fowkes FG, Murray GD, Butcher I, et al. Ankle brachial index combined with Framingham Risk Score to predict cardiovascular events and mortality: A meta-analysis. *JAMA.* 2008;300(2):197–208.

420. Greenland P, Abrams J, Aurigemma GP, et al. Prevention Conference V: Beyond secondary prevention: Identifying the high-risk patient for primary prevention: Noninvasive tests of atherosclerotic burden: Writing Group III. *Circulation.* 2000;101(1):E16–E22.

421. Espinola-Klein C, Rupprecht HJ, Bickel C, et al. Different calculations of ankle-brachial index and their impact on cardiovascular risk prediction. *Circulation.* 2008;118(9):961–967.

422. McDermott MM, Criqui MH, Liu K, et al. Lower ankle/brachial index, as calculated by averaging the dorsalis pedis and posterior tibial arterial pressures, and association with leg functioning in peripheral arterial disease. *J Vasc Surg.* 2000;32(6):1164–1171.

423. Resnick HE, Lindsay RS, McDermott MM, et al. Relationship of high and low ankle brachial index to all-cause and cardiovascular disease mortality: The Strong Heart Study. *Circulation.* 2004;109(6):733–739.

Atherosclerotic Plaque Activity

23

Zahi A. Fayad
James H.F. Rudd
Javier Sanz
Venkatesh Mani

1. INTRODUCTION

Despite considerable therapeutic advances over the past 50 years, cardiovascular disease is the leading cause of death worldwide. This is mainly a result of the increasing prevalence of atherosclerosis, due to the aging population, the improved survival of patients with atherosclerotic cardiovascular disease, and, above all, the widespread underrecognition and undertreatment of individuals with risk factors for atherosclerosis.

Atherosclerosis is characterized by the thickening of the arterial wall to form an atherosclerotic plaque, a process in which cholesterol deposition, inflammation, extracellular-matrix formation, and thrombosis have important roles (Fig. 23.1).[1] Symptoms occur late in the course of disease and are usually caused by the narrowing of the lumen of the artery, which can happen gradually (as a result of progressive plaque growth) or suddenly (as a result of plaque rupture and, subsequently, thrombosis). The resultant decrease in blood supply can affect almost any organ, although coronary heart disease and stroke are the most common consequences.

Traditionally, diagnosis of atherosclerosis was possible only at advanced stages of disease, either by directly revealing the narrowing of the arterial lumen (stenosis) or by evaluating the effect of arterial stenosis on organ perfusion. However, new imaging approaches allow the assessment not only of the morphology of blood vessels but also of the composition of the vessel walls, enabling atherosclerosis-associated abnormalities in the arteries (including the coronary arteries) to be observed, down to the cellular and molecular levels in some cases. Some of these approaches are now in clinical use or are being tested in clinical trials, whereas others are better suited to basic and translational research. Here, we discuss recent advances in molecular activity imaging of cardiovascular atherosclerotic disease.

2. ATHEROSCLEROTIC PLAQUE ACTIVITY IMAGING

Molecular activity imaging not only has the ability to image cardiovascular anatomy and physiology on a macroscopic scale (as has been discussed so far), but it has also become increasingly possible to detect biological processes at the cellular or even molecular level. Molecular imaging relies on the use of contrast agents that target specific cells or molecular pathways of relevance to disease. In addition to the various imaging techniques being developed, contrast agents for tracking potentially important components of atherosclerotic disease are at various stages of development (Fig. 23.1 and Table 23.1).[2–7]

Most of the available probes are in experimental testing, although some have already advanced to clinical evaluation. Imaging probes typically include a moiety (such as an antibody or specific ligand) with high affinity for the desired target molecule. Alternatively, the probe can be modified to facilitate uptake by specific cells. In addition, probes are designed to be detected by various modalities, including ultrasound (which detects microbubbles), single photon emission computed tomography (SPECT) and positron emission tomography (PET) (radioactive isotopes), magnetic resonance imaging (MRI) (paramagnetic and superparamagnetic compounds), computed tomography (CT) (iodinated compounds), or optical imaging (fluorochromes). Many of the targets of interest are located in deep organs and are present at very low (nanomolar) concentrations; imaging modalities therefore need to be highly sensitive as well as safe and economically viable.

Ultrasound is widely available, safe, and inexpensive, but has insufficient penetration for noninvasive imaging of deep vessels (including the coronary arteries) with high spatial resolution or sensitivity. SPECT and PET have a high sensitivity, but also have limited spatial resolution and the additional disadvantage of requiring the use of radioactive agents. By contrast, MRI has a somewhat lower sensitivity than SPECT and PET and requires prolonged imaging times, but it is safe and provides excellent resolution (~10 μm with high-field magnets). CT, conversely, offers the advantages of fast scanning time and superior performance for coronary angiography, at the expense of limited sensitivity and the use of nephrotoxic agents and ionizing radiation. Optical imaging techniques—for example, near infrared fluorescence reflectance or fluorescence molecular tomography—have excellent sensitivity and temporal resolution and allow the tissue distribution of the probe to be precisely determined with ex vivo fluorescence microscopy. So far, however, such techniques could be used noninvasively only to monitor superficial structures because of the limited ability of light to penetrate tissue. Optical imaging techniques and some SPECT and MRI techniques have the advantage of being able to detect more than one molecular signature at a time.

The choice of target for imaging is also clearly important. Because inflammation has a crucial role at all stages of atherosclerosis (Fig. 23.1), macrophages are currently one of the most appealing targets. Ultra-small paramagnetic iron oxide particles are engulfed by macrophages in vivo, and this causes a detectable decrease in the MRI signal in proportion to the degree of atherosclerotic plaque inflammation, as shown in human studies.[8]

A strong correlation between macrophage density and MRI signal was also found recently in a mouse model of atherosclerosis,

Figure 23.1 The development of an atherosclerotic lesion. The progression of an atherosclerotic lesion is shown in a simplified form, developing from a normal blood vessel (**far left**) to a vessel with an atherosclerotic plaque and superimposed thrombus (**far right**). Potential targets for molecular imaging at each stage are also listed. ICAM1, intercellular adhesion molecule 1; LDL, low-density lipoprotein; MMP, matrix metalloproteinase; VCAM1, vascular cell-adhesion molecule 1. (Adapted from Sanz J, Fayad ZA. Imaging of atherosclerotic cardiovascular disease. *Nature.* 2008;451(7181):953–957.)

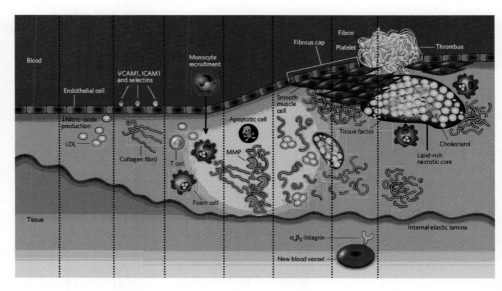

TABLE 23.1

REPRESENTATIVE EFFECT OF SEQUENCE PARAMETERS ON THE ENHANCEMENT OF VARIOUS PLAQUE COMPONENTS. SIGNAL INTENSITIES ARE EXPRESSED RELATIVE TO ADJACENT MUSCLE

Tissue	Sequence weighting		
	T1-W	T2-W	PDW
Media	−	−	±
Fibrocellular	+	+	+
Lipid	±	+	+
Necrotic core	±	+	+
Thrombus	−	−	−
Dense fibrous	±	−	±

+, hyperintense; ±, isointense; −, hypointense
Source: Adapted from Sanz J, Fayad ZA. Imaging of atherosclerotic cardiovascular disease. *Nature.* 2008;451(7181):953–957.

by using a contrast agent consisting of Gd^{3+}-loaded micelles targeted at the macrophage scavenger receptor.[9] Similarly, in rabbits, specific uptake of an iodine containing contrast agent by macrophages allows atherosclerotic lesions to be detected by using CT (Fig. 23.2A & B).[10] Also, with PET, the signal from [18F] fluorodeoxyglucose (FDG) correlates with the concentration of macrophages in human atherosclerotic plaques.[11] Moreover, by using specialized equipment, several imaging techniques can be used concurrently—for example, PET together with CT or, recently, MRI (Fig. 23.2C & D) for the sensitive and reproducible detection of vascular inflammation.[12] This combination approach allows the most appropriate technique(s) for a particular patient, vascular region, and/or disease stage to be chosen, and takes advantage of the particular strengths of each modality. Thrombi are another attractive target for imaging, because acute clinical events often occur as a result of thrombosis triggered by plaque rupture (Fig. 23.1). In animal models, thrombi of different ages and in

different vascular regions have been detected with MRI,[13] and this approach is now being investigated in humans.[5] At the other end of the timeline of atherosclerotic-plaque progression (Fig. 23.1), cell adhesion molecules participate in the early development of lesions by facilitating the recruitment of leukocytes into the vessel wall. In an animal model, increased amounts of vascular cell adhesion molecule 1 (VCAM1) were found in aortic plaques by using a dual contrast agent detectable by both MRI and optical imaging.[14] A similar approach, which used ultrasound detection of microbubbles, found increased expression of endothelial selectins in the heart of rats that had been subjected to transient myocardial ischemia followed by reperfusion.[15] Development of such probes for clinical use could allow the identification of atherosclerosis at early stages and the detection of plaque rupture (which, even when clinically silent, indicates disease instability).

Another possibility is to use probes that emit a detectable signal only after they have been activated by the target. For example, in a recent study of an experimental model of atherosclerosis, a fluorescent probe activated by enzymatic degradation was used to reveal intraplaque protease activity with near-infrared fluorescence.[16]

In addition to being diagnostic and prognostic indicators, probes could also be used for therapeutic purposes, to deliver drugs in a targeted manner. An example of this is a study in which rabbits were administered paramagnetic nanoparticles loaded with an antiangiogenic drug, resulting in a reduction in the extent of atherosclerotic plaques in blood vessels, as observed by noninvasive tracking with MRI.[17] In addition, hematopoietic or cardiac stem cells for use in cell-based therapy could be tagged with appropriate imaging probes, providing insights into the role and fate of these cells after their administration.[18]

3. POSITRON EMISSION IMAGING OF INFLAMMATION

Inflammation is crucial at all stages of atherosclerotic plaque development. The use of imaging might allow early testing of novel antiatherosclerosis drugs, identification of patients at risk of plaque rupture, and insights into the biology of the disease. Imaging modalities are discussed in relation to their potential use in these areas.

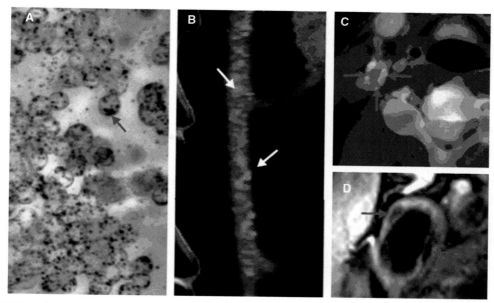

Figure 23.2 Multimodal imaging of inflammation and atherosclerosis. **A:** Molecular imaging of macrophages by using CT, with the iodinated contrast agent N1177. After in vitro incubation of mouse macrophages with N1177, light microscopy in a phase-contrast mode shows the presence of multiple cytoplasmic granules (*red arrow*), confirming uptake of the contrast agent by macrophages. **B:** Three-dimensional reconstruction of a rabbit's abdominal aorta at 2 h after intravenous administration of N1177. A false-color image of N1177 staining is shown overlaid on an angiogram. Intense red spots indicate areas of N1177 accumulation in aortic plaques, which are rich in macrophages (*white arrows*). Organs with high macrophage density are also visible, including the spleen (**top right**). **C:** A combined PET and CT image of a human neck (**axial view**). Atherosclerotic pathology is present at the bifurcation of the right common carotid artery (*red arrows*), as determined by the presence of heavy calcification and large amounts of [18F]fluorodeoxyglucose, which is indicative of inflammatory activity. **D:** Black-blood MRI of the same artery. Carotid arterial wall thickening is evident, as are two areas of signal drop (red arrows), which correspond to calcified regions. (Reproduced from Sanz J, Fayad ZA. Imaging of atherosclerotic cardiovascular disease. *Nature.* 2008;451(7181):953–957, with permission.)

PET imaging is the gold standard oncological imaging technique for monitoring the response to cancer therapy and for the detection of metastatic disease. Arterial FDG uptake was first noted in the aorta of patients undergoing PET imaging for cancer.[19,20] It was soon demonstrated that the degree of FDG uptake was greater in older patients[21] and those with cardiovascular risk factors.[22]

The basis for FDG uptake into the arterial wall is likely due to accumulation within plaque macrophages. Supporting evidence comes from cell culture work, where both leucocytes and macrophages demonstrate increases in both oxidative metabolism and glucose use in response to cellular activating agents and thereby, a dramatic increase in FDG uptake.[23,24]

In the first prospective study of FDG PET atherosclerosis imaging, patients with transient ischemic attack (TIA) were imaged shortly after symptom onset. PET revealed that symptomatic carotid plaque accumulated approximately 30% more FDG at 3 h compared to the asymptomatic artery.[25] This finding was in keeping with the hypothesis that symptomatic plaques contain more highly activated macrophages than asymptomatic lesions.

FDG PET imaging has been proven effective at quantifying inflammation within the aorta[26,27] and vertebral arteries,[28] where it can differentiate carotid artery from vertebral FDG uptake in patients with posterior circulation syndromes. Uptake in patients with peripheral artery disease is also feasible.[29,30] The degree of FDG uptake within arteries is also determined by the number of risk factors for vascular disease that the patient possesses.[31,32]

In parallel with these proofs of principal studies, strong relationships have been documented between the degree of arterial FDG uptake and the density of macrophages determined histologically in both animal models of atherosclerosis and in patients with carotid disease. For example, Tawakol showed a positive correlation between plaque FDG uptake and macrophage density in patients with TIA awaiting surgery ($r = 0.85$, $p < 0.01$).[11]

In addition to being a marker of inflammation, arterial FDG uptake may also predict plaque rupture and clinical events. In a recent study using a rabbit model of atherosclerosis, plaque rupture was promoted by venom injection. Only those aortic plaques with the highest preinjection FDG uptake progressed to rupture and thrombosis.[33] In a long-term oncology study, involving 2,242 patients who underwent multiple PET/CT studies over several years, investigators identified those with ($n = 45$) and without ($n = 56$) arterial FDG uptake. Patients with high FDG uptake were far more likely to have suffered a prior vascular event, or to go on to experience one in the 6 months following the scan.[34]

The short-term interscan reproducibility of FDG PET imaging for atherosclerosis has recently been established in carotid, aorta, and peripheral arteries.[12,30] This is important as a precursor to intervention studies (Fig. 23.2). The first study to investigate whether arterial FDG signal could change after therapy was conducted by Ogawa et al.[35] They used a rabbit model of atherosclerosis, and demonstrated that PET could highlight reduction in FDG uptake after 3 months' therapy with probucol (a lipid lowering antioxidant agent). More recently, a cohort of 43 cancer patients was imaged with FDG PET before and after 3 months of low-dose statin therapy. Compared to placebo group, there was a significant reduction in carotid artery FDG uptake that paralleled the degree of high-density lipoprotein (HDL) elevation.[36] A more recent study[37] examined the effect of risk factor modification on arterial FDG uptake in a group of 60 asymptomatic subjects. Interestingly, with 17 months of dietary and lifestyle modifications, there was a 65% reduction in the number of vascular regions that accumulated FDG. The magnitude of the reduction closely paralleled the rise in HDL seen in the patient group.

A limitation of all FDG studies is the relatively nonspecific nature of FDG uptake. Although several histological studies described here have shown that there is a strong correlation between FDG uptake and macrophage content of plaque, it is also known that FDG can accumulate within other cells that are involved in the initiation and pathogenesis of atherosclerosis. These include endothelial cells[38] and lymphocytes.[39] Tracers more specific for macrophages include ligands for the peripheral benzodiazepine receptor such as [10]C PK11195[40] and PBR28.[41]

Other limitations of PET include errors related to the partial volume effect. This occurs when imaging objects whose size is below the spatial resolution of PET. The result is an inaccurate quantification of the FDG signal. Partial volume errors can be addressed using high resolution magnetic resonance (MR) imaging,[42] where the exact volume of each tissue element within the PET field is determined and used to correct the observed FDG uptake value. The recent introduction of combined PET/MRI scanners will accelerate this effort.[43] Finally, coronary artery imaging presents special problems: cardiac and respiratory movement, myocardial FDG uptake, and the small size (3 to 4 mm) of the coronary arteries. Suppression of myocardial FDG uptake might be possible using a high-fat diet with β-blockade and could be a promising approach.[44]

4. MAGNETIC RESONANCE IMAGING

MRI offers high resolution imaging of the arterial wall without ionizing radiation. Spatial resolutions of 250 ∝m are possible for aorta[45] and carotid plaque imaging.[46] MRI can evaluate the extent of atherosclerosis,[47] and can monitor the efficacy of antiatherosclerotic treatments on plaque volume.[48] In addition, the composition of atherosclerotic plaques (fibrous cap, lipid core, hemorrhage) can be detected using MRI.[47,49] However, identification of inflammation within atherosclerotic plaques requires the injection of MR contrast agents. MR contrast agents can be divided into two main categories, paramagnetic and superparamagnetic, depending on the properties of their contrast moiety and their effect on signal intensity.

4.1. Multicontrast magnetic resonance imaging

By taking advantage of intrinsic differences in the relaxation properties and proton densities between atherosclerotic plaque components, MRI can provide high resolution imaging of plaques without injecting any contrast agent.[50–52] The noncontrast agent approach has been referred to as multicontrast MRI. The small size of the vessels and adjacent lumen requires the acquisition of high spatial and contrast resolutions for atherosclerosis imaging. Atherosclerotic plaques are usually imaged using high-resolution black blood fast spin echo MR sequences. Black blood sequences improve the contrast between atherosclerotic plaques and the lumen and therefore offer a better delineation of the contours of the plaque. These sequences null the signal of the flowing blood by using preparatory pulses (double inversion recovery or parallel saturations bands). New black blood techniques have recently been introduced for the simultaneous acquisition of multiple slices and allow the analysis of a full-length arterial segment with a reduced total examination time. Using these techniques, clinical

studies demonstrated that MRI provides excellent quantitative capabilities for the measurement of total plaque volume with an error in vessel wall area measurement as low as 2.6% for the aorta[53] and 3.5% in the carotids.[48,54]

Signal intensities detected with MRI are influenced by the relaxation times of protons (T1 and T2) and the proton density present in the different components of atherosclerotic plaques. The timing of the excitation pulses of an MR sequence will determine the weight of T1 and T2 relaxation times or proton density in the image contrast. Multicontrast MRI is based on successive T1, T2, and proton density weighted (PDW) sequences. Analysis of signal intensities detected on each of these sequences allows to differentiate each of atherosclerotic plaque components (lipid core, fibrous tissue, hemorrhage, calcification) by their different relaxation properties on MRI (Table 23.1). Development of dedicated software, which analyses the signal intensities of multicontrast MRI on a pixel-by-pixel basis, has further improved the identification of atherosclerotic plaques components.[52] An example of multicontrast MRI showing different plaque components and automatic segmentation of these plaques using a *k*-means cluster algorithm is shown in Figure 23.3.

Multicontrast MRI studies have primarily focused on carotid atherosclerotic plaques. The superficial location of carotid arteries and their relative absence of motion represent less of a technical challenge for imaging than the aorta or the coronary arteries. In

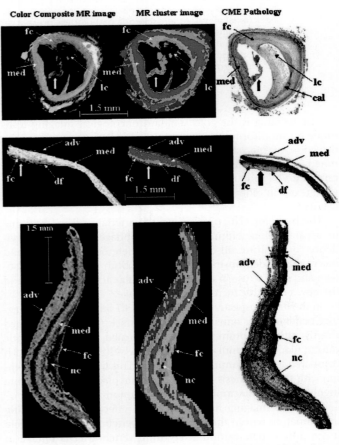

Figure 23.3 Cluster analysis of human atherosclerotic plaque based upon the relative change in signal enhancement after application of T1, T2, and PDW spin echo sequences. Adv, adventitia; nc, necrotic tissue; fc, fibrous cap; med, media. (Reproduced from Nahrendorf M, Jaffer FA, Kelly KA, et al. Noninvasive vascular cell adhesion molecule-1 imaging identifies inflammatory activation of cells in atherosclerosis. *Circulation.* 2006;114(14):1504–1511, with permission.)

this location, multicontrast MRI could also be compared to corresponding histology of atherosclerotic plaques from endarterectomy specimens. For example, studies have demonstrated that in vivo multicontrast MR of human carotid arteries had a sensitivity of 85% and specificity of 92% for the identification of a lipid core and acute intraplaque hemorrhage.[55] Recent histopathological studies suggest that intraplaque hemorrhage may play a role in plaque rupture and also represent a potent atherogenic stimulus. Preliminary studies have shown that[56] multicontrast MRI can also accurately detect intraplaque hemorrhages in carotid atherosclerotic plaques using T_2^*-weighted sequences. Interestingly, a recent study[57] found that the detection of these hemorrhages in carotid atherosclerotic plaques with MRI was associated with an accelerated increase of plaque volume in the next 18 months.

In summary, multicontrast MRI allows for the detection of the different components of atherosclerotic plaques with high accuracy and is particularly promising for the study of carotid atherosclerotic plaques. However, due to low signal-to-noise ratios and partial voluming effects, application of multicontrast MRI is limited to large arteries such as the carotids or aorta. Contrast agents targeted at specific molecules present in atherosclerotic lesions are needed to further improve the detection and characterization of vulnerable plaques using MRI.

4.2. Dynamic contrast-enhanced magnetic resonance imaging

Paramagnetic contrast agents are composed of lanthanide metals such as gadolinium and enhance the longitudinal magnetization (T1) of nearby water protons that results in a greater positive signal in the MR image. One approach to evaluate inflammatory activity in plaque is based on the detection of the degree of plaque neovascularization—a phenomenon closely aligned with inflammation. This can be achieved by dynamic contrast-enhanced MRI (DCE–MRI) using low-molecular-weight gadolinium chelates. DCE–MRI can estimate vessel density and permeability in plaque with high spatial and temporal resolution. The concept was pioneered in oncology, but preliminary studies in atherosclerotic plaques of rabbits[58] and in human carotid plaques[59] showed good correlations between permeability of neovessels measured with DCE–MRI and density of macrophages on immunohistology. Although giving only an indirect evaluation of inflammatory activity in atherosclerotic plaques, DCE–MRI offers the advantage of using readily available, FDA-approved MR contrast agents.

4.3. Molecular imaging with magnetic resonance

Analogous to nuclear and CT, targeted MR contrast agents against molecules involved in inflammation are being developed. Molecular imaging with MRI is challenging because contrast agents need to reach micromolar concentrations in tissues to be detectable. For example, the contrast agent P947 is composed of peptide that specifically binds to matrix metalloproteinases (MMPs) linked covalently to a molecule of gadolinium chelate.[60] One hour after injection of P947, a significantly stronger enhancement was detected with MRI in MMP-rich atherosclerotic plaques of ApoE−/− mice as compared to the aortic wall of wild type mice (95% vs. 10%, respectively). The major advantage of this type of contrast agent is its low molecular weight. This means rapid diffusion into the plaque and the ability to detect specific binding early after injection. For greater amplification, specific peptides or antibodies can be attached to lipid-based nanoparticles (such as micelles, liposomes, and lipoproteins) containing a high payload of gadolinium.[2] For example, immunomicelles composed of monoclonal antibodies against the macrophage scavenger

receptor (MSR) bound covalently to micelles, each containing around 5,900 molecules of gadolinium (MSR-immunomicelles).[9] MSR are strongly expressed by foam cells present in atherosclerotic plaques. MSR-immunomicelles provided a 79% increase in signal intensity of atherosclerotic aortas of ApoE−/− mice 24 h after injection (Fig. 23.3). In addition, a strong correlation was demonstrated between the intensity of signal enhancement measured in plaques with MRI and macrophage content of corresponding histological sections. Although immunomicelles represent an attractive imaging platform to evaluate in vivo the expression of various molecules involved in plaque inflammation, clinical developments are hampered by the need for high concentrations of monoclonal antibodies. As an alternative, small peptides have been bound to gadolinium containing micelles. In a recent study, a peptide mimicking the domain of apolipoprotein ApoA-1 that binds to the macrophage HDL receptor was linked to the micelles. After injection, a 94% signal increase was measured by MRI in atherosclerotic plaque of ApoE−/− mice.[61] Colocalization of micelles with lesional macrophages was demonstrated using confocal microscopy by tracking a fluorescent lipid incorporated into the contrast agent. In addition to gadolinium, micelles can also be loaded with active drugs to target therapeutic molecules to specific cells. For example, nanoparticles or liposomes targeting $\alpha V-\beta 3$ integrins expressed on immature endothelial cells have been previously described for the specific delivery of angiostatic drugs to neovessels.[17,62] Extension of this approach to specific drug delivery to reduce inflammation in atherosclerotic plaques might hold promise.

5. FUTURE DIRECTIONS

Rapid technological progress is transforming the imaging of atherosclerotic cardiovascular disease from a method of diagnosis in symptomatic patients to a tool for the noninvasive detection of early subclinical abnormalities. In addition, a new generation of hybrid technology is now becoming available; this technology combines multiple imaging modalities in a single platform, using one machine for more than one type of imaging (Fig. 23.2C). And new probes designed to be detected by several modalities can take advantage of the strengths of each.

The availability of more powerful imaging techniques has the potential to improve our understanding of the biology of atherosclerosis. Much of the current knowledge has been inferred from static histopathological observations of animal models or human tissue samples studied at different disease stages or after various therapeutic interventions. By using molecular imaging, it is now becoming increasingly possible to obtain noninvasively—from living experimental animals and even humans—the type of information that was previously available only through immunohistochemistry. Improved imaging technologies also hold promise for aiding drug development. Rather than relying on the plasma concentrations of a specific therapeutic agent to infer that it has been delivered to the target organ, imaging might be able to provide a direct readout of the agent's local concentration and activity. Such information could be enormously helpful for deciding which therapies are the best candidates for proceeding to clinical trials.[5]

REFERENCES

1. Lusis AJ. Atherosclerosis. *Nature*. 2000;407(6801):233–241.
2. Briley-Saebo KC, Mulder WJ, Mani V, et al. Magnetic resonance imaging of vulnerable atherosclerotic plaques: Current imaging strategies and molecular imaging probes. *J Magn Reson Imaging*. 2007;26(3):460–479.
3. Choudhury RP, Fuster V, Fayad ZA. Molecular, cellular and functional imaging of atherothrombosis. *Nat Rev Drug Discov*. 2004;3(11):913–925.

4. Wu JC, Bengel FM, Gambhir SS. Cardiovascular molecular imaging. *Radiology.* 2007;244(2):337–355.

5. Jaffer FA, Libby P, Weissleder R. Molecular imaging of cardiovascular disease. *Circulation.* 2007;116(9):1052–1061.

6. Wickline SA, Neubauer AM, Winter PM, et al. Molecular imaging and therapy of atherosclerosis with targeted nanoparticles. *J Magn Reson Imaging.* 2007;25(4):667–680.

7. Sosnovik DE, Nahrendorf M, Weissleder R. Molecular magnetic resonance imaging in cardiovascular medicine. *Circulation.* 2007;115(15):2076–2086.

8. Trivedi RA, Mallawarachi C, JM UK-I, et al. Identifying inflamed carotid plaques using in vivo USPIO-enhanced MR imaging to label plaque macrophages. *Arterioscler Thromb Vasc Biol.* 2006;26(7):1601–1606.

9. Amirbekian V, Lipinski MJ, Briley-Saebo KC, et al. Detecting and assessing macrophages in vivo to evaluate atherosclerosis noninvasively using molecular MRI. *Proc Natl Acad Sci USA.* 2007;104(3):961–966.

10. Hyafil F, Cornily JC, Feig JE, et al. Noninvasive detection of macrophages using a nanoparticulate contrast agent for computed tomography. *Nat Med.* 2007;13(5):636–641.

11. Tawakol A, Migrino RQ, Bashian GG, et al. In vivo 18F-fluorodeoxyglucose positron emission tomography imaging provides a noninvasive measure of carotid plaque inflammation in patients. *J Am Coll Cardiol.* 2006;48(9):1818–1824.

12. Rudd JH, Myers KS, Bansilal S, et al. (18)Fluorodeoxyglucose positron emission tomography imaging of atherosclerotic plaque inflammation is highly reproducible: Implications for atherosclerosis therapy trials. *J Am Coll Cardiol.* 2007;50(9):892–896.

13. Sirol M, Fuster V, Badimon JJ, et al. Chronic thrombus detection with in vivo magnetic resonance imaging and a fibrin-targeted contrast agent. *Circulation.* 2005;112(11):1594–1600.

14. Nahrendorf M, Jaffer FA, Kelly KA, et al. Noninvasive vascular cell adhesion molecule-1 imaging identifies inflammatory activation of cells in atherosclerosis. *Circulation.* 2006;114(14):1504–1511.

15. Villanueva FS, Lu E, Bowry S, et al. Myocardial ischemic memory imaging with molecular echocardiography. *Circulation.* 2007;115(3):345–352.

16. Jaffer FA, Kim DE, Quinti L, et al. Optical visualization of cathepsin K activity in atherosclerosis with a novel, protease-activatable fluorescence sensor. *Circulation.* 2007;115(17):2292–2298.

17. Winter PM, Neubauer AM, Caruthers SD, et al. Endothelial alpha(v)beta3 integrin-targeted fumagillin nanoparticles inhibit angiogenesis in atherosclerosis. *Arterioscler Thromb Vasc Biol.* 2006;26(9):2103–2109.

18. Beeres SL, Bengel FM, Bartunek J, et al. Role of imaging in cardiac stem cell therapy. *J Am Coll Cardiol.* 2007;49(11):1137–1148.

19. Yun M, Yeh D, Araujo LI, et al. F-18 FDG uptake in the large arteries: a new observation. *Clin Nucl Med.* 2001;26(4):314–319.

20. Yun M, Yeh D, Araujo LI, et al. F-18 FDG uptake in the large arteries: a new observation. *Clin Nucl Med.* 2001;26(4):314–319.

21. Yun M, Jang S, Cucchiara A, et al. 18F FDG uptake in the large arteries: A correlation study with the atherogenic risk factors. *Semin Nucl Med.* 2002;32(1):70–76.

22. Tatsumi M, Cohade C, Nakamoto Y, et al. Fluorodeoxyglucose uptake in the aortic wall at PET/CT: Possible finding for active atherosclerosis. *Radiology.* 2003;229(3):831–837.

23. Deichen JT, Prante O, Gack M, et al. Uptake of [(18)F]fluorodeoxyglucose in human monocyte-macrophages in vitro. *Eur J Nucl Med Mol Imaging.* 2003;30(2):267–273.

24. Forstrom LA, Dunn WL, Mullan BP, et al. Biodistribution and dosimetry of [(18)F]fluorodeoxyglucose labelled leukocytes in normal human subjects. *Nucl Med Commun.* 2002;23(8):721–725.

25. Rudd JHF, Warburton EA, Fryer TD, et al. Imaging atherosclerotic plaque inflammation with [18F]-fluorodeoxyglucose positron emission tomography. *Circulation.* 2002;105(23):2708–2711.

26. Dunphy MP, Freiman A, Larson SM, et al. Association of vascular 18F-FDG uptake with vascular calcification. *J Nucl Med.* 2005;46(8):1278–1284.

27. Rudd J, Hyafil F, Cornily JC, et al. Molecular imaging of atherosclerosis using FDG PET/CT with a novel, macrophage-specific CT contrast agent. *J Nucl Med Ann Meet Abstr.* 2007;48(MeetingAbstracts_2):1P-1b.

28. Davies JR, Rudd JH, Fryer TD, et al. Identification of culprit lesions after transient ischemic attack by combined 18F fluorodeoxyglucose positron-emission tomography and high-resolution magnetic resonance imaging. *Stroke.* 2005;36(12):2642–2647.

29. Basu S, Zhuang H, Alavi A. Imaging of lower extremity artery atherosclerosis in diabetic foot: FDG-PET imaging and histopathological correlates. *Clin Nucl Med.* 2007;32(7):567–568.

30. Rudd JH, Myers KS, Bansilal S, et al. Atherosclerosis inflammation imaging with 18F-FDG PET: Carotid, iliac, and femoral uptake reproducibility, quantification methods, and recommendations. *J Nucl Med.* 2008;49(6):871–878.

31. Tahara N, Kai H, Yamagishi S, et al. Vascular inflammation evaluated by [18F]-fluorodeoxyglucose positron emission tomography is associated with the metabolic syndrome. *J Am Coll Cardiol.* 2007;49(14):1533–1539.

32. Tahara N, Kai H, Nakaura H, et al. The prevalence of inflammation in carotid atherosclerosis: Analysis with fluorodeoxyglucose positron emission tomography. *Eur Heart J.* 2007;28(18):2243–2248. EPub 2007 Aug.

33. Aziz K, Berger K, Claycombe K, et al. Noninvasive detection and localization of vulnerable plaque and arterial thrombosis with computed tomography angiography/positron emission tomography. *Circulation.* 2008;117(16):2061–2070.

34. Paulmier B, Duet M, Khayat R, et al. Arterial wall uptake of fluorodeoxyglucose on PET imaging in stable cancer disease patients indicates higher risk for cardiovascular events. *J Nucl Cardiol.* 2008;15:209–217.

35. Ogawa M, Magata Y, Kato T, et al. Application of 18F-FDG PET for monitoring the therapeutic effect of antiinflammatory drugs on stabilization of vulnerable atherosclerotic plaques. *J Nucl Med.* 2006;47(11):1845–1850.

36. Tahara N, Kai H, Ishibashi M, et al. Simvastatin attenuates plaque inflammation: Evaluation by fluorodeoxyglucose positron emission tomography. *J Am Coll Cardiol.* 2006;48(9):1825–1831.

37. Lee SJ, On YK, Lee EJ, et al. Reversal of vascular 18F-FDG uptake with plasma high-density lipoprotein elevation by atherogenic risk reduction. *J Nucl Med.* 2008;49(8):1277–1282.

38. Maschauer S, Prante O, Hoffmann M, et al. Characterization of 18F-FDG uptake in human endothelial cells in vitro. *J Nucl Med.* 2004;45(3):455–460.

39. Ishimori T, Saga T, Mamede M, et al. Increased (18)F-FDG uptake in a model of inflammation: Concanavalin A-mediated lymphocyte activation. *J Nucl Med.* 2002;43(5):658–663.

40. Anholt RR, Pedersen PL, De Souza EB, et al. The peripheral-type benzodiazepine receptor. Localization to the mitochondrial outer membrane. *J Biol Chem.* 1986;261(2):576–583.

41. Fujimura Y, Hwang P, Trout III H, et al. Increased peripheral benzodiazepine receptors in arterial plaque of patients with atherosclerosis: An autoradiographic study with [(3)H]PK 11195. *Atherosclerosis.* 2008. [Epub ahead of print]

42. Izquierdo-Garcia D, Davies JR, Graves MJ, et al. Comparison of methods for magnetic resonance-guided [18-F]fluorodeoxyglucose positron emission tomography in human carotid arteries. Reproducibility, partial volume correction, and correlation between methods. *Stroke.* 2008;40(1):86–93.

43. Pichler B, Judenhofer M, Wehrl H. PET/MRI hybrid imaging: Devices and initial results. *Eur Radiol.* 2008;18(6):1077–1086.

44. Williams G, Kolodny GM. Suppression of myocardial 18F-FDG uptake by preparing patients with a high-fat, low-carbohydrate diet. *Am J Roentgenol.* 2008;190(2):W151–W156.

45. Yonemura A, Momiyama Y, Fayad ZA, et al. Effect of lipid-lowering therapy with atorvastatin on atherosclerotic aortic plaques detected by noninvasive magnetic resonance imaging. *J Am Coll Cardiol.* 2005;45(5):733–742.

46. Yuan C, Beach KW, Smith LH, Jr, et al. Measurement of atherosclerotic carotid plaque size in vivo using high resolution magnetic resonance imaging. *Circulation.* 1998;98(24):2666–2671.

47. Fayad Z, Fuster V. Characterization of atherosclerotic plaques by magnetic resonance imaging. *Ann NY Acad Sci.* 2000;902:173–186.

48. Corti R, Fuster V, Fayad ZA, et al. Lipid lowering by simvastatin induces regression of human atherosclerotic lesions: Two years' follow-up by high-resolution noninvasive magnetic resonance imaging. *Circulation.* 2002;106(23):2884–2887.

49. Yuan C, Mitsumori LM, Beach KW, et al. Carotid atherosclerotic plaque: noninvasive MR characterization and identification of vulnerable lesions. *Radiology.* 2001;221(2):285–299.

50. Choudhury R, Fuster V, Fayad Z. Molecular, cellular and functional imaging of atherosclerosis. *Nat Rev Drug Discov.* 2004;3(11):913–925.

51. Yuan C, Kerwin WS. MRI of atherosclerosis. *J Magn Reson Imaging.* 2004;19(6):710–719.

52. Itskovich V, Samber D, Mani V, et al. Quantification of human atherosclerotic plaques using spatially enhanced cluster analysis of multicontrast-weighted magnetic resonance images. *Magn Reson Med.* 2004;52(3):515–523.

53. Summers R, Andrasko-Bourgeois J, Feuerstein I, et al. Evaluation of the aortic root by MRI: Insights from patients with homozygous familial hypercholesterolemia. *Circulation.* 1998;98(6):509–518.

54. Corti R, Fuster V, Badimon J, et al. New understanding of atherosclerosis (clinically and experimentally) with evolving MRI technology in vivo. *Ann NY Acad Sci.* 2001;947:181–195.

55. Yuan C, Mitsumori LM, Ferguson MS, et al. In vivo accuracy of multispectral magnetic resonance imaging for identifying lipid-rich necrotic cores and intraplaque hemorrhage in advanced human carotid plaques. *Circulation.* 2001;104(17):2051–2056.

56. Chu B, Hatsukami TS, Polissar NL, et al. Determination of carotid artery atherosclerotic lesion type and distribution in hypercholesterolemic patients with moderate carotid stenosis using noninvasive magnetic resonance imaging. *Stroke.* 2004;35(11):2444–2448.

57. Takaya N, Yuan C, Chu B, et al. Presence of intraplaque hemorrhage stimulates progression of carotid atherosclerotic plaques: A high-resolution magnetic resonance imaging study. *Circulation.* 2005;111(21):2768–2775.

58. Calcagno C, Cornily J, Hyafil F, et al. Detection of neovessels in atherosclerotic plaques of rabbits using dynamic contrast enhanced MRI and 18F-FDG PET. *Arterioscler Thromb Vasc Biol.* 2008;28(7):1311–1317.

59. Kerwin WS, Oikawa M, Yuan C, et al. MR imaging of adventitial vasa vasorum in carotid atherosclerosis. *Magn Reson Med.* 2008;59(3):507–514.

60. Lancelot E, Amirbekian V, Brigger I, et al. Evaluation of matrix metalloproteinases in atherosclerosis using a novel noninvasive imaging approach. *Arteriosler Thromb Vasc Biol.* 2008;28(3):425–432.

61. Cormode DP, Briley-Saebo KC, Mulder WJ, et al. An ApoA-I mimetic peptide high-density-lipoprotein-based MRI contrast agent for atherosclerotic plaque composition detection. *Small (Weinheim an der Bergstrasse, Germany).* 2008;4(9):1437–1444.

62. Mulder WJ, Strijkers GJ, Vucic E, et al. Magnetic resonance molecular imaging contrast agents and their application in atherosclerosis. *Top Magn Reson Imaging.* 2007;18(5):409–417.

63. Sanz J, Fayad ZA. Imaging of atherosclerotic cardiovascular disease. *Nature.* 2008;451(7181):953–957.

Vascular Thrombosis

24

Juan J. Badimon
Borja Ibanez
Antonio De Miguel

1. INTRODUCTION

Atherothrombosis is the major cause of mortality and morbidity in Western countries, and it is predicted that coronary artery disease (CAD) will be the dominant cause of mortality worldwide by 2020. The major reasons for the increase are aging of the population, increase in certain risk factors (obesity and diabetes) especially among the youth, and the adoption of an unhealthy lifestyle by developing countries. From the clinical point of view, atherosclerosis is seen as a single diffuse pathologic entity (affecting almost all vascular territories) that progresses silently but with focal clinical manifestations.[1] This chapter is focused on vascular thrombosis. More specifically, we will center on the formation and progression of atherosclerotic lesions leading to high risk/vulnerable plaques, and the triggers for plaque disruption and thrombus formation.

2. PATHOPHYSIOLOGY

2.1. The atherosclerotic plaque

Atherosclerosis is a systemic disease involving the intima of large- and medium-sized arteries (including the aorta, carotids, coronaries, and peripheral arteries) characterized by intimal thickening due to the accumulation of cells and lipids.[2] The deposition of these materials and the subsequent thickening of the wall may significantly compromise the residual lumen leading to ischemic events distal to the arterial stenosis.[3] Rupture or erosion of advanced lesions in coronary arteries initiates platelet activation and aggregation on the surface of the plaque and coagulation cascade activation resulting in acute thrombus formation and subsequent clinical manifestations: unstable angina, non-ST segment elevation acute coronary syndrome, ST elevation myocardial infarction, and sudden cardiac death. These thrombotic episodes largely occur in response to atherosclerotic lesions that have progressed to a high-risk inflammatory/prothrombotic stage. Thus, atherothrombosis is a complex, multifactorial process that involves the two major components (atherosclerosis plus thrombosis) from the pathogenesis of cardiovascular diseases; although distinct from one another, they appear to be closely interrelated (Fig. 24.1).

The main components of atherothrombotic plaques are (a) connective tissue extracellular matrix, including collagen, proteoglycans, and fibronectin elastic fibers; (b) crystalline cholesterol, cholesterol esters, and phospholipids; (c) cells such as monocyte-derived macrophages, T-lymphocytes, and smooth-muscle cells; and (d) thrombotic material with platelets and fibrin deposition. Varying proportions of these components occur in different plaques, thus giving rise to a heterogeneity or spectrum of lesions.

Until recently, atherosclerosis development was seen as a constant progressive process irreversibly associated to aging. However, new evidence indicates that atherosclerotic plaque homeostasis is not necessarily a constant progressing process, and atherosclerotic plaque formation can be slowed, stopped, or even reversed (Fig. 24.2).[4]

2.1.1. Endothelial dysfunction

The initial pathological manifestation of atherosclerosis is a dysfunctional endothelium. Under "healthy" circumstances, the normally functional endothelium is a dynamic autocrine and paracrine organ that creates an antiatherogenic environment protecting against atherogenesis, since endothelial cells constantly secrete substances into the vascular lumen not only to maintain vascular tone and to avoid abnormal platelet adhesion/activation and clot formation, but also for anti-inflammatory and mitogenic regulation activities.[5] This protection is achieved by releasing a series of antithrombotic and vasoactive substances. It is widely accepted that metabolic endothelial dysfunction (even without any mechanical damage) is enough to trigger the pathologic processes leading to plaque formation.

Endothelial dysfunction is often the result of a disturbance in the physiological pattern of blood flow (flow reversal or oscillating shear stress) at bending points and near bifurcations,[6,7] and therefore, there are areas of endothelium more prone to suffer lesion development, leading to the hypothesis that endothelial activity is regulated by different rheologic conditions in vascular bed. Shear stress and local hemodynamics modulate not only the clinical manifestations of the disease (thrombotic complications), but also the progression of the atherosclerotic plaques. Other than biomechanical shear stress forces (enhanced by hypertension), the coexistence of other cardiovascular risk factors is strongly correlated with the development of endothelial dysfunction.

Endothelial dysfunction is characterized by a change in the pattern of synthesis and secretion of different substances, mainly nitric oxide and prostaglandin (PG) I_2, unleashing not only the internalization and oxidation of circulating lipids into the intimal layer, but also the recruitment of inflammatory cells into the vessel wall, smooth muscle cells proliferation, extracellular matrix deposition, vasoconstriction, in addition to a prothrombotic state within the vessel lumen initiating the atherosclerotic process[8,9] (Fig. 24.3); as a result, there are consequences at the systemic level (promoting the activation, adhesion, and aggregation of platelets to the dysfunctional area) and vascular level (endothelial synthesis and exposure of cell adhesive proteins from the selectin superfamily [E- and P-selectins]). These proteins facilitate the homing and internalization of the circulating monocytes into the subendothelial space where they become macrophages.

331

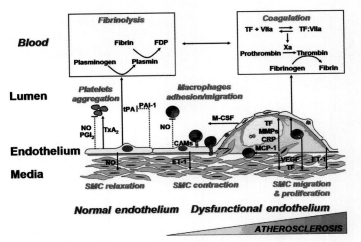

Figure 24.1 Diagram of dysfunctional endothelium and subsequent atherosclerotic lesion development. NO, nitric oxide; ET-1, endothelin; MMP, matrix metalloproteinase; PAI-1, plasminogen activator inhibitor type 1; TF, tissue factor; tPA, tissue plasminogen activator; TXA$_2$, thromboxane A$_2$; CAM, cell adhesion molecule; CRP, C-reactive protein; MCP, monocyte chemotactic protein; M-CSF, monocyte colony stimulating factor; PGI$_2$, prostacyclin; SMC, smooth muscle cell; VEGF, vascular endothelial growth factor. (Adapted from Fuster V, Fayad ZA, Moreno PR, et al. Atherothrombosis and high-risk plaque: Part II: approaches by noninvasive computed tomographic/magnetic resonance imaging. *J Am Coll Cardiol.* 2005;46(7):1209–1218.)

Until recently, it was believed that endothelial repair after an injury was carried out only by neighboring cells; however, recent data suggest that the endothelium can be repopulated and repaired by circulating endothelial progenitor cells. The number of these "endothelial repairing" cells is believed to be a marker of arterial injury in vascular disease,[10] an area of intensive ongoing research.

2.1.2. Lipid Deposition
Lipid accumulation results from an imbalance between the mechanisms responsible for the influx and efflux of lipids into

the arterial wall. Cholesterol accumulation plays a central role in the atherogenesis process. Low-density lipoprotein cholesterol (LDL-C) infiltrates through the arterial endothelium into the intima and binds to different matrix proteins of the subendothelial space, where it undergoes an oxidative process; this binding seems to be related to an ionic interaction of apolipoprotein (apo) B with matrix proteins including proteoglycans, collagen, and fibronectin[11]; secondary changes may occur in the underlying media and adventitia, particularly in advanced disease stages.

LDL is a heterogeneous group of particles that vary in their core content of cholesterol. LDL-C does not reflect the atherogenicity of all of the apo B-containing lipoproteins nor does it necessarily represent the total number of low-density lipoprotein particles (LDL-P) or the distribution of size within those particles. A greater amount of cholesterol in LDL creates larger, more buoyant particles (sometimes referred to as LDL subclass A). A lower amount of cholesterol in LDL generates smaller, denser particles (sometimes referred to as LDL subclass B). Small dense particles of LDL-C are the ones that participate in cholesterol accumulation in atherosclerotic plaques so that, for two patients with the same LDL-C level, the one with a preponderance of small dense LDL-P will have a greater number of LDL-P and more importantly a significantly greater risk of cardiovascular disease.

There is one molecule of apo B for each LDL-C molecule.[12] Apo B level reflects the total number of atherogenic apo B-containing lipoproteins, however, 90% of total plasma apo B is contained within the LDL-C particles.[12] Thus, for a given LDL-C level, a higher apo-B level indicates higher content of LDL-P. In addition, apo B also appears to be a better predictor of subsequent CAD events in patients on treatment with statins.[13,14]

Oxidized cholesterol is highly toxic, and as part of a mechanism of defense, it is phagocytized by the vessel wall macrophages. The presence of the oxidized lipids triggers a series of proinflammatory reactions via different mediators, perpetuating the activation and recruitment of monocytes, macrophages, and inflammatory cells. Macrophages, by engulfing the lipid material, become foam cells. Failure of macrophages to remove cholesterol from

Figure 24.2 Schematic view of cholesterol metabolism and reverse cholesterol transport. LDL, low-density lipoprotein; HDL, high-density lipoprotein. (Reproduced from Choi BG, Vilahur G, Yadegar D, et al. The role of high density lipoprotein cholesterol in the prevention and possible treatment of cardiovascular diseases. *Curr Mol Med.* 2006; 6(5):571–587, with permission.)

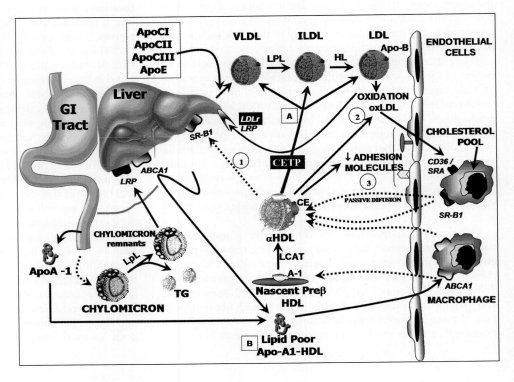

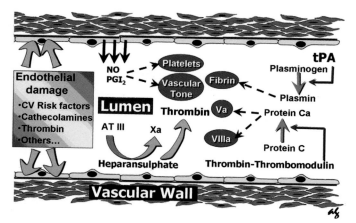

Figure 24.3 Endothelial dysfunction as hallmark of atherothrombotic disease. Simplified diagram of the role of endothelium and the physiologic anticoagulation system. tPA, tissue plasmnogen activator; PGI₂, prostacyclin; NO, nitric oxide. (Reproduced from Badimon JJ, Ibanez B, Fuster V, et al. Coronary Thrombosis: Local and Systemic factors. Chapter 53. In Hurst's the Heart. Edited by McGraw-Hill Professional, with permission.)

the vessel wall promotes its apoptotic death, releasing cholesterol into the vessel wall and, more importantly, inflammatory substances like tissue factor (TF)[15] and metalloproteinases (enzymes able to digest the matrix scaffold), making atherosclerotic lesions more prone to rupture (the so-called vulnerable plaque).[16]

2.1.3. Inflammation and atherosclerosis

Inflammation is another important process playing a dual role (both at the vascular and circulating levels) on affecting plaque progression, vulnerability, and subsequent thrombus formation, and could be considered as the link between atherosclerosis and thrombosis. In fact, the relation of inflammation and atherothrombosis could represent different faces of the same disease.

Development of atherosclerosis is influenced by innate and adaptive immune responses. In the first line of innate immunity, scavenger receptors (SR)-A and CD-36 are responsible for the uptake of oxidized LDL, transforming the macrophage into a foam cell,[17] which produces cytokines that activate neighboring smooth muscle cells, resulting in extracellular matrix formation

and fibrosis. In the second line of innate immunity, toll-like receptors have a significant role and are involved not only in the initiation but also in progression and expansive remodeling of atherothrombosis (fibroblast and macrophages location in the intima and adventitia, neointimal formation, intimal lesions).[18] Adaptive immunity is much more specific than innate immunity, and involves an organized immune response leading to generation of T and B cell receptors and immunoglobulins.

Different inflammatory markers stand out the link between atherosclerosis and inflammation: C-reactive protein (CRP), CD40 Ligand (CD40L), interleukin (IL)-6, IL-1, and tumor necrosis factor (TNF). CRP plays a proinflammatory role in activating monocyte chemotactic protein-1; CRP levels are high in patients with acute coronary syndromes and can be used to predict outcome in those patients.[19,20] CD40L is implicated in the various stages of atherogenesis, including the initiation and progression of atherosclerotic lesions as well as acute complications. Increased levels of soluble CD40L has been observed in unstable angina[21] and hypercholesterolemia,[22] and circulating levels have strong independent prognostic value among apparently healthy individuals.[23]

2.1.4. The high-risk (vulnerable) plaque

Continuous exposure to the systemic, proatherogenic environment increases chemotaxis of monocytes leading to lipid accumulation, necrotic core, and fibrous cap formation, evolving into advanced atherosclerosis. Vulnerability to rupture depends on several factors: (a) circumferential wall stress or cap fatigue; (b) location, size, and consistency of the atheromatous core; and (c) blood flow characteristics, particularly the impact of flow on the proximal aspect of the plaque (i.e., configuration and angulation of the plaque); another important fact is that not all ruptured plaques lead to occlusive thrombus.[16] This observation lead to the concept of vulnerable blood in addition to high risk plaque as a modulator of the clinical manifestations of the disease (Fig. 24.4).[24]

Structural and functional features characterizing these lesions also include eccentric plaque growth with compensatory enlargement of the vessel wall (known as vascular remodeling), vasa vasorum neovascularization leading to lipid core expansion and intraplaque hemorrhage. In addition, inflammation and metalloproteinase expression leads to plaque rupture, often found at the shoulder of large lipid-rich plaques.[16]

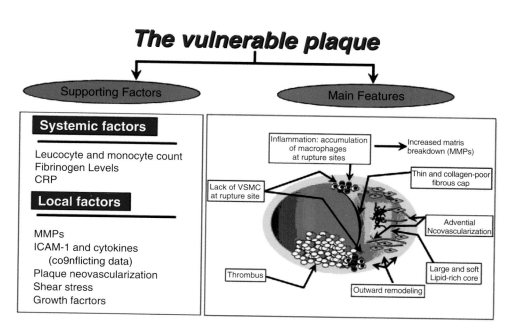

Figure 24.4 The vulnerable plaque. Features and factors associated with plaque vulnerability. MMPs, matrix metalloproteinases; ICAM, intercellular cell adhesion molecule; CRP, C-reactive protein; VSMC, vascular smooth muscle cells. (Reproduced from Vilahur G, Ibanez B, Badimon J. Characteristic features of atherosclerotic plaques that are vulnerable to rupture. Brief review. *Int J Atheroscler.* 2006;1(2):143–148, with permission.)

Atherosclerotic plaques undergoing remodeling are characterized by a larger lipid core, fewer smooth muscle cells, and increased macrophage infiltration.[25] As the plaque grows eccentrically within the vessel wall, remodeling triggers crucial changes within the tunica media and the adventitia (the increased activity of metalloproteinases-2 and -9 digests the internal elastic lamina, modulating the process of remodeling).

Neovascularization and blood extravasation are involved in plaque destabilization and plaque growth.[26–28] Leaky vasa vasorum with the subsequent red blood cell extravasation has been postulated as a major source for intraplaque cholesterol deposition. This change in composition, characterized by increased extracellular cholesterol within the lipid core and excessive macrophage infiltration, increases the vulnerability of the atherosclerotic lesions. In fact, there is a strong correlation between macrophage infiltration and increased vasa vasorum in human atherosclerotic lesions. Pre-existing vasa vasorum in the adventitia are thought to spread into the intima, prompting intimal neovascularization,[27] but intimal disease is considered a prerequisite for vessel wall and plaque neovascularization, since neovessels from adventitial vasa vasorum proliferate in response to vessel wall thickness growth derived from atherosclerosis. It is well known that intraplaque hemorrhage is an event leading to plaque rupture and thrombosis. In addition, stable (fibrocalcific) plaques show reduced microvasculature compared with lipid-rich and ruptured plaques.

Importantly, lipid-rich lesions leading to acute coronary syndromes are often mildly stenotic due to significant positive remodeling and therefore, are not detectable by contrast angiography.[29] This is very important in understanding the concept that early detection of atherosclerosis implies the use of novel imaging modalities that can visualize not only the vessel lumen, but also the entire arterial wall (Fig. 24.5).

On the other hand, the risk of suffering a thrombotic complication depends more on the biochemical and cell composition of the lesions rather than their stenotic severity. At the histologic level, these lesions are mildly stenotic; they have a significant lipid-rich necrotic core separated from the circulating blood by a thin fibrotic cap. At the cellular level, the high-risk lesions show a higher content of macrophages and inflammatory cells; the core is acellular, without the mechanical support of the collagen fibers and delimited by macrophages and cholesterol-loaded cells. The disposition of two zones with different densities (fibrotic cap and lipid-rich core) makes these plaques highly unstable and prone to rupture.[16] In addition, in disrupted lesions the inflammatory cells seem to selectively concentrate in the ruptured areas: macrophages and mast cells through phagocytosis and proteolytic enzymes secretion such as plasminogen activators and matrix metalloproteinases (i.e., collagenases, elastases, and gelatinases) degrade the components of extracellular matrix, contributing significantly to plaque rupture.

2.2. Cellular and molecular mechanisms implicated in vascular thrombosis

Rupture of a high-risk vulnerable plaque changes plaque geometry and triggers coronary thrombosis, resulting in acute occlusion or subocclusion with subsequent clinical manifestations: unstable angina, acute coronary syndrome, and sudden cardiac death; however, it is known that endothelial denudation/disruption is not an absolute prerequisite to allow platelet activation and attachment to the arterial wall,[30] even under high shear rate conditions.[31]

Thrombus organization mediated by repaired collagen heals the rupture site, but increases plaque volume, contributing to the progression of atherothrombosis. More specifically, different

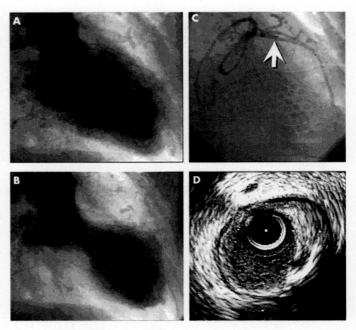

Figure 24.5 Disruption of a nonstenotic plaque leading to acute coronary syndrome. (**A**) End-diastolic and; (**B**) end-systolic cine-ventriculographic frames showing anteroapical akineis. (**C**) Direct left coronary contrast injection showing mild narrowing in the proximal left anterior descending coronary artery. (**D**) The cross sectional IVUS view of LAD clearly shows a disrupted eccentric plaque with positive remodelling from 12 to 5 o'clock. At 4 o'clock there is an image of ulceration, with a cavity inside the plaque. (Reproduced from Ibanez B, Navarro F, Cordoba M, et al. Tako-tsubo transient left ventricular ballooning: is intravascular ultrasound the key to resolve the enigma? *Heart*. 2005;91:102–104, with permission.)

factors (plaque-dependent thrombogenic substrate, rheology, and systemic procoagulant activity) may influence the magnitude and stability of the resulting thrombus and thus, the severity of the acute coronary syndrome.

2.2.1. Platelet activation and aggregation processes
Platelets are the first blood components to arrive at the scene of vascular damage, and they can adhere directly to the dysfunctional endothelial monolayer (even in the absence of endothelial disruption), exposed collagen, and/or macrophages. Accordingly, platelets can also be activated in early stages of the atherosclerotic process. It has been postulated that platelet activation may be attributed to: (a) reduction in the mechanisms implicated in maintaining endothelial antithrombotic properties; (b) reactive oxygen species generated by atherosclerotic risk factors (in fact, the presence of hypertension, hypercholesterolemia, cigarette smoking, and diabetes correlates with a higher number of circulating activated platelets); and (c) an increase in prothrombotic and proinflammatory mediators in the circulation or immobilized on the endothelium.[32] Adhered platelets, in concert with dysfunctional endothelial cells, secrete chemotactic and growth factors, which in turn stimulate migration, accumulation, and proliferation of smooth muscle cells and leukocytes in the intima layer (Fig. 24.6).

The initial recognition of damaged vessel wall by platelets involves (a) adhesion, activation, and adherence to recognition sites on the thromboactive substrate (extracellular matrix proteins such as von Willebrand Factor [vWF], collagen, fibronectin, vitronectin, and laminin), (b) spreading of the platelet on the surface, and (c) aggregation of platelets to form a platelet plug or white thrombus.[33] The efficiency of platelet recruitment will

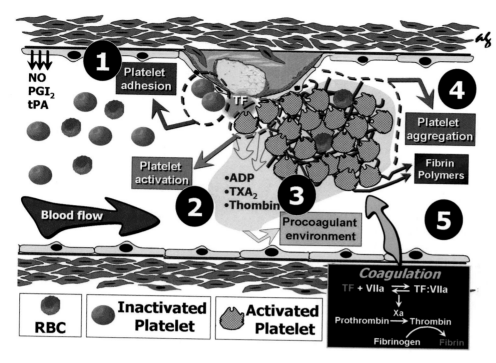

Figure 24.6 Mechanism involved in thrombus formation. Healthy endothelium (**left**) presents antithrombotic properties, since it is able to release vascular protective substances such as nitric oxide (NO), prostacyclin (PGI$_2$), tissue plaminogen activator (tPA) and tissue factor pathway inhibitor (TFPi). On the contrary, dysfunctional endothelium (**right**) not only favors platelet adhesion, activation, and aggregation, but also promotes vascular lipid deposition, macrophage migration, and tissue factor (TF) expression (activation of the coagulation cascade). Following platelet adhesion, activation is characterized by platelet shape change. Activated platelets secrete different agonists prompting activation of circulating platelets, and a procoagulant environment. This prothrombotic milieu will favor thrombus formation and the subsequent clinical manifestations. NO, nitric oxide; PGI$_2$, prostacyclin; tPA, tissue plasminogen activator; TF, tissue factor; TXA$_2$, thromboxane A$_2$. (Reproduced from Ibanez B, Vilahur G, Badimon J. Pharmacology of thienopyridines: Rationale for dual pathway inhibition. *Eur Heart J Suppl.* 2006;8:G3–G9, with permission.)

depend on the underlying substrate and local geometry (local factors). A final step involving the recruitment of other blood cells also occurs; erythrocytes, neutrophils, and occasionally monocytes are found on evolving mixed thrombus. Plaque rupture facilitates the interaction of inner plaque components with the circulating blood; among these components, TF exhibits a potent activating effect on platelets and coagulation.

Platelet function depends on the adhesive interaction of several compounds. Most of the glycoproteins in the platelet membrane surface are receptors for adhesive proteins or mediate cellular interactions. At the site of vascular lesions, circulating vWF binds to the exposed collagen, which subsequently binds to the glycoprotein (GP) Ib/IX receptor on the platelet membrane.[34-36] Under pathological conditions and in response to changes in shear stress, vWF can be secreted from the storage organelles in platelets or endothelial cells, reinforcing the activation process. Although GPIb/IX-vWF interaction is enough to promote binding of platelets to subendothelium, it is highly transient, resulting in rapid dislocation of platelets to the site of injury. GPVI binding to matrix collagen has slower binding kinetics, but once initiated, promotes a firm adhesion of platelets to the vessel surface.[37] Finally, both GPIb/IX and GPVI also regulate platelet–leukocyte adhesion and thereby, are implicated in other vascular processes, such as inflammation and atherosclerosis.[38-40] Perfusion studies conducted at high shear rates have shown that vWF binds to platelet membrane glycoproteins both in adhesion (platelet-substrate interaction) and aggregation (platelet–platelet interaction), leading to thrombus formation.[41-43]

Circulating agents such as epinephrine, thrombin, serotonin, thromboxane A$_2$ (TXA$_2$), and adenosine diphosphate (ADP) are powerful platelet agonists and can also activate platelets via specific platelet surface receptors; these agonists stimulate different membrane receptors promoting subsequent platelet free-ionic Ca^{2+} release of platelet granule components in a process, namely platelet degranulation (discharge of platelet granule contents from the platelet dense granules). Once activated, platelets suffer a considerable shape change and ensuing calcium translocation (Fig. 24.7).

ADP plays a key role in platelet function because it amplifies the platelet response induced by other platelet agonists.[44] This ADP release from platelet granules has an autocrine effect promoting stable platelet aggregation by interacting with specific ADP receptors in the membrane (P2Y$_1$ and P2Y$_{12}$), but also promotes a paracrine effect by binding to ADP receptors of neighboring platelets, amplifying the activation process: intracellular signaling events that result in activation of the GP IIb/IIIa receptor, dense granule release, amplification of platelet aggregation, platelet shape change, and stabilization of the platelet aggregate. Although not activated by ADP, platelets possess a third purinergic receptor (P2X1), which is a fast adenosine triphosphate (ATP)-gated calcium channel receptor mainly involved in platelet shape change.

On the other hand, platelet activation also induces phospholipase-A$_2$ activation that triggers arachidonic acid metabolism; platelet cyclooxygenase (COX)-1 catalyzes the conversion of arachidonic acid to PG G$_2$/H$_2$, and the latter is converted to TXA$_2$, which is released to the circulation where it binds to thromboxane receptors, thus enhancing platelet activation and vasoconstriction. Therefore, platelet activation triggers intracellular signaling and expression of platelet membrane receptors for adhesion and initiation of cell contractile processes that induce shape change and secretion of the granular contents.

On activated platelets, the expression of the integrin IIb/IIIa (αIIbβ_3) receptors for adhesive glycoprotein ligands (mainly fibrinogen and vWF) in the circulation initiates platelet–platelet interaction. The process is perpetuated by the arrival of platelets from the circulation. The initial binding of fibrinogen to IIb/IIIa receptor is a reversible process that is followed seconds to minutes later by an irreversible stabilization of the fibrinogen linkage to the IIb/IIIa complex. This not only results in the binding of fibrinogen, but once fibrinogen is bound "in-side out" signaling also occurs causing amplification of the initial signal and further platelet activation. This leads to further aggregation of platelets and accumulation at the site of vessel injury resulting in thrombus formation.

Figure 24.7 Mechanisms and agonists involved in platelet adhesion, activation, and aggregation. PAR, protease-activated receptor; GP, glycoprotein; vWF, Von Willebrand factor; TP, thromboxane receptor; TXA, thromboxane. (Reproduced from Ibanez B, Vilahur G, Badimon J. Pharmacology of thienopyridines: Rationale for dual pathway inhibition. *Eur Heart J Suppl.* 2006;8:G3–G9, with permission.)

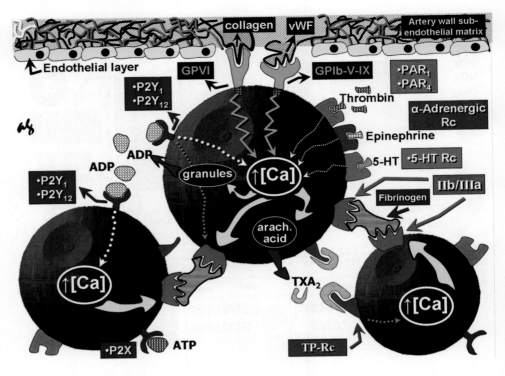

2.2.2. Coagulation cascade activation

During plaque rupture, in addition to platelet deposition in the injured area, the clotting mechanism is activated by the exposure of the plaque contents. The activation of coagulation leads to the generation of thrombin, which is a powerful platelet agonist in addition to being an enzyme that catalyzes the formation and polymerization of fibrin. Fibrin is essential in the stabilization of the platelet thrombus and its ability to withstand removal forces by flow, shear, and high intravascular pressure. The efficacy of fibrinolytic agents demonstrates the importance of fibrin in thrombosis associated with myocardial infarction.

The blood coagulation system involves a sequence of reactions integrating zymogens (proteins susceptible to activation into enzymes via limited proteolysis) and cofactors (nonproteolytic enzyme activators) into three groups: (a) contact activation (generation of factor XIa via the Hageman factor) and TF-dependent activation pathways; (b) the conversion of factor X to factor Xa in a complex reaction requiring the participation of factors IX and VIII; and (c) the conversion of prothrombin to thrombin and fibrin formation.[45] Platelets may provide the membrane requirements for the activation of factor X, although the participation of cells of the vessel wall (in exposed injured vessels) has not been excluded.[46]

Activated factor XI induces the activation of factor IX in the presence of Ca^{2+}. Factor IXa forms a catalytic complex with factor VIII on a membrane surface and efficiently activates factor X in the presence of Ca^{2+} (factors II, VII, IX and are vitamin K–dependent enzymes). Factor VIII forms a noncovalent complex with vWF in plasma, and its function in coagulation is the acceleration of the effects of IXa on the activation of X to Xa.

The TF pathway, previously known as the extrinsic coagulation pathway, through the TF-factor VIIa complex in the presence of Ca^{2+}, induces the formation of Xa. A second TF-dependent reaction catalyzes the transformation of IX into IXa. TF is an integral membrane protein that serves to initiate the activation of factors IX and X and to localize the reaction to cells on which TF is expressed. Other cofactors include factor VIIIa, which binds to platelets and forms the binding site for IXa, thereby forming the machinery for the activation of X; and factor Va, which binds to platelets and provides a binding site for Xa.

Activated platelets provide a procoagulant surface for the assembly and expression of both intrinsic Xase and prothrombinase enzymatic complexes. These complexes respectively catalyze the activation of factor X to factor Xa and prothrombin to thrombin. The expression of activity is associated with the binding of both of the proteases, factor IXa and factor Xa, and the cofactors, VIIIa and Va, to procoagulant surfaces. The binding of IXa and Xa is promoted by VIIIa and Va, respectively, such that Va and likely VIIIa provide the equivalent of receptors for the proteolytic enzymes. The surface of the platelet expresses the procoagulant phospholipids that bind coagulation factors and contribute to the procoagulant activity of the cell.[47]

Activated Xa converts prothrombin into thrombin. The complex that catalyzes the formation of thrombin consists of factors Xa and Va in a 1:1 complex. The interaction of the four components of the "prothrombinase complex" (Xa, Va, phospholipid, and Ca^{2+}) enhances the efficiency of the reaction.[47] Thrombin acts on multiple substrates, including fibrinogen, factor XIII, factors V and VIII, and protein C in addition to its effects on platelets. It plays a central role in hemostasis and thrombosis. The catalytic transformation of fibrinogen into fibrin is essential in the formation of the hemostatic plug and in the formation of arterial thrombi. Thrombin binds to the fibrinogen central domain and cleaves fibrinopeptides A and B, resulting in the formation of fibrin monomer and polymer formation.[48] The fibrin mesh holds the platelets together and contributes to the attachment of the thrombus to the vessel wall.

2.2.3. Role of local factors in the regulation of coronary thrombosis

The cellular and molecular mechanisms of platelet deposition and thrombus formation following vascular damage are modulated by the type of injury, the local geometry at the damaged site (degree of stenosis), and local hemodynamic conditions.[49–52] Similarly, three major factors also determine the vulnerability of the fibrous cap: (a) circumferential wall stress, or cap "fatigue"; (b) lesion characteristics (location, size, and consistency); and (c) blood flow.[53]

2.2.4. Effects derived from the severity of vessel wall damage

Exposure of de-endothelialized vessel wall, native fibrillar collagen type I bundles with a rough surface, or atherosclerotic plaque components at similar blood shear rate conditions leads to increasing degree of platelet deposition.[49] Thromboplastin or TF, readily available in the atherosclerotic intimal space exposed by endothelial loss, contributes to the high thrombogenicity of atherosclerotic plaques.[54] Overall, it is likely that when injury to the vessel wall is mild, the thrombogenic stimulus is relatively limited and the resulting thrombotic occlusion is transient, as occurs in unstable angina. On the other hand, deep vessel injury secondary to plaque rupture or ulceration results in exposure of collagen, TF, and other elements of the vessel matrix, leading to relatively persistent thrombotic occlusion and subsequent acute myocardial infarction. The analysis of the relative contribution of different components of human atherosclerotic plaques show that atheromatous core is up to sixfold more active than the other substrates in triggering thrombosis.[55] Other common features directly related to higher plaque thrombogenicity are high density of activated inflammatory (monocytes/macrophages) T cells, downregulation expression of lysyl oxidase in vascular wall cells due to LDL, cell apoptosis and microparticles with procoagulant activity and postulated apoptotic origin, and matrix metalloproteinases secretion.

2.2.5. Effects derived from geometry

The degree of stenosis caused by the ruptured plaque and the overlying mural thrombi are also key factors for determining thrombogenicity at the local arterial site. Acute platelet deposition after plaque rupture is highly modulated by the degree of narrowing after rupture; thus, changes in geometry may increase platelet deposition, whereas sudden growth

of thrombus at the injury site may create further stenosis and thrombotic occlusion.[51,56]

Spontaneous lysis of thrombus does occur, but the presence of a residual mural thrombus predisposes to recurrent thrombotic vessel occlusion. Two main contributing factors for the development of rethrombosis have been identified: (a) platelet deposition increases with increasing degrees of vessel stenosis; and (b) fragmented thrombus appears to present one of the most powerful thrombogenic surfaces. The fact that a clear predilection exists for lesion formation at arterial branch points strongly indicates the important influence of local hemodynamics and rheologic conditions on atherosclerosis.

2.2.6. Role of systemic factors in the regulation of coronary thrombosis

The severity of coronary thrombosis and associated acute coronary syndrome is modulated by the magnitude and/or stability of the formed thrombus. Once a plaque ruptures, in addition to the local factors, there are circulating systemic factors that modulate, predispose, or lead to acute coronary syndrome. This knowledge leads to the concept of vulnerable patient as a composite of vulnerable plaque plus vulnerable blood.[57,58] Two major pathways are deeply involved in systemic procoagulant activity: coronary risk factors and circulating tissue factor (hyperthrombotic state triggered by systemic factors).

Systemic factors, including elevated LDL, decreased high-density lipoprotein cholesterol (HDL-C), cigarette smoking, diabetes, and disregulated hemostasis, are associated with increased thrombotic complications.[58–61]

TF is a major local player in the vulnerability and thrombogenicity of atherosclerotic plaques, is highly expressed in atherosclerotic plaques, and its content has been related to plaque thrombogenicity.[62] Increased levels of circulating TF activity seems to be associated with cardiovascular risk factors, and improvement in glycemic control showed a reduction in circulating TF, suggesting that circulating TF may be the mechanism of action responsible for the increased thrombotic complications associated with the presence of these cardiovascular risk factors (Fig. 24.8).[63]

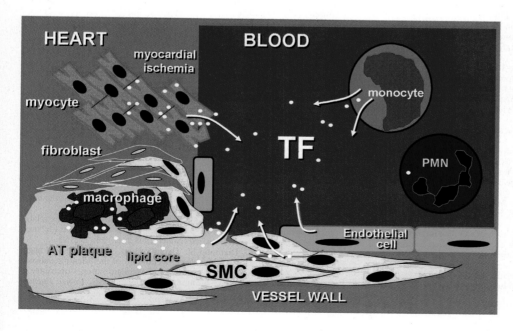

Figure 24.8 Suggested sources of circulating tissue factor. SMC, smooth muscle cell; TF, tissue factor. (Reproduced from Badimon JJ, Ibanez B, Fuster V, et al. Coronary Thrombosis: Local and Systemic factors. Chapter 53. In Hurst's the Heart. Edited by McGraw-Hill Professional, with permission.)

3. FUTURE DIRECTIONS

Thrombogenic systemic factors can be modulated by controlling the cardiovascular risk factors and by dietary and pharmacologic strategies. Currently, it is well known that inflammatory circulating markers correlate with cardiovascular events and severity of the disease, therefore, atherosclerosis and inflammation could represent different faces of the same disease. Several inflammatory markers are postulated as having a significant prognostic value for recurrent cardiovascular events.[64] However, it is clear that the best weapon to treat inflammation in cardiovascular disease is an aggressive management of all the cardiovascular risk factors (i.e., statins, angiotensin converting enzyme-inhibitor, hypoglycemic agents, and antiplatelet agents); interestingly, the use of these therapeutic interventions has been demonstrated to not only offer significant benefits but also reduce the systemic levels of proinflammatory markers.[64]

REFERENCES

1. Badimon JJ, Ibanez B, Fuster V, et al. *Coronary Thrombosis: Local and Systemic Factors.* 12th Ed. New York, NY: McGraw-Hill; 2007.
2. Corti R, Badimon JJ. Biologic aspects of vulnerable plaque. *Curr Opin Cardiol.* 2002;17(6):616–625.
3. Fuster V, Fayad ZA, Moreno PR, et al. Atherothrombosis and high-risk plaque: Part II: Approaches by noninvasive computed tomographic/magnetic resonance imaging. *J Am Coll Cardiol.* 2005;46(7):1209–1218.
4. Badimon JJ, Badimon L, Galvez A, et al. High density lipoprotein plasma fractions inhibit aortic fatty streaks in cholesterol-fed rabbits. *Lab Invest.* 1989;60(3):455–461.
5. Bonetti PO, Lerman LO, Lerman A. Endothelial dysfunction: A marker of atherosclerotic risk. *Arterioscler Thromb Vasc Biol.* 2003;23(2):168–175.
6. Ravensbergen J, Ravensbergen JW, Krijger JK, et al. Localizing role of hemodynamics in atherosclerosis in several human vertebrobasilar junction geometries. *Arterioscler Thromb Vasc Biol.* 1998;18(5):708–716.
7. Nerem RM. Vascular fluid mechanics, the arterial wall, and atherosclerosis. *J Biomech Eng.* 1992;114(3):274–282.
8. Ignarro LJ, Napoli C. Novel features of nitric oxide, endothelial nitric oxide synthase, and atherosclerosis. *Curr Atheroscler Rep.* 2004;6(4):281–287.
9. Voetsch B, Jin RC, Loscalzo J. Nitric oxide insufficiency and atherothrombosis. *Histochem Cell Biol.* 2004;122(4):353–367.
10. Hill JM, Zalos G, Halcox JP, et al. Circulating endothelial progenitor cells, vascular function, and cardiovascular risk. *N Engl J Med.* 2003;348(7):593–600.
11. Khalil MF, Wagner WD, Goldberg IJ. Molecular interactions leading to lipoprotein retention and the initiation of atherosclerosis. *Arterioscler Thromb Vasc Biol.* 2004;24(12):2211–2218.
12. Sniderman AD. How, when, and why to use apolipoprotein B in clinical practice. *Am J Cardiol.* 2002;90(8A):48i–54i.
13. Barter PJ, Ballantyne CM, Carmena R, et al. Apo B versus cholesterol in estimating cardiovascular risk and in guiding therapy: Report of the thirty-person/ten-country panel. *J Intern Med.* 2006;259(3):247–258.
14. Gotto AM, Jr, Whitney E, Stein EA, et al. Relation between baseline and on-treatment lipid parameters and first acute major coronary events in the Air Force/Texas Coronary Atherosclerosis Prevention Study (AFCAPS/TexCAPS). *Circulation.* 2000;101(5):477–484.
15. Hutter R, Valdiviezo C, Sauter BV, et al. Caspase-3 and tissue factor expression in lipid-rich plaque macrophages: Evidence for apoptosis as link between inflammation and atherothrombosis. *Circulation.* 2004;109(16):2001–2008.
16. Vilahur G, Ibanez B, Badimon J. Characteristic features of atherosclerotic plaques that are vulnerable to rupture. Brief review. *Int J Atheroscler.* 2006;1(2):143–148.
17. Hansson GK. Immune mechanisms in atherosclerosis. *Arterioscler Thromb Vasc Biol.* 2001;21(12):1876–1890.
18. Hollestelle SC, De Vries MR, Van Keulen JK, et al. Toll-like receptor 4 is involved in outward arterial remodeling. *Circulation.* 2004;109(3):393–398.
19. Liuzzo G, Biasucci LM, Gallimore JR, et al. The prognostic value of C-reactive protein and serum amyloid a protein in severe unstable angina. *N Engl J Med.* 1994;331(7):417–424.
20. Ridker PM, Cushman M, Stampfer MJ, et al. Inflammation, aspirin, and the risk of cardiovascular disease in apparently healthy men. *N Engl J Med.* 1997;336(14):973–979.
21. Aukrust P, Muller F, Ueland T, et al. Enhanced levels of soluble and membrane-bound CD40 ligand in patients with unstable angina. Possible reflection of T lymphocyte and platelet involvement in the pathogenesis of acute coronary syndromes. *Circulation.* 1999;100(6):614–620.
22. Cipollone F, Mezzetti A, Porreca E, et al. Association between enhanced soluble CD40L and prothrombotic state in hypercholesterolemia: Effects of statin therapy. *Circulation.* 2002;106(4):399–402.
23. Schonbeck U, Varo N, Libby P, et al. Soluble CD40L and cardiovascular risk in women. *Circulation.* 2001;104(19):2266–2268.
24. Naghavi M, Falk E, Hecht HS, et al. From vulnerable plaque to vulnerable patient–Part III: Executive summary of the Screening for Heart Attack Prevention and Education (SHAPE) Task Force report. *Am J Cardiol.* 2006;98(2A):2H–15H.
25. Ward MR, Pasterkamp G, Yeung AC, et al. Arterial remodeling. Mechanisms and clinical implications. *Circulation.* 2000;102(10):1186–1191.
26. Moreno PR, Purushothaman KR, Fuster V, et al. Plaque neovascularization is increased in ruptured atherosclerotic lesions of human aorta: Implications for plaque vulnerability. *Circulation.* 2004;110(14):2032–2038.
27. Virmani R, Kolodgie FD, Burke AP, et al. Atherosclerotic plaque progression and vulnerability to rupture: Angiogenesis as a source of intraplaque hemorrhage. *Arterioscler Thromb Vasc Biol.* 2005;25(10):2054–2061.
28. Fuster V, Moreno PR, Fayad ZA, et al. Atherothrombosis and high-risk plaque: Part I: Evolving concepts. *J Am Coll Cardiol.* 2005;46(6):937–954.
29. Ibanez B, Navarro F, Cordoba M, et al. Tako-tsubo transient left ventricular apical ballooning: Is intravascular ultrasound the key to resolve the enigma? *Heart.* 2005;91(1):102–104.
30. Massberg S, Brand K, Gruner S, et al. A critical role of platelet adhesion in the initiation of atherosclerotic lesion formation. *J Exp Med.* 2002;196(7):887–896.
31. Massberg S, Gruner S, Konrad I, et al. Enhanced in vivo platelet adhesion in vasodilator-stimulated phosphoprotein (VASP)-deficient mice. *Blood.* 2004;103(1):136–142.
32. Huo Y, Ley KF. Role of platelets in the development of atherosclerosis. *Trends Cardiovasc Med.* 2004;14(1):18–22.
33. Ibanez B, Vilahur G, Badimon J. Pharmacology of thienopyridines: Rationale for dual pathway inhibition. *Eur Heart J Suppl.* 2006;8:G3–G9.
34. Ruggeri ZM. Mechanisms initiating platelet thrombus formation. *Thromb Haemost.* 1997;78(1):611–616.
35. Ruggeri ZM. Platelets in atherothrombosis. *Nat Med.* 2002;8(11):1227–1234.
36. Alevriadou BR, Moake JL, Turner NA, et al. Real-time analysis of shear-dependent thrombus formation and its blockade by inhibitors of von Willebrand factor binding to platelets. *Blood.* 1993;81(5):1263–1276.
37. Nieswandt B, Watson SP. Platelet-collagen interaction: Is GPVI the central receptor? *Blood.* 2003;102(2):449–461.
38. Gawaz M. Role of platelets in coronary thrombosis and reperfusion of ischemic myocardium. *Cardiovasc Res.* 2004;61(3):498–511.
39. Andrews RK, Gardiner EE, Shen Y, et al. Platelet interactions in thrombosis. *IUBMB life.* 2004;56(1):13–18.
40. Weyrich AS, Lindemann S, Zimmerman GA. The evolving role of platelets in inflammation. *J Thromb Haemost.* 2003;1(9):1897–1905.
41. Coughlin SR. Thrombin receptor structure and function. *Thromb Haemost.* 1993;70(1):184–187.
42. Sakariassen KS, Bolhuis PA, Sixma JJ. Human blood platelet adhesion to artery subendothelium is mediated by factor VIII-Von Willebrand factor bound to the subendothelium. *Nature.* 1979;279(5714):636–638.
43. Badimon L, Badimon JJ, Turitto VT, et al. Role of von Willebrand factor in mediating platelet-vessel wall interaction at low shear rate; the importance of perfusion conditions. *Blood.* 1989;73(4):961–967.
44. Cattaneo M, Gachet C. ADP receptors and clinical bleeding disorders. *Arterioscler Thromb Vasc Biol.* 1999;19(10):2281–2285.
45. Viles-Gonzalez JF, Badimon JJ. Atherothrombosis: The role of tissue factor. *Int J Biochem Cell Biol.* 2004;36(1):25–30.
46. Nemerson Y. *Mechanisms of Coagulation.* New York: McGraw-Hill; 1990.
47. Mann KG. *Membrane-bound Enzyme Complexes in Blood Coagulation.* New York: Grunne & Stratton; 1984.
48. Comp PC. *Kinetics of Plasma Coagulation Factors.* New York: McGraw-Hill; 1990.
49. Badimon L, Badimon JJ, Turitto VT, et al. Platelet thrombus formation on collagen type I. A model of deep vessel injury. Influence of blood rheology, von Willebrand factor, and blood coagulation. *Circulation.* 1988;78(6):1431–1442.
50. Badimon L, Badimon JJ, Galvez A, et al. Influence of arterial damage and wall shear rate on platelet deposition. Ex vivo study in a swine model. *Arteriosclerosis.* 1986;6(3):312–320.
51. Badimon L, Badimon JJ. Mechanisms of arterial thrombosis in nonparallel streamlines: Platelet thrombi grow on the apex of stenotic severely injured vessel wall. Experimental study in the pig model. *J Clin Invest.* 1989;84(4):1134–1144.
52. Lassila R, Badimon JJ, Vallabhajosula S, et al. Dynamic monitoring of platelet deposition on severely damaged vessel wall in flowing blood. Effects of different stenoses on thrombus growth. *Arteriosclerosis.* 1990;10(2):306–315.
53. Fuster V, Badimon L, Badimon JJ, et al. The pathogenesis of coronary artery disease and the acute coronary syndromes (1). *N Engl J Med.* 1992;326(4):242–250.
54. Mackman N. Role of tissue factor in hemostasis, thrombosis, and vascular development. *Arterioscler Thromb Vasc Biol.* 2004;24(6):1015–1022.
55. Fernandez-Ortiz A, Badimon JJ, Falk E, et al. Characterization of the relative thrombogenicity of atherosclerotic plaque components: Implications for consequences of plaque rupture. *J Am Coll Cardiol.* 1994;23(7):1562–1569.
56. Frojmovic M, Nash G, Diamond SL. Definitions in biorheology: Cell aggregation and cell adhesion in flow. Recommendation of the Scientific Subcommittee on Biorheology of the Scientific and Standardisation Committee of the International Society on Thrombosis and Haemostasis. *Thromb Haemost.* 2002;87(4):771.

57. Naghavi M, Libby P, Falk E, et al. From vulnerable plaque to vulnerable patient: A call for new definitions and risk assessment strategies: Part I. *Circulation.* 2003;108(14):1664–1672.

58. Naghavi M, Libby P, Falk E, et al. From vulnerable plaque to vulnerable patient: A call for new definitions and risk assessment strategies: Part II. *Circulation.* 2003;108(15):1772–1778.

59. Shah PK. Thrombogenic risk factors for atherothrombosis. *Rev Cardiovasc Med.* 2006;7(1):10–16.

60. Markovitz JH, Tolbert L, Winders SE. Increased serotonin receptor density and platelet GPIIb/IIIa activation among smokers. *Arterioscler Thromb Vasc Biol.* 1999;19(3):762–766.

61. Badimon JJ, Badimon L, Turitto VT, et al. Platelet deposition at high shear rates is enhanced by high plasma cholesterol levels. In vivo study in the rabbit model. *Arterioscler Thromb.* 1991;11(2):395–402.

62. Badimon JJ, Lettino M, Toschi V, et al. Local inhibition of tissue factor reduces the thrombogenicity of disrupted human atherosclerotic plaques: Effects of tissue factor pathway inhibitor on plaque thrombogenicity under flow conditions. *Circulation.* 1999;99(14):1780–1787.

63. Sambola A, Osende J, Hathcock J, et al. Role of risk factors in the modulation of tissue factor activity and blood thrombogenicity. *Circulation.* 2003;107(7):973–977.

64. Jaffe AS, Babuin L, Apple FS. Biomarkers in acute cardiac disease: The present and the future. *J Am Coll Cardiol.* 2006;48(1):1–11.

Acute Coronary Syndromes

Kevin Wei
Michael Shapiro

25

1. INTRODUCTION

Each year, over 5 million people present with acute chest pain (CP) to the emergency department (ED) in the United States. The incidence of ST-elevation myocardial infarction (STEMI) has been estimated at 500,000 cases annually in the United States.[1] In the majority who present without diagnostic electrocardiographic (ECG) changes, however, determining the exact etiology of their symptoms continues to present a diagnostic dilemma to physicians. Although the majority of patients have minor causes of CP, most of them will undergo extensive work-ups to exclude non-ST elevation myocardial infarction (NSTEMI), pulmonary embolism, or aortic dissection. The annual incidences of these syndromes have been estimated at 422, 66, and 4 per 100,000 patients respectively,[2-4] making acute myocardial infarction (AMI) the most common serious cause of CP by far. Due to the unreliability of the clinical history, physical exam, chest X-ray (CXR) and early laboratory studies for diagnosing these conditions, ancillary imaging is frequently required. The use of noninvasive imaging techniques including echocardiography, single photon emission computed tomography (SPECT), computed tomography (CT), and cardiac magnetic resonance (CMR) has been shown to be of diagnostic and prognostic utility in patients with suspected acute coronary syndromes (ACS)—making early collaboration between the ED and cardiologists important in the evaluation and triage of patients with CP.

The use of imaging for pulmonary embolism and aortic dissection will be covered in other chapters, while this chapter will focus on ACS—a term that encompasses a wide array of diagnoses from unstable angina pectoris (UAP) to STEMI.

2. PATHOPHYSIOLOGY

An ACS is the clinical manifestation of myocardial ischemia, which is defined as "a decrease in blood flow that results in tissue hypoxia." The sudden decrease in resting myocardial blood flow (MBF) that results in an ACS is usually caused by plaque rupture or erosion, with thrombus formation in the coronary artery.[5] Rarely, an ACS could be the result of coronary artery spasm or dissection, or by increases in myocardial oxygen demand in the setting of hyperthyroidism, severe hypertension, anemia, and so forth.

The degree to which resting MBF is compromised accounts for the wide spectrum of presentations ranging from UAP (which may develop in the setting of an incomplete occlusion of the epicardial coronary artery or in patients with extensive collateralization) to STEMI (complete occlusion with transmural ischemia).

Due to the autoregulatory capacity of the coronary microcirculation, resting MBF remains constant over a wide range of coronary driving pressures.[6] Consequently, MBF does not fall below normal resting levels until a coronary obstruction exceeds 85% to 90% of the luminal area of an epicardial coronary artery.[7] A reduction in resting MBF (and the development of supply/demand mismatch) could result in angina occurring at rest, which is one of the three principal presentations of UAP.[5] Other manifestations of UAP include accelerated angina (increased frequency, duration, or onset at a lower threshold) or new onset angina of at least Canadian Cardiovascular Class III severity (Table 25.1), which may develop in the presence of a severe but noncritical obstruction of the coronary artery.[8] UAP and NSTEMI are part of the same continuum and share the same pathophysiology. With the latter, there is even more profound or prolonged reduction of resting MBF, resulting in more sustained and intense symptoms, coupled with myocardial injury den oted by elevations of biomarkers of necrosis.[5]

3. CLINICAL PRESENTATION AND EVALUATION

Patients presenting to an ED with CP or other symptoms suggestive of an ACS (such as lower jaw or arm discomfort, dyspnea, and diaphoresis) should be rapidly evaluated with the objective of classifying the patient as definite ACS, which is further subdivided into (a) STEMI, (b) NSTEMI, or (c) UAP. Patients with new left bundle branch block on the 12-lead ECG, 0.2 mV ST elevation in anteroseptal leads, or 0.1 mV elevation in other leads can be classified as STEMI and are candidates for immediate reperfusion therapy with fibrinolysis or percutaneous coronary intervention (Fig. 25.1).[1]

In patients who do not appear to be presenting with an ACS, other important provisional diagnoses for the cause of their CP that need to be considered include non-ACS cardiac conditions (such as acute pericarditis), life-threatening noncardiac conditions (such as acute pulmonary embolism, aortic dissection, perforating ulcer, and Boerhaave syndrome), other noncardiac conditions with another specific disease (e.g., esophageal spasm), and undefined noncardiac conditions.

The history, physical examination, ECG, and cardiac markers are currently the main tools used to determine if a patient is presenting with an ACS. These findings are also used to provide initial risk stratification. Features that suggest a high likelihood of ACS secondary to acute plaque rupture include patients whose chief symptom is chest or left arm pain similar to previously documented angina, especially in those with a known history of coronary disease or myocardial infarction; findings on examination of hemodynamic compromise (hypotension) or heart failure (pulmonary edema, rales, and new mitral regurgitation); ECG

TABLE 25.1

CANADIAN CARDIOVASCULAR SOCIETY CLASSIFICATION OF ANGINA

Class	Activity provoking angina	Limitation of activity
I	Prolonged or strenuous exertion	None
II	Walking >2 blocks on the level or climbing >1 flight of stairs	Mild
III	Walking 1–2 blocks on the level or 1 flight of stairs	Marked
IV	Minimal activities or at rest	Severe

abnormalities such as new or dynamic ST-segment depression or deep T-wave inversion; or elevated cardiac serum markers.[5] Most patients in whom a definitive diagnosis of ACS is established are not initially evaluated by noninvasive imaging in order to avoid unnecessary delay in myocardial reperfusion.

Unfortunately, the majority of patients with an ACS do not manifest the symptoms or findings noted above. In a study of 3,814 patients presenting with CP to the ED, 93% of the presenting ECGs were called normal or nondiagnostic. In those patients whose presenting ECG showed only early repolarization, nondiagnostic changes, or was normal, the rate of death, AMI, or revascularization at 30 days was as high as 23%.[9] Thus, a benign ECG at the time of presentation does not confer a good prognosis. Furthermore, as shown in Figure 25.2, the sensitivity of serum cardiac markers for an AMI is very poor until many hours after the onset of symptoms.[10] Because of the time dependent nature of ACS, this delay in the diagnosis and risk stratification of patients may worsen their outcome because definitive treatment is not initiated promptly.

Even though a cardiac event is the most common "serious" etiology of CP, an ACS is eventually diagnosed in only 10% to 30% of patients.[11-13] In the Acute Cardiac Ischemia Time-Insensitive Predictive Instrument (ACI-TIPI) study that included 10,689 patients at least 30 years in age, presenting with chest, left arm, jaw or epigastric pain or discomfort, dyspnea, or other symptoms suggestive of acute ischemia—an ACS was diagnosed in only 17% of patients (AMI in 8% and UAP in 9%), and 6% of patients were considered

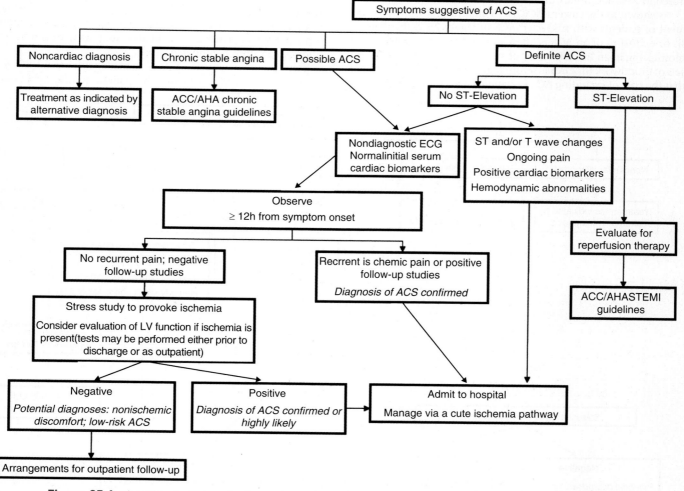

Figure 25.1 Algorithm for the evaluation and management of patients suspected of having ACS. (Redrawn from Anderson JL, Adams CD, Antman EM, et al. ACC/AHA 2007 guidelines for the management of patients with unstable angina/non-ST-elevation myocardial infarction: A report of the American College of Cardiology/American Heart Association Task Force on practice guidelines (Writing committee to Revise the 2002 Guidelines for the Management of Patients with Unstable Angina/Non-ST-Elevation Myocardial Infarction): Developed in collaboration with the American College of Physicians, Society for Academic Emergency Medicine, Society for Cardiovascular Angiography and Interventions, and Society of Thoracic Surgeons. *J Am Coll Cardiol.* 2007;50:e1–e157.)

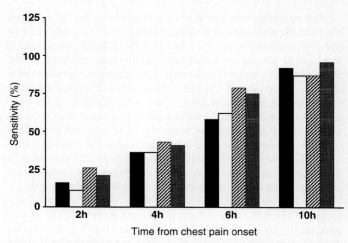

Figure 25.2 Sensitivity of various cardiac serum markers for diagnosis of AMI by time from onset of CP. Troponin T *(white bars)*, Troponin I *(black bars)*, Myoglobin *(hatched bars)*, and CK-MB *(gray bars)*.

to have stable angina. Nonischemic cardiac conditions were diagnosed in 21% and noncardiac problems in 55%.

As shown in the current ACC/AHA algorithm for the management of patients with suspected ACS in Figure 25.2, the diagnosis or exclusion of an ACS is often a prolonged process requiring monitoring in an ED, CP center or step-down unit, with repeated sets of bloodwork for cardiac serum markers. It has been estimated that the cost of excluding ACS in patients with CP represents 8 to

10 billion dollars annually in the United States alone. This process is not only expensive, but time consuming for both physicians and patients.

On the other end of the spectrum, up to 11% of patients are inadvertently discharged from the ED with a missed AMI (average 2.1%), and UAP is missed in up to 4%.[10,14-16] This misdiagnosis and inappropriate discharge leads to increased mortality for those patients who have an AMI outside the hospital.[16]

Thus, in patients with CP but without definitive evidence of ACS at the time of presentation (usually denoted by the presence of ST-elevation, ST-depression or deep T-inversions on the initial ECG, or elevated cardiac serum markers) a diagnostic tool that could improve our diagnostic acumen for ACS and help exclude cardiac CP in all other patients would be invaluable. Such a tool would need to detect either anatomically significant coronary artery disease (CAD), reduced perfusion to myocytes, or the consequences of abnormal perfusion (e.g., abnormal cardiac function). Ideally, such a tool would also have to be rapid, noninvasive, highly accurate, safe, and portable. In recent years, a variety of cardiac imaging modalities that can assess left ventricular (LV) systolic function, myocardial perfusion, or coronary anatomy have been evaluated for this purpose. These include 2D echocardiography, SPECT, CMR, and electron beam or multidetector computed tomography (EBCT or MDCT). An alternative algorithm that utilizes ancillary imaging can therefore be considered in patients without definitive ACS as shown in Figure 25.3, with areas that deviate from the traditional algorithm highlighted in red.

Even after a diagnosis of ACS is made, risk stratification is required to determine whether the patient should be referred

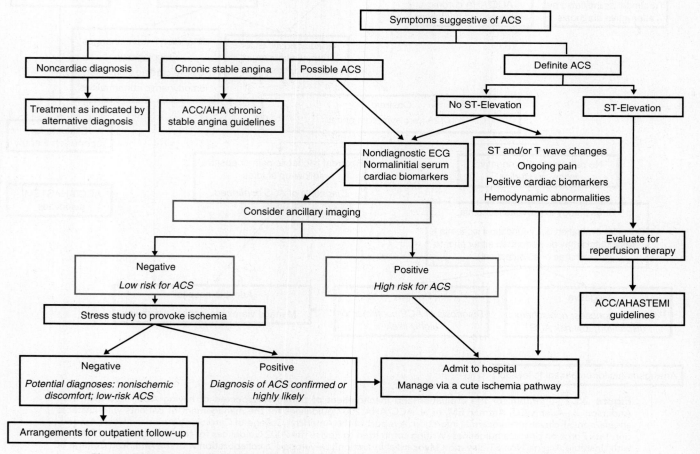

Figure 25.3 Alternative algorithm incorporating ancillary imaging into the evaluation and management of patients suspected of having ACS with a nondiagnostic presenting ECG. ACS, acute coronary syndrome; ECG, electrocardiogram.

for early invasive evaluation or whether the patient can be managed conservatively. High risk clinical features that help earmark patients who are most likely to benefit from early cardiac catheterization include recurrent angina or ischemia at rest or with low-level exertion; elevated cardiac biomarkers; dynamic ST segment depression; congestive heart failure; hemodynamic instability; high grade ventricular arrhythmias; or a history of recent revascularization.[5] Most patients with suspected ACS, however, are clinically at low risk—so ancillary imaging that could risk stratify patients quickly and help determine which patients could benefit from early angiography would also be invaluable.

4. IMAGING IN CHEST PAIN PATIENTS

4.1. Echocardiography

The use of 2D echocardiography to detect NSTEMI or UAP is based on a close relationship between resting MBF and regional wall thickening (WT). Because myocardial contractility is a major determinant of myocardial oxygen consumption, reductions in resting MBF are followed within seconds by the development of hypokinesis. Figure 25.4 illustrates the close coupling that exists between resting MBF and WT.[17] Normal resting MBF (1 mL/kg/min) is associated with WT of ~30%. With acute reductions in resting MBF, WT abnormalities develop within seconds. Thus, the assessment of WT provides an indirect measure of the presence of myocardial ischemia.

In patients who suffer only transient ischemia, even a brief coronary occlusion (5 to 15 min) results in severely reduced regional systolic function.[17] These functional changes occur briskly and are evident for hours after the initial insult, despite reperfusion, and may take up to 48 h to normalize.[18–20] The duration and severity of systolic dysfunction (myocardial stunning) directly relates to the duration of ischemic insult, the severity of the insult, and the adequacy of reperfusion.[18–20]

Early studies evaluating echocardiography in patients presenting to the ED with CP and a nondiagnostic ECG found that analyses of WT had a high sensitivity for detecting AMI (92% to 93%) and cardiac ischemia (88%); however, the specificity was limited to 53% to 57% for AMI and 78% for cardiac ischemia.[21,22]

One of the limitations sited in these early studies was that for optimal sensitivity, the patient must be having active CP. It has

more recently been demonstrated that WT abnormalities can be detected even if patients present many hours after their index event.[23] In patients who suffer an NSTEMI with subendocardial or even patchy myocellular necrosis, WT abnormalities are persistent since WT is derived mainly from the inner 20% to 30% of the myocardium.[24] Although wall motion abnormalities may be present in patients with remote myocardial infarction, abnormal WT in the setting of an ACS is associated with preserved wall thickness, whereas thickness is usually reduced in old scarred segments.

The use of echocardiography to evaluate for WT abnormalities is a Class I indication in patients with suspected myocardial ischemia but nondiagnostic ECG and cardiac serum markers.[25]

4.1.1. Contrast echocardiography

Another limitation of echocardiography includes poor image quality in patients with suboptimal windows, which results in an inability to evaluate WT of all segments accurately. False-negative studies have also been reported in up to 1% of patients with a small AMI detected by serum cardiac markers.[21,22] The former issue has essentially been resolved by the advent of microbubble contrast agents to enhance assessment of left ventricular endocardial borders (LVEBD).[26,27] The two agents currently available for LVEBD in the United States are Optison (GE Healthcare, Princeton, NJ) and Definity (Lantheus Medical Imaging, North Billerica, MA), both of which are composed of high molecular weight gases (perfluoropropane) encapsulated by a thin shell. The low solubility and diffusibility of these gases permit the agents to persist after intravenous administration and opacify the systemic circulation. Their size (smaller than red blood cells) allows the microbubbles to transit unimpeded through the microvasculature.[28]

The microbubble agents used during myocardial contrast echocardiography (MCE) are effective scatterers of ultrasound because they are compressible and oscillate within the sound field. In fact, at the acoustic powers used clinically, microbubbles are easily destroyed by ultrasound. Thus, in order to successfully opacify the LV cavity for LVEBD during high frame rate imaging, the transmit power (as denoted by the mechanical index (MI) on the system) has to be reduced in order to minimize microbubble destruction.

Nonlinear oscillation and destruction of microbubbles by ultrasound produces microbubble signals that are unique from myocardial tissue. These signals can be selectively received by novel imaging modalities designed specifically for MCE. The first MCE modality developed was harmonic imaging, where ultrasound at the fundamental frequency is transmitted, and a high pass filter is used to selectively receive signals at double the transmit frequency (second harmonic). Harmonic imaging is an excellent modality for LVEBD because it is available on all current systems and provides a high frame rate. As noted above, it is important to reduce the MI (to between 0.3 and 0.6) with harmonic imaging to avoid microbubble destruction in the cavity—especially at the apex. The associated reduction in signal can be accommodated by increasing receive gain, which should be adjusted to allow both the endocardial and the epicardial border to be seen. This allows assessment of WT, and not merely endocardial excursion, which can be affected by tethering from adjacent segments. More recently, low MI MCE techniques (see below) that were designed for perfusion imaging have been used for LVEBD, but the frame rates are invariably lower as all these techniques rely on the transmission of multiple ultrasound pulses per line (multipulse techniques).

These imaging modalities allow endocardial borders to be defined with much greater clarity—making even small WT defects identifiable, improving confidence of interpretation, and decreasing inter- and intra-observer variability.[26,27]

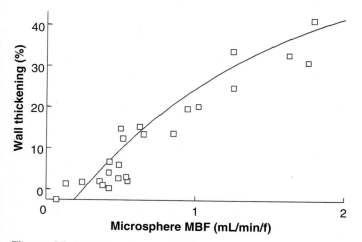

Figure 25.4 Relation between MBF and WT. See text for details. (Redrawn from Leong-Poi, Coggins MP, Sklenar J, et al. Role of collateral blood flow in the apparent disparity between the extent of abnormal wall thickening and perfusion defect size during acute myocardial infarction and demand ischemia. *J Am Coll Cardiol.* 2005;45:565–572.)

Perfusion imaging with echocardiography. MCE can also be used to assess microvascular perfusion (MP). Thus, MCE can directly detect reduced resting MBF (which underlies the development of myocardial ischemia), as well as its consequences on WT.

Unlike the tracers used with CT, CMR, or SPECT, microbubbles remain entirely intravascular, are hemodynamically inert, and have a microvascular rheology identical to that of red blood cells. These properties make microbubbles unique perfusion agents and obviate the need for complex modeling, which is required with many other technologies for quantifying MBF.

For perfusion imaging, sequential ultrasound pulses of differing phase and/or power are transmitted to both generate unique "nonlinear" microbubble signals and suppress tissue signals. Various receive filters are used to selectively receive these nonlinear signals. The ultimate objective of these modalities is to fully optimize the signal (from microbubbles)-to-noise (from tissue) ratio. As shown in Figure 25.5, microbubble backscatter signals (*dotted line,* "a") are of equal intensity to tissue signals (*solid line,* "b") with fundamental imaging, where the transmit and receive frequencies are identical (f_o). With second harmonic imaging (transmit at f_o with receive only at $2f_o$), improvement in the signal-to-noise ratio ("c" vs. "d") is achieved, but strong tissue clutter ("d") is still present. With the recent development of broader band transducers, further improvement in the signal-to-noise ratio ("e" vs. "f") has been accomplished with ultraharmonic imaging (transmit at f_o with receive only at $5/2f_o$), which takes advantage of low tissue noise ("f") at the ultraharmonic while microbubble destruction produces strong microbubble signals ("e") (Fig. 25.5). Harmonic and ultraharmonic imaging use B-mode processing techniques to suppress tissue noise, but Doppler processing can also be used. With the latter, received signals from tissue show little spectral decorrelation compared to the transmitted signal, which can then be suppressed by an appropriate wall filter. Conversely, microbubble destruction produces received signals that are markedly different from those transmitted—consequently, only the power spectrum of microbubbles is displayed (power harmonic Doppler).

Tissue clutter can also be suppressed using multipulse schemes where the amplitude (power modulation) or phase (pulse inversion) of sequential pulses is altered. With power modulation

(Fig. 25.6), pulses at half-height ("a") and full-height amplitude ("b") are transmitted sequentially. The received signals from a linear scatterer such as tissue (Panel A, Fig. 25.6) are identical to the transmitted pulses. Subsequently, the received echoes from the half-height transmitted pulses are scaled and subtracted from the full-height signal, which results in effective removal of tissue clutter. On the other hand, nonlinear scatterers such as microbubbles (Panel B) produce received signals that are different from the transmitted pulses (especially the full-height pulse), resulting in residual microbubble signal even after subtraction. With pulse inversion (Fig. 25.7), sequential pulses of inverted phase are transmitted. Again, linear scatterers (Panel A, Fig. 25.7) produce received signals identical to the transmitted pulses, and summation of the received signals results in cancelation of tissue noise. Nonlinear scatterers (Panel B, Fig. 25.7), however, generate signals that cannot be summed. Both power

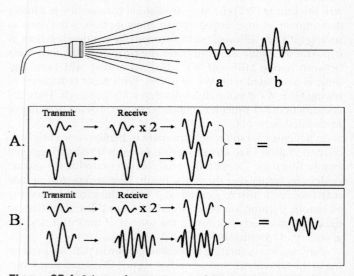

Figure 25.6 Scheme for imaging modalities using power modulation. See text for details. (Redrawn from Wei et al., *Critical Care Med.* 2007;35:S280–S289.)

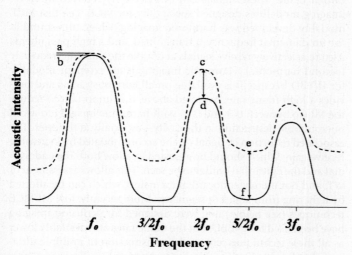

Figure 25.5 Backscatter AI from microbubbles (*dotted line*) and tissue (*solid line*) at the fundamental, harmonic, and ultraharmonic frequencies. See text for details. (Redrawn from Wei et al., *Critical Care Med.* 2007;35:S280–S289.)

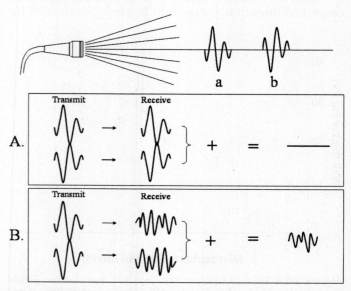

Figure 25.7 Scheme for imaging modalities using pulse inversion. See text for details. (Redrawn from Wei et al., *Critical Care Med.* 2007;35:S280–S289.)

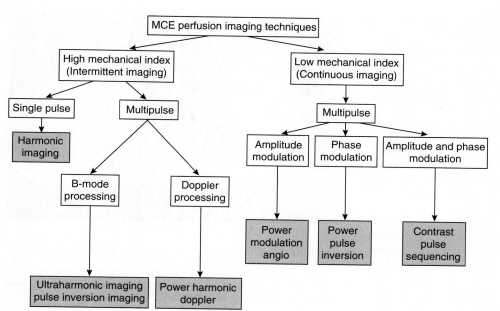

Figure 25.8 Organizational chart for commercially available perfusion imaging modalities. (Redrawn from Wei et al., *Critical Care Med.* 2007;35:S280–S289.)

modulation and pulse inversion have also been combined into a single modality (contrast pulse sequencing) where alternate ultrasound pulses have differing amplitude and phase. As noted above, the ability of these multipulse algorithms to suppress tissue depends on a linear response to the insonating ultrasound, which occurs mainly at low MIs. At high MIs, nonlinear propagation of ultrasound through tissue generates harmonic signals. Thus, these algorithms are incorporated mainly into low MI imaging modes.

The wide array of imaging modalities provides the user with great range and flexibility, and if any particular mode is inadequate for a patient, a different one can be used. A schema is provided in Figure 25.8 to help organize the various imaging modalities currently available on commercial systems.

Quantification of myocardial blood flow with echocardiography. MCE provides a unique solution to the evaluation of MBF because both MBF velocity and myocardial blood volume (MBV) can be determined independently. Microbubbles reside exclusively within the vascular space, so they act as blood pool agents, and their concentration in the myocardium reflects the MBV—90% of which is in capillaries. Thus, steady state contrast enhancement provides an assessment of capillary blood volume.[29]

Flow velocity can be assessed with MCE because microbubbles have the same intravascular rheology as red blood cells.[30,31] Evaluating their transit through the microcirculation provides information regarding red blood cell kinetics. At steady state during a continuous intravenous infusion of microbubbles, the number of microbubbles entering or leaving any microcirculatory unit is constant and will depend on the flow rate. By destroying microbubbles with an ultrasound pulse and then determining the rate of replenishment of microbubbles into tissue, microbubble (or red blood cell) velocity can be determined.[32]

This concept is diagrammatically represented in Figure 25.9. After microbubbles are destroyed by a pulse of ultrasound within the beam elevation (Panel A), the degree of microbubble replenishment into the elevation increases as the pulsing interval is increased since there is more time for replenishment to occur between each

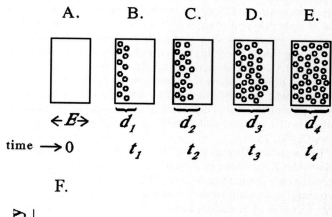

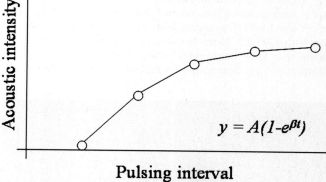

$$y = A(1 - e^{\beta t})$$

Pulsing interval

Figure 25.9 The elevation of the ultrasound beam (*E*), and the degree of replenishment of microbubbles into the elevation (*d*) at different pulsing intervals (*t*) (**Panels A–E**). **Panel F**: Relation between pulsing interval and AI. See text for details. (Redrawn from Wei et al., *Critical Care Med.*)

destructive pulse of ultrasound (Panels B–E). As long as the relation between microbubble concentration and myocardial acoustic intensity (AI) is linear, progressively higher tissue AI is seen at longer pulsing intervals (Panel F). When the pulsing interval is long enough for the entire ultrasound beam elevation to be completely replenished with microbubbles (Panel E), further increases in pulsing interval do not result in any further increases in tissue AI and the pulsing interval versus AI relation plateaus. Plateau myocardial AI represents myocardial (or capillary) blood volume. Since the normal resting blood flow velocity within the capillaries is very low (~1 mm/s) and the ultrasound beam elevation measures approximately 5 mm in thickness, more than 5 s are required between pulses of ultrasound to allow complete replenishment for estimation of capillary blood volume. The pulsing interval versus myocardial AI relation (Panel F) can be fitted to an exponential function: $y = A(1-e^{-\beta t})$, where A is the plateau AI representing capillary blood volume, and β represents the mean microbubble (or red blood cell) velocity. MCE can therefore be used to determine both specific components of MBF—flow velocity (β) and blood volume (A, which is proportional to cross-sectional area).[32]

Perfusion imaging with myocardial contrast echocardiography in chest pain patients. Figure 25.10 shows echocardiographic images from a woman with no prior cardiac history presenting with dyspnea to the ED and a nondiagnostic ECG, demonstrating akinesis of the mid to distal septum, anterior wall, and apex. Perfusion imaging (Fig. 25.11) using harmonic power Doppler imaging was also performed to evaluate resting MBF and the extent of residual viability in the anterior territory since the patient's presentation to the ED was delayed. This demonstrated a slow rate of replenishment of microbubbles into the anterior territory (denoting either very slow antegrade flow in the left anterior descending (LAD) artery due to a critical stenosis, or a completely occluded LAD with slow collateral flow, Panel A, Fig. 25.11). There was, however, nearly complete contrast enhancement of the entire akinetic territory, except for a small subendocardial rim at a long pulsing interval of eight cardiac cycles—denoting extensive microvascular integrity and viability despite prolonged ischemia (Panel B, Fig. 25.11).

The accuracy, clinical utility, and diagnostic and prognostic value of MCE have been evaluated in the ED setting.[33–35] In a multicenter study comparing MCE to SPECT, it was found that the two imaging modalities were equal in their ability to diagnose AMI. In terms of predicting future cardiac events, MCE provided a 17% increase in incremental information for predicting future events which was comparable with the 23% increase in information with SPECT.[33] More recently, MBF assessed with MCE was shown in a large single-center study to increase the diagnostic information over demographic variables, clinical risk factors and

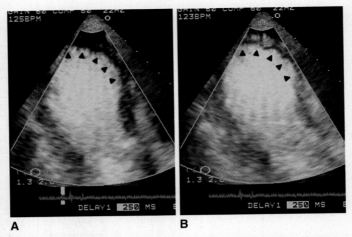

Figure 25.11 Perfusion images from the same patient shown in Figure 25.10, demonstrating slow microbubble replenishment into akinetic zones from the apical three-chamber view (**Panel A**, *arrowheads*), with nearly complete contrast enhancement at long pulsing intervals (**Panel B**, *arrowheads*). See text for details.

ECG data significantly (Bonferroni corrected $p < 0.0001$) for predicting cardiac-related death, AMI, UAP, congestive heart failure, and revascularization within 48 h of ED presentation.[34] When MP was added, significant additional diagnostic information was obtained (Bonferroni corrected $p = 0.0002$).[34]

Apart from the identification of ischemia, accurate risk stratification of CP patients is also important. Those who are intermediate or high risk for an adverse outcome may require admission to a coronary care unit (CCU) or telemetry unit, treatment with potent antiplatelet agents,[36–38] or early referral for cardiac catheterization.[39] MCE can be used to provide earlier and more accurate triage of these patients than clinical evaluation with the thrombolysis in myocardial infarction (TIMI) risk score,[40] which is derived from multiple clinical variables including cardiac troponin-I (cTNI). Because cTNI may not be elevated or immediately available at the time of patient presentation, complete risk stratification and initiation of therapy may be unnecessarily delayed.

The prognostic utility of a score derived only from variables that are available immediately at the time of a patient's presentation to the ED was evaluated.[35] Because laboratory results may not be received for many hours after the initial presentation, a modified TIMI risk score (mTIMI) that excluded cTNI was derived (maximum score of 6). Based on their mTIMI scores, patients were categorized as either low (score ≤ 2), intermediate (score of 3 or 4), or high (score ≥ 5) risk. Although patients with a low mTIMI score had the lowest incidence of primary events, 4.1% of patients still had an early AMI within 24 h of enrollment. Patients with an intermediate score had a similar event rate as those with a high risk score (11% vs. 8.9%, $p = 0.71$). Thus, the mTIMI score was unable to discriminate between these groups.[35]

With MCE, on the other hand, the incidence of a primary (nonfatal AMI or total mortality) event within 24 h of enrollment was only 0.4% in patients with normal RF and MP. In comparison, a 2.3% AMI rate has been reported for patients with CP discharged from the ED based on routine evaluation.[14] The negative predictive value of MCE is therefore excellent. Even in patients with a low mTIMI score, MCE provides further risk stratification. Those patients with abnormal regional function and MP had a significantly worse cardiac outcome than patients with normal MCE (Fig. 25.12).[35] The ability of MCE to provide incremental

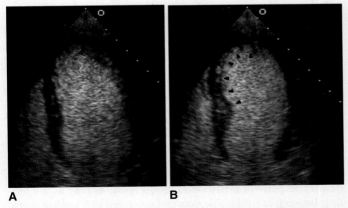

Figure 25.10 Diastolic (**Panel A**) and systolic frames (**Panel B**) from the apical four-chamber view demonstrating the presence of a segmental septal and apical wall motion abnormality (**Panel B**, *arrowheads*) in a patient presenting to the ED with acute dyspnea. See text for details.

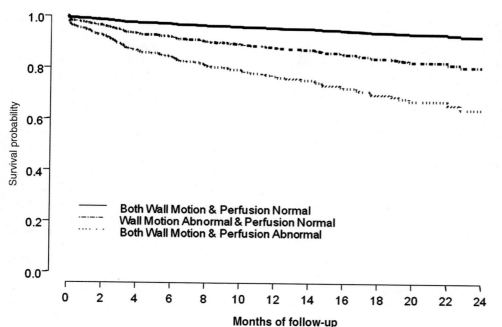

Figure 25.12 Patients at low clinical risk based on a mTIMI score can be further risk stratified using MCE. See text for details. (Reproduced from Tong KL, Kaul S, Wei K, et al. Myocardial contrast echocardiography versus thrombolysis in myocardial infarction score in patients presenting to the emergency department with chest pain and a nondiagnostic electrocardiogram. *J Am Coll Cardiol.* 2005;46:920–927, with permission.)

intermediate (30 day) and late (2 year) prognostic information was also shown in these studies.[34,35]

MCE therefore meets most of the requirements of an ideal tool for the assessment of suspected cardiac CP—it can directly assess the degree and adequacy of MP as well as the presence of WT abnormalities. It is rapid, noninvasive, highly accurate, safe, and portable. For many centers (who would perform and interpret studies after hours, etc.), logistical issues still need to be resolved. The assessment of WT and MP also relies mainly on subjective interpretation, which is associated with well-known limitations. Whether robust and rapid quantitative methods to assess WT (e.g., strain and strain rate imaging) or MP can be developed, or whether these will provide further benefits, remains unclear.

4.2. Nuclear perfusion imaging

The use of nuclear perfusion techniques to evaluate patients with CP is based on the premise that a reduction of resting MBF is associated with a proportional decrease in the uptake of nuclear perfusion tracers.[41,42] Thus, nuclear perfusion techniques provide a direct assessment of reduced resting MBF—the underlying cause of myocardial ischemia.

The first studies utilizing nuclear techniques to diagnose AMI were performed with planar imaging and [201]Thallium.[43] Currently, [201]Thallium has been largely replaced with [99m]Technetium, (^{99m}Tc) sestamibi, or tetrofosmin because of improved energy characteristics and their lack of rapid redistribution (which was a limitation of [201]Thallium).[44] These characteristics make it possible for patients in the ED to be injected with ^{99m}Tc-sestamibi at the time of CP and then imaged hours later to show MP at the time of the patient's symptoms. Planar imaging has also been replaced by SPECT for its improved spatial resolution.

Table 25.2 shows a list of the nuclear studies and their overall sensitivity, specificity, and negative predictive value for diagnosing AMI in patients in the ED.[45-51] The sensitivity for detecting AMI ranged from 90% to 100% with a negative predictive value of 99% to 100%. The limited specificity found in these studies is from the inability of SPECT to distinguish between new and old infarctions—a limitation which is common with other imaging modalities as well.

TABLE 25.2
NUCLEAR IMAGING IN PATIENTS PRESENTING TO THE ED WITH CP AND A NONDIAGNOSTIC ECG

Study	Agent	N	Sensitivity (%)	Specificity (%)	NPV (%)	Endpoint
Varetto et al.[45]	MIBI	62	100	92	100	CAD
Hilton et al.[46]	MIBI	102	94	83	99	CAD/AMI
Tatum et al.[47]	MIBI	438	100	78	100	AMI
Kontos et al.[48]	MIBI	532	93	71	99	AMI
Heller et al.[49]	Tetro-fosmin	357	90	60	99	AMI
Kontos et al.[50]	MIBI	620	92	67	99	AMI
Udelson et al.[51]	MIBI	1215	96	NR	99	AMI

MIBI, ^{99m}Tc-sestamibi Tetrofosmin, ^{99m}Tc-tetrofosmin

In a randomized controlled trial done using SPECT, over 2,400 patients presenting to the ED with CP and nondiagnostic ECGs were randomly assigned to either standard ED evaluation and treatment or SPECT. SPECT imaging was associated with a 32% reduction in the odds of being admitted to hospital for a "rule out."[51] Thus, SPECT may be able to identify low risk patients in the ED who are suitable for discharge, potentially helping to reduce the cost of CP evaluation.

In addition to detecting perfusion defects, ^{99m}Tc-sestamibi SPECT using gated acquisition and reconstruction have the added advantage of assessing regional and global ventricular function.[52-54] This ability to evaluate ventricular function allows SPECT to give prognostic as well as diagnostic information of patients. A recent multicenter study showed that the evaluation of regional function and perfusion provided greater diagnostic and prognostic value than perfusion alone.[33] Their data showed that those patients who had both abnormal wall motion and perfusion defects were significantly more likely to have an AMI compared to those with perfusion defects alone.

Despite the favorable data portrayed in these studies, the diagnostic accuracy of nuclear perfusion studies to detect AMI in CP patients must be interpreted with some caution. Most of the studies enrolled mainly low risk patients—with the low incidence of events, the estimation of the negative predictive value of SPECT may be imprecise. Secondly, most of these studies used CK or CK-MB as the gold standard for the diagnosis of AMI rather than the more sensitive cardiac troponins. It is known that around 3% to 4% of the LV myocardium must be ischemic for a perfusion defect to appear on SPECT,[52] thus, smaller ischemic events detectable only with troponins may not be detected by SPECT, making sensitivity lower. This limitation has been supported by a study that showed normal perfusion by SPECT in 34% of CP patients who were eventually diagnosed with ACS.[49] This study highlighted the limited ability of SPECT to detect unstable angina and smaller ischemic events that are troponin positive but CK-MB negative. Some of these smaller events, however, may be detectable using abnormal RF from gated SPECT.[33]

SPECT has many obvious advantages such as time tested durability, high sensitivity, the combined benefits of evaluating both MP and ventricular function, standardized imaging protocols, and well-established quantitative methods. SPECT is recommended as an appropriate test to consider in patients with suspected cardiac CP and nondiagnostic ECG.[53] An expert panel, however, recently outlined the difficulties of nuclear perfusion imaging, which included decay and license issues, the need for isotope preparation, relative inaccessibility of nuclear laboratories in many hospitals, difficulties with single-image interpretation rather than the usual stress/rest images for comparison, and low spatial resolution.[55]

4.3. Cardiac magnetic resonance imaging

CMR has recently shown promising results in the evaluation of patients with CP. CMR does not expose the patient to ionizing radiation or iodinated contrast agents. CMR has excellent spatial resolution, excellent temporal resolution, intrinsic blood—tissue contrast without the need for administration of an exogenous agent, and can be used to evaluate global and regional wall-motion abnormalities.[56] Valve structure and function, as well as regurgitant lesions, can be assessed with dynamic cine (bright blood) imaging, and the severity of regurgitation can be semi-quantitatively assessed from jet appearance or quantified volumetrically using velocity phase maps.[57] Gadolinium-DTPA can be utilized to assess myocardial perfusion, and the introduction

of delayed-enhancement can determine the presence of viable versus infarcted myocardium.[58-60] The spatial distribution of delayed enhancement may also assist in differentiating ischemic heart disease from other cardiac pathologies (see below). Newer pulse sequences (T2 fast spin echo) allow imaging of myocardial edema, which is particularly useful when evaluating patients with acute CP. The presence of myocardial edema in a patient presenting with acute CP is highly suggestive of ACS.[61]

Although not as advanced in development as MDCT, magnetic resonance angiography can assess proximal and mid coronary artery segments and exclude significant CAD.[62] A recent metaanalysis comparing CMR to MDCT showed MDCT to be superior to CMR in evaluating coronary anatomy; however, CMR still had moderate results including a sensitivity of 72% and specificity of 87% when compared with angiography.[62] It is worth pointing out that as with MDCT, a number of the coronary segments evaluated with CMR were excluded because of motion artifact. Thus, CMR possesses many attributes that make it a potentially excellent method for assessment of patients with suspected ACS.

Similar to echocardiography, CMR can potentially detect acutely ischemic myocardium by identifying segmental RF abnormalities. The reproducibility of CMR for evaluation of LV systolic function is high, with low inter- and intra-observer variability.[63] Figure 25.13 shows short axis images obtained from a 63-year-old man who presented to the ED with exertional CP. His initial evaluation in the ED was negative for myocardial ischemia and infarction. He was referred for a cardiac MRI, which detected a RF abnormality of the inferior wall (end-diastole, Panel A; and end-systole, Panel B).

MP imaging with CMR can be achieved using sequences that demonstrate contrast enhancement within the myocardium after a bolus of contrast.[64,65] The spatial resolution of CMR allows assessment of the transmural extent of a perfusion defect, which is denoted by a subendocardial region that is relatively hypo-enhanced. Figure 25.14 shows a short-axis image obtained using true fast imaging with steady-state precession (FISP) from the same patient in Figure 25.13. A perfusion defect that corresponds to the same territory as the RF abnormality was noted.

The use of CMR in the acute setting of the ED to evaluate patients with CP is less well-established than other modalities presented above. In one study, 161 CP patients presenting to the ED with a nondiagnostic ECG underwent CMR within 12 h of presentation for evaluation of MP and RF. CMR was shown to have a sensitivity of 84% and a specificity of 85% for detection of patients who were having an AMI or unstable angina.[66] The authors pointed out the many advantages of CMR including the high spatial resolution that is able to pick up subtle wall motion abnormalities, which would be undetected by other methods.

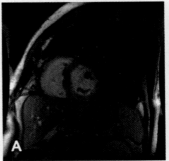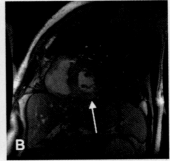

Figure 25.13 End-diastolic and systolic short axis images obtained using CMR in a patient presenting with CP. See text for details.

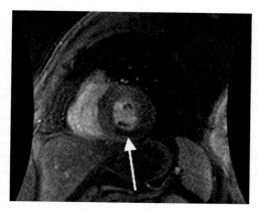

Figure 25.14 Myocardial perfusion imaging on CMR using FISP from the same patient in Figure 25.16. See text for details.

Similar to MCE, CMR has the ability to detect postischemic myocardial stunning by identifying segments with abnormal RF but normal MP. CMR does not expose patients to ionizing radiation or nephrotoxic contrast, it has superior spatial resolution compared to echocardiography and SPECT, can evaluate coronary anatomy, as well as assess MP and RF similar to SPECT and MCE. Thus, CMR is a true "one-stop-shop," but a number of obstacles prevent CMR from becoming a widely accepted tool due to various factors such as cost, limited availability, high complexity, and length of the studies, as well as inability to image patients with claustrophobia, dyspnea, arrhythmias, and metallic implants. Further studies are still needed to evaluate CMR in the acute setting to see if there is a practical application for this technology.

4.4. Computed Tomography

4.4.1. Calcium scoring

The use of EBCT to detect ACS in patients presenting to the ED with CP is based on the measurement of coronary calcium, which has been associated with CAD.[67] Coronary artery calcium scoring by EBCT is performed using 3 mm consecutive slices over the entire heart. Every scan is triggered prospectively by the ECG signal to mid-diastole. Coronary calcium is identified as lesions with a density of 130 HU or above.[68] A score can be calculated using a dedicated algorithm that incorporates the peak density and the area of calcified lesions in all three coronary arteries.[68] Coronary calcium may also be assessed using MDCT—the best reproducibility is obtained using overlapping slice reconstruction, with propectively triggered sequential imaging to help minimize the dose of radiation.[69] Increased coronary calcium has been shown to have an odds ratio of 10.3 for obstructive CAD[70]; however, this data must be weighed against a metaanalysis that showed only a slightly increased risk of cardiac events in an asymptomatic population.[71] There have been a few studies evaluating the use of EBCT to evaluate for coronary calcium as a marker of CAD in patients presenting to the ED with CP.[71–73] These studies showed a high sensitivity (88% to 97%), with a negative predictive value (NPV) of 97% to 98%. However EBCT was limited by a very low specificity of 55% to 59% because the high calcium burden identifies patients who likely have CAD but are not acutely having an ACS in the ED. Moreover, recent studies indicate that a significant number of patients presenting with acute CP, particularly those of younger age, may have a very low calcium score or even a calcium score of 0 and yet have severe coronary stenosis caused by noncalcified plaques.[74] Thus, coronary calcium scoring has really been superseded by the ability

of contrast-enhanced cardiovascular CT angiography (CCTA) to evaluate coronary anatomy and is rarely used alone for the assessment of CP patients today. More detailed discussions about the use of the calcium score scan in symptomatic and asymptomatic patients are available in Chapters 15 and 22.

4.4.2. Contrast enhanced-CT coronary angiography

The use of CCTA in the ED for the evaluation of patients with CP and nondiagnostic ECGs has been increasing over the last few years as newer technology improves the diagnostic quality of the images. The use of 64-slice multidetector CT (MDCT) scanners has shown excellent accuracy for diagnosing CAD. Newer dual-source 64-slice MDCT and 256-slice detectors may further improve temporal resolution and volume coverage, respectively.[69] Cardiac MDCT offers submillimeter isotropic resolution, typically in the range of $400 \mu m$. These advances allow MDCT to evaluate coronary anatomy, ventricular function, and potentially myocardial perfusion—making it an attractive option for the evaluation of patients with suspected ACS. CT also has the added advantage of having a high sensitivity for detecting other serious causes of CP such as aortic dissection and pulmonary embolism.

A typical CCTA can be performed with 60 to 80 mL of contrast media and a breath hold of <10 s. In order to achieve high contrast enhancement in this short time, a contrast agent with a high concentration of iodine (e.g., 370 mgI/mL) should be used along with a test injection or automated threshold-based bolus to ensure proper timing.[69] A saline flush should be performed immediately after administration of contrast to maintain a tight contrast bolus and decrease the total volume of contrast that is needed for the study.[75] The techniques and protocols for CCTA are extensively reviewed in Chapter 9.

The ability to detect and quantify the severity of a coronary stenosis gives MDCT an added benefit over the other imaging modalities discussed so far. A recent metaanalysis showed that MDCT had an 85% sensitivity and a 95% specificity for detecting a stenosis >50% in severity.[76] It is important to point out, however, that a significant number of coronary segments were excluded from analysis in many of these studies because of motion artifact or size <2 mm. Other limitations in MDCT coronary angiography include patients with tachycardia despite the use of betablockade and poor visualization of segments with previous stent placement.

The use of MDCT in the evaluation of acute CP patients in the ED has been evaluated in only small single center studies at this time. Because little data demonstrating CCTA findings in patients with and without ACS are available, there is the potential for inappropriate use of MDCT from additional testing rather than preventing admissions or cost.[69] The North American Society for Cardiac Imaging and the European Society for Cardiac Radiology therefore convened an expert panel to review the literature, identify areas that require more research, and provide interim summary recommendations in preparation for the development of comprehensive guidelines. If ancillary imaging is being considered for a patient with CP as delineated in Figure 25.2, CCTA could be utilized as shown in the algorithm in Figure 25.15.[69]

As discussed above, most patients with CP are admitted to hospital or undergo prolonged observation prior to discharge, and most will not turn out to have an ACS. The powerful negative predictive value of MDCT makes it an attractive option for exclusion of significant CAD in low-risk patients, who can potentially be discharged expediently from the ED. In three recent studies, all of which enrolled adult patients with acute CP that was suspected to be cardiac in etiology, but without initial ECG or

Figure 25.15 Algorithm for use of CCTA in ancillary imaging is considered in a patient with CP.

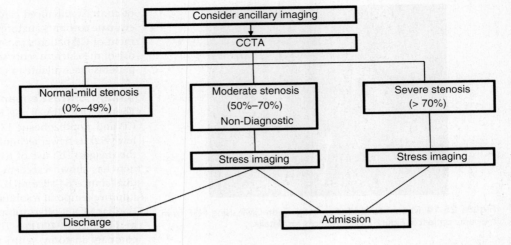

serum biomarker evidence of ischemia—significant CAD (stenosis >50%) was excluded in 60% to 71% of patients.[77–79] The negative predictive value of MDCT for ACS was found to range from 97% to 100%.[77–79] Cardiac events rates (cardiac death, AMI, UAP, etc.,) over a period of 6 to 15 months were very low in patients with minimal abnormalities on MDCT after discharge from the ED.[77,79] Figure 25.16 shows images from a 43-year-old woman who presented to the ED with atypical CP, normal ECG, and negative serum biomarkers. She was referred to cardiac MDCT from the ED. A 3-dimensional volume-rendered image (Panel A), curved multiplanar reformat of LAD coronary artery (Panel B), and multiplanar reformat of right coronary artery (Panel C), demonstrated entirely normal coronary arteries, without evidence of coronary plaque or stenosis. The patient was therefore reassured that her CP was noncardiac in etiology, and she was discharged from the ED without any recommendations for further cardiac testing.

Multivariate regression logistic analyses have shown that MDCT can provide independent incremental risk stratification for the development of an ACS over the clinical evaluation. For every additional segment (total of 17 segments) with plaque, the average increase in odds of having ACS was 1.58 (95% CI, 1.18 to 1.87).[78] Figure 25.17 shows images from a 57-year-old man who presented to the ED with acute CP and an equivocal ECG. Serum biomarkers were initially negative. On cardiac MDCT, a significant stenosis of the midright coronary artery associated with noncalcified plaque [arrow; multiplanar reformat (Panel A) and curved multiplanar reformat (Panel B)] was noted. This lesion was associated with an area of hypoattenuation of the inferior wall, consistent with a perfusion defect (arrow, Panel C). The patient was therefore referred to invasive coronary angiography, which confirmed a hemodynamically significant stenosis of the midright coronary

artery, which was sucessfully revascularized. Although patients, who have significant CAD identified on MDCT, presenting with acute CP are at much higher risk, the positive predictive value of an abnormal CCTA for the development of an ACS is much lower than its negative predictive value (47% to 52%).[78,79] Even though higher noncalcified plaque burden and eccentric remodeling have been found more frequently in patients with ACS, the ability to differentiate "acute" versus "stable" coronary lesions by CCTA is limited.[80] Therefore patients with previously documented CAD or those at high risk probably will not be evaluated by CCTA in the ED. Currently, many patients (up to 25%) may be ineligible for MDCT due to renal insufficiency, tachyarrhythmias, asthma, or inability to comply with breath-hold requirements. In a recent study, significant coronary stenosis could not be excluded in ~17% of studies due to the presence of a prior stent, severe calcification, poor signal-to-noise ratio, or tachycardia.[78]

An important consideration for the use of CT is the exposure to a moderate amount of radiation. This is an increasingly important point of discussion as we further investigate the implications of the vast amount of radiation we expose our patients to in today's highly technological world of medicine. However, with radiation dose reducing strategies, such as prospective triggering, radiation dose has been reduced considerably (~3 to 5 mSv), similar to that of an invasive coronary angiogram. Also, the need for radiographic contrast adds some risk of renal toxicity and hypersensitivity reactions. Similar to SPECT, there is also some potential danger in transporting a patient who is potentially unstable for an imaging study away from a closely monitored setting.

4.5. Detecting mechanical complications of AMI

Differentiation of cardiogenic shock due to extensive myocardial necrosis from mechanical complications such as acute mitral

Figure 25.16 CCTA images from a patient presenting with CP. See text for details.

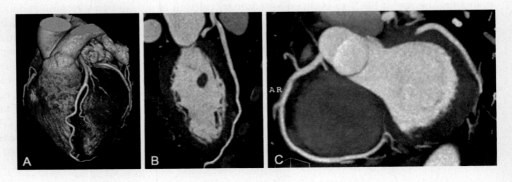

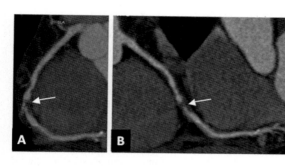
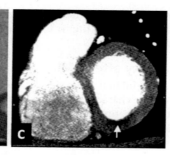

Figure 25.17 CCTA images from a patient presenting with CP. See text for details.

regurgitation due to papillary muscle rupture, ventricular septal rupture, or free wall rupture and tamponade—is critical as recognition of the latter may lead to prompt hemodynamic support and early surgical or other intervention (e.g., percutaneous device closure). Case reports for the detection of mechanical complications of AMI with CT and magnetic resonance are emerging, but the excellent spatial resolution, noninvasive nature, and portability of echocardiography makes it the method of choice for detecting mechanical complications of AMI.[81]

Papillary muscle necrosis and rupture lead to the development of a flail mitral valve leaflet, severe regurgitation, and acute pulmonary edema. It is the least common mechanical complication of AMI.[82] Risk factors for the development of papillary muscle rupture include first infarction, older age, and female gender. Rupture of the anterolateral papillary muscle is less frequent due to its dual blood supply from the diagonal and left circumflex coronary arteries, and rupture of the posteromedial muscle occurs three to six times more frequently.[82] Echocardiographic features may include prolapse or flail mitral valve leaflets, and often identification of the torn papillary muscle as a mobile mass attached to the chordae. Spectral and color Doppler will reveal mitral insufficiency, which may be brief in duration due to noncompliance of the left atrium (LA). Identification of mitral regurgitation may be more difficult if the jet is extremely eccentric. Transesophageal echocardiography may have superior sensitivity in this situation.[83]

Ventricular septal rupture usually presents 3 to 6 days after the index infarction and presents with recurrent CP, heart failure, or shock. Risk factors for its development are similar to those for papillary muscle rupture. The most common site for ventricular septal rupture is the apical posterior septum, and visualization of the defect on transthoracic echocardiography is possible in 40% to 70% of patients.[81] Due to the posterior location of the defect,

off-axis views or apical short axis views may be needed to visualize the defect and the associated left to right shunt. Figure 25.18 shows parasternal long axis images from a patient who developed cardiogenic shock and pulmonary edema with a recent anteroseptal infarct. The echocardiogram demonstrates a large septal rupture in the apical anterior septum (Panel A). Color flow Doppler demonstrates the presence of a large left-to-right shunt (Panel B). Transthoracic echocardiography may not detect all cases of septal rupture as the defect may be a mere serpiginous tunnel or a jagged laceration between the ventricles.[83] However, the sensitivity and specificity of transesophageal echocardiography has been reported to be 100%.[84]

Ventricular free wall rupture occurs equally between the anterior, posterior, and lateral walls.[81] This complication presents with recurrent CP, shock, electromechanical dissociation, and sudden death often during the early convalescent phase after AMI. In the less common subacute form of rupture, adherent pericardium adjacent to the site of rupture may lead to containment of the hemopericardium, which may be recognized echocardiographically as a pseudoaneurysm. Figure 25.19 shows parasternal long axis images from a patient with a huge inferoposterior pseudoaneurysm (PsA, Fig. 25.19). The site of free wall rupture is noted at the base of the papillary muscle. This patient actually developed the pseudoaneurysm as a complication of his or her inferoposterior infarction 2 years prior to presenting for surgical repair.

Apart from the appearance of a thin-walled aneurysm with a narrow neck, color flow Doppler may demonstrate blood flow between the LV and the pseudoaneurysm. In patients with

Figure 25.18 Parasternal long-axis views of a patient with a recent anteroseptal infarct complicated by a ventricular septal defect (VSD) (*green hatch marks*) in the distal septum (**Panel A**). Color flow (**Panel B**) demonstrates a significant left to right shunt. See text for details.

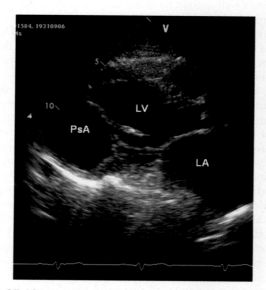

Figure 25.19 Parasternal long-axis image of a patient demonstrating a large apical posterior pseudoaneurysm. LV, left ventricle; LA, left atrium; PsA, pseudoaneurysm. See text for details.

technically limited windows or those with near field noise, the use of contrast for LV border delineation has been shown to improve the detection of apical pseudoaneurysms.[85]

4.6. Assessment of myocardial viability after AMI

Both morbidity and mortality from myocardial infarction are significantly affected by infarct size, which can be characterized by its endocardial length and transmural extent. Experimental studies in dogs have shown that the time course of cell death begins ~30 to 40 min after acute coronary occlusion and occurs initially in the subendocardium where ischemia is most severe.[86] Necrosis extends toward the subepicardium over time and becomes transmural after 6 h. Reperfusion within 2 h can result in functional recovery of the ischemic tissue. This forms the basis for achieving early reperfusion of the infarct-related artery to salvage viable myocardium within the infarct bed and is the primary goal of therapy for patients presenting with AMI.

4.6.1. Assessment of the success of reperfusion and determination of infarct size

Clinical markers of successful reperfusion include resolution of ST-segment elevation, alleviation of angina, and ventricular arrhythmias such as an accelerated idioventricular rhythm. None of these parameters are sensitive or specific for successful reperfusion. The ability of clinical markers to identify successful thrombolysis was previously compared to patency of the infarct-related artery at 90 min after therapy.[87] None of the clinical markers either independently or in combination adequately predicted failure of thrombolytic therapy to open the infarct-related artery.[87] Apart from assessing the success of therapy, identifying patients with unsuccessful thrombolysis may be beneficial, as they may require further interventions such as rescue angioplasty.[88,89]

Even in patients receiving primary angioplasty, it is now recognized that simple recanalization of the infarct-related artery does not ensure a good outcome. Despite patency of the infarct-related artery, microvascular flow may be abnormal due to small vessel spasm, or plugging from thrombi, inflammatory cells, or debris. WT on echocardiography cannot reliably determine the success of reperfusion either, due to the presence of stunning after prolonged ischemia. Global LV segmental wall motion quantified using a wall motion score has been used to define the extent of dysfunctional myocardium within 12 h of presentation of an AMI, and has been shown to correlate with outcome.[89] However, akinesis develops with injury of even the inner 30% of the myocardium, so WT cannot be used to evaluate the transmural extent of viability.[24]

The use of Doppler strain techniques to evaluate regional myocardial deformation can demonstrate abnormal myocardial function from ischemia.[90] This technology has recently been applied to evaluate infarct size early after reperfusion and was compared to contrast-enhanced CMR (see below). The peak negative strain from each of 16 myocardial segments was found to correlate inversely with the transmural extent of infarction on contrast-enhanced CMR. Peak negative strains from all 16 segments were also averaged to obtain an assessment of global strain for the entire LV and was found to have a good inverse relationship with infarct size determined using CMR ($r = 0.77$, $p < 0.0001$).[91]

Another approach to evaluate the success of reperfusion and infarct size is to directly assess MP using MCE. After blood flow is restored to an occluded bed, myocardial opacification should be seen within regions with successful reperfusion. Physiologically, flow within the reperfused bed is heterogeneous and exhibits dynamic fluctuations over time.[92] Using MCE, regions of

significant myocellular injury (necrosis) have microvascular disruption, and show no myocardial contrast enhancement—or "no reflow." These regions may be admixed with others that have normal flow or even reactive hyperemia. Due to the spatial heterogeneity of perfusion in the reperfused myocardium, the extent of the "no reflow" zone on MCE may underestimate the actual infarct size if assessed very early after reperfusion[92,93] but is very accurate by 24 h.[94,95] Figure 25.20 illustrates a subendocardial apical perfusion defect (no-reflow zone) obtained in the apical four-chamber view from a patient who presented with an anterior STEMI that was successfully reperfused with primary angioplasty. The spatial extent of the perfusion defect has been shown to closely match areas of infarction (e.g., using 2,3,5-triphenyltetrazolium chloride staining of pathologic slices), while conversely, areas that demonstrate myocardial contrast enhancement are viable.

Clinical studies have evaluated the relationship between antegrade epicardial flow using the TIMI study group grading system, and the adequacy of MP on MCE. A number of landmark studies have now shown that patients with TIMI grades 1 and 2 flow have a higher incidence of microvascular injury, or "no-reflow" on MCE, than those with TIMI grade 3 flow.[96,97] Even in patients with TIMI grade 3 flow, however, 16% had microvascular no-reflow on MCE,[93] and other studies have found even higher incidences.[98]

The extent of no-reflow on MCE has been shown to have significant consequences. Patients with low- or no-reflow had poor recovery of LV function, greater infarct expansion, remodeling, and LV dilation.[99–101] The relation between recovery of wall motion at 1 month after revascularization in patients with different degrees of no-reflow (contrast score index) are shown in Figure 25.21. At baseline, wall motion was equivalent in all groups. At follow-up, patients with the lowest contrast scores (more no reflow injury) had no significant decrease in the wall motion scores, indicating no improvement in function, while those with significant viability on MCE were much more likely to recover normal resting function. Segments with partial or patchy necrosis had intermediate likelihood of improvement in resting function, but demonstrated contractile reserve with low-dose dobutamine challenge.[101] Moreover, it has been shown that patients with poor microvascular reperfusion have a significantly higher incidence of cardiac events including cardiac death, nonfatal myocardial infarction, and congestive heart failure over a 1 year follow-up period.[99] More recent studies done with intravenously administered contrast agents

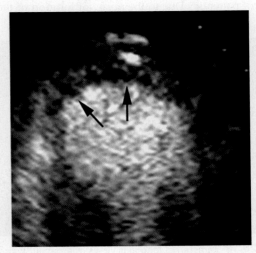

Figure 25.20 Apical four-chamber view obtained using intermittent ultraharmonic imaging. A thin subendocardial area of no-contrast enhancement is noted at the apex. See text for details.

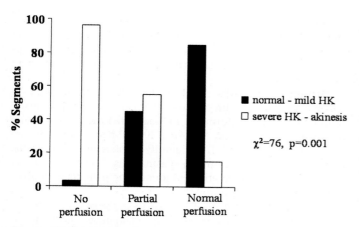

Figure 25.21 Relation between the degree of contrast enhancement on MCE post infarct, and regional segmental function on follow-up echocardiography. See text for details. (Reproduced from Balcells E, Powers E, Lepper W, et al. Detection of myocardial viability by contrast echocardiography in acute infarction predicts recovery of resting function and contractile reserve. *J Am Coll Cardiol.* 2003;41:827–833, with permission.)

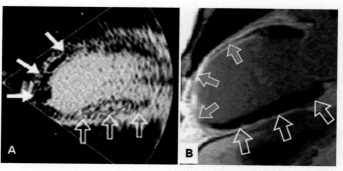

Figure 25.22 Contrast-enhanced MCE image (**Panel A**) and the corresponding delayed hyperenhancement CMR image (**Panel B**) from a patient with prior anteroapical infarction. See text for details. (Reproduced from Janardhanan R, Moon JCC, Pennell DJ, et al. Myocardial contrast echocardiography accurately reflects transmurality of myocardial necrosis and predicts contractile reserve after acute myocardial infarction. *Am Heart J.* 2005;149:355–362, with permission.)

show good concordance between MCE and SPECT for detection of viability, and dysfunctional segments that demonstrated myocardial contrast enhancement had better recovery of wall motion than segments with no-reflow.[102] The presence of reflow defined by MCE 24 h after reperfusion has been found to be associated with higher coronary flow reserve than patients with no-reflow, and these authors also found that these segments had better improvement in regional and global ventricular function at follow-up.[103] Currently, neither strain nor MCE are used routinely for the assessment of infarct size or viability early after AMI.

SPECT imaging with Thallium has been used extensively for identifying viable myocardium.[104,105] Thallium behaves as a potassium analogue and is transported into myocytes with an intact sarcolemmal membrane—thus Thallium uptake denotes the presence of both perfusion and myocellular integrity. ^{99m}Tc has some advantages over thallium due to its shorter half-life, the presence of higher-energy gamma emission which reduces soft-tissue attenuation, and the ability to perform ECG-gated acquisition.[106] SPECT imaging can identify viable tissue and can predict improvement of function after revascularization.[107] Some inherent limitations of SPECT include its poor spatial resolution and the inability to determine the transmural extent of viability, exposure of patients to ionizing radiation, and underestimation of the extent of viability in thinned akinetic segments due to the partial volume effect.[108]

An assessment of myocardial wall thickness and MP imaging with CMR can be used to assess myocardial viability, but delayed-enhancement imaging has become the main method for evaluation of the transmural extent of necrosis and viability. The use of segmented T_1-weighted inversion-recovery-prepared, fast, low-angle-shot imaging performed 5 to 20 min after intravenous administration of 0.1 to 0.2 mmol/kg gadolinium contrast medium demonstrates hyperenhancement of nonviable myocardium, while viable tissue appears hypointense.[109] The excellent spatial resolution of CMR provides a precise estimate of the location and extent of necrotic myocardium. Improvement of regional myocardial function after revascularization has been shown to correlate with the transmural extent of hyperenhancement.[109,110]

Gadolinium-based contrast agents used with CMR diffuse into the interstitial space, and hyperenhancement imaging represents a measure of the increased interstitial space from myocyte loss. Since myocyte loss is accompanied by microvascular loss, perfusion defects on MCE should correlate spatially with areas of hyperenhancement on CMR.[111] Figure 25.22 shows MCE and contrast-enhanced CMR images from a patient who sustained an anterior AMI. A transmural zone of no-reflow is denoted by the lack of contrast enhancement in the mid to distal anterior wall and apex on MCE images from the apical two-chamber view (re-oriented to match CMR images, Panel A). The CMR images from the same patient demonstrated >75% transmural delayed hyperenhancement in the same segments showing no-reflow on MCE (Panel B). Qualitative assessment of MCE showed that absence of opacification was associated with >50% transmural delayed hyperenhancement in 92% of patients. Quantitative assessment of an abnormal rate of myocardial replenishment of microbubbles (β) on MCE provided the best correlation with CMR.[111]

A more extensive discussion of the application of noninvasive imaging methods for evaluation of myocardial viability in patients with chronic ischemic heart disease is available in Chapter 26.

5. FUTURE DIRECTIONS FOR NONINVASIVE IMAGING IN ACS

Active research is ongoing with many of the above imaging modalities to address issues such as how to separate acute from chronic injury and how to detect recent ischemia in patients who have had spontaneous reperfusion and re-establishment of normal perfusion.

For MCE, the ability of microbubbles to detect specific molecular events within the circulation is an area of vigorous research at this time. In ischemia-reperfusion injury, inflammation is a prominent feature. By changing the rheology of microbubbles in the circulation—microbubbles can be made to accumulate at sites of inflammation by attaching to upregulated molecules there. Initial methods for imaging inflammation by microbubble retention relied on nonspecific interactions between microbubbles and activated leukocytes. For example, the denatured albumin shell of Optison could attach to leukocytes via the β_2-integrin Mac-1 and lipid microbubbles such as Definity attached by opsonization with serum complement.[112] More recently, specific "targeted" microbubbles have been developed with more robust attachment to activated leukocytes, or even to the endothelial surface itself.

Strategies that have been used include the addition of phosphatidylserine to the lipid shell to increase complement deposition[113] or the conjugation of specific ligands (such as monoclonal antibodies or peptides) to the microbubble surface.[114,115] This technique has been used to specifically image the molecular mediators of leukocyte recruitment such as the selectins, ICAM-1, VCAM-1, and MAdCAM-1.

The ability of MCE to detect regional myocardial inflammation was tested in an animal experimental model of LAD coronary artery occlusion for 90 min followed by reperfusion. Phosphatidylserine-lipid-shelled microbubbles targeted to activated leukocytes were injected 60 min after reperfusion followed by imaging 15 min later. Figure 25.23 shows the MCE images (Panel A) and a 2,3,5-triphenyl tetrazolium chloride-stained slice of myocardium (to delineate infarction, Panel B). The short-axis background-subtracted color-coded MCE image demonstrates an area of contrast enhancement (green and red) from retained targeted microbubbles. The location and spatial extent of inflammation on MCE includes not only the area of myocardial necrosis (Panel B), but also the surrounding ischemic myocardium that was salvaged by reperfusion. Even up to 120 min after reperfusion, such MCE images of "ischemic memory" should be able to define the presence of recent ischemia, but significant delays between the event and imaging may limit the sensitivity of even MCE. Such issues still require further study.

Real time 3D echocardiography is an emerging technique that has the potential to enhance cardiac functional assessment.[116] 2D echocardiography and MCE can be limited by the inability to visualize all wall segments and the necessity of mentally reconstructing multiple images in the 2D plane. 3D echocardiography makes it possible to instantly obtain 3D imaging of the heart. This technique ensures identification of all wall segments and is potentially more sensitive in identifying small wall motion abnormalities. The role of 3D echo and its benefits over MCE have not been evaluated in patients with CP.

As noted above, many patients continue to present to the ED late after the onset of CP. The detection of myocardial ischemia may not be possible with the assessment of MP if spontaneous reperfusion and restoration of normal MBF has occurred or with RF if stunning has resolved. In the setting of myocardial ischemia, the myocardium shifts high energy ATP production from fatty acid metabolism (which is the preferred metabolic pathway) to glucose utilization.[117] Studies have shown, however, that imaging of an iodinated fatty acid analogue, 15-(p-[iodine-123] iodophenyl-3-(R,S) methylpentadecanoic acid (BMIPP)) using SPECT can identify previous severe ischemia as areas of reduced tracer uptake.

BMIPP is trapped in cardiomyocytes with limited catabolism[118] and can be imaged clinically with labeling using [123]I. Myocardial uptake of BMIPP after an ischemic insult is diminished due to reduced activation of fatty acids by coenzyme A and less fatty acid metabolism.[117]

The ability of BMIPP SPECT to identify recent ischemia in patients presenting with CP was evaluated in 111 patients.[119] BMIPP SPECT was performed 1 to 5 days after the disappearance of the last episode of CP. Abnormal BMIPP had greater sensitivity than tetrofosmin SPECT for identifying patients with ischemia due to fixed CAD or vasomotor spasm. Thus, "ischemic memory imaging" may be one method of identifying patients with acute cardiac causes of CP but no MI.

Metabolic derangements develop early in the ischemic cascade, and maintenance of cellular levels of high-energy phosphates is needed to preserve myocardial function. With severe myocardial ischemia, there is a rapid loss of phosphocreatine and a decrease in the ratio of phosphocreatine to ATP.[120] Using CMR, myocardial energy metabolism can be assessed with Phosphorus 31 nuclear magnetic resonance [^{31}P-nuclear magnetic resonance (NMR)] spectroscopy. ^{31}P spectra using NMR spectroscopy can therefore potentially be used to detect one of the earliest metabolic derangements due to myocardial ischemia.

The use of the phosphocreatine:ATP ratio to detect ischemia using ^{31}P-NMR spectroscopy was evaluated in women admitted to hospital with CP who were found to have no significant CAD on angiography.[121] The change in phosphocreatine:ATP ratio in this group was compared to normal controls and to patients with known severe stenosis (>70%) of the LAD coronary artery. Isometric hand-grip exercise at 30% of maximal grip strength was used as the stressor. In the reference group, the phosphocreatine:ATP ratio decreased by 2.6 ± 10% during stress. The decrease was significantly greater in patients with CAD, where the phosphocreatine:ATP ratio dropped by 20 ± 11%. In patients with CP but normal coronary arteries, 7 of the 35 women had a significant decrease in phosphocreatine:ATP ratio of 29 ± 5.1%—presumably due to diffuse CAD with no focal luminal stenosis or microvascular disease. In the Women's Ischemia Syndrome Evaluation (WISE) study, the detection of ischemia using the phosphocreatine:ATP ratio has been found to predict outcome in women with CP despite the absence of epicardial CAD. Patients with an abnormal ratio had significantly higher rates of hospitalization for angina, catheterization, and treatment costs.[122]

6. FUTURE DIRECTIONS

The diagnosis of ACS, and the differentiation of patients presenting with ACS from benign causes of CP remains a challenge. Echocardiography, SPECT, CT, and CMR have all been used to assist in the assessment of these patients, and all of them have their own strengths and weaknesses when compared to the others. SPECT and echocardiography are well-established technologies that can directly assess the presence of myocardial ischemia and its functional consequence on RF; newer and more expensive techniques such as MDCT and CMR can directly assess coronary anatomy and have just started to be evaluated in the acute CP setting. There are no studies that directly compare these technologies, and more data are clearly needed before the question of whether anatomic imaging or perfusion/function imaging is the better approach can be determined. Other comparisons such as relative safety, availability, logistics, and cost-effectiveness between the various technologies are also lacking.

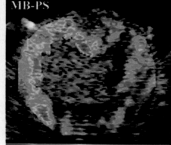
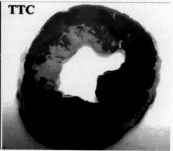

Figure 25.23 Contrast-enhanced MCE image obtained using phosphatidylserine (PS)-labeled microbubbles after reperfusion (**Panel A**) and the 2,3,5-triphenyltetrazolium chloride stained image (**Panel B**). See text for details.

Of all the imaging modalities, MCE is the only one that is portable. The images do not require expensive software or other technology for off-line processing prior to interpretation, and any trained cardiologist can read the study at the bedside or potentially over the internet, providing near-instantaneous results in the acute cardiac setting where time is of the essence. MCE is also relatively cheap compared to other technologies. However, in comparison to SPECT, CMR, or CT where an imaging protocol can be fairly easily standardized, MCE relies most heavily on the skill and expertise of the sonographer and is probably the technology most affected by patient habitus (and the adequacy of the acoustic window). Apart from these issues, the choice of which modality to use depends on personnel and infrastructure available at each institution—to accommodate imaging after normal working hours, for studies to be interpreted rapidly, and for results to be communicated quickly to the ordering physician.

Despite these and other questions that need to be answered before any one technique will be used exclusively, the future of noninvasive cardiac imaging remains an exciting and ever changing field. The adaptation of any one of these techniques into their proper role in ED will take considerably more time and effort in terms of research, money, and clinical experience.

REFERENCES

1. Antman EM, Anbe DT, Armstrong PW, et al. ACC/AHA guidelines for the management of patients with ST-elevation myocardial infarction: A report of the American College of Cardiology/American Heart Association Task Force on Practice Guidelines (Committee to Revise the 1999 Guidelines for the Management of Patients with Acute Myocardial Infarction). 2004. Available at www.acc.org/clinical/guidelines/stemi/index.pdf.
2. American Heart Association. *Heart Disease and Stroke Statistics—2008 Update.* Dallas, TX: American Heart Association; 2008.
3. Silverstein MD, Heit JA, Mohr DN, et al. Trends in the incidence of deep vein thrombosis and pulmonary embolism. A 25-year population-based study. *Arch Intern Med.* 1998;158:585–593.
4. Tsai TT, Nienaber CA, Eagle KA. Acute aortic syndromes. *Circulation.* 2005;112: 3802–3813.
5. Anderson JL, Adams CD, Antman EM, et al. ACC/AHA 2007 guidelines for the management of patients with unstable angina/non-ST-elevation myocardial infarction: a report of the American College of Cardiology/American Heart Association Task Force on practice guidelines (Writing committee to Revise the 2002 Guidelines for the Management of Patients with Unstable Angina/Non-ST-Elevation Myocardial Infarction): Developed in collaboration with the American College of Physicians, Society for Academic Emergency Medicine, Society for Cardiovascular Angiography and Interventions, and Society of Thoracic Surgeons. *J Am Coll Cardiol.* 2007;50:e1–e157.
6. Rouleau J, Boerboom LE, Surjadhana A, et al. The role of autoregulation and tissue diastolic pressures in the transmural distribution of left ventricular blood flow in anesthetized dogs. *Circ Res.* 1979;45:804–815.
7. Gould KL, Lipscomb K. Effects on coronary stenoses on coronary flow reserve and resistance. *Am J Cardiol.* 1974;34:48–55.
8. Campeau L. Grading of angina pectoris (letter). *Circulation.* 1976;54:522–523.
9. Forest RS, Shofer FS, Sease KL, et al. Assessment of the standardized reporting guidelines ECG classification system: The presenting ECG predicts 30 day outcomes. *Ann Emerg Med.* 2004;44:206–212.
10. Pope JH, Ruthazer R, Beshansky JR, et al. The clinical presentation of patients with acute cardiac ischemia in the emergency department: A multicenter controlled clinical trial. *J Thromb Thrombolysis.* 1998;6:63–74.
11. Strussman BJ. National Hospital Ambulatory Medicine Care Survey: 1995 Emergency Department Summary. *Advance Data from Vital and Health Statistics of the Center for Disease Control Prevention/National Center for Health Statistics.*1997;285:1–18.
12. Gilber WB, Lewis LM, Erb RE, et al. Early detection of acute myocardial infarction in patients presenting with chest pain and nondiagnostic ECGs: Serial CK-MB sampling in the emergency department. *Ann Emerg Med.* 1990;9:1359–1366.
13. Gilber WB, Young CP, Hedges JR, et al. Acute myocardial infarction in chest pain patients with non-diagnostic ECG's: Serial CK-MB sampling in the emergency department. *Ann Emerg Med.* 1992;21:504–512.
14. Pope JH, Aufderheide TP, Ruthazer R, et al. Missed diagnosis of acute cardiac ischemia in the emergency department. *N Eng J Med.* 2000;342: 1163–1170.
15. McCarthy BD, Beshansky JR, D'Agostino RB, et al. Missed diagnoses of acute myocardial infarction in the emergency department: Results from a multicenter study. *Ann Emerg Med.* 1993;22:579–582.
16. Lee TH, Rouan GW, Weisberg MC, et al. Clinical characteristics and natural history of patients with acute myocardial infarction sent home from the emergency room. *Am J Cardiol.* 1987;60:219–224.
17. Leong-Poi, Coggins MP, Sklenar J, et al. Role of collateral blood flow in the apparent disparity between the extent of abnormal wall thickening and perfusion defect size during acute myocardial infarction and demand ischemia. *J Am Coll Cardiol.* 2005;45:565–572.
18. Heyndrickx GR, Baig H, Nellens P, et al. Depression of regional blood flow and wall thickening after brief coronary occlusions. *Am J Physiol.* 1978;234:H653–H659.
19. Kloner RA, Jennings RB. Consequences of brief ischemia: Stunning, preconditioning, and their clinical implications: Part 1. *Circulation.* 2001;104: 2981–2989.
20. Nixon JV, Brown CN, Smitherman TC. Identification of transient and persistent segmental wall motion abnormalities in patients with unstable angina by two-dimensional echocardiography. *Circulation.* 1982;65:1497–1503.
21. Sabia P, Afrookteh A, Touchstone D, et al. Value of regional wall motion abnormality in the emergency room diagnosis of acute myocardial infarction. *Circulation.* 1991;84:I85–I92.
22. Villanueva FS, Sabia PJ, Afrookteh A, et al. Value and limitations of current methods of evaluating patients presenting to the emergency room with cardiac-related symptoms for determining long-term prognosis. *Am J Cardiol.* 1992;69:746–750.
23. Kalvaitis S, Kaul S, Tong KL, et al. Effect of time delay on the diagnostic use of contrast echocardiography in patients presenting to the emergency department with chest pain and no S-T segment elevation. *J Am Soc Echocardiogr.* 2006;19:1488–1493.
24. Lieberman AN, Weiss JL, Jugdutt BI, et al. Two-dimensional echocardiography and infarct size: relationship of regional wall motion and thinning to the extent of myocardial infarction in the dog. *Circulation.* 1981;63:739–746.
25. Douglas PS, Khandheria B, Strainback RF, et al. ACCF/ASE/ACEP/ASNC/SCAI/SCCT/SCMR 2007 appropriateness criteria for transthoracic and transesophageal echocardiography. *J Am Coll Cardiol.* 2007;50:187–204.
26. Mulvagh SL, DeMaria AN, Feinstein SB, et al. Contrast echocardiography: Current and future applications. *J Am Soc Echocardiogr.* 2000;12:331–342.
27. Ward RP, Mor-Avi V, Lang, RM. Assessment of left ventricular function with contrast echocardiography. *Cardiol Clin.* 2004;22:211–219.
28. Keller MW, Segal SS, Kaul S. The behaviour of sonicated albumin microbubbles within the microcirculation: A basis for their use during myocardial contrast echocardiography. *Circ Res.* 1989;65:458–467.
29. Jayaweera AR, Wei K, Coggins M, et al. Role of capillaries in determining coronary blood flow reserve: New insights using myocardial contrast echocardiography. *Am J Physiol.* 1999;277:H2363–H2372.
30. Keller MW, Segal SS, Kaul S. The behaviour of sonicated albumin microbubbles within the microcirculation: A basis for their use during myocardial contrast echocardiography. *Circ Res.* 1989;65:458–467.
31. Jayaweera AR, Edwards N, Glasheen WP, et al. In vivo myocardial kinetics of air-filled albumin microbubbles during myocardial contrast echocardiography. Comparison with radiolabeled red blood cells. *Circ Res.* 1994;74:1157–1165.
32. Wei K, Jayaweera AR, Firoozan S, et al. Quantification of myocardial blood flow using ultrasound-induced destruction of microbubbles administered as a constant venous infusion. *Circulation.* 1998;97:473–483.
33. Kaul S, Senior R, Harrel FE, et al. Incremental value of cardiac imaging in patients presenting to the emergency department with chest pain and without ST-segment elevation: A multicenter study. *Am Heart J.* 2004;148:129–136.
34. Rinkevich D, Kaul S, Wang XQ, et al. Regional left ventricular perfusion and function in patients presenting to the emergency department with chest pain and no ST-segment elevation. *Eur Heart J.* 2005;26:1606–1611.
35. Tong KL, Kaul S, Wei K, et al. Myocardial contrast echocardiography versus thrombolysis in myocardial infarction score in patients presenting to the emergency department with chest pain and a nondiagnostic electrocardiogram. *J Am Coll Cardiol.* 2005;46:920–927.
36. A comparison of aspirin plus tirofiban with aspirin plus heparin for unstable angina. Platelet Receptor Inhibition in Ischemic Syndrome Management (PRISM) Study Investigators. *N Engl J Med.* 1998;338:1498–1505.
37. Inhibition of the platelet glycoprotein IIb/IIIa receptor with tirofiban in unstable angina and non-Q-wave myocardial infarction. Platelet Receptor Inhibition in Ischemic Syndrome Management in Patients Limited by Unstable Signs and Symptoms. (PRISM-PLUS) Study Investigators. *N Engl J Med.* 1998;338: 1488–1497.
38. Inhibition of platelet glycoprotein IIb/IIIa with eptifibatide in patients with acute coronary syndromes. The PURSUIT Trial Investigators. Platelet Glycoprotein IIb/IIIa in Unstable Angina: Receptor Suppression Using Integrilin Therapy. *N Engl J Med.* 1998;339:436–443.
39. Cannon CP, Weintraub WS, Demopoulos LA, et al. TACTICS (Treat Angina with Aggrastat and Determine Cost of Therapy with an Invasive or Conservative Strategy)—Thrombolysis in Myocardial Infarction 18 Investigators: Comparison of early invasive and conservative strategies in patients with unstable coronary syndromes treated with the glycoprotein IIb/IIIa inhibitor tirofiban. *N Engl J Med.* 2001;344:1879–1887.
40. Antman E, Cohen M, Bernink PJL, et al. The TIMI risk score for unstable angina/non-ST elevation MI. A method for prognostication and therapeutic decision making. *JAMA.* 2000; 284:835–842.
41. Glover DK. Ruiz M. Edwards NC, et al. Comparison between ^{201}Tl and ^{99m}Tc sestamibi uptake during adenosine-induced vasodilation as a function of coronary stenosis severity. *Circulation.* 1995;91:813–820.
42. Okada RD, Glover D, Gaffney T, et al. Myocardial kinetics of technetium-99 m-hexakis-2-methoxy-2-methlpropyl-isonitrile. *Circulation.* 1988;77: 491–498.

43. Wackers FJ, Lie KI, Liem KL, et al. Potential value of thallium-201 scintigraphy as a means of selecting patients for the coronary care unit. *Br Heart J.* 1979;41:111–117.

44. Beller GA, Glover DK, Edwards NC, et al. Watson DD. ^{99m}Tc-sestamibi uptake and retention during myocardial ischemia and reperfusion. *Circulation.* 1993;87:2033–2042.

45. Varetto T, Cantalupi D, Altieri A, et al. Emergency room technetium-99 m sestamibi imaging to rule out acute myocardial ischemic events in patients with nondiagnostic electrocardiograms. *J Am Coll Cardiol.* 1993;22:1804–1808.

46. Hilton TC, Thompson RC, Williams HJ, et al. Technetium-99 m sestamibi myocardial perfusion imaging in the emergency room evaluation of chest pain. *J Am Coll Cardiol.* 1994;23:1016–1022.

47. Tatum JL, Jesse RL, Kontos MC, et al. Comprehensive strategy for the evaluation and triage of the chest pain patient. *Ann Emerg Med.* 1997;29:116–123.

48. Kontos MC, Jesse RL, Schmidt KL, et al. Value of acute rest sestamibi perfusion imaging for evaluation of patients admitted to the emergency department with chest pain. *J Am Coll Cardiol.* 1997;30:976–982.

49. Heller GV, Stowers SA, Hendel RC, et al. Clinical value of acute rest technetium-99 m tetrofosmin tomographic myocardial perfusion imaging in patients with acute chest pain and nondiagnostic electrocardiograms. *J Am Coll Cardiol.* 1998;31:1011–1017.

50. Kontos MC, Jesse RL, Anderson FP, et al. Comparison of myocardial perfusion imaging and cardiac troponin I in patients admitted to the emergency department with chest pain. *Circulation.* 1999;99:2073–2078.

51. Udelson JE, Beshansky JR, Ballin DS, et al. Myocardial perfusion imaging for evaluation and triage of patients with suspected acute cardiac ischemia: A randomized controlled trial. *JAMA.* 2002;288:2693–2700.

52. O'Connor MK, Hammell T, Gibbons RJ. In vitro validation of a simple tomographic technique for estimation of percentage myocardium at risk using methoxyisobutyl isonitrile technetium 99 m (sestamibi). *Eur J Nucl Med.* 1990;17:69–76.

53. Brindis RG, Douglas PS, Hendel RC, et al. ACCF/ASNC appropriateness criteria for single-photon emission computed tomography myocardial perfusion imaging (SPECT MPI): A report of the American College of Cardiology Foundation Quality Strategic Directions Committee Appropriateness Criteria Working Group and the American Society of Nuclear Cardiology. *J Am Coll Cardiol.* 2005;46:1587–1605.

54. Mannting F, Morgan-Mannting MG. Gated SPECT with technetium-99 m-sestamibi for assessment of myocardial perfusion abnormalities. *J Nucl Med.* 1993;34:601–608.

55. Heller GV, Udelson JE, Ziffer J, et al. Assessing suspected acute cardiac ischemia in the emergency department: Logistics, testing modalities, implications for perfusion imaging. *J Nucl Cardiol.* 2001;8:274–285.

56. Wagner S, Auffermann W, Buser P, et al. Functional description of the left ventricle in patients with volume overload, pressure overload, and myocardial disease using cine magnetic resonance imaging. *Am J Cardiac Imag.* 1991;5:87–97.

57. Lotz J, Meier C, Leppert A, et al. Cardiovascular flow measurement with phase-contrast MR imaging: basic facts and implementation. *Radiographics.* 2002;22:651–671.

58. Kim RJ, Chen EL, Lima JA, et al. Myocardial Gd-DTPA kinetics determine MRI contrast enhancement and reflect the extent and severity of myocardial injury after acute reperfused infarction. *Circulation.* 1996;94:3318–3326.

59. Kim RJ, Fieno DS, Parrish TB, et al. Relationship of MRI delayed contrast enhancement to irreversible injury, infarct age, and contractile function. *Circulation.* 1999;100:1992–2002.

60. Setser RM, Bexell DG, O'Donnell TP, et al. Quantitative assessment of myocardial scar in delayed enhancement magnetic resonance imaging. *J Magn Reson Imag.* 2003;18:434–441.

61. Aletras AH, Tilak GS, Natanzon A, et al. Retrospective determination of the area at risk for reperfused acute myocardial infarction with T2-weighted cardiac magnetic resonance imaging: histopathological and displacement encoding with stimulated echoes (DENSE) functional validations. *Circulation.* 2006;113:1865–1870.

62. Kaandorp TAM, Lamb HF, Bax JJ, et al. Magnetic resonance imaging of coronary arteries, the ischemic cascade, and myocardial infarction. *Am Heart J.* 2005;149:200–208.

63. Barkhausen J, Ruehm SG, Goyen M, et al. MR evaluation of ventricular function: true fast imaging with steady- state precession versus fast low-angle shot cine MR imaging: feasibility study. *Radiology.* 2001;219:264–269.

64. Chiu CW, So NM, Lam WW, et al. Combined first-pass perfusion and viability study at MR imaging in patients with non-ST segment-elevation acute coronary syndromes: feasibility study. *Radiology.* 2003;226:717–722.

65. Bellenger NG, Davies LC, Francis JM, et al. Reduction in sample size for studies of remodeling in heart failure by the use of cardiovascular magnetic resonance. *J Cardiovasc Magn Reson.* 2000;2:271–278.

66. Kwong RY, Schussheim AE, Rekhraj S, et al. Detecting acute coronary syndrome in the emergency department with cardiac magnetic resonance imaging. *Circulation.* 2003;107:531–537.

67. White CS, Kuo D, Keleman M, et al. Chest pain evaluation in the emergency room: can multi-slice CT provide a comprehensive evaluation? *AJR Am J Roentgenol.* 2005;185(2):533–540.

68. Agatston AS, Janowitz WR, Hildner FJ, et al. Quantification of coronary artery calcium using ultrafast computed tomography. *J Am Coll Cardiol.* 1990;15:827–832.

69. Wintersperger BJ, Nikolaou K, von Ziegler F, et al. Image quality, motion artifacts, and reconstruction timing of 64-slice coronary computed tomography angiography with 0.33-s rotation speed. *Invest Radiol.* 2006;41:436–442.

70. Rumberger JA, Sheedy PF II, Breen JF, et al. Electron beam computed tomography and coronary artery disease: Scanning for coronary artery calcification. *Mayo Clin Proc.* 1996;71(4):369–377.

71. O'Malley PG, Taylor AJ, Jackson JL, et al. Prognostic value of coronary electron-beam computed tomography for coronary heart disease events in asymptomatic populations. *Am J Cardiol.* 2000;85(8):945–948.

72. Georgiou D, Budoff MJ, Kaufer E, et al. Screening patients with chest pain in the emergency department using electron beam tomography: A follow-up study. *J Am Coll Cardiol.* 2001;38:105–110.

73. McLaughlin VV, Balogh T, Rich S. Utility of electron beam computed tomography to stratify patients presenting to the emergency room with chest pain. *Am J Cardiol.* 1999;84:327–328.

74. Rubinshtein R, Gaspar T, Halon DA, et al. Prevalence and extent of obstructive coronary artery disease in patients with zero or low calcium score undergoing 64-slice cardiac multidetector computed tomography for evaluation of a chest pain syndrome. *Am J Cardiol.* 2007;99:472–475.

75. Stillman AE, Oudkerk M, Ackerman M, et al. Use of multidetector computed tomography for the assessment of acute chest pain: A consensus statement of the North American Society of Cardiac Imaging and the European Society of Cardiac Radiology. *Int J Cardiovasc Imaging.* 2007;23:415–427.

76. Schuijf JD, Bax JJ, Wijns W, et al. Meta-analysis of comparative diagnostic performance of magnetic resonance imaging and multislice computed tomography for noninvasive coronary angiography. *Am Heart J.* 2006;15:404–411.

77. Rubinshtein R, Halon DA, Gaspar T, et al. Usefulness of 64-slice cardiac computed tomographic angiography for diagnosing acute coronary syndromes and predicting clinical outcome in emergency department patients with chest pain of uncertain origin. *Circulation.* 2007;115(13):1762–1768.

78. Hoffmann U, Nagurney JT, Moselewski F, et al. Coronary multidetector computed tomography in the assessment of patients with acute chest pain. *Circulation.* 2006;114(21):2251–2260.

79. Goldstein JA, Gallagher MJ, O'Neill WW, et al. A randomized controlled trial of multi-slice coronary computed tomography for evaluation of acute chest pain. *J Am Coll Cardiol.* 2007;49(8):863–871.

80. Motoyama S, Kondo T, Sarai M, et al. Multislice computed tomographic characteristics of coronary lesions in acute coronary syndromes. *J Am Coll Cardiol.* 2007;50:319–326.

81. Buda AJ. The role of echocardiography in the evaluation of mechanical complications of acute myocardial infarction. *Circulation.* 1991;84(Suppl. I):I-109–I-121.

82. Zotz RJ, Dohmen G, Genth S, et al. Diagnosis of papillary muscle rupture after acute myocardial infarction by transthoracic and transesophageal echocardiography. *Clin Cardiol.* 1993;16:665–670.

83. Edwards BS, Edwards WD, Edwards JE. Ventricular septal rupture complicating acute myocardial infarction: Identification of simple and complex types in 53 autopsied hearts. *Am J Cardiol.* 1984;54:1201–1205.

84. Birnbaum Y, Fishbein MC, Blanche C, et al. Ventricular septal rupture after acute myocardial infarction. *N Engl J Med.* 2002;347:1426–1432.

85. Thanigaraj S, Perez JE. Diagnosis of cardiac rupture with the use of contrast-enhanced echocardiography. *J Am Soc Echocardiogr.* 2000;13(9):862–865.

86. Reimer KA, Jennings RB. The "wavefront phenomenon" of myocardial ischemic cell death. II. Transmural progression of necrosis within the framework of ischemic bed size (myocardium at risk) and collateral flow. *Lab Invest.* 1979;40:633–644.

87. Califf RM, O'Neill W, Stacks RS, et al. Failure of simple clinical measurements to predict perfusion status after intravenous thrombolysis. *Ann Intern Med.* 1988;108:658–662.

88. Belenkie I, Trabousi M, Hall C, et al. Rescue angioplasty during myocardial infarction has a beneficial effect on mortality: A tenable hypothesis. *Can J Cardiol.* 1992;8:357–362.

89. Kan G, Visser CA, Koolen JJ, et al. Short and long term predictive value of admission wall motion score in acute myocardial infarction. A cross sectional echocardiographic study of 345 patients. *Br Heart J.* 1986;56:422–427.

90. Edvardsen T, Skulstad H, Aakuhs S, et al. Regional myocardial systolic function during acute myocardial ischemia assessed by strain Doppler echocardiography. *J Am Coll Cardiol.* 2001;37:726–730.

91. Vartdal T, Brunvand H, Pettersen E, et al. Early prediction of infarct size by strain Doppler echocardiography after coronary reperfusion. *J Am Coll Cardiol.* 2007;49:1715–1721.

92. Villanueva FS, Glasheen WP, Sklenar J, et al. Characterization of spatial patterns of flow within the reperfused myocardium by myocardial contrast echocardiography. Implications in determining extent of myocardial salvage. *Circulation.* 1993;88:2562–2569.

93. Sklenar J, Ismail S, Villanueva FS, et al. Dobutamine echocardiography for determining the extent of myocardial salvage after reperfusion. An experimental evaluation. *Circulation.* 1994;90:1502–1512.

94. Kamp O, Lepper W, Vanoverschelde JL, et al. Serial evaluation of perfusion defects in patients with a first acute myocardial infarction referred for primary PTCA using myocardial contrast echocardiography. *Eur Heart J.* 2001;22:1485–1495.

95. Main ML, Magalski A, Chee NK, et al. Full-motion pulse inversion power Doppler contrast echocardiography differentiates stunning from necrosis and predicts recovery of left ventricular function after acute myocardial infarction. *J Am Coll Cardiol.* 2001;38:1390–1394.

96. Ito H, Okamura A, Iwakura K, et al. Myocardial perfusion patterns related to thrombolysis in myocardial infarction perfusion grades after coronary angioplasty in patients with acute anterior wall myocardial infarction. *Circulation.* 1996;93:1993–1999.

97. Iwakura K, Ito H, Takiuchi S, et al. Alternation in the coronary blood flow velocity pattern in patients with no reflow and reperfused acute myocardial infarction. *Circulation.* 1996;94:1269–1275.

98. Porter TR, Li S, Oster R, et al. The clinical implications of no reflow demonstrated with intravenous perfluorocarbon containing microbubbles following restoration of thrombolysis in myocardial infarction (TIMI) 3 flow in patients with acute myocardial infarction. *Am J Cardiol.* 1998;82:1173–1177.

99. Ito H, Maruyama A, Iwakura K, et al. Clinical implications of the 'no reflow' phenomenon. A predictor of complications and left ventricular remodeling in reperfused anterior wall myocardial infarction. *Circulation.* 1996;93:223–228.

100. Ragosta M, Camarano G, Kaul S, et al. Microvascular integrity indicates myocellular viability in patients with recent myocardial infarction. New insights using myocardial contrast echocardiography. *Circulation.* 1994;89:2562–2569.

101. Balcells E, Powers E, Lepper W, et al. Detection of myocardial viability by contrast echocardiography in acute infarction predicts recovery of resting function and contractile reserve. *J Am Coll Cardiol.* 2003;41:827–833.

102. Sakuma T, Hayashi Y, Sumii K, et al. Prediction of short- and intermediate-term prognoses of patients with acute myocardial infarction using myocardial contrast echocardiography one day after recanalization. *J Am Coll Cardiol.* 1998;32:890–897.

103. Rocchi G, Kasprzak JD, Galema TW, et al. Usefulness of power Doppler contrast echocardiography to identify reperfusion after acute myocardial infarction. *Am J Cardiol.* 2001;87:278–282.

104. Mori T, Minamiji K, Kurogane H. Rest injected thallium-201 imaging for assessing viability of severe asynergic regions. *J Nucl Med.* 1991;32:1718–1724.

105. Ragosta M, Beller GA, Watson DD. Quantitative planar rest-redistribution Tl-201 imaging in detection of myocardial viability and prediction of improvement in left ventricular function after coronary bypass surgery in patients with severely depressed left ventricular function. *Circulation.* 1993;87:1630–1641.

106. Senior R. Diagnostic and imaging considerations: Role of viability. *Heart Failure Rev.* 2006;11:125–134.

107. Bonow RO. Identification of viable myocardium. *Circulation.* 1996;94:2674–2680.

108. Smith WH, Kastner RJ, Calnon DA, et al. Quantitative gated single photon emission computed tomography imaging: A counts-based method for display and measurement of regional and global ventricular systolic function. *J Nucl Cardiol.* 1997;4:451–463.

109. Krombach GA, Niendorf T, Gunther RW, et al. Characterization of myocardial viability using MR and CT imaging. *Eur Radiol.* 207(17):1433–1444.

110. Choi KM, Kim RJ, Gubernikoff G, et al. Transmural extent of acute myocardial infarction predicts long-term improvement in contractile function. *Circulation.* 2001;104:1101–1107.

111. Janardhanan R, Moon JCC, Pennell DJ, et al. Myocardial contrast echocardiography accurately reflects transmurality of myocardial necrosis and predicts contractile reserve after acute myocardial infarction. *Am Heart J.* 2005;149:355–362.

112. Lindner JR, Coggins MP, Kaul S, et al. Microbubble persistence in the microcirculation during ischemia-reperfusion and inflammation: Integrin- and complement-mediated adherence to activated leukocytes. *Circulation.* 2000;101:668–675.

113. Christiansen JP, Leong-Poi H, Klibanov AL, et al. Noninvasive imaging of myocardial reperfusion injury using leukocyte-targeted contrast echocardiography. *Circulation.* 2002;105:1764–1767.

114. Weller GE, Lu E, Csikari MM, et al. Ultrasound imaging of acute cardiac transplant rejection with microbubbles targeted to intercellular adhesion molecule-1. *Circulation.* 2003;108:218–224.

115. Lindner JR, Song J, Christiansen J, et al. Ultrasound assessment of inflammation and renal tissue injury with microbubbles targeted to P-selectin. *Circulation.* 2001;104:2107–2112.

116. Monaghan MJ. Role of real time 3D echocardiography in evaluating the left ventricle. *Heart.* 2006;92:131–136.

117. Dilsizian V, Bateman TM, Bergmann SR, et al. Metabolic imaging with beta-methyl-*p*-[(123)I]-iodophenyl-pentadecanoic acid identifies ischemic memory after demand ischemia. *Circulation.* 2005;112:2169–2174.

118. Goodman MM, Kirsch G, Knapp FF Jr. Synthesis and evaluation of radioiodinated terminal *p*-iodophenyl substituted a- and b-methyl branched fatty acids. *J Med Chem.* 1984;27:390–397.

119. Cave AC, Ingwall JS, Friedrich J, et al. ATP synthesis during low-flow ischemia: Influence of increased glycolytic substrate. *Circulation.* 2000;101:2090–2096.

120. Kawai Y, Tsukamoto E, Nozaki Y, et al. Significance of reduced uptake of iodinated fatty acid analogue for the evaluation of patients with acute chest pain. *J Am Coll Cardiol.* 2001;38:1888–1894.

121. Buchthal SD, den Hollander JA, Merz CN, et al. Abnormal myocardial phosphorus-31 nuclear magnetic resonance spectroscopy in women with chest pain but normal coronary angiograms. *N Engl J Med.* 2000;342:829–835.

122. Johnson BD, Shaw LJ, Buchthal SD, et al. National Institutes of Health-National Heart, Lung, and Blood Institute. Prognosis in women with myocardial ischemia in the absence of obstructive coronary disease: results from the National Institutes of Health-National Heart, Lung, and Blood Institute-Sponsored Women's Ischemia Syndrome Evaluation (WISE). *Circulation.* 2004;109:2993–2999.

Chronic Ischemic Heart Disease

26

Wael A. Jaber

1. INTRODUCTION

Over the last two decades tremendous advances in the diagnosis and treatment of cardiovascular disease led to increased survival, and therefore prevalence of patients with chronic ischemic heart disease (IHD). The increase in the incidence of cardiovascular disease risk factors namely obesity, diabetes mellitus, physical inactivity, and chronic kidney disease played a key role in increasing the incidence of IHD in the United States and most of the industrialized world.[1] In addition, the increasing age of the US population contributed to this ever growing epidemic. On the other hand, positive development on the medical front of statins, aspirin, ACE inhibitors, interventional therapies (PCI, Stents), and surgery (CABG) attenuated the acute mortality from IHD. These transformational forces led to a reclassification of IHD into mostly a chronic medical condition.

In this chapter, we will summarize the pathophysiology, diagnosis, and treatment options of chronic IHD; in addition, we will discuss the various imaging modalities used to assess the different aspects of the disease as well as the ones used for diagnosis and follow-up of patients.

1.1. Epidemiology

In the United States, the prevalence of IHD in 2005 was 7.3%, with men (8.9%) having higher prevalence of MI, angina, and IHD than women (6.1%) (Table 26.1). Prevalence increased as the age of the population surveyed increased and was higher in groups with lower education level. No prevalence difference was noted among whites and African-Americans; however, the prevalence of IHD was higher among American Indians/Alaska natives and people of multiracial origin as compared to the nonHispanic white population.[1] In patients 45 to 64 years of age, the average age-adjusted IHD incidence rates per 1,000 person-years were 12.5 and 10.6 in white men and black men respectively, while they were 4 and 5.1 in white women and black women. The annual incidence of myocardial infarction (MI) was estimated at 600,000 new and 320,000 recurrent MIs.[1]

Due to improvement in the diagnosis and treatment of IHD, the mortality from IHD decreased by 59% from 1950 to 1999. However, IHD is still the number one killer in the United States and most developed countries in both genders. For instance, IHD claimed the life of one of every five Americans who died in 2004. IHD led to around 451,000 deaths, while MI was responsible for 157,000 deaths. IHD is also rapidly becoming a leading mortality cause in the fast developing countries of Asia and Arab Gulf.

The improvement in IHD treatment (PCI, CABG, lipid lowering drugs, and antihypertensive medications) was responsible

for 47% of the observed decrease in mortality between the years 1980 and 2000. Improvement in IHD risk factors, namely lowering cholesterol levels, smoking cessation, controlling systolic blood pressure, and increase in physical activity, led to 44% of the reduction in mortality in the same period.[1] However, due to its higher prevalence, the number of inpatient discharges after short-stay hospital admissions with IHD as the first-listed diagnosis increased by 5% to 1,828,000 from 1979 to 2005. The increased prevalence of IHD and the increased cost of treatment led to an estimated 156.4 billion dollars in direct and indirect health care costs of IHD in 2008.[1]

1.2. Clinical presentation

The clinical presentation of patients with chronic IHD varies depending on the gender of the patient, the age of the patient, as well as on his or her comorbid illnesses. Ischemia might masquerade as a symptom related to a specific organ system (digestive system such as epigastric pain or indigestion, musculoskeletal system such as shoulder or elbow pain...) especially in the elderly, diabetics, women, as well as people with psychological/psychiatric diseases.

The physician should consider first if the patients signs and symptoms are suggestive of coronary ischemia. Once ischemia and other life-threatening conditions are ruled out by appropriate diagnostic means, other conditions can be considered and treated.

1.2.1. Symptoms

The most common symptom of coronary artery disease is chest pain or angina pectoris. Typical angina is defined as a retrosternally located chest pain, precipitated by exertion and relieved by rest or nitroglycerin. Atypical angina satisfies two of the previously mentioned criteria; nonspecific chest pain satisfies one or none of the aforementioned criteria.[2] One of the defining features of stable angina is the fact that it is reversible upon reversal of the causative agent (exercise, emotional stress,etc.); in addition, the angina attacks tend to repeat themselves in the same way over a long period of time (months to years).[3] The prevalence of chronic stable angina was higher among women in the 40 to 74 years age group compared to men.[1] Men tended to present more frequently with MI as the first manifestation of coronary artery disease (CAD).[4]

In a study of patients suffering from stable coronary artery disease undergoing screening or follow-up myocardial perfusion imaging (MPI), investigators collected information at baseline, then after the exercise portion of the MPI and before the images were taken in patients who suffered from angina.[2] Women more commonly described their pain as sharp and hot

TABLE 26.1

RISK OF STROKE, CHF, SUDDEN DEATH, RECURRENT MI OR FATAL CHD, AND MORTALITY 5 YEARS AFTER A FIRST MI STRATIFIED BY GENDER, RACE, AND AGE GROUP

		White		Black	
		Female	*Male*	*Female*	*Male*
40–69	Stroke risk	5.00	3.00	9.00	8.00
	CHF risk	11.00	7.00	14.00	11.00
	Sudden death	1.90	1.10	1.40	2.50
	Recurrent MI and Fatal CHD	18.00	14.00	29.00	27.00
	Mortality	12.00	8.00	11.00	14.00
>70	Stroke risk	10.00	6.00	17.00	7.00
	CHF risk	25.00	21.00	24.00	29.00
	Sudden death	3.50	6.00	4.80	14.90
	Recurrent MI and Fatal CHD	24.00	24.00	32.00	30.00
	Mortality	32.00	27.00	28.00	26.00

Source: Rosamond W, Flegal K, Furie K, et al. Heart disease and stroke statistics–2008 update: A report from the American Heart Association Statistics Committee and Stroke Statistics Subcommittee. *Circulation.* 2008;117(4):e25–e146.

burning. Both males and females described the pain as throbbing, aching, heavy, tiring, exhausting, tender, and fearful. Women were more likely to suffer from nonpain-related symptoms than men; for instance, more women suffered from trembling, numbness in face/throat, palpitation, knot in throat, and tight in neck and throat. Women with more perfusion defects on myocardial perfusion scan reported more atypical symptoms.[2] Women tended to suffer from pain in the neck area more frequently while men suffered from pain in the shoulder and arm area more often.[2]

Nausea/vomiting, dyspnea, and indigestion tend to occur more frequently in women than men; however, in the above study, the difference between genders was not significant once the investigators adjusted for the higher incidence of anxiety symptoms in women.[2] In women, the extent of the myocardial perfusion defect was not related to the severity of the symptoms.[2] The difference in the way women with angina describe their symptoms leads to under diagnosis of heart disease in the female population. Physicians tend to look for alternative diagnoses to their symptoms, leading to serious consequences of missing and undertreating myocardial ischemia. Awareness of heart disease as the leading cause of death among women increased in 2006 in a survey of females done by the American Heart Association as compared to previous years. White women were more aware of the impact of heart disease on their prognosis as compared to black and Hispanic women.[1]

1.2.2. Outcome

Not surprisingly, age, gender, and race are major determinants of morbidity and mortality. Patients who survive the acute stage of MI will have a 1.5 to 15 times higher risk of illness and death than the general population. Within 1 year of a first MI, 18% of men above 40 years and 23% of women will die; in the 40 to 69 age group, the mortality of men ranged from 8% to 14% while women mortality ranged from 11% to 12% depending on the race; the mortality was worse in the older age groups; in patients above 70 years, around 27% of men died while women mortality ranged from 28% to 32% depending on race.[1]

This grim outlook persists even 5 years after MI. In the 40 to 69 years age group, the mortality increased to 15% to 27% in men and 22% to 32% in women; in the age group of above 70 years, the mortality was 50% to 56% in men and 56% to 62% in women depending on race (Table 26.1).[1]

The percentage of patients who will suffer from recurrent MI or fatal IHD within 5 years after an MI ranged from 14% to 30% in men and 18% to 32% in women depending on the race and the age group; in general, more women than men tended to have recurrent MI or fatal IHD in the 5 years period after MI. The percentage of persons who progress to heart failure (HF) within 5 years of a first MI ranged from 7% to 29% in men and 12% to 25% in women depending on the race and the age group; women tended to progress more to HF than men except black men in the age group of above 70 years who progressed to HF more than black women (Table 26.1).[1]

The percentage of patients who will suffer from a stroke 5 years after a first MI ranged from 4% to 6% in men and 6% to 11% in women depending on race and age group. Women fared worse as far as stroke is concerned in all the age groups considered as compared to men (Table 26.1).[1]

The percentage of patients who suffered from sudden cardiac death (SCD) 5 years after a first MI ranged from 1.1% to 2.5% in men in the 40 to 69 years age group as opposed to 1.4% to 1.9% in women in the same age group. In the age group of above 70 years, the percentage of men dying from SCD ranged from 6% to 14.9%, while in women, the incidence of SCD ranged from 3.5% to 4.8% depending on race (Table 26.1).

2. PATHOPHYSIOLOGY

2.1. Chronic stable angina

2.1.1. Molecular basis for atherosclerosis formation

In animal models of atherosclerosis, it was shown that normal endothelium does not bind white blood cells with affinity. However, as soon as the animals are started on an atherogenic diet, the endothelial cells start expressing surface adhesion molecules, vascular cell adhesion molecule-1 (VCAM-1), which can bind monocytes and lymphocytes involved in atheroma development.[5] The expression of these molecules is mostly in areas most prone to develop atherosclerosis such as the bifurcation of arteries. In these areas, the absence of laminar flow leads to decreased production of NO, which suppresses production of other leukocyte adhesion molecules such as intercellular adhesion molecule-1 (ICAM-1). Once the endothelium expresses the adequate receptors for attachment of the white blood cells, the WBCs would attach and cross the endothelial layer into the intima.[6] In the early stages of human atherosclerosis, lipid deposition occurs in the outer layers of the intima and to a lesser extent in the inner layers and in the media in the walls of the coronary arteries; this leads to the formation of fatty streaks.[7]

The fatty streak represents the modification of the lipids in the plaque by oxidation and glycation; this leads to a local inflammatory response.[5] This local inflammatory response results in an increase in the production of local adhesion molecules on the surface of endothelial cells. In response to the modified lipoproteins in the vascular wall, the endothelial cells start producing macrophage chemoattractant protein-1 (MCP-1). The monocytes infiltrate into the lesion and achieve maturation into macrophages in response to the macrophage colony stimulating factor produced by the inflamed intima.[5] Macrophages increase the expression on their surfaces of scavenger receptors; they engulf lipoproteins and transform into foam cells.[5] They start proliferating and secreting proinflammatory cytokines such as TNF-α and IL-1β.[5] This atherosclerotic lesion induces the migration of CD4+ T cells in response to many cytokines including chemokine-inducible protein 10, IFN-inducible T-cell α-chemoattractant. In humans, the CD4+ T cells react to antigens associated with oxidized LDL. The T lymphocytes in response to cytokines available in the plaque switch to T helper 1 (Th1) phenotype. These cells amplify the inflammatory response further by producing IFN-γ and CD40 ligand (CD40L).[5] The receptor of this ligand, CD40, is expressed by all the cells involved in the atherosclerotic lesion development, including macrophages, endothelial cells, smooth muscle cells (SMCs), T cells, and platelets.[5] Activation of CD40 leads to expression of adhesion molecules, matrix metalloproteinases, and amplification of the immune response. This leads to plaque progression. A particular feature of human atheroma is the expression of IL-18 and its receptor. This receptor is found on the surface of macrophages, endothelial cells, and SMCs.[5] Activation of IL-18 receptor leads to the production of various molecules involved in atherogenesis in humans including VCAM1, IL-6, and matrix metalloproteinases (1, 9, and 13) as well as IFN-γ. The activation of various cytokines leads to the amplification of the inflammatory response and thus progression of atheromas.[5] As the T cells and activated macrophages accumulate in the progressing atheroma, the growth of this atheroma occurs as a result of the activity of SMCs. SMCs, in response to PDGF released by endothelial cells and matrix metalloproteinase 9 (MMP9) produced by activated macrophages, migrate from the media into the intima. In response to PDGF and TGF-β, the SMCs secrete collagen, which leads to the growth of the atherosclerotic plaque and its stabilization.[5] This process leads to the transformation of the plaque from an unstable, lipid rich plaque into a stable, fibrotic, and eventually calcific plaque; the calcific plaque might cause significant flow-limiting stenosis. As the atherosclerotic lesion progresses, the limitation to coronary blood flow becomes more severe; the patient will become symptomatic partly secondary to flow limitation and partly due to inability of the distal vascular bed to vasodilate in response to ischemic stress due to endothelial dysfunction.[8] This leads to anginal symptoms developing in response to various demand/supply stimuli.

2.1.2. Plaque anatomy

The plaque composition differs in patients with stable versus unstable angina/MI. Plaques in unstable angina patients tend to have less fibrous tissue, more inflammatory cell infiltration, and larger atheroma burden as compared to stable coronary artery disease plaques. Unstable, vulnerable plaques tend to have a complex ulcerated appearance with yellow discoloration, ragged edges, and thrombi formation; plaques in stable IHD, on the other hand, had a more smooth surface, white color, and no thrombi formation.[9]

A study using three-vessel virtual histology IVUS (VH-IVUS) to compare plaque composition in patients with ACS versus patients with stable angina found greater necrotic core areas, more thin cap fibroatheromas, multiple ruptured plaques, and smaller fibrofatty plaque areas in patients with ACS as compared to patients with stable angina. In addition, ACS patients had more ruptured plaques as compared to stable angina patients.[10]

In addition, remodeling of the vessel wall tends to be different in stable versus unstable angina. This difference in remodeling contributes to the pathophysiology of stable angina. For instance, the vessel in stable angina tends to undergo negative remodeling, which is defined as a decrease in the vessel size as the plaque accumulates; in unstable angina, the vessel increases in its cross-sectional area as atherosclerosis worsens; this is known as positive remodeling. In addition, the plaque area is smaller in the patients with stable angina versus patients with unstable angina (Figs. 26.1–26.3).[11] The reduction in the size of the vessel in stable angina and the inability of the vessel to autoregulate due to endothelial dysfunction worsen flow limitation by plaque accumulation; this leads to angina in such patients.

2.2. Myocardial stunning and hibernation

Myocardial stunning is the acute ischemic injury that the living cardiac myocytes in the border zone of an MI sustain as a consequence of the decrease in coronary perfusion. The ischemic injury results in a loss of contractile function of these cardiac myocytes. However, the contractile function theoretically returns to normal once the acute ischemic phase resolves. The likelihood of this theoretical recovery is inversely related to the duration of the ischemic injury and the time to resolve normal blood flow. The resting myocardial perfusion to these myocytes is normal.[12] If normal myocardial blood flow/ flow reserve is not restored, patients develop a chronic state called myocardial hibernation; this state is secondary to repetitive episodes of decreased perfusion and of myocardial stunning as a consequence. Areas of hibernating myocardium mixed with scar tissue are thought to be present in up to 50% of patients with previous MI.[13] This leads the myocytes into a chronic postischemic contractile dysfunction. This process is characterized by decreased blood flow to the myocardium at risk, a blunted response to the administration of vasodilators and an intact glucose uptake by the myocytes as measured by labeled fluoro-deoxyglucose (FDG).[14] This state may partially or completely resolve as soon as the blood flow resumes to ischemic areas by revascularization.[12]

In addition to the functional impairment of the cardiac myocytes, the intracellular morphology of the cells is affected by the ischemia.[15] After the onset of the ischemic injury, capillaries become leaky and fluid diffuses into the interstitial spaces making the interstitium hypotonic. This hypotonic environment leads to swelling of myocytes secondary to migration of fluid into the cytoplasm of myocytes by osmosis.[15] The myocytes' edema leads to an increase in the distance between the actin and myosin filaments. This reduces the traction force that the myosin filaments exert on the actin filaments to induce individual myocyte contraction. As a result of the decrease in the contractile work of the

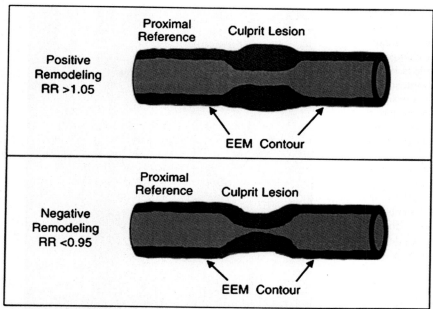

Figure 26.1 Definitions of vessel remodeling and types. (Reproduced from Schoenhagen P, et al. Extent and direction of arterial remodeling in stable versus unstable coronary syndromes: An intravascular ultrasound study. *Circulation*. 2000;101(6): 598–603, with permission.)

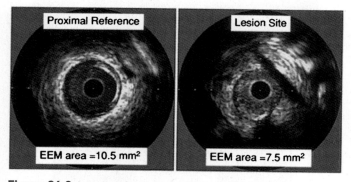

Figure 26.2 Intravascular ultrasound image from patient with stable clinical presentation. (Reproduced from Schoenhagen P, et al. Extent and direction of arterial remodeling in stable versus unstable coronary syndromes: An intravascular ultrasound study. *Circulation*. 2000;101(6): 598–603, with permission.)

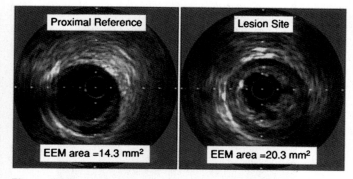

Figure 26.3 Intravascular ultrasound image from patient with unstable clinical presentation. (Reproduced from Schoenhagen P, et al. Extent and direction of arterial remodeling in stable versus unstable coronary syndromes: An intravascular ultrasound study. *Circulation*. 2000;101(6):598–603, with permission.)

individual myocytes in the ischemic border zone, contractile dysfunction ensues. This edema resolves with resolution of ischemia and contractile function improves as a consequence.[15]

Hibernating myocytes tend to suffer from loss and disarray of their contractile proteins, upregulation of glucose transporters, accumulation of glycogen, and depletion of the sarcoplasmic reticulum. In addition, areas of interstitial fibrosis were noted in some patients with hibernating myocardium.[14] In one study, patients with myocardial hibernation were divided into two groups based on the response to dobutamine, patients with inotropic contractile reserve and patients without inotropic contractile reserve. The patients without contractile reserve had more myofibrillar loss and glycogen-laden myocytes; however, the amount of interstitial fibrosis did not differ between the two groups.[14] The group that had a higher inotropic contractile reserve had a greater improvement in regional myocardial function as compared to the group that had no inotropic contractile reserve 6 months after CABG.[14] However, the global ejection fraction improved in both groups indicating the benefit of revascularization in such patients. A study done on hibernating myocardium in pigs subjected to left anterior descending coronary artery (LAD) ligation showed that a multitude of enzymes are affected by the chronic ischemic state leading to hibernation.[16] The enzymes were mainly downregulated at 3 months after LAD ligation; however, some returned to normal after 5 months of the ischemic injury; all the enzymes of the citric acid cycle, the electron transport chain, and the ATP-synthase subunits were downregulated at 3 months. Among glycolysis enzymes, pyruvate dehydrogenase was downregulated. Other enzymes reduced were cytoplasmic creatine kinase, myoglobin, and long chain acid CoA dehydrogenase.[16] In contrast, other proteins important in stress conditions were upregulated including HSP 27 (heat shock protein 27), HSP20-B6, desmin, and vimentin. Other proteins, important in protecting against oxygen free radicals, such as superoxide dismutase and peroxiredoxin-2 were increased as well at 3 months.[16] At 5 months, acyl-CoA dehydrogenase long chain acyl-CoA dehydrogenase, ATP synthase, mitochondrial CK, and mitochondrial aspartate aminotransferase returned to normal. In addition, cytoskeletal proteins, desmin and vimentin, returned to normal after 5 months of inducing ischemia. The changes that affected the rest of the enzymes got accentuated even further at 5 months of chronic ischemia.[16] These changes are aimed at protecting the cardiac myocytes from chronic ischemia. They serve to protect the cells from progression to apoptosis. The level of apoptosis detected at 3 months of ischemia was significantly higher than normal; however, this level was equivalent to apoptosis seen in normal conditions 5 months after the ischemic injury, indicating the protective and adaptive effect of the aforementioned molecular changes on the myocardium.[16]

In the literature, functional recovery of hibernating myocardial tissue ranges from 24% to 82% of all dysfunctional segments.[13] This translated in improvement of global LV function in 38% to 88% of patients in a published metaanalysis of studies of patients with hibernating myocardium treated with revascularization.[12] In both stunned and hibernating myocardium, however, there is a decrease in coronary flow reserve; functional recovery of hibernating myocardium depends on timely restoration of an adequate coronary flow reserve.[12] In most of these studies, segments less than 6 mm in thickness did not show marked improvement after revascularization.[12]

The recovery of the myocardium after revascularization depends on the chronicity of the ischemic injury and the structural damage sustained by the myocardium and may last up to 14 months after injury.[12] Baseline myocardial blood flow before revascularization is not the best predictor of the extent of improvement expected after revascularization; the improvement rather depends on the amount of injury sustained by the myocytes over time. Myocytes which were subjected to repetitive episodes of ischemia and stunning are less likely to improve significantly.[17] A metaanalysis of the value of viability assessment in predicting mortality after revascularization showed a trend of improvement in survival of patients who underwent revascularization provided that they have viable myocardium as compared to patients who underwent medical therapy. This trend was not noted in patients who did not have a viable myocardium.[12] In addition, the longer the waiting time between assessment of viability and revascularization, the worse the mortality.[12] However, this metaanalysis included only nonrandomized studies; currently, some randomized studies are ongoing to clarify the survival benefit from revascularization in patients with viable myocardium.

2.3. Ischemic mitral insufficiency

Ischemic mitral valve insufficiency occurs in many patients after MI or chronic ischemia. Contrary to other causes of organic mitral insufficiency, in ischemic mitral insufficiency valvular anatomy is normal.[18] Ischemic mitral valve insufficiency develops in 15% of patients after acute MI. Given the morbidity and mortality associated with this condition, the appropriate diagnostic technique should be chosen to assess the extent of the improvement expected after repair and whether the possibility for improvement exists.[18] The mechanism of development of ischemic mitral valve insufficiency is related to left ventricular (LV) remodeling leading to displacement of the papillary muscles posteriorly, laterally, and apically, resulting in apical tethering and restricted systolic motion and therefore closure/coaptation of the valve (Fig. 26.4). The distance of separation between the papillary muscles and the mitral annulus might play a role in the pathogenesis of ischemic mitral valve insufficiency. Patients with ischemic mitral valve insufficiency had a larger distance between the papillary muscles as compared to normal control subjects and to subjects with MI but without ischemic mitral valve insufficiency.[19] In extreme cases, a papillary muscle could rupture, leading to severe MR (Fig. 26.5A & B).

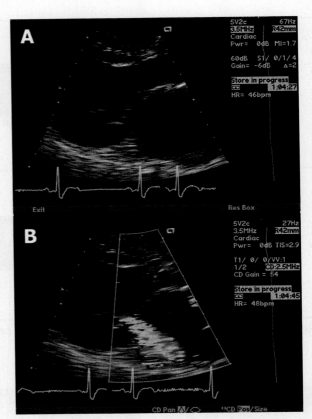

Figure 26.4 Parasternal long axis TTE showing a restricted posterior leaflet and mitral regurgitation. (**A**) 2 D imaging; (**B**) Color Doppler.

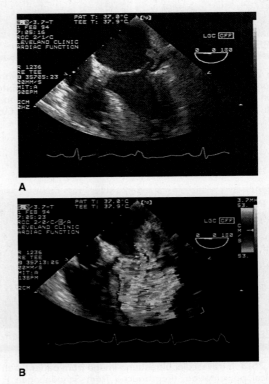

Figure 26.5 A: Mid-esophageal TEE view of ruptured papillary muscle in a patient with recent infarct; **B:** Mitral regurgitation in the setting of ischemic ruptured papillary muscle.

When associated with IHD, severe ischemic mitral regurgitation independently predicts worse outcome including more death and more frequent hospitalization for heart failure as compared to patients with IHD and no ischemic mitral valve insufficiency regardless of ejection fraction (EF), according to a study by Okura et al.[20]

The conventional approach for treating ischemic mitral valve insufficiency is mitral valve annuloplasty and CABG. However, continuous LV remodeling after surgery can lead to recurrent MR. Furthermore, annuloplasty might lead to the development of functional mitral stenosis in some patients. Magne et al.[21] studied patients with moderate to severe ischemic mitral valve insufficiency who underwent MV annuloplasty and CABG and had a decrease in functional capacity. Although mitral insufficiency resolved completely in these patients after surgery, peak systolic pulmonary artery pressure increased significantly. More than 50% of the patients with ischemic mitral valve insufficiency involved in this study had symptoms suggestive of moderate to severe mitral stenosis after the annuloplasty.[21] In addition, recurrent mitral insufficiency after annuloplasty is common and associated with worse outcome.[21]

3. DIAGNOSTIC EVALUATION

The timely diagnosis and appropriate management of IHD reduces mortality and improves quality of life of the affected patients. The evaluation of IHD includes assessment of ventricular function,

coronary anatomy, ischemic burden, and the amount of stunned and hibernating myocardium; the latter information helps elucidate the amount of improvement expected upon revascularization of the patient in question. A diagnostic algorithm is presented in Figure 26.6.

3.1. Evaluation of ventricular function

The evaluation of the LV function is an integral part of the assessment of the patient with IHD (see Chapter 16). The amount of LV dysfunction, both systolic and diastolic, dictates the prognosis and medical therapy, and defines the risk of recurrent hospitalizations.[22, 23] Many techniques are available to assess ventricular function; 2D echocardiography is the most widely used method. However, it is limited in accuracy by geometric assumptions of LV shape and by being highly operator and observer dependent.[23] Other techniques are available as well including contrast biplane cineventriculography (CVG), Single photon emission computed tomography (SPECT), MUGA, multislice computed tomography (MSCT), 3D Echocardiography, and MRI.[22,24] MRI is considered the clinical gold standard to assess cardiac volumes and left and right ventricular ejection fraction.[22] In a study comparing the aforementioned procedures in 88 patients with suspected IHD, Dewey et al.[22] found a good correlation between 2D echocardiography, CVG, and MSCT with MRI results. The correlation was most significant for MSCT.[22] Inability to visualize the apex is an important limitation of 2D echocardiography. An important

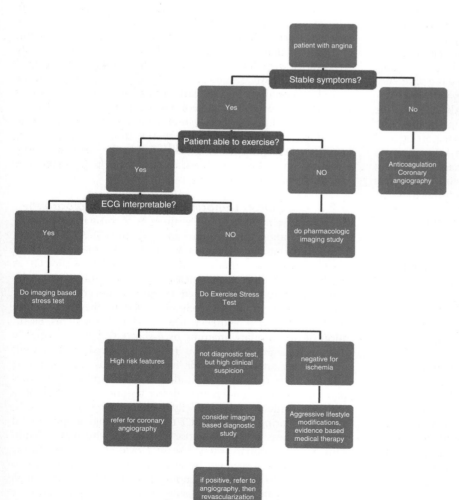

Figure 26.6 Evaluation of patients with angina. (From Gibbons RJ, Balady GJ, Bricker JT, et al. ACC/AHA 2002 guideline update for exercise testing: Summary article. A report of the American College of Cardiology/American Heart Association task force on practice guidelines (committee to update the 1997 exercise testing guidelines). *J Am Coll Cardiol.* 2002;40(8):1531–1540.)

Figure 26.7 Standard apical 4 (**A**) and 2 (**B**) chamber views of the LV and contrast enhanced (**C, D**) TTE apical images showing the improvement in endocardial border definition with use of contrast.

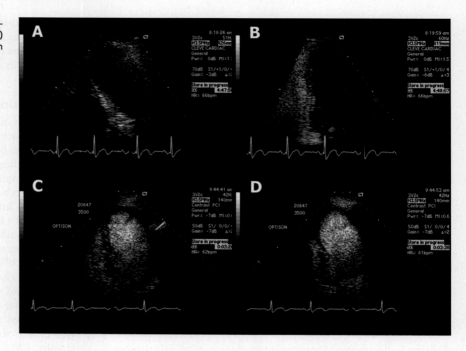

limitation of CVG is its limited ability to assess septal and lateral wall motion abnormalities.[22] The drawbacks to the use of MSCT are the radiation exposure and the need for contrast administration.[22] The major limitation of 3D echocardiography is the inability to image excessively dilated hearts with acceptable accuracy. In addition, the image quality is an important limitation in this technique. The image quality improves significantly once contrast agents are used (Fig. 26.7).[23] In a study comparing the difference between images obtained by 3D echocardiography with and without the use of contrast agents in patients with cardiac disease, the authors found marked improvement in the image quality after contrast administration. The scoring given to the images obtained rose from 2.4 ± 1.0 to 3.0 ± 0.9 ($p < 0.001$) with a 0 score given to an invisible image and 4 score given to an image of excellent quality; in addition, the number of segments with a score less than 2 dropped from 28% to 11% after contrast administration.[23] The evaluation of LV function with contrast echocardiography was similar to the evaluation of LV function using MRI.[23]

3.2. Evaluation of coronary anatomy

The evaluation of coronary anatomy is important in patients with IHD in order to assess the feasibility of revascularization; this is most beneficial especially in patients with hibernating myocardium where the benefit from restoring blood flow might result in tangible improvement in LVEF and thus quality of life of these patients. The assessment of the coronary arteries can be done by multiple methods including invasive coronary angiography (ICA), and more recently intravascular ultrasound (IVUS) and MSCT.

3.2.1. Invasive coronary angiography

ICA is the gold standard for the diagnosis of IHD in patients suspected of having clinically significant atherosclerosis. Clinically significant CAD is defined as intraluminal stenosis of at least 50% (some angiographers prefer to use 70% to define clinically significant stenosis).[25] It is used to delineate coronary anatomy and the extent of luminal obstruction of the coronary arteries. It provides information about the length, diameter, location, and eccentricity of the coronary stenosis as well as the presence of collateral

circulation. In addition, it reveals the cause of the obstruction (atheroma vs. spasm vs. dissection).[25] The limitations of the procedures include its inability to differentiate stable from unstable atheromas and its inability to detect nonobstructive coronary lesions. Other limitations include exposure to ionizing radiation and the fact that the procedure involves injection of potentially nephrotoxic dye which limits its application in the end stage renal disease population.[25] Some of the risks inherent in the procedure include a mortality of 0.11%, arrhythmias risk of 0.38%, vascular complications of 0.43%, and contrast reaction risk of 0.37%.[25]

This procedure has no absolute contraindications. The relative contraindications include but are not limited to renal impairment, severe anemia, active bleeding or bleeding predisposition, infection, and refusal of patient to undergo further treatment if the angiography revealed significant disease.[25]

3.2.2. Computed tomography coronary angiography

A less invasive method for the evaluation of coronary anatomy is computed tomography coronary angiography (CTCA). The advent of 4-slice computed tomography constituted a breakthrough in the evaluation of coronary anatomy. However, the 4-slice CTCA machines had difficulty in measuring with good accuracy the coronary anatomy and tended to miss some critical lesions. The improvement in this technology led to the introduction of 16 slice followed by the 64, 128, and 256 slice systems. Evaluation of the coronary anatomy by 4-slice CTCA led to correctly diagnosing significant stenosis (>50%) in proximal and middle coronary arteries. However, it had difficulties in diagnosing lesions in the right and circumflex coronary arteries.[26] In comparison, 16-slice scanners may detect lesions greater than 50% with a sensitivity and specificity higher than 85%.[27] A recent study comparing 64-slice MSCT to coronary angiography found that MSCT was able to diagnose all patients who had a significant stenotic coronary artery disease. However, upon comparing the accuracy on a segment by segment basis, MSCT was able to detect only 126 out of 144 stenotic segments.[28] MSCT has a high prevalence of false positive results, whereby patients who have one vessel disease by angiography are frequently diagnosed with multivessel disease with MSCT. The main limitation of the MSCT is its inability to visualize the artery lumen in patients with severe vessel calcifications. In addition, the need to reduce heart rate and sustain a prolonged breathhold to ensure good image quality limit the accuracy of this method in patients with advanced IHD, LV dysfunction and heart failure.[29] Similarly to invasive angiography, ionizing radiation exposure is a consideration when using CTA to define coronary anatomy.

3.2.3. Intravascular ultrasound

ICA permits the imaging of the lumen of the coronary artery while giving little information about the walls of the coronary artery; however, atheroma formation results in reverse remodeling of the coronary artery resulting in a diseased coronary artery but normal lumen early on. As atherosclerosis progresses, the lumen of the artery starts to narrow to levels detectable by coronary angiography. Consequently, use of IVUS results in earlier detection of the atheroma. In most cases, nevertheless, the information derived from IVUS is not necessary to make clinical decisions about revascularization in patients with IHD. Generalized clinical use of this technique remained elusive and limited to highly specialized heart centers.

3.3. Detection and quantification of ischemia

The failure to detect myocardial ischemia is an important public health issue. In the United States, 2.1% of cases of MI who present to the emergency departments are discharged, resulting in 11,000 missed diagnoses of MI/year.[30] The nonhospitalized MI patients had a risk of death that was 1.9 more than hospitalized MI patients.[30] Various techniques with variable sensitivities and specificities to detect ischemia will be discussed in the following sections.

3.3.1. ECG

The ECG is one of the earliest and most basic noninvasive techniques used to detect the presence of ischemia. It helps in the timely detection of ischemia, guides therapy, and helps decrease mortality and morbidity in patients presenting to the emergency departments with complaints of chest pain. Failure to recognize ischemia on ECG was the most common cause of complications in patients discharged from the emergency room presenting with symptoms suggestive of coronary disease.[30] Ischemia is diagnosed by ST segment elevation of ≥ 0.2 mV in leads V1, V2, and V3 or ≥ 0.1 mV in the other leads or ST segment depression of ≥ 0.1 mV in any lead; the ischemic changes should be present in at least two contiguous leads.[31] The sensitivity of these criteria to diagnose MI ranges from 45% to 50% and the specificity from 92% to 97%.[32,33] However, reliance on these criteria alone leads to a missed diagnosis of myocardial ischemia in around a third of patients presenting to the emergency departments with MI.[30,31] One study suggested using criteria to identify STEMI-equivalent patients based on finding of ST segment depression of ≥ 0.1 mV in ≥ 2 contiguous leads or in one lead that is contiguous to a lead meeting the ST segment elevation criteria. This resulted in an increase in the sensitivity, however, at the expense of a decrease in specificity of the ECG.[32] Another study suggested the addition of seven additional leads to the 12-lead ECG (–V1, –V2, –V3, –aVL, –I, aVR, (in Europe –aVR and –III are frequently included in the ECG). In some studies, this led to a marked increase in sensitivity from 45% to 80% for LAD and right coronary artery (RCA) ischemia and from 32% to 64% for Cx ischemia.[34] A study comparing 24 leads (inverting all leads), 19 leads (inverting only the aforementioned seven leads), and 16 leads (adding V4R, V5R, V8,

and V9) found that the more leads used, the higher the sensitivity and the lower the specificity to detect AMI. For instance, the sensitivities of the 12-, 16-, and 24-lead ECG were 28.1%, 33.1%, and 36.8%, respectively. The specificities, however, were 97%, 93.2%, and 94.5%, respectively.[35]

3.3.2. Stress ECG

Stress ECG is among the first tests used for assessing the presence of ischemia in patients at risk of IHD. The procedure is generally safe. However, the risks of death and MI have been reported to occur at the rate of 1 per 2,500 tests done.[36] Monitoring should include measurement of HR, ECG, and blood pressure during all the stages of the test. The patient should be monitored for signs and symptoms of ischemia throughout the test. The type of the protocol used and the type of exercise capacity in metabolic equivalents should be reported in the test as well.[36] Exercise stress test is terminated when the patient reaches 85% of the maximum predicted heart rate. The limitations inherent in this approach are evident in patients on β-blockers, patients with impaired heart rate response, and patients with excessive heart rate response. Other indications to stop the test include hemodynamic instability, acute neurologic signs and symptoms, and moderate to severe angina and arrhythmias (sustained ventricular tachycardia, SVT, high degree heart block) as well as ST segment elevation ≥ 1 mm or ST segment depression ≥ 2 mm. A stress test is positive when ST segment depression or ST segment elevation occurs 60 to 80 ms after the end of the QRS. The sensitivity of the exercise stress test is 67% and the specificity 72% for detecting obstructive CAD.[36] The presence of LVH and resting ST depression lowers the specificity of the exercise stress test. Drugs affecting the interpretation of a stress test include Digoxin, β-blockers, and nitrates. Heart block might affect the interpretation of stress tests; both left bundle branch block (LBBB) and right bundle branch block (RBBB) might cause exercise induced ST depression regardless of the presence of ischemia. Impaired heart rate recovery after exercise treadmill test is an independent predictor of mortality.[37] In a study of 1,959 patients, the heart rate increase at peak exercise was the most powerful and accurate predictor of all cause and cardiovascular mortality.[38] Stress ECG is usually advisable for patients who have stable chest pain or patients with unstable chest pain stabilized by aggressive medical therapy or patients who underwent prior revascularization. Patients post MI benefit from stress ECG as well.[39] Patients who are not able to exercise or have ECG changes which mask the interpretation of stress ECG need to undergo an imaging study to evaluate the possibility of CAD and predict their prognosis in the presence of CAD.[39]

3.3.3. Stress echocardiography

Another modality used for detection and quantification of ischemia is stress echocardiography. Both dobutamine and dipyridamole stress echocardiography (at this time used mainly in Europe) have similar accuracy for detecting the presence of CAD (Table 26.2). However, the side effect profile is higher with the use of dobutamine as compared to the use of dipyridamole. The sensitivity of stress echocardiography varies with the agent used with higher specificities achieved with the use of dipyridamole as compared to dobutamine. For instance, the sensitivity and specificity with dobutamine use are 81% and 84.1% respectively, as compared to 71.9% and 94.6% for dipyridamole.[40] A study done on patients undergoing dobutamine stress echo showed that the occurrence of severe hypotensive response (defined as a drop in systolic blood pressure >20 mm Hg at peak exercise) during the testing was associated with increased risk of cardiac death.

TABLE 26.2
SENSITIVITY AND SPECIFICITY OF DIFFERENT IMAGING MODALITIES

	Patients, n	Sensitivity, Mean (95% CI)	Specificity, Mean (95% CI)	PPV, Mean (95% CI)	NPV, Mean (95% CI)
Conventional nuclear					
99mTc-sestamibi	19	71(51–91)	40(18–62)	—	—
SPECT FDG	94	86(79–93)	93(88–98)	—	—
201Tl rest, reinjection	211	84(79–89)	70(64–76)	97(92–100)	93(86–100)
201Tl rest, redistribution + FDG	47	86(76–96)	92(84–100)	90(81–99)	89(80–98)
Total	371	84(80–88)	77(73–81)	94(89–98)	91(85–97)
Echocardiography					
DSE	408	76(71–80)	81(77–85)	84(77–91)	91(85–96)
DSE + Strain rate	55	67(55–79)	89(81–97)	—	—
End-diastolic wall thickness	43	63(49–77)	68(54–82)	—	—
Total	506	74(70–77)	81(77–84)	84(77–91)	91(85–96)
PET					
FDG	205	81(75–96)	65(59–72)	—	—
Total	205	81(75–86)	65(59–72)	—	—

PPV, positive predictive value; NPV, negative predictive value.
Source: Camici PG, Prasad SK, Rimoldi OE. Stunning, hibernation, and assessment of myocardial viability. *Circulation*. 2008;117(1):103–114.

Patients who had a smaller reduction in their BP <20 mm Hg did not have a significant reduction in their survival as compared to patients with no drop in their blood pressure during the dobutamine stress echocardiography (DSE).[41] While the sensitivity and specificity of stress ECG are lower for women as compared to the values for men, they are comparable for stress echocardiography in both genders.[42] In patients with stable angina, stress echocardiography performs best in patients who have an intermediate pretest probability of CAD and have uninterpretable ECG and are unable to exercise. However, in patients who have low pretest probability of CAD with ECG changes and inability to exercise, stress echocardiography is considered appropriate as well. It is recommended as well in patients with high pretest probability of CAD regardless of ECG and functional status. In patients suffering from acute chest pain with no ECG changes and negative serial cardiac enzymes, stress echocardiography is also recommended.[43]

3.3.4. Stress myocardial perfusion imaging
In addition to detecting ischemia by ECG abnormalities and wall motion abnormalities, ischemia can be detected by myocardial perfusion abnormalities. Nuclear myocardial perfusion tests are based on differential myocardial uptake of a radioactive tracer (thallium, Tc-99, Rb-82) (Table 26.3) by different regions of the LV during pharmacologic (dipyridamole, dobutamine) - or exercise-induced stress (Fig. 26.8). The uptake of the tracer will be reduced across stenotic coronary lesions. Resting images are taken to differentiate between scar and stress-induced reduction in tracer uptake. The lower attenuation of the signals detected with the positron emission tomography (PET) scanners and the higher resolutions obtained makes the PET scanners more desirable than the SPECT scanners.[44] The sensitivity and specificity of gated SPECT for detection of occlusive IHD is 91% and 72%, respectively. The use of PET results in improving the specificity of diagnosing significant stenosis to 90% (Table 26.2).[44] Patients with normal SPECT and Rb PET have

TABLE 26.3
RADIOTRACERS USED FOR MYOCARDIAL IMAGING: CHARACTERISTICS OF SPECT AND PET RADIOPHARMACEUTICALS

Modality	Tracer	Usual dose (MBq)	Photon energy (keV)	Time to imaging from injection	Physical half-life	Comments
SPECT	201Tl	111–166.5	80	1–15 min	73 h	Potassium analog Redistribution with time
	99mTc-Sestamibi	296–1,480	140	15–45 min	6 h	Mitochondrial uptake Cationic and lipophilic
	99mTc-Tetrofosmin					No significant redistribution
PET	82Rb	1,110–2,220	511	80 s	75 s	Potassium analog Generator produced
	13N-Ammonia	370–740	511	6 min	10 min	ATP-dependent trapping in cytoplasm Requires on-site cyclotron

Source: Vesely MR, Dilsizian V. Nuclear cardiac stress testing in the era of molecular medicine. *J Nucl Med*. 2008;49(3):399–413.

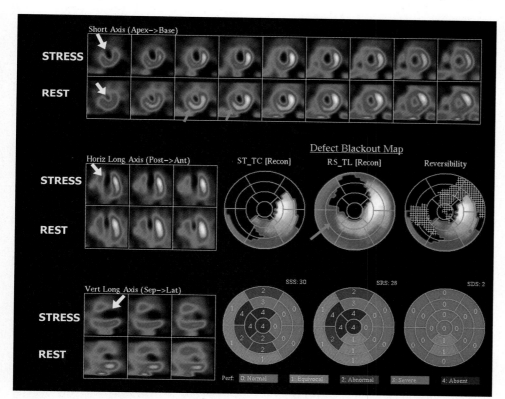

Figure 26.8 A SPECT study showing left anterior descending artery territory scar (*white arrows*) and right coronary artery territory exercise-induced ischemia (*green arrows*).

<1% and 0.4% probability respectively of cardiac events annually.[44] The use of stress nuclear studies is recommended in patients with an intermediate probability of CAD based on risk factors. It is recommended as well in patients with NSTEMI and unstable angina that are stabilized medically to assess the extent of inducible ischemia. In patients who have coronary lesions established by prior CAD, it is recommended to do stress nuclear studies to assess the hemodynamic significance of the stenosis (Figs. 26.9 and 26.10).[45]

3.3.5. Stress perfusion MRI

Another noninvasive method to diagnose CAD and quantify the ischemic burden is stress MRI. Stress MRI may use dobutamine to induce wall motion abnormalities imaging or adenosine or dipyridamole with gadolinium to evaluate myocardial perfusion. The sensitivity of MRI differs according to the technique used. For dobutamine stress MRI, a metaanalysis found sensitivity and specificity of 83% and 86%, respectively.[46] For MRI MPI, the sensitivity and specificity were 91% and 81%, respectively. MRI was compared to coronary angiography as the gold standard in this meta-analysis. The prevalence of CAD in the population studied was 57.4% in the perfusion imaging group and 71% in the dobutamine imaging group. The use of MRI, however, is limited by claustrophobia, limited availability, obesity, and motion artifact among other limitations. It is recommended to use it in intermediate risk patients who cannot exercise and who have baseline ECG abnormalities.[46]

3.4. Assessment of contractile reserve

3.4.1. Dobutamine echocardiography

The presence of hibernating myocardium can be assessed by DSE. Low dose (5 to 10 µg/kg/min) dobutamine leads to increased contractility in the hibernating segments and increase in myocardial wall thickening. Higher doses of dobutamine (40 µg/kg/min) and atropine can be used to elicit either further improvement or decline in function due to the supply-demand mismatch.[12] The

improvement in contractility and myocardial wall thickening with low doses followed by worsening in function and decrease in wall thickening ischemia at high doses is the most specific predictor on DSE for improvement after revascularization—this is known as the biphasic response. Thus, patients with this finding on DSE benefit from revascularization. In contrast, segments with impaired function and thickening at rest which show improvement in contractility and wall thickening at low and high doses of dobutamine have a uniphasic response; this is mostly seen in cases of reperfused MI and is less predictive than the biphasic response of myocardial viability after revascularization. Patients exhibiting the uniphasic response might need further viability assessment to see if they would improve with revascularization. Scarred myocardium does not react to dobutamine infusion at any dose.[12] The wall motion scoring index (WMSI) is computed at rest and after the infusion. If Δ WMSI is ≥0.4, indicating inotropic response to dobutamine, the possibility of improvement after revascularization is high.[47] Patients who have viable myocardium treated by revascularization have higher survival rates as compared to patients treated by medical therapy alone.[48] In addition, the lower the EF, the higher the survival benefit in patients with viable myocardium who have revascularization. Mortality does not differ in the patients who have no viable myocardium regardless of the treatment received and of the EF.[48]

3.4.2. Dobutamine MRI

Contractile reserve as a measure of viability can be assessed as well using dobutamine MRI. Analysis is based on the difference between maximal thickening at any dobutamine infusion rate and at rest. Low contractile reserve in response to dobutamine is a reflection of myocardial ischemia and necrosis; a positive response, however, is a sign of myocardial stunning/hibernation. MRI allows the determination of the response of the myocardium to dobutamine stress. It allows as well assessment of viable

Figure 26.9 Rest/Stress SPECT images showing left anterior descending artery ischemia and post-stress left ventricular cavity dilation.

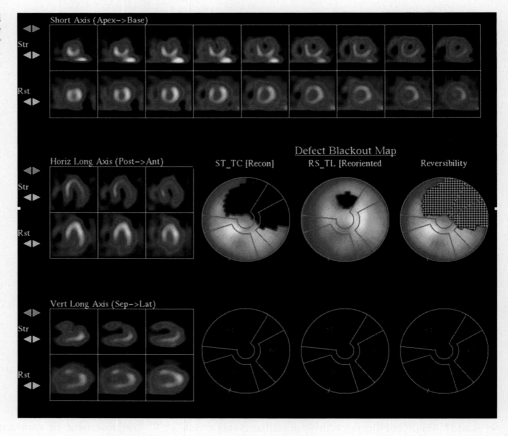

Figure 26.10 Rest/Stress SPECT perfusion images showing left anterior descending artery territory and circumflex coronary artery territory ischemia with post stress cavity dilation in a patient with severe left main coronary disease.

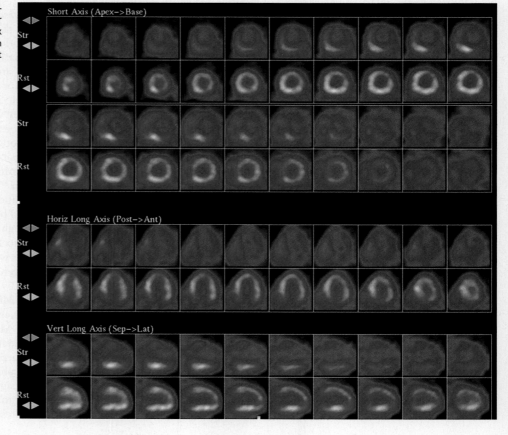

myocardial segments using delayed contrast enhancement. The optimal dose of dobutamine has been investigated in order to assess the contractile reserve following an MI.[49] Contractile reserve of dysfunctional segments is assessed at rest and at dobutamine doses from 5 to 20 µg/kg/min. Infusion of dobutamine at a dose of 20 µg/kg/min results in the highest amount of thickening and the most decrease in the amount of dysfunctional segments as compared with the other doses infused. Some suggest that 20 µg/kg/min is the optimal dose to assess the contractile reserve and to avoid missing segments that might be viable.[49]

3.5. Myocardial perfusion/metabolic imaging

SPECT may be used for the determination of hibernating myocardium. It depends on the uptake of tracers such as Thallium and Technetium labeled tracers by myocardial tissue. The uptake of these tracers at physiologic levels depends on blood flow and sarcolemmal integrity. Thallium tracers can be detected in the myocardium after injection in areas with normal blood flow having a fast redistribution time after 4 to 24 h of the injection. Imaging of the heart late after injection can demonstrate the presence of Thallium in myocardial segments where the tracer was absent at baseline. This finding can be interpreted as a marker of sarcolemmal integrity and tissue viability.[12] ^{99m}Tc-sestamibi and ^{99m}Tc-tetrofosmin, the most commonly used tracers, on the other hand have a slower redistribution time, higher energy-photon emission, and reduced amount of soft tissue attenuation than Thallium.[12] The resulting images using these tracers have better quality, less artifacts, and less radiation exposure as compared to Thallium. SPECT has a higher sensitivity and lower specificity than echocardiography based techniques. The main limitations of SPECT include the high amount of ionizing radiation, low spatial resolution, and attenuation artifacts.[12]

Myocardial metabolism plays an important role in IHD as well as in multiple disease states, especially diseases that involve the whole myocardium (e.g., Diabetes Mellitus, heart failure). Hence the importance of imaging techniques that assess the myocardial metabolism in this setting.

Positron emission tomography (PET) is the most sensitive and possibly the gold standard for viability assessment when used to decide on the amount of improvement after revascularization.

In PET, there are perfusion tracers to quantify myocardial blood flow and metabolic tracers to assess energy utilization patterns and thus viability (Table 26.3). Simply stated, regions showing decreased flow and decreased FDG uptake are considered scarred tissues; tissues with reduced blood flow and normal FDG uptake are considered hibernating.[12]

3.6. Myocardial scar imaging

Scar imaging is essential in order to distinguish between patients who will benefit from revascularization procedures and patients who will not. This will ensure improved function in patients with little scar and spares patients with high amount of scar the burden of revascularization.

3.6.1. FDG-Positron emission tomography

The gold standard to assess the amount of scar and myocardial tissue viability is FDG-PET. A discrepancy between the uptake of FDG and Ammonia or Rubidium (flow-metabolism mismatch) predicts tissue viability. Many variables come into play when using FDG to assess for viability. For instance, fasting period, age, hospitalization status all affect FDG uptake by the myocardium. Two protocols are followed to assess viability. Imaging is done under either low (fasting) or high glucose metabolism (oral glucose loading or euglycemic insulin clamp technique).[50]

The normal myocardium depends on FFA for metabolism and takes up FDG minimally; however, ischemic myocardium takes up FDG avidly and appears as hot spots. However, during imaging under fasting conditions there is heterogeneous uptake of FDG by normal myocardium which causes interpretation difficulty.

Imaging under high glucose metabolism is done by ingestion of a glucose load (50 to 75 g) which leads to increased insulin in the body and increases the uptake of FDG by normal myocardium. Under these conditions, the normal and ischemic myocardium will show marked enhancement secondary to FDG uptake. The hibernating myocardium will show normal or near normal FDG uptake (PET uptake scores ranging from 0 to 2) with reduced ammonia myocardial blood flow (<2.5 standard deviations) as compared to normal tissue.[51] Scar tissue will show absence of enhancement; the FDG uptake score of scar tissue will be 3 to 4 with reduced myocardial blood flow (Figs. 26.11 & 26.12).[50,51]

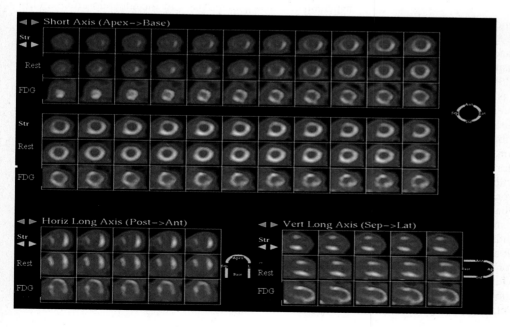

Figure 26.11 A PET scan with rest and stress Rubidium followed by FDG images. There is evidence of LAD ischemia (rest/stress images) and perfusion/metabolic mismatch (Rst/FDG images) indicating myocardial hibernation.

Figure 26.12 A PET scan with rest and stress Rubidium followed by FDG images. There is evidence of LAD territory fixed perfusion defect (Rest/stress) with a matched perfusion metabolic defect (Rest/FDG) indicating myocardial scar.

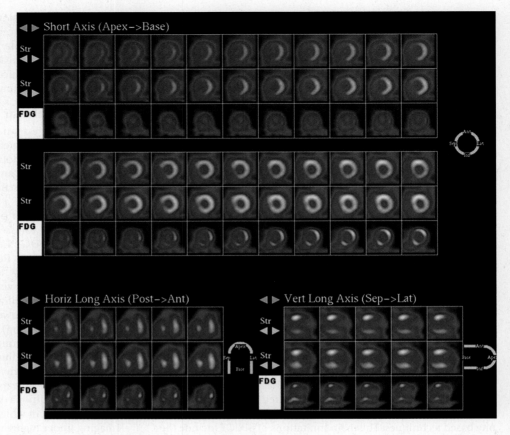

The amount of scar assessed by FDG uptake was shown to be an independent negative predictor of functional recovery. For instance in a study of patients with chronic IHD (history of previous MI and Ejection Fraction <40%), comparison of hibernating versus scar segments of the myocardium by PET-FDG showed that patients with myocardial scar and lower glucose metabolic rate had higher rates of cardiovascular events (cardiac death, recurrent MI or worsening heart failure).[51]

3.6.2. MRI

Another technique used to assess the amount of scar in the myocardium is contrast- enhanced MRI (ce-MRI). The contrast used is gadolinium-diethylenetriamine pentaacetic acid (Gd-DTPA). It is a biologically inert, and diffuses passively in the extracellular spaces; it has a 20 min half life in blood.[52] It tends to concentrate more in acutely infarcted myocardium as well as in scarred areas as compared to normal myocardial tissue. In acute MI, it tends to distribute itself in cells that lost membrane integrity. In chronically scarred areas, it tends to redistribute in the extracellular spaces. Images of infarcted myocardium appear enhanced relative to normal myocardium when performed after a delay (5 to 20 min) after intravenous contrast injection; areas with reversible ischemia appear similar to normal myocardium. Studies in animals showed, however, that delayed enhancement as a marker of infarcted myocardium overestimates infarct size by around 10%.[52] The extent of delayed enhancement tends to be stable over time once the procedure is optimized, and it ranges from 7 to 42 min after contrast injection; this time range provided excellent correlation with infarct size estimation done with SPECT. One advantage of the MRI compared with SPECT is the high spatial resolution with MRI; this makes MRI the most suitable imaging technique

for the detection of subendocardial infarction.[52] In addition, MRI is useful in differentiating ischemic cardiomyopathy (ICM) from Non-ICM (NICM). The main ways MRI helps in differentiating the two forms of cardiomyopathy are by detecting the presence of CAD by MRI angiography, wall motion abnormalities by stress MRI, and the location of scar tissue (Figs. 26.13A & B and 26.14). In addition, delayed hyperenhancement is usually found in the majority of patients (around 100%) with ICM, as compared to 12% of patients with NICM. Moreover, ICM patients' delayed hyperenhancement pattern starts in the subendocardial and/or transmyocardial areas depending on the infarct size and it follows the distribution of a coronary artery; while the NICM patients' hyperenhancement pattern does not. Hyperenhancement may be found as well in myocarditis patients. However, the pattern in these patients is very similar to the pattern found in patients with NICM.[53] The involvement is mainly in the epicardial areas of

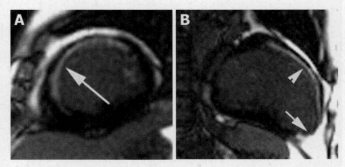

Figure 26.13 MRI short axis (**A**) and long axis (**B**) images post-gadolinium injection showing 50% transmural delayed hyperenhancement in a patient with previous LAD territory infarct.

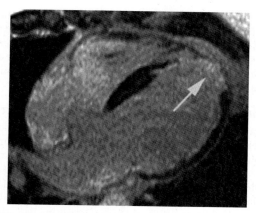

Figure 26.14 MRI 4-chamber image postgadolinium injection showing full thickness infarct involving the distal LAD territory.

the myocardium. It decreases with improvement of the myocarditis and disappears almost completely with recovery. The hyperenhancement seen on MRI has been used to guide biopsy and resulted in improved yield of the biopsy as compared to blind biopsies. In cases of Chagas disease, ce-MRI is able to detect cardiac involvement even before the onset of symptoms by finding delayed enhancement; the pattern is similar to NICM pattern.[53] The main limitation of this technique is the fact that it is difficult to apply in dyspneic, noncooperative patients, patients with end-stage renal disease, and those with implantable metal devices such as pacemakers and defibrillators.[12]

In a comparison done between contrast enhanced MRI and low dose dobutamine MRI in patients with chronic coronary artery disease,[54] the two techniques were comparable when the extent of scarring was mild or severe. However, in patients with intermediate amount of transmural infarct (hyperenhancement score 3), 42% had contractile reserve, whereas 58% did not have contractile reserve. Therefore, both techniques were comparable when the infarct was small or large; in intermediate cases, dobutamine MRI is needed to assess contractile reserve.[54]

3.6.3. Myocardial contrast echocardiography
Another in-vivo method to assess flow and cellular integrity is contrast echocardiography. However, currently this method has not gained attraction clinically due to issues related to reproducibility of data. Myocardial contrast echocardiography uses contrast agent consisting of acoustically active gas filled microbubbles that remain within the confines of the microcirculation. After constant intravenous infusion of the bubbles, they reach a steady state concentration in the blood; a burst of high intensity ultrasound is used to destroy the microbubbles within the myocardium. Subsequent filling of the myocardium with microbubbles occurs after 5 to 15 cardiac cycles; this determines the velocity of blood flow in the myocardium. Viable segments will have homogeneous contrast enhancement; scarred areas where the microcirculation is absent, absence of contrast enhancement is noticed.[12] This method has high sensitivity and low specificity for predicting recovery after revascularization as compared to DSE wall motion assessment; it shares the advantages of safety, low cost, portability, and wide spread availability with DSE.[12] The limitations are shared as well by both techniques and they include being operator dependent with high interobserver variability. In addition, patient related factors such as poor acoustic windows and significant LV dysfunction lead to poor resolution and low diagnostic accuracy.[12] To date, this method remains largely confined to the

research field. Application of this modality to patients was faced with major difficulties which led to its limited applicability to experimental medicine.

4. SELECTING AND GUIDING THERAPY

4.1. Patients with preserved EF
One way to select therapy is to stratify patients with CAD according to their heart function. Patients with preserved ejection fraction can be treated with evidence based medical therapy according to the guidelines set forth by the ACC and AHA.[55] A treatment algorithm is shown in Figure 26.15.

4.1.1. Medical therapy
Aspirin. The optimal dose of aspirin to be used in IHD patients was not definitely studied in a randomized control trial comparing two aspirin doses. Patients with established IHD should be on Aspirin 75 to 162 mg/day therapy indefinitely. In patients who are allergic to aspirin, clopidogrel 75 mg/day therapy is recommended.[56] Combined aspirin and clopidogrel therapy was studied in high risk patients for atherosclerosis and in patients with established cardiovascular disease (defined as patients with multiple atherothrombotic risk factors, documented coronary disease, documented cerebrovascular disease, or documented symptomatic peripheral arterial disease). There was no difference in the primary end point (first occurrence of MI, stroke (of any cause), or death from cardiovascular causes) between the groups that received aspirin and clopidogrel and the group that received only aspirin.[57] Patients on combination therapy had less

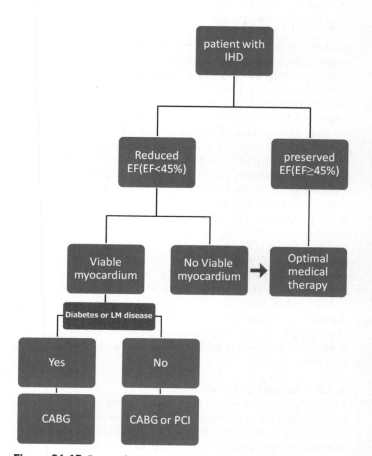

Figure 26.15 Revascularization algorithm in patients with chronic IHD.

revascularization, less hospitalization for unstable angina, and less transient ischemic attacks. However, the risk of moderate bleeding (bleeding that led to transfusion but was not life threatening) with the combination was significantly higher as compared to treatment with aspirin alone.[57] Subgroup analysis of patients with prior MI, stroke, or peripheral arterial disease in the CHARISMA trial showed that they derive significant benefit from combination therapy. The rate of cardiovascular death, MI, and stroke was significantly decreased in the combination group. The analysis showed similar increased moderate bleeding in the combination group while the severe bleeding was similar in both groups. The results of this subgroup analysis need to be validated in a clinical trial.[58]

Statins. Statins are indicated in patients with coronary artery disease in order to reduce the LDL <100 mg/dL. However, in studies where LDL was lowered below 100 mg/dL down to 62 mg/dL, further cardiovascular benefit was obtained.[59] Thus, in very high risk patients defined as patients with IHD, and multiple major risk factors including Diabetes, severe and poorly controlled risk factors (e.g., smoking) and elevated TG >200, HDL <40, and non-HDL cholesterol >130, the LDL target is <70 mg/dL.[59] A metaanalysis compared the safety and efficacy of more intensive statin treatment with less intensive therapy in patients with CAD.[60] No difference in overall mortality was noted in the group with more intensive lipid lowering therapy as compared to the less intensive therapy group in stable coronary artery disease patients; a 25% reduction in mortality was noted in patients with ACS who had a more aggressive lipid lowering regimen. In addition, a significant reduction in coronary mortality, reinfarction, stroke, and major cardiovascular events were noted in patients on the more intensive therapy arm.[60]

β-blockers. Treatment with β-blockers in patients with an MI results in decreased mortality and reduced recurrent infarction. A study comparing atheroma size and progression in patients with MI that were treated with β-blockers compared with patients who were not treated found a decrease in the size of the atheroma in patients who received β-blocker therapy compared to patients not receiving this treatment. Follow-up of atheroma volume by IVUS showed a decrease in the size of the atheroma in patients that were treated with β-blockers as compared to patients who did not receive this treatment. Similarly, a study done on patients with coronary artery disease with preserved EF and who did not suffer from MI showed that β-blocker therapy resulted in better survival; however, no effect was seen on the end point of reinfarction and combination of death and nonfatal MI.[61]

ACE inhibitors. ACE inhibitors are indicated in secondary prevention in patients with stable coronary artery disease.[62] A combined analysis of three trials (HOPE, EUROPA, AND PEACE) investigating the effect of ACEI in patients with stable coronary artery disease showed that treatment with ACEI resulted in reduced total and cardiovascular mortality, recurrent or new nonfatal MI, fatal and nonfatal strokes, and heart failure requiring hospitalization.[63]

4.1.2. Patients with reduced EF

Patients with dysfunctional myocardium need to be assessed for revascularization in addition to optimal medical therapy (OMT). These patients might benefit from revascularization if they have hibernating myocardium as opposed to scar tissue. The proper selection of patients to undergo revascularization by PCI or CABG

results in marked improvement in the heart function; this might lead to a significant impact on the quality of life of these patients and avoids the morbidity/mortality of unnecessary surgery/intervention in patients with scarred myocardium. To be able to select the patients that will benefit most from revascularization, viability assessment should be done.

4.2. Viability studies and relationship to outcome

Investigators assessed the role of PET with FDG in predicting tissue viability and the relationship of viability assessment by PET to the outcome of patients. PET with FDG is considered the most sensitive method for predicting recovery of dysfunctional myocardium after revascularization.[64] The PARR-2 study assessed whether the inclusion of FDG-PET in the decision tree to revascularize patients with IHD and EF ≤ 35% myocardium had an impact on their outcome. There was no difference in the two groups in the primary outcome of cardiac death. However, around 25% of patients in the PET group did not adhere to the recommendations of revascularization provided by the results of the PET imaging. Post hoc analysis of patients who adhered to the PET imaging recommendation showed significant reduction in events as opposed to the standard therapy group.[64] Similarly, analysis of patients who did not undergo catheterization prior to the PET in both groups showed significant benefit of PET assisted decision making as opposed to standard therapy in reducing cardiac events.[64] However, these analyses violate the intention to treat principle and might have an inherent bias.[64]

In addition to the role of PET in viability assessment, ce-MRI has emerged over the past few years as a reliable method for viability assessment and its relationship to outcome.

Knuesel et al.[65] assessed the value of ce-MRI alongside FDG-PET in assessment of viability and the relationship of the findings to outcome in 19 patients with IHD. They stratified myocardial segments into segments which are thin or thick by ce-MRI (≤4.5 mm wall thickness or >4.5 mm, respectively) or metabolically viable or nonviable according to FDG uptake by PET (≥50% uptake or <50% uptake, respectively).[65] Patients with thin, metabolically nonviable segments were deemed to have the highest amount of scar. In this type of segments, 87% of the segments did not regain function after revascularization; however, 85% of segments which were metabolically viable and had a thickness greater than 4.5 mm, recovered function after revascularization. Patients who underwent revascularization had a nonsignificant increase in their EF from 41.6% ± 10.9% to 45.3% ± 9.8% ($p = 0.08$); patients on medical therapy had no change in their EF (30.0% ± 12.8% at baseline, 29.8% ± 11.1% at follow-up). The assessment of viability by PET and MRI correlated closely in this study.[65] A study done by Bondarenko et al. assessing the value of MRI prior to revascularization in predicting the regain of function of revascularized segments according to the extent of hyperenhancement found that segments with the highest hyperenhancement (75% to 100% transmurality, with hyperenhancement defined as enhancement ≥5 SD than remote normal myocardial segments in the same slice) tended to be the least likely to recover function; segments which displayed lower level of transmural hyperenhancement 1% to 25%, 26% to 50%, and 51% to 75% were 4, 8, and 20 times less likely to have functional improvement as compared with segments with no hyperenhancement ($p < 0.001$).[66] The ejection fraction improved in 20 of the revascularized patients while it remained stable or worsened in 25 of the patients. However, the patients who had worsening in their EF had periprocedural hyperenhancement indicating new loss of function of myocardial segments after revascularization found by follow-up ce-MRI.[66] The importance of assessment of myocardial viability in patients with myocardial dysfunction who have planned to undergo revascularization stems from the aforementioned findings.

Although the evidence provided by the PARR-2 study is inconclusive and there was no randomized double blind trial indicating the benefit of viability assessment in patients with IHD and reduced ejection fraction, viability assessment provides a guide to the prognosis of the patients and the possibility of improvement by revascularization. The options that are available for revascularization are either by CABG or PCI.

4.3. Myocardial revascularization

Revascularization (CABG, PCI) in patients with IHD is vital in a subset of patients who have stunned or hibernating myocardium. In this subset of patients, revascularization was proven to improve outcome and prognosis as well as quality of life. In patients who do not have hibernating myocardium, no benefit from revascularization was found as compared to medical therapy.

4.3.1. CABG

In patients with multivessel coronary artery disease, CABG was shown to be superior to PCI as a revascularization strategy. A study done by Kohsaka et al.[67] randomized patients with multivessel disease to either CABG or PCI. They followed the patients up for 9 years. CABG resulted in better long term survival as compared to PCI (hazard ratio 0.7, 95% confidence interval 0.6 to 0.9; $p = 0.004$). However, in this study, more patients in the CABG group had triple vessel disease (76%) as compared to 27% with triple vessel disease in the PCI group.[67] Six-year follow-up data analysis from the SoS (Stent or Surgery) trial showed similarly a higher survival in patients randomized to undergo CABG (6.8% of patients died) versus PCI (10.9% of patients died) ($p = 0.022$).[68]

In patients with Stable CAD (multivessel disease with documented >70% occlusion and preserved EF) enrolled in the MASSII trial medical therapy, PCI and CABG were compared.[69] No difference in overall mortality, cardiovascular mortality, or recurrent MI was noted between the three groups. However, the CABG group needed significantly less additional intervention (3.5%) as compared to the medical therapy (24.2%) and PCI (32.2%) groups.[69] Anginal symptoms were more prevalent in the medical therapy group as compared to the PCI and CABG groups (no difference in anginal symptoms was found between the last two groups).[69]

4.3.2. PCI

Primary angioplasty with stent implantation is considered the standard of care in patients with acute MI. The use of PCI in these patients results in improvement in survival, better vessel patency, and reduced reinfarction rates as compared to medical therapy.[70] Different types of stents may be used for revascularization including bare metal stents (BMS) and drug eluting stents (DES). A comparison between DES and BMS in patients with MI showed that patients who received a DES had better survival at 2 years after MI as compared to a matched cohort of patients who received BMS (10.7% vs. 12.8%, $p = 0.02$). While there was no significant difference in the reinfarction rate at 2 years, need for target vessel revascularization was higher in the subgroup that received BMS versus DES group (14.5% vs. 9.6%, $p <0.001$).[70]

The INSPIRE clinical trial[71] investigated the use of aggressive medical therapy as compared to revascularization in reducing scintigraphic ischemia in patients with IHD (large total (≥20%) and ischemic (≥10%) LV perfusion defect size (PDS) and an LVEF ≥35% by adenosine SPECT. There was no difference in cardiac mortality and reinfarction in the two groups investigated.[71] However, one limitation of the INSPIRE trial is the fact that it was designed before drug-eluting stents use. This might have affected the improvement in ischemia suppression seen in the revascularization group.[71] The COURAGE trial investigated the use of PCI plus medical therapy versus medical therapy alone in patients with stable coronary artery disease. Patients who were randomized to PCI plus medical therapy had no improvement in the primary end point, defined as death from any cause and nonfatal MI during a follow-up period reaching up to 7 years.[72] The secondary endpoint defined as a composite of death, MI, stroke, and hospitalization for unstable angina with negative biomarkers was not different between the two groups studied, either.[72] A substudy from the courage trial found that PCI with OMT compared to OMT alone resulted in a significantly greater reduction in ischemia at 18 months follow-up as assessed by MPI (33.3% of patients on medical therapy + PCI with >5% ischemia reduction vs. 18.9% of patients on therapy alone). Similarly, moderate to severe ischemia patients (defined as >10% ischemic myocardium on pretreatment MPS) treated with PCI + therapy had a greater reduction in ischemia at 18 months of follow-up (78% vs. 55% respectively). Patients with >5% ischemic myocardium had worse outcome than patients with <5% ischemia by MPS; hence, the importance of PCI + therapy lies in reducing the ischemic burden as opposed to therapy alone. In addition, patients who underwent PCI + therapy had smaller LV end-systolic volumes and higher EF at 18 months of follow-up as compared to the group that received medical therapy alone.[73]

The management outlined above is for patients with IHD who are stable. However, in patients presenting with IHD and decompensated heart failure, the treatment options are to stabilize the patient with a series of interventions including medical therapy (as discussed above), as well as mechanical interventions in patients refractory to acute medical management. These include mechanical support devices (IABP, ECMO). The use of mechanical assist devices including LVADs helps as a bridge in patients with advanced stage heart failure for heart transplantation. Some patients referred for heart transplantation who were worked up by viability assessment and who were revascularized after finding viable myocardium demonstrated improvement in symptoms after the revascularization. These patients' status and their candidacy for heart transplantation were reviewed.

4.4. Mechanical support devices

Mechanical support devices have been used extensively to restore organ perfusion in cases of acute heart failure (cardiogenic shock) and in patients with end stage heart failure as a bridge to heart transplantation. Other indications for the LV assist devices include high risk revascularization procedures (CABG in high risk patients, percutaneous closure of a VSD). The immediate benefit of mechanical support devices is the fact that they help restoring organ perfusion in cases of acute heart failure.

4.4.1. Intra aortic balloon pump

The intra aortic balloon pump (IABP) use reduces myocardial oxygen demand and increases coronary blood flow velocity. In patients presenting to the GUSTO I trial with cardiogenic shock, patients who received IABP were compared to those who did not.[74] Patients who received IABP tended to have more anterior MI, higher CKs, and higher CKMB fractions as compared to the control group. Patients in the IABP group were more likely to have inotropic support, intubation, and monitoring. There was no significant improvement in mortality in patients that received IABP as compared to the control group at 30 days.[74] However, the mortality at 1 year was lower in the group that received early IABP as compared to the control group. The rates of recurrent ischemia and reinfarction were higher, however, in patients who had early implantation of the IABP. There was no difference in the incidence of severe or life-threatening bleeding in the group who received IABP and the group who did not. However, there was more moderate bleeding in the IABP group.[74]

4.4.2. Left ventricular assist devices

The left ventricular assist devices (LVAD) help maintain circulation in cases of severe LV failure. One of the advantages of LVADs over IABP is the fact that they restore cardiac output while the function of IABP is to decrease afterload.[75] Another advantage of LVAD is that they do not need extracorporeal oxygenation since they aspirate blood directly from the atrium or ventricle. Two LVADs widely used are the TandemHeart, which aspirates the blood from the left atrium and injects it into the femoral artery, and the impella recover system, which aspirates blood from the left ventricle and injects it into the ascending aorta.[75] A multicenter randomized controlled trial compared TandemHeart with the IABP in 42 patients with cardiogenic shock.[76] The duration of support was 2.5 days. Patients in the TandemHeart group had greater increases in the cardiac index and lower PCWP as compared to patients on the IABP. The percentage of patients on the TandemHeart that suffered from adverse events was similar to that of IABP patient group.[76] There was no significant difference in mortality between the two patients groups (53% in the TandemHeart as compared to 64% in the IABP group).[76]

4.4.3. Extra corporeal membrane oxygenation

Extra corporeal membrane oxygenation (ECMO) is used in cases of severe cardiopulmonary failure, failure to wean from cardiopulmonary bypass and from decompensated end stage heart failure.[77] ECMO should be initiated prior to complete cardiopulmonary collapse in patients with anticipated deterioration. Risk factors for death from ECMO include female sex, age >55 years, shorter height, thoracic aortic operation, decompensated heart failure, and cardiogenic shock.[77] Complications of ECMO use include infection, dialysis, and stroke. ECMO with IABP support yielded better results when compared to patients with IABP; patients with IABP were more likely to be weaned as compared to patients who did not have IABP. A study assessed the 5 years survival of patients receiving ECMO. Survival after 1 week and 4 weeks of ECMO was 58% and 38%, respectively. Sixty-three percent of patients who survived to the 4 weeks time point achieved 5 years survival. Survival after being bridged from ECMO to LVAD or to transplantation was 67% at 30 days and 44% at 5 years.[77]

4.4.4. Heart transplantation

Coronary artery disease is the most common cause of heart failure. In addition to the treatment modalities outlined above, the treatment of end stage HF is heart transplantation. However, this treatment modality is limited by the low number of donors. Among the relative contraindications of heart transplantation is advanced age, cachexia, and morbid obesity.[78] The modalities discussed above, especially LVADs, are used most often as a bridge to transplantation. A study investigating the impact of age on the outcome of advanced HF patients undergoing heart transplantation showed that increasing age did not predict a worse outcome after 5 years of follow-up. The factor that resulted in statistically significant mortality difference in heart transplant recipients by multivariate analysis was ischemic etiology of the heart failure.[79] One year survival following heart transplantation is 77% to 85%; 5 year survival ranges from 61% to 76%.[78,79] A study investigating the effect of body weight on survival in heart transplant recipients showed no adverse effect on survival in heart transplant recipients due to weight. They assessed as well the effect of any weight gain following cardiac transplantation. Patients who gained >5 kg had better survival than patients who gained from 0 to 5 kg; both of these groups had better survival than patients who lost any weight during the first year after transplantation.[78]

5. IMAGING AND PROGNOSIS

5.1. Echocardiography

Stress echocardiography is a useful tool for risk stratification in patients with coronary artery disease. It is an independent predictor of cardiac events in patients with established CAD. Patients with normal DSE have a markedly reduced risk of cardiac events during the 3 years following the study.[80] In patients known to have CAD, the presence of wall motion abnormality was shown to confer bad prognosis. WMSI abnormality at peak stress conferred a hazard ratio of 2.3 for events (death and nonfatal MI) as compared to CFR abnormality (HR 4.9).[81] The addition of inflammatory markers such as IL6 and tissue factor result in improvement in the ability of the stress echocardiography in risk assessment of IHD patients. IL6 and TF increased in patients with ischemia undergoing DSE as compared to patients without ischemia. IL6 was elevated in patients who had cardiac events as compared to patients who did not suffer from cardiac events; tissue factor did not differ between these two patient groups. Patients with IL6 value >3.15 pg/mL at peak DSE had a 2.7 risk of events as compared to patients with IL6 <3.15 pg/mL.[80]

The prognostic value of wall thickness has been recently investigated in patients with chronic stable coronary artery disease.[82] Patients with LVH (higher posterior wall thickness and septal thickness as compared to patients with no LVH) tended to be older, men, diabetics, with a history of DM and CHF. The increased LV mass in the patients studied was shown to be an adverse prognostic indicator. Patients with abnormal relative wall thickness and LVH had significantly higher all cause mortality and higher death from sudden and arrhythmic causes as compared to patients with normal wall thickness after adjustment for all confounding variables.[82, 83]

5.2. Nuclear perfusion imaging

Stress gated myocardial perfusion scanning (MPS) is the most commonly used method for risk stratification.[84] Patients with normal MPS are at low risk for subsequent cardiac events. On the other hand, patients with extensive perfusion defects need to undergo coronary angiography and be treated accordingly. Ejection fraction and end systolic volume measurements were shown to add value to the risk assessment using MPS.[84] In a retrospective study of patients with angiographic CAD who underwent ^{99m}Tc-Sestamibi SPECT imaging, there were only three nonfatal MI in the CAD group as compared to normal control subjects over a period of 50 months of follow-up; this difference was not statistically significant. However, the rate of soft cardiac events (late revascularization) was higher in the CAD group as compared to the control group.[85]

5.3. Magnetic resonance imaging

Characterization of the scar tissue by magnetic resonance imaging was shown to carry important prognostic information. In a study by Yokota et al., patients with cardiovascular events had a larger scar volume and higher scar percentage of the myocardium as compared to patients with no cardiovascular events even though both groups had a similar ejection fraction.[86] Comparison between assessment of left ventricular end-systolic volume (LVESV), left ventricular end-diastolic volume (LVEDV), and LVEF and between the volume of the scar tissue and the percentage of scar in the myocardium quantitation by MRI showed that LVESV, LVEDV, and LVEF have less correlation than scar quantitation in predicting the risk of cardiovascular events.[86] In another study, the amount of peri-infarct ischemia by magnetic resonance imaging was shown to correlate with cardiovascular outcome in patients with severe ICM. For instance, patients with higher amounts of peri-infarct ischemia were found to have higher percentage of cardiovascular events as compared to patients with less ischemic peri-infarct zone.[87]

5.4. Computed tomography

A study comparing the prognostic implications of MSCT findings in patients with known coronary artery disease was undertaken by Pundziute et al.[88] Patients with more extensive atherosclerosis on MSCT had a higher incidence of cardiac events as compared to patients with less segments involvement on MSCT.[88] Multivariate analysis showed that the independent predictors of adverse cardiac events by MSCT included the presence of coronary plaques, obstructive CAD, LM/LAD disease, number of coronary segments with plaques, number of coronary segments with obstructive plaques, and number of coronary segments with mixed (calcified, noncalcified) plaques. Conversely patients with normal MSCT had an excellent prognosis, while patients with evidence of CAD on MSCT had a 30% increase in cardiac events.[88]

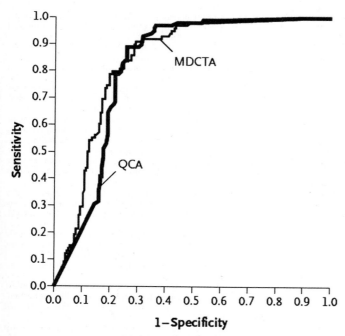

Figure 26.16 Receiver-operating-characteristic (ROC) curve (solid line) describing the performance of CTA (AUC, 0.84; 95% CI, 0.79 to 0.88) versus quantitative coronary angiography (QCA, AUC, 0.82; 95% CI, 0.77 to 0.86) to predict which patients would undergo surgical or catheter-based coronary revascularization within 30 days after conventional coronary angiography. (Adapted from Miller JM, et al. Diagnostic performance of coronary angiography by 64-row CT. *N Engl J Med.* 2008;359:2324–2336.)

6. FUTURE DIRECTIONS

The value of cardiac imaging for the evaluation of patients with chronic IHD is undeniable. Contrast-enhanced CT is capable of detecting the presence of CAD with high sensitivity and specificity. A recent multicenter study[89] demonstrated that CT angiography was similar to conventional angiography in its ability to identify patients who will require revascularization with an area under the curve (AUC) of 0.84 (95% CI, 0.79 to 0.88) for multidetector CT angiography versus 0.82 (95% CI, 0.77 to 0.86) for conventional angiography (Fig. 26.16). Viability assessment by SPECT, PECG, dobutamine echocardiography, and CMR delayed-enhancement identify patients who are more likely to derive benefit from revascularization. Nevertheless, these tests have not been compared head-to-head in large clinical trials. Even more, although several studies demonstrate that patients with IHD and viable myocardium treated medically have worse outcomes compared to those undergoing revascularization, these studies have been largely retrospective and patients have not been randomized to treatment groups. As we approach a new era of economic constraints, outcome studies will need to be conducted to establish the clinical utility of imaging studies for selecting appropriate candidates for medical therapy, revascularization, and devices.

REFERENCES

1. Rosamond W, et al. Heart disease and stroke statistics–2008 update: A report from the American Heart Association Statistics Committee and Stroke Statistics Subcommittee. *Circulation.* 2008;117(4):e25–e146.
2. D'Antono B, et al. Angina symptoms in men and women with stable coronary artery disease and evidence of exercise-induced myocardial perfusion defects. *Am Heart J.* 2006;151(4):813–819.
3. Abrams J. Clinical practice. Chronic stable angina. *N Engl J Med.* 2005;352(24):2524–2533.
4. Friedewald VE, et al. The editor's roundtable: Chronic stable angina pectoris. *Am J Cardiol.* 2007;100(11):1635–1643.
5. Packard RR, Libby P. Inflammation in atherosclerosis: From vascular biology to biomarker discovery and risk prediction. *Clin Chem.* 2008;54(1):24–38.
6. Libby P, Ridker PM, Maseri A. Inflammation and atherosclerosis. *Circulation.* 2002;105(9):1135–1143.
7. Nakashima Y, et al. Early human atherosclerosis: Accumulation of lipid and proteoglycans in intimal thickenings followed by macrophage infiltration. *Arterioscler Thromb Vasc Biol.* 2007;27(5):1159–1165.
8. Halcox JP, et al. Prognostic value of coronary vascular endothelial dysfunction. *Circulation.* 2002;106(6):653–658.
9. Pasterkamp G, Fitzgerald PF, de Kleijn DP. Atherosclerotic expansive remodeled plaques: A wolf in sheep's clothing. *J Vasc Res.* 2002;39(6):514–523.
10. Hong MK, et al. A three-vessel virtual histology intravascular ultrasound analysis of frequency and distribution of thin-cap fibroatheromas in patients with acute coronary syndrome or stable angina pectoris. *Am J Cardiol.* 2008;101(5):568–572.
11. Schoenhagen P, et al. Extent and direction of arterial remodeling in stable versus unstable coronary syndromes: An intravascular ultrasound study. *Circulation.* 2000;101(6):598–603.
12. Camici PG, Prasad SK, Rimoldi OE. Stunning, hibernation, and assessment of myocardial viability. *Circulation.* 2008;117(1):103–114.
13. Wijns W, Vatner SF, Camici PG. Hibernating myocardium. *N Engl J Med.* 1998;339(3):173–181.
14. Pagano D, et al. Hibernating myocardium: Morphological correlates of inotropic stimulation and glucose uptake. *Heart.* 2000;83(4):456–461.
15. Bragadeesh T, et al. Post-ischaemic myocardial dysfunction (stunning) results from myofibrillar oedema. *Heart.* 2008;94(2):166–171.
16. Page B, et al. Persistent regional downregulation in mitochondrial enzymes and upregulation of stress proteins in swine with chronic hibernating myocardium. *Circ Res.* 2008;102(1):103–112.
17. Camici PG, Rimoldi OE. Myocardial blood flow in patients with hibernating myocardium. *Cardiovasc Res.* 2003;57(2):302–311.
18. Canty JM Jr, et al. Hibernating myocardium: Chronically adapted to ischemia but vulnerable to sudden death. *Circ Res.* 2004;94(8):1142–1149.
19. D'Ancona G, et al. Ischemic mitral valve regurgitation: The new challenge for magnetic resonance imaging. *Eur J Cardiothorac Surg.* 2007;32(3):475–480.
20. Okura H, et al. Functional mitral regurgitation predicts prognosis independent of left ventricular systolic and diastolic indices in patients with ischemic heart disease. *J Am Soc Echocardiogr.* 2008;21(4):355–360.
21. Magne J, et al. Restrictive annuloplasty for ischemic mitral regurgitation may induce functional mitral stenosis. *J Am Coll Cardiol.* 2008;51(17):1692–1701.
22. Dewey M, et al. Evaluation of global and regional left ventricular function with 16-slice computed tomography, biplane cineventriculography, and

two-dimensional transthoracic echocardiography: Comparison with magnetic resonance imaging. *J Am Coll Cardiol.* 2006;48(10):2034–2044.

23. Krenning BJ, et al. Comparison of contrast agent-enhanced versus non-contrast agent-enhanced real-time three-dimensional echocardiography for analysis of left ventricular systolic function. *Am J Cardiol.* 2007;100(9):1485–1489.

24. Jenkins C, et al. Comparison of two- and three-dimensional echocardiography with sequential magnetic resonance imaging for evaluating left ventricular volume and ejection fraction over time in patients with healed myocardial infarction. *Am J Cardiol.* 2007;99(3):300–306.

25. Scanlon PJ, et al. ACC/AHA guidelines for coronary angiography. A report of the American College of Cardiology/American Heart Association Task Force on practice guidelines (committee on coronary angiography). Developed in collaboration with the Society for Cardiac Angiography and Interventions. *J Am Coll Cardiol.* 1999;33(6):1756–1824.

26. Nieman K, et al. Coronary angiography with multi-slice computed tomography. *Lancet.* 2001;357(9256):599–603.

27. Garcia MJ, Lessick J, Hoffmann MH. Accuracy of 16-row multidetector computed tomography for the assessment of coronary artery stenosis. *JAMA.* 2006;296(4):403–411.

28. Bayrak F, et al. Diagnostic performance of 64-slice computed tomography coronary angiography to detect significant coronary artery stenosis. *Acta Cardiol.* 2008;63(1):11–17.

29. Dill T, et al. Radiation dose exposure in multislice computed tomography of the coronaries in comparison with conventional coronary angiography. *Int J Cardiol.* 2008;124(3):307–311.

30. Pope JH, et al. Missed diagnoses of acute cardiac ischemia in the emergency department. *N Engl J Med.* 2000;342(16):1163–1170.

31. Fayn J, et al. Improvement of the detection of myocardial ischemia thanks to information technologies. *Int J Cardiol.* 2007;120(2):172–180.

32. Martin TN, et al. ST-segment deviation analysis of the admission 12-lead electrocardiogram as an aid to early diagnosis of acute myocardial infarction with a cardiac magnetic resonance imaging gold standard. *J Am Coll Cardiol.* 2007;50(11):1021–1028.

33. Owens C, et al. Comparison of value of leads from body surface maps to 12-lead electrocardiogram for diagnosis of acute myocardial infarction. *Am J Cardiol.* 2008;102(3):257–265.

34. Perron A, et al. Maximal increase in sensitivity with minimal loss of specificity for diagnosis of acute coronary occlusion achieved by sequentially adding leads from the 24-lead electrocardiogram to the orderly sequenced 12-lead electrocardiogram. *J Electrocardiol.* 2007;40(6):463–469.

35. Tragardh E, et al. Detection of acute myocardial infarction using the 12-lead ECG plus inverted leads versus the 16-lead ECG (with additional posterior and right-sided chest electrodes). *Clin Physiol Funct Imaging.* 2007;27(6):368–374.

36. Gibbons RJ, et al. ACC/AHA guidelines for exercise testing. A report of the American College of Cardiology/American Heart Association Task Force on practice guidelines (committee on exercise testing). *J Am Coll Cardiol.* 1997;30(1):260–311.

37. Nishime EO, et al. Heart rate recovery and treadmill exercise score as predictors of mortality in patients referred for exercise ECG. *JAMA.* 2000;284(11):1392–1398.

38. Leeper NJ, et al. Prognostic value of heart rate increase at onset of exercise testing. *Circulation.* 2007;115(4):468–474.

39. Gibbons RJ, et al. ACC/AHA 2002 guideline update for exercise testing: Summary article. A report of the American College of Cardiology/American Heart Association task force on practice guidelines (committee to update the 1997 exercise testing guidelines). *J Am Coll Cardiol.* 2002;40(8):1531–1540.

40. Picano E, Molinaro S, Pasanisi E. The diagnostic accuracy of pharmacological stress echocardiography for the assessment of coronary artery disease: A meta-analysis. *Cardiovasc Ultrasound.* 2008;6(30).

41. Dunkelgrun M, et al. Significance of hypotensive response during dobutamine stress echocardiography. *Int J Cardiol.* 2008;125(3):358–363.

42. McKeogh JR. The diagnostic role of stress echocardiography in women with coronary artery disease: Evidence based review. *Curr Opin Cardiol.* 2007;22(5):429–433.

43. Douglas PS, et al. ACCF/ASE/ACEP/AHA/ASNC/SCAI/SCCT/SCMR 2008 appropriateness criteria for stress echocardiography: A report of the American College of Cardiology Foundation Appropriateness Criteria Task Force, American Society of Echocardiography, American College of Emergency Physicians, American Heart Association, American Society of Nuclear Cardiology, Society for Cardiovascular Angiography and Interventions, Society of Cardiovascular Computed Tomography, and Society for Cardiovascular Magnetic Resonance: Endorsed by the Heart Rhythm Society and the Society of Critical Care Medicine. *Circulation.* 2008;117(11):1478–1497.

44. Vesely MR, Dilsizian V. Nuclear cardiac stress testing in the era of molecular medicine. *J Nucl Med.* 2008;49(3):399–413.

45. Klocke FJ, et al. ACC/AHA/ASNC guidelines for the clinical use of cardiac radionuclide imaging–executive summary: A report of the American College of Cardiology/American Heart Association Task Force on practice guidelines (ACC/AHA/ASNC committee to revise the 1995 guidelines for the clinical use of cardiac radionuclide imaging). *Circulation.* 2003;108(11):1404–1418.

46. Nandalur KR, et al. Diagnostic performance of stress cardiac magnetic resonance imaging in the detection of coronary artery disease: A meta-analysis. *J Am Coll Cardiol.* 2007;50(14):1343–1353.

47. Sicari R, et al. Prognostic value of myocardial viability recognized by low-dose dobutamine echocardiography in chronic ischemic left ventricular dysfunction. *Am J Cardiol.* 2003;92(11):1263–1266.

48. Allman KC, et al. Myocardial viability testing and impact of revascularization on prognosis in patients with coronary artery disease and left ventricular dysfunction: A meta-analysis. *J Am Coll Cardiol.* 2002;39(7):1151–1158.

49. Barmeyer AA, et al. Myocardial contractile response to increasing doses of dobutamine in patients with reperfused acute myocardial infarction by cardiac magnetic resonance imaging. *Cardiology.* 2008;110(3):153–159.

50. Kudo T. Metabolic imaging using PET. *Eur J Nucl Med Mol Imaging.* 2007;34(1):S49–S61.

51. Feola M, et al. Myocardial scar and insulin resistance predict cardiovascular events in severe ischaemic myocardial dysfunction: A perfusion-metabolism positron emission tomography study. *Nucl Med Commun.* 2008;29(5):448–454.

52. Saraste A, Nekolla S, Schwaiger M. Contrast-enhanced magnetic resonance imaging in the assessment of myocardial infarction and viability. *J Nucl Cardiol.* 2008;15(1):105–117.

53. Gottlieb I, et al. Magnetic resonance imaging in the evaluation of non-ischemic cardiomyopathies: Current applications and future perspectives. *Heart Fail Rev.* 2006;11(4):313–323.

54. Kaandorp TA, et al. Head-to-head comparison between contrast-enhanced magnetic resonance imaging and dobutamine magnetic resonance imaging in men with ischemic cardiomyopathy. *Am J Cardiol.* 2004;93(12):1461–1464.

55. Fraker TD Jr, et al. 2007 chronic angina focused update of the ACC/AHA 2002 Guidelines for the management of patients with chronic stable angina: A report of the American College of Cardiology/American Heart Association Task Force on practice guidelines writing group to develop the focused update of the 2002 Guidelines for the management of patients with chronic stable angina. *Circulation.* 2007;116(23):2762–2772.

56. Becker RC, et al. The primary and secondary prevention of coronary artery disease: American College of Chest Physicians evidence-based clinical practice guidelines (8th Edition). *Chest.* 2008;133(6):776S–814S.

57. Bhatt DL, et al. Clopidogrel and aspirin versus aspirin alone for the prevention of atherothrombotic events. *N Engl J Med.* 2006;354(16):1706–1717.

58. Bhatt DL, et al. Patients with prior myocardial infarction, stroke, or symptomatic peripheral arterial disease in the CHARISMA trial. *J Am Coll Cardiol.* 2007;49(19):1982–1988.

59. Grundy SM, et al. Implications of recent clinical trials for the National Cholesterol Education Program Adult Treatment Panel III guidelines. *Circulation.* 2004;110(2):227–239.

60. Josan K, Majumdar SR, McAlister FA. The efficacy and safety of intensive statin therapy: A meta-analysis of randomized trials. *CMAJ.* 2008;178(5):576–584.

61. Bunch TJ, et al. Effect of beta-blocker therapy on mortality rates and future myocardial infarction rates in patients with coronary artery disease but no history of myocardial infarction or congestive heart failure. *Am J Cardiol.* 2005;95(7):827–831.

62. Brugts JJ, et al. Pharmacogenetics of ACE inhibition in stable coronary artery disease: Steps towards tailored drug therapy. *Curr Opin Cardiol.* 2008;23(4):296–301.

63. Dagenais GR, et al. Angiotensin-converting-enzyme inhibitors in stable vascular disease without left ventricular systolic dysfunction or heart failure: A combined analysis of three trials. *Lancet.* 2006;368(9535):581–588.

64. Beanlands RS, et al. F-18-fluorodeoxyglucose positron emission tomography imaging-assisted management of patients with severe left ventricular dysfunction and suspected coronary disease: A randomized, controlled trial (PARR-2). *J Am Coll Cardiol.* 2007;50(20):2002–2012.

65. Knuesel PR, et al. Characterization of dysfunctional myocardium by positron emission tomography and magnetic resonance: Relation to functional outcome after revascularization. *Circulation.* 2003;108(9):1095–1100.

66. Bondarenko O, et al. Functional outcome after revascularization in patients with chronic ischemic heart disease: A quantitative late gadolinium enhancement CMR study evaluating transmural scar extent, wall thickness and periprocedural necrosis. *J Cardiovasc Magn Reson.* 2007;9(5):815–821.

67. Kohsaka S, et al. Long-term clinical outcome of coronary artery stenting or coronary artery bypass grafting in patients with multiple-vessel disease. *J Thorac Cardiovasc Surg.* 2008;136(2):500–506.

68. Booth J, et al. Randomized, controlled trial of coronary artery bypass surgery versus percutaneous coronary intervention in patients with multivessel coronary artery disease: Six-year follow-up from the Stent or Surgery Trial (SoS). *Circulation.* 2008;118(4):381–388.

69. Hueb W, et al. Five-year follow-up of the medicine, angioplasty, or surgery study (MASS II): A randomized controlled clinical trial of 3 therapeutic strategies for multivessel coronary artery disease. *Circulation.* 2007;115(9):1082–1089.

70. Mauri L, et al. Drug-eluting or bare-metal stents for acute myocardial infarction. *N Engl J Med.* 2008;359(13):1330–1342.

71. Mahmarian JJ, et al. An initial strategy of intensive medical therapy is comparable to that of coronary revascularization for suppression of scintigraphic ischemia in high-risk but stable survivors of acute myocardial infarction. *J Am Coll Cardiol.* 2006;48(12):2458–2467.

72. Boden WE, et al. Optimal medical therapy with or without PCI for stable coronary disease. *N Engl J Med.* 2007;356(15):1503–1516.

73. Shaw LJ, et al. Optimal medical therapy with or without percutaneous coronary intervention to reduce ischemic burden: Results from the clinical outcomes utilizing revascularization and aggressive drug evaluation (COURAGE) trial nuclear substudy. *Circulation.* 2008;117(10):1283–1291.

74. Anderson RD, et al. Use of intraaortic balloon counterpulsation in patients presenting with cardiogenic shock: Observations from the GUSTO-I Study. Global utilization of streptokinase and TPA for occluded coronary arteries. *J Am Coll Cardiol.* 1997;30(3):708–715.

75. Windecker S. Percutaneous left ventricular assist devices for treatment of patients with cardiogenic shock. *Curr Opin Crit Care.* 2007;13(5):521–527.
76. Burkhoff D, et al. A randomized multicenter clinical study to evaluate the safety and efficacy of the TandemHeart percutaneous ventricular assist device versus conventional therapy with intraaortic balloon pumping for treatment of cardiogenic shock. *Am Heart J.* 2006;152(3):469 e1–e8.
77. Smedira NG, et al. Clinical experience with 202 adults receiving extracorporeal membrane oxygenation for cardiac failure: Survival at five years. *J Thorac Cardiovasc Surg.* 2001;122(1):92–102.
78. Clark AL, et al. Heart transplantation in heart failure: The prognostic importance of body mass index at time of surgery and subsequent weight changes. *Eur J Heart Fail.* 2007;9(8):839–844.
79. Grigioni F, et al. Age and heart transplantation: Results from a heart failure management unit. *Clin Transplant.* 2008;22(2):150–155.
80. Ikonomidis I, et al. Additive prognostic value of interleukin-6 at peak phase of dobutamine stress echocardiography in patients with coronary artery disease. A 6-year follow-up study. *Am Heart J.* 2008;156(2):269–276.
81. Rigo F, et al. The additive prognostic value of wall motion abnormalities and coronary flow reserve during dipyridamole stress echo. *Eur Heart J.* 2008;29(1):79–88.
82. Turakhia MP, Schiller NB, Whooley MA. Prognostic significance of increased left ventricular mass index to mortality and sudden death in patients with stable coronary heart disease (from the Heart and Soul Study). *Am J Cardiol.* 2008;102(9):1131–1135.
83. Ghali JK, Liao Y, Cooper RS. Influence of left ventricular geometric patterns on prognosis in patients with or without coronary artery disease. *J Am Coll Cardiol.* 1998;31(7):1635–1640.
84. Berman DS, et al. Roles of nuclear cardiology, cardiac computed tomography, and cardiac magnetic resonance: Noninvasive risk stratification and a conceptual framework for the selection of noninvasive imaging tests in patients with known or suspected coronary artery disease. *J Nucl Med.* 2006;47(7):1107–1118.
85. Yang MF, et al. Prognostic value of normal exercise 99mTc-sestamibi myocardial tomography in patients with angiographic coronary artery disease. *Nucl Med Commun.* 2006;27(4):333–338.
86. Yokota H, et al. Quantitative characterization of myocardial infarction by cardiovascular magnetic resonance predicts future cardiovascular events in patients with ischemic cardiomyopathy. *J Cardiovasc Magn Reson.* 2008;10(1):17.
87. Tsukiji M, et al. Peri-infarct ischemia determined by cardiovascular magnetic resonance evaluation of myocardial viability and stress perfusion predicts future cardiovascular events in patients with severe ischemic cardiomyopathy. *J Cardiovasc Magn Reson.* 2006;8(6):773–779.
88. Pundziute G, et al. Prognostic value of multislice computed tomography coronary angiography in patients with known or suspected coronary artery disease. *J Am Coll Cardiol.* 2007;49(1):62–70.
89. Miller JM, et al. Diagnostic performance of coronary angiography by 64-row CT. *N Engl J Med.* 2008;359:2324–2336.

Aortic Stenosis

27

L. Leonardo Rodriguez and Ruvin Gabriel

1. INTRODUCTION

Comprehensive evaluation of aortic stenosis (AS) has been a remarkable success of noninvasive cardiovascular imaging. The use of echocardiography has allowed evaluation of left ventricular (LV) function and degree of hypertrophy, transvalvular gradients, aortic valve morphology, and degree of associated aortic regurgitation (AR). It has also provided knowledge of the natural history of the disease and prognosis. The advent of multislice computed tomography (CT) has provided additional information about the degree of calcification and precise measurements of the ascending aorta and, more recently, diagnostic images of the coronary anatomy.[1] The routine use of these techniques has decreased the need for cardiac catheterization and, in particular, to cross the valve to quantify stenosis severity.[2]

1.1. Epidemiology

AS is the most common single valvular lesion seen in the adult population. In the Euro Heart Survey, AS accounted for 43.1% of single native left-sided valve disease.[3] The age at presentation depends on the etiology of the lesion. Unicuspid valves are infrequent in the adult population (approximately 0.02%)[4] and present in the third decade of life. Patients with bicuspid present in the fifth and sixth decades of life.[5] Patients with degenerative aortic disease present after the seventh decade of life. In the Helsinki Aging Study, severe aortic calcification was seen in 13% of patients 75 years or older. Critical AS was seen in 2.2% of the same population.[6]

Although rheumatic heart disease is prevalent in the developing world, in the United States, rheumatic AS now represents the least common form of AS. In Europe, rheumatic AS accounts for 11% of the cases[3] (Table 27.1). Rheumatic AS typically presents in the fifth and sixth decades of life and is seen often associated with AR and mitral valve disease.

1.2. Clinical presentation

1.2.1. Symptoms

The normal area of the adult aortic valve measures, on average, 3.0 to $4.0\,cm^2$; reduction of valve area usually does not produce symptoms until the valve reaches one fourth of its normal dimension, typically $<1.0\,cm^2$

Patients with AS may remain asymptomatic for many years. As the disease progresses, symptoms associated with physical activities will appear. The classic triad of angina, syncope and heart failure and its prognostic significance was described by Ross and Braunwald in 1968[7] and confirmed recently.[8–10] In a study of 622 patients with asymptomatic, significant AS, a third of the patients developed symptoms in the following 2 years and two thirds in

5 years.[9] Once symptoms develop, the prognosis without intervention is poor, particularly in those with congestive heart failure (CHF) with a mean survival of <2 years. The incidence of sudden death is relatively rare in asymptomatic patients (1% to 4%)[9,11] but increases dramatically in symptomatic patients (up to 34%).[12]

2. PATHOGENESIS

2.1. Acquired aortic stenosis

Degenerative calcification of the aortic valve is the most common cause of AS accounting for 82% of the cases in The Euro Heart Survey on Valvular Heart Disease.[3] Traditionally considered to be the result of chronic mechanical stress on normal valves, degenerative AS is now believed to be caused by proliferative and inflammatory changes (Fig. 27.1).[13] The histological features in acquired AS have received considerable attention lately.[14–19]

The stenotic aortic valve shows a series of abnormalities that include:

1. Inflammation
2. Angiogenesis
3. Extracellular matrix remodeling
4. Biomineralization (calcification)[13]

The early lesion of calcific aortic disease involves basement membrane disruption, upregulation of angiotensin-converting enzyme activity, macrophage and T-lymphocyte migration, and lipid infiltration. Increased bone-regulatory protein expression results in calcification and bone formation.[20] A recent study used thermography in valves of patients with nonrheumatic AS undergoing aortic valve replacement (AVR). It showed that thermal heterogeneity correlated with inflammatory infiltrates and neovessels, supporting the hypothesis of an active inflammatory process being involved in these patients.[21]

There has also been significant progress in the understanding of the molecular mechanisms of aortic valve calcification. The role of oxidative stress in calcified, stenotic aortic valves has been elegantly studied.[22] It appears that oxidative stress is increased in calcified regions of human stenotic aortic valves. Increased oxidative stress is due at least in part to reduction in expression and activity of antioxidant enzymes and perhaps to uncoupled NOS activity. These mechanisms of oxidative stress are different from the ones occurring in atherosclerotic arteries.[22]

Calcific AS is also observed in a number of conditions with increased calcium turnover, including Paget disease of bone and end-stage renal disease. Radiation heart disease also affects the aortic valve with heavy leaflet calcification and is commonly associated with severe coronary artery disease and mitral valve calcification.

TABLE 27.1
ETIOLOGY OF AORTIC STENOSIS

Degenerative	81.9
Rheumatic	11.2
Congenital	5.4
Endocarditis	0.8
Inflammatory	0.1
Other	0.6

Source: Iung B, et al. A prospective survey of patients with valvular heart disease in Europe: The Euro heart survey on valvular heart disease. *Eur Heart J.* 2003;24(13):1231–1243.

2.2. Bicuspid aortic stenosis

Bicuspid aortic valve (BAV) represents the most common form of congenital AS. BAVs are present in 1% to 2% of the population and are more common in males; and many of these patients will develop stenosis.[23] In a large group of adults with BAVs, 22% had moderate or severe AS.[24] BAVs were found in 28% of surgical excised valves at one institution.[25] Progressive fibrosis and calcification of the bicuspid leaflets results in significant stenosis most commonly in the fifth and sixth decades of life. Unicommissural valves usually calcify earlier. The abnormal anatomy of the unicommissural or BAV causes turbulent flow, leading to fibrosis and calcification.

Bicuspid valves can be truly bileaflet valves with two sinus of Valsalva or they can be the result of congenital fusion of two of the leaflets. The most common morphological variant is the fusion of the left and right coronary cusps seen in around 60% of the cases.[26] Bicuspid valves often are associated with dilatation of the ascending aorta that may progress to aneurysm formation. Approximately 10% of the patients with BAV have sinus dilatation >40 mm at the time of presentation[24] but it may increase to

40% on follow-up.[27] Although bicuspid valve has been reported to have up to ninefold risk of dissection,[28–31] this complication has been seen in <1% of patients in recent prospective and population studies.[24,27]

The pathogenesis of BAV remains unclear and many factors are of importance in the formation of the semilunar valves. Several genes or gene products have been implicated in formation of BAV and some forms of BAV appear to be heritable.[26] Recent research suggests that a DNA transcriptional error, possibly for the gene encoding endothelial nitric oxide synthetase, may be implicated in the genetic abnormality that leads to BAV. It appears that the microfibrils within the aortic valve and the aortic root are defective in structure in patients with BAV disease.[32]

2.3. Rheumatic aortic stenosis

Rheumatic AS is rarely an isolated disease and usually occurs in conjunction with mitral valve stenosis. Rheumatic AS is characterized by diffuse fibrous leaflet thickening with variable degree of commissural fusion. The early stage of rheumatic AS is characterized by edema, lymphocytic infiltration, and revascularization of the leaflets. Thickening, commissural fusion, and scarred leaflet edges are present in the later stages.[33]

2.4. Pathophysiology

Normal aortic valves have an area of 3 to 4 cm^2 and offer little resistance to forward flow. A systolic gradient between the left ventricle and the aorta develops when the valve area has decreased to less than half of its initial area. Worsening AS leads to progressive increments in the transvalvular gradient and LV pressure overload. The left ventricle adapts to the systolic pressure overload developing concentric hypertrophy that results in increased LV wall thickness with normal chamber volume.[34]

According to Laplace's equation, the increased wall thickness allows normalization of wall stress:

$$\text{Stress} = \text{pressure} \times \text{radius}/2(\text{wall thickness}) \qquad (\text{Eq. 27.1})$$

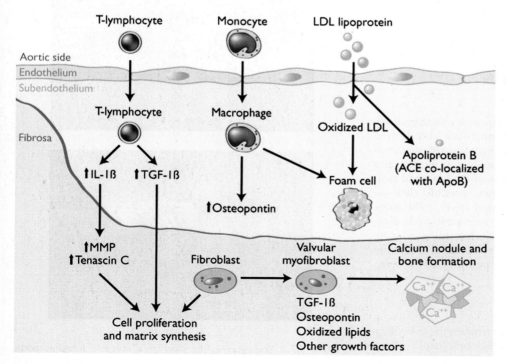

Figure 27.1 Potential pathways involved in calcific aortic valve disease. T lymphocytes and macrophages infiltrate endothelium and release cytokines that act on valvular fibroblasts to promote cellular proliferation and extracellular matrix remodeling. LDL is oxidized and taken up by macrophages to become foam cells. ACE is colocalized with apolipoprotein B (ApoB) and facilitates conversion of angiotensin II (AngII). A subset of valvular myofibroblasts differentiate into osteoblast phenotype that is capable of promoting bone formation. IL, interleukin; TGF, Transforming growth factor; MMP, matrix metalloproteinases.

Thus, the increased pressure in the left ventricle is offset by the augmented wall thickness, but wall stress remains normal. However, the development of hypertrophy may have negative consequences. With increased myocardial mass there is more oxygen demand that cannot be met by inadequate capillary growth. There is increased interstitial fibrosis with alteration of ventricular filling. In patients with AS and severe LV hypertrophy, there is delayed relaxation and increased myocardial stiffness, both of which contribute to increased LV filling pressures. Because of impaired early filling, the contribution of atrial contraction augments. This explains why patients with significant AS tolerate the development of atrial fibrillation poorly. Diastolic dysfunction has an important role in patient's symptoms and poor exercise tolerance.

In cases when the hypertrophic process is inadequate and wall thickness does not increase proportional to the intraventricular pressure, afterload mismatch may result leading to decrease in ejection fraction (EF).

The response to pressure overload in not uniform, with women more frequently showing smaller, hypertrophied, stiffer ventricles than men.[35] It has been described that one in ten patients with severe AS do not develop hypertrophy by mass criteria.[36]

Systemic arterial compliance is reduced in approximately 40% of patients with moderate or severe AS.[37] Systemic vascular resistance contributes to global LV afterload in adults with AS, a fact that needs to be kept in mind when evaluating patients with AS. Some authors have recommended evaluating valvulo-arterial impedance using the formula:

$$ZVA = (SAP + DP)/SVi, \qquad \text{(Eq. 27.2)}$$

where SAP is the systolic arterial pressure measured by sphygmomanometry; DP is the mean transvalvular gradient; and SVi is the stroke volume index for prediction of LV dysfunction and patient outcomes.[37]

The physiopathologic abnormalities seen in AS are reflected in the fundamental findings of noninvasive imaging tests:

1. Concentric LV hypertrophy with preserved EF in most of the patients
2. High transaortic valve gradients
3. Abnormal diastolic function

3. DIAGNOSTIC EVALUATION

3.1. Clinical diagnosis

The physical exam in patients with moderate or severe AS typically reveals peripheral pulses with reduced amplitude and delayed upstroke. The apical impulse is usually vigorous and sustained and not displaced. A crescendo–decrescendo systolic murmur with late peaking is prominent at the base of the heart and radiates to the carotids and often to the LV apex. A systolic click can be heard in a third of patients with bicuspid valves.[27] The aortic component is diminished or absent and may exhibit paradoxical splitting. However, when compared to echocardiography, no single physical examination finding or combination of findings appears to have both high sensitivity and specificity for the detection of severe valvular AS.[38]

3.2. Echocardiography

Ultrasound evaluation of the aortic valves remains the main diagnostic modality in patients with AS. Echocardiography allows evaluation of leaflet morphology and peak instantaneous and mean transvalvular gradients. In addition, this technique provides information on the presence and severity of AR and other associated valvular lesions, LV function, right ventricular systolic pressure, and proximal ascending aorta dimensions.

Although most of the information can be obtained from transthoracic echocardiography (TTE), transesophageal echo provides more detailed information on valve anatomy and the ascending aorta.

The recommendations for the diagnostic use of echocardiography were established by an American College of Cardiology/American Heart Association (ACC/AHA) task force in 2008.[39]

1. Echocardiography is recommended for the diagnosis and assessment of AS severity. (Level of Evidence: B)
2. Echocardiography is recommended in patients with AS for the assessment of LV wall thickness, size, and function. (Level of Evidence: B)
3. Echocardiography is recommended for re-evaluation of patients with known AS and changing symptoms or signs. (Level of Evidence: B)
4. Echocardiography is recommended for the assessment of changes in hemodynamic severity and LV function in patients with known AS during pregnancy. (Level of Evidence: B)[40]
5. TTE is recommended for re-evaluation of asymptomatic patients: every year for severe AS; every 1 to 2 years for moderate AS; and every 3 to 5 years for mild AS. (Level of Evidence: B)

3.2.1. Two-dimensional echocardiography

Two-dimensional echo (2DE) provides anatomical information of the aortic valve. For morphologic assessment, the parasternal window offers the best diagnostic images. From the parasternal long axis, the degree of leaflet mobility and thickening can be evaluated as well as annular diameter and calcification (Figs. 27.2 and 27.3). The ascending aorta is also evaluated from this window usually

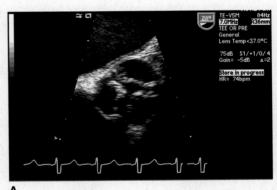

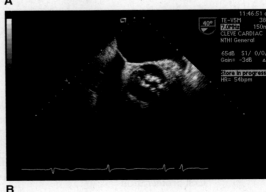

Figure 27.2 Transesophageal view of a stenotic trileaflet aortic valve. **A:** Notice the triangular configuration. **B:** A bicuspid valve, with elongated opening.

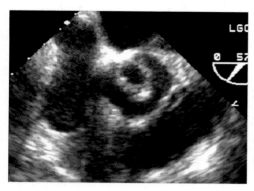

Figure 27.3 Unicuspid, unicommissural valve.

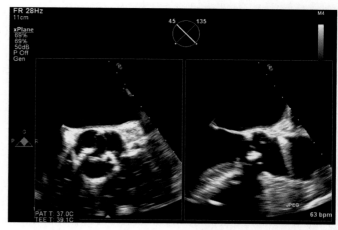

Figure 27.4 Simultaneous biplane, real time acquisition of short axis and long axis transesophageal views in patient with trileaflet aortic stenosis.

from higher intercostal space. Associated AR, when present, is also detected from this view. The parasternal short axis is optimal to evaluate the number of leaflets, fusion of the commissures, and degree of leaflet opening. Leaflet morphology should be evaluated in late systole when the leaflets are fully opened. The normal trileaflet valve has a triangular shape while bicuspid valves typically have an oval opening (Fig. 27.2). Bicuspid valves have a raphe formed by leaflet fusion and found in around 60% to 80% of the cases between the left and right coronary cusps.[26] Unicuspid valves have a unique morphology with an eccentric valvular orifice during systole and a single commissural zone of attachment. These valves can also lack a commissural attachment (acommissural valve), and have one aortic leaflet with or without visualization of raphe.[4]

In adult patients, the morphology of the valve cannot always be determined by TTE particularly when heavily calcified and TEE provides superior definition. Short axis view (45° to 60°) during TEE examination typically shows high-quality images that greatly facilitates the anatomical assessment in adult patients. The long axis view (120° to 150°) is ideal to evaluate leaflet opening and AR. From this view, the aortic dimension should be obtained typically at the annulus, sinus of valsalva, sinotubular junction, and ascending aorta. Transvalvular gradients by TEE are not easy to obtain. They require deep transgastric views from 0° or 100° for proper CW Doppler alignment.

Planimetry of aortic valve area. With good quality short-axis views by TTE or TEE, planimetry of the valve opening during systole can be used as a measure of the severity of the AS.[41-46] Although planimetry appears easy to obtain, some have reported poor correlation with catheterization and Doppler derived valve area.[47] Planimetry of the valve requires meticulous imaging ensuring that the cross section of the valve is at the tip of the leaflets. Planimetry provides data on the anatomical size of the valve and therefore may be larger than the calculated effective orifice area (EOA) obtained by Doppler methods (see 3.3.2). Heavily calcified valves make planimetry challenging and often unreliable.

The advent of real time 3D echo (RT3DE) has allowed simultaneous acquisition of biplane images that facilitate obtaining true short axis views of the aortic valve (Fig. 27.4).[48] RT3DE planimetry was feasible in 92.7% of cases by TTE in patients with trileaflet valves.[48] Direct aortic valve orifice measurement using intracardiac echo has also been described but is rarely used in clinical practice.[49]

3.2.2. Doppler examination

While 2DE provides anatomical information, Doppler echocardiography provides physiological assessment. Estimation of pressure gradients and valve area is the foundation of clinical assessment of the hemodynamic severity of AS.

Using the maximal velocity of the blood flow across the valve, it is possible to calculate pressure gradients using the modified Bernoulli equation.[50-54]

$$\Delta P = 4V^2 \qquad \text{(Eq. 27.3)}$$

Maximal transvalvular velocities are obtained using continuous wave (CW) Doppler. Because of the angle dependence of Doppler signals, it is of critical importance to interrogate the aortic valve from multiple windows. These windows should include the apical, suprasternal, and right sternal windows. The best one to record signals varies from patient-to-patient and with age. In younger patients, velocities from the right sternal border are easier to obtain.[54] The audio of the Doppler signal may be helpful when obtaining maximal Doppler velocities.

The peak gradient derived from the maximal velocities corresponds to the maximal instantaneous pressure difference between the LV and the aorta. This is different from the peak-to-peak gradients routinely measured in the catheterization laboratory. Significant differences between these two measurements can occur particularly in patients with associated AR or when the catheter is placed too far upstream from the aortic valve.

The correlation between transvalvular gradients measured by CW Doppler and direct catheter measured gradients is very good. In a study of simultaneous catheter and Doppler gradients, the correlation between maximal and mean gradients were 0.92 and 0.93, respectively. However, when measurements are not obtained simultaneously the correlation is not as good (Tables 27.2 and 27.3). This is explained by the flow dependence of jet velocities and gradients and therefore different hemodynamic conditions may affect the results.

TABLE 27.2

CORRELATION BETWEEN AVA BY GORLIN AND CONTINUITY EQUATION IN STUDIES WITH SIMULTANEOUS DATA ACQUISITION

Author	No of patients	Correlation
Stamm[158]	35	0.94
Berger[159]	24	0.79
Currie[160]	100	0.92 (peak);0.93 (mean)
Oh[161]	100	0.86

TABLE 27.3

CORRELATION BETWEEN AVA BY GORLIN AND CONTINUITY EQUATION IN STUDIES WITHOUT SIMULTANEOUS DATA ACQUISITION

Author	No of patients	R
Otto[162]	48	0.86
Zoghbi[163]	39	0.95
Teirstein[164]	30	0.88
Oh[161]	100	0.83

It is recognized that a number of sources of error may impact the accuracy of Doppler gradients and should be considered in clinical practice. Some are related to the technique of data acquisition, in particular an inappropriate recording angle and failure to account for an increased subvalvular velocity and velocity variability when arrhythmias are present (Fig. 27.5). The clinical significance of high aortic Doppler velocities/high gradients has been reported in a large number of patients with longitudinal follow-up.[9,55] A maximal velocity >4 m/s correlates with severe AS and an increased incidence of adverse events.[9,55,56] This velocity threshold has been incorporated in the ACC/AHA guidelines for clinical management of patients with AS. Although a velocity >4.0 to 4.5 m/s is highly specific for severe AS, it should be remembered that it is not too sensitive (44% to 48%).[56] Transvalvular velocities/gradients are flow dependent and some patients with severe AS and low flow may exhibit lower velocities. Therefore, reliable assessment of the severity of AS requires estimates of the aortic valve area (AVA), particularly in patients with LV dysfunction.

In addition to technical factors, another source of discrepancy between direct catheter measurements and Doppler derived gradients is pressure recovery that will be discussed below.

AVA:

According to the continuity equation, the product of flow area and flow velocity is constant before and at the level of a restrictive orifice:

$$A_1 \times V_1 = A_2 \times V_2 \qquad \text{(Eq. 27.4)}$$

This can be applied to calculate the area of a stenotic orifice. For the AVA:

$$\text{VTI}_{LVOT} \times \text{area}_{LVOT} = \text{VTI}_{aortic\ valve} \times \text{area}_{aortic\ valve} \qquad \text{(Eq. 27.5)}$$

$$\text{AoVA} = \text{VIT}_{LVOT} \times \text{area}_{LVOT}/\text{VTI}_{aortic\ valve} \qquad \text{(Eq. 27.6)}$$

where

VTI = velocity time integral

LVOT = left ventricular outflow tract

There are then three important components (Fig. 27.6):

— VTI of LVOT: Obtained from pulsed Doppler at the lLV outflow from the apical window. Typically, the sample volume is placed just distal to the aortic annulus. However, in some patients there is already flow acceleration at this place and spectral Doppler shows velocity dispersion. In these patients, the sample volume needs to be moved more apically until a smooth, laminar flow is obtained (Fig. 27.7). In the early description of the calculation of AoVA by continuity, variation in the LVOT velocities up to 14% were reported.[57]

— LVOT diameter: Measured in the parasternal long axis view. As this diameter is squared to calculate LVOT area, small errors are magnified. In patients with heavy calcification, this measurement is challenging. When compared to TEE, a difference up to 4 mm has been reported.[58] Obviously, these differences have a significant impact on the calculation of valve area. Recent 3D studies suggest that some patients may have an elliptical LVOT, leading to over or underestimation of LVOT area when using 2D measurements.

— CW Doppler: Another source of error when the velocity is not properly recorded. Interrogation from multiple windows is essential to ensure that the maximal velocity is obtained.

It needs to be clearly understood that the continuity equation provides the EOA. This is the smallest cross section of the flow across the stenosis at the level of the vena contracta. This is different from the anatomical area that can be obtained by direct planimetry of the orifice or during direct anatomical inspection. The ratio of effective to anatomical area (coefficient of orifice contraction) depends on the orifice morphology.[59,60]

The calculation of Aortic valve area (AoVA) by continuity implies several assumptions:

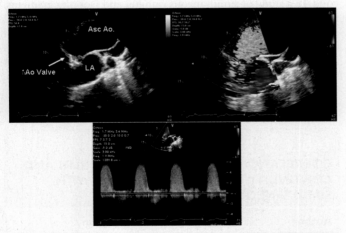

Figure 27.5 Imaging from the right sternal window in a patient with severe aortic stenosis. Note the excellent alignment of the Doppler and the direction of the jet. The maximal jet velocity from this window was 6 m/s and only 3.5 m/s from the apical window.

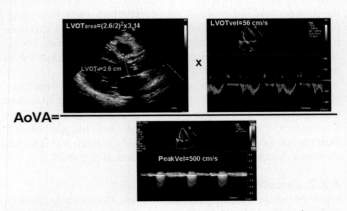

Figure 27.6 Components of the continuity equation. In this example the calculated aortic valve area is 0.6 cm².

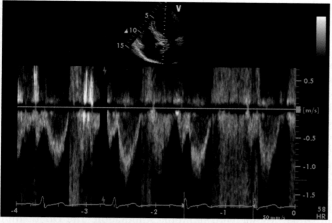

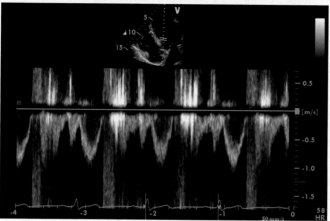

Figure 27.7 Beat to beat variation and dispersion of LVOT Doppler velocities when the sample volume is placed too close to the aortic valve (**top**). Velocities become more constant and better define modal velocities when the sample volume is placed farther from the aortic valve (**bottom**).

1. The flow before the obstruction is laminar with a flat profile. The flow at the LVOT is not flat but skewed with higher anteroseptal velocities.[61]
2. The LVOT is circular and does not change in shape and size during systole.
3. The LVOT is oval when visualized with multiplanar CT.
4. The velocity and diameter of LVOT are measured at the same location. Because LVOT diameter and velocities are measured from different windows, this is sometimes difficult to achieve.

The Doppler application of the continuity equation has been clinically validated and compared to valve area obtained by the Gorlin equation. Correlations as a high as 0.95 have been reported[62] (Tables 27.2 and 27.3). A simplified method using peak LVOT and aortic velocities (instead of VTI) has also been shown to be clinically accurate[57,62] ($r = 0.89–0.95$) and is easier to calculate.

The EOA is also flow dependent,[63] a phenomenon that has been described even in rigid orifices. At low flow rates, the reduction in kinetic energy may facilitate vortex formation beyond the anatomical orifice, which then tends to squeeze the flow jet and reduce the vena contracta, resulting in a smaller EOA. The importance of this observation may become clinically relevant in moderately severe AS and impaired ventricular function and low flow state. The presence of significant AR on the calculation

of valve area may have limited impact on the accuracy of the continuity equation.[57,64]

Pressure recovery. The use of Bernoulli's simplified equation is based on an additional assumption that all potential energy converted into kinetic energy at the level of the stenosis is completely lost downstream in turbulent friction, vortex formation, and heat (Fig. 27.8).[65] Pressure recovery depends on the gradual deceleration of flow with reattachment of streamlines as poststenotic jet expands, allowing the conversion of kinetic energy back into potential energy (velocity decreases, and pressure is recovered). When this fluid dynamic phenomenon is present, the LV pressure required to maintain a given systemic pressure and therefore the actual hemodynamic burden are significantly overestimated by the Doppler measurement.[65–78]

Pressure recovery is a source of discrepancy between valve area calculated invasively and the one obtained by continuity. The peak Doppler velocity used in the denominator of the continuity equation corresponds to the velocity at the maximal pressure drop and minimal jet area (vena contracta). The direct pressure gradient measured by catheterization (used in Gorlin's equation) is measured downstream when some degree of pressure recovery has occurred (Fig. 27.8). In patients with small valve areas and dilated aorta, this is not a problem because the jet energy is dissipated in vortex formation and heat. For patients with smaller aortas (<3 cm in diameter), a formula to correct for pressure recovery (energy loss) has been proposed.

$$EOA_{corrected} = EOA_{Doppler} \times AA/EOA_{Doppler} - AA \qquad (Eq.\ 27.6)$$

where, $EOA_{Doppler}$ is the effective orifice by continuity equation and AA is the cross-sectional area of the aorta at the sinotubular junction. Some authors have proposed the routine use of this formula to achieve better correlation with invasive measurements.[69,78,79]

A practical consequence of the overestimation of valve area by continuity is the potential for misclassifying patients with moderate AS as severe.[70] The guidelines definition of severe AS as

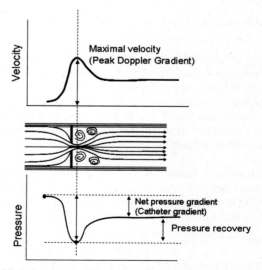

Figure 27.8 Schematic of flow through a stenotic orifice. Flow accelerates on approaching the orifice, converting potential energy (pressure) into kinetic energy (velocity). After exiting the orifice, flow converges into the narrowest area (vena contract). Part of the energy of the jet is lost in turbulence and heat. Downstream the streamlines of flow reattach as jet expands, allowing the conversion of kinetic energy back into potential energy (velocity decreases, and pressure is recovered).

TABLE 27.4

ACC/AHA GUIDELINES INCORPORATING AORTIC VALVE AREA, PEAK AORTIC JET VELOCITY AND MEAN TRANSVALVULAR GRADIENTS TO GRADE THE SEVERITY OF AORTIC STENOSIS

	Mild	Moderate	Severe
Peak jet velocity (m/s)	<3.0	3.0–4.0	>4.0
Mean gradient (mm Hg)	<25	25–40	>40
Valve area (cm²)	>1.5	1.0–1.5	<1.0
Valve area index (cm²/m²)			<0.6

Source: Bonow RO, et al. ACC/AHA 2006 guidelines for the management of patients with valvular heart disease: A report of the American College of Cardiology/American Heart Association task force on practice guidelines (writing committee to revise the 1998 guidelines for the management of patients with valvular heart disease). Developed in collaboration with the society of cardiovascular anesthesiologists: Endorsed by the society for cardiovascular angiography and interventions and the society of thoracic surgeons. *Circulation.* 2006;114(5):e84–e231.

AVA <1.0 was based mostly on catheterization data. In practice, patients with valve area calculated by echo-Doppler of ≥1.0 cm² rarely have significant gradients.[70] Using a Doppler valve area of <0.8 cm² appears to be more clinically relevant to define severe AS.

The ACC/AHA guidelines incorporate AVA, peak aortic jet velocity, and mean transvalvular gradients to grade the severity of AS (Table 27.4).[40]

Valve resistance. In the search for indices of AS severity that are less flow dependent the concept of valve resistance (resistance = gradient/flow) has been proposed. Initially obtained from catheterization data, this index can also be calculated from Doppler data:

$$\text{Valve resistance} = 1.333 \times 4\,V_{max}^2 / \text{ area LVOT} \times \text{ velocity LVOT} \qquad \text{(Eq. 27.7)}$$

or

$$\text{Valve resistance} = 1.333 \times \text{Peak aortic gradient} / \text{ stroke volume} \qquad \text{(Eq. 27.8)}$$

The main difference between valve area and valve resistance is that in calculated area, the pressure gradient is proportional to the square of flow, and in valve resistance, the pressure gradient is proportional to the first power of flow.[80–83]

In practice, this index is also flow dependent and has not replaced calculation of valve area in the clinical diagnosis and management of patients with AS.[84]

Doppler velocity index. Because one of the sources of error in calculating valve area is the measurement of LVOT diameter, the ratio of LVOT velocity to peak aortic velocity has been proposed as another index of severity:

$$\text{Doppler velocity index} = \text{LVOT velocity (pulsed wave Doppler)} / \text{maximal aortic velocity (CW Doppler)} \qquad \text{(Eq. 27.9)}$$

This, also called dimensionless index, is useful when measurement of the LVOT diameter is inaccurate and was described to evaluate prosthetic stenosis.[85] The cutoff for severe AS is < 0.25.

Aortic stenosis with left ventricular dysfunction. Patients with severe AS usually present with normal or hyperdynamic LV function.

A relatively small number of patients, however, have profound systolic dysfunction at the time of diagnosis. This can be the result of associated coronary disease, primary contractile dysfunction or afterload mismatch. Two important clinical questions are associated to this condition. First, is the reduced valve area due to true calcific stenosis or is it the result of low stroke volume and reduced opening forces (pseudostenosis)? Patients with LV dysfunction and high gradients do not present a major diagnostic or therapeutic dilemma. These patients should be operated promptly. On the other hand, patients with suspected severe AS and low gradients (mean gradient <30 mm Hg), although uncommon, remain a formidable diagnostic and therapeutic challenge.

Dobutamine echocardiography is an important tool in the diagnosis and management of these patients.[84,86–93] Dobutamine is used to evaluate the presence of contractile reserve: increase in stroke volume with inotropic stimulation. The Dobutamine infusion rate in this particular echocardiographic stress protocol is usually started at 5 mg/kg/min and increased up to 20 mg/kg/min. Criteria for terminating the test are reaching maximal dose or an increase in heart rate > 10 to 20 beats/min above resting levels. At each stage, LVOT and peak aortic velocities are obtained and AVA calculated. Patients with truly severe AS show a fixed valve area with increasing gradients during Dobutamine stress test (DbST). If Dobutamine infusion augments valve area >0.2 cm² (with a final valve area >1 cm²) with little change in gradient, the patient is unlikely to have severe AS. The incorrect overestimation of the severity of AS in patients with low stroke volume has been called pseudosevere stenosis and is the result of reduced opening forces. The incidence of this condition has been reported between 5% and 30% of patients with suspected AS and low EF[84] but is a very small part of the total population of patients with AS. Those patients with no inotropic response to Db (absence of contractile reserve) remain a diagnostic and therapeutic challenge. Additional parameters such as degree of valvular calcification and levels of brain natriuretic peptide (BNP)[94,95] may have incremental diagnostic value. Elevated BNP of >550 pg/mL indicates a poor outcome for patients treated either surgically or medically, with only 47% of such patients surviving for 1 year compared with 97% survival in patients with lower BNP values.[95]

Monin et al.[90,91,96] have extensively studied the role of Db echo for prognosis in patients with severe AS and LV dysfunction. From their data, it is clear that those patients with no or minimal contractile reserve (increase in stroke volume of ≥20% compared to baseline values) have a poor prognosis and very high surgical mortality compared to those with contractile reserve (6% vs. 33%).[97] However, in those who survive surgery symptoms and EF improve over time. Based on these findings, surgery should not be contraindicated on the basis of absence of contractile reserve alone.[97] In centers with low surgical mortality, AVR should be offered to patients with low flow/low gradient AS that are otherwise reasonably good surgical candidates.[98–100] The use of BNP as mentioned above to deny surgery to the difficult group of patients needs to be tested in larger prospective studies.

The ACC/AHA gives a IIaB indication for Db echo in patients with AS and LV dysfunction. In the ESC guidelines, patients with AS, low gradient (<40 mm Hg), and LV dysfunction *with* contractile reserve have a IIaC indication for aortic valve surgery and *without* contractile reserve a IIbC indication.[40]

Low flow severe AS in patients with normal ejection fraction. It has been described that an important proportion of patients with severe AS and normal EF have low transvalvular flow rates (SVI ≤35 mL/m²) and low transvalvular gradients. These patients are usually older and predominantly females and have more pronounced concentric LVH with smaller ventricles. Prognosis of these patients appears to be worse with lower survival when compared to similar patients with normal flow rates. The clinical importance of identifying this subgroup of patients is that they may be misdiagnosed and surgery may be denied or delayed. Medical treatment of these patients carries a poor prognosis.[101]

Evaluation of diastolic function in patients with aortic stenosis. Patients with AS develop concentric LVH as an adaptive mechanism to normalize wall stress of the pressure-overloaded ventricle. In these patients, LV filling dynamics are not uniform but vary depending on the degree of LV hypertrophy and the contractile state.[102,103] In patients with a moderate hypertrophy, Doppler mitral inflow pattern shows decreased early velocity and a predominant A-wave filling.[104] This delayed relaxation pattern is seen in the majority of patients. However, it is not clear that LV relaxation is abnormal as some have reported a normal time constant of LV relaxation and the Doppler findings could be just related to age.[105] These patients have, in general, normal filling pressures. In patients with severe LV hypertrophy, relaxation is delayed and left ventricle chamber stiffness is increased. Elevation of filling pressures is manifested by increased E wave velocity, short deceleration time, and reduced atrial contribution.[103] In patients with AS, isometric exercise decreases relaxation rate and increases left ventricular end-diastolic pressure (LVEDP).[106] In a study of 399 patients that underwent AVR, 42% had moderate to severe preoperative diastolic dysfunction defined by a combination of mitral inflow and pulmonary vein flow abnormalities. The severity of diastolic dysfunction had an important impact in long-term mortality after AVR.[107]

Tissue Doppler velocities have also been evaluated in patients with AS.[108,109] In patients with AS and normal EF, septal annular A' velocity < 9.6 cm/s appears to be associated with reduced event-free survival.[109] LV torsion has been studied in patients with AS with magnetic resonance (MR) imaging using myocardial tagging techniques.[110,111]. In AS patients, there is a reduction in basal and an increase in apical rotation resulting in increased torsion of the ventricle. Diastolic untwisting is delayed and prolonged.[110,111] Ventricular torsion has also been assessed using echocardiographic 2D speckle tracking.[112-115]. This new technique may allow the

study of ventricular torsion in a larger population of patients with AS and establish its clinical utility and prognostic value.

Pulmonary hypertension in patients with severe aortic stenosis. The prevalence of severe pulmonary hypertension in patients with severe aortic valve stenosis has been reported to be 19% to 29%[116,117] in patients undergoing preoperative invasive hemodynamic evaluation. This condition has been associated with end-stage AS and sudden death.[118] However, when other causes of pulmonary hypertension, such as mitral regurgitation, are excluded, the prevalence drops to around 2.5%.[119] These patients are older and 40% have EF ≤35%.[117,119] The presence of severe pulmonary hypertension increases perioperative mortality.[119] The fact that in these patients the *E/Ea* ratio is a predictor of pulmonary artery pressure.[108] is suggestive that diastolic dysfunction plays an important role in the development of pulmonary hypertension.

3.3. Magnetic resonance

Cardiac magnetic resonance (CMR) imaging is more accurate and reproducible in measuring LV volumes, function, and mass compared to echocardiography. CMR imaging is particularly useful when acoustic windows in the echocardiogram are poor or when there are discordant imaging and catheterization results. A variety of CMR imaging sequences can also enable a comprehensive evaluation of all aspects of AS. Balanced steady-state free precession (SSFP) "bright blood" cine sequences offer a higher contrast between blood and surrounding structures, allowing visualization of restricted cusp opening in stenotic aortic valves and planimetry of AVA (Fig. 27.9). The presence of turbulent blood flow through the stenotic valve can be visualized as a lower intensity "signal void" on cine CMR images. Phase contrast or velocity encoded cine CMR allows noninvasive quantification of blood flow and peak velocities through the stenotic valve allowing an estimate of transvalvular gradients and AVA using the continuity equation. CMR is the imaging modality of choice for assessing the impact of AS on LV size, mass, and function. Delayed contrast-enhanced CMR using inversion recovery gradient echo sequences can assess preoperative presence of myocardial scar from concomitant coronary

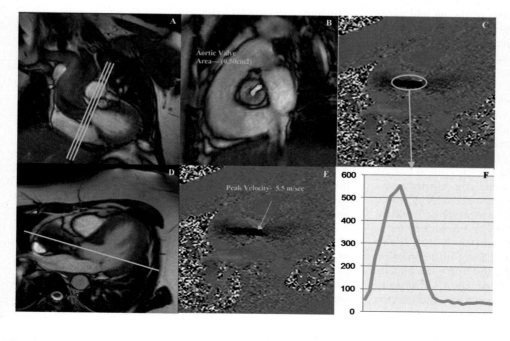

Figure 27.9 Cine SSFP series through the LV outflow tract in two orthogonal planes (**Panel A**—oblique coronal basal short axis, **Panel D**—oblique transverse long axis of the left ventricular outflow tract) allows the assessment of valve leaflet doming and visualization of the stenotic jet. Planimetry of the valve orifice is planned at the valve leaflet tips at the maximum excursion of the aortic annular plane during early to mid systole. An off-center shift of 3 mm above and below this plane can ensure that the minimum valve area is obtained (**Panel B**). Planimetry of this unicuspid valve confirms an aortic valve area of 0.5 cm². An in-plane velocity encoded image is aligned with the jet direction in two orthogonal planes to identify the peak velocity (**Panels C, E**), and is plotted versus time (**Panel F**). A peak velocity of 5.5 m/s equates to a peak gradient of 121 mm Hg consistent with severe aortic stenosis.

artery disease and gadolinium contrast enhanced MR angiography allows an assessment of aortic morphology and dimensions.

CMR is useful in quantifying the severity of AS.[120–124] Valve area can be assessed by direct planimetry using a cross-sectional plane.[121,123,125–129]. The stenotic aortic valve typically appears thickened on longitudinal three-chamber and oblique coronal LV outflow tract balanced SSFP cine CMR images and typical asymmetric doming of the leaflets can be seen in congenitally bicuspid and unicuspid valves. Planimetry of the stenotic valve orifice is also feasible from breathhold balanced SSFP cine MRI images. Planning of an imaging slice to acquire the true stenotic aortic valve orifice at the leaflet tips may require several contiguous slices perpendicular to valve plane, commencing at the aortic valve annulus.

The presence of a "signal void" from turbulent flow in the aortic root on balanced SSFP cine images is often a clue to the presence of AS. Balanced SSFP cine sequences are relatively flow insensitive compared to gradient echo cine sequences. The use of echo planar imaging gradient echo cine images has greater sensitivity to flow and may be a useful additional sequence for evaluating the severity of the point of maximum flow acceleration or concomitant regurgitation.

An alternative approach to calculate valve area involves applying the "continuity equation" to calculate AVA, utilizing measurements of the LVOT area and VTI of systolic forward flow in the LVOT and at the aortic valve leaflet tips by velocity encoded cine CMR images.[130] Care must be taken as systematic underestimation of VTI measurements have been noted as the $VTI_{LVOT}/VTI_{Aortic\ valve}$ ratio approaches 1:4.[127]

3.3.1. Assessment of transvalvular gradients using cardiac magnetic resonance

Velocity encoded cine CMR assessment of the peak and mean velocities through the stenotic aortic valve allows calculation of transvalvular gradients using the modified Bernoulli's equation. Correct alignment of the imaging plane and an appropriate choice of encoding velocity (V_{ENC}) are required for reliable estimation of the peak velocity.[131] A combination of both through-plane (velocity jet perpendicular to the imaging plane) and in-plane (velocity jet parallel to the imaging plane) velocity mapping can ensure that the true peak velocity within the jet is acquired, especially in the setting of eccentric jets with congenital AS (Fig. 27.10). At least two orthogonal in-plane velocity mapping planes aligned through the axis of the jet will allow visualization of the entire jet, enabling points of peak velocity to be identified. However, in narrower jets associated with severe AS, movement of the jet within the imaging slice during systole can make acquisition of the peak velocity difficult.[132,133] Through-plane velocity mapping perpendicular to the jet direction can also be used to acquire velocity measurements. An imaging plane positioned 10 mm distal to the aortic valve annulus appears to correlate best with peak and mean velocities acquired with Doppler echocardiography. Slice tracking techniques to compensate for motion of the aortic valve annular plane during systole have been evaluated but are not available for routine clinical use. An appropriate choice of V_{ENC} is crucial for accurate velocity assessment. The better the V_{ENC} matches the true peak velocity within the region of interest, the more precise the measurement will be. Setting of the V_{ENC} below the peak velocity will result in aliasing and wrapping of the velocity information (Fig. 27.10). Setting of the V_{ENC} too high will increase the impact of noise on velocity cine imaging by potentially masking the true peak velocity. Several groups have used velocity encoded cine CMR imaging to determine peak velocity, transvalvular gradients and effective

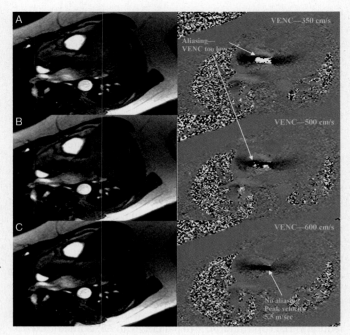

Figure 27.10 Information from velocity-encoded measurements is processed into two sets of images. A magnitude image (**left column**) which is a bright blood image used for anatomic orientation and a phase (velocity) image (**right column**) in which the gray value of each pixel represents the velocity information of each voxel. In these in-plane velocity encoded images, the stenotic jet is encoded with flow to the left in black and to the right in white. In **Panels A and B** aliasing is seen in the phase image because the encoding velocity (V_{ENC}) is set too low, resulting in wrapping around of the velocity information within voxels with velocities higher than the V_{ENC}. In **Panel C** the peak velocity is displayed using an appropriate V_{ENC}.

valve area in patients with AS. All have reported good agreement between velocity-encoded cine CMR imaging and echocardiography. However, many of these studies have included few patients and mostly evaluated patients with mild or moderate stenosis. Technical factors may limit the assessment of peak velocities in turbulent jets in patients with severe AS. Appropriate shortening of the echo time (TE) to <3.5 can reduce underestimation of velocities due to the effects of higher order motion such as acceleration in stenotic jets.[134]

After AVR, CMR can be used to demonstrate improvement in LV function, myocardial metabolism, and diastolic function as well as reduced hypertrophy.[135,136] Animal experiments have explored the role of MRI in guiding percutaneous implantation of aortic prosthetic valves.[137]

3.4. Computed tomography

Advances in spatial and temporal resolution of the latest CT scanners (64-slice and greater) and the development of electrocardiographic (ECG) gating algorithms have enabled the acquisition of multiphase image data. The ability of CT to detect calcium in the aorta can assist planning of surgery[138–142] and has been applied recently to the evaluation of aortic valve stenosis. Similar to the evaluation of coronary artery calcification, aortic valve calcification can be measured by volumetric methods (e.g., the Agatston method and calcium mass). The amount of calcium correlates with the severity of disease and has been linked to risk for coronary atherosclerosis. Serial CT scans can be used to assess AS disease progression.[143] Over 18 to 24 months of follow-up, the aortic valve calcium score predicted short-term adverse clinical outcome in patients with asymptomatic AS.[144] However,

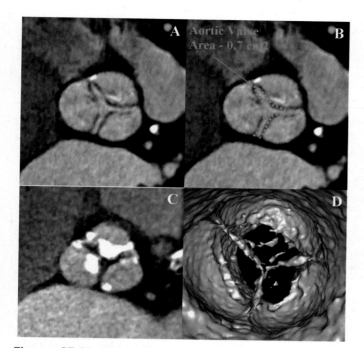

Figure 27.11 Multiplanar reconstruction of transverse planes through the aortic valve during the systolic phases (0% to 40%) allows planimetry of the aortic valve area (**Panels A, B**) by CT. Calcification of the aortic valve leaflets is clearly demonstrated and can be quantified (**Panel C**). Volume rendered imaging can allow characterization of leaflet and sinus morphology (**Panel D**).

given the potential for excess radiation exposure from serial imaging, this presently remains a research application.

CT imaging software can be utilized to reconstruct retrospectively gated multiphase images into cine loops to assess valve morphology and motion. Volume rendering techniques can produce high-resolution 3D imaging of the valve apparatus (Fig. 27.11). Using these techniques it is possible to directly measure the orifice area by planimetry.[120,138,140,144–148] The correlation is good (Table 27.5) and, as expected, there is a trend for overestimation of AVA by CT compared to continuity equation (anatomical vs EOA).

Preoperative evaluation of patients with AS prior to AVR with CT has the potential to exclude significant coronary artery disease in selected low atherosclerotic risk patients.[149] A normal CT angiogram with 64 slice multidetector scanners has a negative predictive value of 97%, providing an alternative to conventional invasive angiography.[150] However, diagnostic assessment of luminal stenosis may be reduced in the setting of calcium deposits and in vessels under 1.5 mm, a common finding in patients with calcific degenerative AS.

In addition, a noncontrast or contrast CT scan of the aortic root and ascending aorta can aid the cardiothoracic surgeon to identify the relationship of cardiac structures prior to median sternotomy, and a description of ascending aorta and arch calcification can assist in the planning of bypass cannulation. The use of CT for a comprehensive examination of patients with AS that includes assessment of AVA, LV EF, and coronary anatomy has been well validated,[151] but once again, exposure to radiation remains a limitation for its routine use.

3.5. Stress testing

Patients with moderate to severe AS have an abnormal exercise physiology, and even asymptomatic patients may exhibit a reduced tolerance to exercise. Cardiac output at rest is within normal limits, but the normal increase in cardiac output with exercise is blunted. The reduced increase in cardiac output with exercise is mediated primarily by increased heart rate with little change in stroke volume. Transvalvular flow rate increases due to the shortened systolic ejection period with proportional increase in transvalvular gradient.

The exercise ST in patient with AS may be abnormal because of the ECG response or hemodynamic changes. The presence of ST changes and ventricular arrhythmias has been linked to unfavorable prognosis. An abnormal hemodynamic response is expressed as blunted (<10 mm Hg increase) or decreased systolic blood pressure with exercise. The relative importance of these parameters for risk stratification has varied among different authors.

Exercise STs have been shown to be safe in asymptomatic patients with moderate to severe AS. It is then of critical importance to obtain a careful medical history in these patients. On the day of test, the patient should be asked again if new symptoms have occurred since the test was requested.

Although the indication for surgery can be done in most patients based on clinical and hemodynamic parameters,[40,152] ST can be very useful in asymptomatic patients. In patients with advanced ventricular dysfunction, ST provides prognostic information. In asymptomatic patients, or those with equivocal symptoms, the test is performed with the intention to unmask symptoms or elicit an abnormal hemodynamic response (i.e., decrease in blood pressure). The relative importance of exercise parameters in evaluating patients with AS is a subject of some controversy (Table 27.6). In asymptomatic patients, Otto et al. found that exercise parameters have no additional value over jet velocity, rate of change in jet velocity, and baseline functional status.[55] Amato et al.[153] reported an unfavorable prognosis (sudden death or symptoms) in patients with an abnormal ST. Others have reported that besides an abnormal ST, an increase in mean transaortic pressure gradient by ≥18 mm Hg during exercise had incremental prognostic value.[154] Exercise-limiting symptoms as the only independent predictors of outcome (symptom-free survival) at 12 months has also been reported and, in that particular study, an abnormal blood pressure response or ST segment depression did not improve the accuracy of the exercise test.[155] The discrepancies may be explained by the different outcomes selected in the studies (Table 27.6).

The ACC/AHA guidelines give a class IIb indication to exercise testing in asymptomatic patients with AS.[39] The ESC guidelines have a different approach and relate the different ST responses to the indications for AVR.[156]

3.6. Differential diagnosis

The differential diagnosis included other causes of nonvalvular LVOT obstruction.

Hypertrophic cardiomyopathy is discussed in another chapter. In these patients, in general, the aortic valve is anatomically

TABLE 27.5
CORRELATION BETWEEN CT AORTIC VALVE AREA AND ECHO-DOPPLER VALVE AREA

Author	N	r
Feuchtner[142]	46	0.89
Tanaka[145]	29	0.96
Laissy[151]	40	0.77
Habis[157]	52	0.76

TABLE 27.6
STRESS TEST STUDIES IN PATIENTS WITH SEVERE AS

Author	No of patients	Severity of AS	Stress test	Outcome	Predictors
Otto et al.[55]	123	Peak vel >2.5 m/s	Symptoms: BPdrop <10 mm Hg, ST >5 mm "significant arrhythmias"	Death or AVR	Jet velocity function status Rate of change of jet velocity
Amato et al.[153]	66, No CAD	AoVA 0.3–1.0 cm^2	ST, symptoms: ventricular Arrhythmias, BP increase <20 mm Hg	Symptoms: Sudden death	Positive stress test (ST or symptoms or hemodynamic response)
Lancellotti et al.[154]	69	AoVA ≤1.0 cm^2	Angina, dyspnea, ST changes, "significant arrhythmias," BP increase <20 mm Hg	Symptoms: CHF cardiac death, AVR	Increase in mean grad >18 mm Hg, Abn stress test AoVA <0.75 cm^2
Das 2005[155]	125	AoVA <1.4 cm^2	Symptoms: ST changes, >3 consecutive premature ventricular complex (PVCs), BP equal or below baseline	Exertional symptoms or cardiac death	Limiting symptoms during stress test

normal and, although it may exhibit midsystolic closure, the valvular opening is unrestricted.

Subvalvular stenosis most commonly presents in childhood and can be seen in adult patients too. These patients typically show a high Doppler velocity in the outflow tract with normal AV on echo. Frequently, AR is present due to aortic valve jet lesion. There are two subtypes of subvalvular AS: discrete subvalvular membrane or ridge and fibromuscular tunnel. Transthoracic, transesophageal echo, and MRI usually provide diagnostic anatomic and functional images.

4. CARDIOVASCULAR IMAGING FOR GUIDANCE OF INTERVENTIONS

According to recent guidelines, AVR is indicated in the presence of symptoms, LV dysfunction, and when there is a need for other cardiovascular surgeries: Coronary artery bypass graft (CABG) or mitral valve surgery. The European and ACC/AHA guidelines also offer some guidance in the management of patients with asymptomatic severe AS (Table 27.7). ST has a role in these patients eliciting symptoms or abnormal ECG or blood pressure response.

4.1. Percutaneous and transapical aortic valve replacement

This is a novel technology with the potential to change the management of patients with severe AS and increased surgical risk. The initial clinical trials are promising and have shown that this new valve provided rapid relief to the aortic valve obstruction with low residual gradients.

It is too early to establish the precise role of imaging in this evolving technique. In the preliminary experience, echo has been used for screening and grading the severity of AS, to provide limited procedural guidance, and more importantly to evaluate presence and severity of AR. The strengths of CT and CMR also lend themselves to preprocedural planning. Sizing of the aortic valve implant is crucial for minimizing the risk of device migration and reducing the potential for paravalvular AR. Image reconstruction of 3D and 4Dimage datasets by CT can accurately define the size of the aortic annulus in the three-chamber and oblique coronal LVOT imaging planes, aiding appropriate sizing of the valve implant (Fig. 27.12). The anatomic relationship between aortic annulus and coronary ostia and the degree of aortic valve and root calcification may identify patients at risk of embolism and preprocedural planning of valve position. Transfemoral percutaneous AVR requires a retrograde approach to the valve via the aorta. Assessing the tortuosity of the thoracic and abdominal aorta and the size of the iliac and femoral arteries, and evaluating the severity of atherosclerotic disease is important for assessing the feasibility of a percutaneous versus a transapical approach.

Postprocedure, both CT and CMR have a role in assessing possible aorta and cardiac complications. CMR assessment of paravalvular AR and LV pseudoaneurysm after transapical AVR can be safely performed. Nonclinical trials have confirmed the safety of Edwards SAPIEN transcatheter heart valves under static magnetic fields of 3 T and spatial gradient fields of 720 G/cm or less.

Hybrid catheterization laboratories with fluoroscopy and CT capabilities are likely to provide optimal information guidance and deployment. As many of these patients have tenuous renal function, an echo-Doppler technique is likely to be necessary to evaluate residual AR. Whether intracardiac echo can provide this information remains unclear.

5. FUTURE DIRECTIONS

The diagnostic techniques for evaluation of AS are mature and well established. However, there is room for refinement. The incremental value of 3DE for anatomic assessment and Doppler tissue for early detection of LV dysfunction need further studies. The role of speckle tracking strain and torsion and the combined use of imaging techniques with biomarkers in low flow/low gradient aortic needs prospective validation likely in a multicentric effort.

The exiting era of percutaneous valvular interventions is in its infancy and will likely require a multi-imaging, multidisciplinary approach. CT provides the best assessment of calcification combined with accurate and reproducible sizing of the ascending aorta and is being incorporated in preoperative assessment of adult patients with degenerative AS. Whether this approach will result in less perioperative morbidity and mortality is currently only speculative. How to utilize this multi-imaging approach in a cost effective manner is an important goal of future research.

TABLE 27.7
INDICATIONS FOR AORTIC VALVE REPLACEMENT IN AORTIC STENOSIS

ACC/AHA guidelines	ESC guidelines
Class I	*Class I*
1. Symptomatic patients with severe AS 2. AVR is indicated for patients with severe AS undergoing coronary artery bypass graft surgery 3. AVR is indicated for patients with severe AS undergoing surgery on the aorta or other heart valves 4. AVR is recommended for patients with severe AS and LV systolic dysfunction (ejection fraction <0.50)	ACC/AHA Indications 1. Symptomatic patients with severe AS 2. AVR is indicated for patients with severe AS undergoing coronary artery bypass graft surgery 3. AVR is indicated for patients with severe AS undergoing surgery on the aorta or other heart valves 4. AVR is recommended for patients with severe AS and LV systolic dysfunction (ejection fraction <0.50) 5. Asymptomatic patients with severe AS and abnormal exercise test showing symptoms on exercise
Class IIa	*Class IIa*
1. AVR is reasonable for patients with moderate AS undergoing CABG or surgery on the aorta or other heart valves	ACC/AHA Indication 1. AVR is reasonable for patients with moderate AS undergoing CABG or surgery on the aorta or other heart valves 2. Asymptomatic patients with severe AS and abnormal exercise test showing fall in blood pressure below baseline 3. Asymptomatic patients with severe AS and moderate-to-severe valve calcification, and a rate of peak velocity progression ≥0.3 m/s/year AS with low gradient (<40 mm Hg) and LV dysfunction with contractile reserve
Class IIb	*Class IIb*
1. AVR may be considered for asymptomatic patients with severe AS and abnormal response to exercise (e.g., development of symptoms or asymptomatic hypotension) 2. AVR may be considered for adults with severe asymptomatic AS if there is a high likelihood of rapid progression (age, calcification, and CAD) or if surgery might be delayed at the time of symptom onset 3. AVR may be considered in patients undergoing CABG who have mild AS when there is evidence, such as moderate to severe valve calcification, that progression may be rapid 4. AVR may be considered for asymptomatic patients with extremely severe AS (AVA<0.6 cm², mean gradient >60 mm Hg, and jet velocity >5.0 m/s) when operative mortality is 1.0% or less	1. Asymptomatic patients with severe AS and abnormal exercise test showing complex ventricular arrhythmias 2. Asymptomatic patients with severe AS and excessive LV hypertrophy (≥15 mm) unless this is due to hypertension AS with low gradient (<40 mm Hg) and LV dysfunction without contractile reserve

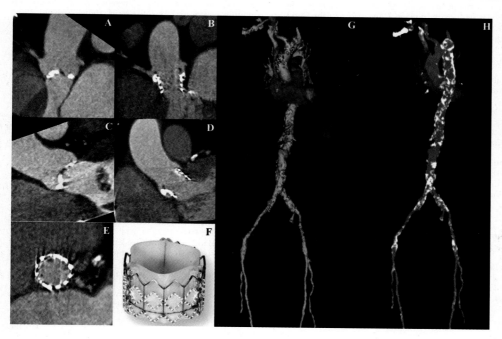

Figure 27.12 Defining the size of the aortic annulus and the distance from the annulus to the coronary ostia by CT is important for planning correct positioning of the transcatheter aortic valve implant (**Panels A, C**—preimplantation and **Panels B, D, E**—postimplantation). An Edwards SAPIEN transcatheter valve is displayed in (**Panel F**). The severity of calcific atherosclerosis and size of iliac vessels can be displayed in volume rendered and maximum intensity projection views of the aorta (**Panels G, H**).

REFERENCES

1. Gilard M, Cornily JC, Pennec PY, et al. Accuracy of multislice computed tomography in the preoperative assessment of coronary disease in patients with aortic valve stenosis. J Am Coll Cardiol. 2006;p. j.jacc.2005.11.085.
2. Popovic AD, et al. Time-related trends in the preoperative evaluation of patients with valvular stenosis. Am J Cardiol. 1997;80(11):1464–1468.
3. Iung B, et al. A prospective survey of patients with valvular heart disease in Europe: The Euro heart survey on valvular heart disease. Eur Heart J. 2003;24(13):1231–1243.
4. Novaro GM, Mishra M, Griffin BP. Incidence and echocardiographic features of congenital unicuspid aortic valve in an adult population. J Heart Valve Dis. 2003;12(6):674–678.
5. Fenoglio JJ, Jr, et al. Congenital bicuspid aortic valve after age 20. Am J Cardiol. 1977;39(2):164–169.
6. Lindroos M, et al. Prevalence of aortic valve abnormalities in the elderly: An echocardiographic study of a random population sample. J Am Coll Cardiol. 1993;21(5):1220–1225.
7. Ross J, Jr, Braunwald E. Aortic stenosis. Circulation. 1968;38(1):61–67.
8. Kelly TA, et al. Comparison of outcome of asymptomatic to symptomatic patients older than 20 years of age with valvular aortic stenosis. Am J Cardiol. 1988;61(1):123–130.
9. Pellikka PA, et al. Outcome of 622 adults with asymptomatic, hemodynamically significant aortic stenosis during prolonged follow-up. Circulation. 2005;111(24):3290–3295.
10. Pellikka PA, et al. The natural history of adults with asymptomatic, hemodynamically significant aortic stenosis. J Am Coll Cardiol. 1990;15(5):1012–1017.
11. Rosenhek R, et al. Predictors of outcome in severe, asymptomatic aortic stenosis. N Engl J Med. 2000;343(9):611–617.
12. Chizner MA, Pearle DL, deLeon AC Jr. The natural history of aortic stenosis in adults. Am Heart J. 1980;99(4):419–424.
13. Akat K, Borggrefe M, Kaden JJ. Aortic valve calcification—basic science to clinical practice. Heart. 2008.
14. Otto CM, et al. Characterization of the early lesion of 'degenerative' valvular aortic stenosis. Histological and immunohistochemical studies. Circulation. 1994;90(2):844–853.
15. Meng X, et al. Expression of functional Toll-like receptors 2 and 4 in human aortic valve interstitial cells: Potential roles in aortic valve inflammation and stenosis. Am J Physiol Cell Physiol. 2008;294(1):C29–C35.
16. Wallby L, et al. T lymphocyte infiltration in non-rheumatic aortic stenosis: A comparative descriptive study between tricuspid and bicuspid aortic valves. Heart. 2002;88(4):348–351.
17. Babu AN, et al. Lipopolysaccharide stimulation of human aortic valve interstitial cells activates inflammation and osteogenesis. Ann Thorac Surg. 2008;86(1):71–76.
18. Olsson M, et al. Accumulation of T lymphocytes and expression of interleukin-2 receptors in nonrheumatic stenotic aortic valves. J Am Coll Cardiol. 1994;23(5):1162–1170.
19. O'Brien KD, et al. Apolipoproteins B, (a), and E accumulate in the morphologically early lesion of 'degenerative' valvular aortic stenosis. Arterioscler Thromb Vasc Biol. 1996;16(4):523–532.
20. Goldbarg SH, et al. Insights into degenerative aortic valve disease. J Am Coll Cardiol. 2007;50(13):1205–13.
21. Toutouzas K, et al. In vivo aortic valve thermal heterogeneity in patients with nonrheumatic aortic valve stenosis the: First in vivo experience in humans. J Am Coll Cardiol. 2008;52(9):758–763.
22. Miller JD, et al. Dysregulation of antioxidant mechanisms contributes to increased oxidative stress in calcific aortic valvular stenosis in humans. J Am Coll Cardiol. 2008;52(10):843–850.
23. Beppu S, et al. Rapidity of progression of aortic stenosis in patients with congenital bicuspid aortic valves. Am J Cardiol. 1993;71(4):322–327.
24. Tzemos N, et al. Outcomes in adults with bicuspid aortic valves. JAMA. 2008;300(11):1317–1325.
25. Sabet HY, et al. Congenitally bicuspid aortic valves: A surgical pathology study of 542 cases (1991 through 1996) and a literature review of 2,715 additional cases. Mayo Clin Proc. 1999;74(1):14–26.
26. Schaefer BM, et al. The bicuspid aortic valve: An integrated phenotypic classification of leaflet morphology and aortic root shape. Heart. 2008.
27. Michelena HI, et al. Natural history of asymptomatic patients with normally functioning or minimally dysfunctional bicuspid aortic valve in the community. Circulation. 2008;117(21):2776–2784.
28. Gurvitz M, et al. Frequency of aortic root dilation in children with a bicuspid aortic valve. Am J Cardiol. 2004;94(10):1337–1340.
29. Ferencik M, Pape LA. Changes in size of ascending aorta and aortic valve function with time in patients with congenitally bicuspid aortic valves. Am J Cardiol. 2003;92(1):43–46.
30. Larson EW, Edwards WD. Risk factors for aortic dissection: A necropsy study of 161 cases. Am J Cardiol. 1984;53(6):849–855.
31. Della Corte A, et al. Echocardiographic anatomy of ascending aorta dilatation: Correlations with aortic valve morphology and function. Int J Cardiol. 2006;113(3):320–326.
32. Fedak PW, et al. Bicuspid aortic valve disease: Recent insights in pathophysiology and treatment. Expert Rev Cardiovasc Ther. 2005;3(2):295–308.
33. Mihaljevic TS, Sayeed MR. Stamou SC, et al. Pathophysiology of aortic valve disease. In: Lh C, ed. Cardiac Surgery in the Adult. New York: McGraw-Hill; 2008; 825–840.
34. Spann JE, et al. Ventricular performance, pump function and compensatory mechanisms in patients with aortic stenosis. Circulation. 1980;62(3):576–582.
35. Carroll JD, et al. Sex-associated differences in left ventricular function in aortic stenosis of the elderly. Circulation. 1992;86(4):1099–1107.
36. Seiler C, Jenni R. Severe aortic stenosis without left ventricular hypertrophy: Prevalence, predictors, and short-term follow up after aortic valve replacement. Heart. 1996;76(3):250–255.
37. Briand M, et al. Reduced systemic arterial compliance impacts significantly on left ventricular afterload and function in aortic stenosis: Implications for diagnosis and treatment. J Am Coll Cardiol. 2005;46(2):291–298.
38. Munt B, et al. Physical examination in valvular aortic stenosis: Correlation with stenosis severity and prediction of clinical outcome. Am Heart J. 1999;137(2):298–306.
39. Bonow RO, et al. 2008 Focused update incorporated into the ACC/AHA 2006 guidelines for the management of patients with valvular heart disease: A report of the American College of Cardiology/American Heart Association task force on practice guidelines (writing committee to revise the 1998 guidelines for the management of patients with valvular heart disease) endorsed by the society of cardiovascular anesthesiologists, society for cardiovascular angiography and interventions, and society of thoracic surgeons. J Am Coll Cardiol. 2008;52(13):e1–e142.
40. Bonow RO, et al. ACC/AHA 2006 guidelines for the management of patients with valvular heart disease: A report of the American College of Cardiology/American Heart Association task force on practice guidelines (writing committee to revise the 1998 guidelines for the management of patients with valvular heart disease): Developed in collaboration with the society of cardiovascular anesthesiologists: Endorsed by the society for cardiovascular angiography and interventions and the society of thoracic surgeons. Circulation. 2006;114(5):e84–e231.
41. Cormier B, et al. Value of multiplane transesophageal echocardiography in determining aortic valve area in aortic stenosis. Am J Cardiol. 1996;77(10):882–885.
42. Hoffmann R, Flachskampf FA, Hanrath P. Planimetry of orifice area in aortic stenosis using multiplane transesophageal echocardiography. J Am Coll Cardiol. 1993;22(2):529–534.
43. Tardif JC, et al. Effects of variations in flow on aortic valve area in aortic stenosis based on in vivo planimetry of aortic valve area by multiplane transesophageal echocardiography. Am J Cardiol. 1995;76(3):193–198.
44. Tardif JC, et al. Simultaneous determination of aortic valve area by the Gorlin formula and by transesophageal echocardiography under different transvalvular flow conditions. Evidence that anatomic aortic valve area does not change with variations in flow in aortic stenosis. J Am Coll Cardiol. 1997;29(6):1296–1302.
45. Kim CJ, et al. Correspondence of aortic valve area determination from transesophageal echocardiography, transthoracic echocardiography, and cardiac catheterization. Am Heart J. 1996;132(6):1163–1172.
46. Arsenault M, et al. Variation of anatomic valve area during ejection in patients with valvular aortic stenosis evaluated by two-dimensional echocardiographic planimetry: Comparison with traditional Doppler data. J Am Coll Cardiol. 1998;32(7):1931–1937.
47. Bernard Y, et al. Planimetry of aortic valve area using multiplane transoesophageal echocardiography is not a reliable method for assessing severity of aortic stenosis. Heart. 1997;78(1):68–73.
48. Blot-Souletie N, et al. Comparison of accuracy of aortic valve area assessment in aortic stenosis by real time three-dimensional echocardiography in biplane mode versus two-dimensional transthoracic and transesophageal echocardiography. Echocardiography. 2007;24(10):1065–1072.
49. Foster GP, et al. Determination of aortic valve area in valvular aortic stenosis by direct measurement using intracardiac echocardiography: A comparison with the Gorlin and continuity equations. J Am Coll Cardiol. 1996;27(2):392–398.
50. Callahan MJ, et al. Validation of instantaneous pressure gradients measured by continuous-wave Doppler in experimentally induced aortic stenosis. Am J Cardiol. 1985;56(15):989–993.
51. Currie PJ, et al. Continuous-wave Doppler echocardiographic assessment of severity of calcific aortic stenosis: A simultaneous Doppler-catheter correlative study in 100 adult patients. Circulation. 1985;71(6):1162–1169.
52. Galan A, Zoghbi WA, Quinones MA. Determination of severity of valvular aortic stenosis by Doppler echocardiography and relation of findings to clinical outcome and agreement with hemodynamic measurements determined at cardiac catheterization. Am J Cardiol. 1991;67(11):1007–1012.
53. Hegrenaes L, Hatle L. Aortic stenosis in adults. Non-invasive estimation of pressure differences by continuous wave Doppler echocardiography. Br Heart J. 1985;54(4):396–404.
54. Hatle L, Angelsen BA, Tromsdal A. Non-invasive assessment of aortic stenosis by Doppler ultrasound. Br Heart J. 1980;43(3):284–292.
55. Otto CM, et al. Prospective study of asymptomatic valvular aortic stenosis. Clinical, echocardiographic, and exercise predictors of outcome. Circulation. 1997;95(9):2262–2270.
56. Oh JK, et al. Prediction of the severity of aortic stenosis by Doppler aortic valve area determination: Prospective Doppler-catheterization correlation in 100 patients. J Am Coll Cardiol. 1988;11(6):1227–1234.
57. Skjaerpe T, Hegrenaes L, Hatle L. Noninvasive estimation of valve area in patients with aortic stenosis by Doppler ultrasound and two-dimensional echocardiography. Circulation. 1985;72(4):810–818.
58. Moss RR, et al. Role of echocardiography in percutaneous aortic valve implantation. J Am Coll Cardiol Img. 2008;1(1):15–24.
59. Flachskampf FA, et al. Influence of orifice geometry and flow rate on effective valve area: An in vitro study. J Am Coll Cardiol. 1990;15(5):1173–1180.

60. Gilon D, et al. Effect of three-dimensional valve shape on the hemodynamics of aortic stenosis: Three-dimensional echocardiographic stereolithography and patient studies. *J Am Coll Cardiol.* 2002;40(8):1479–1486.
61. Zhou YQ, Faerestrand S, Matre K. Velocity distributions in the left ventricular outflow tract in patients with valvular aortic stenosis. Effect on the measurement of aortic valve area by using the continuity equation. *Eur Heart J.* 1995;16(3):383–393.
62. Zoghbi WA, et al. Accurate noninvasive quantification of stenotic aortic valve area by Doppler echocardiography. *Circulation.* 1986;73(3):452–459.
63. Burwash IG, et al. Dependence of Gorlin formula and continuity equation valve areas on transvalvular volume flow rate in valvular aortic stenosis. *Circulation.* 1994;89(2):827–835.
64. Grayburn PA, et al. Pivotal role of aortic valve area calculation by the continuity equation for Doppler assessment of aortic stenosis in patients with combined aortic stenosis and regurgitation. *Am J Cardiol.* 1988;61(4):376–381.
65. Vandervoort PM, et al. Pressure recovery in bileaflet heart valve prostheses. Localized high velocities and gradients in central and side orifices with implications for Doppler-catheter gradient relation in aortic and mitral position. *Circulation.* 1995;92(12):3464–3472.
66. Razzolini R, et al. Discrepancies between catheter and Doppler estimates of aortic stenosis: The role of pressure recovery evaluated 'in vivo'. *J Heart Valve Dis.* 2007;16(3):225–229.
67. Rhodes KD, et al. Prediction of pressure recovery location in aortic valve stenosis: An in-vitro validation study. *J Heart Valve Dis.* 2007;16(5):489–494.
68. Isaaz K, et al. How important is the impact of pressure recovery on routine evaluation of aortic stenosis? A clinical study in 91 patients. *J Heart Valve Dis.* 2004;13(3):347–356.
69. Garcia D, et al. Discrepancies between catheter and Doppler estimates of valve effective orifice area can be predicted from the pressure recovery phenomenon: Practical implications with regard to quantification of aortic stenosis severity. *J Am Coll Cardiol.* 2003;41(3):435–442.
70. Levine RA, Schwammenthal E. Stenosis is in the eye of the observer: Impact of pressure recovery on assessing aortic valve area. *J Am Coll Cardiol.* 2003;41(3):443–445.
71. Villavicencio RE, et al. Pressure recovery in pediatric aortic valve stenosis. *Pediatr Cardiol.* 2003;24(5):457–462.
72. Gjertsson P, et al. Important pressure recovery in patients with aortic stenosis and high Doppler gradients. *Am J Cardiol.* 2001;88(2):139–144.
73. DeGroff CG, Shandas R, Valdes-Cruz L. Pressure recovery and aortic stenosis. *J Am Coll Cardiol.* 2000;35(1):260–261.
74. Baumgartner H, et al. "Overestimation" of catheter gradients by Doppler ultrasound in patients with aortic stenosis: A predictable manifestation of pressure recovery. *J Am Coll Cardiol.* 1999;33(6):1655–1661.
75. Niederberger J, et al. Importance of pressure recovery for the assessment of aortic stenosis by Doppler ultrasound. Role of aortic size, aortic valve area, and direction of the stenotic jet in vitro. *Circulation.* 1996;94(8):1934–1940.
76. Chambers J. Is pressure recovery an important cause of "Doppler aortic stenosis" with no gradient at cardiac catheterization? *Heart.* 1996;76(5):381–383.
77. Voelker W, et al. Pressure recovery in aortic stenosis: An in vitro study in a pulsatile flow model. *J Am Coll Cardiol.* 1992;20(7):1585–1593.
78. Spevack DM, et al. Routine adjustment of Doppler echocardiographically derived aortic valve area using a previously derived equation to account for the effect of pressure recovery. *J Am Soc Echocardiogr.* 2008;21(1):34–37.
79. Garcia D, et al. Assessment of aortic valve stenosis severity: A new index based on the energy loss concept. *Circulation.* 2000;101(7):765–771.
80. Isaaz K, et al. Demonstration of postvalvuloplasty hemodynamic improvement in aortic stenosis based on Doppler measurement of valvular resistance. *J Am Coll Cardiol.* 1991;18(7):1661–1670.
81. Voelker W, et al. Comparison of valvular resistance, stroke work loss, and Gorlin valve area for quantification of aortic stenosis. An in vitro study in a pulsatile aortic flow model. *Circulation.* 1995;91(4):1196–1204.
82. Roger VL, et al. Aortic valve resistance in aortic stenosis: Doppler echocardiographic study and surgical correlation. *Am Heart J.* 1997;134(5 Pt 1):924–929.
83. Antonini-Canterin F, et al. Is aortic valve resistance more clinically meaningful than valve area in aortic stenosis? *Heart.* 1999;82(1):9–10.
84. Bermejo J, Yotti R. Low-gradient aortic valve stenosis: Value and limitations of dobutamine stress testing. *Heart.* 2007;93(3):298–302.
85. Chafizadeh ER, Zoghbi WA. Doppler echocardiographic assessment of the St. Jude Medical prosthetic valve in the aortic position using the continuity equation. *Circulation.* 1991;83(1):213–223.
86. Bountioukos M, et al. Safety of dobutamine stress echocardiography in patients with aortic stenosis. *J Heart Valve Dis.* 2003;12(4):441–446.
87. deFilippi CR, et al. Usefulness of dobutamine echocardiography in distinguishing severe from nonsevere valvular aortic stenosis in patients with depressed left ventricular function and low transvalvular gradients. *Am J Cardiol.* 1995;75(2):191–194.
88. Grayburn PA. Assessment of low-gradient aortic stenosis with dobutamine. *Circulation.* 2006;113(5):604–606.
89. Lange RA, Hillis LD. Dobutamine stress echocardiography in patients with low-gradient aortic stenosis. *Circulation.* 2006;113(14):1718–1720.
90. Monin JL, et al. Aortic stenosis with severe left ventricular dysfunction and low transvalvular pressure gradients: Risk stratification by low-dose dobutamine echocardiography. *J Am Coll Cardiol.* 2001;37(8):2101–2107.
91. Monin JL, et al. Low-gradient aortic stenosis: Operative risk stratification and predictors for long-term outcome: A multicenter study using dobutamine stress hemodynamics. *Circulation.* 2003;108(3):319–324.
92. Schwammenthal E, et al. Dobutamine echocardiography in patients with aortic stenosis and left ventricular dysfunction: Predicting outcome as a function of management strategy. *Chest.* 2001;119(6):1766–1777.
93. Zuppiroli A, et al. Therapeutic implications of contractile reserve elicited by dobutamine echocardiography in symptomatic, low-gradient aortic stenosis. *Ital Heart J.* 2003;4(4):264–270.
94. Bergler-Klein J, et al. Natriuretic peptides predict symptom-free survival and postoperative outcome in severe aortic stenosis. *Circulation.* 2004;109(19):2302–2308.
95. Bergler-Klein J, et al. B-type natriuretic peptide in low-flow, low-gradient aortic stenosis: Relationship to hemodynamics and clinical outcome: Results from the multicenter Truly or Pseudo-Severe Aortic Stenosis (TOPAS) study. *Circulation.* 2007;115(22):2848–2855.
96. Monin JL, et al. Low-gradient aortic stenosis: Impact of prosthesis-patient mismatch on survival. *Eur Heart J.* 2007;28(21):2620–2626.
97. Quere JP, et al. Influence of preoperative left ventricular contractile reserve on postoperative ejection fraction in low-gradient aortic stenosis. *Circulation.* 2006;113(14):1738–1744.
98. Pereira JJ, et al. Survival after aortic valve replacement for severe aortic stenosis with low transvalvular gradients and severe left ventricular dysfunction. *J Am Coll Cardiol.* 2002;39(8):1356–1363.
99. Connolly HM, et al. Severe aortic stenosis with low transvalvular gradient and severe left ventricular dysfunction: Result of aortic valve replacement in 52 patients. *Circulation.* 2000;101(16):1940–1946.
100. Levy F, et al. Aortic valve replacement for low-flow/low-gradient aortic stenosis: Operative risk stratification and long-term outcome: A European Multicenter Study. *J Am Coll Cardiol.* 2008;51(15):1466–1472.
101. Hachicha Z, et al. Paradoxical low-flow, low-gradient severe aortic stenosis despite preserved ejection fraction is associated with higher afterload and reduced survival. *Circulation.* 2007;115(22):2856–2864.
102. Murakami T, et al. Diastolic filling dynamics in patients with aortic stenosis. *Circulation.* 1986;73(6):1162–1174.
103. Vanoverschelde JL, et al. Hemodynamic and volume correlates of left ventricular diastolic relaxation and filling in patients with aortic stenosis. *J Am Coll Cardiol.* 1992;20(4):813–821.
104. Sheikh KH, et al. Doppler left ventricular diastolic filling abnormalities in aortic stenosis and their relation to hemodynamic parameters. *Am J Cardiol.* 1989;63(18):1360–1368.
105. Otto CM, Pearlman AS, Amsler LC. Doppler echocardiographic evaluation of left ventricular diastolic filling in isolated valvular aortic stenosis. *Am J Cardiol.* 1989;63(5):313–316.
106. Gabay J, et al. Effects of isometric exercise on the diastolic function in patients with severe aortic stenosis with or without coronary lesion. *Int J Cardiol.* 2005;104(1):52–58.
107. Gjertsson P, et al. Preoperative moderate to severe diastolic dysfunction: A novel Doppler echocardiographic long-term prognostic factor in patients with severe aortic stenosis. *J Thorac Cardiovasc Surg.* 2005;129(4):890–896.
108. Casaclang-Verzosa G, et al. E/Ea is the major determinant of pulmonary artery pressure in moderate to severe aortic stenosis. *J Am Soc Echocardiogr.* 2008;21(7):824–827.
109. Poh KK, et al. Prognostication of valvular aortic stenosis using tissue Doppler echocardiography: Underappreciated importance of late diastolic mitral annular velocity. *J Am Soc Echocardiogr.* 2008;21(5):475–481.
110. Stuber M, et al. Alterations in the local myocardial motion pattern in patients suffering from pressure overload due to aortic stenosis. *Circulation.* 1999;100(4):361–368.
111. Nagel E, et al. Cardiac rotation and relaxation in patients with aortic valve stenosis. *Eur Heart J.* 2000;21(7):582–589.
112. Notomi Y, et al. Measurement of ventricular torsion by two-dimensional ultrasound speckle tracking imaging. *J Am Coll Cardiol.* 2005;45(12):2034–2041.
113. Helle-Valle T, et al. New noninvasive method for assessment of left ventricular rotation: Speckle tracking echocardiography. *Circulation.* 2005;112(20):3149–3156.
114. Kim HK, et al. Assessment of left ventricular rotation and torsion with two-dimensional speckle tracking echocardiography. *J Am Soc Echocardiogr.* 2007;20(1):45–53.
115. Sengupta PP, et al. Twist mechanics of the left ventricle: Principles and application. *J Am Coll Cardiol Img.* 2008;1(3):366–376.
116. Silver K, et al. Pulmonary artery hypertension in severe aortic stenosis: Incidence and mechanism. *Am Heart J.* 1993;125(1):146–150.
117. Kapoor N, Varadarajan P, Pai RG. Echocardiographic predictors of pulmonary hypertension in patients with severe aortic stenosis. *Eur J Echocardiogr.* 2008;9(1):31–33.
118. McHenry MM, et al. Pulmonary hypertension and sudden death in aortic stenosis. *Br Heart J.* 1979;41(4):463–467.
119. Malouf JF, et al. Severe pulmonary hypertension in patients with severe aortic valve stenosis: Clinical profile and prognostic implications. *J Am Coll Cardiol.* 2002;40(4):789–795.
120. Malyar NM, et al. Assessment of aortic valve area in aortic stenosis using cardiac magnetic resonance tomography: Comparison with echocardiography. *Cardiology.* 2008;109(2):126–134.
121. Schlosser T, et al. Quantification of aortic valve stenosis in MRI-comparison of steady-state free precession and fast low-angle shot sequences. *Eur Radiol.* 2007;17(5):1284–1290.
122. Meave-Gonzalez A, et al. Pure aortic stenosis and magnetic resonance in adult patients. *Arch Cardiol Mex.* 2007;77(4):308–312.
123. Debl K, et al. Planimetry of aortic valve area in aortic stenosis by magnetic resonance imaging. *Invest Radiol.* 2005;40(10):631–636.

124. Hartiala JJ, et al. Evaluation of left atrial contribution to left ventricular filling in aortic stenosis by velocity-encoded cine MRI. *Am Heart J.* 1994;127(3):593–600.

125. Reant P, et al. Absolute assessment of aortic valve stenosis by planimetry using cardiovascular magnetic resonance imaging: Comparison with transesophageal echocardiography, transthoracic echocardiography, and cardiac catheterisation. *Eur J Radiol.* 2006;59(2):276–283.

126. Kupfahl C, et al. Evaluation of aortic stenosis by cardiovascular magnetic resonance imaging: Comparison with established routine clinical techniques. *Heart.* 2004;90(8):893–901.

127. Caruthers SD, et al. Practical value of cardiac magnetic resonance imaging for clinical quantification of aortic valve stenosis: Comparison with echocardiography. *Circulation.* 2003;108(18):2236–2243.

128. John AS, et al. Magnetic resonance to assess the aortic valve area in aortic stenosis: How does it compare to current diagnostic standards? *J Am Coll Cardiol.* 2003;42(3):519–526.

129. Sondergaard L, et al. Valve area and cardiac output in aortic stenosis: Quantification by magnetic resonance velocity mapping. *Am Heart J.* 1993;126(5):1156–1164.

130. Tanaka K, Makaryus AN, Wolff SD. Correlation of aortic valve area obtained by the velocity-encoded phase contrast continuity method to direct planimetry using cardiovascular magnetic resonance. *J Cardiovasc Magn Reson.* 2007;9(5):799–805.

131. Lotz J, et al. Cardiovascular flow measurement with phase-contrast MR imaging: Basic facts and implementation. *Radiographics.* 2002;22(3):651–671.

132. Masci PG, Dymarkowski S, Bogaert J. Valvular heart disease: What does cardiovascular MRI add? *Eur Radiol.* 2008;18(2):197–208.

133. Gatehouse PD, et al. Applications of phase-contrast flow and velocity imaging in cardiovascular MRI. *Eur Radiol.* 2005;15(10):2172–2184.

134. O'Brien KR, et al. MRI phase contrast velocity and flow errors in turbulent stenotic jets. *J Magn Reson Imaging.* 2008;28(1):210–218.

135. Biederman RW, et al. Physiologic compensation is supranormal in compensated aortic stenosis: Does it return to normal after aortic valve replacement or is it blunted by coexistent coronary artery disease? An intramyocardial magnetic resonance imaging study. *Circulation.* 2005;112(9):I429–I436.

136. Rajappan K, et al. Assessment of left ventricular mass regression after aortic valve replacement—cardiovascular magnetic resonance versus M-mode echocardiography. *Eur J Cardiothorac Surg.* 2003;24(1):59–65.

137. Kuehne T, et al. Magnetic resonance imaging-guided transcatheter implantation of a prosthetic valve in aortic valve position: Feasibility study in swine. *J Am Coll Cardiol.* 2004;44(11):2247–2249.

138. Shavelle DM, et al. Usefulness of aortic valve calcium scores by electron beam computed tomography as a marker for aortic stenosis. *Am J Cardiol.* 2003;92(3):349–353.

139. Ruhl KM, et al. Variability of aortic valve calcification measurement with multislice spiral computed tomography. *Invest Radiol.* 2006;41(4):370–373.

140. Cowell SJ, et al. Aortic valve calcification on computed tomography predicts the severity of aortic stenosis. *Clin Radiol.* 2003;58(9):712–716.

141. Kaden JJ, et al. Correlation of degree of aortic valve stenosis by Doppler echocardiogram to quantity of calcium in the valve by electron beam tomography. *Am J Cardiol.* 2002;90(5):554–557.

142. Feuchtner GM, et al. Multislice computed tomography for detection of patients with aortic valve stenosis and quantification of severity. *J Am Coll Cardiol.* 2006;47(7):1410–1417.

143. Pohle K, et al. Progression of aortic valve calcification: Association with coronary atherosclerosis and cardiovascular risk factors. *Circulation.* 2001;104(16):1927–1932.

144. Feuchtner GM, et al. Aortic valve calcification as quantified with multislice computed tomography predicts short-term clinical outcome in patients with asymptomatic aortic stenosis. *J Heart Valve Dis.* 2006;15(4):494–498.

145. Tanaka H, et al. The simultaneous assessment of aortic valve area and coronary artery stenosis using 16-slice multidetector-row computed tomography in patients with aortic stenosis comparison with echocardiography. *Circ J.* 2007;71(10):1593–1598.

146. Demirkol MO, et al. Dipyridamole myocardial perfusion tomography in patients with severe aortic stenosis. *Cardiology.* 2002;97(1):37–42.

147. Kapila A, Hart R. Calcific cerebral emboli and aortic stenosis: Detection of computed tomography. *Stroke.* 1986;17(4):619–621.

148. Janson R, et al. Computer-cardio-tomography in idiopathic hypertrophic subvalvular aortic stenosis—A new contribution to non-invasive diagnosis (author's transl). *Rofo.* 1979;130(5):536–542.

149. Meijboom WB, et al. Pre-operative computed tomography coronary angiography to detect significant coronary artery disease in patients referred for cardiac valve surgery. *J Am Coll Cardiol.* 2006;48(8):1658–1665.

150. Shrivastava V, et al. Is cardiac computed tomography a reliable alternative to percutaneous coronary angiography for patients awaiting valve surgery? *Interact Cardiovasc Thorac Surg.* 2007;6(1):105–109.

151. Laissy JP, et al. Comprehensive evaluation of preoperative patients with aortic valve stenosis: Usefulness of cardiac multidetector computed tomography. *Heart.* 2007;93(9):1121–1125.

152. Vahanian A, et al. Guidelines on the management of valvular heart disease. *Rev Esp Cardiol.* 2007;60(6):1e–50e.

153. Amato MC, et al. Treatment decision in asymptomatic aortic valve stenosis: Role of exercise testing. *Heart.* 2001;86(4):381–386.

154. Lancellotti P, et al. Prognostic importance of quantitative exercise Doppler echocardiography in asymptomatic valvular aortic stenosis. *Circulation.* 2005;112(9):1377–I382.

155. Das P, Rimington H, Chambers J. Exercise testing to stratify risk in aortic stenosis. *Eur Heart J.* 2005;26(13):1309–1313.

156. Vahanian A, et al. Guidelines on the management of valvular heart disease: The task force on the management of valvular heart disease of the European Society of Cardiology. *Eur Heart J.* 2007;28(2):230–268.

157. Habis M, et al. Comparison of 64-slice computed tomography planimetry and Doppler echocardiography in the assessment of aortic valve stenosis. *J Heart Valve Dis.* 2007;16(3):216–224.

158. Stamm RB, Martin RP. Quatification of pressure gradients across stenotic valves by Doppler ultrasound. *J Am Coll Cardiol.* 1983;2(4):707–718.

159. Berger M, Hecht SR. Doppler echocardiographic assessment of aortic stenosis using the peak velocity ratio. *Am J Cardiol.* 1992;70(4):536–537.

160. Currie PJ, Seward JB, Reeder GS, et al. Continuous-wave Doppler echocardiographic assessment of severity of calcific aortic stenosis: a simultaneous Doppler-catheter correlative study in 100 adult patients. *Circulation.* 1985;71(6):1162–1169.

161. Oh JK, Taliercio CP, Holmes DR Jr, et al. Prediction of the severity of aortic stenosis by Doppler aortic valve area determination: prospective Doppler-catheterization correlation in 100 patients. *J Am Coll Cardiol.* 1988;11(6):1227–1234.

162. Otto CM, Pearlman AS, Comess KA, et al. Determination of the stenotic aortic valve area in adults using Doppler echocardiography. *J Am Coll Cardiol.* 1986;7(3):509–517.

163. Zoghbi WA, Galan A, Quinones MA. Accurate assessment of aortic stenosis severity by Doppler echocardiography independent of aortic jet velocity. *Am Heart J.* 1988;116(3):855–863.

164. Teirstein P, Yeager M, Yock PG, et al. Doppler echocardiographic measurement of aortic valve area in aortic stenosis: a noninvasive application of the Gorlin formula. *J Am Coll Cardiol.* 1986;8(5):1059–1065.

Aortic Regurgitation

28

Kameswari Maganti
Vera H. Rigolin
Robert O. Bonow

1. INTRODUCTION

Aortic regurgitation (AR) is characterized by a reflux of blood from the aorta into the left ventricle during diastole, due to malcoaptation of the aortic cusps. The clinical presentation of AR is determined by the acuity of presentation, severity of regurgitation, aortic and left ventricular (LV) compliance, and LV end-diastolic volume. Although chronic AR is insidious and well tolerated for decades, acute AR may lead to a rapid cardiac decompensation and is a surgical emergency with high fatality rates if left untreated.[1-3]

1.1. Epidemiology

AR is a common worldwide disorder although the precise incidence and prevalence of AR is not known. In the Framingham Offspring Study,[4] the prevalence of chronic AR as detected by color Doppler echocardiography in a large unselected adult population was 13% in men and 8.5% in women. However, trace to mild AR was much more common in this population. Age and male gender were noted to be predictors of AR in this study. Hypertension did not predict AR but rather was associated with modest increases in aortic root size when age was included in a multivariate model; confirming what was noted in earlier observations,[5] the Strong Heart Study[6] reported an overall prevalence of AR of 10% in a native American population. Age and aortic root diameter rather than gender were independent predictors of AR. Most cases were of mild severity. The prevalence of moderate or greater AR was 0.5% and 2.7% respectively. Severe AR seems to affect men more than women.[7,8]

1.2. Clinical presentation

In acute AR, patients generally have a sudden onset of severe dyspnea from acutely elevated LV filling pressures, hypotension, and compensatory tachycardia. By contrast, in chronic AR, the volume and pressure overload follows a long insidious course that may span decades. There is an excess afterload with recruitment of preload reserve and compensatory hypertrophy to maintain a compensated state. Once this balance is shifted, patients become symptomatic and may experience dyspnea from LV dysfunction and angina from diminished coronary flow reserve.

2. PATHOPHYSIOLOGY

AR results from abnormalities of the aortic leaflets or their supporting structures, aortic root and annulus, or both. Figure 28.1 demonstrates a normal, trileaflet aortic valve. There are numerous causes of AR. Rheumatic heart disease still remains the most common cause of severe AR worldwide. However, diseases involving the aortic root and ascending aorta are now becoming more frequent causes of AR in the western hemisphere.[9]

Abnormalities of the aortic cusps that may result in AR include congenital leaflet abnormalities such as bicuspid (Fig. 28.2), unicuspid (Fig. 28.3), or quadricuspid (Fig. 28.4) valves or rupture of a congenitally fenestrated valve; other congenital defects such as large ventricular septal defects and subaortic membranes (Fig. 28.5); rheumatic heart disease with fusion of the commissures and retraction of the aortic valve leaflets due to scarring and fibrosis; infective endocarditis(Fig. 28.6); atherosclerotic degeneration; myxomatous infiltration of aortic valve, tumors (Fig. 28.7), connective tissue disorders such as Marfan syndrome, inflammatory diseases such as aortitis, antiphospholipid syndrome, and use of anorectic drugs.[8,10-15] Other systemic disorders that may affect the aortic valve include lupus erythematosus, giant cell arteritis, Takayasu arteritis, ankylosing spondylitis, Jaccoud arthropathy, Whipple disease, and Crohn disease.

Diseases that primarily affect the annulus or aortic root include idiopathic aortic root dilation, degeneration of the extracellular matrix as an isolated condition or associated with Marfan syndrome or congenitally bicuspid aortic valves, Ehlers–Danlos syndrome, and osteogenesis imperfecta.[16] AR may also arise from inflammatory aortitis, such as syphilitic aortitis, aortitis noted with other connective tissue diseases such as ankylosing spondylitis, giant cell arteritis, the Behçet syndrome, psoriatic arthritis, and other forms of arthritis associated with ulcerative colitis, relapsing polychondritis, and Reiter syndrome.[16] Aortic root enlargement causes AR due to annular dilatation, resulting in leaflet separation and loss of coaptation. A bicuspid aortic valve is commonly associated with dilation of the aortic root in addition to the congenital leaflet abnormality because of abnormalities in the aortic matrix[2,17-20] Similarly, ankylosing spondylitis can result in abnormalities of both the leaflets and the aortic root. It is important to note that chronic AR by itself may lead to progressive aortic root dilatation over time.

Acute AR, a surgical emergency, is fortunately rare. It is most commonly caused by endocarditis.[2,21,22] Figure 28.8 shows an echocardiogram of a patient with acute AR due to endocarditis causing prolapse of the right coronary cusp. Another common cause of acute AR is aortic dissection,[23] which may present in patients with hypertension, connective tissue disorders such as Marfan syndrome,[8,9,24] syphilitic aortitis, and occasionally during/due to pregnancy.[25] Infrequently, acute AR may be the result of aortic laceration or blunt chest trauma.[24,26-28] It rarely occurs due to complications of invasive procedures such as aortic balloon valvuloplasty, percutaneous balloon dilatation for aortic coarctation, and radiofrequency catheter ablation.[29]

393

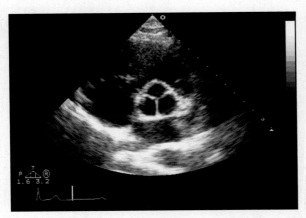

Figure 28.1 Parasternal short-axis view of a normal, trileaflet aortic valve is shown.

Bicuspid aortic valves. Bicuspid aortic valves are of particular interest due to their unique pathology and association with aortic root enlargement[2,17-20] The incidence of bicuspid valve disease in general population is 1% to 2% with male preponderance. There appears to be familial clustering; therefore, echocardiographic screening of first degree relatives is warranted. Bicuspid valves develop from abnormal cusp formation during valvulogenesis. Mutations in the signaling and transcriptional regulator NOTCH1 cause a spectrum of developmental aortic valve anomalies such as bicuspid aortic valves.[17,30] Inadequate production of fibrillin-1 during valvulogenesis may disrupt formation of the aortic cusps and also weaken the aortic root. Although aortic stenosis is the most common complication of bicuspid valves, varying degrees of AR can result from incomplete closure, cusp prolapse, fibrotic retraction, or dilatation of the sinotubular junction.[12,13,15,17-19] Patients with bicuspid aortic valves are also at risk of developing aortic aneurysms that are prone to rupture and dissection.[19,20] Even after aortic valve replacement (AVR), progressive aortic root enlargement can be noted in these patients.[31,32] Thus, diligent routine screening of the aortic root in patients with bicuspid valves is imperative.

Marfan syndrome. The Marfan syndrome also deserves a special mention due to its unique characteristics. Marfan syndrome is an autosomal dominant disorder and is relatively frequent in the order of 2 to 3 per 10,000. It occurs in all races and genetic groups and is caused by a defect in the gene that encodes fibrillin-1(*FBN1*).[33] A defect in the microfibrils explains all of the pleiotropic manifestations of Marfan syndrome. Mutations in fibrillin may result in inappropriate or excessive activation of transforming growth factor-β (TGF-β) receptors. Similar aortic pathology occurs in genetic disorders related to TGF-β receptors, such as the Loeys–Dietz syndrome.[34] In these conditions, dilatation of the aortic root and aortic dissection is the major cause of morbidity and mortality.[35,36] Management of these patients is complex since predicting long term risks of aortic dissection is difficult.

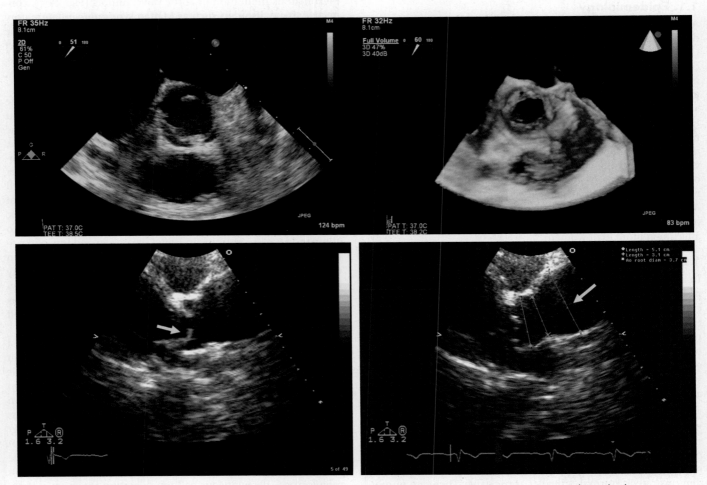

Figure 28.2 A short axis view of a bicuspid aortic valve is shown. Images were acquired using a transesophageal echo system. The right upper panel shows a 2D echo image of the valve. The left upper panel shows a 3D image of the same valve. The left lower panel shows doming of the leaflets during systole (*arrow*). The right lower panel shows an ascending aortic aneurysm (*arrow*), a finding often seen in patients with bicuspid aortic valves.

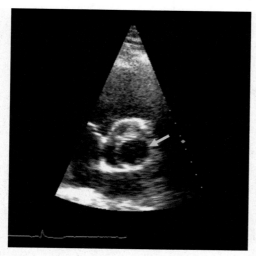

Figure 28.3 An example of a unicuspid aortic valve is shown. Note the circular appearance of the valve when it is fully opened (*arrow*).

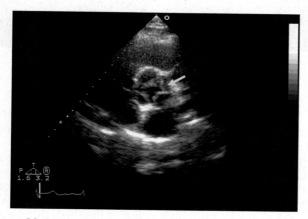

Figure 28.4 A 2D echo of a quadricuspid aortic valve is shown. Note the four visible leaflets (*arrow*).

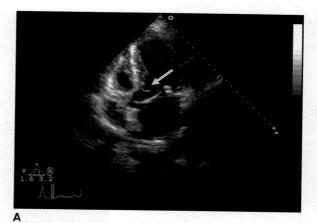

A

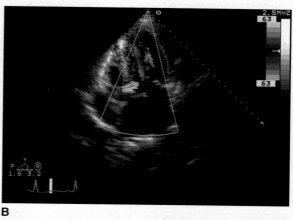

B

Figure 28.5 **Panel A** shows a subaortic membrane (*arrow*). **Panel B** demonstrates the resultant AR.

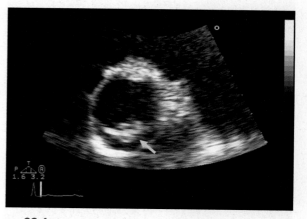

Figure 28.6 A vegetation (*arrow*) is demonstrated on a bicuspid aortic valve.

Children with Marfan syndrome tend to have more mitral valve disease, whereas aortic problems are more often noted in adolescence and beyond. Characteristic findings on echocardiography include dilatation of the aortic root and ascending aorta with effacement of the sinotubular junction. AR results from incomplete central coaptation of the stretched leaflets due to annular dilatation. The anterior leaflet of the mitral valve is often elongated and redundant, and prolapses into the left atrium. Hence, there is often some degree of mitral regurgitation.[37] The risk factors for aortic dissection include a family history of aortic dissection, the severity of aortic root dilatation, and the ratio of the actual to predicted sinus dimension. A ratio less than or equal to 1.3 is a predictor of good long term outcome.[35] Patients with a ratio less than 1.5 times the mean predicted diameter for their body size can be monitored annually, whereas more frequent evaluation is necessary if the diameter increases.

2.1. Hemodynamic alterations

Chronic AR. In chronic AR, there is combined preload and afterload excess imposed on the left ventricle. The excess preload reflects the volume overload that is directly related to the severity of AR, with only minimal volume overload in mild AR but massive volume overload with severe AR. The afterload excess is due to the combination of the increase in LV wall stress from the regurgitant volume and the elevated systolic blood pressure that results from the increase in total forward LV stroke volume, representing the regurgitant volume as well as the LV forward flow that is ejected into the aorta during systole.[38,39] In addition, systolic hypertension contributes to progressive aortic root dilatation, which in turn can contribute further to worsening severity of AR. The combination of preload and afterload excess with severe AR leads ultimately to progressive LV dilatation with resultant systolic dysfunction. With LV dysfunction, symptoms of heart failure

Figure 28.7 A 2D and associated 3D echo image of a trileaflet aortic valve with a papillary fibroelastoma (*arrow*).

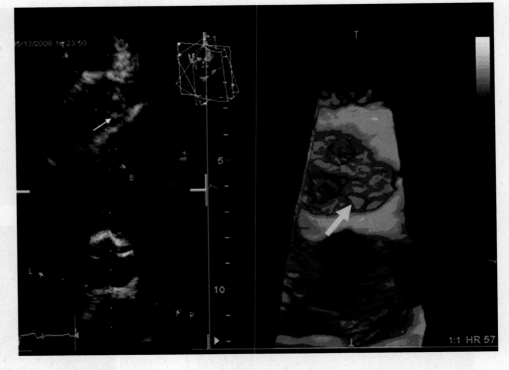

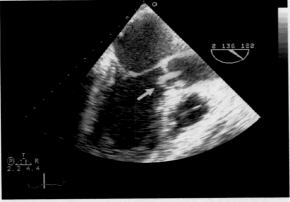

A

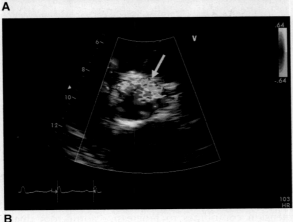

B

Figure 28.8 Panel A shows the echo from a patient with acute AR due to endocarditis causing prolapse of the right coronary cusp (*arrow*). The resultant severe AR is shown in **Panel B**.

such as dyspnea on exertion, orthopnea, and paroxysmal nocturnal dyspnea may develop.

In early, compensated severe AR, the left ventricle adapts to the volume overload by development of eccentric hypertrophy with replication of sarcomeres in series and elongation of myocytes and myofibers.[38–45] This eccentric hypertrophy helps to maintain the ratio of the LV cavity radius to wall thickness, thereby regulating the LV wall stress to normal levels (*Laplace's law*, which is the product of ventricular pressure and radius divided by twice the wall thickness). Increased systolic wall stress and afterload are stimuli for further concentric hypertrophy. The systolic function is thus preserved due to the combination of chamber dilatation and hypertrophy. Thus, despite an increase in preload and afterload, the above compensatory changes seek to maintain normal LV systolic function despite a large regurgitant volume and allow patients to remain asymptomatic for many years. The slope of the LV pressure–volume relationship, a load-independent measure of myocardial function, is normal in these early stages.[45] With the large end-diastolic volumes and increased wall thickness, patients with AR often have extreme cardiomegaly, resulting in the so-called cor bovinum.

Over time, progressive LV dilation and systolic hypertension increase LV wall stress. As this occurs, there is a phase during which LV ejection fraction is still normal, but early myocardial dysfunction develops that is largely masked by increased preload. Peak elastance (E_{max}) on the LV pressure volume relationship is decreased at this stage. The LV ejection fraction is likely to increase after successful AVR despite the early myocardial dysfunction. Eventually, if preload reserve or compensatory hypertrophy is insufficient, further afterload mismatch will result in a decline in systolic function and ejection fraction.[40] There is an increase in the interstitial fibrosis, a decrease in the LV compliance, and an increase in the LV end-diastolic pressure accompanying this stage of LV decompensation. With progression of LV dysfunction, there is an increase in left atrial, pulmonary artery wedge, and right sided pressures with a decrease in forward cardiac output, first noted with exercise and then at rest. This ultimately results in heart failure if left untreated.

Exertional dyspnea is the most common manifestation, but angina can also occur because of a reduction in coronary flow reserve predominantly with systolic coronary flow.[46,47] This reduced oxygen supply coupled with the increased oxygen demand results in myocardial ischemia that in turn may contribute further to the deterioration of LV systolic function. Figure 28.9 demonstrates the hemodynamic alterations in chronic AR.

Acute AR. In contrast to the pathophysiologic changes in chronic AR noted above, in acute AR the regurgitant volume fills a normal sized left ventricle that has no time to adapt to the large regurgitant volume as well as the left atrial inflow. The forward stroke volume thereby decreases with an abrupt increase in LV diastolic pressures. Cardiac output is maintained by obligate tachycardia, but this may be insufficient to prevent hypotension or overt cardiogenic shock.[2] The heightened LV diastolic pressure may cause early closure of mitral valve (Fig. 28.10). This has the effect to protect the pulmonary venous bed from the excessive end-diastolic pressure unless there is coexistent diastolic mitral regurgitation. Premature closure of the mitral valve in combination with tachycardia also contributes to the shortened diastole.[48]

2.2. Natural history

The natural history of AR is dependent upon multiple variables such as the etiology and severity of the AR, coexistent aortic root pathology, and the adaptive response of the left ventricle. AR severity may worsen as a result of progressive leaflet pathology and/or involvement of the aortic root. It is likely that many if not most patients with mild AR do not progress to more severe regurgitation.[37] In chronic AR, LV dilation occurs gradually and progressively, depending on the severity of AR, hemodynamic

factors, and the degree of eccentric hypertrophy and remodeling, which may vary from patient to patient. As noted previously, patients with chronic AR usually remain asymptomatic for many years.

The natural history of severe AR is limited by studies with small sample sizes as well as inconsistent reporting of symptoms and parameters of LV function. The current treatment guidelines for AR from the American Heart Association (AHA) and the American College of Cardiology (ACC)[2] are based on nine published studies with a total of 593 patients and a mean follow-up of 6.6 years.[49–57] Table 28.1 outlines the results from these pooled studies. Five of the natural history studies were consistent in identifying age, end-systolic dimension (or volume), end-diastolic dimension (or volume), and exercise ejection fraction in patients with severe AR as markers of progression to symptoms and/or LV systolic dysfunction with time.[51–53,56,57] In one study,[52] an end-systolic dimension of greater than 50 mm resulted in a risk of death, symptoms, or LV dysfunction of 19% per year; this risk was 6% per year in patients with end-systolic dimensions between 40 and 50 mm, and no patients with an end-systolic dimension below 40 mm developed an adverse cardiac event during the 8-year follow-up period. In aggregate, among asymptomatic patients with normal LV systolic function, the rate of progression to asymptomatic LV dysfunction is less than 3.5% per year, development of symptoms or LV dysfunction averages less than 6% per year, and the risk of sudden death is less than 0.2% per year.[2] By contrast, among asymptomatic patient with LV systolic dysfunction, progression of symptoms is greater than 25% per year.[2] These outcomes are depicted in Table 28.2.

As noted in Table 28.2, severe symptoms, including dyspnea or angina, identify a high risk population with an annual mortality of almost 25%,[2] with independent predictors of survival being age, functional class, comorbidity index, atrial fibrillation, LV end-systolic diameter, and ejection fraction.[58,59] Patients with Class II symptoms have an annual mortality of 6.3%.[58] However,

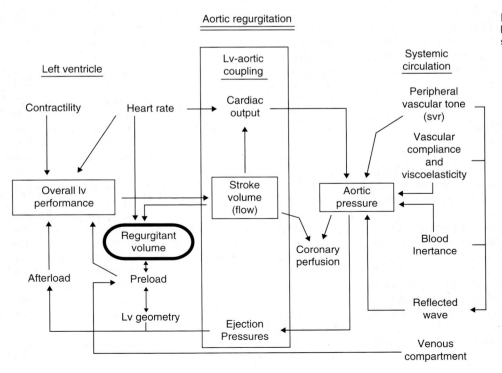

Figure 28.9 A flowchart outlining the hemodynamic alterations of chronic AR is shown.

Figure 28.10 An M-mode tracing of the mitral valve is shown. Note the early closure of the mitral valve (*arrow*) suggesting severe, acute AR.

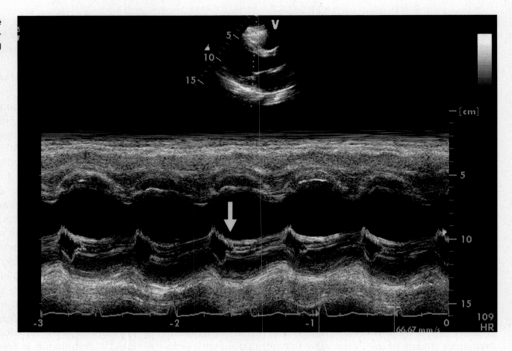

some patients may develop LV dysfunction in the absence of symptoms. The majority of such patients will become symptomatic, requiring AVR within 2 to 3 years.[2,60-62] In addition, more than 25% of initially asymptomatic patients who die or develop LV systolic dysfunction do so without warning signs.[50-53,56] LV dysfunction is often reversible with surgical correction if detected early before symptoms or severe depression of ejection fraction and/or marked LV dilatation. However, long standing LV dysfunction reduces the chances of LV recovery following surgery.[63]

Taken together, these studies indicate that asymptomatic patients with normal LV function generally have a favorable prognosis and also indicate that decline in LV ejection fraction with exercise or decline in resting ejection fraction during serial follow-up may identify patients who are likely to require surgical intervention. Patients with even moderate symptoms or evidence of severe LV dilation are at higher risk and should be considered for early intervention. These findings emphasize the importance of noninvasive imaging in the assessment of these patients, including, in particular, the asymptomatic patients.

3. DIAGNOSTIC EVALUATION

3.1. Echocardiography

Quantification of regurgitant severity provides not only prognostic data but also determines the timing of intervention.[2,64] Echocardiography is the most widely used diagnostic tool to assess LV dimensions, volumes, and ejection fraction. It allows the assessment of LV size and function, morphologic assessment of the aortic valve, aortic annulus, and the aortic root. In assessing the morphology of the aortic valve and the aortic root, echocardiography aids in determining the etiology of AR. Finally, echocardiography is well suited to quantifying the severity of AR. The American Society of Echocardiography guidelines for quantification of valvular regurgitation emphasize the need to integrate all the above information to properly evaluate patients with AR.[64] Table 28.3 provides an outline of this diagnostic evaluation.

Despite the success of 2D echocardiography for the accurate detection of LV volumes and ejection fraction, this technique is limited due to the geometric assumptions that must be applied. LV volume and ejection fraction measurements have been extensively studied using real-time three-dimensional echocardiography (RT3D). The major advantage to this technique is the freedom from geometric assumptions. This technique therefore results in improved accuracy, particularly in abnormally shaped hearts (See Chapter 11). RT3D now allows for rapid full-volume acquisitions of the left ventricle. Off-line semiautomated software has been developed for accurate calculation of global and regional wall motion, volumes and ejection fraction. Although not specifically studied in patients with AR, LV volume assessment using RT3D has been shown to be accurate, rapid, and superior to standard 2D echocardiographic techniques.[42] The major limitation to this technique is the reduced accuracy in patients with poor acoustic windows. Figure 28.11 demonstrates the utility of RT3D in a patient with AR due to a bicuspid aortic valve.

In cases in which the echocardiogram is technically suboptimal, other techniques such as radionuclide angiography or cardiac magnetic resonance (CMR) imaging may be useful. In general, patients with mild AR and normal LV size and function should undergo a clinical evaluation at least once per year. Routine echocardiography can be performed every 2 to 3 years unless there is evidence of progression of disease before that time.[2] However, the likelihood of progression will depend on the etiology of the disorder.

Asymptomatic patients with severe AR and normal LV size and function should undergo clinical exams and echocardiography yearly unless symptoms arise beforehand. Patients with significant LV dilatation (end-diastolic dimension greater than 60 mm) require clinical evaluations every 6 months and echocardiographic imaging every 6 to 12 months. Patients with very severe LV dilatation (end-diastolic dimension greater than 70 mm or end-systolic dimension greater than 50 mm) may require serial echoes every 4 to 6 months.[40]

2D echocardiographic assessment of cardiac anatomy. Echocardiographic evaluation of the anatomy of the aortic leaflets, annulus,

TABLE 28.1
STUDIES OF THE NATURAL HISTORY OF ASYMPTOMATIC PATIENTS WITH AORTIC REGURGITATION

Study, (Year)	No. of patients	Mean follow-up, y	Progression to symptoms, death, or LV dysfunction, rate per y (%)	Progression to asymptomatic LV dysfunction		Mortality, No. of patients	Comments
				n	Rate per y (%)		
Bonow et al. (1983, 1991)[49,52]	104	8.0	3.8	4	0.5	2	Outcome predicted by LV ESD, EDD change in EF with exercise, and rate of change in ESD and EF at rest with time
Scognamiglio et al. (1986)[a,50]	30	4.7	2.1	3	2.1	0	3 patients who developed asymptomati LV dysfunction initially had lower PAP/ESV ratios and trended towarD higher LV ESD and EDD and lower FS
Siemienczuk et al. (1989)[51]	50	3.7	4.0	1	0.5	0	Patients included those receiving placebo and medical dropouts in a randomized drug trial; included some patients with NYHA FC II symptoms, outcome predicted by LV, ESV, EDV, change in EF with exercise, and end-systolic wall stress
Scognamiglio et al. (1994)[a,53]	74	6.0	5.7	15	3.4	0	All patients received digoxin as part of a randomized trial
Tornos et al. (1995)[54]	101	4.6	3.0	6	1.3	0	Outcome predicted by pulse pressure, LV ESD, EDD, and EF at least
Ishii et al. (1996)[55]	27	14.2	3.6	—	—	0	Development of symptoms predicted by systolic BP, LV ESD, EDD, mass index, and wall thickness. LV function not reported in all patients
Borer et al. (1998)[56]	104	7.3	6.2	7	0.9	4	20% Of patients in NYHA FC II; outcome predicted by initial FC II symptoms, change in LV EF with exercise, LV ESD, and LV FS
Tarasoutchi et al. (2003)[57]	72	10	4.7	1	0.1	0	Development of symptoms predicted by LV ESD and EDD. LV function not reported in all patients
Evangelista et al. (2005)[88]	31	7	3.6	—	—	1	Placebo control group in 7-year vasodilator clinical trial
Average	593	6.6	4.3	37	1.2	0.18% / y	

— indicates that data were not available.
[a]Two studies by the same authors involved separate patient groups.
BP, blood pressure; EDD, end-diastolic dimension; EDV, end-diastolic volume; EF, ejection fraction; ESD, end-systolic dimension; ESV, end-systolic volume; FC, functional class; FS, fractional shortening; LV, left ventricular; NYHA, New York Heart Association; PAP, pulmonary artery pressure.

and aortic root is important in defining the etiology and severity of AR. Disorders such as valvular endocarditis, bicuspid aortic valve, degenerative valve disease, aortic root dilation, and dissection of the ascending aorta have different implications with regard to treatment. In contrast to mild AR that is sometimes observed in the setting of a structurally normal aortic valve, it is unusual for severe AR to develop without any abnormalities of aortic valve or aortic root.

Color Doppler evaluation. Color Doppler flow mapping is widely used to identify the presence of AR and estimate its severity. In general, color flow jets are composed of three distinct segments. These are the proximal isovelocity surface area (PISA) or flow convergence zone, which is the area of flow acceleration into the aortic valve orifice; the vena contracta, which is the narrowest and highest-velocity region of the jet at or just downstream from the orifice; and the jet itself, which extends from the aortic valve into

TABLE 28.2
NATURAL HISTORY OF AORTIC REGURGITATION

Asymptomatic patients with normal LV systolic function	
Progression to symptoms and/or LV dysfunction	<6% / y
Progression to asymptomatic LV dysfunction	<3.5% / y
Sudden death	<0.2% / y
Asymptomatic patients with LV dysfunction	
Progression to cardiac symptoms	>25% / y
Symptomatic patients	
Mortality rate	>10% / y

LV, left ventricular.

the LV cavity. Comparison of ratio of the width of the AR jet to the width of the LV outflow tract (LVOT) in the parasternal long axis view is one semiquantitative measure of AR severity. A jet width/LVOT width ratio of less than 25% is consistent with mild AR, whereas a ratio of 65% or greater is consistent with severe AR.[65] This works best when the regurgitant orifice is relatively round

in shape and when the direction of the regurgitant jet is central. When the regurgitant orifice is elliptical, as in bicuspid aortic valves, this ratio can lead to underestimation of AR severity.[66] The short-axis view is helpful for quantification in such cases. Figure 28.12 demonstrates color Doppler evaluation of an eccentric jet of AR in the parasternal long axis view.

Vena contracta width. The vena contracta is defined as the narrowest central flow region of a jet. In the case of AR, this can be measured in a parasternal long-axis or short-axis view. There is good validity of this measurement in assessing the severity of AR.[67-69] A vena contracta width greater than 6 mm has been shown to correlate well with severe AR, having a sensitivity of 95% and a specificity of 90%. Conversely, a vena contracta width less than 0.3 cm is more consistent with mild AR.[68] Figure 28.13 shows measurement of vena contracta width in a patient with severe AR.

Jet eccentricity. Eccentricity of the regurgitant jet may contribute to the understanding of mechanisms of aortic valve dysfunction.[70] There is entrainment of fluid on all sides with a centrally directed jet, which therefore appears larger and wider as opposed to an eccentrically directed jet. This should be taken into account when AR severity is graded.

3.1.5. PISA method
The PISA method is ideally used for calculating regurgitant volume and effective regurgitant orifice. However, it is not always

TABLE 28.3
ECHOCARDIOGRAPHIC PARAMETERS OF AR SEVERITY

	Mild	Moderate	Severe
Structural parameters			
1. LA size	Normal[a]	Normal or dilated	Usually dilated[b]
2. Aortic leaflets	Normal or abnormal	Normal or abnormal	Abnormal/flail, or wide coaptation defect
Doppler parameters			
1. Jet width in LVOT–Color Flow[c]	Small in central jets	Intermediate	Large in central jets; variable in eccentric jets
2. Jet density–CW	Incomplete or faint	Dense	Dense
3. Jet deceleration rate–CW (PHT, ms)[d]	Slow > 500	Medium 500–200	Steep < 200
4. Diastolic flow reversal in descending aorta–PW	Brief, early diastolic reversal	Intermediate	Prominent holodiastolic reversal
Quantitative parameters[e]			
1. VC width, cm[c]	<0.3	0.3–0.60	≥0.6
2. Jet width/LVOT width, %[c]	<25	25–45, 46–64	≥65
3. Jet CSA/LVOT CSA, %[c]	<5	5–20, 21–59	≥60
4. R Vol, ml/beat	<30	30–44, 45–59	≥60
5. RF, %	<30	30–39, 40–49	≥50
6. EROA, cm²	<0.10	0.10–0.19, 0.20–0.29	≥0.30

AR, Aortic regurgitation; CSA, cross sectional area; CW, continuous wave Doppler; EROA, effective regurgitant orifice area; LV, left ventricle; LVOT, left ventricular outflow tract; PHT, pressure half-time; PW, pulsed wave Doppler; *R* Vol, regurgitant volume; RF, regurgitant fraction; VC, vena contracta.
[a] Unless there are other reasons for LV dilation. Normal 2D measurements: LV minor axis ≤ 2.8 cm/m², LV end-diastolic volume ≤ 82 ml/m² (2).
[b] Exception: would be acute AR, in which chambers have not had time to dilate.
[c] At a Nyquist limit of 50–60 cm/s. Quantitative parameters can sub-classify the moderate regurgitation group into mild-to-moderate and moderate-to-severe regurgitation as shown.
[d] PHT is shortened with increasing LV diastolic pressure and vasodilator therapy, and may be lengthened in chronic adaptation to severe AR
[e] Quantitative parameters can subclassify the moderate regurgitation group into mild-to-moderate and moderate-to-severe regurgitation as shown.

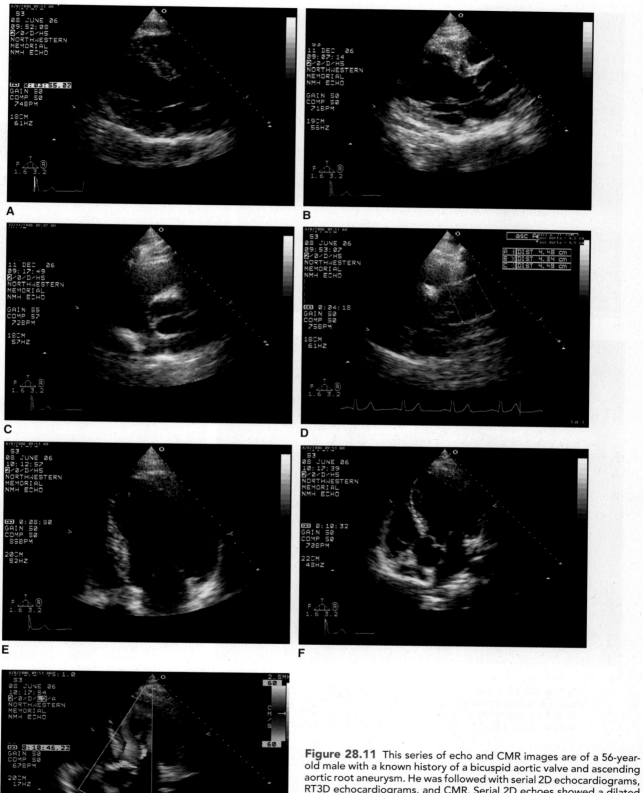

Figure 28.11 This series of echo and CMR images are of a 56-year-old male with a known history of a bicuspid aortic valve and ascending aortic root aneurysm. He was followed with serial 2D echocardiograms, RT3D echocardiograms, and CMR. Serial 2D echoes showed a dilated LV with no change in dimensions on serial follow-up. LV end-diastolic dimension was 6.4 cm and the end-systolic dimension was 4.0 cm (**A,B**). The 2D echo shows the bicuspid nature of the aortic valve (**C**) as well as the ascending aortic aneurysm (**D**). The 2D apical views confirm that the LV is dilated but the ejection fraction is preserved (**E**). The apical five-chamber view shows that the mechanism of aortic insufficiency is a prolapsing leaflet (**F**).There is an eccentric jet of AR (**G**).

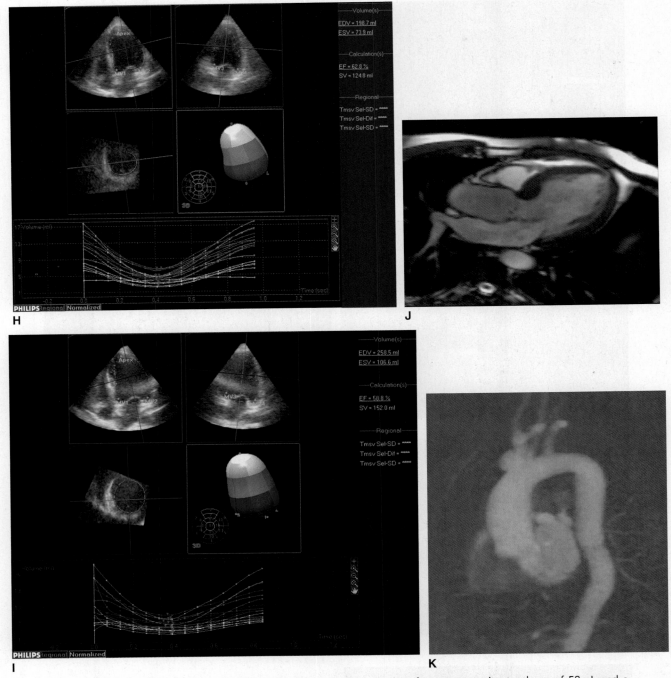

Figure 28.11 *(continued)* Quantification using the continuity equation shows a regurgitant volume of 52 mL and a regurgitant fraction of 32%. Despite the lack of change in LV volumes and ejection fraction by 2D echo, serial RT3D echocardiography showed an increase in volumes and a decline in ejection fraction that was similar to what was seen in the CMR (**H,I**). **J,K**: Demonstrate CMR images of the dilated LV and the dilated aorta.

possible to use this method for quantification of AR as it is less common to identify a clear proximal flow convergence in patients with AR compared with those with mitral regurgitation. To obtain these measurements, the Nyquist velocity should be shifted toward the direction of the jet to produce a clearly visible, hemispheric PISA region that is as large as possible. The surface area of the PISA region is $2\pi r^2$, where r is the radius from the aliasing line to the orifice. Peak regurgitant flow is obtained by multiplying this value by the aliasing velocity. The effective regurgitant orifice

area is then calculated as the peak regurgitant flow divided by the peak velocity of the AR jet obtained by continuous wave Doppler, as shown in Figure 28.14. The PISA method has been shown to work in quantifying central AR jets but is less accurate in eccentric jets or with aortic root dilation.[71]

Quantitative Doppler flow measurements. Regurgitant volume and regurgitant fraction can be calculated by comparing flow at the aortic level with that at the mitral valve level.[64] The total stroke volume is generally measured in the LVOT by multiplying

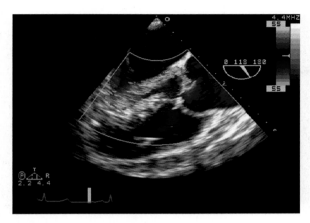

Figure 28.12 A color Doppler image is shown of an eccentric jet of AR.

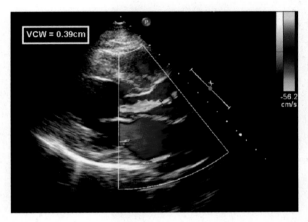

Figure 28.13 Parasternal long axis view is shown to demonstrate the vena contracta measurement in a patient with severe AR. Please note that the vena contracta is the narrowest waist of the jet just downstream from the aortic orifice.

the LVOT area times the velocity time integral of the pulsed Doppler LVOT flow. The mitral stroke volume is measured in a similar fashion but is more prone to error because of difficulty in accurately measuring the mitral annulus and placing the pulsed Doppler sample volume at the level of the annulus. Effective regurgitant orifice area can be calculated by dividing the regurgitant volume by the velocity time integral of the AR jet obtained from continuous wave Doppler signal. This method provides quantitative measures of AR severity but is tedious and prone to error.[2,64]

Supportive findings on echocardiography. There are a number of echocardiographic findings that provide supporting evidence to accurately assess AR severity. By M-mode echocardiography, early mitral valve closure indicates increased LV filling pressures and is often present in severe AR, unless there is coexisting tachycardia.[72] Occasionally, fine fibrillatory motion of the anterior mitral leaflet is discerned on the M-mode echocardiogram if the jet of AR impinges on the anterior mitral leaflet (Fig. 28.15).

The continuous wave Doppler spectral signal of the AR jet also provides clues to the severity of the leak (Fig. 28.16). The density of signal provides a clue if it can be accurately evaluated, with greater density of the signal strength indicating more severe AR. The pressure half-time is another important parameter to assess. With severe AR, diastolic pressure will decrease rapidly in the aorta, thus leading to a shorter pressure half-time or a more rapid deceleration slope. In general, an AR pressure half-time

less than 250 ms indicates severe AR, between 250 to 500 ms reflects moderate AR (Fig. 28.17), whereas a pressure half-time greater than 500 ms suggests mild AR.[64] LV end-diastolic pressure can be calculated as the diastolic blood pressure minus the end-diastolic pressure gradient calculated from the modified Bernoulli equation.[73] However, it is important to emphasize that the rate of deceleration of AR velocities is a reflection of equilibration of the diastolic pressure gradient between the aorta and left ventricle in addition to the size of the regurgitant orifice. Therefore, a change in LV pressure or aortic pressure may influence the pressure half-time value, irrespective of the degree of AR. In chronic AR, a large regurgitant volume may not significantly shorten the pressure half-time.[74] Conversely, moderate AR into a stiff left ventricle, especially in the acute or subacute setting, may significantly shorten the pressure half-time. Thus, pressure half-time and early mitral valve closure are considered markers of the hemodynamic consequences of AR rather than the regurgitant volume itself.

Another important supportive sign of severe AR is diastolic flow reversal in the descending aorta. Although brief early diastolic flow reversal is often seen in normal subjects, holodiastolic flow reversal usually indicates at least moderate AR.[75] Figure 28.18 Panels A and B shows the holodiastolic flow reversal in the abdominal aorta on transthoracic and transesophageal echocardiography.

LV size and geometry. Echocardiography is useful in measuring LV dimensions, volumes, and ejection fraction, all of which are important determinants of the timing of surgery in chronic severe AR. Serial progression of LV dilation predicts the need for surgery.[52] Careful measurement of LV dimensions, volumes, and ejection fraction is therefore imperative and should be done in a consistent and uniform fashion. Figure 28.19 shows an example of a patient with severe LV enlargement, which is a marker for chronic, severe AR. Serial echocardiograms to assess progression of LV dilation and severity of AR are recommended every 2 to 3 years in stable asymptomatic patients with mild AR and normal LV size and function.[2] In asymptomatic patients with LV dilation, more frequent echocardiograms (every 6 to 12 months) are indicated.[2] Table 28.3 outlines the echocardiographic signs to quantify the severity of AR.

3.2. Cardiac catheterization

Cardiac catheterization is reserved for selected patients in whom noninvasive imaging is inconclusive. It is most often used to assess coronary anatomy prior to surgery in patients in whom coronary artery disease is suspected.

Supravalvular aortography provides a semiquantitative approach to grade AR during cardiac catheterization. Visual grading of AR severity is based on the amount of contrast that appears in the left ventricle after aortography. Mild or 1+ AR is defined as contrast appearing in the left ventricle but clearing with each beat. Moderate or 2+ AR represents faint opacification of the entire left ventricle over several cardiac cycles. Moderately severe or 3+ AR is defined as opacification of the entire left ventricle with the same intensity as in the aorta. Severe or 4+ AR is opacification of the entire left ventricle on the first heart beat with intensity higher than in the aorta. Unfortunately, this method is highly subjective and depends on the amount of contrast injected as well as the size of the left ventricle. It correlates poorly with regurgitant volume, particularly in patients with a dilated left ventricle.[76]

3.3. Radionuclide imaging

Radionuclide angiography is useful when echocardiographic imaging is suboptimal, when there is a discrepancy between

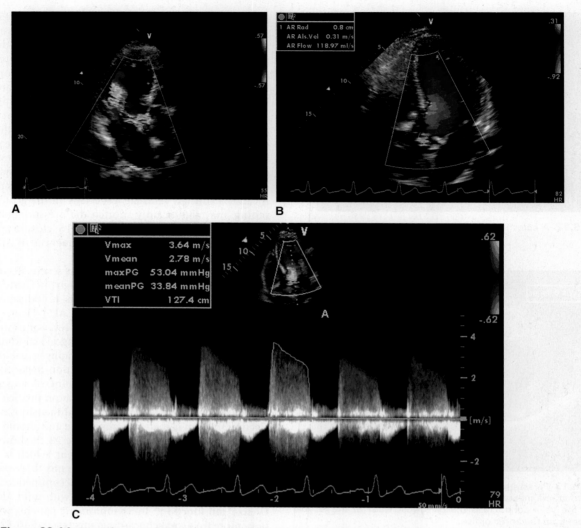

Figure 28.14 Quantification of AR severity using the PISA method is shown. **Panel A** shows the color flow image of the AR jet. **Panel B** shows the measurement of the radius. **Panel C** shows the spectral Doppler signal of the AR jet. The velocity time integral and peak velocity values are used in the PISA calculation. In this case the effective regurgitant orifice is calculated to be 0.34 cm² and the regurgitant volume is calculated to be 43.5 mL.

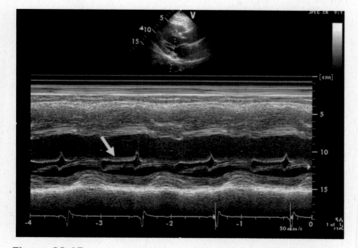

Figure 28.15 An M-mode tracing of the mitral valve is shown. Note the fine fibrillatory motion of the anterior leaflet of the mitral valve (*arrow*) due to the jet of AR directed at the valve.

clinical and echocardiographic findings or when more accurate assessment of LV ejection fraction is needed. This technique provides accurate ejection fraction, measurement of the ratio of LV and right ventricular (RV) stroke volume as a measure of AR severity, and the assessment of LV systolic function before and during exercise.[37,56,62,77] A LV/RV stroke volume greater than 2.0 is a measure of severe AR, provided there is no associated valvular regurgitation such as mitral, tricuspid, or pulmonic regurgitation.[77]

3.4. Cardiac magnetic resonance

CMR provides highly accurate assessment of LV volumes, mass, and ejection fraction, particularly when echocardiography is suboptimal or unable to provide this information.[78–80] In addition to providing well delineated anatomic information, accurate information about regurgitant volumes and flow can also be obtained using CMR using a variety of techniques.[81]

Total LV and RV stroke volume can be determined from LV end-diastolic and end-systolic volumes, which are measured by summing the volumes of a stack of slices of known thickness (typically 1 cm)

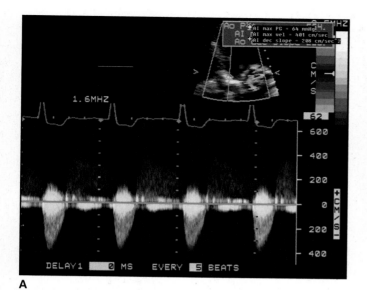

A

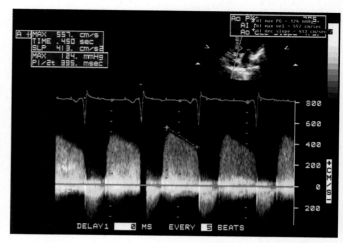

Figure 28.17 The pressure–half time measurement of a patient with moderate AR is shown.

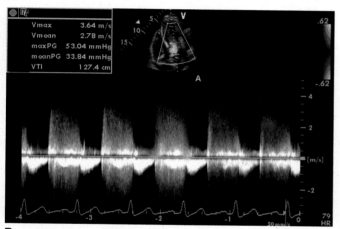

B

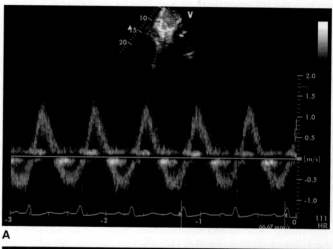

A

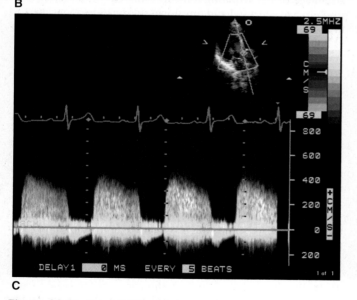

C

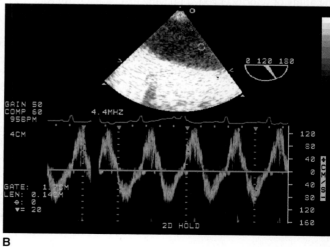

B

Figure 28.16 Panel A shows the spectral Doppler signal of the AR jet. Note the faint signal density suggesting mild AR. **Panel B** shows the spectral Doppler signal of a patient with moderate AR. Note the stronger signal density. **Panel C** shows the spectral Doppler signal of a patient with severe AR. Note that the signal density of the AR jet is equally as strong as the one for the forward flow across the aortic valve.

Figure 28.18 Spectral Doppler images of the descending thoracic aorta by transthoracic echo **(Panel A)** and of the abdominal aorta by transesopheageal echo **(Panel B)** are shown. Note that the spectral signal during diastole lasts throughout diastole and is equal in strength to the forward flow in systole. These findings suggest severe AR.

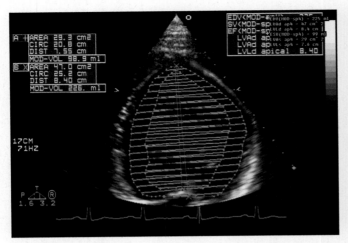

Figure 28.19 Calculation of LV volumes using 2D echocardiography is shown. In this example the LV volume is increased. LV end-diastolic volume index was calculated to be 99.8 mL/m², which is consistent with severe LV enlargement.

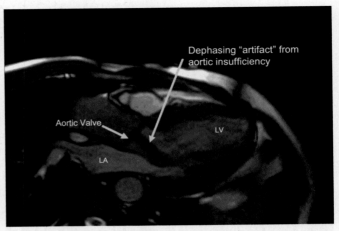

Figure 28.20 A CMR image of a patient with AR is shown. Note the dephasing artifact caused by the AR jet. LA, left atrium; LV, left ventricle.

through the left ventricle from base to apex. Regurgitant volume is then computed as the difference between the LV and RV stroke volumes. Although CMR has not been used as extensively as echocardiography in AR patients, it can be useful for detecting progressive LV dilation and planning timing of operation for asymptomatic patients with severe AR. In addition, this technique provides important information about the size and structure of the aorta. Figure 28.20 demonstrates CMR image of a patient with AR.

Velocity encoded imaging is a very useful technique that allows quantification of flow using CMR. This method is based on the principle that the phase angle or the spin of moving protons changes in proportion to their velocity. A magnetic gradient is then used to quantify the velocity of flow. This technique allows for the accurate calculation of forward and regurgitant flows and volumes.[82] A potential limitation of this technique is that flow calculation may be inaccurate in the presence of severe turbulence, such as in patients with mixed stenosis and regurgitation. Figure 28.21 demonstrates the utility of velocity encoded imaging in a patient with AR.

3.5. Role of exercise testing

Exercise testing may be useful to identify asymptomatic patients with varying degrees of LV systolic dysfunction when such information is not readily available by history or by noninvasive imaging. In this subset of patients, exercise testing may be very useful in eliciting symptoms or determining functional capacity. Some studies have suggested that an exercise-induced decrease in LV ejection fraction is a predictor of poor outcome that warrants surgery.[56] However, others have demonstrated that this index is also influenced importantly by LV wall stress and other loading conditions, which themselves are altered during exercise.[83-85] Thus, it is not clear that exercise LV ejection fraction provides independent information that is helpful in determining the need for surgery in asymptomatic patients with normal LV systolic function at rest.[2]

3.6. Evaluation of the aortic root and ascending aorta

An important consideration in patients with AR is the presence and severity of dilatation of the aortic root and ascending aorta. Bicuspid aortic valve disease is most often associated with aortic aneurysms and an increased propensity for aortic dissection both before

and after AVR.[16] The ACC/AHA guidelines for management of patients with valvular heart disease recommend that replacement of the aortic root or ascending aorta be performed in adults with a bicuspid aortic valve when the aortic root dimension is greater than 5.0 cm, the rate of dilation is 0.05 cm/year or greater, or the aortic root is greater than 4.5 cm in patients who have met the criteria for AVR based on the criteria noted above.[2] When aortic root dilatation is noted on echocardiography, CMR or computed tomography (CT) of the aorta can be performed to provide additional 3-dimensional assessment of the extent and severity of dilatation. If there are changes noted on annual serial echocardiographic surveillance, CMR, or CT studies may be repeated. Although CT measurements are in general easier to compare in serial studies, CMR has the advantage of not requiring ionizing radiation. In addition CMR may provide structural and functional information about the aortic wall, abnormal aortic compliance, increased wall edema and/or inflammation, which may be evaluated using various cine SSFP, and edema-weighted spin echo sequences.

4. DETERMINING THE OPTIMAL INTERVENTION

Table 28.4 outlines the indications for surgery in patients with AR. Echocardiography is the most widely used noninvasive tool to assess LV dimensions, volumes, and ejection fraction in patients with AR to aid in this decision-making process. Figure 28.22 outlines the management strategy for patients with chronic, severe AR.

Symptomatic severe AR. Severe symptoms (New York Heart Association [NYHA] functional class III or IV) and LV dysfunction with an ejection fraction less than 50% are independent risk factors for poor postoperative survival, and therefore surgery is recommended when a patient is in NYHA class II before severe LV dysfunction has developed.[2,52,54,77,85,86] This is shown in Figure 28.23. Patients with LV systolic dysfunction and/or any degree of symptoms related to the valve disorder are candidates for surgery and need to be counseled against strenuous exertion.

Asymptomatic severe AR. Asymptomatic patients with severe AR and normal LV systolic function should undergo clinical reevaluation and echocardiography yearly unless symptoms arise beforehand. Patients with significant LV dilatation (end-diastolic dimension greater than 60 mm) require clinical evaluations every

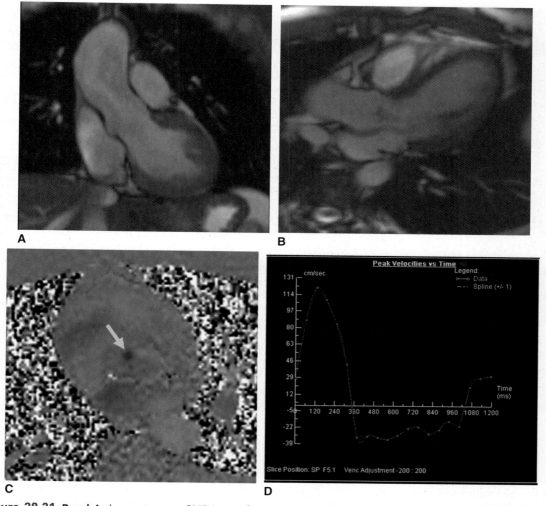

Figure 28.21 **Panel A** demonstrates a CMR image from a patient with AR and ascending aortic aneurysm. **Panel B** shows an image of the AR as well as the aortic aneurysm. **Panel C** shows the velocity-encoded images of the AR. The central jet of AR is seen as black (*arrow*). **Panel D** shows the velocity time curve generated from these images. The regurgitant volume was calculated to be 12%.

6 months and echocardiographic imaging every 6 to 12 months. Patients with very severe LV dilatation (end-diastolic dimension greater than 70 mm or end-systolic dimension greater than 50 mm) may require serial echoes every 4 to 6 months,[2] although these latter patients may also be considered for surgery (a class IIb ACC/AHA guidelines recommendation). Patients with more severe dilatation (end-diastolic dimension 75 mm or greater and/or end-systolic dimension 55 mm or greater) should be considered for AVR (a class IIa recommendation). Asymptomatic patients with severe AR, normal resting LV ejection fraction, and mild to moderate LV dilatation have an excellent prognosis and do not need prophylactic surgery. Similarly, normal resting LV ejection fraction that fails to rise with exercise is not a definite indication for surgery but is a warning sign that predicts future resting LV dysfunction.[2,77] The exercise ejection fraction is a relatively nonspecific response related to the degree of volume overload as well as exercise induced changes in preload, heart rate, and peripheral resistance.[83–85] Exercise testing may therefore be best used to assess functional status in patients with unclear symptoms or borderline LV dysfunction.[2,87]

Severe AR secondary to ascending aortic or aortic root disease. The indications for AVR in these patients are similar to those in patients with primary AR, but one must also assess severity of ascending aorta

and aortic root dilatation. Aortic root or ascending aortic replacement should be considered when the aortic or aortic root dimension is greater than 5.0 cm, the rate of dilation is 0.05 cm/year or greater, or the aortic root is greater than 4.5 cm and the patient is undergoing AVR.[2]

Symptomatic patients with moderate AR. Surgical intervention is recommended for these patients if it is certain that the symptoms are cardiac in etiology. Exercise testing may be helpful in determining functional status. Every attempt must be made to accurately quantify the severity of regurgitation, as eccentric jets of AR may be falsely downgraded in severity.[70]

4.1. Selecting and guiding therapy

Medical therapy. The role of medical therapy for chronic severe AR is not well defined. It has been hypothesized that a treatment to reduce afterload will reduce LV wall stress and improve forward cardiac output, thus decreasing LV dilation and delaying the need for surgical intervention. Data supporting this approach have been inconclusive.[53,88] There is consensus, however, that patients with AR who have systemic arterial hypertension should be treated as hypertension worsens the regurgitant flow. Vasodilators such as nifedipine or angiotensin converting

TABLE 28.4
INDICATIONS FOR SURGERY IN PATIENTS WITH AORTIC INSUFFICIENCY

Class I

1. AVR is indicated for symptomatic patients with severe AR irrespective of LV systolic function (*level of evidence: B*).
2. AVR is indicated for asymptomatic patients with chronic severe AR and LV systolic dysfunction (ejection fraction 0.50 or less) at rest (*level of evidence: B*).
3. AVR is indicated for patients with chronic severe AR while undergoing CABG or surgery on the aorta or other heart valves (*level of evidence: C*).

Class IIa

AVR is reasonable for asymptomatic patients with severe AR with normal LV systolic function (ejection fraction > 0.50) but with severe LV dilatation (end-diastolic dimension > 75 mm or end-systolic dimension > 55 mm)[a] (*level of evidence: B*).

Class IIb

1. AVR may be considered in patients with moderate AR while undergoing surgery on the ascending aorta (*level of evidence: C*).
2. AVR may be considered in patients with moderate AR while undergoing CABG (*level of evidence: C*).
3. AVR may be considered for asymptomatic patients with severe AR and normal LV systolic function at rest (ejection fraction > 0.50) when the degree of LV dilatation exceeds an end-diastolic dimension of 70 mm or end-systolic dimension of 50 mm, when there is evidence of progressive LV dilatation, declining exercise tolerance, or abnormal hemodynamic responses to exercise[a] (*level of evidence: C*).

Class III

AVR is not indicated for asymptomatic patients with mild, moderate, or severe AR and normal LV systolic function at rest (ejection fraction > 0.50) when degree of dilatation is not moderate or severe (end-diastolic dimension < 70 mm, end-systolic dimension < 50 mm)[a] (*level of evidence: B*).

[a]Consider lower threshold values for patients of small stature of either gender.

enzyme (ACE) inhibitors are preferred, and beta-blocking agents should be used with great caution. Vasodilator therapy is not recommended in patients with mild or moderate AR and normal LV function in the absence of systemic hypertension since the prognosis in this group is excellent without treatment. Atrial fibrillation and bradyarrhythmias are poorly tolerated and should be prevented if possible and aggressively treated if they develop.

Chronic medical therapy is not a substitute for surgery in patients who are surgical candidates. However, medications may be useful in some symptomatic patients who refuse surgery or are considered inoperable due to coexisting severe comorbidities. These patients should receive an aggressive regimen including vasodilators, digoxin, diuretics, and salt restriction to combat their heart failure symptoms. Beta blockers should be avoided. Nitrates are usually not beneficial in relieving anginal symptoms in these patients.

Short term studies spanning 6 months to 2 years have demonstrated beneficial effects of vasodilator drugs on some indexes of LV function.[53,89–92] However, the long-term benefits of chronic vasodilator therapy in asymptomatic patients with severe AR and normal LV ejection fraction remain controversial. A prospective trial of nifedipine showed clinical benefit,[53] but a subsequent trial comparing placebo, nifedipine, and the ACE inhibitor enalapril showed no difference in clinical outcomes between groups.[88] In light of these findings, definitive recommendations for the use of chronic long-acting nifedipine or ACE inhibitors in asymptomatic patients with severe AR are not possible.[2]

Patients with AR are at risk for endocarditis. Therefore meticulous dental care and routine dental exams and cleanings are imperative. However, not every patient with AR needs prophylactic antibiotics. According to the updated AHA guidelines,[93] only the following individuals who are at the highest risk of developing endocarditis should receive prophylactic antibiotics prior to dental and other procedures: those with artificial heart valves or a prior history of endocarditis, certain specific, serious congenital lesions (such as unrepaired or incompletely repaired cyanotic congenital heart disease, including palliative shunts and conduits, completely repaired congenital heart defects with prosthetic material or device, and any repaired congenital heart defect with residual defect at the site or adjacent to the site of a prosthetic patch or prosthetic device), and those who have undergone a cardiac transplant and develop a problem in a heart valve.

Surgical valve replacement. The definitive therapy remains AVR with or without replacement of the aortic root. Emergency surgery is the definitive treatment for acute severe AR because the acute volume overload results in life-threatening hypotension and pulmonary edema.[1–3] Vasodilator therapy with sodium nitroprusside may stabilize the patient during transport to surgery. Beta blockers are contraindicated since cardiac output is maintained through an increase in heart rate, and lowering the heart rate may precipitate life-threatening hypotension and even shock. Atrial pacing to increase heart rate might be of theoretical benefit,[94] but this does not have an established role in clinical practice. Intra-aortic balloon counterpulsation is absolutely contraindicated. Antibiotics should be given if endocarditis is suspected.

In contrast to acute AR, patients with chronic AR may be asymptomatic for many years or even their entire life. Therefore, the critical issue is to determine if and when surgical intervention

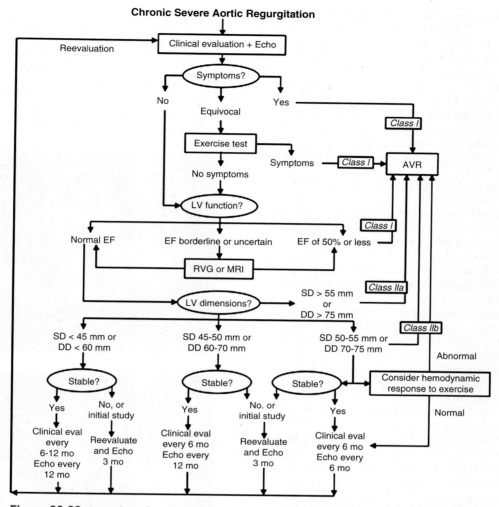

Figure 28.22 An outline of management strategy for patients with chronic, severe AR is shown.

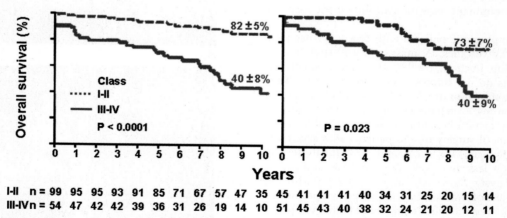

Figure 28.23 Survival curves for patients with severe, chronic AR stratified according to New York Heart Associate classification LVEF ≥ 50% (left panel) and 50% without CAD (right panel). Note that survival is worse for patients with advanced heart failure.

is required. There are no randomized controlled trials to guide surgical decision making. However, reasonable guidelines have been proposed on the basis of the aforementioned natural history of AR, retrospective studies, and expert opinion.[2] Patients with mild AR are not candidates for surgery due to their excellent long term prognosis. AVR is recommended in severe AR for all symptomatic patients irrespective of LV function, and conversely,

AVR is recommended when resting ejection fraction is less than 50% regardless of the presence of symptoms. Surgery is also reasonable when the left ventricle is markedly dilated (end-diastolic dimension greater than 75 mm or end-systolic dimension greater than 55 mm, a IIa recommendation in the ACC/AHA guidelines) and in patients with moderate AR who are undergoing coronary artery bypass grafting surgery or repair of an aortic root aneurysm. Finally, surgery may also be considered in asymptomatic patients with normal ejection fraction (greater than 50%), a dilated left ventricle (end-diastolic dimension greater than 70 mm or end-systolic dimension greater than 50 mm) when there is evidence of progressive LV dilatation, declining exercise tolerance, or abnormal hemodynamic response to exercise (a IIb recommendation in the ACC/AHA guidelines).[2] As noted previously, surgical repair of the aorta or aortic root should be considered when the aortic or aortic root dimension is greater than 5.0 cm, the rate of dilation 0.05 cm/year or greater, or the aortic root is greater than 4.5 cm in patients who have met the criteria for AVR noted above.[2]

The LV dimensions used to determine cut off values for surgical referral must be interpreted with caution in women and men of small stature. Surgical correction of AR may need to be considered at an earlier stage in women as they may develop more severe symptoms despite similar LV dimensions as men when corrected for body surface area.[7] However, the data supporting the use of cardiac dimensions corrected for body surface area are limited. Thus clinical judgment is needed when treating women and men of small stature.[2]

Aortic valve repair is possible in experienced centers in selected patients such as those with bicuspid valves with prolapsing leaflets with minimal sclerosis[95-96] or those undergoing repair of aneurysms of the aorta or aortic root.[97] However, outcomes have generally been less favorable than repair of the mitral valve.[98]

According to the Society of Thoracic Surgeons national database,[99] the overall risk of AVR is roughly 4% when performed in isolation and 6.8% when performed in conjunction with CABG. This risk is considerably lower in high volume centers and in patients with no symptoms (1% to 2%) and in those with better preoperative LV function (2% for ejection fraction 50% or greater but 8% for ejection fraction of 35% or less). For patients with ascending aortic aneurysms, an ascending aortic graft with prosthesis is associated with a mortality of 1% to 10%, depending on symptoms, LV size and function, and severity of AR,[2] with the most important determinant being the skill and experience of the surgical team.

Surgery for symptomatic patients with severe AR has been shown to reduce LV volumes, LV mass, and wall stress and to increase LV ejection fraction.[43,55,100-102] However, a small percentage of patients do not improve. Such patients have either preoperative LV dysfunction or NYHA functional class III or IV heart failure symptoms. Even patients with dilated left ventricles or low LV ejection fraction benefit from surgery. Chaliki et al[102] reported the results of surgery in 450 patients with severe AR. Operative mortality was 14%, 6.7%, and 3.7% for those with LV ejection fraction less than 35%, 36% to 49%, and greater than 50%, respectively. Moreover, surgical survivors with low preoperative LV ejection fraction had improved symptoms and LV function. Thus, even though it is highly desirable to operate on patients before irreversible LV changes have occurred, it is almost never "too late" to operate in chronic severe AR, although patients with severe LV dysfunction and a systolic blood pressure less than 120 mm Hg may be at particularly high risk.[103]

Clinical monitoring is continued following surgery. An echocardiogram should be obtained prior to hospital discharge or at the first postoperative outpatient visit in order to establish a baseline with which to compare future studies. In general, there is usually a rapid decline in LV diastolic volume following surgery, and the initial decline in LV end-diastolic dimension is predictive of long-term LV systolic function and survival.[100] On the other hand, the LV ejection fraction often declines immediately following AVR due to the reduced preload and may take several months to improve. After the initial postoperative evaluation, the patient should be seen and examined again at 6 and 12 months following surgery, then yearly thereafter. If the postoperative echocardiogram in an asymptomatic patient indicates that LV systolic function is normal and there has been a substantial reduction in LV volumes, follow-up echocardiograms are only needed if there is a new murmur, suspicion of valve dysfunction, (Fig. 28.24) or concerns about LV function.[2]

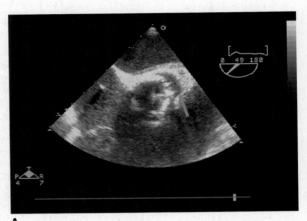

A

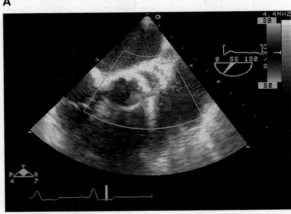

B

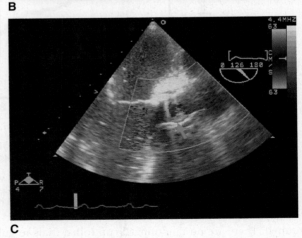

C

Figure 28.24 Transesophageal echo images of a patient and bioprosthetic aortic valve endocarditis are shown. **Panel A** shows a short axis image of the prosthesis. Note the large cavity formed by dehiscence of the valve (*arrow*). **Panel B** shows the same short axis image with color Doppler demonstrating flow into this cavity (*arrow*). **Panel C** is a long axis view showing the perivalvular flow into the left ventricle (*arrow*).

Patients with persistent postoperative LV dysfunction should be treated with ACE inhibitors, beta blockers, and other evidence-based measures for all patients with LV systolic dysfunction. These patients should undergo repeat echocardiography at 6 and 12 month postoperative visits and then as clinically indicated thereafter.[2]

5. FUTURE DIRECTIONS

It is conceivable that further insights into molecular mechanisms of myocardial adaptation to volume overload may yield new therapeutic targets to reduce myocardial fibrosis and hypertrophy and help preserve LV size and function. Future developments in interventional cardiology may offer new alternatives for patients with severe AR who are not considered surgical candidates. Percutaneous implantation of heart valve prosthesis may be possible in such patients, although this is still investigational at this time.[104–106]

On the basis of available evidence and consensus opinion, surgery is indicated for patients with severe AR who either[1] are symptomatic or[2] have evidence of decreasing LV ejection fraction or markedly increasing degree of LV dilatation. It appears that it is best to operate before LV end-systolic diameter increases to greater than 55 mm or 25 mm/m^2 or before LV ejection fraction falls to less than 50%. The role of medical therapy, particularly vasodilators, is primarily to decrease systolic hypertension in asymptomatic patients, with inconclusive evidence that this will delay the onset of LV dysfunction. Medical therapy is not a substitute for surgery in patients who are surgical candidates. The clinical implications of the change in size and function of the left ventricle emphasize the critical role of echocardiography in patients with AR. Careful attention to accurate assessment of LV dilatation and systolic function, size of the ascending aorta and aortic root, and etiology of AR, plus accurate quantification of the severity of AR, are imperative to the successful management of patients with this condition.

REFERENCES

1. Cohn LH, Birjiniuk V. Therapy of acute aortic regurgitation. *Cardiol Clin.* 1991;9:339–352.
2. Bonow RO, Carabello BA, Chatterjee K, et al. ACC/AHA 2006 guidelines for the management of patients with valvular heart disease: A report of the American College of Cardiology/American Heart Association Task Force on Practice Guidelines (writing committee to revise the 1998 guidelines for the management of patients with valvular heart disease): Developed in collaboration with the Society of Cardiovascular Anesthesiologists: Endorsed by the Society for Cardiovascular Angiography and Interventions and the Society of Thoracic Surgeons. *Circulation.* 2006;114:e1–e148.
3. Otto CM, Bonow RO. Valvular heart disease. In: Libby P, Bonow RO, Mann DL, Zipes DP, eds. *Braunwald's Heart Disease: A Textbook of Cardiovascular Medicine.* 8th Ed. Philadelphia, Pa: Elsevier Science; 2007:1625–1693.
4. Singh JP, Evans JC, Levy D, et al. Prevalence and clinical determinants of mitral, tricuspid, and aortic regurgitation (the Framingham Heart Study) (published correction appears in *Am J Cardiol.* 1999;84:1143). *Am J Cardiol.* 1999;83:897–902.
5. Kim M, Roman MJ, Cavallini MC, et al. Effect of hypertension on aortic root size and prevalence of aortic regurgitation. *Hypertension.* 1996;28:47–52.
6. Lebowitz NE, Bella JN, Roman MJ, et al. Prevalence and correlates of aortic regurgitation in American Indians: The Strong Heart Study. *J Am Coll Cardiol.* 2000;36:461–467.
7. Klodas E, Enriquez-Sarano M, Tajik JA et al. Surgery for aortic regurgitation in women: Contrasting indications and outcomes as compared with men. *Circulation.* 1996;94:2472–2478.
8. Olson LJ, Subramanian R, Edwards WD. Surgical pathology of pure aortic insufficiency: A study of 225 cases. *Mayo Clin Proc.* 1984;5:835–841.
9. Roberts WC, Ko JM, Moore TR, et al. Causes of pure aortic regurgitation in patients having isolated aortic valve replacement at a single US tertiary hospital (1993 to 2005). *Circulation.* 2006;114:422–429.
10. Waller BF, Howard J, Fess S. Pathology of aortic valve stenosis and pure aortic regurgitation: A clinical-morphologic assessment: part II. *Clin Cardiol.* 1994;17:15–16.
11. Waller BF, Taliercio CP, Dickos DK, et al. Rare or unusual causes of chronic, isolated, pure aortic regurgitation. *Clin Cardiol.* 1990;1:577–581.
12. Guiney TE, Davies MJ, Parker DJ, et al. The aetiology and course of isolated severe aortic regurgitation: a clinical, pathological, and echocardiographic study. *Br Heart J.* 1987;58:358–368.
13. Roberts WC, Morrow AG, McIntosh CL, et al. Congenitally bicuspid aortic valve causing severe, pure aortic regurgitation without superimposed infective endocarditis. *Am J Cardiol.* 1981;47:206–209.
14. Michel PL, Acar J, Chomette G, et al. Degenerative aortic regurgitation. *Eur Heart J.* 1991;12:875–882.
15. Roberts WC, Ko JM. Frequency by decades of unicuspid, bicuspid, and tricuspid aortic valves in adults having isolated aortic valve replacement for aortic stenosis, with or without associated aortic regurgitation. *Circulation.* 2005;11:920–925.
16. Roman MJ, Devereux RB, Niles NW, et al. Aortic root dilatation as a cause of isolated, severe aortic regurgitation. *Ann Intern Med.* 1987;106:800–807.
17. Fedak PWM, Verma S, David TE, et al. Clinical and pathophysiological implications of a bicuspid aortic valve. *Circulation.* 2002;106:900–904.
18. Roberts WC, Morrow AG, McIntosh CL, et al. Congenitally bicuspid aortic valve causing severe, pure aortic regurgitation without superimposed infective endocarditis. Analysis of 13 patients requiring aortic valve replacement. *Am J Cardiol.* 1981;47:206–209.
19. Braverman AC, Guven H, Beardslee MA, et al. The bicuspid aortic valve. *Curr Probl Cardiol.* 2005;30:470–522.
20. Bonow RO. Bicuspid aortic valves and dilated aortas: A critical review of the critical review of the ACC/AHA guidelines recommendations. *Am J Cardiol.* 2008;102:111–114.
21. Mann T, McLaurin L, Grossman W, et al. Assessing the hemodynamic severity of acute aortic regurgitation due to infective endocarditis. *N Engl J Med.* 1975;293:108–113.
22. Kardaras FG, Kardara DF, Rontogiani DP, et al. Acute aortic regurgitation caused by non-bacterial thrombotic endocarditis. *Eur Heart J.* 1995;6:1152–1154.
23. Gustavsson CG, Gustafson A, Albrechtsson U, et al. Diagnosis and management of aortic dissection, clinical and radiological follow-up. *Acta Med Scand.* 1988;223:247–253.
24. Onorati F, De Santo LS, Carozza A, et al. Marfan syndrome as a predisposing factor for traumatic aortic insufficiency. *Ann Thorac Surg.* 2004;77:2192–2194.
25. Elkayam U, Bitar F. Valvular heart disease and pregnancy. Part I: Native valves. *J Am Coll Cardiol.* 2005;46:223–230.
26. Yeo TC, Ling LH, Ng WL, et al. Spontaneous aortic laceration causing flail aortic valve and acute aortic regurgitation. *J Am Soc Echocardiogr.* 1999;12:76–78.
27. Pretre R, Faidutti B. Surgical management of aortic valve injury after nonpenetrating trauma. *Ann Thorac Surg.* 1993;56:1426.
28. Obadia JF, Tatou E, David M. Aortic valve regurgitation caused by blunt chest injury. *Br Heart J.* 1995;74:545–547.
29. McCrindle BW. Independent predictors of immediate results of percutaneous balloon aortic valvotomy in children: Valvuloplasty and angioplasty of congenital anomalies (VACA) registry investigators. *Am J Cardiol.* 1996;77:286–293.
30. Garg V, Muth AN, Ransom JF, et al. Mutations in NOTCH1 cause aortic valve disease. *Nature.* 2005;437:270–274.
31. Russo CF, Mazzetti S, Garatti A, et al. Aortic complications after bicuspid aortic valve replacement: Long-term results. *Ann Thorac Surg.* 2002;74:S1773–S1776.
32. Yasuda H, Nakatani S, Stugaard M, et al. Failure to prevent progressive dilation of ascending aorta by aortic valve replacement in patients with bicuspid aortic valve: Comparison with tricuspid aortic valve. *Circulation.* 2003;108(Suppl II):II-291–II-294.
33. Francke U, Furthmayr H. Marfan's syndrome and other disorders of fibrillin. *N Engl J Med.* 1994;330:1384–1385.
34. Loeys BL, Schwarze U, Holm T, et al. Aneurysm syndromes caused by mutations in the TGF-β receptor. *N Engl J Med.* 2006;355:788–798.
35. Legget ME, Unger TA, O'Sullivan CK, et al. Aortic root complications in Marfan's syndrome: Identification of a lower risk group. *Heart.* 1996;75(4):389–395.
36. Januzzi JL, Isselbacher EM, Fattori R, et al. Characterizing the young patient with aortic dissection: Results from the International Registry of Aortic Dissection (IRAD). *J Am Coll Cardiol.* 2004;43:665–669.
37. Otto CM. Aortic regurgitation. In: Otto CM, ed. *Valvular Heart Disease.* 2nd Ed. Philadelphia, Pa: WB Saunders; 2004:302–335.
38. Carabello BA. Aortic regurgitation: A lesion with similarities to both aortic stenosis and mitral regurgitation. *Circulation.* 1990;82:1051–1053.
39. Rigolin VH, Bonow RO. Hemodynamic characteristics and progression to heart failure in regurgitant lesions. *Heart Failure Clin.* 2007;2:453–460.
40. Ricci DR. Afterload mismatch and preload reserve in chronic aortic regurgitation. *Circulation.* 1982;66:826–834.
41. Ross J Jr, McCullagh WH. Nature of enhanced performance of the dilated left ventricle during chronic volume overloading. *Circ Res.* 1972;30:549–556.
42. Starling MR, Kirsh MM, Montgomery DG, et al. Mechanism for left ventricular systolic dysfunction in aortic regurgitation: Importance for predicting the functional response to aortic valve replacement. *J Am Coll Cardiol.* 1991;17:887–897.
43. Taniguchi K, Nakanos S, Kawashima Y, et al. Left ventricular ejection performance, wall stress and contractile state in aortic regurgitation before and after aortic valve replacement. *Circulation.* 1990;82:798–807.

44. Wisenbaugh T, Spann JF, Carabello BA. Differences in myocardial performance and load between patients with similar amounts of chronic aortic versus chronic mitral regurgitation. *J Am Coll Cardiol.* 1984;3:916–923.

45. Magid NM, Young MS, Wallerson DC, et al. Hypertrophic and functional response to experimental chronic aortic regurgitation. *J Mol Cell Cardiol.* 1988;20:239–246.

46. Nitenberg A, Foult JM, Antony I, et al. Coronary flow and resistance reserve in patients with chronic aortic regurgitation, angina pectoris and normal coronary arteries. *J Am Coll Cardiol.* 1988;11:478–486.

47. Ardehali A, Segal J, Cheitlin MD. Coronary blood flow reserve in acute aortic regurgitation. *J Am Coll Cardiol.* 1995;25:1387–1392.

48. Eusebio J, Louie EK, Edwards DC, et al. Alterations in transmitral flow dynamics in patients with early mitral valve closure and aortic regurgitation. *Am Heart J.* 1994;128:941–947.

49. Bonow RO, Rosing DR, McIntosh CL, et al. The natural history of asymptomatic patients with aortic regurgitation and normal left ventricular function. *Circulation.* 1983;68:509–517.

50. Scognamiglio R, Fasoli G, Dalla VS. Progression of myocardial dysfunction in asymptomatic patients with severe aortic insufficiency. *Clin Cardiol.* 1986;9:151–156.

51. Siemienczuk D, Greenberg B, Morris C, et al. Chronic aortic insufficiency: Factors associated with progression to aortic valve replacement. *Ann Intern Med.* 1989;110:587–592

52. Bonow RO, Lakatos E, Maron BJ, et al. Serial long term assessment of the natural history of asymptomatic patients with chronic aortic regurgitation and normal left ventricular systolic function. *Circulation.* 1991;84:1625–1635.

53. Scognamiglio R, Rahimtoola SH, Fasoli G, et al. Nifedipine in asymptomatic patients with severe aortic regurgitation and normal left ventricular function. *N Engl J Med.* 1994;331:689–694.

54. Tornos MP, Olona M, Permanyer-Miralda G, et al. Clinical outcome of severe asymptomatic chronic aortic regurgitation: A long term prospective follow-up study. *Am Heart J.* 1995;130:333–339.

55. Ishii K, Hirota Y, Suwa M, et al. Natural history and left ventricular response in chronic aortic regurgitation. *Am J Cardiol.* 1996;78:357–361.

56. Borer JS, Hochreiter C, Herrold EM, et al. Prediction of indications for valve replacement among symptomatic patients with chronic aortic regurgitation and normal left ventricular performance. *Circulation.* 1998;97:525–534.

57. Tarasoutchi F, Grinberg M, Spina GS, et al. Ten-year clinical laboratory follow-up after application of a symptom-based therapeutic strategy to patients with severe chronic aortic regurgitation of predominant rheumatic etiology. *J Am Coll Cardiol.* 2003;41:1316–1324.

58. Dujardin KS, Enriquez-Sarano M, Schaff HV, et al. Mortality and morbidity of chronic aortic regurgitation in clinical practice: A long term follow-up study. *Circulation.* 1999;99:1851–1857.

59. Enriquez-Sarano M, Tajik AJ. Clinical practice: Aortic regurgitation. *N Engl J Med.* 2004;351:1539–1546.

60. Henry WL, Bonow RO, Rosing DR, et al. Observations on the optimum time for operative intervention for aortic regurgitation II: Serial echocardiographic evaluation of asymptomatic patients. *Circulation.* 1980;61:484–492.

61. McDonald IG, Jelinek VM. Serial M-mode echocardiography in severe chronic aortic regurgitation. *Circulation.* 1980;62:1291–1296.

62. Bonow RO. Radionuclide angiography in the management of asymptomatic aortic regurgitation. *Circulation.* 1991;84(suppl I):I-296–Ixx302.

63. Bonow RO, Rosing DR, Maron BJ, et al. Reversal of left ventricular dysfunction after aortic valve replacement for chronic aortic regurgitation: Influence of duration of preoperative left ventricular dysfunction. *Circulation.* 1984;70:570–579.

64. Zoghbi WA, Enriquez-Sarano M, Foster E, et al. Recommendations for evaluation of the severity of native valvular regurgitation with two-dimensional and Doppler echocardiography. *J Am Soc Echocardiogr.* 2003;16:777–802.

65. Perry GJ, Helmcke F, Nanda NC, et al. Evaluation of aortic insufficiency by Doppler color flow mapping. *J Am Coll Cardiol.* 1987;9:952–959.

66. Taylor AL, Eichhorn EJ, Brickner ME, et al. Aortic valve morphology: An important in vitro determinant of proximal regurgitant jet width by Doppler color flow mapping. *J Am Coll Cardiol.* 1990;16:405–412.

67. Ishii M, Jones M, Shiota T, et al. Quantifying aortic regurgitation by using the color Doppler-imaged vena contracta: A chronic animal model study. *Circulation.* 1997;96:2009–2015.

68. Tribouilloy CM, Enriquez-Sarano M, Bailey KR, et al. Assessment of severity of aortic regurgitation using the width of the vena contracta: A clinical color Doppler imaging study. *Circulation.* 2000;102:558–564.

69. Willett DL, Hall SA, Jessen ME, et al. Assessment of aortic regurgitation by transesophageal color Doppler imaging of the vena contracta: Validation against an intraoperative aortic flow probe. *J Am Coll Cardiol.* 2001;37:1450–1455.

70. Cohen GI, Duffy CI, Klein AL, et al. Color Doppler and two-dimensional echocardiographic determination of the mechanism of aortic regurgitation with surgical correlation. *J Am Soc Echocardiogr.* 1996;9:508–515.

71. Tribouilloy CM, Enriquez-Sarano M, Fett SL, et al. Application of the proximal flow convergence method to calculate the effective regurgitant orifice area in aortic regurgitation. *J Am Coll Cardiol.* 1998;32:1032–1039.

72. Meyer T, Sareli P, Pocock WA, et al. Echocardiographic and hemodynamic correlates of diastolic closure of mitral valve and diastolic opening of aortic valve in severe aortic regurgitation. *Am J Cardiol.* 1987;59:1144–1148.

73. Grayburn PA, Handshoe R, Smith MD, et al. Quantitative assessment of the hemodynamic consequences of aortic regurgitation by means of continuous wave Doppler recordings. *J Am Coll Cardiol.* 1987;10:135–141.

74. Teague SM, Heinsimer JA, Anderson JL, et al. Quantification of aortic regurgitation utilizing continuous wave Doppler ultrasound. *J Am Coll Cardiol.* 1986;8:592–599.

75. Touche T, Prasquier R, Nitenberg A, et al. Assessment and follow-up of patients with aortic regurgitation by an updated Doppler echocardiographic measurement of the regurgitant fraction in the aortic arch. *Circulation.* 1985;72:819–824.

76. Croft CH, Lipscomb K, Mathis K, et al. Limitations of qualitative angiographic grading in aortic or mitral regurgitation. *Am J Cardiol.* 1984;53:1593–1598.

77. Borer JS, Bonow RO. Contemporary approach to aortic and mitral regurgitation. *Circulation.* 2003;108:2432–2438.

78. Kozerke S, Schwitter J, Pedersen EM, et al. Aortic and mitral regurgitation: Quantification using moving slice velocity mapping. *J Magn Reson Imaging.* 2001;14:106–112.

79. Chatzimavroudis GP, Oshinski JN, Franch RH, et al. Quantification of the aortic regurgitant volume with magnetic resonance phase velocity mapping: A clinical investigation of the importance of imaging slice location. *J Heart Valve Dis.* 1998;7:94–101.

80. Krombach GA, Kuhl H, Bucker A, et al. Cine MR imaging of heart valve dysfunction with segmented true fast imaging with steady state free precession. *J Magn Reson Imaging.* 2004;19:59–67.

81. Higgins CB, Wagner S, Kondo C, et al. Evaluation of valvular heart disease using cine gradient echo magnetic resonance imaging. *Circulation.* 1991;84(suppl I): I-198–I-207.

82. Underwood SR, Firmin DN, Klipstein RH, et al. Magnetic resonance velocity mapping: Clinical application of a new technique. *Br Heart J.* 1987;57(5):404–412.

83. Lewis SM, Riba AL, Berger HJ, et al. Radionuclide angiographic exercise left ventricular performance in chronic aortic regurgitation: Relationship to resting echographic ventricular dimensions and systolic wall stress index. *Am Heart J.* 1982;103:498–504.

84. Goldman ME, Packer M, Horowitz SF, et al. Relation between exercise-induced changes in ejection fraction and systolic loading conditions at rest in aortic regurgitation. *J Am Coll Cardiol.* 1984;3:924–929.

85. Greenberg B, Massie B, Thomas D, et al. Association between the exercise ejection fraction response and systolic wall stress in patients with chronic aortic insufficiency. *Circulation.* 1985;7:458–465.

86. Klodas E, Enriquez-Sarano M, Tajik AJ, et al. Optimizing timing of surgical correction in patients with severe aortic regurgitation: Role of symptoms. *J Am Coll Cardiol.* 1997;30:746–752.

87. Borer JS. Aortic valve replacement for the asymptomatic patient with aortic regurgitation: A new piece of the strategic puzzle. *Circulation.* 2002;106:2637–2639.

88. Evangelista A, Tornos P, Sambola A, et al. Long-term vasodilator therapy in patients with severe aortic regurgitation. *N Engl J Med.* 2005;353:1342–1349.

89. Dumesnil JG, Tran K, Dagenais GR. Beneficial long-term effects of hydralazine in aortic regurgitation. *Arch Intern Med.* 1990;150:757–760.

90. Lin M, Chiang HT, Lin SL, et al. Vasodilator therapy in chronic asymptomatic aortic regurgitation: Enalapril versus hydralazine therapy. *J Am Coll Cardiol.* 1994;24:1046–1053.

91. Wisenbaugh T, Sinovich V, Dullabh A, et al. Six month pilot study of captopril for mildly symptomatic, severe isolated mitral and isolated aortic regurgitation. *J Heart Valve Dis.* 1994;3:197–204.

92. Schon HR, Dorn R, Barthel P, et al. Effects of 12 months quinapril therapy in asymptomatic patients with chronic aortic regurgitation. *J Heart Valve Dis.* 1994;3:500–509.

93. Wilson W, Taubert KA, Gewitz M, et al. Prevention of infective endocarditis. Guidelines from the American Heart Association. A guideline from the American Heart Association Rheumatic Fever, Endocarditis, and Kawasaki Disease Committee, Council on Cardiovascular Disease in the Young, and the Council on Clinical Cardiology, Council on Cardiovascular Surgery and Anesthesia, and the Quality of Care and Outcomes Research Interdisciplinary Working Group. *Circulation.* 2007. (www.americanheart.org)

94. Meyer TE, Sareli P, Marcus RH, et al. Beneficial effect of atrial pacing in severe acute aortic regurgitation and role of M-mode echocardiography in determining the optimal pacing interval. *Am J Cardiol.* 1991;67:398–403.

95. Casselman FP, Gillinov AM, Akhrass R, et al. Intermediate-term durability of bicuspid aortic valve repair for prolapsing leaflet. *Eur J Cardiothorac Surg.* 1999;15:302–308.

96. Minakata K, Schaff HV, Zehr KJ, et al. Is repair of aortic valve regurgitation a safe alternative to valve replacement? *J Thorac Cardiovasc Surg.* 2004;127:645–653.

97. David TE, Feindel CM, Webb GD, et al. Aortic valve preservation in aortic root aneurysm: Results of the reimplantation technique. *Ann Thorac Surg.* 2007;83:S732–S735.

98. Maurer G. Aortic regurgitation. *Heart.* 2006;92:994–1000.

99. Society of thoracic surgeons national cardiac surgery database. Available at: http://www.sts.org/documents/pdf/

100. Bonow RO, Dodd JT, Maron BJ, et al. Long-term serial changes in left ventricular function and reversal of ventricular dilatation after valve replacement for chronic aortic regurgitation. *Circulation.* 1988;78:1108–1120.

101. Roman MJ, Klein L, Devereux RB, et al. Reversal of left ventricular dilatation, hypertrophy, and dysfunction by valve replacement in aortic regurgitation. *Am Heart J.* 1989;118:553–563.
102. Chaliki HP, Mohty D, Avierinos JF, et al. Outcomes after aortic valve replacement in patients with severe aortic regurgitation and markedly reduced left ventricular function. *Circulation.* 2002;106:2687–2693.
103. Carabello BA. Is it ever too late to operate on the patient with valvular heart disease? *J Am Coll Cardiol.* 2004;44:376–383.
104. Boudjemline Y, Bonhoeffer P. Steps toward percutaneous aortic valve replacement. *Circulation.* 2002;105:775–778.
105. Webb JG, Chandavimol M, Thompson CR, et al. Percutaneous aortic valve implantation retrograde from the femoral artery. *Circulation.* 2006;113:842–850.
106. Rosengart TK, Feldman T, Borger MA, et al. Percutaneous and minimally invasive valve procedures. A scientific statement from the American Heart Association Council on Cardiovascular Surgery and Anesthesia, Council on Clinical Cardiology, Functional Genomics and Translational Biology Interdisciplinary Working Group, and Quality of Care and Outcomes Research Interdisciplinary Working Group. *Circulation.* 2008;117:1750–1767.

Mitral Stenosis

29

José Alberto de Agustín
José Luis Zamorano

1. INTRODUCTION

1.1. Epidemiology

Mitral stenosis (MS) is an obstruction to left ventricular (LV) inflow at the level of the mitral valve (MV) as a result of a structural abnormality of the MV apparatus, which prevents proper opening during diastolic filling of the left ventricle. In the great majority of cases, MS has resulted from rheumatic involvement of the MV,[1,2] although only 50% to 70% of patients report a history of rheumatic fever.[3-5] The ratio of women to men presenting with isolated MS is 2:1. Congenital malformation of the MV occurs rarely and is observed mainly in infants and children. Acquired causes of MV obstruction, other than rheumatic heart disease, are rare. These include left atrial myxoma (Fig. 29.1), ball valve thrombus, mucopolysaccharidosis, systemic lupus erythematosus, carcinoid heart disease, endomyocardial fibrosis, and severe annular calcification.[6,7]

1.2. Clinical presentation
1.2.1. Symptoms

The symptoms induced by MS are primarily related to the severity of the valvular stenosis as reflected by the left atrial pressure, pulmonary pressures, pulmonary vascular resistance, and cardiac output. However, many patients with severe MS deny symptoms because slow progression of the disease is "matched" by a gradual reduction in physical activity. As a result, a careful history regarding maximum levels of exertion is often required to document a slow decline in exercise tolerance. Any situation that increases the cardiac output, which raises transmitral flow, or causes tachycardia, which decreases diastolic filling time can markedly increase the transmitral pressure gradient and precipitate symptoms such as fatigue, dyspnea, or frank pulmonary edema. In others, the initial manifestation of MS is the onset of atrial fibrillation (AF) or an embolic event.[3] Rarely, patients may present with hemoptysis, hoarseness, or dysphagia.

1.2.2. Physical examination

The characteristic auscultatory findings of rheumatic MS are accentuated first heart sound (S1), opening snap (OS), low-pitched middiastolic rumble, and a presystolic murmur. These findings, however, may be absent with severe pulmonary hypertension, low cardiac output, and a heavily calcified immobile MV. A shorter A2–OS interval and longer duration of diastolic rumble indicates more severe MS. An A2–OS interval of less than 0.08 s implies severe MS.[8] Physical findings of pulmonary hypertension, such as a loud P2 or right ventricular heave, also suggest severe MS.

1.2.3. Outcome

MS is a continuous, progressive, lifelong disease, usually consisting of a slow, stable course in the early years followed by a progressive acceleration later in life.[4] There is a long latent period of 20 to 40 years from the occurrence of rheumatic fever to the onset of symptoms. In the asymptomatic or minimally symptomatic patient, survival is greater than 80% at 10 years. Once symptoms develop, there is another period of almost a decade before symptoms become disabling. However, once significant limiting symptoms occur, there is a dismal 5% to 15% 10-year survival rate.[9] With the development of severe pulmonary hypertension, mean survival drops to less than 3 years.[10] The mortality of untreated patients with MS is due to progressive pulmonary and systemic congestion in 60% to 70%, systemic embolism in 20% to 30%, pulmonary embolism in 10%, and infection in 1% to 5%.[7]

2. PATHOPHYSIOLOGY

2.1. Congenital

In countries that have a low prevalence of rheumatic valve disease, MS in nonimmigrant adolescents and young adults is often congenital.[11] The anatomy of congenital MS is variable, and can be the result of any or all of combinations of a supravalvular ring (cor triatriatum), annular hypoplasia, and abnormalities of the leaflets, chordae tendineae, and papillary muscles.[11-13] Affected patients may have a number of other congenital abnormalities involving the left side of the heart, including a bicuspid aortic valve and coarctation of the aorta. A wide spectrum of papillary muscle abnormalities can exist. They may be underdeveloped with a reduced interpapillary distance in some cases, the muscles being very close or fused (parachute MV). A single papillary muscle is often seen; the anterolateral one being absent in many cases, but a variable array is possible. In some cases where two papillary muscles are present, the chordae from the mitral leaflets insert totally into only one. Many of the above cases are associated with thickened and short chordae, which play a major role in the pathogenesis of the stenosis.

2.2. Rheumatic

Once begun, the rheumatic process leads to inflammation in all three layers of the heart: endocardium, myocardium, and pericardium. However, the disease primarily affects the endocardium, leading to inflammation and scarring of the cardiac valves. Mitral disease begins with the formation of tiny nodules located along the coapting portions of the valve leaflets. The leaflets thicken with eventual deposition of fibrin on the cusps and loss of normal valve morphology. Disease progression results in a number of pathologic

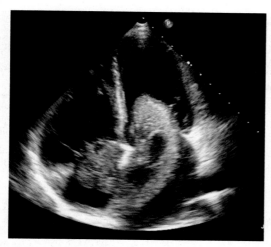

Figure 29.1 Atrial myxoma causing severe mitral stenosis.

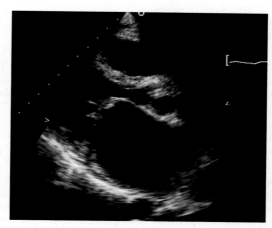

Figure 29.3 Paraexternal long axis view. Classic pattern of "doming" of the leaflets in diastole due to fusion of the leaflet tips at the commissures.

changes affecting the MV apparatus, which are diagnostic for rheumatic valve disease.[14] These include fusion of the leaflet commissures, thickening, fusion and shortening of the chordae tendineae. In addition, there may be superimposed thickening, fibrosis, and calcification of the leaflets.[15] These degenerative changes often develop over the span of decades. The net effect is a stenotic MV with a symmetric, central, oval-shaped orifice (Fig. 29.2) and a classic pattern of "doming" of the leaflets in diastole due to fusion of the leaflet tips at the commissures (Fig. 29.3).

2.3. Functional

MS in the absence of rheumatic involvement has been attributed in some instances to mitral annular calcification. Annular calcification leads to rigidity of the mitral annulus, which in turn prevents normal function of the ring during systole and diastole. The absence or reduction of normal annular dilatation during diastole results in functional MS and its failure to contract at end-diastole helps produce mitral regurgitation (MR). A small, thickwalled, noncompliant left ventricle with a restricted inflow tract is an important contributing cause of the mitral diastolic pressure difference.

2.4. Hemodynamic alterations

The normal MV area is 4 to 5 cm². Narrowing of the valve area to less than 2.5 cm² typically occurs before the development of symptoms.[16] The primary hemodynamic consequence of MS is a pressure gradient between the left atrium (LA) and left ventricle in diastole. The elevated left atrial pressure is reflected backward, causing an increase in pulmonary venous, capillary, and arterial pressures and resistance. With mild to moderate MS, these abnormalities are often only apparent with exercise, emotional stress, infection, pregnancy, or AF with a rapid ventricular response; symptoms eventually are seen at rest as the severity of the stenosis increases. Increased pressure and distension of the pulmonary veins and capillaries can lead to pulmonary edema. In patients with chronic severe MS, however, pulmonary edema may not occur owing to a marked decrease in pulmonary microvascular permeability. The pulmonary arterioles may react with vasoconstriction, intimal hyperplasia, and medial hypertrophy, which lead to pulmonary arterial hypertension and protect the lungs from pulmonary edema.[17,18] These functional and structural changes contribute to the ability of a patient with severe MS to remain minimally symptomatic for prolonged periods of time.[19] Doppler-echocardiographic studies have reported annual loss of MV area ranging from 0.09 to 0.32 cm².[20,21] With isolated MS, the LV systolic and diastolic pressures are usually normal. However, when the stenosis is very severe, there may be a decrease in LV filling and end-diastolic volume, leading to reductions in stroke volume and cardiac output.

3. DIAGNOSTIC EVALUATION

The diagnostic tools of choice in the evaluation of a patient with MS are 2D and Doppler echocardiography.[22–27] Echocardiographic imaging provides determination of the etiology of stenosis, evaluation of the detailed morphology of the valve apparatus, measurement of valve orifice, and evaluation of subvalvular structures, particularly the chordae and papillary muscles. Doppler echocardiography provides accurate assessment of the transvalvular gradient and valve area. Cardiac magnetic resonance (CMR) and cardiac computed tomography rarely provide additional information but it is important to recognize that the anatomic and hemodynamic features of MS may be incidentally detected by these imaging modalities in patients previously undiagnosed.

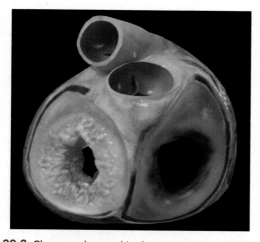

Figure 29.2 Changes observed in rheumatic MS, virtual reconstruction. Note leaflet thickening, calcification, and fusion of the commissures. The net effect is a stenotic mitral valve with a symmetric, central oval-shaped orifice.

3.1. Morphologic valve and subvalvular assessment

With transthoracic two-dimensional echocardiography (2DE), the mitral leaflets are thickened, have reduced motion during diastole, and show doming (Fig. 29.3), which is indicative of commissural fusion. 2DE can be used to assess the morphologic appearance of the MV apparatus.[28–32] Wilkins score (Table 29.1) is an echocardiographic grouping based on valve flexibility, subvalvular fusion, leaflet calcification, and the absence or presence of commissural calcium, grading the severity of involvement of elements of the MV on a scale of 1 through 4, with a score of 1 representing normal.[33] The value for each of these four scores is added together for a total "splitability index" of 4 to 16. Others authors like Cormier (Table 29.2), use a more general assessment of valve anatomy. These features may be important when one considers the timing and type of intervention to be performed.[34] Patients with a Wilkins score of <8 (mobile noncalcified leaflets, no commissural calcification, and little subvalvular fusion) may be candidates for either balloon catheter or surgical commissurotomy.

The typical morphologic features of MS may be recognized also by CCT and CMR (Figs. 29.4–29.7). Cardiac CT may be particularly useful to determine the extent, severity, and location of leaflet and subvalvular calcification.

3.2. Estimation of stenosis severity

3.2.1. M-mode echocardiography

MS alters the appearance of the M-mode tracing of the MV, so its normal early diastolic closure is delayed or abolished (Fig. 29.8). The early diastolic closure slope produces an easily recognized pattern and can also be quantitated to separate normal atrial inflow from obstructed and to differentiate among the degrees of obstruction. Although this method is the least reliable means

TABLE 29.1

ANATOMIC CLASSIFICATION OF THE MITRAL VALVE: WILKINS' SCORE

Leaflet mobility
1. Highly mobile valve with restriction of only the leaflet tips
2. Middle portion and base of leaflets have reduced mobility
3. Valve leaflets move forward in diastole mainly at the base
4. No or minimal forward movement of the leaflets in diastole

Valvular thickening
1. Leaflets near normal (4–5 mm)
2. Mid-leaflet thickening, marked thickening of the margins
3. Thickening extends through the entire leaflets (5–8 mm)
4. Marked thickening of all leaflet tissue (>8–10 mm)

Subvalvular thickening
1. Minimal thickening of chordal structures just below the valve
2. Thickening of chordae extending up to one third of chordal length
3. Thickening extending to the distal third of the chordae
4. Extensive thickening and shortening of all chordae extending down to the papillary muscle

Valvular calcification
1. A single area of increased echo brightness
2. Scattered areas of brightness confined to leaflet margins
3. Brightness extending into the midportion of leaflets
4. Extensive brightness through most of the leaflet tissue

TABLE 29.2

ANATOMIC CLASSIFICATION OF THE MITRAL VALVE: CORMIER'S SCORE

Echocardiographic group	Mitral valve anatomy
Group 1	Pliable noncalcified anterior mitral leaflet and mild subvalvular disease, i.e., thin chordae ≥10 mm long
Group 2	Pliable noncalcified anterior mitral leaflet and severe subvalvular disease, i.e., thickened chordae <10 mm long
Group 3	Calcification of mitral valve of any extent, as assessed by fluoroscopy, whatever the subvalvular apparatus

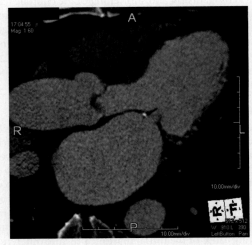

Figure 29.4 Cardiac CT long axis image of the mitral valve orifice.

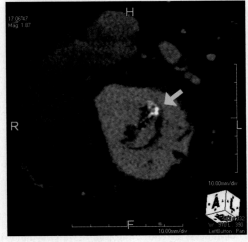

Figure 29.5 Cardiac CT short axis image of the mitral valve orifice. Commissural calcification is noted (*arrow*).

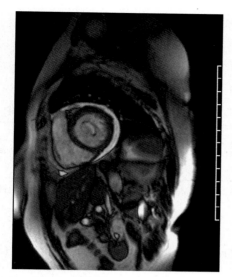

Figure 29.6 Cardiac magnetic resonance SSFP short axis image of a moderately stenotic mitral valve.

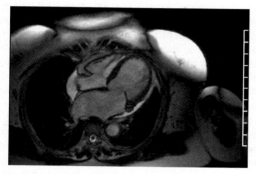

Figure 29.7 Cardiac magnetic resonance SSFP four-chamber image of a moderately stenotic mitral valve.

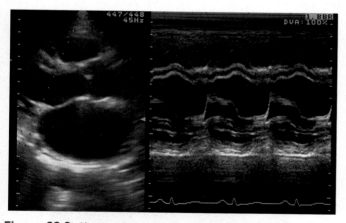

Figure 29.8 Classic pattern of the M-mode tracing of the mitral valve in patients with mitral stenosis. Early diastolic closure is delayed or abolished.

orientation, its maximum diastolic opening area can be measured by direct planimetry of the two-dimensional image (Fig. 29.9). This method is a reliable means of judging the severity of obstruction. Planimetry of the valve orifice has the advantage of being relatively hemodynamically independent. The greatest limitation is that measurements of the MV orifice area are made in the short axis view with no simultaneous independent imaging to verify that the imaging plane corresponds to the smallest and most perpendicular view of the mitral orifice. Because of this disadvantage, it requires significant experience and operator skill to obtain the correct imaging plane that displays the true MV orifice. As the disease process progresses, the border of the valve orifice becomes more calcified and irregular, making the tracing of the orifice more challenging. Likewise, after percutaneous mitral valvuloplasty (PMV), the commissural fusion can split in an asymmetric fashion, again making the tracing of the orifice less reproducible between observers. Typically, a valve orifice area of <1 cm² is considered severe, regardless of the method used to calculate its size. Indirect methods to identify the severity of MS include observing the degree of foreshortening of the chordae tendineae, estimating the extent of leaflet calcification, and noting the degree of left atrial enlargement (Fig. 29.10), the degree of LV underloading, and the presence of right ventricular and atrial dilatation.

3.2.3. Doppler echocardiography[23,25,35]

The mean transmitral gradient can be accurately and reproducibly measured from the continuous-wave Doppler signal across

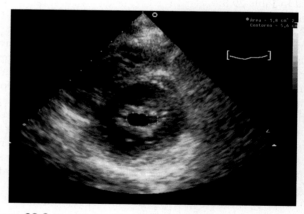

Figure 29.9 Two-dimensional planimetry of the valve orifice.

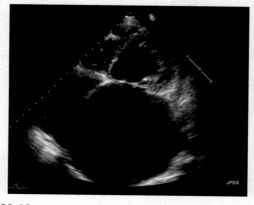

Figure 29.10 Severe left atrial enlargement in a patient with severe mitral stenosis.

of quantitating the severity of obstruction, a slope of less than 10 mm/s (normal is >60 mm/s) is evidence for severe MS.

3.2.2. Two-dimensional echocardiography

In the parasternal short axis plane, the opening of the valve can be imaged just above the tips of the papillary muscles. From this the MV with the modified Bernoulli equation ($4V^2$). Also, the mean transmitral gradient can be measured by tracing the area under the curve of the mitral E and A waves obtained by continuous wave Doppler.[23,25] Severe MS is defined by a mean transmitral gradient greater than 10 mm Hg. The MV area can be noninvasively derived from Doppler echocardiography with either the diastolic pressure half-time method (Fig. 29.11) or the continuity equation.[36] The pressure half-time[35–38] is the time required for the gradient between the LA and the LV to fall to one-half of its initial value. A pressure half-time of 220 ms is equivalent to an MV area (MVA) of 1 cm²[35–38]; therefore:

$$MVA = 220 \div \text{pressure half-time} \qquad \text{(Eq. 29.1)}$$

PHT-derived MVA may be influenced by hemodynamic factors (heart rate, cardiac index, cardiac rhythm, LV systolic and diastolic dysfunction, left ventricular and atrial compliance, LV hypertrophy, and concomitant valvular disease).[39] These factors need to be considered in patients with severe MS and elevated left atrial pressure, since the presence of reduced left atrial compliance will reduce the pressure half-time, yielding a false, larger MVA. These hemodynamic factors change rapidly during the immediate post-PMV period, which may explain the significant discrepancies observed in earlier studies between the PHT-derived MVA and the Gorlin's-derived MVA. Doppler echocardiography may also be used to estimate pulmonary artery systolic pressure from the tricuspid regurgitation velocity signal[40] and to assess severity of concomitant MR. The criteria for the assessment of the severity of MS using mean gradient, pulmonary artery systolic pressure, and valve area are summarized in Table 29.3.

3.2.4. Stress echocardiography

Formal hemodynamic exercise testing can be done noninvasively with either a supine bicycle or upright treadmill with Doppler recordings of transmitral and tricuspid velocities.[41–44] During exercise, the increase in heart rate reduces diastolic filling. Documentation of a transmitral gradient pulmonary pressure elevation during exercise is useful in patients whose symptoms do not seem concordant with the degree of MS at rest. A right ventricular systolic pressure >60 mm Hg and/or a mean MV gradient >15 mm Hg at peak or immediate postexercise are indicative of severe MS. In patients who cannot exercise, dobutamine has been used to increase heart rate.

TABLE 29.3

CRITERIA FOR THE ASSESSMENT OF THE SEVERITY OF MITRAL STENOSIS

	Mean gradient, mm Hg	MVA, cm²	PASP, mm Hg
Mild	< 5	> 1.5	< 30
Moderate	5–10	1.0–1.5	30–50
Severe	> 10	< 1.0	> 50

MVA, mitral valve area; PASP, pulmonary artery systolic pressure.

3.2.5. Three-dimensional echocardiography (3DE)

One of the most significant developments of the last decade, particularly in the field of cardiac imaging, has been real-time three-dimensional echocardiography (RT3DE). 3DE provides unique orientations of the cardiac structures not obtainable by standard 2DE. 3DE has evolved from a research tool to having practical utility, one of them being the accurate planimetry of the MVA in rheumatic MS. 3DE can provide not only adequate imaging of the anatomic structure of the MV orifice (commissural splitting and leaflet tears),[45] but also information on the optimal plane of the smallest MV orifice area (Figs. 29.12 and 29.13). RT3DE offers the possibility of accurately measuring the MV orifice area because of its ability to crop the volume data set in any position in space, and therefore select the en-face view that includes the smallest MV area. In addition, planimetry using RT3DE is not limited to the parasternal window as 2DE is, rather, it can also be performed from the apical window. The utility of RT3DE in the evaluation of patients with MS, and, in particular, the assessment of MVA have been established by multiple studies.[46–52] Currently, it can be argued that sufficient evidence has been compiled to prove that RT3DE is superior to traditional 2DE and should be used routinely to quantify the MVA in MS, particularly in the immediate post-PMV period, where other methods have been proven to be inaccurate.[53–55]

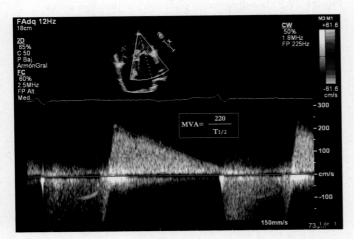

Figure 29.11 Calculating MVA by means of the pressure half-time: time it takes from peak pressure gradient to fall by 50%.

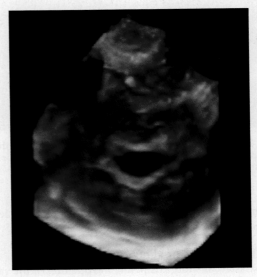

Figure 29.12 RT3DE short axis image of a rheumatic mitral valve.

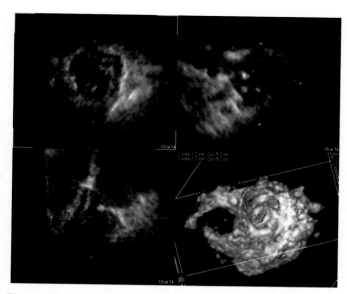

Figure 29.13 The figure shows the accurate way that RT3DE provides to localize the mitral valvular orifice in three orthogonal planes.

3.2.6. Cardiac magnetic resonance and computed tomography

CMR imaging allows direct visualization of valve area with good image quality. CMR can easily demonstrate the thickened leaflets and reduced diastolic opening of the valve in patients with MS. The maximal extent of leaflet opening determined by CMR correlates with stenosis severity.[56] Cine gradient-echo CMR can identify turbulent flow, creating a signal void in the high intensity blood pool.[57] This signal void may allow identification of the site of obstruction, for example, differentiating subvalvular from valvular stenosis.[58] The quantitative assessment of stenotic valves with CMR primarily involves: (1) evaluating valve area using direct planimetry, and (2) determining peak and average velocities across the valve in order to estimate MVA by the pressure half-time method and pressure gradients with the modified Bernoulli equation (Fig. 29.14).

It has been shown that the MVA, as assessed by CMR planimetry, closely corresponds to the echo-derived MVA and the invasively assessed MVA by cardiac catheterization.[59] Thus, planimetry of the MV area by CMR offers an alternative non-invasive method in the diagnosis of MS for patients with technically inadequate echo images. Planimetry of mitral opening by CCT has also been shown to provide accurate assessment of stenosis severity.[60]

In-plane as well as through-plane velocity mapping by CMR has been used to measure the transmitral peak velocity in MS. In order to obtain the maximal velocity, the plane of interrogation must be set perpendicular to the direction of flow and then several phase contrast sections are obtained near the vena contracta of the jet to identify the maximum velocity. The velocity-encoding gradient needs to be often adjusted to encompass the predicted velocity range. Compared to Doppler echocardiography, an accuracy rate of 87% has been reported, with an inter-observer reproducibility rate of 96%.[61,62] CMR-determined Peak early filling (E, $r = 0.99$) and atrial contraction (A, $r = 0.99$) velocities and estimated MV area by the pressure half-time (PHT, $r = 0.94$) method have been validated against Doppler echocardiography.[63]

The presence of calcium in the mitral annulus is associated with systemic atherosclerosis and carries negative prognostic implications. The amount of mitral annular calcium can also be quantified with CCT, although reproducibility appears to be somewhat lower than that for the aortic valve. In rheumatic MS, calcification can extend to the leaflets, commissures, subvalvular apparatus or even the left atrial wall. CCT has been reported to be useful in evaluating MV morphology in patients undergoing balloon mitral commissurotomy.[64]

However, the accuracy of CMR and CCT may be limited in AF since most imaging protocols with these techniques currently require data from multiple cardiac cycles.

3.2.7. Catheterization

Catheterization including left ventriculography (to evaluate the severity of MR) is indicated to assess hemodynamics when there is a discrepancy between Doppler-derived hemodynamics and the clinical status of a symptomatic patient or between the Doppler-derived mean gradient and valve area. Absolute left- and right-side pressure measurements should be obtained by catheterization when there is elevation of pulmonary artery pressure out of proportion to mean gradient and valve area. Invasive hemodynamic evaluation is also necessary to assess the severity and the hemodynamic cause of increased pulmonary vascular resistance, because pulmonary vasodilator therapy may be of benefit in such patients. If symptoms appear to be out of proportion

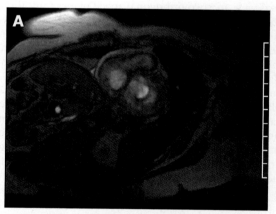
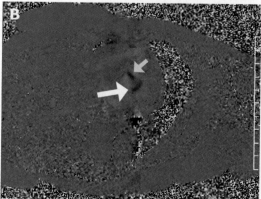

Figure 29.14 Cine SSFP (**A**) and phase contrast (**B**) images of a stenotic mitral valve. Gradients and pressure half-time are determined from the phase-encoded velocity determinations, using Bernoulli's equation. The white arrow indicates mitral flow whereas the yellow arrow shows a jet of aortic insufficiency.

to noninvasive assessment of resting hemodynamics, right- and left-heart catheterization with exercise may be useful. Transseptal catheterization may rarely be required for direct measurement of left atrial pressure if there is doubt about the accuracy of pulmonary artery wedge pressure. The indications for coronary angiography in patients who need intervention are showed in Table 29.4. Cardiac CT may be a suitable alternative to invasive cardiac surgery in patients undergoing MV replacement, although this application has not yet been validated in this setting. Imaging of the coronary arteries may be difficult in patients with AF if there is inadequate heart rate control.

3.3. Evaluation of the left atrium and LA appendage

Imaging of the right and left atria and their appendages can provide important information, particularly in patients with AF who are at increased risk for thromboembolic events resulting from left atrial or atrial appendage thrombus. The LA is a slightly tapered, pillow-shaped structure, which can be easily imaged from a number of echocardiographic windows and views (Fig. 29.6). Left atrial volume and function can be estimated from the M-mode echocardiogram from the long axis precordial window and represent the anterior to posterior dimension of that structure. This dimension is the least sensitive to left atrial enlargement[65] but, when increased, is a highly specific indicator of dilation. Because of the irregular shape of the LA and the single and largely unrepresentative dimension represented by the M-mode image, volume estimates are preferred for evaluating the LA. These measurements require two-dimensional images, preferably obtained from the long axis view and two orthogonal apical planes (apical four and two-chamber view). The same algorithms used for LV measurements can be used to extrapolate volume estimations from area and length measurements.[66,67] The value of measuring left atrial volume to recognize pathology requires knowledge of normal population parameters. In males the volume is 41 to 50 mL while in females it is 34 to 36 mL; the volume index is 21 to 24 mL/m[2].[68] By measuring the atrium during both systole and diastole, one can gain a concept of normal atrial function. Mean end-systolic left atrial volume in a group of normal males and females is 40 mL and its smallest volume at end-diastole (after emptying both passively and actively) is 25 mL; the fractional change per cardiac cycle is 65%. Atrial contraction accounts for only about 10 mL of atrial transport in the healthy young heart; this value more than doubles with aging.[69] Two-dimensional atrial dimensions, measured serially, show that lone AF results in progressive enlargement of the atria,[70] while cardioversion to sinus rhythm prevents these changes.[71] In rheumatic disease, left atrial diameter

predicts the occurrence of AF and the rapidity of restoration of atrial function after cardioversion.[72] In paroxysmal lone AF, atrial "size" at the onset of the arrhythmia does not seem to predict recurrence, but maintenance of sinus rhythm prevents progressive enlargement.[73]

The ability of transthoracic echocardiography to identify or exclude left atrial or atrial appendage thrombi is limited. Transesophageal echocardiography (TEE) is the preferred technique for detection of left atrial thrombi. TEE permits examination of most of the LA, including excellent views of the left atrial appendage. The left atrial appendage is long and thin with a narrow point of origin from the body of the LA. During atrial systole, the appendage cavity becomes very small. Doppler echocardiography permits measurement of flow into and out of the left atrial appendage during sinus rhythm and during AF or flutter. Left atrial thrombi are present on TEE in approximately 13% of nonanticoagulated patients with AF[74,75] and more often (33% in one series) in patients with rheumatic MS.[76] In patients with AF who have had an acute thromboembolic event, residual thrombus can be detected by TEE in approximately ≥ 45% of cases.[77] Atrial thrombi infrequently occur in the setting of sinus rhythm. Small thrombi must be distinguished from the normal trabeculations (pectinate muscles) of the left atrial appendage. Left-sided contrast agents as such can be useful in distinguishing left atrial appendage thrombi from trabeculation because thrombi appear as a filling defect, but trabeculations do not. Other features on the TEE may be helpful in assessing thrombi: the almost ubiquitous finding of spontaneous echo contrast indicative of predisposing stasis almost always accompanies thrombus and may be helpful in differentiating thrombi from tumor or normal anatomy. Older, organized thrombi may show an echogenic series of layers, representing the lines of Zahn. The function of the left atrial appendage on TEE has been studied in patients at risk for the development of left atrial thrombi.[78] The presence or absence of thrombus can be determined by CCT after contrast administration with very high sensitivity although lower specificity, since slow flow may often impair contrast opacification in the left atrial appendage.

A pulsed Doppler sample, placed within the left atrial appendage, reveals a characteristic pattern that is dependent upon the patient's underlying rhythm and atrial function. In patients with sinus rhythm, there are well-defined filling and emptying waves (peak filling velocity >25 cm/s), appropriately timed with atrial contraction; there is a decrease in filling and emptying velocity of 2 and 4 cm/s for each 10 year increase in age. However, among patients with AF, some have well-defined wave forms while others have low velocity, poorly defined wave forms. Thrombi and spontaneous echo contrast are significantly more likely to occur in the latter group with low velocity wave forms.

4. DETERMINING OPTIMAL TIME OF INTERVENTION

4.1. Symptomatic severe mitral stenosis

The prognosis dramatically worsens once the patient with MS develops symptoms. Two-dimensional and Doppler echocardiography is indicated to evaluate MV morphology, hemodynamics, and pulmonary artery pressure. Patients who have New York Heart Association (NYHA) functional class ≥ II and evidence of severe MS have a poor prognosis if left untreated[3-6] and should be considered for intervention with either balloon valvotomy or surgery (Fig. 29.15).

TABLE 29.4

INDICATIONS OF CORONARY ANGIOGRAPHY IN PATIENTS SCHEDULED FOR VALVULAR SURGERY

History of coronary artery disease
Suspected myocardial ischemia (Chest pain, abnormal noninvasive testing)
LV systolic dysfunction
In men aged over 40 and postmenopausal women
≥1 cardiovascular risk factor

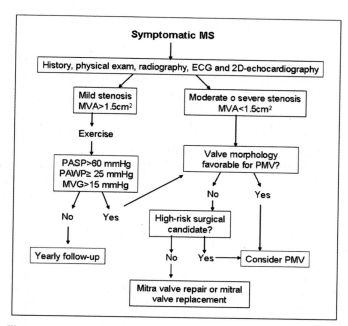

Figure 29.15 Management strategy for patients with symptomatic severe MS. MS, mitral stenosis; MVA, mitral valve area; PASP, pulmonary artery systolic pressure; PAWP, pulmonary artery wedge pressure; MVG, mean mitral valve pressure gradient; PMV, percutaneous mitral valvuloplasty.

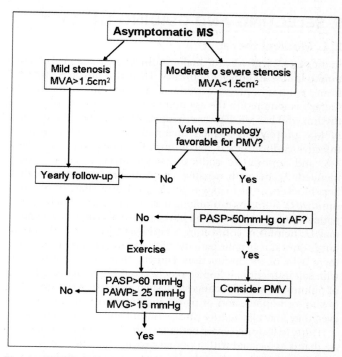

Figure 29.16 Management strategy for patients with asymptomatic severe MS. MS, mitral stenosis; MVA, mitral valve area; PASP, pulmonary artery systolic pressure; PAWP, pulmonary artery wedge pressure; MVG, mean mitral valve pressure gradient; PMV, percutaneous mitral valvuloplasty; AF, atrial fibrillation.

4.2. Asymptomatic severe mitral stenosis

Patients with MS usually have years without symptoms before the onset of deterioration. All patients should be informed that any change in symptoms warrants reevaluation. In the asymptomatic patient, yearly reevaluation is recommended (Fig. 29.16). At the time of the yearly evaluation, a history, physical examination, chest X-ray, and ECG should be obtained. Physical examination is useful to assess the progression of the severity of MS. A shortening of the A2-OS interval, longer duration of the mid-diastolic murmur, and the presence of findings of pulmonary hypertension indicates more severe MS. An echocardiogram is not recommended yearly unless there is a change in clinical status or the patient has severe MS. Ambulatory ECG monitoring (Holter or event recorder) to detect paroxysmal AF is indicated in patients with palpitations. Because of the slowly progressive course of MS, patients may remain "asymptomatic" with severe stenosis merely by readjusting their lifestyles to a more sedentary level. Elevated pulmonary vascular resistance and/or low cardiac output may also play an adaptive role in preventing congestive symptoms from occurring in patients with severe MS. Elevation of pulmonary vascular resistance is an important physiologic event in MS, and the level of pulmonary pressure is an indicator of the overall hemodynamic sequelae. Patients with moderate pulmonary hypertension at rest (pulmonary artery systolic pressure greater than 50 mm Hg) and pliable MV leaflets may be considered for percutaneous mitral valvotomy even if they deny symptoms. In patients who lead a sedentary lifestyle, a hemodynamic exercise test with Doppler echocardiography is useful. Objective limitation of exercise tolerance with a rise in transmitral gradient above 15 mm Hg and a rise in pulmonary artery systolic pressure above 60 mm Hg may be an indication for percutaneous valvotomy if the MV morphology is suitable. There is a subset of asymptomatic patients with severe MS (valve area less than 1.0 cm²) and severe pulmonary hypertension (pulmonary artery systolic pressure greater than 75% of systemic pressure either at rest or with exercise). If these patients do not have a valve morphology favorable for percutaneous mitral balloon valvotomy or surgical valve repair, it is controversial whether MV replacement should be performed in the absence of symptoms to prevent RV failure, but surgery is generally recommended in such patients. However, the patient should be involved in the decision regarding intervention.

4.3. Symptomatic moderate mitral stenosis

A subset of patients have significant limiting symptoms, yet clinical and Doppler echocardiographic evaluation do not indicate severe MS. In such patients, formal exercise testing or dobutamine stress may be useful to differentiate symptoms due to MS from other causes of symptoms. Exercise tolerance, heart rate and blood pressure response, transmitral gradient, and pulmonary artery pressure can be obtained at rest and during exercise. Right and left heart catheterization with exercise may be helpful and occasionally necessary.[79] Patients who are symptomatic with a significant elevation of pulmonary artery pressure (greater than 60 mm Hg), mean transmitral gradient (greater than 15 mm Hg), or pulmonary artery wedge pressure (greater than 25 mm Hg) during exercise[80–82] have hemodynamically significant MS and should be considered for further intervention. Alternatively, patients who do not manifest elevation in pulmonary artery, pulmonary artery wedge, or transmitral pressures coincident with development of exertional symptoms most likely would not benefit from intervention on the MV. Hemodynamic measurements by cardiac catheterization can be used to determine the severity of MS. Direct measurements of left atrial and LV pressure determine the transmitral gradient, which is the fundamental expression of severity of MS.[83] Thus, the transmitral gradient derived by Doppler echocardiography may be more accurate than that obtained by cardiac catheterization with pulmonary artery wedge pressure.[84]

5. SELECTING AND GUIDING THERAPY

5.1. Medical therapy

In the patient with MS, the major problem is mechanical obstruction to inflow at the level of the MV. The left ventricle is protected from a volume or pressure overload, and thus, no specific medical therapy is required in the asymptomatic patient in normal sinus rhythm who has MS. Because rheumatic fever is the primary cause of MS, prophylaxis against rheumatic fever is recommended. Infective endocarditis is uncommon but does occur in isolated MS, and appropriate endocarditis prophylaxis is also recommended. Agents with negative chronotropic properties, such as beta-blockers or heart rate-regulating calcium channel blockers, improve LV filling by prolonging diastole and may be of benefit in patients in sinus rhythm who have exertional symptoms. Digoxin may be helpful in controlling a rapid ventricular rate during AF but it does not benefit patients with MS in sinus rhythm unless there is LV or RV dysfunction. Diuretic therapy, in combination with salt restriction, is appropriate when there are manifestations of pulmonary vascular congestion such as exertional shortness of breath, orthopnea, and/or paroxysmal nocturnal dyspnea. However, they may also reduce cardiac output and worsen fatigue.

Thirty to forty percent of patients with symptomatic MS develop AF that is associated with a poorer prognosis, with a 10-year survival rate of 25% compared with 46% in patients who remain in sinus rhythm.[6] The risk of arterial embolization, especially stroke, is significantly increased.[85] Patients with MS who have chronic AF have a stroke risk of 7% to 15% per year. Long-term oral anticoagulation (target INR 2.5, range 2 to 3) is recommended in patients with MS who have either a prior embolic event or paroxysmal, persistent, or permanent AF, since all forms of AF carry a similar risk for thromboembolism. A rate control strategy is generally preferred because outcomes are as good as or perhaps better than those with a rhythm control strategy; and, with a rhythm control strategy, long-term anticoagulation is still required in most patients. Nevertheless, conversion to sinus rhythm should be considered in patients with a contraindication to long-term anticoagulation and in those who are symptomatic with AF, have had previous thromboembolism despite adequate anticoagulation, or whose AF is of short duration. Although radiofrequency ablation has been increasingly studied in patients without structural heart disease, its role in those with rheumatic heart disease is uncertain. Recurrent paroxysmal AF may be treated for maintenance of sinus rhythm in selected patients with class IC antiarrhythmic drugs (in conjunction with negative dromotropic agent) or class III antiarrhythmic drugs.

Patients with mild MS will remain asymptomatic even with strenuous exercise. In more severe MS, exercise can cause sudden marked increases in pulmonary venous pressure from the increase in heart rate and cardiac output, at times resulting in pulmonary edema.[63] The long-term effects of repeated exertion-related increases in pulmonary venous and pulmonary artery pressures on the lung or right ventricle remain unknown. MS rarely causes sudden death. These factors must be considered when recommending physical activity and exercise for the patient with MS. In the majority of patients with MS, recommendations for exercise are symptom limited. This will prevent extreme elevations in the transmitral gradient that may lead to pulmonary edema.

5.2. Percutaneous mitral valvuloplasty

PMV was first performed in the early 1980s and became a clinically approved technique in 1994. There is a higher success rate and lower complication rate in experienced, high-volume centers. The immediate results of PMV are similar to those of mitral commissurotomy.[86–89] The mean valve area usually doubles (from 1 to 2 cm²), with a 50% to 60% reduction in transmitral gradient. Overall, 80% to 95% of patients may have a successful procedure, which is defined as an MV area greater than 1.5 cm² and a decrease in left atrial pressure to less than 18 mm Hg in the absence of complications. The most common acute complications reported in large series include severe MR, which occurs in 2% to 10%, and a residual atrial septal defect. The majority of small left-to-right shunts at the atrial level will close spontaneously over the course of 6 months. Less frequent complications include perforation of the left ventricle (0.5% to 4.0%), embolic events (0.5% to 3%), and myocardial infarction (0.3% to 0.5%). The mortality rate with balloon valvotomy in larger series has ranged from 1% to 2%.[90] TEE has been used during the procedure to guide transseptal puncture and balloon placement (Fig. 29.17). It has also been used after the procedure to allow for prompt recognition of major complications (LV or left atrial perforation with tamponade, and severe MR and creation of a large atrial septal defect) and to assess the following parameters of response to the procedure: the resolution of spontaneous echo contrast in response to relief of obstruction, and the hemodynamic impact of the residual atrial septal defect resulting from the transseptal puncture. However, TEE has the disadvantage that general anesthesia may be required due to the length of the procedure. Most centers use transthoracic and/or intracardiac echocardiography. Intracardiac echocardiography employs an ultrasound-tipped catheter inserted intravenously

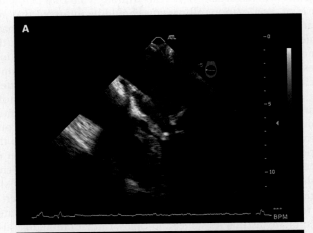

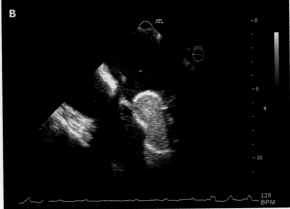

Figure 29.17. Percutaneous mitral valvulotomy: Transesophageal four-chamber views before (**A**) and during (**B**) balloon inflation.

and manipulated within the heart, and can delineate the extent of valvular deformity and may also be useful in visualizing several key steps of the valvotomy procedure, including[91] transseptal puncture of the interatrial septum, exclusion of thrombus from the left atrial appendage, optimizing balloon placement across the valve orifice, and initial assessment of the results of dilatation. Disadvantages of this approach are increased cost and, with current transducers, an inability to accurately measure MV area or adequately assess MR. In centers with skilled, experienced operators, PMV should be considered the initial procedure of choice for patients who have a favorable valve morphology. The underlying MV morphology is the factor of greatest importance in determining outcome.[92] Patients with valvular calcification, thickened fibrotic leaflets with decreased mobility, and subvalvular fusion have a higher incidence of acute complications and a higher rate of recurrent stenosis on follow-up. Relative contraindications to percutaneous balloon valvotomy are summarized in Table 29.5.

5.3. Surgical valve replacement

MV replacement is an accepted surgical procedure for patients with severe MS who are not candidates for PMV. The perioperative mortality of MV replacement is dependent on multiple factors, including functional status, age, LV function, cardiac output, concomitant medical problems, and concomitant CAD. In the young, healthy person, MV replacement can be performed with a risk of less than 5%; however, in the older patient with concomitant medical problems or pulmonary hypertension at systemic levels, the perioperative mortality of MV replacement may be as high as 10% to 20%.[93] The choice of prosthesis is based on patient age, the risk of anticoagulation, and patient and surgeon preference. MV replacement with preservation of subvalvular apparatus aids in maintaining LV function,[94] but this can be particularly difficult in patients with rheumatic involvement. Complications of MV replacement include valve thrombosis, valve dehiscence, valve infection, valve malfunction, and embolic events. There is also the known risk of long-term anticoagulation in patients receiving mechanical prostheses. In the patient with NYHA functional class III symptoms due to severe MS or combined MS/MR, MV replacement results in excellent symptomatic improvement.

5.4. Pregnancy

MS is primarily a disease of women, in whom the pathophysiology is often exacerbated by the physiologic demands of pregnancy. During the second trimester, cardiac output increases by 70%, thereby increasing the resting transmitral gradient. During pregnancy, the patient's symptomatic status will increase by 1 NYHA class. For pregravid patients in class I, pregnancy poses few problems; however, for more symptomatic patients, pregnancy may cause serious clinical difficulties. Mild symptoms may be managed with the use of diuretics. However, in advanced disease, relief of MS during pregnancy may be advisable. It seems wise to proceed with PMV when the pregnant patient is obviously failing medical therapy. Alternatively, it might be wise to provide PMV before pregnancy in symptomatic women or in women who already have asymptomatic pulmonary hypertension.

6. FUTURE DIRECTIONS

Rheumatic MV stenosis still remains an important public health concern in developed countries. To define the best therapeutic strategy in patients with rheumatic MV stenosis, accurate measurements of the MVA are necessary. Doppler-based methods are heavily influenced by hemodynamic variables, LV hypertrophy, and associated valvular disease. Accordingly, methods based on direct measurement of the valvular orifice should be more accurate. 2D-traced planimetry has multiple limitations, the major one being the correct image plane orientation. RT3D provides a unique "en-face" view of the complete MV apparatus and has shown that it can improve the accuracy of 2D echo MVA planimetry. Until now, 3DE has not been routinely performed due to the cumbersome nature of older platforms, prolonged data acquisition and off-line processing time. With the advent of the new transthoracic 3D matrix array probes that allow real-time 3D rendering, many of the above limitations could be circumvented. Compared to all other echo-Doppler methods, RT3D agrees best with the invasively determined MVA, the usual gold standard. RT3D has also shown its superiority in evaluating the MVA in the most difficult scenario for the traditional noninvasive methods: the immediate postvalvuloplasty period. Thus, we can conclude that RT3D is a feasible and accurate technique for measuring MVA in patients with rheumatic MV stenosis and that it is still useful under the conditions where other noninvasive methods fail. Perhaps, in the near future, it should replace Gorlin method as the reference method to quantify the MVA in rheumatic MV stenosis.

REFERENCES

1. Olson LJ, Subramanian R, Ackermann DM, et al. Surgical pathology of the mitral valve: A study of 712 cases spanning 21 years. *Mayo Clin Proc.* 1987;62:22–34.
2. Horstkotte D, Niehues R, Strauer BE. Pathomorphological aspects, aetiology and natural history of acquired mitral valve stenosis. *Eur Heart J.* 1991;12(Suppl B):55–60.
3. Wood P. An appreciation of mitral stenosis. I. Clinical features. *Br Med J.* 1954;4870:1051–1063.
4. Selzer A, Cohn KE. Natural history of mitral stenosis: A review. *Circulation.* 1972;45:878–890.
5. Rowe JC, Bland EF, Sprague HB, et al. The course of mitral stenosis without surgery: Ten- and twenty-year perspectives. *Ann Intern Med.* 1960;52:741–749.
6. Olesen KH. The natural history of 271 patients with mitral stenosis under medical treatment. *Br Heart J.* 1962;24:349–357.
7. Roberts WC, Perloff JK. Mitral valvular disease: A clinicopathologic survey of the conditions causing the mitral valve to function abnormally. *Ann Intern Med.* 1972;77:939–975.
8. Craige E. Phonocardiographic studies in mitral stenosis. *N Engl J Med.* 1957;257:650–654.
9. Munoz S, Gallardo J, Diaz-Gorrin JR, et al. Influence of surgery on the natural history of rheumatic mitral and aortic valve disease. *Am J Cardiol.* 1975;35:234–242.
10. Ward C, Hancock BW. Extreme pulmonary hypertension caused by mitral valve disease: Natural history and results of surgery. *Br Heart J.* 1975;37:74–78.
11. Bonow RO, Carabello BA, Chatterjee K, et al. ACC/AHA 2006 guidelines for the management of patients with valvular heart disease. A report of the American College of Cardiology/American Heart Association Task Force on Practice Guidelines (Writing committee to revise the 1998 guidelines for the management of patients with valvular heart disease). *J Am Coll Cardiol.* 2006; 48:e1–e148.

TABLE 29.5

CONTRAINDICATIONS FOR PERCUTANEOUS MITRAL VALVULOPLASTY

Mild mitral stenosis (valve area >1.5 cm²)
Left atrial thrombus
More than mild mitral regurgitation
Massive or bicommissural calcification
Need for open-heart surgery on another valve, or coronary arteries, or ascending aorta
Contraindications for transseptal catheterization

12. Ruckman RN, Van PR. Anatomic types of congenital mitral stenosis: Report of 49 autopsy cases with consideration of diagnosis and surgical implications. *Am J Cardiol.* 1978;42:592–601.

13. Moore P, Adatia I, Spevak PJ, et al. Severe congenital mitral stenosis in infants. *Circulation.* 1994;89:2099–2106.

14. Marcus RH, Sareli P, Pocock WA, et al. The spectrum of severe rheumatic valve disease in a developing country. *Ann Intern Med.* 1994;120:177.

15. Rajamannan NM, Nealis TB, Subramaniam M, et al. Calcified rheumatic valve neoangiogenesis is associated with vascular endothelial growth factor expression and osteoblast-like bone formation. *Circulation.* 2005;111:3296–3301.

16. Gorlin R, Gorlin SG. Hydraulic formula for calculation of the area of the stenotic mitral valve, other cardiac valves, and central circulatory shunts. *Am Heart J.* 1951;41:1–29.

17. Gorlin R. The mechanism of the signs and symptoms of mitral valve disease. *Br Heart J.* 1954;16:375–380.

18. Wood P. An appreciation of mitral stenosis, II: Investigations and results. *Br Med J.* 1954;4871:1113–1124.

19. Hugenholtz PG, Ryan TJ, Stein SW, et al. The spectrum of pure mitral stenosis: Hemodynamic studies in relation to clinical disability. *Am J Cardiol.* 1962;10:773–784.

20. Dubin AA, March HW, Cohn K, et al. Longitudinal hemodynamic and clinical study of mitral stenosis. *Circulation.* 1971;44:381–389.

21. Gordon SP, Douglas PS, Come PC, et al. Two-dimensional and Doppler echocardiographic determinants of the natural history of mitral valve narrowing in patients with rheumatic mitral stenosis: Implications for follow-up. *J Am Coll Cardiol.* 1992;19:968–973.

22. Henry WL, Griffith JM, Michaelis LL, et al. Measurement of mitral orifice area in patients with mitral valve disease by real-time, two-dimensional echocardiography. *Circulation.* 1975;51:827–831.

23. Holen J, Aaslid R, Landmark K, et al. Determination of pressure gradient in mitral stenosis with a non-invasive ultrasound Doppler technique. *Acta Med Scand.* 1976;199:455–460.

24. Nichol PM, Gilbert BW, Kisslo JA. Two-dimensional echocardiographic assessment of mitral stenosis. *Circulation.* 1977;55:120–128.

25. Hatle L, Brubakk A, Tromsdal A, et al. Noninvasive assessment of pressure drop in mitral stenosis by Doppler ultrasound. *Br Heart J.* 1978;40:131–140.

26. Wann LS, Weyman AE, Feigenbaum H, et al. Determination of mitral valve area by cross-sectional echocardiography. *Ann Intern Med.* 1978;88:337–341.

27. Martin RP, Rakowski H, Kleiman JH, et al. Reliability and reproducibility of two dimensional echocardiograph measurement of the stenotic mitral valve orifice area. *Am J Cardiol.* 1979;43:560–568.

28. Reid CL, McKay CR, Chandraratna PA, et al. Mechanisms of increase in mitral valve area and influence of anatomic features in double-balloon, catheter balloon valvuloplasty in adults with rheumatic mitral stenosis: A Doppler and two-dimensional echocardiographic study. *Circulation.* 1987;76:628–636.

29. Rediker DE, Block PC, Abascal VM, et al. Mitral balloon valvuloplasty for mitral restenosis after surgical commissurotomy. *J Am Coll Cardiol.* 1988;11: 252–256.

30. Fatkin D, Roy P, Morgan JJ, et al. Percutaneous balloon mitral valvotomy with the Inoue single-balloon catheter: Commissural morphology as a determinant of outcome. *J Am Coll Cardiol.* 1993;21:390–397.

31. Iung B, Cormier B, Ducimetiere P, et al. Functional results 5 years after successful percutaneous mitral commissurotomy in a series of 528 patients and analysis of predictive factors. *J Am Coll Cardiol.* 1996;27:407–414.

32. Cannan CR, Nishimura RA, Reeder GS, et al. Echocardiographic assessment of commissural calcium: A simple predictor of outcome after percutaneous mitral balloon valvotomy. *J Am Coll Cardiol.* 1997;29:175–180.

33. Wilkins GT, Weyman AE, Abascal VM, et al. Percutaneous balloon dilatation of the mitral valve: An analysis of echocardiographic variables related to outcome and the mechanism of dilatation. *Br Heart J.* 1988;60:299–308.

34. Reid CL, Chandraratna PA, Kawanishi DT, et al. Influence of mitral valve morphology on double-balloon catheter balloon valvuloplasty in patients with mitral stenosis: Analysis of factors predicting immediate and 3-month results. *Circulation.* 1989;80:515–524.

35. Hatle L, Angelsen B, Tromsdal A. Noninvasive assessment of atrioventricular pressure half-time by Doppler ultrasound. *Circulation.* 1979;60:1096–1104.

36. Nakatani S, Masuyama T, Kodama K, et al. Value and limitations of Doppler echocardiography in the quantification of stenotic mitral valve area: Comparison of the pressure half-time and the continuity equation methods. *Circulation.* 1988;77:78–85.

37. Thomas JD, Wilkins GT, Choong CY, et al. Inaccuracy of mitral pressure half-time immediately after percutaneous mitral valvotomy. Dependence on transmitral gradient and left atrial and ventricular compliance. *Circulation.* 1988;78: 980–993.

38. Flachskampf FA, Weyman AE, Guerrero JL, et al. Influence of orifice geometry and flow rate on effective valve area: An in vitro study. *J Am Coll Cardiol.* 1990;15:1173–1180.

39. Rodriguez L, Thomas JD, Monterroso V, et al. Validation of the proximal flow convergence method: Calculation of orifice area in patients with mitral stenosis. *Circulation.* 1993;88:1157–1165.

40. Currie PJ, Seward JB, Chan KL, et al. Continuous wave Doppler determination of right ventricular pressure: A simultaneous Doppler catheterization study in 127 patients. *J Am Coll Cardiol.* 1985;6:750–756.

41. Himelman RB, Stulbarg M, Kircher B, et al. Noninvasive evaluation of pulmonary artery pressure during exercise by saline-enhanced Doppler echocardiography in chronic pulmonary disease. *Circulation.* 1989;79:863–871.

42. Tamai J, Nagata S, Akaike M, et al. Improvement in mitral flow dynamics during exercise after percutaneous transvenous mitral commissurotomy: Noninvasive evaluation using continuous wave Doppler technique. *Circulation.* 1990;81: 46–51.

43. Leavitt JI, Coats MH, Falk RH. Effects of exercise on transmitral gradient and pulmonary artery pressure in patients with mitral stenosis or a prosthetic mitral valve: A Doppler echocardiographic study. *J Am Coll Cardiol.* 1991;17:1520–1526.

44. Cheriex EC, Pieters FA, Janssen JH, et al. Value of exercise Doppler-echocardiography in patients with mitral stenosis. *Int J Cardiol.* 1994;45:219–226.

45. Applebaum RM, Kasliwal RR, Kanojia A, et al. Utility of three-dimensional echocardiography during balloon mitral valvuloplasty. *J Am Coll Cardiol.* 1998;32(5):1405–1409.

46. Zamorano J, Cordeiro P, Sugeng L, et al. Real-time three-dimensional echocardiography for rheumatic mitral valve stenosis evaluation: An accurate and novel approach. *J Am Coll Cardiol.* 2004;43:2091–2096.

47. Zamorano J, Perez de Isla L, Sugeng L, et al. Non-invasive assessment of mitral valve area during percutaneous balloon mitral valvuloplasty: Role of real-time 3D echocardiography. *Eur Heart J.* 2004;25:2086–2091.

48. Binder TM, Rosenhek R, Porenta G, et al. Improved assessment of mitral valve stenosis by volumetric real-time three-dimensional echocardiography. *J Am Coll Cardiol.* 2000;36:1355–1361.

49. Chen Q, Nosir YF, Vletter WB, et al. Accurate assessment of mitral valve area in patients with mitral stenosis by three-dimensional echocardiography. *J Am Soc Echocardiogr.* 1997;10:133–140.

50. Applebaum RM, Kasliwal RR, Kanojia A, et al. Utility of three-dimensional echocardiography during balloon mitral valvuloplasty. *J Am Coll Cardiol.* 1998;32:1405–1409.

51. Limbu YR, Shen X, Pan C, et al. Assessment of mitral valve volume by quantitative three-dimensional echocardiography in patients with rheumatic mitral valve stenosis. *Clin Cardiol.* 1998;21:415–418.

52. Sugeng L, Weinert L, Lammertin G, et al. Accuracy of mitral valve area measurements using transthoracic rapid freehand 3-dimensional scanning: Comparison with noninvasive and invasive methods. *J Am Soc Echocardiogr.* 2003;16: 1292–1300.

53. Sebag IA, Morgan JG, Handschumacher MD, et al. Usefulness of three-dimensionally guided assessment of mitral stenosis using matrix array ultrasound. *Am J Cardiol.* 2005;96(8):1151–1156.

54. Perez de Isla L, Casanova C, Almeria C, et al. Which method should be the reference method to evaluate the severity of rheumatic mitral stenosis? Gorlin's method versus 3D echo. *Eur J Echocardiogr.* 8:470–473.

55. Mannaerts HFJ, Kamp O, Visser CA. Should mitral valve area assessment in patients with mitral stenosis be based on anatomical or on functional evaluation? A plea for 3D echocardiography as the new clinical standard. *Eur Heart J.* 2004;25:2073–2074.

56. Casolo GC, Zampa V, Rega L, et al. Evaluation of mitral stenosis by cine magnetic resonance imaging. *Am Heart J.* 1992;123(5):1252–1260.

57. Evans AJ, Blinder RA, Herfkens RJ, et al. Effects of turbulence on signal intensity in gradient echo images. *Invest Radiol.* 1988;23(7):512–518.

58. Globits S, Higgins CB. Assessment of valvular heart disease by magnetic resonance imaging. *Am Heart J.* 1995;129(2):369–381.

59. Djavidani B, Debl K, Lenhart M, et al. Planimetry of mitral valve stenosis by magnetic resonance imaging. *J Am Coll Cardiol.* 2005;45:2048–2053.

60. Messika-Zeitoun D, Serfaty JM, Laissy JP, et al. Assessment of the mitral valve area in patients with mitral stenosis by multislice computed tomography. *J Am Coll Cardiol.* 2006;48:411–413.

61. Kilner PJ, Manzara CC, Mohiaddin RH, et al. Magnetic resonance jet velocity mapping in mitral and aortic valve stenosis. *Circulation.* 1993;87:1239–1248.

62. Heidenreich PA, Steffens J, Fujita N, et al. Evaluation of mitral stenosis with velocity-encoded cine-magnetic resonance imaging. *Am J Cardiol.* 1995;75:365–369.

63. Lin SJ, Brown PA, Watkins MP, et al. Quantification of stenotic mitral valve area with magnetic resonance imaging and comparison with Doppler ultrasound. *J Am Coll Cardiol.* 2004;44:133–137.

64. White ML, Grover MM, Weiss RM, et al. Prediction of change in mitral valve area after mitral balloon commissurotomy using cine computed tomography. *Invest Radiol.* 1994;29(9):827–833.

65. Lester SJ, Ryan EW, Schiller NB, et al. Best method in clinical practice and in research studies to determine left atrial size. *Am J Cardiol.* 1999;84:829–832.

66. Schabelman S, Schiller NB, Silverman NH, et al. Left atrial volume estimation by two-dimensional echocardiography. *Cathet Cardiovasc Diagn.* 1981;7:165–178.

67. Kircher B, Abbott JA, Pau S, et al. Left atrial volume determination by biplane two-dimensional echocardiography: Validation by cine computed tomography. *Am Heart J.* 1991;121:864.

68. Wang Y, Gutman JM, Heilbron D, et al. Atrial volume in a normal adult population by two-dimensional echocardiography. *Chest.* 1984;86:595–601.

69. Thomas L, Levett K, Boyd A, et al. Compensatory changes in atrial volumes with normal aging: Is atrial enlargement inevitable? *J Am Coll Cardiol.* 2002;40: 1630–1635.

70. Sanfilippo AJ, Abascal VM, Sheehan M, et al. Atrial enlargement as a consequence of atrial fibrillation. A prospective echocardiographic study. *Circulation.* 1990;82:792–797.

71. Welikovitch L, Lafreniere G, Burggraf GW, et al. Change in atrial volume following restoration of sinus rhythm in patients with atrial fibrillation: A prospective echocardiographic study. *Can J Cardiol.* 1994;10:993–996.

72. Thomas L, Thomas SP, Hoy M, et al. Comparison of left atrial volume and function after linear ablation and after cardioversion for chronic atrial fibrillation. *Am J Cardiol.* 2004;93:165–170.

73. Rostagno C, Olivo G, Comeglio M, et al. Left atrial size changes in patients with paroxysmal lone atrial fibrillation. An echocardiographic follow-up. *Angiology.* 1996;47:797–801.

74. Manning WJ, Silverman DI, Keighley CS, et al. Transesophageal echocardiographically facilitated early cardioversion from atrial fibrillation using short-term anticoagulation: Final results of a prospective 4.5 year study. *J Am Coll Cardiol.* 1995;25:1354–1361.

75. Klein AL, Grimm RA, Murray D, et al. Use of transesophageal echocardiography to guide cardioversion in patients with atrial fibrillation. *N Engl J Med.* 2001;344:1411–1420.

76. Srimannarayana J, Varma RS, Satheesh S, et al. Prevalence of left atrial thrombus in rheumatic mitral stenosis with atrial fibrillation and its response to anticoagulation: A transesophageal echocardiographic study. *Indian Heart J.* 2003;55:358–361.

77. Zabalgoitia M, Halperin JL, Pearce LA, et al. Transesophageal echocardiographic correlates of clinical risk of thromboembolism in nonvalvular atrial fibrillation. Stroke prevention in atrial fibrillation III investigators. *J Am Coll Cardiol.* 1998;31:1622–1626.

78. Agmon Y, Khandheria BK, Gentile F, et al. Echocardiographic assessment of the left atrial appendage. *J Am Coll Cardiol.* 1999;34:1867–1877.

79. Gorlin R, Sawyer CG, Haynes FW, et al. Effects of exercise on circulatory dynamics in mitral stenosis, III. *Am Heart J.* 1951;41:192–203.

80. Kasalicky J, Hurych J, Widimsky J, et al. Left heart haemodynamics at rest and during exercise in patients with mitral stenosis. *Br Heart J.* 1968;30: 188–195.

81. Harvey RM, Ferrer I, Samet P, et al. Mechanical and myocardial factors in rheumatic heart disease with mitral stenosis. *Circulation.* 1955;11:531–551.

82. Aviles RJ, Nishimura RA, Pellikka PA, et al. Utility of stress Doppler echocardiography in patients undergoing percutaneous mitral balloon valvotomy. *J Am Soc Echocardiogr.* 2001;14:676–681.

83. Braunwald E, Moscovitz HL, Mram SS, et al. The hemodynamics of the left side of the heart as studied by simultaneous left atrial, left ventricular, and aortic pressures; particular reference to mitral stenosis. *Circulation.* 1955;12:69–81.

84. Nishimura RA, Rihal CS, Tajik AJ, et al. Accurate measurement of the transmitral gradient in patients with mitral stenosis: A simultaneous catheterization and Doppler echocardiographic study. *J Am Coll Cardiol.* 1994;24:152–158.

85. Daley R, Mattingly TW, Holt CL, et al. Systemic arterial embolism in rheumatic heart disease. *Am Heart J.* 1951;42:566–581

86. Multicenter experience with balloon mitral commissurotomy: NHLBI Balloon Valvuloplasty Registry Report on immediate and 30-day follow-up results: The National Heart, Lung, and Blood Institute Balloon Valvuloplasty Registry Participants. *Circulation.* 1992;85:448–461.

87. Cohen DJ, Kuntz RE, Gordon SP, et al. Predictors of long-term outcome after percutaneous balloon mitral valvuloplasty. *N Engl J Med.* 1992;327:1329–1335.

88. Dean LS, Mickel M, Bonan R, et al. Four-year follow-up of patients undergoing percutaneous balloon mitral commissurotomy: A report from the National Heart, Lung, and Blood Institute Balloon Valvuloplasty Registry. *J Am Coll Cardiol.* 1996;28:1452–1457.

89. Palacios IF, Sanchez PL, Harrell LC, et al. Which patients benefit from percutaneous mitral balloon valvuloplasty? Prevalvuloplasty and postvalvuloplasty variables that predict long-term outcome. *Circulation.* 2002;105:1465–1471.

90. Complications and mortality of percutaneous balloon mitral commissurotomy: A report from the national heart, lung, and blood institute balloon valvuloplasty registry. *Circulation.* 1992;85:2014–2024.

91. Green NE, Hansgen AR, Carroll JD. Initial clinical experience with intracardiac echocardiography in guiding balloon mitral valvuloplasty: Technique, safety, utility, and limitations. *Catheter Cardiovasc Interv.* 2004;63:385–394.

92. Padial LR, Freitas N, Sagie A, et al. Echocardiography can predict which patients will develop severe mitral regurgitation after percutaneous mitral valvulotomy. *J Am Coll Cardiol.* 1996;27:1225–1231.

93. Birkmeyer JD, Siewers AE, Finlayson EV, et al. Hospital volume and surgical mortality in the United States. *N Engl J Med.* 2002;346:1128–1137.

94. Wu ZK, Sun PW, Zhang X, et al. Superiority of mitral valve replacement with preservation of subvalvular structure to conventional replacement in severe rheumatic mitral valve disease: A modified technique and results of one-year follow up. *J Heart Valve Dis.* 2000;9:616–622.

Mitral Insufficiency

30

Takahiro Shiota

1. INTRODUCTION

Mitral insufficiency or regurgitation (MR) may occur as a primary condition or as a functional disorder in patients with different forms of cardiomyopathy, is the second most primary MR, is defined by the presence of structural valvular abnormalities, and is the second most prevalent valve disorder after aortic stenosis. The most common etiologies of primary MR in the western world are mitral valve prolapse and flail due to myxomatous mitral valve disease (Barlow's) and fibroelastic deficiency followed by infective endocarditis, rheumatic valve disease, and congenital cleft of the anterior leaflet.[1] Other more rare causes include radiation therapy, carcinoid syndrome, systemic lupus erythematosus (Libman–Sacks lesions), rheumatoid arthritis, and trauma, which may cause damage to the mitral valve leaflet. Functional MR is associated with extravalvular abnormalities, including left ventricular (LV) dilation, annular dilation, and LV dysfunction. In this category, the mitral valve itself is morphologically normal. Functional MR can be further subdivided into ischemic and nonischemic MR. The former is caused by coronary artery disease (CAD) with/without papillary muscle dysfunction and LV wall motion abnormality, while the latter is seen in patients with nonischemic dilated cardiomyopathy and annular dilation due to chronic atrial fibrillation.[2] Both ischemic and nonischemic MR show restrictive motion of the posterior leaflet with/without annular dilation.[3-5]

Carpientier et al.[6] classified mechanisms of MR based on the mobility of the mitral valve as:

Type 1: normal valvular movement (such as annular dilation and perforation)
Type II: excessive movement (such as prolapse, flail, and ruptured papillary muscle)
Type III: restrictive motion
Type IIIa: diastolic restriction (such as rheumatic disease and leaflet thickening)
Type IIIb: systolic restriction (such as ischemic MR)

Echocardiography is the most powerful clinical tool to investigate and differentiate the cause of mitral valve regurgitation, although in recent years, cardiac magnetic resonance (CMR) has also been validated for assessing the cause and severity of MR.[7,8]

2. CLINICAL PRESENTATION

Patients with acute severe MR often present with severe shortness of breath due to acute pulmonary congestion. Careful history taking and echocardiography can reveal the cause of acute MR, such as infective endocarditis, rupture of the chordae and tendon with/

without myocardial infraction, or trauma. On the other hand, patients with chronic severe MR may not have any symptoms for a long time. These patients are often found to have a heart murmur incidentally or during a routine physical exam and may not be aware of the cause. Fatigue, decrease in the activity level, and weakness may be initial signs of decreased forward stroke volume or low cardiac output due to severe MR and LV dysfunction. When LV dysfunction and MR severity worsen, patients may develop clear signs of congestive heart failure, including dyspnea and orthopnea.

On physical examination, most patients with severe MR have a holosystolic murmur best heard at the apex, typically radiating toward the axilla. A midsystolic click followed by late systolic murmur may be heard in a typical patient with myxomatous mitral valve prolapse without flail. The murmur may radiate to the anterior precordium or to the back, depending on the leaflet involved and direction of the regurgitant jet. When the transmitral flow is increased due to volume overload in the left atrium, a short diastolic rumble or a third heart sound may be noted at the apex. This heart sound suggests a severe degree of MR. However, many patients with severe chronic ischemic MR and LV dilation may present with subtle systolic murmurs.

The electrocardiogram is not specific for the diagnosis of MR although premature ventricular contractions are frequently noted in patients with mitral valve prolapse.[9] Chest X-ray has been used to identify cardiomegaly and pulmonary congestion. Echocardiography is the imaging modality of choice for definitive diagnosis in patients with suspected MR.

2.1. Outcomes

Without intervention, acute MR is poorly tolerated and has a poor prognosis. As for chronic MR, patients with mild to moderate MR may remain asymptomatic without any significant alteration of hemodynamics. The progression of MR severity has been studied with serial echocardiography.[10] Independent predictors of progression of mitral regurgitant severity are a new flail leaflet and dilation of the mitral annulus. Regression of MR is associated with marked changes in afterload, particularly decreased blood pressure.[10] However, effectiveness of medical management of blood pressure for improving MR remains controversial.[10,11]

In a clinical follow-up study of 456 asymptomatic patients with chronic organic MR in which echocardiography was used to quantify MR volume and effective regurgitant orifice area (EROA), the estimated 5-year rate of death was reportedly 22% ± 3% from any cause and 14% ± 3% from cardiac causes.[12] The 5-year rate of cardiac events (death from cardiac causes, heart failure, or new atrial fibrillation) was 33% ± 3%.[12] Among patients with medically managed chronic MR, the 5-year survival rate was highest (91% ± 3%) among those with a regurgitant orifice <20 mm² (mild MR) and lowest (58% ± 9%) among those with an effective orifice area of >40 mm² (severe MR). Not only the degree of MR but also age, atrial fibrillation, left atrial dilation, LV dilation, and low LV ejection fraction (LVEF) have been reported to be predictors of poor prognosis.[12,13] Overall survival in patients with severe asymptomatic organic MR undergoing mitral valve repair or replacement has been shown to be higher than the expected cumulative survival with medical therapy.[13]

As for ischemic MR, there is a body of evidence of the negative impact of chronic ischemic MR on survival in patients with CAD; the greater the degree of MR, the worse the prognosis, even in those patients with mild to moderate MR.[14–16]

3. PATHOPHYSIOLOGY

3.1. Mitral valve prolapse and flail

Mitral valve prolapse and flail are caused by myxomatous mitral valve disease and fibroelastic deficiency.[6,17] Characteristic echocardiographic features of myxomatous mitral valve are thickened, redundant leaflets and chordae with excessive motion of the leaflet into the left atrium (Figs. 30.1 and 30.2).

This condition may vary in severity and in cases with a milder degree or borderline prolapse; no significant MR is found by echocardiography. Severe prolapse or bowing of the leaflet with the tip toward the left ventricle is caused by excessive elongation of the chordae, resulting in the incompetent closure of the mitral orifice during systole and severe MR. Fibroelastic deficiency is characterized by thinner leaflets and chords. These are however histologically abnormal and typically present with chordal rupture and prolapse of the posterior leaflet, most commonly the middle scallop.[6,17,18] A large regurgitant flow convergence (FC) zone is seen in patients with severe MR (Fig. 30.3). Because of severe volume overload in such a patient, LA and LV dilation (Figs. 30.1–30.3) with high velocity of early transmitral flow (Fig. 30.4) and systolic reversal flow in the pulmonary vein (Fig. 30.5) are almost always noted by echocardiographic examination. Flail of the leaflet is caused by rupture of the chordae with the tip of the leaflet moving away from the ventricle into the left atrium during systole (Fig. 30.6). The flail condition almost always causes severe holosystolic MR.[12,19,20]

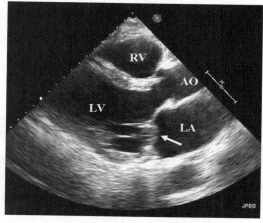

Figure 30.1 Example of transthoracic echocardiography from a patient with severe MR due to severe prolapse of the posterior leaflet *(white arrow)*. This is a parasternal long-axis view. AO, aorta; LA, left atrium; LV, left ventricle; RV, right ventricle.

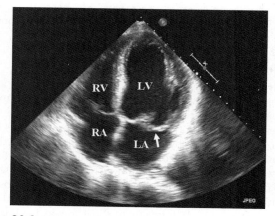

Figure 30.2 Example of a transthoracic echocardiography from a patient with severe MR due to severe prolapse of the posterior leaflet *(white arrow)*. This is an apical four-chamber view. LA, left atrium; LV, left ventricle; RA, right atrium; RV, right ventricle.

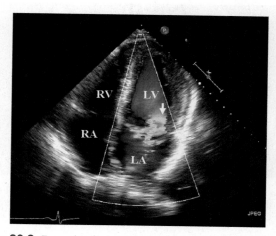

Figure 30.3 Example of a transthoracic color Doppler echocardiography from a patient with severe MR due to severe prolapse of the posterior leaflet, showing a large FC zone *(white arrow)*. This is an apical four-chamber view. LA, left atrium; LV, left ventricle; RA, right atrium; RV, right ventricle.

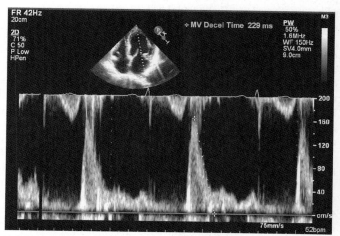

Figure 30.4 Example of pulsed Doppler echocardiography from a patient with severe MR due to severe prolapse of the posterior leaflet, showing a high early diastolic transmitral inflow velocity (160 cm/s).

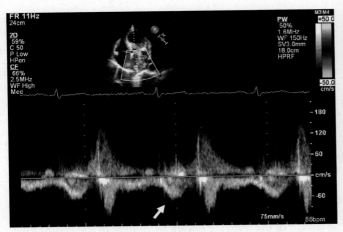

Figure 30.5 Example of pulsed Doppler echocardiography from a patient with severe MR due to severe prolapse of the posterior leaflet, showing systolic flow reversal in the right upper pulmonary vein.

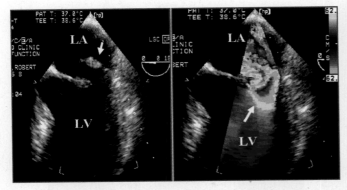

Figure 30.6 Example of TEE from a patient with severe MR due to flail of the posterior leaflet (*white arrow*, **left panel**), demonstrating a large FC zone (*white arrow*, **right panel**).

Multiplane transesophageal echocardiography (TEE) can demonstrate clear images of typical findings of mitral valve flail (Fig. 30.6) and prolapse.[21,22] Patients with severe prolapse, as well as patients with leaflet flail, show a large FC zone, which is evidence of severe MR. Two-dimensional echocardiographic images are usually sufficient to establish the anatomical diagnosis. Although prolapse may be detected in cardiac computed tomography (CCT) and CMR, the higher spatial and temporal resolution of echocardiography make it the superior imaging modality (Fig. 30.7, Movie 30.1). In selected patients, however, CMR may be useful to quantify the severity of LV dilation and MR regurgitant volume.[23] Regurgitant jets may be visualized in cine "bright-blood" images as a region of signal void produced by dephasing of the spins caused by turbulence (Figs. 30.8 and 30.9, Movies 30.2–30.5). The presence of a signal void provide accurate identification of the presence of aortic or MR with a sensitivity >93% and a specificity >89% compared to Doppler flow imaging or angiography. As with color Doppler flow imaging, the spatial distribution of the region of signal void is related to regurgitant severity, allowing separation of mild from severe degrees of regurgitation. However, the magnitude of signal void is dependent on multiple imaging parameters such as echo time and flip angle used on the acquisition sequence. Moreover, turbulence may actually decrease in the presence of severe regurgitation, where the flow becomes laminar.

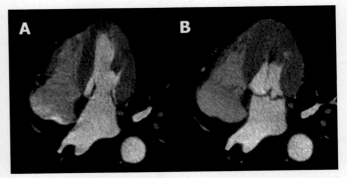

Figure 30.7 (**Movie 30.1**). End-diastolic (**A**) and end-systolic (**B**) contrast-enhanced cardiac CT images obtained from a patient with mitral valve prolapse.

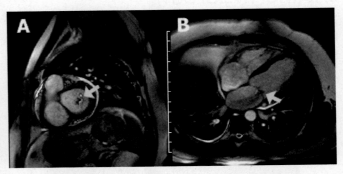

Figure 30.8 (**Movies 30.2, 30.3**). Cine-SSFP short-axis (**A**) and four-chamber CMR images (**B**) obtained from a patient with moderate MR.

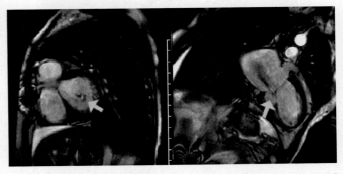

Figure 30.9 (**Movies 30.4, 30.5**). Cine-SSFP short-axis (**left panel**) and two-chamber CMR images (**right panel**) obtained from a patient with severe MR.

3.2. Infective endocarditis

Infective endocarditis is potentially one of the most fatal among all causes of MR. Echocardiography is the best imaging tool for the diagnosis of infective endocarditis along with positive blood cultures (see Chapter 32).[24–26] When infective endocarditis is suspected, echocardiography should be performed immediately. Vegetations are the most common echocardiographic findings in endocarditis of the mitral valve followed by valve prolapse secondary to chordal rupture, leaflet perforation, and annular abscess.[27] Vegetations are seen in the path of MR. However, transthoracic echocardiography is often unable to show convincing images of such abnormalities, including vegetations, especially when the vegetations are small (<3 mm).[28] TEE has been proven to be a better tool to detect and establish the existence of vegetations and abscesses.[11,28–32] When the suspicion of infective endocarditis is

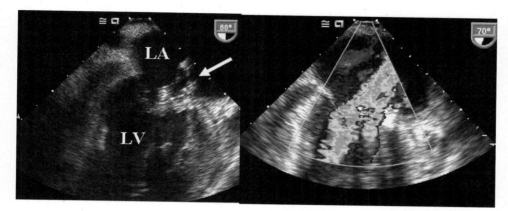

Figure 30.10 Example of TEE from a patient with severe MR due to infective endocarditis, demonstrating vegetations (*white arrow*) and multiple regurgitant jets (**right panel**). LA, left atrium, LV, left ventricle.

high, such as in patients with a prosthetic valve, previous endocarditis, new heart murmurs, intravenous drug use, and congenital heart disease, TEE is indicated as the first imaging test.[26] It is critical to demonstrate vegetations, annular abscess, and dehiscence of a prosthetic valve and new valvular regurgitation with echocardiography because these are considered to be major criteria in the diagnosis of infective endocarditis and have important implications for surgical management.[26] Even without the evidence of positive blood cultures, it is possible to establish the diagnosis of infective endocarditis with echocardiographic demonstration of the above mentioned findings with three minor criteria, including fever (body temperature > 38 °C), predisposition to endocarditis such as a predisposing heart condition or intravenous drug use, vascular phenomena such as embolism, and immunologic phenomena such as glomerulonephritis, Osler nodes, and Roth spots.[26] Considering the potentially fatal clinical scenario, early treatment with antibiotics and/or surgery based on the echocardiography findings may make the difference between life or death while awaiting confirmation with positive blood cultures.

Figure 30.10 shows the irregular shape of a large vegetation attached to the mitral valve and associated severe MR, originating from the area of the vegetation. Figure 30.11 demonstrates images of a small vegetation by 2D TEE and Figure 30.12 shows the same vegetation seen by 3D TEE. The location, size, and motion of the vegetation are more clearly visualized by 3D TEE.

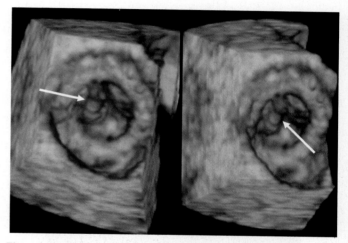

Figure 30.12 Examples of real-time 3D TEE, showing a vegetation (*white arrows*) and an annuloplasty ring. These images are from the same patient as in Figure 30.11.

3.3. Rheumatic mitral valve disease

Doming of the anterior mitral valve leaflet is the characteristic feature of rheumatic mitral valve disease. MR in patients with rheumatic mitral valve disease is caused by scarring, shortening, focal nodular formation and rigidity of the mitral valve leaflets and fusion of the chordae.[33] Dilation of the left ventricle is also reported to be a contributing factor in rheumatic MR.[34] MR is the predominant lesion in the first and second decades following an episode of rheumatic carditis, whereas the relative prevalence of stenosis increases with age.[35] Figure 30.13 demonstrates the anatomical abnormalities that are commonly found in rheumatic MR. However, it is sometimes difficult to discern the etiology because the dominant feature of the leaflet abnormality in rheumatic MR can be prolapse.[6] The presence of nodules in the anterior leaflet is a sign of rheumatic origin in patients with rheumatic MR with leaflet prolapse.[36]

3.4. Congenital anomalies

A mitral valve cleft (Fig. 30.14) is the most common congenital defect causing MR and is associated with endocardial cushion defect (see Chapter 40). In partial endocardial cushion defect, which is the combination of ostium primum atrial septal defect and mitral cleft, the degree of MR is the major determinant of symptoms. Echocardiographically there are unique features, including a posteriorly directed MR jet, as seen in Figure 30.15. The short-axis view shows a defect at the mid-part of the anterior

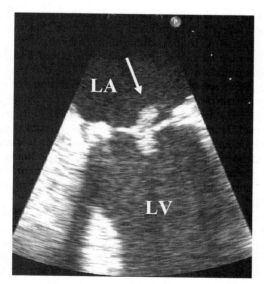

Figure 30.11 Example of TEE from a patient with infective endocarditis, demonstrating a vegetation (*white arrow*). LA, left atrium; LV, left ventricle.

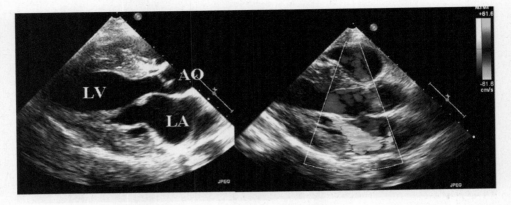

Figure 30.13 Example of transthoracic echocardiography from a patient with severe MR due to rheumatic mitral valve disease with (**right**) and without (**left**) color Doppler imaging (*white arrow*). This is a parasternal long-axis view. AO, aorta; LA, left atrium; LV, left ventricle.

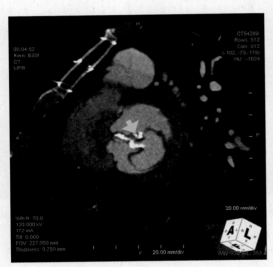

Figure 30.14 Contrast-enhanced cardiac CT short-axis image obtained from a patient with a mitral valve cleft.

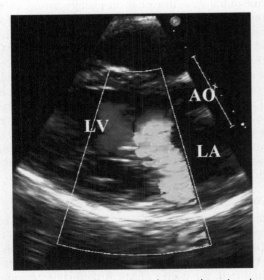

Figure 30.15 Example of color Doppler transthoracic echocardiography from a patient with severe MR due to cleft of the anterior leaflet. This is a parasternal long-axis view. AO, aorta; LA, left atrium; LV, left ventricle.

leaflet and associated severe MR, originating from the area of the cleft, as seen in Figure 30.16. Early repair is recommended for this condition.[37–39] Ostium primum atrial septal defects are better visualized with TEE than with transthoracic echocardiography as seen in Figure 30.17. Although multivariate analysis showed no predictors for MV surgery in patients with atrioventricular canal, long-term echocardiographic follow-up is warranted.[40]

3.5. Functional mitral regurgitation

3.5.1. Ischemic mitral regurgitation

As previously mentioned, ischemic MR is defined as MR caused by CAD without any anatomical abnormality of the mitral valve leaflets.[4,5] Thus, ischemic MR should be distinguished from ischemic CAD and concomitant MR due to other organic mitral valve diseases, such as myxomatous prolapse/flail, rheumatic disease, endocarditis, and severe fibrosis or calcification as mentioned above. Echocardiography can demonstrate such organic mitral valve abnormalities with ease and thus is the most powerful tool for characterizing ischemic MR. As a matter of fact, before echocardiography gained widespread popularity in the clinical setting, there were unclear or heterogeneous concepts of this entity, resulting in confusions in medical and surgical literature on the nature and prognosis or survival rate of patients with ischemic MR. Ischemic MR may have either an acute or a chronic, insidious presentation.

Acute ischemic mitral regurgitation. Acute ischemic MR is often associated with elongation or rupture of a papillary muscle following a myocardial infarction. Rupture of the papillary muscle is a rare complication of myocardial infarction, but once it occurs, the prognosis is very poor and often fatal.[41] This occurs more frequently in elderly, hypertensive patients and has significant association with ischemia/infarction of the right coronary artery and/or the left circumflex coronary artery territories, probably due to single blood supply to the posteromedial papillary muscle.[42] Without surgery, the mortality rate is 75% within 24 h and 95% within 2 weeks. Prompt recognition of this critical condition after myocardial infarction by echocardiography is thus extremely important and indeed lifesaving. Transthoracic echocardiography can show a mobile echo density attached to the LV, but these critically ill patients often have a very poor transthoracic window. Therefore, TEE is a more reliable imaging method to clearly identify a ruptured papillary muscle (Fig. 30.18).[42–45] Color Doppler echocardiography demonstrates severe MR due to the rupture of a papillary muscle.

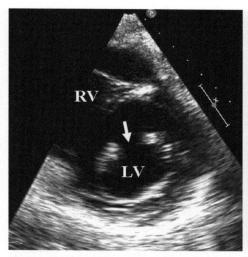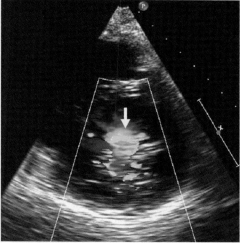

Figure 30.16 Example of transthoracic echocardiography from a patient with severe MR due to cleft of the anterior leaflet with (**right**) and without (**left**) color Doppler imaging. Cleft (*white arrow*, **left panel**) and a large FC zone (*white arrow*, **right panel**) are well appreciated. This is a parasternal short-axis view. LV, left ventricle; RV, right ventricle.

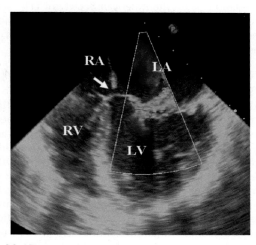

Figure 30.17 Example of TEE from a patient with severe MR due to cleft of the anterior leaflet, demonstrating a primum atrial septal defect (*white arrow*). LA, left atrium; LV, left ventricle; RA, right atrium; RV, right ventricle.

Chronic ischemic mitral regurgitation. Chronic ischemic MR is usually caused by ischemia of the right coronary artery or left circumflex artery, which causes papillary muscle dysfunction and postero–inferior LV wall motion abnormalities and LV dilation.[5] Figure 30.19 shows a typical patient with chronic ischemic MR.[46] Apically displaced mitral valve leaflets due to displaced or dysfunctional papillary muscles and hypo or akinetic inferior–posterior LV wall motion as well as mitral annular dilation are the major features.[4,5] The MR jet is usually directed posteriorly or centrally.[47] One study reported overestimation of the severity of ischemic or functional MR by the use of the color Doppler jet area method[48] while others revealed underestimation of MR volumes by the FC zone method.[49] These studies may suggest that it is imperative to use both color Doppler jet area method and the FC method to evaluate ischemic or functional MR.

3.5.2. Nonischemic functional mitral regurgitation

Functional MR in patients with dilated cardiomyopathy is caused by or associated with annular dilation, LV dilation, LV dysfunction, and apically displaced or tethered mitral valve leaflets.[5,50,51]

While the pattern of MV deformation from the medial to the lateral side was asymmetrical in some patients with ischemic MR, it is symmetrical in patients with idiopathic dilated cardiomyopathy.[5] In patients with chronic atrial fibrillation, dilated annulus may cause moderate functional MR.[2]

4. DETERMINATION OF MITRAL REGURGITATION SEVERITY

There are several echocardiographic methods for determining the severity of MR, including color Doppler jet area, proximal isovelocity surface area (PISA) or FC method, vena contracta (VC) (proximal jet width) method, and pulmonary venous flow pattern method.[52–69] MRI is also used to determine the severity of MR.[23]

4.1. Color Doppler jet area method

Many echocardiographic methods for assessing the severity of MR have been proposed and published in a variety of cardiology and ultrasound journals. Among them, the color Doppler regurgitant jet area method is most widely used for judging the severity of MR.[52,59] This visual method is historically the first one and most importantly, is very simple (Fig. 30.20).

In a previous study,[52] the best correlation with angiography was obtained when the maximal MR jet area (MJA) was expressed as a percentage of the left atrial area (LAA) obtained in the same plane. The maximum MJA/LAA was under 20% in 34 of 36 patients with angiographic grade I MR, between 20% and 40% in 17 of 18 patients with grade II MR, and over 40% in 26 of 28 patients with severe MR. Another study,[59] which also used angiography as a gold standard, demonstrated that an MJA > 8 cm² predicted severe MR with a sensitivity of 82% and specificity of 94%, whereas an MJA < 4 cm² predicted mild MR with a sensitivity and specificity of 85% and 75%, respectively. In this study, the authors also reported that the ratio of MJA/LAA provided similar sensitivity or specificity; MJA/LAA > 40% predicts severe MR with sensitivity of 73% and specificity of 92%. MJA/LAA < 20% predicts mild MR with sensitivity of 65% and specificity of 93%.

The aliasing velocity (Nyquist limit) is one of the most important factors when evaluating MJA and should be set at 50 to 60 cm/s.[70] Multiplane 2D views, including parasternal long/

Figure 30.18 Example of TEE from a patient with rupture of the papillary muscle (*white arrow*) with severe MR (**right panel**). AO, aorta; LA, left atrium; LV, left ventricle.

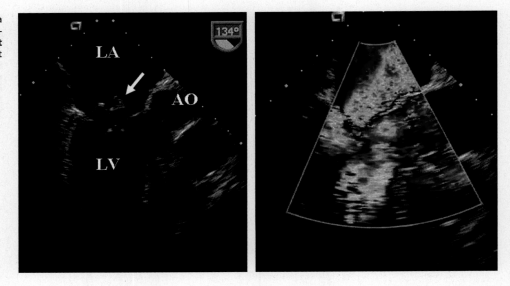

short-axis and apical views, should be used to image MR jets. However, this color Doppler method cannot be properly used in certain patients, including those with artificial valves because of significant acoustic shielding. Thus, in such patients, TEE often needs to be employed to evaluate the severity of MR. The jet area value depends on many instrumental factors such as pulse repetition frequency, aliasing velocity, imaging field, color gain, priority of tissue, and color imaging.[62] Because of these factors, especially the proximity of the imaging with less attenuation of the ultrasound, TEE may overestimate the jet area as compared to TTE imaging of the MR color jet.[71] As a matter of fact, in a previous study comparing valvular regurgitant severity by TTE and TEE, 6 patients of 13 with moderate regurgitation judged by TTE were graded as severe by TEE. Even some cases of mild or absent MR by TTE were graded as severe by TEE in this study.[71] Therefore, one cannot apply the criteria for TTE when using TEE for imaging.

Another common pitfall of the jet area method is jet eccentricity. An eccentric jet or wall impinging jet appears to be much smaller (as much as 40%) than a central jet area even when the regurgitant volume/fraction is the same as that of a central jet.[57] Accordingly, only weak correlations have been reported between jet area and regurgitant volumes in previous echocardiographic studies.[62] An eccentric, wall-impinging jet swirling in the LA is considered to be severe irrespective of its jet area according to the

recommendations from the American Society of Echocardiography.[57,70] Color Doppler 3D echocardiography may demonstrate the entire jet extension without requiring multiple planes or mental reconstruction (Fig. 30.21).[49,72,73]

4.2. Proximal isovelocity surface area or flow convergence method

Major advantages of the PISA or the FC method, over the color jet area method are as follows. First, this method is not influenced by color gain. Thus, one can increase color gain as much as needed to see the FC surface. Secondly, this method is not significantly affected by eccentricity of the MR jet. Once one optimizes the PISA or the FC region, one can judge the severity of MR irrespective of pattern or size of jet extension (Fig. 30.22). More importantly, this method can provide a truly quantitative assessment of regurgitant volume and regurgitant orifice area, while the color jet area method cannot. When we assume the shape of the FC zone is a hemisphere, the maximal area of the FC zone (S) is calculated as $2\pi r^2$ (r, maximal aliasing distance from the regurgitant orifice, cm). Thus, the peak regurgitant flow rate Q (mL/s) is calculated as S (cm^2) × V (aliasing velocity cm/s) = $2\pi r^2$ × V. The duration of the peak regurgitant flow rate T is calculated as T = VTI/V_{max} (VTI, the velocity time integral of MR jet, cm; V_{max}, the peak regurgitant velocity, cm/s). The regurgitant volume is calculated as (the peak regurgitant flow rate) ×

Figure 30.19 Example of TEE from a patient with severe MR due to the restrictive motion of the posterior leaflet (*white arrow*, **left panel**). The regurgitant jet is eccentric and directed posteriorly. Note a large FC toward the regurgitant orifice (*white arrow*, **right panel**).

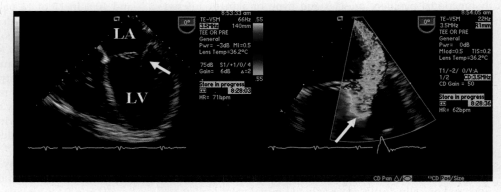

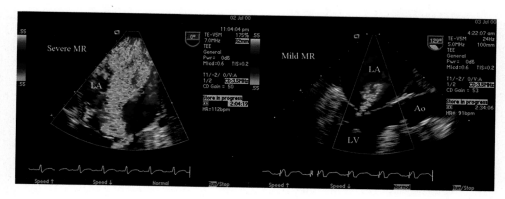

Figure 30.20 Pre (**left panel**) and post (**right panel**) repair of the mitral valve in a patient with severe MR due to a restrictive motion of the mitral valve leaflets and dilated annulus. Note the remarkable reduction of the color jet area of the regurgitation after the repair (**from left panel to right panel**).

(the duration of the peak regurgitant flow rate) which is $Q \times T = S \times V \times T = 2\pi r^2 \times V \times VTI/V_{max}$ (mL). The EROA (in square centimeter) = regurgitant volume/VTI = $2\pi r^2 \times V/V_{max}$. When the aliasing velocity is selected 40 cm/s and V_{max} (CW peak velocity of MR jet) is assumed to be 5 or 500 cm/s, EROA = $2 \times 3.14 \times 40$ (cm/s) r^2/500 cm/s = $0.5 \times r^2$ (cm^2) = $r^2/2$. However, when MR is severe, the shape and size of the PISA may not be very clear with 40 cm/s of aliasing velocity. Higher aliasing velocities such as 60 cm/s may be more appropriate to determine the maximal size of the PISA for accurate measurement of EROA and regurgitant volume with the use of the general equation.

Even when we do not apply a quantitative assessment of valvular regurgitation, the maximal size of FC aliasing distance may be sufficient to judge MR severity. When one does not see an FC diameter >4 mm at a Nyquist of 40 cm/s, the regurgitation is trivial or at most mild (or effective regurgitant orifice, EROA < 0.2 cm^2). When we see an FC diameter larger than 8 mm at an aliasing velocity > 50 cm/s (EROA > 0.4 cm^2), the regurgitation is severe.[63] All regurgitation in between are deemed moderate.[70]

This conventional 2D FC method is easy to apply and thus is recommended when one only needs to judge the severity of valvular regurgitation quantitatively as recommended by the American Society of Echocardiography.[70]

The 2D FC method assumes a hemispheric shape of the FC surface to assess MR severity, and thus the method has limitations when the FC shape is not hemispheric. Real-time 3D color Doppler echocardiography, which is now available, can overcome this limitation, allowing a more accurate assessment of MR severity. In one recent investigation with real-time 3D echocardiography with color Doppler capability, the geometry of the FC surface in functional MR was elongated, distinctly different from the more focal pathology of mitral valve prolapse (Figs. 30.23 to 30.25), leading to underestimation of the severity of MR when using the PISA method.[49]

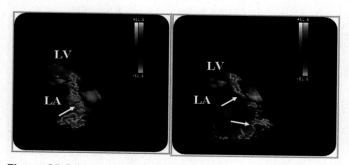

Figure 30.21 Examples of transthoracic color Doppler 3D echocardiography from a patient with severe MR. MR jet extensions viewed from the left atrium in two different cardiac phases. Note that the jet extension changes during the cardiac cycle.

4.3. Vena contracta (proximal jet width) method

This method is another echo/Doppler technique for grading and quantifying the severity of MR (Fig. 30.26).[67,61,68] Color Doppler VC is defined as the diameter at the connection of the regurgitant jet and the flow acceleration zone. In order to find the VC, one may start to see FC and look for a regurgitant jet while still keeping the FC image on the monitor. In this manner, one can find the connection between the FC and regurgitant jet. Width of the VC < 0.3 cm is considered to be mild MR and ≥0.7 cm is considered severe.[70] This method is not quite as easy as the jet area or FC method in day-to-day practice probably because of the technical difficulty to demonstrate a clear VC. However, when a high resolution image of VC is available, especially by TEE, as seen in Figure 30.25, this may be a useful alternative to the FC and color jet area methods. In a clinical TEE study, a diameter > 0.55 cm was suggestive of severe MR although the authors did not express their "regurgitant jet width at its origin" as VC.[65] Accuracy of the measurement of VC depends on how the VC is cut in the 2D plane. Therefore, color Doppler 3D echocardiography can potentially provide a more precise location, shape, and size of VC.

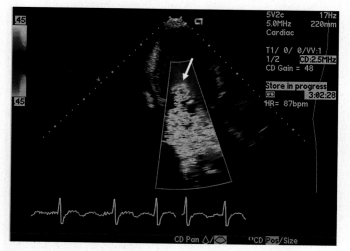

Figure 30.22 Example of the FC (*arrow*) toward the mitral regurgitant orifice or PISA from a patient with severe MR due to mitral valve prolapse.

Figure 30.23 Examples of transthoracic color Doppler 3D echocardiography from a patient with severe ischemic MR. Rotated views of an FC zone. Note the rounded shape of FC in the **left panel** and the elongated shape in the **mid** and **right panels**. LA, left atrium; LV, left ventricle.

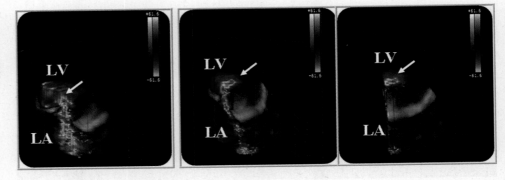

Figure 30.24 Examples of transthoracic color Doppler 3D echocardiography from a patient with severe MR due to prolapse. Note a rounded shape of the FC zone in all views.

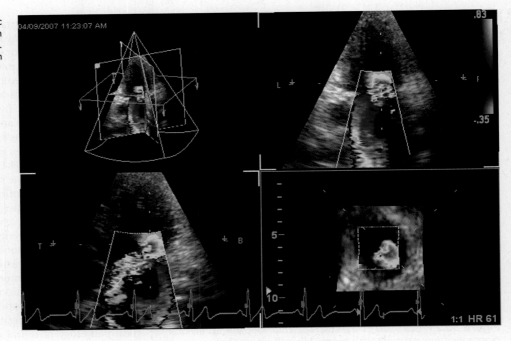

Figure 30.25 Examples of transthoracic color Doppler 3D echocardiography from a patient with severe ischemic MR. Note an elongated shape of the FC zone, especially on the right upper panel.

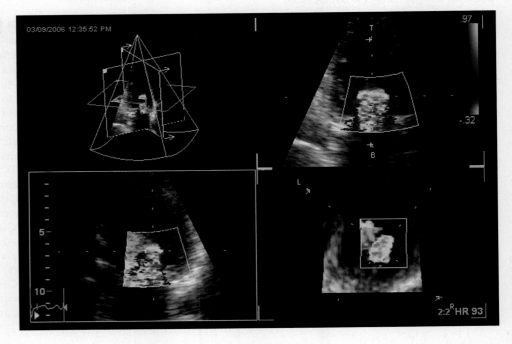

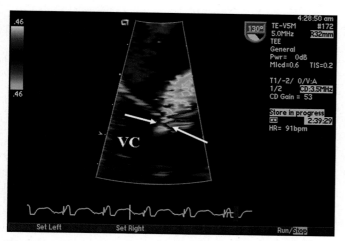

Figure 30.26 An example of VC imaging (*arrow*) from a patient with mild MR.

4.4. Pulmonary venous flow

Pulmonary venous flow patterns recorded by the pulsed Doppler method are another aid for grading the severity of MR. In one of the earliest clinical studies, 26 (93%) of 28 patients with severe regurgitation by transesophageal color flow mapping had reversed systolic flow (Fig. 30.27). The sensitivity of reversed systolic flow in detecting severe 4+ MR by transesophageal color flow mapping was 93% and the specificity was 100%.[58] However, this flow pattern may be influenced by the location of the sampling site or selection of the four pulmonary vein interrogated and LV performance.[66] Pulmonary venous flow reversal is more common in acute than in chronic MR, since LA size and compliance also determine the presence and magnitude of flow reversal.

4.5. Other imaging methods

As a result of volume overloading, in patients with severe MR, LV and LA sizes are increased and early diastolic trans-mitral flow (E wave) velocity is also increased.[69] Dense CW Doppler signal of MR is also expected in severe MR.[74] Such echo indices should be sought and systematically assessed when one finalizes the judgment of the severity of MR. Also CMR can determine the location

and severity of MR. In the presence of isolated MR, regurgitant volume may be calculated as the difference between left and right ventricular stroke volumes and regurgitant fraction as the ratio of LV to RV stroke volumes. Most commonly, MR regurgitant volume is determined as the difference between ventricular stroke volume and phase-contrast velocity determined forward trans-valvular flow (Figs. 30.28 and 30.29). From a stack of 10 to 20 contiguous 5 to 10 mm thick short-axis images acquired from the base to the apex of the LV, during breath-holding, the images are traced off-line for volumetric quantification based on Simpson's rule. CMR has been shown to determine regurgitant fractions with 90% accuracy compared with radionuclide ventriculography and echocardiography.

The evaluation of regurgitant lesions by CCT is limited since regurgitant flow cannot be visualized. However, in isolated MR, regurgitant volume and fraction can be derived from the difference between the left and right ventricular stroke volumes.

5. TREATMENT

5.1. Medical management

Clinical studies in patients with organic MR reported decrease in MR severity with the use of angiotensin converting enzyme inhibitor.[75–77] However, these studies were relatively small (the number of patients studied were between 11 and 23) and follow-up was limited to 52 weeks. Thus, due to lack of large and long-term follow-up studies, no medical therapy seems definitively indicated or effective in asymptomatic patients with chronic organic MR and normal LV function except in the presence of systemic hypertension.[11] In recent studies, carvedilol[78] and cardiac resynchronization therapy have reportedly decreased functional MR in patients with LV dysfunction.[79–82]

5.2. Surgical management

As a general rule, surgery is indicated when echocardiography shows severe MR and the patient has symptoms or when he or she is hemodynamically unstable.[11,83] In symptomatic (NYHA class III/VI) patients with organic MR, postoperative survival rate was reportedly much worse (48% ± 4% in 10 years) than that (76% ± 5% in 10 years) in asymptomatic or minimally symptomatic (NYHA class I/II) patients.[84] Thus, even when the patient is asymptomatic and hemodynamically stable, surgery may be

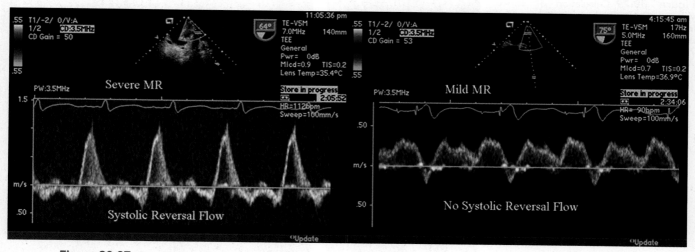

Figure 30.27 Comparison of pulmonary venous flow pattern between pre (**left panel**) and post (**right panel**) repair of the mitral valve in a patient with severe MR. Note the remarkable change of the pattern (see text) after the repair. From the same patient as in Figure 30.24.

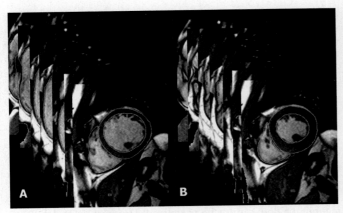

Figure 30.28 Stacked end-diastolic **(A)** and end-systolic **(B)** cine SSFP short-axis images used to calculate LV volumes.

considered when successful mitral valve repair is expected for severe MR.[11,84] For example, surgical repair for mitral valve prolapse and flail is often successful in major reference heart centers[85,86] while successful valve repair is less likely in cases that are rheumatic, infective, ischemic, or when significant calcification is present.

5.2.1. Surgical consideration for asymptomatic patients

One of the major concerns in asymptomatic MR patients who are followed medically is latent LV dysfunction that is predictive of poor prognosis after MV surgery but may not be detected with resting echocardiography. Thus, stress echocardiography may be of value in disclosing latent LV dysfunction in minimally symptomatic patients with MR.[87–89] Latent LV dysfunction reportedly manifests only at exercise as an inadequate increase in ejection fraction and a larger end-systolic volume. These variables may also be useful to predict LV dysfunction after repair.[89]

Figure 30.30 shows the recommendation of the AHA/ACC and European guidelines for asymptomatic chronic severe MR. Based on these guidelines, surgical correction, whether mitral valve

repair or replacement, should be considered when echocardiography shows dilated LV (endosystolic diameter > 40 to 45 mm) or LVEF < 60% in asymptomatic patients with chronic severe MR. When LVEF is >60% with LVESD < 40 to 45 mm, surgery should be considered only when the patient has new onset of atrial fibrillation or pulmonary hypertension (systolic pulmonary artery pressure > 50 or > 60 mmHg with exercise) and also when mitral valve repair is likely to be successful.[11,83]

However, Enriquez-Sarano et al.[12] reported that cardiac surgery was independently associated with improved survival in 232 asymptomatic patients with organic MR and normal LV function (mitral valve repair in 209 patients). Considering the poor 5-year survival rate in patients with an effective regurgitant orifice of at least 40 mm², they concluded that such severe MR patients should promptly be considered for cardiac surgery.[12] This recommendation naturally leads to earlier surgery than the conditions of the ACC/AHA and European guidelines (namely, LVEF < 60%, LVESD > 40 to 45 mm, atrial fibrillation, and pulmonary hypertension).[11,83] Also when the patient has flail mitral valve, the group from Mayo Clinic recommended early surgery independent of the guidelines because of an improved long-term survival rate, decreased cardiac mortality, and decreased morbidity by mitral valve repair.[90,91]

By contrast, Rosenhek et al.[13] studied 132 consecutive asymptomatic MR patients prospectively and reported extremely high overall survival rate of 91% ± 3% at 8 years without surgery. This study included patients with flail and even in the group with flail, 52% of patients did not reach the defined criteria for surgery at 8 years.[13] Thus, they recommended adherence (not earlier surgery) to the ACC/AHA and European guidelines.[13]

5.2.2. Other factors affecting surgical results

It is imperative to remember that surgical result is heavily dependent on the level of experience of surgeons, cardiologists, and cardiac anesthesiologists.[92] Intraoperative TEE is widely used in reference heart centers for monitoring the result of the surgery and reportedly improves surgical outcomes.[86,93,94] When MR with at least moderate degree is found in the operating room by TEE, a second pump run to redo repair may be attempted to ensure success.

Figure 30.29 Calculation of stroke volume **(C)** from the velocity-encoded images **(B)** obtained at the level of the ascending aorta **(A)**. (See Chapters 6 and 7 for details).

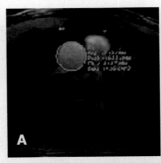

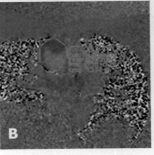

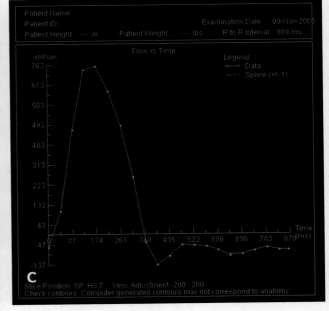

Asymptomatic Chronic Severe MR

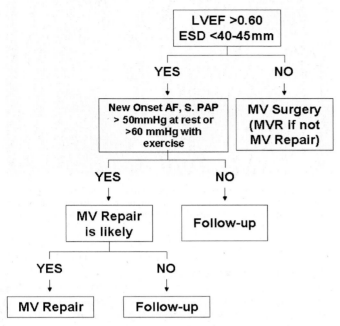

Figure 30.30 Management strategy for patients with asymptomatic chronic severe MR. AF, atrial fibrillation; ESD, end-systolic diameter; LVEF, left ventricular ejection fraction; MR, mitral regurgitation; MVR, mitral valve replacement; sPAP, systolic pulmonary artery pressure.

Recently developed real-time 3D TEE provides unprecedented clear images of the mitral valve, both of normal (Fig. 30.31) and mitral valve prolapse (MVP) (Fig. 30.32).[95] Figure 30.33 demonstrates successful mitral valve repair with an annuloplasty ring. With such technological developments in echocardiography and MRI/CT, specialized cardiologists will be able to obtain detailed anatomical information of more complex mitral valve pathologies and share patient experiences with skilled valve surgeons. With technological advancement and the combined efforts of skilled cardiologists and surgeons, mitral valve repair will surely be more successful in the near future.[18,92]

5.2.3. Mitral regurgitation due to degenerative disease (prolapse and flail)

Expected survival rate after mitral valve repair in patients with mitral valve prolapse and flail is excellent in "reference" heart centers.[85,86,96] In particular, mitral valve repair for posterior leaflet prolapse is more successful (10 years durability is 98%) than anterior leaflet prolapse.[86] Failure of mitral valve repair is usually attributed to the absence of an annuloplasty ring (on initial or earlier surgery), residual prolapse, suture dehiscence, interscallop

malcoaptation, and occurrence of postoperative systolic anterior motion of the mitral valve.[94,97,98]

5.2.4. Mitral regurgitation due to infective endocarditis

Valve surgery for patients with complicated, left-sided native valve endocarditis (namely, not only mitral valve disease but also

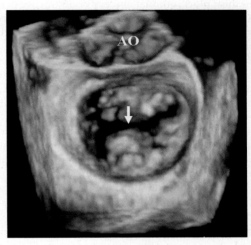

Figure 30.32 Example of real-time 3D TEE, showing a large segment of prolapse of the posterior leaflet (*white arrow*). This is the so-called surgical or *en face* view from the left atrium.

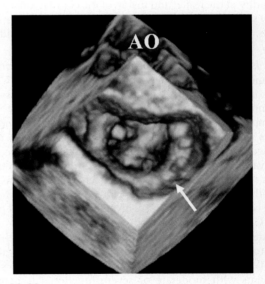

Figure 30.33 Example of real-time 3D TEE, showing an annuloplasty ring after mitral valve repair. This is the so-called surgical or *en face* view from the left atrium. AO, aorta.

Figure 30.31 Example of real-time 3D TEE, showing a normal mitral valve during three different cardiac timings. This is the so-called surgical or *en face* view from the left atrium.

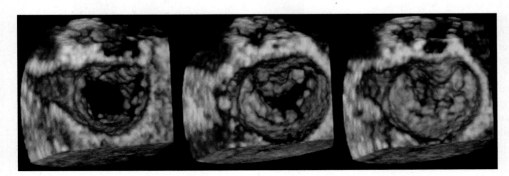

aortic valve disease) was independently associated with reduced 6-month mortality. The reduced mortality was particularly evident among patients with moderate to severe congestive heart failure.[99] Thus, surgery should not be delayed in patients with acute endocarditis when congestive heart failure develops.[26] Also surgery is indicated for native valve endocarditis patients with elevated LV end-diastolic or left atrial pressure or moderate or severe pulmonary hypertension with fungal or highly resistant organisms, heat block, annular abscess, or destructive penetrating lesions (Class I).[11] In prosthetic valve endocarditis, surgery is indicated for patients with dehiscence, worsening MR, and abscess formation (all Class I).[11]

Mitral valve replacement is performed in most patients with infective endocarditis and severe MR.[99,100] However, mitral valve repair using Carpentier's techniques in patients with active endocarditis has reportedly had very good long-term results with a low rate of recurrence or reoperation.[27]

The size of the vegetation seems to predict the occurrence of complications.[101] In one echocardiographic study, patients with a vegetation diameter >10 mm had a significantly higher incidence of embolic events than did those with a vegetation diameter ≤10 mm.[31] However, surgical indication simply due to the size of the vegetation remains controversial.

5.2.5. Rheumatic mitral regurgitation

As for surgical intervention in patients with rheumatic MR, the results of mitral valve repair are often satisfactory.[102] However, severe leaflet and chordal deformation, including calcification and rigidity of the leaflet and fusion of the chordae, are predictive of early surgical failure and late recurrence, and therefore in such patients, replacement of the mitral valve should be considered.[102]

5.2.6. Ischemic or functional mitral regurgitation

Percutaneous coronary intervention, CABG, or CABG with MV surgery in patients with ischemic MR was reportedly associated with improved survival compared with medical therapy.[103] Studies comparing CABG with and without mitral valve surgery in patients with significant ischemic MR with decreased EF showed improved survival rate in patients who underwent concomitant mitral valve surgery.[104] In another study, moderate ischemic MR did not reliably resolve with CABG surgery alone and was associated with reduced survival.[105] Therefore, a mitral valve procedure may be considered for patients with at least moderate MR presenting for CABG.[105]

In another study, however, mitral valve surgery with CABG was not associated with improved survival versus CABG alone.[103] Also, MV repair with CABG did not improve long-term survival in patients with moderate or severe functional ischemic MR although it may reduce postoperative MR and improve early symptoms compared with CABG alone.[106,107] MV annuloplasty alone without addressing fundamental ventricular pathology may be insufficient to improve long-term clinical outcomes.[107] Thus, new approaches to ischemic MR that address LV remodeling have been proposed recently.[108,109] As an alternative to surgical correction, percutaneous catheter-based procedures for eliminating or reducing ischemic or functional MR have been reported recently.[110–112]

As for residual MR after restrictive annuloplasty, echocardiography was used to predict the result of surgical repair for functional or ischemic MR.[47,51] A higher mitral annular diameter, larger tethering area, and greater MR severity are identified as independent predictors for failure of MV repair.[47,51]

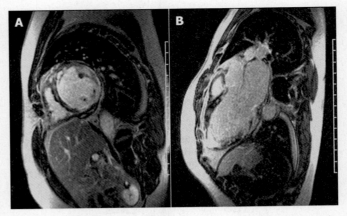

Figure 30.34 CMR turbo-spin echo images obtained post gadolinium injection demonstrating extensive myocardial fibrosis in a patient with cardiomyopathy and severe MR. (**A**) short axis; (**B**) long axis view.

CMR has been proven to be useful in patients with ischemic MR to detect viable myocardium.[113,114] Because the recurrence of ischemic MR is associated with LV dysfunction or remodeling after surgery,[115] the ability of CMR to detect myocardial viability and predict the recovery of myocardial function after CABG is of quintessential value (Fig. 30.34).

6. FUTURE DIRECTIONS

New 3D imaging technologies, including real-time 3D TEE, are gaining widespread acceptance not only in the field of noninvasive cardiology but also in invasive cardiology and surgery. Further developments of real-time 3D technology with color Doppler capability along with refined high temporal resolution CCT and CMR, demonstrating virtual reality of the mitral valve anatomy, certainly enhance diagnostic capabilities (Fig. 30.35). As for management of MR patients, less invasive approaches of surgery are now available, including robotic approaches. Also, multiple percutaneous catheter-based approaches are on the horizon. In the near future, these new less invasive management strategies may change the timing of surgery in asymptomatic patients, which is currently quite controversial.

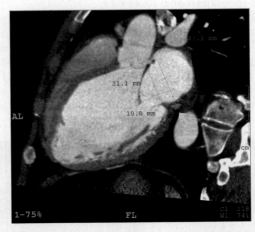

Figure 30.35 Contrast-enhanced CT long-axis image obtained from a patient with dilated cardiomyopathy being considered for percutaneous mitral annuloplasty demonstrating the anatomic relationship of the coronary sinus.

REFERENCES

1. Olson LJ, Subramanian R, Ackermann DM, et al. Surgical pathology of the mitral valve: A study of 712 cases spanning 21 years. *Mayo Clin Proc.* 1987;62:22–34.
2. Tanimoto M, Pai RG. Effect of isolated left atrial enlargement on mitral annular size and valve competence. *Am J Cardiol.* 1996;77:769–774.
3. Otsuji Y, Handschumacher MD, Schwammenthal E, et al. Insights from three-dimensional echocardiography into the mechanism of functional mitral regurgitation: Direct in vivo demonstration of altered leaflet tethering geometry. *Circulation.* 1997;96:1999–2008.
4. Otsuji Y, Handschumacher MD, Liel-Cohen N, et al. Mechanism of ischemic mitral regurgitation with segmental left ventricular dysfunction: Three-dimensional echocardiographic studies in models of acute and chronic progressive regurgitation. *J Am Coll Cardiol.* 2001;37:641–648.
5. Kwan J, Shiota T, Agler DA, et al. Geometric differences of the mitral apparatus between ischemic and dilated cardiomyopathy with significant mitral regurgitation: Real-time three-dimensional echocardiography study. *Circulation.* 2003;107:1135–1140.
6. Carpentier A, Chauvaud S, Fabiani JN, et al. Reconstructive surgery of mitral valve incompetence: Ten-year appraisal. *J Thorac Cardiovasc Surg.* 1980;79:338–348.
7. D'Ancona G, Biondo D, Mamone G, et al. Ischemic mitral valve regurgitation in patients with depressed ventricular function: Cardiac geometrical and myocardial perfusion evaluation with magnetic resonance imaging. *Eur J Cardiothorac Surg.* 2008;34:964–968.
8. D'Ancona G, Mamone G, Marrone G, et al. Ischemic mitral valve regurgitation: The new challenge for magnetic resonance imaging. *Eur J Cardiothorac Surg.* 2007;32:475–480.
9. Shiota T, Sakamoto T, Hada Y, et al. Prevalence of mitral valve prolapse in patients with premature ventricular contractions and the relationship between the prolapse and the types of premature contractions. *J Cardiol.* 1989;19:499–504.
10. Enriquez-Sarano M, Basmadjian AJ, Rossi A, et al. Progression of mitral regurgitation: A prospective Doppler echocardiographic study. *J Am Coll Cardiol.* 1999;34:1137–1144.
11. Bonow RO, Carabello BA, Chatterjee K, et al. 2008 Focused Update Incorporated Into the ACC/AHA 2006 Guidelines for the Management of Patients With Valvular Heart Disease A Report of the American College of Cardiology/American Heart Association Task Force on Practice Guidelines (Writing Committee to Revise the 1998 Guidelines for the Management of Patients With Valvular Heart Disease) Endorsed by the Society of Cardiovascular Anesthesiologists, Society for Cardiovascular Angiography and Interventions, and Society of Thoracic Surgeons. *J Am Coll Cardiol.* 2008;52:e1–e142.
12. Enriquez-Sarano M, Avierinos JF, Messika-Zeitoun D, et al. Quantitative determinants of the outcome of asymptomatic mitral regurgitation. *N Engl J Med.* 2005;352:875–883.
13. Rosenhek R, Rader F, Klaar U, et al. Outcome of watchful waiting in asymptomatic severe mitral regurgitation. *Circulation.* 2006;113:2238–2244.
14. Grigioni F, Enriquez-Sarano M, Zehr KJ, et al. Ischemic mitral regurgitation: Long-term outcome and prognostic implications with quantitative Doppler assessment. *Circulation.* 2001;103:1759–1764.
15. Trichon BH, Felker GM, Shaw LK, et al. Relation of frequency and severity of mitral regurgitation to survival among patients with left ventricular systolic dysfunction and heart failure. *Am J Cardiol.* 2003;91:538–543.
16. Grigioni F, Detaint D, Avierinos JF, et al. Contribution of ischemic mitral regurgitation to congestive heart failure after myocardial infarction. *J Am Coll Cardiol.* 2005;45:260–267.
17. Anyanwu AC, Adams DH. Etiologic classification of degenerative mitral valve disease: Barlow's disease and fibroelastic deficiency. *Semin Thorac Cardiovasc Surg.* 2007;19:90–96.
18. Adams DH, Anyanwu AC, Sugeng L, et al. Degenerative mitral valve regurgitation: Surgical echocardiography. *Curr Cardiol Rep.* 2008;10:226–232.
19. Grigioni F, Enriquez-Sarano M, Ling LH, et al. Sudden death in mitral regurgitation due to flail leaflet. *J Am Coll Cardiol.* 1999;34:2078–2085.
20. Enriquez-Sarano M, Tajik AJ. Natural history of mitral regurgitation due to flail leaflets. *Eur Heart J.* 1997;18:705–707.
21. Fehske W, Grayburn PA, Omran H, et al. Morphology of the mitral valve as displayed by multiplane transesophageal echocardiography. *J Am Soc Echocardiogr.* 1994;7:472–479.
22. Chaudhry FA, Upadya SP, Singh VP, et al. Identifying patients with degenerative mitral regurgitation for mitral valve repair and replacement: A transesophageal echocardiographic study. *J Am Soc Echocardiogr.* 2004;17:988–994.
23. Sechtem U, Pflugfelder PW, Cassidy MM, et al. Mitral or aortic regurgitation: Quantification of regurgitant volumes with cine MR imaging. *Radiology.* 1988;167:425–430.
24. Durack DT, Lukes AS, Bright DK. New criteria for diagnosis of infective endocarditis: Utilization of specific echocardiographic findings. Duke Endocarditis Service. *Am J Med.* 1994;96:200–209.
25. Lukes AS, Bright DK, Durack DT. Diagnosis of infective endocarditis. *Infect Dis Clin North Am.* 1993;7:1–8.
26. Baddour LM, Wilson WR, Bayer AS, et al. Infective endocarditis: Diagnosis, antimicrobial therapy, and management of complications: A statement for healthcare professionals from the Committee on Rheumatic Fever, Endocarditis, and Kawasaki Disease, Council on Cardiovascular Disease in the Young, and the Councils on Clinical Cardiology, Stroke, and Cardiovascular Surgery and Anesthesia, American Heart Association: Endorsed by the Infectious Diseases Society of America. *Circulation.* 2005;111:e394–e434.
27. Zegdi R, Debieche M, Latremouille C, et al. Long-term results of mitral valve repair in active endocarditis. *Circulation.* 2005;111:2532–2536.
28. Daniel WG, Mugge A, Martin RP, et al. Improvement in the diagnosis of abscesses associated with endocarditis by transesophageal echocardiography. *N Engl J Med.* 1991;324:795–800.
29. Matsuzaki M, Toma Y, Kusukawa R. Clinical applications of transesophageal echocardiography. *Circulation.* 1990;82:709–722.
30. Hill EE, Herijgers P, Claus P, et al. Abscess in infective endocarditis: The value of transesophageal echocardiography and outcome: A 5-year study. *Am Heart J.* 2007;154:923–928.
31. Mugge A, Daniel WG, Frank G, et al. Echocardiography in infective endocarditis: Reassessment of prognostic implications of vegetation size determined by the transthoracic and the transesophageal approach. *J Am Coll Cardiol.* 1989;14:631–638.
32. Taams MA, Gussenhoven EJ, Bos E, et al. Enhanced morphological diagnosis in infective endocarditis by transoesophageal echocardiography. *Br Heart J.* 1990;63:109–113.
33. Ortiz E, Somerville J. Assessment by cross sectional echocardiography of surgical "mitral valve" disease in children and adolescents. *Br Heart J.* 1986;56:267–271.
34. Vasan RS, Shrivastava S, Vijayakumar M, et al. Echocardiographic evaluation of patients with acute rheumatic fever and rheumatic carditis. *Circulation.* 1996;94:73–82.
35. Marcus RH, Sareli P, Pocock WA, et al. The spectrum of severe rheumatic mitral valve disease in a developing country: Correlations among clinical presentation, surgical pathologic findings, and hemodynamic sequelae. *Ann Intern Med.* 1994;120:177–183.
36. Atalay S, Ucar T, Ozcelik N, et al. Echocardiographic evaluation of mitral valve in patients with pure rheumatic mitral regurgitation. *Turk J Pediatr.* 2007;49:148–153.
37. Bender HW Jr, Hammon JW Jr, Hubbard SG, et al. Repair of atrioventricular canal malformation in the first year of life. *J Thorac Cardiovasc Surg.* 1982;84:515–522.
38. Abbruzzese PA, Livermore J, Sunderland CO, et al. Mitral repair in complete atrioventricular canal: Ease of correction in early infancy. *J Thorac Cardiovasc Surg.* 1983;85:388–395.
39. Michielon G, Stellin G, Rizzoli G, et al. Left atrioventricular valve incompetence after repair of common atrioventricular canal defects. *Ann Thorac Surg.* 1995;60:S604–S609.
40. Fraisse A, Massih TA, Kreitmann B, et al. Characteristics and management of cleft mitral valve. *J Am Coll Cardiol.* 2003;42:1988–1993.
41. Replogle RL, Campbell CD. Surgery for mitral regurgitation associated with ischemic heart disease: Results and strategies. *Circulation.* 1989;79:I122–I125.
42. Manning WJ, Waksmonski CA, Boyle NG. Papillary muscle rupture complicating inferior myocardial infarction: Identification with transesophageal echocardiography. *Am Heart J.* 1995;129:191–193.
43. Patel AM, Miller FA Jr, Khandheria BK, et al. Role of transesophageal echocardiography in the diagnosis of papillary muscle rupture secondary to myocardial infarction. *Am Heart J.* 1989;118:1330–1333.
44. Stoddard MF, Keedy DL, Kupersmith J. Transesophageal echocardiographic diagnosis of papillary muscle rupture complicating acute myocardial infarction. *Am Heart J.* 1990;120:690–692.
45. Moursi MH, Bhatnagar SK, Vilacosta I, et al. Transesophageal echocardiographic assessment of papillary muscle rupture. *Circulation.* 1996;94:1003–1009.
46. Levine RA, Hung J, Otsuji Y, et al. Mechanistic insights into functional mitral regurgitation. *Curr Cardiol Rep.* 2002;4:125–129.
47. Kongsaerepong V, Shiota M, Gillinov AM, et al. Echocardiographic predictors of successful versus unsuccessful mitral valve repair in ischemic mitral regurgitation. *Am J Cardiol.* 2006;98:504–508.
48. McCully RB, Enriquez-Sarano M, Tajik AJ, et al. Overestimation of severity of ischemic/functional mitral regurgitation by color Doppler jet area. *Am J Cardiol.* 1994;74:790–793.
49. Matsumura Y, Fukuda S, Tran H, et al. Geometry of the proximal isovelocity surface area in mitral regurgitation by 3-dimensional color Doppler echocardiography: Difference between functional mitral regurgitation and prolapse regurgitation. *Am Heart J.* 2008;155:231–238.
50. Boltwood CM, Tei C, Wong M, et al. Quantitative echocardiography of the mitral complex in dilated cardiomyopathy: The mechanism of functional mitral regurgitation. *Circulation.* 1983;68:498–508.
51. Calafiore AM, Gallina S, Di Mauro M, et al. Mitral valve procedure in dilated cardiomyopathy: Repair or replacement? *Ann Thorac Surg.* 2001;71:1146–1152; Discussion 1152–1153.
52. Helmcke F, Nanda NC, Hsiung MC, et al. Color Doppler assessment of mitral regurgitation with orthogonal planes. *Circulation.* 1987;75:175–183.
53. Bargiggia GS, Tronconi L, Sahn DJ, et al. A new method for quantitation of mitral regurgitation based on color flow Doppler imaging of flow convergence proximal to regurgitant orifice. *Circulation.* 1991;84:1481–1489.
54. Recusani F, Bargiggia GS, Yoganathan AP, et al. A new method for quantification of regurgitant flow rate using color Doppler flow imaging of the flow convergence region proximal to a discrete orifice: An in vitro study. *Circulation.* 1991;83:594–604.
55. Utsunomiya T, Ogawa T, Tang HA, et al. Doppler color flow mapping of the proximal isovelocity surface area: A new method for measuring volume flow rate across a narrowed orifice. *J Am Soc Echocardiogr.* 1991;4:338–348.
56. Utsunomiya T, Ogawa T, Doshi R, et al. Doppler color flow "proximal isovelocity surface area" method for estimating volume flow rate: Effects of orifice shape and machine factors. *J Am Coll Cardiol.* 1991;17:1103–1111.

57. Chen CG, Thomas JD, Anconina J, et al. Impact of impinging wall jet on color Doppler quantification of mitral regurgitation. *Circulation*. 1991;84:712–720.

58. Klein AL, Obarski TP, Stewart WJ, et al. Transesophageal Doppler echocardiography of pulmonary venous flow: A new marker of mitral regurgitation severity. *J Am Coll Cardiol*. 1991;18:518–526.

59. Spain MG, Smith MD, Grayburn PA, et al. Quantitative assessment of mitral regurgitation by Doppler color flow imaging: Angiographic and hemodynamic correlations. *J Am Coll Cardiol*. 1989;13:585–590.

60. Vandervoort PM, Rivera JM, Mele D, et al. Application of color Doppler flow mapping to calculate effective regurgitant orifice area: An in vitro study and initial clinical observations. *Circulation*. 1993;88:1150–1156.

61. Fehske W, Omran H, Manz M, et al. Color-coded Doppler imaging of the vena contracta as a basis for quantification of pure mitral regurgitation. *Am J Cardiol*. 1994;73:268–274.

62. Shiota T, Jones M, Teien D, et al. Color Doppler regurgitant jet area for evaluating eccentric mitral regurgitation: An animal study with quantified mitral regurgitation. *J Am Coll Cardiol*. 1994;24:813–819.

63. Shiota T, Jones M, Teien DE, et al. Evaluation of mitral regurgitation using a digitally determined color Doppler flow convergence 'centerline' acceleration method. Studies in an animal model with quantified mitral regurgitation. *Circulation*. 1994;89:2879–2887.

64. Grayburn PA, Fehske W, Omran H, et al. Multiplane transesophageal echocardiographic assessment of mitral regurgitation by Doppler color flow mapping of the vena contracta. *Am J Cardiol*. 1994;74:912–917.

65. Mele D, Vandervoort P, Palacios I, et al. Proximal jet size by Doppler color flow mapping predicts severity of mitral regurgitation: Clinical studies. *Circulation*. 1995;91:746–754.

66. Passafini A, Shiota T, Depp M, et al. Factors influencing pulmonary venous flow velocity patterns in mitral regurgitation: An in vitro study. *J Am Coll Cardiol*. 1995;26:1333–1339.

67. Hall SA, Brickner ME, Willett DL, et al. Assessment of mitral regurgitation severity by Doppler color flow mapping of the vena contracta. *Circulation*. 1997;95:636–642.

68. Zhou X, Jones M, Shiota T, et al. Vena contracta imaged by Doppler color flow mapping predicts the severity of eccentric mitral regurgitation better than color jet area: A chronic animal study. *J Am Coll Cardiol*. 1997;30:1393–1398.

69. Thomas L, Foster E, Hoffman JI, et al. The mitral regurgitation index: An echocardiographic guide to severity. *J Am Coll Cardiol*. 1999;33:2016–2022.

70. Zoghbi WA, Enriquez-Sarano M, Foster E, et al. Recommendations for evaluation of the severity of native valvular regurgitation with two-dimensional and Doppler echocardiography. *J Am Soc Echocardiogr*. 2003;16:777–802.

71. Smith MD, Harrison MR, Pinton R, et al. Regurgitant jet size by transesophageal compared with transthoracic Doppler color flow imaging. *Circulation*. 1991;83:79–86.

72. De Simone R, Glombitza G, Vahl CF, et al. Three-dimensional color Doppler: A clinical study in patients with mitral regurgitation. *J Am Coll Cardiol*. 1999;33:1646–1654.

73. Sugeng L, Weinert L, Lang RM. Real-time 3-dimensional color Doppler flow of mitral and tricuspid regurgitation: Feasibility and initial quantitative comparison with 2-dimensional methods. *J Am Soc Echocardiogr*. 2007;20:1050–1057.

74. Utsunomiya T, Patel D, Doshi R, et al. Can signal intensity of the continuous wave Doppler regurgitant jet estimate severity of mitral regurgitation? *Am Heart J*. 1992;123:166–171.

75. Marcotte F, Honos GN, Walling AD, et al. Effect of angiotensin-converting enzyme inhibitor therapy in mitral regurgitation with normal left ventricular function. *Can J Cardiol*. 1997;13:479–485.

76. Host U, Kelbaek H, Hildebrandt P, et al. Effect of ramipril on mitral regurgitation secondary to mitral valve prolapse. *Am J Cardiol*. 1997;80:655–658.

77. Tischler MD, Rowan M, LeWinter MM. Effect of enalapril therapy on left ventricular mass and volumes in asymptomatic chronic, severe mitral regurgitation secondary to mitral valve prolapse. *Am J Cardiol*. 1998;82:242–245.

78. Capomolla S, Febo O, Gnemmi M, et al. Beta-blockade therapy in chronic heart failure: diastolic function and mitral regurgitation improvement by carvedilol. *Am Heart J*. 2000;139:596–608.

79. Linde C, Leclercq C, Rex S, et al. Long-term benefits of biventricular pacing in congestive heart failure: Results from the MUltisite STimulation in cardiomyopathy (MUSTIC) study. *J Am Coll Cardiol*. 2002;40:111–118.

80. Breithardt OA, Sinha AM, Schwammenthal E, et al. Acute effects of cardiac resynchronization therapy on functional mitral regurgitation in advanced systolic heart failure. *J Am Coll Cardiol*. 2003;41:765–770.

81. St John Sutton MG, Plappert T, Abraham WT, et al. Effect of cardiac resynchronization therapy on left ventricular size and function in chronic heart failure. *Circulation*. 2003;107:1985–1990.

82. Fukuda S, Grimm R, Song JM, et al. Electrical conduction disturbance effects on dynamic changes of functional mitral regurgitation. *J Am Coll Cardiol*. 2005;46:2270–2276.

83. Vahanian A, Baumgartner H, Bax J, et al. Guidelines on the management of valvular heart disease: The Task Force on the Management of Valvular Heart Disease of the European Society of Cardiology. *Eur Heart J*. 2007;28:230–268.

84. Tribouilloy CM, Enriquez-Sarano M, Schaff HV, et al. Impact of preoperative symptoms on survival after surgical correction of organic mitral regurgitation: Rationale for optimizing surgical indications. *Circulation*. 1999;99:400–405.

85. David TE, Armstrong S, Sun Z, et al. Late results of mitral valve repair for mitral regurgitation due to degenerative disease. *Ann Thorac Surg*. 1993;56:7–12; Discussion 13–14.

86. Gillinov AM, Cosgrove DM. Mitral valve repair for degenerative disease. *J Heart Valve Dis*. 2002;11(Suppl 1):S15–S20.

87. Leung DY, Armstrong G, Griffin BP, et al. Latent left ventricular dysfunction in patients with mitral regurgitation: Feasibility of measuring diminished contractile reserve from a simplified model of noninvasively derived left ventricular pressure-volume loops. *Am Heart J*. 1999;137:427–434.

88. Leung DY, Griffin BP, Snader CE, et al. Determinants of functional capacity in chronic mitral regurgitation unassociated with coronary artery disease or left ventricular dysfunction. *Am J Cardiol*. 1997;79:914–920.

89. Leung DY, Griffin BP, Stewart WJ, et al. Left ventricular function after valve repair for chronic mitral regurgitation: Predictive value of preoperative assessment of contractile reserve by exercise echocardiography. *J Am Coll Cardiol*. 1996;28:1198–1205.

90. Ling LH, Enriquez-Sarano M, Seward JB, et al. Clinical outcome of mitral regurgitation due to flail leaflet. *N Engl J Med*. 1996;335:1417–1423.

91. Ling LH, Enriquez-Sarano M, Seward JB, et al. Early surgery in patients with mitral regurgitation due to flail leaflets: A long-term outcome study. *Circulation*. 1997;96:1819–1825.

92. Adams DH, Anyanwu AC. The cardiologist's role in increasing the rate of mitral valve repair in degenerative disease. *Curr Opin Cardiol*. 2008;23:105–110.

93. Nifong LW, Chitwood WR, Pappas PS, et al. Robotic mitral valve surgery: A United States multicenter trial. *J Thorac Cardiovasc Surg*. 2005;129:1395–1404.

94. Agricola E, Oppizzi M, Maisano F, et al. Detection of mechanisms of immediate failure by transesophageal echocardiography in quadrangular resection mitral valve repair technique for severe mitral regurgitation. *Am J Cardiol*. 2003;91:175–179.

95. Sugeng L, Shernan SK, Salgo IS, et al. Live 3-dimensional transesophageal echocardiography initial experience using the fully-sampled matrix array probe. *J Am Coll Cardiol*. 2008;52:446–449.

96. Gillinov AM, Blackstone EH, Rajeswaran J, et al. Ischemic versus degenerative mitral regurgitation: Does etiology affect survival? *Ann Thorac Surg*. 2005;80:811–819; Discussion 809.

97. Marwick TH, Stewart WJ, Currie PJ, et al. Mechanisms of failure of mitral valve repair: An echocardiographic study. *Am Heart J*. 1991;122:149–156.

98. Freeman WK, Schaff HV, Khandheria BK, et al. Intraoperative evaluation of mitral valve regurgitation and repair by transesophageal echocardiography: Incidence and significance of systolic anterior motion. *J Am Coll Cardiol*. 1992;20:599–609.

99. Vikram HR, Buenconsejo J, Hasbun R, et al. Impact of valve surgery on 6-month mortality in adults with complicated, left-sided native valve endocarditis: A propensity analysis. *JAMA*. 2003;290:3207–3214.

100. Mullany CJ, Chua YL, Schaff HV, et al. Early and late survival after surgical treatment of culture-positive active endocarditis. *Mayo Clin Proc*. 1995;70:517–525.

101. Sanfilippo AJ, Picard MH, Newell JB, et al. Echocardiographic assessment of patients with infectious endocarditis: Prediction of risk for complications. *J Am Coll Cardiol*. 1991;18:1191–1199.

102. Pomerantzeff PM, Brandao CM, Faber CM, et al. Mitral valve repair in rheumatic patients. *Heart Surg Forum*. 2000;3:273–276.

103. Trichon BH, Glower DD, Shaw LK, et al. Survival after coronary revascularization, with and without mitral valve surgery, in patients with ischemic mitral regurgitation. *Circulation*. 2003;108(Suppl 1):II103–II110.

104. Prifti E, Bonacchi M, Frati G, et al. Ischemic mitral valve regurgitation grade II-III: Correction in patients with impaired left ventricular function undergoing simultaneous coronary revascularization. *J Heart Valve Dis*. 2001;10:754–762.

105. Lam BK, Gillinov AM, Blackstone EH, et al. Importance of moderate ischemic mitral regurgitation. *Ann Thorac Surg*. 2005;79:462–470; Discussion 462–470.

106. Wong DR, Agnihotri AK, Hung JW, et al. Long-term survival after surgical revascularization for moderate ischemic mitral regurgitation. *Ann Thorac Surg*. 2005;80:570–577.

107. Mihaljevic T, Lam BK, Rajeswaran J, et al. Impact of mitral valve annuloplasty combined with revascularization in patients with functional ischemic mitral regurgitation. *J Am Coll Cardiol*. 2007;49:2191–2201.

108. Hung J, Chaput M, Guerrero JL, et al. Persistent reduction of ischemic mitral regurgitation by papillary muscle repositioning: Structural stabilization of the papillary muscle-ventricular wall complex. *Circulation*. 2007;116:I259–I263.

109. Hung J, Solis J, Guerrero JL, et al. A novel approach for reducing ischemic mitral regurgitation by injection of a polymer to reverse remodel and reposition displaced papillary muscles. *Circulation*. 2008;118:S263–S269.

110. Foster E, Wasserman HS, Gray W, et al. Quantitative assessment of severity of mitral regurgitation by serial echocardiography in a multicenter clinical trial of percutaneous mitral valve repair. *Am J Cardiol*. 2007;100:1577–1583.

111. Silvestry FE, Rodriguez LL, Herrmann HC, et al. Echocardiographic guidance and assessment of percutaneous repair for mitral regurgitation with the Evalve MitraClip: Lessons learned from EVEREST I. *J Am Soc Echocardiogr*. 2007;20:1131–1140.

112. Condado JA, Acquatella H, Rodriguez L, et al. Percutaneous edge-to-edge mitral valve repair: 2-Year follow-up in the first human case. *Catheter Cardiovasc Interv*. 2006;67:323–325.

113. Bax JJ. Assessment of myocardial viability in ischemic cardiomyopathy. *Heart Lung Circ*. 2005;14(Suppl 2):S8–S13.

114. Isbell DC, Kramer CM. Magnetic resonance for the assessment of myocardial viability. *Curr Opin Cardiol*. 2006;21:469–472.

115. Hung J, Papakostas L, Tahta SA, et al. Mechanism of recurrent ischemic mitral regurgitation after annuloplasty: Continued LV remodeling as a moving target. *Circulation*. 2004;110:II85–II90.

31

Tricuspid and Pulmonary Valve Disease

Deborah Kwon
Brian Griffin

1. INTRODUCTION

The tricuspid valve is the inflow valve to the right ventricle (RV) whereas the pulmonary valve is the RV outflow valve. Both tend to be less involved in conditions such as rheumatic disease than the left-sided valves but tend to be more affected by congenital diseases of the heart. Imaging of these valves is usually best performed by transthoracic echocardiography (TTE) initially followed by transesophageal echocardiography (TEE) when necessary. Other imaging modalities such as MRI are useful in the assessment of specific congenital anomalies but have limited value in the assessment of valvular pathology of the right-sided valves. Three-dimensional (3D) echocardiography provides incremental information with regard to right ventricular size and function and in the assessment of pathology of individual leaflets of the tricuspid valve.

2. NORMAL TRICUSPID VALVE ANATOMY AND PHYSIOLOGY

The tricuspid valve separates the right atrium from the RV and typically comprises three leaflets, anterior, septal, and posterior leaflets. In comparison to the mitral valve annulus, the tricuspid valve annulus is slightly apically displaced. This anatomical finding can help distinguish the tricuspid valve from the mitral valve in many complex congenital diseases where situs is uncertain. The apical displacement of the tricuspid valve creates a small area in which the left ventricle is separated from the right atrium by the membranous septum. Disruption of this space can result in a left ventricular to right atrial shunt (Gerbode defect).

The tricuspid valve opens during diastole when the right atrial pressure exceeds the right ventricular pressure. The tricuspid valve closes during ventricular systole when the right ventricular pressure exceeds the right atrial pressure and prevents regurgitation into the right atrium while the RV contracts. This facilitates blood passing through the pulmonic valve and into the pulmonary circulation.

3. NORMAL PULMONARY VALVE ANATOMY AND PHYSIOLOGY

The pulmonary valve is a semilunar valve that separates the RV from the pulmonary artery and has three cusps. The pulmonic valve opens at the onset of ventricular systole when the intraventricular pressure in the RV exceeds the pressure in the pulmonary artery. The pulmonic valve closes when the pressure in the RV falls below the pulmonary artery pressure, the end of ventricular systole.

4. IMAGING OF THE NORMAL VALVES

4.1. Tricuspid valve

4.1.1. Transthoracic echocardiogram

The tricuspid valve is best visualized from the long and short axis parasternal, apical four-chamber, and subcostal views. The tricuspid valve leaflet anatomy can be quite variable, but the anterior leaflet is typically the most anatomically constant.

The septal and anterior leaflets typically are best seen in the parasternal long axis (right ventricular inflow) view. The posterior leaflet is best seen in the parasternal short axis view at the level of the aortic valve and is the leaflet adjacent to the RV free wall. The leaflet imaged adjacent to the aortic root can be either the septal or anterior leaflet. The anterior and septal leaflets are also seen in the apical four-chamber view, with the anterior leaflet adjacent to the RV free wall and the septal leaflet adjacent to the interventricular septum. Doppler echocardiography can be used to determine the presence of regurgitation or stenosis.

4.1.2. Transesophageal echocardiogram

The tricuspid valve is usually more difficult to visualize with TEE than with TTE since it is a thinner structure that is farther from the TEE transducer than the TTE probe. In addition, aortic or mitral valve prostheses or calcium can result in shadowing artifacts, further obscuring optimal visualization of the tricuspid valve by TEE.

The best imaging planes to visualize the tricuspid valve are the midesophageal view at 0°, 30°, 60°, and transgastric views. Similar to the apical four-chamber view with TTE, the septal and anterior leaflets are usually seen at the midesophageal view at 0°. Retroflexion of the probe can bring the posterior leaflet into view. The tricuspid valve can also be seen in the transgastric view by turning the probe clockwise from the mitral valve short axis view (0°) or from the left ventricular long axis view (90°).

4.2. Pulmonic valve

The pulmonic valve is technically the most difficult valve to visualize by echocardiography. Typically the best view to see the pulmonic valve with TTE is in the parasternal short axis view. The pulmonic valve can also be visualized in the high esophageal view between 45° and 90° at the short axis view of the aorta on TEE. The pulmonic valve as well as the main pulmonary artery can also be seen by withdrawing the probe slightly from the level of the aorta in the horizontal (0°) plane. Doppler echocardiography can be used to determine the presence of significant regurgitation or stenosis.

4.3. Epidemiology

4.3.1. Tricuspid regurgitation

Mild tricuspid regurgitation (TR) is present in approximately 70% of normal adults. This is not associated with clinical symptoms or abnormalities on physical exam or on electrocardiography. More severe TR may result from leaflet abnormalities or from dilatation of the annulus.[1-3] Clinically significant TR occurs in 0.9% of the population. Functional TR (due to annular dilatation) predominates.

In a study of 5,223 adults with TR (predominantly male with a mean age of 67),[3] only 8% had primary tricuspid valve pathology. Of the 92% of patients who had functional TR, 72% had significant pulmonary hypertension. The remaining patients had functional TR secondary to mitral disease or severe ventricular dysfunction. No gender difference in prevalence of TR was reported. TR more commonly results from congenital conditions such as Ebstein anomaly or rheumatic disease at a younger age whereas in older patients functional causes predominate.

The morbidity and mortality of the disease process are secondary to the underlying cause. In rheumatic disease, mortality rates with treatment are <3%. In Ebstein anomaly, mortality depends upon the severity of the valvular deformity and the feasibility of correction. Mortality rates with correction are approximately 10%. TR resulting from myocardial dysfunction or dilatation has a mortality of up to 50% in 5 years.

4.3.2. Tricuspid stenosis

Tricuspid stenosis (TS) occurs in <1% of the United States population. Although 15% of patients with rheumatic heart disease have TS at autopsy, it is estimated to be clinically significant in only 5% of these patients. TS occurs in approximately 3% of the international population. It is more prevalent in areas with a high incidence of rheumatic fever. TS is more common in women than in men. Congenital TS has a slightly higher male predominance.

4.3.3. Pulmonic regurgitation

Trivial or mild pulmonic regurgitation (PR) is physiologic and is present on Doppler echocardiography in nearly all individuals, particularly in older patients. More severe PR is rare. When it is present, it is usually secondary to an underlying process such as pulmonary hypertension or results from surgical or catheter intervention for congenital narrowing of the pulmonary valve or RV outflow tract. Rarely, it results from congenital absence of the valve or severe endocarditis.

The morbidity and mortality associated with PR secondary to pulmonary hypertension depends upon the underlying cause of the pulmonary hypertension as well as the right ventricular function. The prognosis of congenital PR depends upon the severity upon diagnosis, the progression of the regurgitation, and the RV's ability to compensate for the volume overload state. One study demonstrated that 29% of patients with significant PR developed symptoms of right heart failure within 40 years.[4]

4.3.4. Pulmonic stenosis

Pulmonic stenosis (PS) usually refers to isolated valvular, subvalvular, or supravalvular obstruction (Figs. 31.1 and 31.2, Movie 31.1). However, it can also be associated with more complicated congenital heart disorders. Valvular pulmonary stenosis is usually an isolated lesion (90%), but supravalvular PS can also coexist. A slight female predominance exists.[5] Significant PS usually presents in infancy or childhood, given the predominance

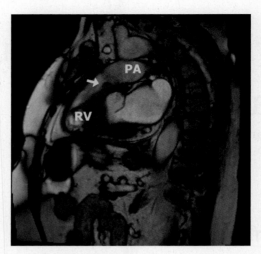

 Figure 31.1 (Movie 31.1). Infundibular pulmonic stenosis seen by CMR. PA, pulmonary artery; RV, right ventricle.

of congenital PS. However, acquired PS can cause symptoms at any age and depends on the underlying process that results in PS.[6] Mild and moderate PS does not affect long-term mortality or morbidity. However, severe PS may lead to right heart failure, arrhythmias, and early death. Mild PS usually does not progress in severity as the pulmonic valve orifice size usually increases with body growth. Therefore, symptoms caused by congenital PS in childhood may resolve by adulthood. Several studies have demonstrated that PS does not progress in 75% of patients with congenital PS. In the Natural History Study of Congenital Heart Defects, for example, patients with valve gradients <25 mm Hg did not experience an increase in gradient during 25 years of follow-up.[7] Progression occurred in 12.5% of the patients, mostly children with gradients >50 mm Hg at initial examination, and 60% of patients with severe PS required intervention within 10 years of diagnosis.[6,7] When PS is corrected during childhood, the patients' long-term survival improves and matches that of an unaffected age- and sex-matched cohort. But the more severe and protracted the course of PS, the less optimal the outcome of intervention. Therefore, death due to RV failure can result in the most severe cases.

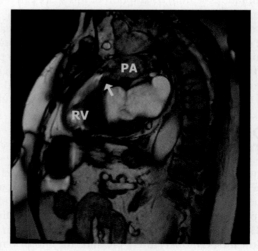

Figure 31.2 Turbulent flow visualized during systole by CMR in the same patient. PA, pulmonary artery; RV, right ventricle.

4.4. Clinical presentation

4.4.1. Symptoms and clinical exam findings

Tricuspid regurgitation. Patients with severe TR may remain asymptomatic for years. Eventually right-sided heart failure ensues causing fatigue from low cardiac output, peripheral edema which may be marked, and in later stages ascites and painful hepatosplenomegaly. Patients may be aware of distended and pulsatile jugular veins. Symptoms due to the primary disorder often predominate in secondary or functional TR.

On physical exam, patients with severe TR have distended, prominent, and pulsatile jugular veins due to elevated right atrial pressures. On close examination of the jugular venous pulsations, large "v" waves are observed due to systolic regurgitation into the right atrium. Jugular venous distension is more evident with inspiration, due to increased venous return. Furthermore, a systolic thrill can occasionally be felt over the jugular veins in patients with severe TR.

A dynamic right ventricular heave due to a dilated RV can be perceived with palpation of the left sternal border. Patients with severe TR may also present with ascites, peripheral edema, and even anasarca in severe disease. The liver is often enlarged and tender and may be pulsatile in severe TR.

On cardiac auscultation, TR results in a holosystolic murmur that is best heard at the right or left mid sternal border. This murmur usually augments with inspiration (Rivero-Carvallo sign) or other maneuvers that increase venous return, such as leg raising, exercise, and hepatic compression. However, if TR is severe, a murmur may not be appreciated. A right-sided S3 is often associated with an extremely dilated RV, and a right-sided S4 may also be heard if there is significant right ventricular hypertrophy. P2 may be increased and a split S2 may be marked in patients with pulmonary hypertension.[8,9]

Tricuspid stenosis. Patients with TS may present with fatigue and signs of systemic venous hypertension. These symptoms usually develop gradually but can occur rapidly if the patient develops atrial fibrillation or flutter. Patients often complain of lower extremity edema and abdominal discomfort and fullness, as a result of hepatomegaly and hepatic congestion. These findings are usually out of proportion to dyspnea if the patient does not have significant concomitant left-sided valvular pathology. However, patients with TS usually also have significant mitral and/or aortic valve disease and this may be the major symptomatic presentation.[10,11]

On physical exam, the jugular venous pulse is prominent and "giant A waves" are often observed. However, if the patient is in atrial fibrillation, the A wave is absent. Patients will often have significant peripheral edema and ascites. A diastolic murmur and opening snap may be auscultated along the left lower sternal border. The intensity of the murmur and opening snap should increase with maneuvers that increase blood flow across the tricuspid valve, such as inspiration (Carvallo sign), leg raising, squatting, or isotonic exercise. TR is also often present, and therefore, a holosystolic murmur may be heard in a similar location. S1 may be split widely, and a single S2 can be present as a result of inaudible closure of the pulmonary valve due to the decrease in blood flow through the stenotic tricuspid valve.

Pulmonic regurgitation. When PR is severe and has resulted in right ventricular enlargement and systolic dysfunction, symptoms of right-sided heart failure occur. Patients complain of shortness of breath, fatigue, light-headedness, peripheral edema, and palpitations. Patients with severe right ventricular failure may also complain of abdominal distension from ascites, right upper quadrant pain due to hepatic distension, and early satiety. Patients with severe PR may have other symptoms specific to the underlying disease process that has resulted in significant PR.

On physical exam, the jugular venous pressure is usually increased. If the RV is enlarged, an RV heave can be palpated at the left lower sternal border. Palpable pulmonary artery pulsation at the left upper sternal border may be present in the setting of significant pulmonary artery dilatation. If there is congenital absence of the pulmonic valve, P2 is inaudible. In other low pulmonary pressure PR states, P2 is delayed due to an increased right ventricular end-diastolic volume, which results in a widened-split S2. A brief decrescendo, low-pitched, early diastolic murmur can be auscultated at the upper left sternal border. The murmur increases in intensity by squatting or inspiration and decreases with Valsalva maneuvers or expiration. An S3 or S4 may be heard at the left mid-to-lower sternal border due to RV hypertrophy or failure and is augmented by inspiration.

In PR secondary to pulmonary hypertension, P2 is accentuated. The Graham Steell murmur of PR in pulmonary hypertension is high-pitched, and early diastolic decrescendo murmur is noted over the left upper-to-left midsternal area as a result of high-velocity regurgitant flow across an incompetent pulmonic valve. This murmur may simulate aortic regurgitation and is heard when the pulmonary artery systolic pressure is >60 mm Hg.[12,13]

Pulmonic stenosis. Most children and adults with mild-to-moderately severe PS are asymptomatic. Patients with severe PS may complain of exertional dyspnea and fatigue. Rarely, patients have presented with exertional angina, syncope, and sudden death. Patients with severe PS may have symptoms of right heart failure that have been outlined previously. On physical exam, a RV heave may be palpated along the left parasternal border. A systolic thrill may also be palpated at the level of the second intercostal space in the left upper sternal border. Upon auscultation, a normal S1 and a widely split S2 are often heard as well as a systolic crescendo-decrescendo ejection murmur in the left upper sternal border that increases with inspiration. As PS becomes more severe, the ejection murmur increases in intensity and duration. A systolic ejection click may precede the murmur and may increase in intensity on expiration.[14,15] A right-sided S4 that augments with inspiration may be present and signifies right ventricular hypertrophy and pressure overload with diminished right ventricular compliance. The murmur of supravalvular PS may be continuous and is softer, and higher pitched than valvular PS.

5. PATHOPHYSIOLOGY

5.1. Tricuspid regurgitation

TR gives rise to a flow of blood back into the right atrium during systole. As the right atrium is usually compliant, there are no significant hemodynamic consequences with mild or moderately severe TR. However, if TR is severe, the right atrial and venous pressure rises and can result in the signs and symptoms of right-sided heart failure such as edema and hepatic congestion. Furthermore, reduced forward flow occurs leading to impaired perfusion of the kidneys and other vital organs.

TR can be classified as (a) primary/intrinsic valve pathology or (b) secondary or functional.[16,17] Secondary TR is due to right ventricular hypertension, dilatation, and dysfunction. TR is usually secondary to conditions affecting the left heart and results in annular dilatation and leaflet tethering. Common causes of functional/secondary TR are listed in Table 31.1.[8,9,16,17]

TABLE 31.1

COMMON CAUSES OF FUNCTIONAL/SECONDARY TRICUSPID REGURGITATION

Left-sided heart failure

    Coronary artery disease

    Mitral stenosis or regurgitation

    Aortic stenosis or regurgitation

Primary pulmonary disease

    Cor pulmonale

    Pulmonary embolism

    Pulmonary hypertension of any cause

Left to right shunt

    Atrial septal defect

    Ventricular septal defect

    Anomalous pulmonary venous return

Eisenmenger syndrome

Stenosis of the pulmonic valve or pulmonary artery

Right ventricular dilatation

Right ventricular dysfunction

    Cardiomyopathy

    Myocarditis

    RV ischemia

    Endomyocardial fibrosis

    Arrhythmogenic right ventricular dysplasia

Hyperthyroidism

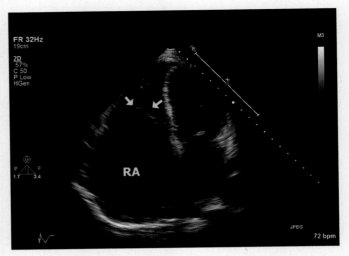

Figure 31.3 (**Movie 31.2**). Dilated right atrium (RA) and apically displaced tricuspid leaflets in a patient with Ebstein anomaly.

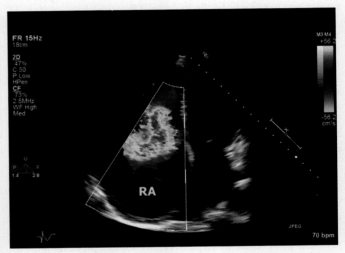

Figure 31.4 (**Movie 31.3**). Color Doppler demonstrating severe tricuspid regurgitation in the same patient. RA, right atrium.

Primary tricuspid valve pathology leading to significant TR is much less common. Various congenital anomalies and acquired diseases can alter the tricuspid valve morphology leading to valve incompetence. These include among others cleft valve generally in association with atrioventricular canal defect and Ebstein anomaly (see Chapter 40). The anatomy of the tricuspid valve in Ebstein anomaly is highly variable. The tricuspid valve leaflets are malformed and are partly attached to the fibrous tricuspid valve annulus and the right ventricular endocardium. The anterior leaflet is the largest leaflet and is usually attached to the tricuspid valve annulus. The posterior and septal leaflets are usually vestigial or absent. If these leaflets are present, the free edges are usually displaced into the body of the RV or the apex, leading to "atrialization" of the RV (Figs. 31.3 and 31.4, Movies 31.2 and 31.3). The tricuspid valve is often referred to as "sail-like" or funnel-shaped and is almost always incompetent, and sometimes stenotic.[18] Ebstein anomaly is classified as mild, moderate, or severe depending on the extent of apical displacement of the valve leaflets, degree of TR, and degree of right-sided cardiac chamber dilation and dysfunction.[19] Such classification helps risk stratify patients with Ebstein anomaly as prognosis has been shown to be dependent upon the degree of apical displacement of the tricuspid annulus and the severity of the regurgitation.[20]

TR due to rheumatic involvement is usually associated with mitral and aortic valve pathology.[8] Diffuse fibrous thickening, commissural fusion, fused chordae, or calcific deposits develop. The subvalvular apparatus may occasionally be mildly thickened by fibrous tissue. Rheumatic involvement of the tricuspid valve usually results in a combination of TR and TS. Rheumatic disease is the most common cause of pure TR due to deformation of the leaflets.

Endocarditis of the tricuspid valve can lead to significant TR. Precipitating factors that contribute to infection of the valve include alcoholism, intravenous drug use, neoplasms, infected indwelling catheters, extensive burns, and immune deficiency disease. Patients with tricuspid valve endocarditis usually present with pneumonia from septic pulmonary emboli rather than with symptoms of right heart failure.

The incidence of myxomatous tricuspid valve varies from 0.3% to 3.2%. Tricuspid valve prolapse is associated with mitral valve prolapse and rarely is isolated to the tricuspid valve.[8,9] Tricuspid valve prolapse may lead to significant TR and even to a flail valve leaflet.

Pure TR can occur as part of the carcinoid heart syndrome. Carcinoid heart disease is characterized by plaquelike deposits of fibrous tissue (Figs. 31.5 and 31.6, Movie 31.4). The valves and endocardium of the right side of the heart are most often affected,[21,22] because inactivation of humoral substances by the

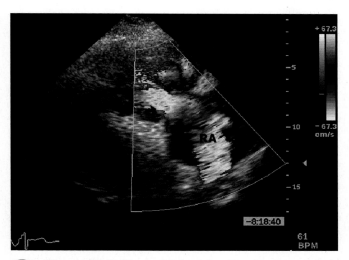

Figure 31.5 (Movie 31.4). Color Doppler image of the restricted tricuspid diastolic flow in a patient with carcinoid. RA, right atrium.

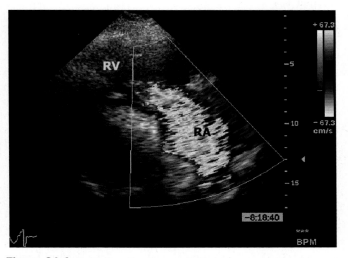

Figure 31.6 Color Doppler demonstration of severe tricuspid regurgitation in the same patient. RV, right ventricle; RA, right atrium.

lung protect the left heart. Fibrous white plaques form on the ventricular aspect of the tricuspid valve and endocardium and cause the valve to adhere to the RV wall. The leaflets become restricted, preventing proper coaptation of the leaflets during systole and resulting in TR.[23]

Papillary muscle dysfunction may result from RV ischemia or infarction, fibrosis, or infiltrative processes.

Trauma to the RV may damage the structures of the tricuspid valve, resulting in insufficiency of the structure.[24] Trauma can be associated with stab wounds or projectile destruction of the valve. However, trauma may be external such as blunt chest wall injury with disruption of chordal structures. Iatrogenic trauma can result from damage with a pacemaker lead, a stiff guide wire, or radiofrequency ablation for treatment of arrhythmias or due to inadvertent damage to the tricuspid apparatus at the time of endomyocardial biopsy. Iatrogenic causes of TR are often unrecognized as the functional consequences are slow to develop and the regurgitation is often progressive.

Patients with Marfan syndrome or other connective-tissue diseases (e.g., osteogenesis imperfecta and Ehlers–Danlos syndrome)

may have TR. Typically, dysfunction of other valves is also observed in the same patient. The etiology of the regurgitation can be attributed to a floppy tricuspid valve and a mildly dilated tricuspid valve annulus.[25-27]

Endocarditis in systemic lupus erythematosus or rheumatoid arthritis can also result in TR.

Medications that activate serotoninergic pathways may cause valvular lesions similar to those observed with carcinoid. Other medications such as methysergide, pergolide, and fenfluramine have also been associated with TR.[28,29]

5.2. Tricuspid stenosis

TS results from inadequate excursion of the valve leaflets due to alterations in the structure of the tricuspid valve. TS leads to a persistent diastolic pressure gradient between the right atrium and RV. This gradient increases when blood flow across the tricuspid valve increases (inspiration and exercise) and decreases when blood flow decreases (expiration). A mean pressure gradient of 2 mm Hg establishes the diagnosis of TS. A gradient as low as 5 mm Hg usually leads to an elevated mean right atrial pressure. As a result, most patients with significant TS have jugular venous distension, ascites, and peripheral edema.

There are four main causes of TS: rheumatic heart disease, carcinoid heart disease, congenital TS or tricuspid atresia, and endocarditis. The most common etiology is rheumatic fever, and tricuspid valve involvement occurs universally with mitral and aortic valve involvement.[30-33]

Rheumatic TS results from diffuse thickening of the leaflets and occurs with or without fusion of the commissures. The chordae tendineae may be thickened and shortened; however, calcification of the valve rarely occurs. The leaflet tissue is composed of dense collagen and elastic fibers and leads to significant distortion of the normal leaflet layers.[10,30,31]

Carcinoid heart disease can occasionally result in TS. The carcinoid fibrous white plaques located on the valvular and mural endocardium lead to thickened, rigid leaflets, which are restricted in mobility. This usually results in significant TR. Fibrous tissue proliferation on the atrial and ventricular surfaces of the valve structure can lead to a reduced valve orifice area.[21,22]

Congenital TS or tricuspid atresia can manifest as incompletely developed leaflets, shortened or malformed chordae, small annuli, abnormal size and number of the papillary muscles, or any combination of these defects.[34,35] Other cardiac anomalies are usually present.[36]

Bacterial endocarditis of the tricuspid valve usually results in significant regurgitation. However, significant TS occasionally results when large vegetations obstruct the orifice usually in the setting of an infected permanent pacemaker lead or a prosthetic valve. Other less common causes of TS include Fabry disease, giant blood cysts, right atrial or metastatic tumor, endomyocardial fibrosis, and systemic lupus erythematosus.[32,33,37]

5.3. Pulmonic regurgitation

PR can be classified by the presence of normal versus abnormal valve leaflet morphology. The most common cause of PR is due to dilation of the valve annulus or pulmonary artery due to pulmonary hypertension. PR is rarely caused by intrinsic valve abnormalities such as infective endocarditis, carcinoid, rheumatic heart disease, or trauma/complications after certain procedures.

In pulmonary regurgitation secondary to pulmonary hypertension, patients have primary lung disease and/or severely elevated pulmonary vascular resistance. Primary pulmonary hypertension occurs rarely mainly in younger women. This diagnosis can be made only after all other causes of pulmonary hypertension have been excluded. Secondary pulmonary hypertension is the most common cause of PR in adults. Other rare causes of significant PR in anatomically normal pulmonic valves due to valve annular dilation include Marfan, rheumatoid arthritis, Takayasu arteritis, and idiopathic dilated pulmonary artery trunk.[38]

Rare congenital causes of pulmonary regurgitation include absence of the pulmonary valve, fenestrated or redundant pulmonary valve leaflets, and bicuspid or quadricuspid pulmonary valves. Patients with Tetralogy of Fallot (TOF) may also develop severe pulmonary regurgitation following surgical repair of this condition (e.g., pulmonary valvotomy). Severe acute PR can result following balloon dilation of critical pulmonary stenosis or perforation of valvar pulmonary atresia.

Infective endocarditis of the pulmonic valve is a rare condition, accounting for <1.5% to 2% of all cases of endocarditis.[39] Most cases of reported pulmonic valve endocarditis occur in children with congenital heart disease or in intravenous drug abusers or in patients with an atrial septal defect and a large left-to-right intracardiac shunt.[40] Rheumatic involvement of the pulmonary valve is rare especially in developed countries and only occurs when the other three valves are also affected. Carcinoid affected the pulmonary valve 88% of one series of 74 patients with carcinoid heart disease. Of these, 49% exhibited significant PS, and 81% had significant PR.[22] Medications that act via serotoninergic pathways (e.g., methysergide, pergolide, and fenfluramine) have been associated to the development of significant PR. Pulmonary artery catheters can cause pulmonary valve damage and significant PR if the catheter tip is withdrawn across the pulmonic valve with the balloon inflated. Pulmonary valvuloplasty of a stenotic pulmonic valve (e.g., pulmonary balloon valvuloplasty) can result in PR. However, the severity of regurgitation is usually clinically insignificant. Complications of surgical repair of PS or congenital heart disease (i.e., TOF) can also result in significant PR.

5.4. Pulmonic stenosis

Pulmonic valvular stenosis (PS) is usually of congenital origin and very rarely is a result of acquired valvular heart disease. PS occurs in roughly 7% to 12% of subjects with congenital heart disease. Valvular PS, as opposed to subvalvular or supravalvular stenosis, is the cause of isolated right ventricular outflow obstruction in 80% of cases. Pulmonic valvular stenosis and pulmonary artery branch stenosis are frequently seen in the congenital rubella syndrome, often associated with a patent ductus.[12,41]

Congenital PS typically occurs in the fetal heart during the first 8 weeks of pregnancy. Valvular PS is the most common form of isolated right ventricular obstruction. Associated congenital anomalies include TOF, double outlet RV, univentricular atrioventricular connection, and atrioventricular canal defect. A bicuspid valve is found in as many as 90% of patients with TOF, whereas it is rare in individuals with isolated valvar PS.[12,13,42]

Congenital valvular PS can be categorized as dome-type or dysplastic. The pulmonic valve is more frequently dome-shaped due to fused cusps of varying thickness and fused commissures in the setting of a normal-sized annulus. Hypertrophy of the septal and parietal bands narrowing the right ventricular infundibulum often accompanies the pulmonic valve lesion, especially if it is severe. However, if the pulmonic valve is dysplastic, the leaflets are thickened and the annulus is small, leading to restricted leaflet mobility.[12,13,43] Although PS is usually an isolated abnormality, it may be associated with ventricular septal defect or lead to secondary right ventricular infundibular hypertrophy. The pulmonic

valve may be dysplastic, as seen in 67% of Noonan syndrome[5] producing obstruction in the absence of adherent leaflets. The leaflets are thickened, rigid, and myxomatous, and they are limited in their lateral movement because of the presence of tissue pads within the pulmonic valve sinuses.

Acquired valvular PS is rare; carcinoid and rheumatic fever are the two most frequent etiologies. Cardiac tumors or aneurysm of the sinus of Valsalva may rarely produce extrinsic obstruction of the RV outflow tract.

6. DIAGNOSTIC EVALUATION

6.1. Evaluation of ventricular function

Careful evaluation of the RV is necessary in determining the chronicity and severity of the right-sided valvular lesions. This involves evaluation of wall thickness, shape, ventricular cavity size and content, as well as regional and global contractile function. The RV presents challenges to imaging with echocardiography due to its anterior position and complex shape. 3D echocardiography allows a fuller evaluation of structure and function as do both MRI and nuclear imaging techniques (see Chapter 16).

6.2. Morphologic valve assessment

6.2.1. Tricuspid valve

Two-dimensional (2D) TTE is usually the best modality to visualize the tricuspid valve. The tricuspid valve is routinely evaluated using the long and short axis parasternal, apical four-chamber, and subcostal views. The normal tricuspid valve thickness is ≤3 mm.[1] In the 2D parasternal long axis view, the septal and anterior leaflets are generally visualized. In the parasternal short axis view at the level of the aortic valve, the posterior leaflet is imaged along the right ventricular free wall and either the septal or anterior leaflet is imaged adjacent to the aortic root. In the apical four-chamber view, the anterior and septal leaflets are visualized.[44-48]

Careful examination of the tricuspid valve annulus and leaflets may identify if the etiology of TR is from primary structural abnormalities of the leaflets and chordae or from secondary myocardial dysfunction and dilatation (Figs. 31.7 and 31.8, Movies 31.5 and 31.6). TTE may reveal prolapse of the tricuspid valve, endocarditis, rheumatic heart disease, or Ebstein anomaly. The tricuspid valve annulus is slightly apically displaced when compared to the mitral valve annulus. This feature is useful in identifying the tricuspid valve in many congenital conditions.

When imaging the tricuspid valve with TEE, it is best visualized in the midesophageal four-chamber view at 0°, 30°, and 60° and from the transgastric view. In the four-chamber view, the septal and anterior leaflets are usually seen, and the posterior leaflet can be seen by retroflexing the probe. TR jet velocity is best measured in a view in which the ultrasound beam and the regurgitant jet are most parallel, often between 30° and 60° in the midesophageal view. In the transgastric position, the tricuspid valve is brought into view by turning the probe clockwise from the mitral valve short axis view (0°) or left ventricular long axis view (90°).

On the 2D echocardiogram (using TTE or TEE), the presence and degree of TR can be evaluated by inspection of RV size and function, right atrial size and function, the tricuspid valve, and the vena cavae.

Ebstein anomaly is confirmed by the presence of apical displacement of the septal tricuspid valve leaflet (by ≥8 mm/m² body surface area compared to the position of the mitral valve) demonstrated in the apical four-chamber view. A dilated RV with

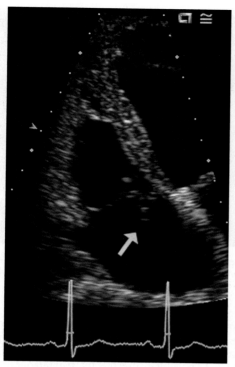

Figure 31.7 (Movie 31.5). Flail tricuspid valve. RA, right atrium.

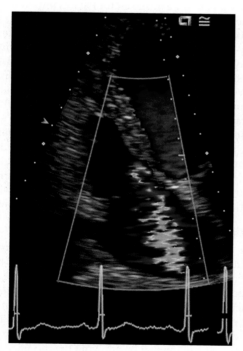

Figure 31.8 (Movie 31.6). Color Doppler demonstrating moderate-to-severe tricuspid regurgitation in the same patient.

an atrialized portion of the ventricle should be identified based upon the position of the tricuspid annulus. Paradoxical septal motion is typically present due to right ventricular volume overload induced by TR.[49,50]

2D echocardiography using TTE or TEE[9] enables identification of the specific features of TS. Doming of the tricuspid valve is

pathognomonic for TS and is seen in the parasternal long-axis view or in the apical four-chamber view. Other 2D echocardiographic features of TS include restricted mobility of the leaflets, reduced separation of the leaflet tips, reduction in the diameter of the tricuspid annulus, and thickening and calcification of the leaflets. Although leaflet thickening is seen, the degree of thickening and calcification is generally less pronounced than in rheumatic mitral stenosis.

Recent studies have demonstrated the utility of real-time 3D echocardiography for more complete and accurate assessment of the tricuspid valve annulus and leaflet morphology. Real-time 3D echo overcomes the inability to correctly identify the three tricuspid leaflets by traditional 2D echocardiography. 3D echo may also prove to be useful in planning surgical tricuspid valve interventions. It has been shown to be highly reproducible, providing real-time anatomical and functional measurements.[44,51,52]

The tricuspid valve is more difficult to appreciate on CT. Intracardiac contrast administration timed to optimize right heart structures (e.g., a CT pulmonary angiogram protocol) in combination with ECG gating can help better visualize the tricuspid valve.[53] Although leaflet morphology and thickening may not be accurately assessed, the presence of right atrial and ventricular dilatation, contrast in the inferior vena cava (IVC) or hepatic veins during first-pass contrast-enhanced CT, is a sensitive CT sign of TR.[54]

6.2.2. Pulmonic valve

Two-dimensional imaging of the pulmonary valve allows inspection of the leaflets for abnormal motion patterns such as systolic doming and noting pulmonary artery dilation. The pulmonic valve is viewed on TEE in the high esophageal view at 50° to 90° near the short axis view of the aorta. Slight withdrawal of the probe from the level of the aorta in the horizontal (0°) plane may improve visualization of the pulmonic valve and main pulmonary artery.

Because PR is almost always secondary to pulmonary hypertension, the morphologic assessment of the pulmonic valve usually does not reveal any intrinsic valve abnormalities. In some cases, pulmonic ring dilatation with poor valve leaflet coaptation may be observed. TEE may be useful in identifying the absence of the pulmonary valve, fenestrated or redundant pulmonary valve leaflets, and bicuspid or quadricuspid pulmonary valves. The pulmonic valve leaflets should be carefully evaluated for leaflet perforation if the patient has had a recent placement of a permanent pacemaker or PA catheter. Infective endocarditis of the pulmonic valve is a rare condition, but careful assessment of pulmonic valve vegetations should be conducted in patients with risk factors and history of fevers and septic pulmonary emboli if there is no evidence of tricuspid valve endocarditis.

Rheumatic involvement of the pulmonary valve is rare and is usually affected following mitral, aortic, and tricuspid valve involvement. Restricted and/or thickened pulmonic valves may suggest carcinoid involvement in the appropriate clinical scenario. Cardiac magnetic resonance (CMR) imaging has shown to have excellent temporal and spatial resolution and can provide visualization of the pulmonic valve morphology, accurate estimation of the severity of regurgitation, the mechanism of regurgitation, and right ventricular size and function.[55,56]

2D echocardiographic findings that may be seen in isolated valvular PS include systolic doming of the valve, thickening of the pulmonic valve (Figs. 31.9–31.11, Movies 31.7 and 31.8), poststenotic dilation of the main pulmonary artery, and variable degrees of right ventricular hypertrophy and pulmonary masses or tumors (Fig. 31.12, Movie 31.9). TEE can also identify PS that

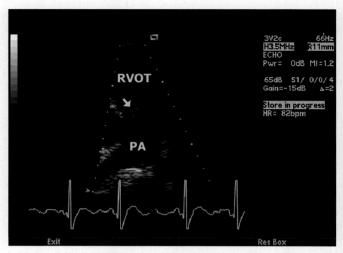

 Figure 31.9 (Movie 31.7). Thickened leaflets in a congenitally bicuspid pulmonic valve. PA, pulmonary artery; RVOT, right ventricular outflow tract.

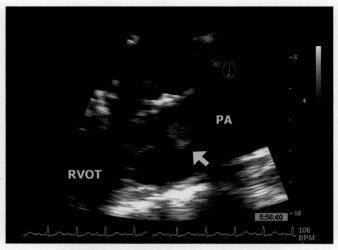 **Figure 31.12 (Movie 31.9).** Pulmonary valve papillary fibroelastoma seen by TEE. RVOT, right ventricular outflow tract; PA, pulmonary artery.

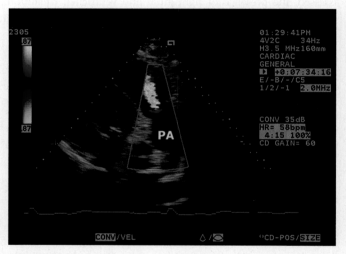

Figure 31.10 (Movie 31.8). Color Doppler demonstrates moderate pulmonary valve insufficiency in the same patient. PA, pulmonary artery.

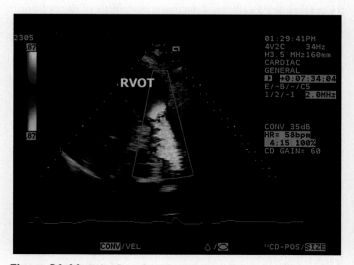

Figure 31.11 Color flow demonstrates restricted systolic flow in the same patient. RVOT, right ventricular outflow tract.

results from extrinsic compression caused by sinus of Valsalva aneurysm, postoperative hematoma, sarcoma, and pericardial cyst.[57] The right ventricular outflow tract (RVOT) should be carefully evaluated for evidence of sub-PS. Patients with ventricular septal defects that fail to close can develop severe RVOT obstruction on rare occasions. The condition is referred to as double chamber RV and may be mistaken for PS. It is important to differentiate these two entities by echocardiography because the double chamber RV is highly amenable to surgery, even late in life. It should be suspected when a systolic jet is seen impinging on the pulmonary valve. CMR may also help to aid in the assessment and characterization of PS.[55] CMR offers improved visualization of the RVOT allowing for better identification of subvalvular lesions. Furthermore, the distal PA as well as segmental PA branch stenosis can also be identified.

Cardiac CT can also provide useful information regarding the pulmonic valve, although PV cusps can be difficult to accurately identify on CT, unless these are thickened. However, the right heart size, the presence of right ventricular and right atrial dilatation/hypertrophy, pulmonary trunk dilatation, and bowing of the interventricular septum to the left can be readily assessed.[53]

6.3. Estimation of stenosis severity

Although 2D echocardiography using TTE or TEE enables the identification and characterization of TS, planimetry of the tricuspid valve area usually cannot be obtained.[58] Therefore, Doppler echocardiography is essential for quantifying the degree of TS.[59] TS is present when there is diastolic flow acceleration on the atrial side of the valve and an increased pressure half-time. The mean tricuspid diastolic gradient can be estimated from the tricuspid inflow time velocity integral by applying the modified Bernoulli equation. Though estimating tricuspid valve area using echocardiography is not as well-established as estimating mitral valve area, the same methods for calculating mitral valve area, such as pressure half-time, the continuity equation, and proximal isovelocity surface area (PISA), can be applied to the tricuspid valve.[60] The severity of TS can also be determined by the mean and end-diastolic gradients. Significant TS results in a mean gradient of 3 to 5 mm Hg and an end-diastolic gradient of 1 to 3 mm Hg.[9] Tricuspid valve area in cm^2 can be calculated by the following equation: 190/pressure half-time.[61] A tricuspid valve with valve area <1 cm, with elevated mean and end-diastolic gradients, is considered severely stenotic and may need surgical intervention.

The severity of pulmonary stenosis is defined by continuous wave Doppler examination by assessing the peak systolic gradient across the valve. Although the valve area calculated by the continuity equation serves as the main variable in judging the severity of aortic stenosis, the peak gradient is the most important value for judging severity in pulmonary stenosis. Peak velocities can be converted into pressure gradients by using the modified Bernoulli equation:

$$\text{Peak gradient, in mm Hg} = 4 \times \text{peak velocity} \qquad \text{(Eq. 31.1)}$$

Severe pulmonary stenosis is defined as a peak jet velocity >4 m/s (peak gradient >60 mm Hg) or valve area <0.5 cm^2.[1] Moderate stenosis is defined as a peak jet velocity of 3 to 4 m/s (peak gradient 36 to 60 mm Hg) or valve area 0.5 to 1.0 cm^2, while in mild stenosis the velocity is <3 m/s (peak gradient <36 mm Hg) or valve area >1.0 cm^2. Severe PS and/or Doppler evidence of right-sided pressures approaching or exceeding systemic pressures or a 2D echocardiogram demonstrating paradoxical septal motion during systole with reversal of the usual right convex curvature of the interventricular septum is an indication for therapeutic intervention.[57,62]

6.4. Estimation of regurgitant severity

6.4.1. Tricuspid regurgitation

The severity of TR is determined using a semi-quantitative approach. Jet area, proximal flow acceleration, and the width of the vena contracta are used to quantify the severity of TR. If the TR jet is central, the Nyquist limit should be set at 50 to 60 cm/s. A jet area of <5 cm^2 suggests mild TR, 5 to 10 cm^2 suggests moderate TR, and >10 cm^2 suggests severe TR.

Proximal flow acceleration refers to the effect of increasing blood velocity as regurgitant blood approaches the regurgitant orifice from the ventricular side of the valve. This phenomenon is seen as a series of concentric roughly hemispheric isovelocity shells of decreasing surface area and increasing surface velocity using color Doppler (see Chapters 2 and 30). The peak measurable blood velocity is limited by the relatively low sampling rate of color Doppler. When flow velocity exceeds the aliasing velocity (V_A, Nyquist limit), color reversal occurs. This convergence signal is referred to as the PISA.[63] At a given aliasing velocity, the radius (r) of PISA increases with increasing regurgitant volume. The effective regurgitant orifice area (EROA) can be calculated by dividing the flow rate through the regurgitant orifice (which is estimated as the product of the surface area of the hemisphere [$2\pi r^2$] and V_A) by the peak velocity of the regurgitant jet [PkV$_{reg}$]:

$$\text{EROA} = (2\pi r^2 \times V_A)/\text{PkV}_{reg} \qquad \text{(Eq. 31.2)}$$

An EROA of ≥40 mm^2 is a criterion of severe regurgitation in both TR and MR.[64–66]

The PISA method is not as accurate in quantifying eccentric jets as compared to central jets. Although PISA is widely used to quantify the severity of MR, it has limitations in its applicability to the assessment of TR due to the greater difficulty in visualizing a measurable contour of flow convergence.[63] The 2003 ASE guideline recommendations include PISA radius as a parameter for grading TR severity, although the guidelines note that such quantification is rarely needed clinically given the availability of other methods, such as the width of the vena contracta.[63] At a Nyquist limit of 28 cm/s, a TR PISA radius of ≤0.5 cm is categorized as mild, a radius of 0.6 to 0.9 cm is moderate, and a radius of >0.9 cm is severe.

The vena contracta is the narrowest width of the color flow regurgitant jet as it flows downstream from the valve orifice. The vena contracta width correlates with other echocardiographic measures of TR severity and with clinical evidence of TR.[66–69] TR is severe if the vena contracta width is >0.7 cm at a Nyquist limit of 50 to 60 cm/s.[63]

Early diastolic peak velocity (peak E) and velocity time integral of right ventricular inflow are increased in proportion to TR severity. A tricuspid peak E of ≥0.65 m/s is consistent with the presence of severe TR.[63,70] The presence of an A-wave dominant tricuspid inflow pattern virtually excludes the likelihood that the TR is severe.

The TR jet contour is also used to grade TR. The continuous Doppler flow pattern of the TR jet is usually symmetric, reflecting the relative equality of rates of flow acceleration and deceleration. However, in severe TR, the large regurgitant volume flows into the right atrium during systole and overwhelms the ability of atrial capacitance or compliance to maintain low pressure. Therefore, a rapid rise in atrial late systolic pressure occurs. This rise or V-wave results in early equilibration of right atrial and right ventricular pressures. This is illustrated by an asymmetric early peaking triangular regurgitant wave form. Therefore, mild TR is associated with a parabolic shape, moderate TR is associated with a variable contour, and severe TR is associated with a triangular early peaking jet.[63,71]

Furthermore, the strength of the Doppler signal is proportional to the number of red blood cells regurgitating into the right atrium. Therefore, the relative density of the regurgitant signal reflects the magnitude of the regurgitant fraction.[72] As a result, sparse TR jets usually indicate mild TR and dense TR jets indicate moderate or severe TR.[63]

Hepatic vein systolic flow reversal is an important criterion for severe TR. However, systolic flow reversal may not be accurate when atrial fibrillation is present. If severe TR is suspected, but the echocardiographic findings are not consistent with this suspicion, agitated saline or other ultrasound contrast agents can be used to enhance the TR jet signal and visualization of hepatic vein flow reversal.[59] Other findings that aid in the confirmation of the presence of severe TR include RV and RA enlargement, dilated tricuspid annulus, paradoxical interventricular septal movement, reflecting the increased volume within the RV (diastolic overload), and a dilated IVC with systolic flow reversal.

The severity of TR can be reliably assessed by CMR by determinations of regurgitant volume, fraction, and orifice. Regurgitant volume is determined as the difference between the RV planimetered-derived stroke volume (RV end-diastolic–RV end-systolic volume) and stroke volume derived from phase-encoded velocities obtained at the proximal pulmonary arteries.

6.4.2. Pulmonic regurgitation

Trivial or trace pulmonary regurgitation is frequently detected by Doppler echocardiography and is normally present in a high percentage of healthy persons.[73,74] Severe pulmonary regurgitation is defined as the color jet filling the RVOT and a dense continuous wave Doppler signal with a steep deceleration slope.[62] The color jet arises centrally at the valve commissure and has a very narrow vena contracta in trivial PR. It penetrates only a short distance into the RVOT. In more severe degrees of regurgitation, the size of the vena contracta and the penetration of the jet into the RVOT increase. Rapid equalization of the end-systolic pressure gradient between the pulmonary artery and RV assessed by pulsed or continuous wave Doppler echocardiography suggests more severe

PR. The Doppler signal is greatly shortened as it returns to the baseline (zero flow) well before the onset of systole. Furthermore, the Doppler signal in severe PR is very dense. However, with wide open PR (usually due to congenitally absent pulmonic valve), the color Doppler may fail to detect the jet altogether due to the brisk and laminar regurgitant flow. The severity of TR may be determined by CMR as the ratio of forward and reversed flow determined from phased-encoded velocities obtained at the proximal main pulmonary artery.[75,76] CMR is particularly useful in the follow-up of patients with severe PR, such as those with previous repair of Fallot tetralogy, given its ability of precisely quantifying regurgitant volume, RV volumes, and ejection fraction (see Chapter 41).

6.5. Evaluation of the pulmonary artery

Assessment of the main pulmonary artery and its branches should be performed in concert with examining the function of the pulmonary valve. The lateral wall of the main pulmonary artery usually cannot be well visualized because of the overlying lung.

Doppler interrogation of the pulmonary artery systolic velocity or the tricuspid valve regurgitation jet peak velocity can provide an estimation of pulmonary artery pressure and pulmonary vascular resistance. This can be used to monitor pulmonary vascular resistance in patients with heart failure due to left ventricular systolic dysfunction.[77]

Patient with patent ductus arteriosus will demonstrate a high velocity jet coming from the left main branch of the pulmonary artery that can be detected during both phases of the cardiac cycle.

6.6. Assessment of the right atrium

Normally, the right and left atria appear to be nearly equal in size and shape. The right atrium enlarges and becomes spherical in isolated TR. The degree of atrial enlargement depends on the duration and severity of TR, intrinsic disease of atrial muscle, as well as the presence and duration of chronic atrial fibrillation. A normal-sized right atrium in setting of severe TR suggests that the valvular disease is relatively acute.[63]

6.7. Assessment of the inferior vena cava

The IVC and hepatic veins can be best imaged in the subcostal view. The IVC size and respiratory variation are used to estimate right atrial pressure.[78,79] In severe TR, the vena cava expands in systole and retrograde V waves are often present. Pulse wave and color Doppler imaging of the IVC can also demonstrate alterations in IVC and hepatic vein flow due to severe TR. Generally, blood flows toward the heart during both phases of the cardiac cycle in these vessels. During inspiration, the normally dominant systolic inflow signal is exaggerated. Retrograde IVC flow occurs only briefly after atrial contraction under normal conditions. However, systolic reversal in these vessels indicates severe TR.[70] The normally dominant systolic component of flow may be blunted or reversed, and this abnormality is accentuated during inspiration.[80,81]

7. DETERMINING OPTIMAL TIME OF INTERVENTION

7.1. Symptomatic tricuspid regurgitation

In patients with severe TR and symptoms of right heart failure, the underlying cause for the TR should be ascertained and optimally treated. If the TR continues to be severe, or patients are undergoing mitral valve repair/replacement, patients can undergo tricuspid annuloplasty. Patients with intrinsic tricuspid valve pathology may require tricuspid valve replacement if the valve is not amenable to repair. Because of the increased incidence of mechanical prosthetic valve thrombosis in this low-flow position, a bioprosthetic valve is preferable. Patients with moderate TR and symptoms of right heart failure should be optimally medically treated. Thorough investigations for other causes of RV failure should be conducted and addressed. There are no current guidelines for surgical intervention in patients with moderate TR regardless of symptoms. Therefore, tricuspid annuloplasty or replacement should only be considered if the patient is undergoing open heart surgery for other reasons or has severe, refractory symptoms despite optimal medical therapy. The indications for surgical intervention for TR in adults and children are listed in Tables 31.2 and 31.3, respectively.

TABLE 31.2
INDICATIONS FOR SURGICAL INTERVENTION FOR TR IN ADULTS

Class I
1. Tricuspid valve repair is beneficial for severe TR in patients with mitral valve (MV) disease requiring MV surgery. (*Level of Evidence: B*)

Class IIa
1. Tricuspid valve replacement or annuloplasty is reasonable for severe primary TR when symptomatic. (*Level of Evidence: C*)
2. Tricuspid valve replacement is reasonable for severe TR secondary to diseased/abnormal tricuspid valve leaflets not amenable to annuloplasty or repair. (*Level of Evidence: C*)

Class IIb
Tricuspid annuloplasty may be considered for less than severe TR in patients undergoing MV surgery when there is pulmonary hypertension or tricuspid annular dilatation. (*Level of Evidence: C*)

Class III
1. Tricuspid valve replacement or annuloplasty is not indicated in asymptomatic patients with TR whose pulmonary artery systolic pressure is less than 60 mm Hg in the presence of a normal MV. (*Level of Evidence: C*)
2. Tricuspid valve replacement or annuloplasty is not indicated in patients with mild primary TR. (*Level of Evidence: C*)

Source: From Bonow RO, et al. 2008 focused update incorporated into the ACC/AHA 2006 guidelines for the management of patients with valvular heart disease: A report of the American College of Cardiology/American Heart Association Task Force on Practice Guidelines (Writing Committee to revise the 1998 guidelines for the management of patients with valvular heart disease). Endorsed by the Society of Cardiovascular Anesthesiologists, Society for Cardiovascular Angiography and Interventions, and Society of Thoracic Surgeons. *J Am Coll Cardiol.* 2008;52(13):el-e142.

TABLE 31.3
INDICATIONS FOR SURGICAL INTERVENTION FOR TR IN ADOLESCENTS OR YOUNG ADULTS

Class I

1. Surgery for severe TR is recommended for adolescent and young adult patients with deteriorating exercise capacity (NYHA functional class III or IV). (*Level of Evidence: C*)
2. Surgery for severe TR is recommended for adolescent and young adult patients with progressive cyanosis and arterial saturation less than 80% at rest or with exercise. (*Level of Evidence: C*)
3. Interventional catheterization closure of the atrial communication is recommended for the adolescent or young adult with TR who is hypoxemic at rest and with exercise intolerance due to increasing hypoxemia with exercise. When the tricuspid valve appears difficult to repair surgically. (*Level of Evidence: C*)

Class IIa

1. Surgery for severe TR is reasonable in adolescent and young adult patients with NYHA functional class II symptoms if the valve appears to be repairable. (*Level of Evidence: C*)
2. Surgery for severe TR is reasonable in adolescent and young adult patients with atrial fibrillation. (*Level of Evidence: C*)

Class IIb

1. Surgery for severe TR may be considered in asymptomatic adolescent and young adult patients with increasing heart size and a cardiothoracic ratio of more than 65%. (*Level of Evidence: C*)
2. Surgery for severe TR may be considered in asymptomatic adolescent and young adult patients with stable heart size and an arterial saturation of less than 85% when the tricuspid valve appears repairable. (*Level of Evidence: C*)
3. In adolescent and young adult patients with TR who are mildly cyanotic at rest but who become very hypoxemic with exercise, closure of the atrial communication by interventional catheterization may be considered when the valve does not appear amenable to repair. (*Level of Evidence: C*)
4. If surgery for Ebstein anomaly is planned in adolescents and young adult patients (tricuspid valve repair or replacement), a preoperative electrophysiological study may be considered to identify accessory pathways. If present, these may be considered for mapping and ablation either preoperatively or at the time of surgery. (*Level of Evidence: C*)

Source: Bonow RO, et al. 2008 focused update incorporated into the ACC/AHA 2006 guidelines for the management of patients with valvular heart disease: A report of the American College of Cardiology/American Heart Association Task Force on Practice Guidelines (Writing Committee to revise the 1998 guidelines for the management of patients with valvular heart disease). Endorsed by the Society of Cardiovascular Anesthesiologists, Society for Cardiovascular Angiography and Interventions, and Society of Thoracic Surgeons. *J Am Coll Cardiol*. 2008;52(13):el-e142.

7.2. Asymptomatic tricuspid regurgitation

Patients with severe TR and no symptoms or echocardiographic signs of right heart failure can be treated medically. The underlying cause for the TR again should be determined and optimally treated. If the patient is undergoing mitral valve repair/replacement, it is reasonable to also repair the tricuspid valve at that time. However, if TR is the sole valvular lesion, the patient can be treated medically with diuretics as needed but will need to be followed closely to look for signs of RV dilation or failure. Once this occurs, the patient may benefit from tricuspid annuloplasty or replacement as patients with severe TR and signs of RV failure have worse outcomes.[82]

7.3. Symptomatic tricuspid regurgitation

Patients with signs and symptoms of systemic venous hypertension and congestion should be considered for balloon valvotomy. Patients with symptoms and transvalvular pressure gradients of ≥3 mm Hg and valve areas <1.5 cm² can be referred for this intervention. Valvotomy is contraindicated in patients with moderate or severe TR. Valve area usually increases from <1.0 cm² to almost 2.0 cm². Residual TS usually still persists; however, the increase in valve area is usually sufficient to produce a significant reduction in the transvalvular pressure gradient and right atrial pressure as well as symptoms.[83,84] Tumor masses, vegetations, and thrombi are also contraindications to valvotomy. Patients with the previously stated conditions or with intrinsic valve disease with severely altered tricuspid valve morphology should undergo a tricuspid replacement with a bioprosthetic valve.

7.4. Asymptomatic tricuspid regurgitation

In the treatment of TS, the underlying cause of the valvular pathology should be assessed and treated appropriately. Bacterial endocarditis should be treated with the appropriate antibiotics as determined by the sensitivity of the organisms cultured. Sinus rhythm should be restored if any cardiac arrhythmias are present. Right atrial volume overload should be corrected with diuresis and salt restriction. If TS remains severe and the patient exhibits echocardiographic signs of right heart failure valvotomy or tricuspid replacement may be reasonable.

7.5. Symptomatic pulmonic regurgitation

PR rarely results in symptoms due to the RV's ability to adapt to low-pressure volume overload without difficulty. It is high-pressure volume overload that leads to right-sided heart failure. The underlying etiology causing severe PR must be treated to prevent right heart failure. Successful treatment of the underlying cause can reverse right-sided heart strain and failure. If PR is a result of severe pulmonary hypertension determining the cause and treating the specific disease appropriately can result in regression of PR and surgical intervention is usually not indicated. Such entities include primary pulmonary hypertension and secondary pulmonary hypertension due to thromboembolism, severe mitral stenosis, and severe intrinsic lung disease, which can all manifest as severe pulmonary hypertension with PR.

If severe PR is a result of an abnormal pulmonic valve, surgical reconstruction or pulmonic valve replacement can be considered if the patient has significant symptoms or has echocardiographic signs of right heart failure.

7.6. Asymptomatic pulmonic regurgitation

PR rarely results in symptoms due to the RV's ability to adapt to low-pressure volume overload without difficulty. It is high-pressure volume overload that leads to right-sided heart failure. In patients with no symptoms or signs of right heart failure, the mainstay of treatment is to treat the underlying cause. Treating the underlying cause can prevent the progression to right heart strain and failure. Patients with severe PR due to intrinsic valve disease should be followed closely as surgical intervention will eventually be necessary to prevent RV failure. Asymptomatic patients with severe PR due to intrinsic valve disease should be referred for surgical intervention only when there are echocardiographic findings suggesting significant RV volume overload and/or failure.

7.7. Symptomatic pulmonic stenosis

Balloon valvotomy is the preferred intervention for PS due to the high success and low complication rates. Favorable long-term hemodynamic and clinical results have been demonstrated in several studies.[7,85–88] Therefore, balloon valvotomy is the treatment of choice in moderate–severe PS. Although PS is only considered severe if the peak gradient is >60 mm Hg, balloon valvotomy is recommended in symptomatic patients with peak systolic gradient >30 mm Hg.[62] Roughly 25% to 50% of patients with pulmonic valvotomy will need a repeat procedure including pulmonary valve replacement for pulmonic insufficiency, open valvotomy, and balloon valvotomy.[85] The studies that evaluated outcomes postvalvotomy demonstrated that most of the reinterventions were performed more than 25 years after the initial procedure. The only predictor of the need for reintervention was closed valvotomy. Moderate to severe pulmonary regurgitation was present in 37%.[89] Balloon valvotomy may be less effective in patients with a dysplastic valve. A surgical repair or replacement may be necessary if the valve is severely dysplastic. The indications for balloon valvotomy in PS are listed in Table 31.4.

7.8. Asymptomatic pulmonic stenosis

Balloon valvotomy is indicated in asymptomatic patients with peak systolic gradient >40 mm Hg (moderate to severe disease). Furthermore, balloon valvotomy may also be considered in asymptomatic patients with a peak systolic gradient of 30 to 39 mm Hg. About 25% of asymptomatic patients with moderate PS will eventually require intervention because of progressive symptoms or right heart failure.[15]

8. SELECTING AND GUIDING THERAPY

8.1. Medical therapy

Mild TR and PR do not warrant medical therapy as these findings are physiologic. More significant regurgitation from either the tricuspid or pulmonic valve are most often secondary to left-sided heart disease or pulmonary hypertension. Therefore, the mainstay of medical therapy is to treat the underlying cause to prevent progression to right ventricular failure. When right heart failure is present, diuretics and restoration of sinus rhythm are the focus of medical therapy.

8.2. Surgical valve replacement

Surgical valve repair is always preferred given the low-flow state of the right side of the heart. Surgical valve replacement should only be performed when the valve cannot be repaired. If the tricuspid or pulmonic valve is replaced, bioprosthetic valves are the valves of choice given the high likelihood of thrombosis of mechanical valves in these positions.

8.3. Percutaneous valve repair

Tricuspid or pulmonic valvotomy is the preferred intervention in patients with tricuspid or PS if it is indicated. Tumor masses, vegetations, and thrombi are contraindications to valvotomy. Patients with the previously stated conditions or with intrinsic valve disease with severely altered tricuspid or pulmonic valve morphology should undergo a valve replacement with a bioprosthetic valve.

A recent study demonstrated the successful use of a percutaneous self-expanding stented bioprosthetic pulmonic valve in TOF patients after primary repair. Further long-term follow-up is needed to determine the viability of this newly available device as an alternative treatment strategy.[90]

8.4. Evaluation of coronary artery disease

Patients with risk factors for coronary artery disease and are being evaluated for percutaneous/surgical intervention should be

---

TABLE 31.4

INDICATIONS FOR BALLOON VALVOTOMY IN PULMONIC STENOSIS

Class I
1. Balloon valvotomy is recommended in adolescent and young adult patients with pulmonic stenosis who have exertional dyspnea, angina, syncope, or presyncope and an RV-to-pulmonary artery peak-to-peak gradient >30 mm Hg at catheterization. (*Level of Evidence: C*)
2. Balloon valvotomy is recommended in asymptomatic adolescent and young adult patients with pulmonic stenosis and RV-to-pulmonary artery peak-to-peak gradient >40 mm Hg at catheterization. (*Level of Evidence: C*)

Class IIb
1. Balloon valvotomy may be reasonable in asymptomatic adolescent and young adult patients with pulmonic stenosis and an RV-to-pulmonary artery peak-to-peak gradient 30 to 39 mm Hg at catheterization. (*Level of Evidence: C*)

Class III
1. Balloon valvotomy is not recommended in asymptomatic adolescent and young adult patients with pulmonic stenosis and RV-to-pulmonary artery peak-to-peak gradient <30 mm Hg at catheterization. (*Level of Evidence: C*)

Source: Bonow RO, et al. 2008 focused update incorporated into the ACC/AHA 2006 guidelines for the management of patients with valvular heart disease: A report of the American College of Cardiology/American Heart Association Task Force on Practice Guidelines (Writing Committee to revise the 1998 guidelines for the management of patients with valvular heart disease). Endorsed by the Society of Cardiovascular Anesthesiologists, Society for Cardiovascular Angiography and Interventions, and Society of Thoracic Surgeons. *J Am Coll Cardiol.* 2008;52(13):el-e142.

evaluated for coronary artery disease with coronary angiogram. The presence of coronary artery disease can help decide between a percutaneous or surgical intervention if it is indicated.

9. FUTURE DIRECTIONS

Imaging currently plays a key role in the detection and management of conditions affecting the tricuspid and pulmonary valve. As percutaneous approaches to right-sided valve conditions advance, there will be a greater need for multimodality imaging as is now occurring with aortic and mitral valve disease. Thus, it is likely that 3D echocardiography, CT, and MRI will all have a role in the selection of patients for percutaneous valve replacement and repair, to allow selection of the appropriate procedure and device and at the time of the procedure to allow optimal device placement.

REFERENCES

1. Hansing CE, Rowe GG. Tricuspid insufficiency. A study of hemodynamics and pathogenesis. *Circulation*. 1972;45(4):793–799.
2. Mutlak D, et al. Echocardiography-based spectrum of severe tricuspid regurgitation: The frequency of apparently idiopathic tricuspid regurgitation. *J Am Soc Echocardiogr*. 2007;20(4):405–408.
3. Nath J, Foster E, Heidenreich PA. Impact of tricuspid regurgitation on long-term survival. *J Am Coll Cardiol*. 2004;43(3):405–409.
4. Shimazaki Y, Blackstone EH, Kirklin JW. The natural history of isolated congenital pulmonary valve incompetence: Surgical implications. *Thorac Cardiovasc Surg*. 1984;32(4):257–259.
5. Burch M, et al. Cardiologic abnormalities in Noonan syndrome: Phenotypic diagnosis and echocardiographic assessment of 118 patients. *J Am Coll Cardiol*. 1993;22(4):1189–1192.
6. Connelly MS, et al. Canadian consensus conference on adult congenital heart disease 1996. *Can J Cardiol*. 1998;14(3):395–452.
7. Chen CR, et al. Percutaneous balloon valvuloplasty for pulmonic stenosis in adolescents and adults. *N Engl J Med*. 1996;335(1):21–25.
8. Frater R. Tricuspid insufficiency. *J Thorac Cardiovasc Surg*. 2001;122(3):427–429.
9. Shah PM, Raney AA. Tricuspid valve disease. *Curr Probl Cardiol*. 2008;33(2):47–84.
10. Roguin A, et al. Long-term follow-up of patients with severe rheumatic tricuspid stenosis. *Am Heart J*. 1998;136(1):103–108.
11. Sharma S, et al. Percutaneous double-valve balloon valvotomy for multivalve stenosis: Immediate results and intermediate-term follow-up. *Am Heart J*. 1997;133(1):64–70.
12. Brickner ME, Hillis LD, Lange RA. Congenital heart disease in adults. First of two parts. *N Engl J Med*. 2000;342(4):256–263.
13. Brickner ME, Hillis LD, Lange RA. Congenital heart disease in adults. Second of two parts. *N Engl J Med*. 2000;342(5):334–342.
14. Hultgren HN, et al. The ejection click of valvular pulmonic stenosis. *Circulation*. 1969;40(5):631–640.
15. Hayes CJ, et al. Second natural history study of congenital heart defects. Results of treatment of patients with pulmonary valvar stenosis. *Circulation*. 1993;87(2 Suppl):I28–I37.
16. Waller BF, Howard J, Fess S. Pathology of tricuspid valve stenosis and pure tricuspid regurgitation–Part III. *Clin Cardiol*. 1995;18(4):225–230.
17. Waller BF, et al. Etiology of pure tricuspid regurgitation based on anular circumference and leaflet area: Analysis of 45 necropsy patients with clinical and morphologic evidence of pure tricuspid regurgitation. *J Am Coll Cardiol*. 1986;7(5):1063–1074.
18. Dearani JA, Danielson GK. Congenital Heart Surgery Nomenclature and Database Project: Ebstein's anomaly and tricuspid valve disease. *Ann Thorac Surg*. 2000;69(4 Suppl):S106–S117.
19. Attenhofer Jost CH, et al. Ebstein's anomaly. *Circulation*. 2007;115(2):277–285.
20. Khan IA. Ebstein's anomaly of the tricuspid valve with associated mitral valve prolapse. *Tex Heart Inst J*. 2001;28(1):72.
21. Lundin L, et al. Carcinoid heart disease: Relationship of circulating vasoactive substances to ultrasound-detectable cardiac abnormalities. *Circulation*. 1988;77(2):264–269.
22. Pellikka PA, et al. Carcinoid heart disease. Clinical and echocardiographic spectrum in 74 patients. *Circulation*. 1993;87(4):1188–1196.
23. Simula DV, et al. Surgical pathology of carcinoid heart disease: A study of 139 valves from 75 patients spanning 20 years. *Mayo Clin Proc*. 2002;77(2):139–147.
24. Luo GH, et al. Correction of traumatic tricuspid insufficiency using the double orifice technique. *Asian Cardiovasc Thorac Ann*. 2005;13(3):238–240.
25. Khashu M, et al. Right-sided cardiac involvement in osteogenesis imperfecta. *J Heart Valve Dis*. 2006;15(4):588–590.
26. McDonnell NB, et al. Echocardiographic findings in classical and hypermobile Ehlers–Danlos syndromes. *Am J Med Genet A*. 2006;140(2):129–136.
27. Petitalot JP, Chaix AF, Barraine R. Echocardiographic features of triple valve prolapse with incompetent foramen ovale in Marfan's syndrome. *Am Heart J*. 1986;111(1):187–189.
28. Baseman DG, et al. Pergolide use in Parkinson disease is associated with cardiac valve regurgitation. *Neurology*. 2004;63(2):301–304.
29. Pritchett AM, et al. Valvular heart disease in patients taking pergolide. *Mayo Clin Proc*. 2002;77(12):1280–1286.
30. Daniels SJ, Mintz GS, Kotler MN. Rheumatic tricuspid valve disease: Two-dimensional echocardiographic, hemodynamic, and angiographic correlations. *Am J Cardiol*. 1983;51(3):492–496.
31. Hauck AJ, et al. Surgical pathology of the tricuspid valve: A study of 363 cases spanning 25 years. *Mayo Clin Proc*. 1988;63(9):851–863.
32. Waller BF. Morphological aspects of valvular heart disease: Part I. *Curr Probl Cardiol*. 1984;9(7):1–66.
33. Waller BF. Morphological aspects of valvular heart disease: Part II. *Curr Probl Cardiol*. 1984;9(8):1–74.
34. Cohen ML, et al. Congenital tricuspid valve stenosis with atrial septal defect and left anterior fascicular block. *Clin Cardiol*. 1990;13(7):497–499.
35. Tennstedt C, et al. Spectrum of congenital heart defects and extracardiac malformations associated with chromosomal abnormalities: Results of a seven year necropsy study. *Heart*. 1999;82(1):34–39.
36. Lev M, et al. The pathologic anatomy of Ebstein's disease. *Arch Pathol*. 1970;90(4):334–343.
37. Acikel M, et al. A case of free-floating ball thrombus in right atrium with tricuspid stenosis. *Int J Cardiol*. 2004;94(2–3):329–330.
38. Waller BF, Howard J, Fess S. Pathology of pulmonic valve stenosis and pure regurgitation. *Clin Cardiol*. 1995;18(1):45–50.
39. Cassling RS, Rogler WC, McManus BM. Isolated pulmonic valve infective endocarditis: A diagnostically elusive entity. *Am Heart J*. 1985;109(3 Pt 1):558–567.
40. Cremieux AC, et al. Clinical and echocardiographic observations in pulmonary valve endocarditis. *Am J Cardiol*. 1985;56(10):610–613.
41. Braunwald E, Douglas P Zipes, Libby P. *Heart Disease: A Textbook of Cardiovascular Medicine*. 8th Ed. Philadelphia, PA: WB Saunders Company; 2007.
42. Cabrera A, et al. Double-chambered right ventricle. *Eur Heart J*. 1995;16(5):682–686.
43. Mack G, Silberbach M. Aortic and pulmonary stenosis. *Pediatr Rev*. 2000;21(3):79–85.
44. Anwar AM, et al. Assessment of normal tricuspid valve anatomy in adults by real-time three-dimensional echocardiography. *Int J Cardiovasc Imaging*. 2007;23(6):717–724.
45. Brown AK, Anderson V. Two dimensional echocardiography and the tricuspid valve. Leaflet definition and prolapse. *Br Heart J*. 1983;49(5):495–500.
46. Otto CM. *Textbook of Clinical Echocardiography*. 3rd Ed. Philadelphia, PA: Elsevier Saunders; 2004.
47. Tajik AJ, et al. Two-dimensional real-time ultrasonic imaging of the heart and great vessels. Technique, image orientation, structure identification, and validation. *Mayo Clin Proc*. 1978;53(5):271–303.
48. Tei C, et al. Echocardiographic evaluation of normal and prolapsed tricuspid valve leaflets. *Am J Cardiol*. 1983;52(7):796–800.
49. Gussenhoven EJ, et al., "Offsetting" of the septal tricuspid leaflet in normal hearts and in hearts with Ebstein's anomaly. Anatomic and echographic correlation. *Am J Cardiol*. 1984;54(1):172–176.
50. Shiina A, et al. Two-dimensional echocardiographic spectrum of Ebstein's anomaly: Detailed anatomic assessment. *J Am Coll Cardiol*. 1984;3(2 Pt 1):356–370.
51. Ahlgrim AA, et al. Three-dimensional echocardiography: An alternative imaging choice for evaluation of tricuspid valve disorders. *Cardiol Clin*. 2007;25(2):305–309.
52. Anwar AM, et al. Value of assessment of tricuspid annulus: Real-time three-dimensional echocardiography and magnetic resonance imaging. *Int J Cardiovasc Imaging*. 2007;23(6):701–705.
53. Manghat NE, et al. Imaging the heart valves using ECG-gated 64-detector row cardiac CT. *Br J Radiol*. 2008;81(964):275–290.
54. Groves AM, et al. Semi-quantitative assessment of tricuspid regurgitation on contrast-enhanced multidetector CT. *Clin Radiol*. 2004;59(8):715–719.
55. Weber OM, Higgins CB. MR evaluation of cardiovascular physiology in congenital heart disease: Flow and function. *J Cardiovasc Magn Reson*. 2006;8(4):607–617.
56. Grothoff M, et al. Evaluation of postoperative pulmonary regurgitation after surgical repair of tetralogy of Fallot: Comparison between Doppler echocardiography and MR velocity mapping. *Pediatr Radiol*. 2008;38(2):186–191.
57. Shively BK. Transesophageal echocardiographic (TEE) evaluation of the aortic valve, left ventricular outflow tract, and pulmonic valve. *Cardiol Clin*. 2000;18(4):711–729.
58. Zaroff JG, Picard MH. Transesophageal echocardiographic (TEE) evaluation of the mitral and tricuspid valves. *Cardiol Clin*. 2000;18(4):731–750.
59. Cheitlin MD, et al. ACC/AHA/ASE 2003 Guideline Update for the Clinical Application of Echocardiography: Summary article. A report of the American College of Cardiology/American Heart Association Task Force on Practice Guidelines (ACC/AHA/ASE Committee to Update the 1997 Guidelines for the Clinical Application of Echocardiography). *J Am Soc Echocardiogr*. 2003;16(10):1091–1110.
60. Fawzy ME, et al. Doppler echocardiography in the evaluation of tricuspid stenosis. *Eur Heart J*. 1989;10(11):985–990.
61. Perez JE, Ludbrook PA, Ahumada GG. Usefulness of Doppler echocardiography in detecting tricuspid valve stenosis. *Am J Cardiol*. 1985;55(5):601–603.

62. Bonow RO, et al. ACC/AHA 2006 guidelines for the management of patients with valvular heart disease: A report of the American College of Cardiology/American Heart Association Task Force on Practice Guidelines (writing committee to revise the 1998 Guidelines for the Management of Patients With Valvular Heart Disease): Developed in collaboration with the Society of Cardiovascular Anesthesiologists: Endorsed by the Society for Cardiovascular Angiography and Interventions and the Society of Thoracic Surgeons. *Circulation.* 2006;114(5):e84–e231.

63. Zoghbi WA, et al. Recommendations for evaluation of the severity of native valvular regurgitation with two-dimensional and Doppler echocardiography. *J Am Soc Echocardiogr.* 2003;16(7):777–802.

64. Gonzalez-Vilchez F, et al. Assessment of tricuspid regurgitation by Doppler color flow imaging: Angiographic correlation. *Int J Cardiol.* 1994;44(3):275–283.

65. Grossmann G, et al. Comparison of the proximal flow convergence method and the jet area method for the assessment of the severity of tricuspid regurgitation. *Eur Heart J.* 1998;19(4):652–659.

66. Tribouilloy CM, et al. Quantification of tricuspid regurgitation by measuring the width of the vena contracta with Doppler color flow imaging: A clinical study. *J Am Coll Cardiol.* 2000;36(2):472–478.

67. Shapira Y, et al. Evaluation of tricuspid regurgitation severity: Echocardiographic and clinical correlation. *J Am Soc Echocardiogr.* 1998;11(6):652–659.

68. Simpson IA, et al. Current status of flow convergence for clinical applications: Is it a leaning tower of "PISA"? *J Am Coll Cardiol.* 1996;27(2):504–509.

69. Utsunomiya T, et al. Regurgitant volume estimation in patients with mitral regurgitation: Initial studies using color Doppler "proximal isovelocity surface area" method. *Echocardiography.* 1992;9(1):63–70.

70. Danicek V, et al. Relation of tricuspid inflow E-wave peak velocity to severity of tricuspid regurgitation. *Am J Cardiol.* 2006;98(3):399–401.

71. Imanishi T, et al. Validation of continuous wave Doppler-determined right ventricular peak positive and negative dp/dt: Effect of right atrial pressure on measurement. *J Am Coll Cardiol.* 1994;23(7):1638–1643.

72. Enriquez-Sarano M, et al. Amplitude-weighted mean velocity: Clinical utilization for quantitation of mitral regurgitation. *J Am Coll Cardiol.* 1993;22(6):1684–1690.

73. Borgeson DD, et al. Frequency of Doppler measurable pulmonary artery pressures. *J Am Soc Echocardiogr.* 1996;9(6):832–837.

74. Ristow B, et al. Pulmonary regurgitation end-diastolic gradient is a Doppler marker of cardiac status: Data from the Heart and Soul Study. *J Am Soc Echocardiogr.* 2005;18(9):885–891.

75. Rebergen SA, et al. Pulmonary regurgitation in the late postoperative follow-up of tetralogy of Fallot. Volumetric quantitation by nuclear magnetic resonance velocity mapping. *Circulation.* 1993;88(5 Pt 1):2257–2266.

76. Chowdhury UK, et al. Noninvasive assessment of repaired tetralogy of Fallot by magnetic resonance imaging and dynamic radionuclide studies. *Ann Thorac Surg.* 2006;81(4):1436–1442.

77. Scapellato F, et al. Accurate noninvasive estimation of pulmonary vascular resistance by Doppler echocardiography in patients with chronic failure heart failure. *J Am Coll Cardiol.* 2001;37(7):1813–1819.

78. Brennan JM, et al. Reappraisal of the use of inferior vena cava for estimating right atrial pressure. *J Am Soc Echocardiogr.* 2007;20(7):857–861.

79. Simonson JS, Schiller NB. Sonospirometry: A new method for noninvasive estimation of mean right atrial pressure based on two-dimensional echographic measurements of the inferior vena cava during measured inspiration. *J Am Coll Cardiol.* 1988;11(3):557–564.

80. Skjaerpe T, Hatle L. Diagnosis of tricuspid regurgitation. Sensitivity of Doppler ultrasound compared with contrast echocardiography. *Eur Heart J.* 1985;6(5):429–436.

81. Thomas L, Foster E, Schiller NB. Peak mitral inflow velocity predicts mitral regurgitation severity. *J Am Coll Cardiol.* 1998;31(1):174–179.

82. Sagie A, et al. Significant tricuspid regurgitation is a marker for adverse outcome in patients undergoing percutaneous balloon mitral valvuloplasty. *J Am Coll Cardiol.* 1994;24(3):696–702.

83. Orbe LC, et al. Initial outcome of percutaneous balloon valvuloplasty in rheumatic tricuspid valve stenosis. *Am J Cardiol.* 1993;71(4):353–354.

84. Ribeiro PA, et al. Percutaneous double balloon valvotomy for rheumatic tricuspid stenosis. *Am J Cardiol.* 1988;61(8):660–662.

85. Earing MG, et al. Long-term follow-up of patients after surgical treatment for isolated pulmonary valve stenosis. *Mayo Clin Proc.* 2005;80(7):871–876.

86. Jarrar M, et al. Long-term invasive and noninvasive results of percutaneous balloon pulmonary valvuloplasty in children, adolescents, and adults. *Am Heart J.* 1999;138(5 Pt 1):950–954.

87. Rao PS, et al. Results of three to 10 year follow up of balloon dilatation of the pulmonary valve. *Heart.* 1998;80(6):591–595.

88. Stanger P, et al. Balloon pulmonary valvuloplasty: Results of the valvuloplasty and angioplasty of congenital anomalies registry. *Am J Cardiol.* 1990;65(11):775–783.

89. Roos-Hesselink JW, et al. Long-term outcome after surgery for pulmonary stenosis (a longitudinal study of 22–33 years). *Eur Heart J.* 2006;27(4):482–488.

90. Schreiber C, et al. A new treatment option for pulmonary valvar insufficiency: First experiences with implantation of a self-expanding stented valve without use of cardiopulmonary bypass. *Eur J Cardiothorac Surg.* 2007;31(1):26–30.

91. Bonow RO, et al. 2008 focused update incorporated into the ACC/AHA 2006 guidelines for the management of patients with valvular heart disease: a report of the American College of Cardiology/American Heart Association Task Force on Practice Guidelines (Writing Committee to revise the 1998 guidelines for the management of patients with valvular heart disease). Endorsed by the Society of Cardiovascular Anesthesiologists, Society for Cardiovascular Angiography and Interventions, and Society of Thoracic Surgeons. *J Am Coll Cardiol.* 2008;52(13):e1–e142.

Infective Endocarditis

32

Marc A. Miller
Martin E. Goldman

1. INTRODUCTION

The first comprehensive description of endocarditis was by Sir William Osler in the Gustonian Lectures of 1885.[1] Defined as an inflammation of the endocardial surfaces of the heart or vascular structures, endocarditis has been classified by rate of progression and severity (acute vs. subacute), whether native valves or prosthetic materials are involved (e.g., prosthetic valve endocarditis and cardiac device infections) and whether it is infectious in origin. A series of events which promote the development of infectious endocarditis (IE) include endothelial trauma, formation of nonbacterial thrombotic endocarditis (NBTE), transient bacteremia, adherence and proliferation of bacteria within a vegetation and a subsequent immune response.[2] The promoter step, endothelial trauma, is often caused by blood flowing with high velocity through a narrow orifice, such as stenotic or regurgitant valvular lesions. This explains why the vegetations in aortic regurgitation are found on the left ventricular valvular surface, while those in patients with an infected ventricular septal defect with left-to-right shunting are found on the right ventricular surface. Jet lesions from valve turbulence produce endothelial damage, while adherence to the damaged valve is mediated by microbial surface components recognizing adhesive matrix molecules. Staphylococcus and Streptococcus avidly bind to fibronectin and platelets.

In the general population, the annual incidence of IE is 5 to 7 per 100,000 people[3] and more than 15,000 new cases are diagnosed each year in the United States.[4] Specific groups, such as those with congenital or rheumatic heart disease, prosthetic heart valves and intravenous drug users (IVDUs) are at greatest risk for developing endocarditis.[5] Responsible for almost 2,500 annual deaths in the United States, IE is associated with significant morbidity and mortality.[6] Prospective observational studies and international registries have reported in-hospital death rates of 22% for patients with prosthetic valve endocarditis,[7] 24% for IE due to non-HACEK Gram-negative bacilli,[8] and at least 20% for native-valve endocarditis due to Staphylococcus aureus.[9] Complications of IE, which develop in up to half of all cases,[10] include congestive heart failure, myocardial infarction, annular abscess, conduction system disease, immune responses, central and peripheral thromboemboli, renal failure and death.

Over the last few decades there appears to have been a change in the microbiological profile of IE. Although Viridans group streptococci appear to remain a common cause of native-valve IE in rural-based communities with a low incidence of injection drug abuse,[3,11] the incidence of S. aureus continues to rise and is now the leading cause of IE (Table 32.1); the latter being especially true in patients with prosthetic valve, intravenous drug abusers, and health care-associated IE.[7,12]

2. DIAGNOSIS OF ENDOCARDITIS

2.1. Transthoracic echocardiography

Clinical suspicion, blood cultures, and cardiac imaging make up the core components of the IE evaluation. However, since the clinical presentation can be quite variable, blood cultures are negative in up to 30% of cases[13] and clinical imaging does not always exclude IE, various diagnostic criteria have been proposed. The most widely utilized and best validated are the Duke criteria; originally published in 1994 and modified in 2000 (Table 32.2).[14,15] Echocardiography, which includes both transthoracic and transesophageal studies, has been the most extensively validated of all imaging modalities and is the only one included in the modified Duke criteria. An echocardiogram positive for IE is defined as an oscillating intracardiac mass on a valve or supporting endocardial structure (Fig. 32.1, Movie 32.1), or on implanted material in the absence of an alternative anatomic explanation, or a new partial dehiscence of a prosthetic heart valve or an intracardiac abscess.[14] A vegetation has distinctive irregular borders and can be sessile or pedunculated with independent motion from the underlying structure. An abscess is defined as an echolucent cavity within the valvular annulus or adjacent myocardial structures in the setting of a valvular infection.[16] Findings suggestive of IE, but not diagnostic, include a nonoscillating mass, nodular valve thickening, and new valvular fenestrations.[17] Minor pathologies frequently seen on valves, such as Lambl excrescences, redundant leaflet tissue, fibrocalcific degenerative changes, and ruptured chordae, can confound the diagnosis.

Two-dimensional (2D) transthoracic echocardiography (TTE) has a sensitivity of 55% to 65% and a specificity of >90% and can be used as an initial screening test in patients with a low-clinical suspicion of IE, good image quality, and absence of prosthetic material (Fig. 32.2).[18,19] Interestingly, despite the multiple innovations which have dramatically improved the resolution of echocardiography, TTE still fails to detect nearly half of all cases of native valve IE in the modern era.[20]

2.2. Transesophageal echocardiography

Transesophageal echocardiography, because of its higher transmit frequency compared to TTE (5 to 8 mHz vs. 1 to 3 mHz) and its retrocardiac position closer to the valves, has a higher sensitivity of 85% to 98% and similar specificity for the detection of IE. TEE should be the initial imaging test for those patients with intermediate to high probability of disease, suspected

455

TABLE 32.1

MICROBIOLOGIC ETIOLOGY IN 1,779 PATIENTS WITH DEFINITE ENDOCARDITIS IN THE INTERNATIONAL COLLABORATION ON ENDOCARDITIS-PROSPECTIVE COHORT STUDY

Staphylococcus	No. (%)
S. aureus	558 (31.6)
Coagulase-negative staphylococci	186 (10.5)
Streptococcus	
Viridans group streptococci	319 (18.0)
Streptococcus bovis	114 (6.5)
Other streptococci	91 (5.1)
Enterococci	188 (10.6)
HACEK	30 (1.7)
Non-HACEK Gram-negative bacteria	38 (2.1)
FUNGI	32 (1.8)
Polymicrobial	23 (1.3)
Other	56 (3.1)
Culture negative	144 (8.1)

Source: From Fowler VG, Jr, Miro JM, Hoen B, et al. Staphylococcus aureus endocarditis: A consequence of medical progress. *JAMA.* 2005;293:3012–3021.

complicated IE or those patients with prosthetic valves, cardiac devices, and indwelling catheters (Table 32.3). A comparison study of TTE versus TEE, in a group of 80 patients who underwent either surgery or necropsy, demonstrated that vegetation detection rate was significantly higher for TEE (90%) than for TTE (58%), especially when prosthetic valves were evaluated.[21] The important incremental value of TEE in patients with prosthetic heart valves was further demonstrated by Roe et al.[17] in a cohort of 112 patients with 114 suspected episodes of IE. Patients were first classified by TTE into a diagnostic category of the Duke criteria (definite, possible, or rejected), and then the diagnostic classification was reassigned using TEE results. Diagnostic reclassification occurred in only 11% of episodes of suspected IE in native cardiac valves, but in more than one third of episodes of prosthetic heart valves. TEE is also especially useful in cases of culture-negative endocarditis, for which it also enhances the diagnostic accuracy of the Duke criteria as compared to TTE.[22] Forgoing an initial TTE and proceeding directly to TEE, in at least intermediate probability cases, also appears to be a cost-effective strategy, especially in patients with prosthetic or repaired heart valves, cardiac devices, and indwelling catheters.[23] Although a negative TEE virtually excludes native-valve endocarditis, if there remains a high clinical suspicion for IE after an initial negative TEE, then it should be repeated after 48 h and within one week.[19] Causes of false-negative TEEs include very small lesions and shadowing from either dense calcium or a prosthetic valve apparatus. As such, off-angle views need to be explored. A repeat TEE after an initial negative examination may be especially useful in patients with cardiac prostheses and implantable intracardiac devices, such as pacemakers and defibrillators. In a prospectively studied cohort of 262 patients, of whom more than half had prosthetic heart valves, repeat TEE led to a reassignment from "possible" endocarditis to "definite" endocarditis in a substantial number of cases.[24] However, there

seems to be little incremental benefit to more than three repeat examinations.

In addition to establishing the diagnosis of IE, echocardiography, especially the high resolution of TEE, also plays a pivotal role in the management of IE. Echocardiography can characterize the vegetation (size, shape, and mobility) and establish the presence of a leaflet perforation, abscess or fistula, features which are strong predictors of mortality and IE-related complications (Figs. 32.3–32.6, Movies 32.2, 32.3, 32.4A, 32.4C, 32.4E, 32.4G).[25,26] Of 178 consecutive patients with definite infective endocarditis who underwent TEE, Di Salvo et al.[27] demonstrated a strong relationship between vegetation characteristics and risk of embolic events. Embolic events occurred far more frequently (60%) in those patients with a vegetation length of ≥10 mm as compared to those patients (23%) with a vegetation length of < 10 mm. In a meta-analysis of ten studies involving almost 750 patients, the risk of embolic complications was almost three times higher in patients with infective endocarditis and large vegetations (defined as > 10 mm) than in patients with either no detectable vegetations or small vegetations.[28] Highly mobile, pedunculated or prolapsing vegetations also increase the risk of heart failure, need for valve replacement and have a greater propensity to embolize.

Echocardiography is also useful to detect the presence of potential indications for surgical intervention, such as paravalvular (prosthetic) leaks and annular or aortic abscess (Table 32.4). An abscess is defined as an area of myocardial or periannular thickening with nonhomogenous or echolucent zone (liquification). A new murmur, pericardial involvement, and new high-degree atrioventricular block suggest myocardial abscess. Although significantly more sensitive than transthoracic, TEE may still miss a significant percentage of IE-associated myocardial abscesses due to shadowing or lack of differentiation from surrounding tissue. In a cohort of 115 patients with definite IE who underwent both

TABLE 32.2
MODIFIED DUKE CRITERIA FOR DIAGNOSIS OF INFECTIVE ENDOCARDITIS

Major criteria

Blood cultures

- ≥2 positive for typical IE microorganisms (viridans *Streptococcus* spp., *Streptococcus bovis*, HACEK group, *Staphylococcus aureus* or enterococci) in the absence of primary focus
- Persistently positive (two sets drawn > 12 h apart, or ≥3 of 4 sets with first and last separated by >1 h)
- One positive for *Coxiella burnettii* or IgG titer against phase I > 1:800

Endocardial involvement

- Positive TTE or TEE (the latter recommended for prosthetic valves, complicated IE, congenital heart disease, or if TTE images inadequate): (1) discrete, echogenic, oscillating intracardiac mass on valve or supporting structure, in the path of regurgitant jets, or on implanted material, in the absence of an alternative anatomic explanation; (2) periannular abscess; or (3) new partial dehiscence of prosthetic valve
- New valvular regurgitation (worsening of or change in pre-existing murmur insufficient)

Minor criteria

Broader clinical findings

- Predisposing cardiac condition or intravenous drug use
- Fever (temperature ≥ 38 °C)
- Vascular phenomena (major arterial emboli, septic pulmonary infarct, mycotic aneurysm, intracranial hemorrhage, conjunctival hemorrhage, and Janeway lesions)
- Immunologic phenomena (glomerulonephritis, Osler's nodes, Roth's spots, and positive rheumatoid factor)
- Microbiological findings of positive blood cultures not meeting major criteria or serologic evidence of active infection with plausible microorganisms (excludes single positive cultures of coagulase-negative staphylococci and organisms that do not cause endocarditis)

Diagnosis

Definite

- Pathology or bacteriology of vegetations, major emboli, or intracardiac abscess specimen, or
- Two major criteria, or
- One major and three minor criteria, or
- Five minor criteria

Possible

- One major and one minor criterion, or
- Three minor criteria

Rejected

- Firm alternative diagnosis, or
- Resolution of syndrome after 4 days of antimicrobial therapy, or
- No pathologic evidence at surgery or autopsy after 4 days of antimicrobial therapy, or
- Does not meet definite or possible criteria

Source: From Haldar SM, et al. Infective endocarditis: Diagnosis and management. *Nat Clin Pract Cardiovasc Med.* 3(6):310–317.

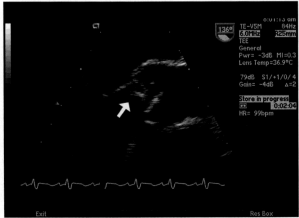
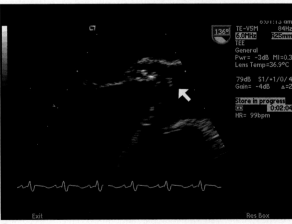

A   B

Figure 32.1 (**Movie 32.1**). Aortic valve vegetation seen by TEE prolapsing into the LV outflow tract during diastole (**A**) and into the aorta during systole (**B**).

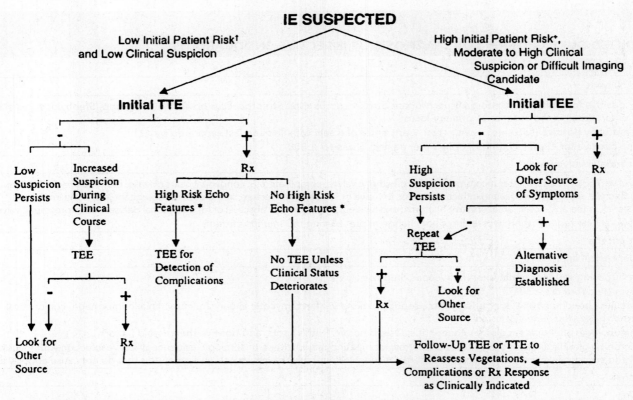

Figure 32.2 Algorithm for the use of transthoracic (TTE) and transesophageal echocardiography (TEE) in suspected infective endocarditis. *High-risk echocardiographic features include large and mobile vegetations, valvular insufficiency, suggestion of perivalvular extension, or secondary ventricular dysfunction (see text). For example, a patient with fever and a previously known heart murmur and no other stigmata of IE. +High initial patient risks include prosthetic heart valves, many congenital heart diseases, previous endocarditis, new murmur, heart failure, or other stigmata of endocarditis. Rx indicates antibiotic treatment for endocarditis. (Reproduced with permission from Bayer AS, Bolger AF, Taubert KA, et al. Diagnosis and management of infective endocarditis and its complications. *Circulation.* 1998;98:2936–2948.)

TABLE 32.3

ACC/AHA RECOMMENDATIONS FOR TRANSESOPHAGEAL ECHOCARDIOGRAPHY IN ENDOCARDITIS

Transesophageal echocardiography	Class of recommendation, level of evidence[a]
To assess severity of valvular lesions in symptomatic patients, if transthoracic echocardiography is nondiagnostic	I, C
To diagnose IE in patients with valvular heart disease and positive blood cultures, if transthoracic echocardiography is nondiagnostic	I, C
To diagnose complications of IE with potential impact on prognosis and management (e.g., abscess, perforation, and shunts).	I, C
First-line diagnostic study to diagnose prosthetic valve endocarditis and assess for complications	I, C
For preoperative evaluation in patients with known infective endocarditis, unless the need for surgery is evident on transthoracic imaging and unless preoperative imaging will delay surgery in urgent cases	I, C
Patients with persistent staphylococcal bacteremia without a known source	IIa, C
To detect IE in patients with nosocomial staphylococcal bacteremia	IIb, C

[a]Classification of Recommendation: Class I: Evidence and/or general agreement that the treatment is beneficial, useful, and effective; Class II: Conflicting evidence and/or divergence of opinion about the usefulness/efficacy; IIa: weight of evidence/opinion is in favor of usefulness/efficacy; IIb: usefulness/efficacy is less well established by evidence/opinion; Class III: Evidence of general agreement that the therapy is not useful or effective and in some cases may be harmful.
Level of Evidence: A: derived from multiple randomized clinical trials or metaanalyses; B: derived from single randomized trial or nonrandomized studies; C: consensus opinion of experts, case studies, or standard of care.
Source: From Bonow RW, et al. *Circulation.* 2006;114(5):e84–e231.

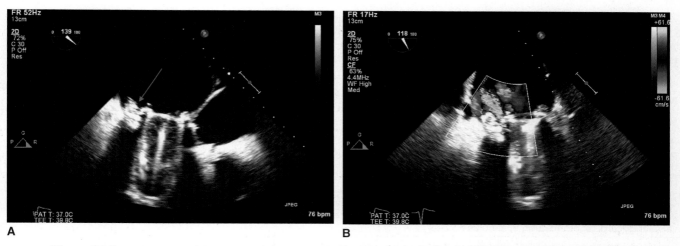

A

B

Figure 32.3 **A:** 2D TEE from a 54-year-old woman with prosthetic mitral valve (double tilting disc) endocarditis complicated by a large paravalvular abscess (*arrow*). **B:** Color flow Doppler demonstrating significant paravalvular mitral regurgitation as a consequence of the abscess.

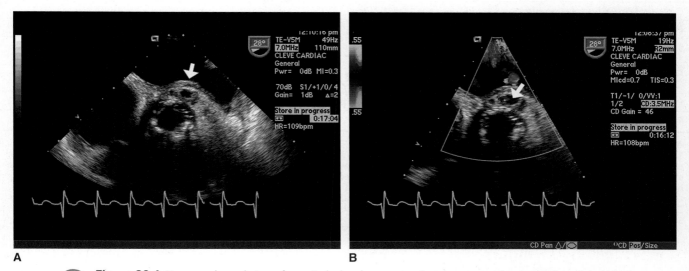

A

B

Figure 32.4 Transesophageal view of a perivalvular abscess seen between an aortic prosthesis and the mitral valve as an echolucent space by 2D **(A, Movie 32.2)** and demonstrating intracavitary flow by color Doppler **(B, Movie 32.3).**

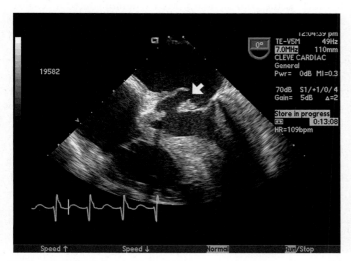

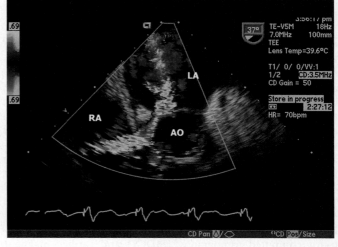

Figure 32.5 Transesophageal view of a perforation at the base of the mitral valve anterior leaflet caused by the regurgitant jet in a patient with aortic valve endocarditis.

Figure 32.6 (Movie 32.4). Aortic valve endocarditis complicated by fistulae into the left atrium (LA) and right atrium (RA).

TABLE 32.4

ACC/AHA GUIDELINES FOR SURGICAL THERAPY OF NATIVE AND PROSTHETIC VALVE INFECTIOUS ENDOCARDITIS

Native valve endocarditis	Class of recommendation, level of evidence[a]
Valve stenosis or regurgitation resulting heart failure	I, B
AR or MR with hemodynamic evidence of elevated LV end-diastolic or left-atrial pressures (e.g., premature closure of MV with AR, rapid decelerating MR signal by continuous-wave Doppler, or moderate to severe pulmonary hypertension)	I, B
Fungal or other highly resistant organisms	I, B
Complicated by heart block, annular or aortic abscess, or destructive penetrating lesions (e.g., sinus of Valsalva to right atrium, right ventricle, or left atrium fistula; mitral leaflet perforation with aortic valve endocarditis; or infection in annulus fibrosa)	I, B
Recurrent emboli and persistent vegetations despite appropriate antibiotic therapy	IIa, C
Mobile vegetations in excess of 10 mm with or without emboli	IIb, C
Prosthetic valve endocarditis	
Consultation with a cardiac surgeon	I, C
Present with heart failure	I, B
Dehiscence evidenced by cine fluoroscopy or echocardiography	I, B
Increasing obstruction or worsening regurgitation	I, C
Complications (e.g., abscess)	I, C
Persistent bacteremia or recurrent emboli despite appropriate antibiotic therapy	IIa, C
Relapsing infection	IIa, C

AR, aortic regurgitation; MR, mitral regurgitation; MV, mitral valve.
[a]Classification of Recommendation: Class I: Evidence and/or general agreement that the treatment is beneficial, useful, and effective; Class II: Conflicting evidence and/or divergence of opinion about the usefulness/efficacy; IIa: weight of evidence/opinion is in favor of usefulness/efficacy; IIb: usefulness/efficacy is less well established by evidence/opinion; Class III: Evidence of general agreement that the therapy is not useful or effective and in some cases may be harmful.
Level of Evidence: A: derived from multiple randomized clinical trials or metaanalyses; B: derived from single randomized trial, or nonrandomized studies; C: consensus opinion of experts, case studies, or standard of care.
Source: From Bonow RW, et al. *Circulation*. 2006;114(5):e84–e231.

TEE and cardiac surgery, an abscess was found intraoperatively in 38% of patients and yet the preoperative TEE missed more than half of them.[29] Of note is that almost two thirds of missed abscesses were localized and potentially masked by calcification in the posterior mitral annulus.

2.3. Real-time three-dimensional echocardiography

Real-time three-dimensional (3D) echocardiography is an emerging technology that has been evaluated for a variety of clinical applications, such as ventricular geometry and valvular anatomy, but its utility for either the diagnosis or management of IE has yet to be firmly established.[30] Transesophageal 3D echo, which can accurately characterize the anatomy and pathology of the mitral valve, may be complimentary to 2D TEE for the assessment of IE-associated complications and may eventually prove to be superior for imaging prosthetic valves, intracardiac devices, and indwelling catheters (Fig. 32.7).

2.4. CT, MRI, and radionuclide imaging

Despite numerous case reports and small series using multidetector computed tomography (MDCT) and cardiac magnetic resonance (CMR) imaging, the diagnostic yield and true clinical utility of these modalities in the diagnosis of IE are unknown.

In a series of 37 consecutive patients with clinically suspected IE who underwent both MDCT and TEE, and using intraoperative findings as the gold standard, MDCT demonstrated a sensitivity of 97%, specificity of 88%, and a negative predictive value of 97%.[31] Multislice CT and CMR appear to be very useful for the assessment of IE-associated complications, such as perivalvular pseudoaneurysms and myocardial abscesses (Fig. 32.8),[32,33] though small (≤2 mm) leaflet perforations may be missed. In one isolated case report, CMR detected an aortic perivalvular abscess secondary to *S. aureus*, which had been missed by two prior TEEs.[34]

Scintigraphies, using Indium-111 labeled leukocytes, Gallium-67, technetium-99 m-labeled antigranulocyte antibodies, and PET/CT with ^{18}F-FDG–Labeled leukocytes, have all been studied for the noninvasive detection of IE. Indium-111 labeled leukocytes, an established means of detecting inflammatory conditions such as chronic osteomyelitis, has questionable utility in the diagnostic workup of acute IE. In a study of seven patients with echocardiographic and microbiological evidence of acute bacterial endocarditis, all Indium-111 scans were negative.[35] More recently, investigators have begun to exploit the platelet activation which occurs during the formation and proliferation of a vegetation. Technetium

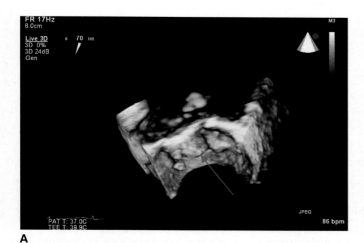

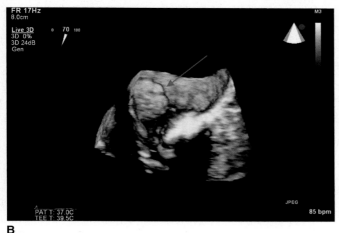

Figure 32.7 Three-dimensional TEE images from a 57-year-old woman with a large mitral annular abscess with highly mobile components on both the atrial (**A**) and ventricular (**B**) sides.

99 m–labeled Annexin V, which binds to phosphatidylserine on the surface of activated platelets, was used to detect thrombotic vegetations in experimental animal models of endocarditis.[36] Although few studies have compared echocardiography with radionuclide imaging for the detection of IE, the lower sensitivity and specificity of scintigraphy have relegated it to an adjunctive test in the setting of equivocal echocardiographic results.[37]

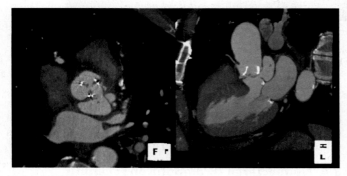

Figure 32.8 Multidetector 64-slice computed tomography short- and long-axis views of a subaortic saccular aneurysm (*arrow*) and a periprosthetic (biological) aortic valve abscess, occurring 12 years after the initial aortic valve replacement.

3. SPECIAL CONSIDERATIONS

3.1. Prosthetic valve endocarditis

The incidence of prosthetic-valve endocarditis (PVE), which carries a high mortality, is greatest within the first 12 months postoperatively (1.4% to 3.1%) and decreases significantly thereafter (3.0% to 5.7% over 5 years). In a prospective, observational cohort study conducted including 556 patients with definite PVE, 71% of health care-associated PVE events occurred within the first year of valve implantation, and *S. aureus* was the most common causative organism (23.0%) followed by coagulase-negative staphylococci (16.9%). Although *Streptococcus viridans* is an uncommon cause of early-onset PVE (<2 months after intervention), it can account for up to 20% of cases of late-onset (>12 months) PVE.[38] TEE is superior to TTE for diagnosing PVE and periannular complications. However, shadowing from valve discs, struts and annular rings, mandates utilizing off-angle views. In patients with both aortic and mitral prosthesis, TEE planes project the mitral shadows which can obscure the aortic valve. As such, a combination of off-angle views, gastric imaging, and TTE may be required to accurately assess for PVE.

3.2. Permanent pacemaker and implantable cardioverter-defibrillator infection

There has been a remarkable increase in the worldwide implantation of permanent pacemakers (PPMs) and implantable cardioverter-defibrillators (ICDs) as well as the number of cardiac device infections (CDIs). In a study of medicare beneficiaries comparing the incidence of CDIs in 1990 to those in 1999, the rate of infection increased by 124%.[39] Although the estimated incidence of CDIs varies widely (0.13% to 19.9%) and is dependent upon the type of device implanted, the site of implantation, and the underlying comorbidities of the patients, CDIs can occur in up to approximately 1% of patients with implantable cardiac devices.[40] CDIs are often classified anatomically—such as localized pocket infections, an isolated infection of the device lead, an isolated infection of the heart valve, or a combination of a device-lead infection and a valvular infection[41]—and by time of onset. "Early" CDIs are those acquired within a month of implantation, "late" CDIs are those which develop from 1 to 12 months after implant, and "delayed" are those beyond the first year. The most common microbial agent in CDIs is staphylococci, and the rate of CDI appears to be higher in patients with defibrillators than in those with pacemakers.[40] In addition to the tremendous additional hospital cost, estimated to range anywhere from $25,000 to $50,000,[42] CDIs are associated with significant morbidity and mortality.[43]

TTE has a low sensitivity (25% to 30%) for detecting lead infections, whereas the high sensitivity (>90%) of TEE, combined with its ability to characterize the morphology of vegetations and detect the presence of IE-associated complications, makes it the initial imaging modality in any patient with suspected CDI.[44] Based upon their own clinical experience and a review of published literature, Sohail et al. have proposed an algorithm for the approach to adults with PPM/ICD infection (Table 32.5). Additionally, TEE can improve the safety and efficacy of transvenous lead extraction.[45] 3D TEE may provide better differentiation between infectious masses versus fibrinous strands; the latter being commonly seen on implanted cardiac devices (Fig. 32.9).

3.3. Intravenous drug users

The annual incidence of IE in IVDUs ranges from 2% to 5%,[46] affects right-sided valves (tricuspid) in up to 50% of cases (compared to less than 10% in non-IV drug users) and is most

TABLE 32.5
MAYO CLINIC GUIDELINES FOR THE DIAGNOSIS AND MANAGEMENT OF CARDIAC DEVICE INFECTIONS
1. All patients should have at least two sets of blood cultures drawn at initial evaluation
2. Generator tissue Gram stain and culture and lead tip culture should be obtained
3. Patients who either have positive blood cultures or have negative blood cultures but had recent antibiotics before obtaining blood cultures should have a transesophageal echocardiogram (TEE) to assess for device-related endocarditis
4. Sensitivity of TTE is low and is not recommended to evaluate for device-related endocarditis
5. Patients with negative blood cultures and recent prior antibiotics and valve vegetations on TEE should be managed in consultation with an infectious diseases expert
6. All patients with device infection should undergo complete device removal, regardless of clinical presentation
7. A large (>1 cm) lead vegetation is not a stand-alone indication for surgical lead removal
8. Blood cultures should be repeated in all patients after device explantation. Patients with persistently positive blood cultures should be treated for at least 4 weeks with antimicrobials even if TEE is negative for vegetations or other evidence of infection
9. Duration of antimicrobial therapy should also be extended to ≥4 weeks in patients with complicated infection (endocarditis, septic venous thrombosis, osteomyelitis, and metastatic seeding)
10. Adequate debridement and control of infection should be achieved at all sites before reimplantation of a new device
11. Re-evaluation for continued need of the device should be performed before new device placement
12. If an infected cardiac device cannot be removed, then long-term suppressive antibiotic therapy should be administered after completing an initial course of treatment and securing a clinical response to therapy. Infectious diseases expert opinion should be sought

Source: From Sohail MR. *J Am Coll Cardiol*. 2007;49:1851–1859.

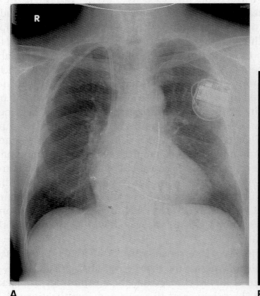

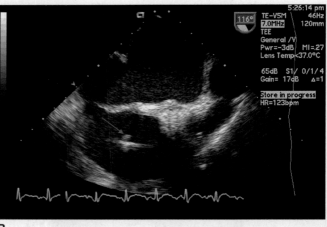

A   **B**

Figure 32.9 A: Chest X-ray from a 56-year-old heart transplant recipient with persistent left superior vena cava, who underwent single-lead ICD implantation. **B:** TEE, performed 6 months later for *Staphylococcus aureus* bacteremia, demonstrating a highly mobile 0.3 cm² echodensity attached to the right atrial portion of the ICD lead.

commonly due to staphylococcus. Left-sided IE in IVDUs is associated with an especially poor prognosis (overall mortality 20% to 30%) and requires prompt recognition and treatment.[46] The presence of HIV does not appear to alter the diagnostic accuracy of the Duke Criteria. In a cohort of 201 consecutive adult IVDUs with a suspected IE, the Duke criteria had a similar sensitivity, specificity, and diagnostic accuracy in IVDUs with and without HIV infection.[47] In addition to their increased risk of developing

polymicrobial and fungal (*Candida* species) IE, unusual forms of right-sided endocarditis, such as pulmonary valve or eustachian valve endocarditis, can occur in IVDUs.[48]

3.4. Nonbacterial thrombotic endocarditis

NBTE characterized by sterile vegetations and consisting primarily of platelets and fibrin can be seen in association with a variety of conditions including autoimmune diseases, connective tissue disorders, hypercoagulable states, and malignancy.[49] In a prospective echocardiographic screening of 200 unselected ambulatory patients with solid tumors, cardiac valvular vegetations were found in 19% of the patients; the most common location being the aortic and mitral valve.[50] Given the high prevalence of NBTE in cancer patients, the relatively small size of the vegetations, and the low sensitivity of TTE to detect NBTE vegetations, TEE should be considered in any patient with malignancy and an unexplained thromboembolic event.[51]

Libman–Sacks endocarditis, originally described in 1924, are noninfective verrucous vegetations found in up to 10% of patients with antiphospholipid syndrome and systemic lupus erythematosus (SLE)[52] and considered by many to be a subset of NBTE.[53] The vegetations can develop anywhere on the endocardial surface of the heart but have a predisposition for the left-sided heart valves, particularly the atrial surface of the mitral valve (Fig. 32.10, Movie 32.5).[54] These lesions typically arise on opposing leaflets (kissing vegetations). Aside from the vegetations characteristic of Libman–Sacks endocarditis, other valvular abnormalities common to SLE patients include isolated valvular thickening, regurgitation, and stenosis.[55] Patients with Libman–Sacks endocarditis are at increased risk of both progression to severe valvular disease (e.g., mitral regurgitation) and thromboembolic events (e.g., stroke). TEE is superior to TTE in detecting Libman–Sacks endocarditis and should be considered in patients who have nondiagnostic TTEs, suspected cardioembolism, or unexplained deterioration in valve function, or those in whom superimposed IE is suspected.[56] The laboratory findings of low to normal white blood cell count, increased levels of C-reactive protein, and the presence of antiphospholipid or anticardiolipin antibody levels strongly suggest Libman–Sacks lesions rather than IE.

3.5. Infective endocarditis in the elderly

Elderly patients (>65 years of age) carry an almost five times greater risk of IE compared younger patients which may be due to their higher prevalence of degenerative valve disease, implanted cardiac devices, and chronic illnesses. Furthermore, compared to younger patients the elderly are less likely to have intracardiac vegetations and more likely to have intracardiac abscesses. TEE should be strongly considered in any elderly patient with

suspected IE, especially if there is an underlying acquired cardiac pathology (e.g., mitral annular calcification) with the potential for a false-negative examination.[57]

4. PREVENTION OF INFECTIVE ENDOCARDITIS: REVISED GUIDELINES

The American Heart Association recently revised its guidelines on the prevention of IE. Notably, the focus of prevention switched from recommending prophylaxis based solely on individuals with increased lifetime risk of acquisition of IE to recommending prophylaxis only for those patients with an underlying cardiac condition associated with the greatest risk of adverse outcome from infective endocarditis. Cardiac conditions associated with the highest risk of adverse outcomes, and for which prophylaxis for dental procedures (which involve manipulation of gingival tissue or the perforation of oral mucosa) is reasonable, are listed in Table 32.6. Furthermore, antibiotic prophylaxis for the prevention of IE is no longer recommended for patients who undergo a genitourinary or gastrointestinal tract procedure.

Prior to the publication of these new guidelines, echocardiography was the single most important factor in endocarditis prophylaxis decision making.[58] If the new guidelines are adopted, then the number of preprocedural echocardiograms ordered solely for the purpose of diagnosing low and intermediate cardiac abnormalities will decrease accordingly. However, the clinician still has the discretion to consider the patient's underlying clinical condition, planned procedure, and risk of bacteremia in deciding whether to prescribe prophylactic antibiotics.

5. FUTURE DIRECTIONS

Echocardiography remains the imaging modality of choice for patients with suspected native or prosthetic valve endocarditis. Transesophageal echocardiography may be considered the initial imaging technique in patients with high clinical suspicion for IE, prosthetic valves, intracardiac devices, indwelling catheters, and the elderly to expedite diagnosis and therapeutic intervention.

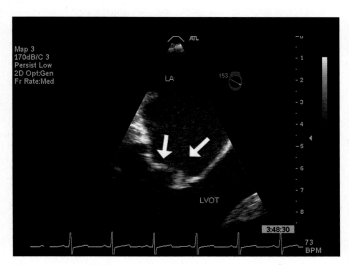

Figure 32.10. (Movie 32.5). Aseptic Liebman–Sacks mitral valve vegetations seen by TEE in a patient with anticardiolipin antibodies and recent stroke.

TABLE 32.6
CARDIAC CONDITIONS ASSOCIATED WITH THE HIGHEST RISK OF ADVERSE OUTCOME FROM ENDOCARDITIS FOR WHICH PROPHYLAXIS WITH DENTAL PROCEDURES IS REASONABLE
Prosthetic cardiac valve or prosthetic material used for cardiac valve repair
Previous IE
Congenital heart disease (CHD)
Unrepaired cyanotic CHD, including palliative shunts and conduits
Completely repaired congenital heart defect with prosthetic material or device, whether placed by surgery or by catheter intervention, during the first 6 months after the procedure
Repaired CHD with residual defects at the site or adjacent to the site of a prosthetic patch or prosthetic device (which inhibit endothelialization)
Cardiac transplantation recipients who develop cardiac valvulopathy

Source: From *Circulation.* 2007 9;116:1736–1754.

REFERENCES

1. Pruitt RD. William Osler and his Gulstonian Lectures on malignant endocarditis. *Mayo Clin Proc.* 1982;57:4–9.
2. Wilson W, Taubert KA, Gewitz M, et al. Prevention of infective endocarditis: Guidelines from the American Heart Association: A guideline from the American Heart Association Rheumatic Fever, Endocarditis, and Kawasaki Disease Committee, Council on Cardiovascular Disease in the Young, and the Council on Clinical Cardiology, Council on Cardiovascular Surgery and Anesthesia, and the Quality of Care and Outcomes Research Interdisciplinary Working Group. *Circulation.* 2007;116:1736–1754.
3. Tleyjeh IM, Steckelberg JM, Murad HS, et al. Temporal trends in infective endocarditis: A population-based study in Olmsted County, Minnesota. *JAMA.* 2005;293:3022–3028.
4. Liao L, Kong DF, Samad Z, et al. Echocardiographic risk stratification for early surgery with endocarditis: A cost-effectiveness analysis. *Heart.* 2008;94:e18.
5. Moreillon P, Que YA. Infective endocarditis. *Lancet.* 2004;363:139–149.
6. Rosamond W, Flegal K, Furie K, et al. Heart disease and stroke statistics–2008 update: A report from the American Heart Association Statistics Committee and Stroke Statistics Subcommittee. *Circulation.* 2008;117:e25–e146.
7. Wang A, Athan E, Pappas PA, et al. Contemporary clinical profile and outcome of prosthetic valve endocarditis. *JAMA.* 2007;297:1354–1361.
8. Morpeth S, Murdoch D, Cabell CH, et al. Non-HACEK gram-negative bacillus endocarditis. *Ann Intern Med.* 2007;147:829–835.
9. Miro JM, Anguera I, Cabell CH, et al. Staphylococcus aureus native valve infective endocarditis: Report of 566 episodes from the International Collaboration on Endocarditis Merged Database. *Clin Infect Dis.* 2005;41:507–514.
10. Hill EE, Herijgers P, Herregods MC, et al. Evolving trends in infective endocarditis. *Clin Microbiol Infect.* 2006;12:5–12.
11. Hoen B, Alla F, Selton-Suty C, et al. Changing profile of infective endocarditis: Results of a 1-year survey in France. *JAMA.* 2002;288:75–81.
12. Fowler VG, Jr, Miro JM, Hoen B, et al. Staphylococcus aureus endocarditis: A consequence of medical progress. *JAMA.* 2005;293:3012–3021.
13. Naber CK, Erbel R. Infective endocarditis with negative blood cultures. *Int J Antimicrob Agents.* 2007;30(Suppl. 1):S32–S36.
14. Durack DT, Lukes AS, Bright DK. New criteria for diagnosis of infective endocarditis: Utilization of specific echocardiographic findings. Duke Endocarditis Service. *Am J Med.* 1994;96:200–209.
15. Li JS, Sexton DJ, Mick N, et al. Proposed modifications to the Duke criteria for the diagnosis of infective endocarditis. *Clin Infect Dis.* 2000;30:633–638.
16. Choussat R, Thomas D, Isnard R, et al. Perivalvular abscesses associated with endocarditis; clinical features and prognostic factors of overall survival in a series of 233 cases. Perivalvular Abscesses French Multicentre Study. *Eur Heart J.* 1999;20:232–241.
17. Roe MT, Abramson MA, Li J, et al. Clinical information determines the impact of transesophageal echocardiography on the diagnosis of infective endocarditis by the duke criteria. *Am Heart J.* 2000;139:945–951.
18. Jacob S, Tong AT. Role of echocardiography in the diagnosis and management of infective endocarditis. *Curr Opin Cardiol.* 2002;17:478–485.
19. Horstkotte D, Follath F, Gutschik E, et al. Guidelines on prevention, diagnosis and treatment of infective endocarditis executive summary; the task force on infective endocarditis of the European society of cardiology. *Eur Heart J.* 2004;25:267–276.
20. Reynolds HR, Jagen MA, Tunick PA, et al. Sensitivity of transthoracic versus transesophageal echocardiography for the detection of native valve vegetations in the modern era. *J Am Soc Echocardiogr.* 2003;16:67–70.
21. Mugge A, Daniel WG, Frank G, et al. Echocardiography in infective endocarditis: Reassessment of prognostic implications of vegetation size determined by the transthoracic and the transesophageal approach. *J Am Coll Cardiol.* 1989;14:631–638.
22. Kupferwasser LI, Darius H, Muller AM, et al. Diagnosis of culture-negative endocarditis: The role of the Duke criteria and the impact of transesophageal echocardiography. *Am Heart J.* 2001;142:146–152.
23. Heidenreich PA, Masoudi FA, Maini B, et al. Echocardiography in patients with suspected endocarditis: A cost-effectiveness analysis. *Am J Med.* 1999;107:198–208.
24. Vieira ML, Grinberg M, Pomerantzeff PM, et al. Repeated echocardiographic examinations of patients with suspected infective endocarditis. *Heart.* 2004;90:1020–1024.
25. Sachdev M, Peterson GE, Jollis JG. Imaging techniques for diagnosis of infective endocarditis. *Cardiol Clin.* 2003;21:185–195.
26. Thuny F, Di Salvo G, Belliard O, et al. Risk of embolism and death in infective endocarditis: Prognostic value of echocardiography: A prospective multicenter study. *Circulation.* 2005;112:69–75.
27. Di Salvo G, Habib G, Pergola V, et al. Echocardiography predicts embolic events in infective endocarditis. *J Am Coll Cardiol.* 2001;37:1069–1076.
28. Tischler MD, Vaitkus PT. The ability of vegetation size on echocardiography to predict clinical complications: A meta-analysis. *J Am Soc Echocardiogr.* 1997;10:562–568.
29. Hill EE, Herijgers P, Claus P, et al. Abscess in infective endocarditis: The value of transesophageal echocardiography and outcome: A 5-year study. *Am Heart J.* 2007;154:923–928.
30. Badano LP, Dall'Armellina E, Monaghan MJ, et al. Real-time three-dimensional echocardiography: Technological gadget or clinical tool? *J Cardiovasc Med (Hagerstown).* 2007;8:144–162.
31. Feuchtner GM, Stolzmann P, Dichtl W, et al. Multislice computed tomography in infective endocarditis: Comparison with transesophageal echocardiography and intraoperative findings. *J Am Coll Cardiol.* 2009;53:436–444.
32. Christiaens L, Ardilouze P, Sorbets E. Aortic valvular endocarditis visualised by 16-row detector multislice computed tomography. *Heart.* 2006;92:1466.
33. Pollak Y, Comeau CR, Wolff SD. Staphylococcus aureus endocarditis of the aortic valve diagnosed on MR imaging. *AJR Am J Roentgenol.* 2002;179:1647.
34. Sverdlov AL, Taylor K, Elkington AG, et al. Images in cardiovascular medicine. Cardiac magnetic resonance imaging identifies the elusive perivalvular abscess. *Circulation.* 2008;118:e1–e3.
35. McDermott BP, Mohan S, Thermidor M, et al. The lack of diagnostic value of the indium scan in acute bacterial endocarditis. *Am J Med.* 2004;117:621–623.
36. Rouzet F, Dominguez Hernandez M, Hervatin F, et al. Technetium 99 m-labeled annexin V scintigraphy of platelet activation in vegetations of experimental endocarditis. *Circulation.* 2008;117:781–789.
37. Morguet AJ, Munz DL, Ivancevic V, et al. Immunoscintigraphy using technetium-99 m-labeled anti-NCA-95 antigranulocyte antibodies as an adjunct to echocardiography in subacute infective endocarditis. *J Am Coll Cardiol.* 1994;23:1171–1178.
38. Lopez J, Revilla A, Vilacosta I, et al. Definition, clinical profile, microbiological spectrum, and prognostic factors of early-onset prosthetic valve endocarditis. *Eur Heart J.* 2007;28:760–765.
39. Cabell CH, Heidenreich PA, Chu VH, et al. Increasing rates of cardiac device infections among Medicare beneficiaries: 1990–1999. *Am Heart J.* 2004;147:582–586.
40. Uslan DZ, Sohail MR, St Sauver JL, et al. Permanent pacemaker and implantable cardioverter defibrillator infection: A population-based study. *Arch Intern Med.* 2007;167:669–675.
41. Duval X, Selton-Suty C, Alla F, et al. Endocarditis in patients with a permanent pacemaker: A 1-year epidemiological survey on infective endocarditis due to valvular and/or pacemaker infection. *Clin Infect Dis.* 2004;39:68–74.
42. Ferguson TB Jr, Ferguson CL, Crites K, et al. The additional hospital costs generated in the management of complications of pacemaker and defibrillator implantations. *J Thorac Cardiovasc Surg.* 1996;111:742–751.
43. Sohail MR, Uslan DZ, Khan AH, et al. Infective endocarditis complicating permanent pacemaker and implantable cardioverter-defibrillator infection. *Mayo Clin Proc.* 2008;83:46–53.
44. Victor F, De Place C, Camus C, et al. Pacemaker lead infection: Echocardiographic features, management, and outcome. *Heart.* 1999;81:82–87.
45. Endo Y, O'Mara JE, Weiner S, et al. Clinical utility of intraprocedural transesophageal echocardiography during transvenous lead extraction. *J Am Soc Echocardiogr.* 2008;21:861–867.
46. Miro JM, del Rio A, Mestres CA. Infective endocarditis in intravenous drug abusers and HIV-1 infected patients. *Infect Dis Clin North Am.* 2002;16:273–295,vii-viii.
47. Cecchi E, Imazio M, Tidu M, et al. Infective endocarditis in drug addicts: Role of HIV infection and the diagnostic accuracy of Duke criteria. *J Cardiovasc Med (Hagerstown).* 2007;8:169–175.
48. Moss R, Munt B. Injection drug use and right sided endocarditis. *Heart.* 2003;89:577–581.
49. Eiken PW, Edwards WD, Tazelaar HD, et al. Surgical pathology of nonbacterial thrombotic endocarditis in 30 patients, 1985–2000. *Mayo Clin Proc.* 2001;76:1204–1212.
50. Edoute Y, Haim N, Rinkevich D, et al. Cardiac valvular vegetations in cancer patients: A prospective echocardiographic study of 200 patients. *Am J Med.* 1997;102:252–258.
51. Dutta T, Karas MG, Segal AZ, et al. Yield of transesophageal echocardiography for nonbacterial thrombotic endocarditis and other cardiac sources of embolism in cancer patients with cerebral ischemia. *Am J Cardiol.* 2006;97:894–898.
52. Moyssakis I, Tektonidou MG, Vassilliou VA, et al. Libman-Sacks endocarditis in systemic lupus erythematosus: Prevalence, associations, and evolution. *Am J Med.* 2007;120:636–642.
53. Asopa S, Patel A, Khan OA, et al. Non-bacterial thrombotic endocarditis. *Eur J Cardiothorac Surg.* 2007;32:696–701.
54. Hojnik M, George J, Ziporen L, et al. Heart valve involvement (Libman-Sacks endocarditis) in the antiphospholipid syndrome. *Circulation.* 1996;93:1579–1587.
55. Roldan CA, Shively BK, Crawford MH. An echocardiographic study of valvular heart disease associated with systemic lupus erythematosus. *N Engl J Med.* 1996;335:1424–1430.
56. Roldan CA, Qualls CR, Sopko KS, et al. Transthoracic versus transesophageal echocardiography for detection of Libman-Sacks endocarditis: A randomized controlled study. *J Rheumatol.* 2008;35:224–229.
57. Durante-Mangoni E, Bradley S, Selton-Suty C, et al. Current features of infective endocarditis in elderly patients: Results of the International Collaboration on Endocarditis Prospective Cohort Study. *Arch Intern Med.* 2008;168:2095–2103.
58. Singh SM, Joyner CD, Alter DA. The importance of echocardiography in physicians' support of endocarditis prophylaxis. *Arch Intern Med.* 2006;166:549–553.

Dilated Cardiomyopathy

33

Richard W. Troughton

1. INTRODUCTION

Dilated cardiomyopathy (DCM) is defined as the presence of left ventricular (LV) dilatation and systolic dysfunction in the absence of macrovascular coronary artery disease or abnormal loading due to hypertension or valvular disease.[1-3] There are multiple causes for DCM (Table 33.1), but all are characterized by abnormal LV myocardial structure and function that can be due either to a primary abnormality of myocardium or secondary to another process, such as drug toxicity or systemic disease.[1,2]

1.1. Epidemiology

The prevalence of DCM is estimated at 30 to 40 per 100,000 of the general population, with an incidence of 5 to 8 new cases per 100,000 annually.[3] DCM is the underlying cause for one third of systolic heart failure cases, although up to half of the subjects with DCM in the community may be asymptomatic.[4-6]

An underlying cause can be identified in half of all cases with DCM. In the remaining cases with idiopathic DCM no definite cause is found.[1-3,7] Previous myocarditis, drug toxicity, stress cardiomyopathy, and tachycardia mediated cardiomyopathy are important definable causes.[3,7] Genetic predisposition is an important factor in 20% to 50% of cases of DCM mainly due to autosomal dominant inheritance of mutations in genes encoding important myocardial proteins, while X-linked, mitochondrial or autosomal recessive inheritance accounts for a small proportion of familial cardiomyopathy.[8,9]

There is significant regional variation in the epidemiology of DCM, with prevalence of trypanosomal disease (Chagas disease) or toxoplasma and nutritional deficiency being more common in developing countries, Africa and South America.[2,10,11]

1.2. Clinical presentation
1.2.1. Symptoms and physical signs
The initial clinical presentation with DCM is diverse reflecting the broad range of underlying etiologies and can vary from asymptomatic to mild, moderate, or severe heart failure. Heart failure symptoms are common and include reduced exercise tolerance, fatigue, orthopnea, paroxysmal nocturnal dyspnea, or features of fluid retention.[12] Palpitations or syncope may be more common in sarcoidosis or Chagas disease. Systemic thromboembolism due to LV thrombus may occur in peripartum cardiomyopathy (PPCM), LV noncompaction, or Chagas disease.[11,13] The diagnosis of DCM is frequently an incidental finding in asymptomatic subjects undergoing cardiac imaging to investigate incidental abnormalities found on electrocardiogram or chest radiology. Examination findings are nonspecific but may include low-volume pulse with tachycardia, elevation of jugular venous pressure (JVP), displaced, hypokinetic LV apical impulse with accompanying third heart sound, basal lung crackles, hepatomegaly, and peripheral edema.[12] The presence of an apical pansystolic murmur may indicate functional mitral regurgitation.

1.2.2. Outcome
The natural history of DCM is variable, reflecting the diversity of underlying etiology.[7] Historical reports indicated high rates of progressive LV dysfunction and mortality in DCM. Modern pharmacotherapy, particularly neurohormonal blockade with angiotensin converting enzyme (ACE) inhibitors, angiotensin type 1 receptor blocker (ARB), mineralocorticoid receptor antagonists, and β-adrenergic receptor blockers, has led to improved clinical outcomes and attenuation or even reversal of LV remodeling.[12] Despite effective drug and device treatments, recent estimates of mortality rates for symptomatic DCM remain relatively high and in the order of 30% at 5 years.[7,14] Survival is strongly influenced by the underlying cause for DCM or by underlying genetic abnormality, with significantly lower mortality in peripartum and idiopathic cardiomyopathy compared to other causes such as infiltrative cardiomyopathies, anthracycline related cardiomyopathies, or those related to specific genetic polymorphisms such as the laminopathies.[7,15]

Although progressive LV dysfunction is common, a significant proportion of subjects with new onset heart failure due to DCM may also experience spontaneous recovery of LV systolic function.[13,16]

2. PATHOPHYSIOLOGY

2.1. Viral myocarditis

Myocarditis, particularly due to viral infection, is the most common identifiable cause of new onset DCM and is also implicated as the underlying cause in many cases of idiopathic DCM.[7,17,18] Persistence of viral genome can be identified in myocardial biopsies from up to 70% of idiopathic DCM patients.[19,20]

Many viruses can cause myocarditis including coxsackievirus, influenza, adenovirus, parvovirus, cytomegalovirus, and human immunodeficiency virus (HIV). Myocardial damage results from direct viral cytopathic effects, including the actions of viral proteases on key structural or functional proteins such as dystrophin.[21,22] Host immune responses largely mediated by lymphocytic infiltration also contribute to myocardial damage.[23]

Most cases of viral myocarditis resolve spontaneously without sequelae even when there is mild LV dysfunction at presentation.[17] Greater LV dysfunction at presentation (LV ejection fraction

TABLE 33.1
CAUSES OF DILATED CARDIOMYOPATHY

Idiopathic
Familial
Sarcomeric proteins
Troponin I,T, and C
Actin
β-Myosin
α-Tropomyosin
Cytoskeletal proteins
Dystrophin (X-linked)
Desmin
Nuclear membrane proteins
Lamin A/C
Mitochondrial
Myocarditis
Viral
Bacterial
Trypanosomal
Inflammatory/autoimmune
Sarcoidosis
Scleroderma
Drug related
Alcohol
Anthracyclines
Trastuzumab
Pregnancy and peripartum related
Endocrine
Thyroid related
Pheochromocytoma
Nutritional
Thiamine
Tachycardia mediated
Unclassified
Stress cardiomyopathy
Isolated noncompaction

Cardiac magnetic resonance (CMR) imaging provides accurate quantification of LV volumes and systolic function and demonstrates characteristic appearances including focal intramural and subepicardial high intensity on T1 images with matching subepicardial or intramural late enhancement of gadolinium, with sparing of the subendocardium.[17,28,29] These findings in combination with the pattern of regional wall motion may be helpful in guiding endomyocardial biopsy.[30] Appearances on CMR predict the likelihood of persisting LV dysfunction, with larger LV end-diastolic volume and greater extent of late postgadolinium enhancement, particularly in the interventricular septum, associated with persisting LV dysfunction.[20]

2.2. Infiltrative and inflammatory disorders

2.2.1. Cardiac amyloid

Although cardiac amyloid is characterized on echocardiography by increased wall thickness (see Chapter 34), advanced diastolic dysfunction, and atrial dilatation, in the late stages up to 25% of subjects may develop significant LV systolic dysfunction and some degree of LV dilatation.[31] Primary (AL) amyloid results from immunoglobulin light chain disease in B-cell related lymphoproliferative conditions such as myeloma or monoclonal gammopathy of uncertain significance.[31] Up to 50% of deaths in primary amyloid result from cardiac involvement due to deposition of AL fibrils in myocardium. Systemic or secondary amyloid (AA) is associated with inflammatory conditions and results in secondary deposition of serum amyloid A in organ beds including the heart. Treatment of the underlying condition may attenuate progression but rarely reverses cardiac amyloid.[31]

Although the echocardiographic appearances of amyloid are well characterized, they are nonspecific and may not differentiate amyloid from other restrictive or infiltrative cardiomyopathies. Appearance on CMR is distinctive and correlates well with biopsy proven cardiac amyloid, thereby allowing accurate noninvasive characterization.[32,33] Hyperintense gadolinium signal soon after injection is followed by a characteristic pattern of ill-defined subendocardial late enhancement that matches amyloid deposition (Fig. 33.1).[32,33]

2.2.2. Sarcoidosis

Sarcoidosis is a noncaseating granulomatous multisystem disease with cardiac involvement in 30% to 60% of cases. Cardiac involvement is associated with conduction block and tachyarrhythmias and may produce a DCM phenotype in up to 30% of

[LVEF] < 40%) is associated with a >50% chance of developing chronic systolic dysfunction and with higher mortality risk.[17,23,24] Persistence of viral genome and extensive immunohistochemical changes are also associated with progressive LV dysfunction and worse survival.[19,24–26] Mortality for subjects with biopsy proven myocarditis is similar to that of DCM as a whole, although paradoxically a better prognosis has been reported for fulminant myocarditis.[27]

Echocardiography is the most common initial imaging modality employed during acute myocarditis or after recovery. In both settings, appearances are nonspecific. LV dilatation may be minimal in the acute form, but systolic function is often impaired and regional wall motion abnormalities may be seen frequently.

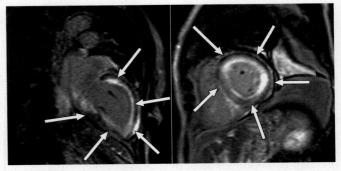

Figure 33.1 Cardiac MRI late-enhancement two-chamber long-axis **(left)** and short-axis **(right)** images showing intense subendocardial enhancement involving all left ventricle walls (*arrows*) in a 76-year-old woman with histologic diagnosis of amyloidosis of periumbilical adipose tissue. (Adapted from Belloni E, et al. *Am J Roentgenol.* 2008;191:1702–1710.)

TABLE 33.2

COMPARISON OF RELATIVE UTILITY OF DIFFERENT IMAGING MODALITIES FOR ASSESSMENT OF KEY VARIABLES IN DILATED CARDIOMYOPATHY

	Echocardiography	CMR	MDCT	Nuclear imaging
LV morphology	+++	+++	++	+
LV volumes and mass	++	+++	+++	++
LV systolic function	+++	+++	++	++
LV diastolic function	+++	+	+/−	+
Synchrony	+++	+	+/−	+/−
RV size and function	+	+++	++	+
Mitral regurgitation	+++	++	+/−	−
Distribution and extent of myocardial scar	+	+++	+	++

LV, left ventricular; RV, right ventricular; CMR, cardiac magnetic resonance imaging; MDCT, multidetector computed tomography.

cases. Cardiac imaging frequently demonstrates increased LV wall thickness. CMR imaging demonstrates characteristic appearances including widespread areas of transmural myocardial hyperenhancement particularly in the septum.[34]

2.2.3. Cardiomyopathy related to Iron overload
Iron overload associated with conditions such as hemochromatosis or β-thalassemia may result in iron deposition in the myocardium leading to injury and eventually to a reduction in LV systolic function that may be irreversible if treatment is delayed.[35] Early treatment with iron chelation may prevent development of systolic dysfunction; however, measurements of serum and hepatic iron correlate poorly with myocardial deposition. Echocardiographic appearances of DCM due to iron overload are nonspecific and may appear late in the clinical course. In contrast, cardiac MR may provide early detection of iron deposition in myocardium, potentially allowing early intervention.[35] Specifically, increased myocardial iron is associated with shorter T2 time and more rapid decay in T2 signal intensity.[36]

2.3. Chagas disease
Cardiomyopathy is seen in 30% to 40% of the suspected 18 million worldwide, mainly Latin American sufferers of chronic Chagas disease.[11,37] Transmission of the protozoan Trypanosoma Cruzi (T. Cruzi) via insect vectors—or less frequently through blood transfusion, contaminated needle, or congenital transmission—leads to acute infection that is frequently subclinical.[37] The chronic phase of the disease develops beyond 2 months and can be confirmed serologically by the presence of IgG antibodies to T. Cruzi present in blood. The chronic form is indeterminate in 60% of sufferers, but causes progressive cardiomyopathy in up to 40%. Cardiomyopathy due to Chagas disease is characterized by cardiac enlargement, with the classical finding of LV apical aneurysm seen in up to half of the patients. Histological findings include mild cellular inflammatory response and diffuse fibrosis involving the myocardium and conducting system, particularly the right bundle. T. Cruzi antigens or gene fragments can be identified in myocardium. The clinical course is characterized

by progressive enlargement of all cardiac chambers, symptomatic heart failure, conduction block—typically of the right bundle, arrhythmias including multifocal ventricular tachycardia, and an increased risk of LV thrombus and pulmonary thromboembolism.[37] In refractory patients, transplantation may be required. Outcome after ventricular aneurysmectomy is variable and this is not routinely advocated. Cardiac pacing or implantable cardioverter devices (ICDs) may be required in the setting of conduction disease or ventricular arrhythmias.

2.4. Peripartum cardiomyopathy
PPCM is defined as new onset LV dilatation and systolic dysfunction occurring in the last month of pregnancy or the first 5 months postpartum and in the absence of other cause for cardiomyopathy.[38] Pregnancy related cardiomyopathy occurring earlier in gestation or beyond 6 months after delivery may be part of the same entity.[13] PPCM occurs in <1 in 300 live births and accounts for only a small proportion (4%) of DCM, but its presentation and acute clinical course may be dramatic. Risk of PPCM is greater in older, multiparous mothers and in the setting of toxemia, gestational hypertension, tocolytic therapy, or twin pregnancy.[13,38] Although inflammatory infiltrate and the presence of viral genome have been seen on endomyocardial biopsy in some series, the cause for PPCM remains unclear and immune or cytokine mediated mechanisms appear to be important.[39] Presentation is with clinical features of LV dysfunction and heart failure symptoms that may be masked in some cases by symptoms of late pregnancy. Echocardiography demonstrates impairment of LV systolic function. Mitral regurgitation is common and when LVEF is low (<35%), LV thrombus is frequently seen and may be accompanied by systemic embolism. Initial treatment is with diuretics and vasodilators—hydralazine can be safely used during pregnancy with ACE inhibitors favored postpartum. Because of LV thrombus and increased systemic and pulmonary thromboembolic risk, heparin is essential during pregnancy and warfarin therapy is advocated postpartum. Improvement in LV function occurs more frequently than for other causes of DCM, but in up to 50% LV dysfunction may persist beyond 6 months.[13] Early mortality rates may be as high as 15%

in some series, but longer-term prognosis appears to be better for PPCM than other causes of DCM.[7] Longer-term treatment with ACE inhibitors and β-blockers is essential and monitoring with 6-monthly echocardiography is advocated as late recovery of LV function has been documented. The risk of recurrent PPCM is significant,[40] with heart failure rates during subsequent pregnancies of 20% in those with normalized LV function and 40% in those with impaired LV function.[38]

2.5. Drug-induced
2.5.1. Alcohol-related cardiomyopathy
Low or moderate alcohol intake (7 to 12 units per week) may lower the risk of cardiovascular and heart failure events, but excessive consumption may impair myocardial structure and function.[41] Risk of alcohol-related DCM increases with higher average daily intake and longer duration of exposure. An intake in excess of 80 g ethanol per day for a minimum of 5 years is typically reported as the threshold for DCM, although female gender and genetic polymorphisms increase susceptibility. Asymptomatic LV dysfunction occurs in up to one third of alcoholic patients and closely mirrors prevalence of cirrhosis in this group. Mechanisms for ethanol-induced cardiomyopathy include increased apoptosis, activation of the renin–angiotensin system, altered myocardial protein synthesis, and adverse actions of acetaldehyde on myocardial contractility, calcium handling, and cellular oxidative status.[41] Nutritional factors including thiamine deficiency may also contribute. Abnormal biochemical or hematological indices may be present, particularly relating to red cell morphology or hepatic function. Pathological changes on endomyocardial biopsy are relatively nonspecific, but early changes in mitochondrial ultrastructure may point to ethanol cardiomyopathy. Appearances on cardiac imaging are nonspecific, although left ventricular hypertrophy (LVH) is frequently present.

2.5.2. Chemotherapy related cardiomyopathy
Anthracycline related cardiotoxicity is responsible for up to 4% of DCM cases. Cardiotoxicity is mediated in part by myocyte injury resulting from increased production of free radical oxygen species.[42] Risk of toxicity is related to cumulative dose with LV dysfunction occurring in up to 25% of subjects receiving doxorubicin doses above 550 g/m² and in 35% of those receiving doses of >600 g/m².[43] However, doses as low as 200 g/m² can cause LV dysfunction, with increased risk of cardiomyopathy associated with greater age, prior radiation therapy, and concomitant chemotherapy.[42] Cardiomyopathy usually occurs within 12 months of anthracycline treatment, but may occur late in up to 40% of cases, particularly after treatment in childhood or with higher doses. Adjunctive use of dexrazoxane may reduce injury, and alternative agents such as epirubicin or mitoxantrone have lesser cardiotoxicity. Noninvasive imaging is recommended to monitor LV systolic function during therapy and to identify late toxicity. Echocardiography and radionuclide ventriculography are methods of choice for monitoring changes in LVEF, with a limited role for CMR imaging.[44] Newer echocardiographic modalities such as 2D speckle tracking imaging can identify changes in regional or global deformation before changes in EF occur, which may facilitate early detection of toxicity.[45]

Trastuzumab (herceptin), a recombinant monoclonal antibody to human epidermal growth factor (also known as ErbB2 or HER-2Neu), is approved for treatment of advanced breast cancer in 20% of patients with overexpression of the HER-2 oncogene.[46,47] Treatment with Trastuzumab is associated with a minor reduction in LVEF measured by echocardiography or multiple-gated acquisition (MUGA) scan. Cardiac toxicity, defined as a fall in LVEF by >10% or from normal to below 40%, has been documented in up to 7% of recipients.[47] Risk of toxicity is up to fourfold greater in subjects receiving concurrent anthracycline therapy. Monitoring of LVEF is recommended during Trastuzumab therapy, and in most instances there is recovery of LV function after withdrawal of Trastuzumab and treatment with ACE inhibitor and β-blocker therapy. The mechanism of Trastuzumab cardiac toxicity is unclear, but experimental studies and animal models demonstrate that HER-2Neu plays a critical role in regulating normal cardiac development.[47]

2.6. Familial cardiomyopathy
One third of DCM cases have a familial genetic basis.[8,9] In 75% of familial cardiomyopathy there is autosomal dominant inheritance of mutations in genes encoding important structural or functional myocardial proteins.[8,9] A range of mutations have been identified, many involving sarcomeric proteins such as actin, myosin, and the troponins.[48,49] The phenotype and natural history of familial cardiomyopathy varies depending on the cardiac protein affected, but typically, there is mild LV dilatation associated with systolic dysfunction. Involvement of the conducting system is seen with some mutations, particularly those affecting Lamin A/C.[15] Mutations with autosomal recessive inheritance occur less frequently but present at an early age with a more aggressive adverse natural history, while mutations of mitochondrial origin account for <1% of documented cases of DCM.[8]

In family members of subjects with DCM, the presence of autoantibodies to cardiac proteins denotes a greater risk of developing LV enlargement or systolic dysfunction.[50]

While cardiac imaging of familial DCM demonstrates nonspecific appearances, preclinical cardiomyopathy may be detected in family members of affected subjects using cardiac MRI[51] or echocardiography with tissue Doppler imaging.[52]

2.7. X-linked familial cardiomyopathy
Familial cardiomyopathy is X-linked in 5% to 10% of cases, resulting from mutations in the Dystrophin gene that also produce the skeletal muscle abnormalities of Becker and Duchenne muscular dystrophy.[53,54] A DCM phenotype and involvement of the conducting system are associated with extensive fibrosis particularly in the lateral wall. Functional mitral regurgitation is frequently seen.[55] Cardiomyopathy occurs at an early age in Duchenne muscular dystrophy and is evident in nearly all subjects by the late teenage years. Heart failure symptoms may be initially masked by physical inactivity due to skeletal muscle abnormalities, but survival beyond the third decade is rare and cardiomyopathy is a common cause of death. Although skeletal muscle abnormalities are less severe in Becker muscular dystrophy, the cardiomyopathy may be more severe possibly reflecting the impact of result of greater physical activity.[53,54]

Findings on cardiac imaging including echocardiography are nonspecific and typically show dilatation of all chambers. Features of noncompaction may also be evident.[55] Diagnosis should be suspected in young men presenting with DCM, especially in the setting of skeletal muscle abnormality or raised serum creatinine kinase levels. The diagnosis can be confirmed by skeletal electromyography or muscle biopsy and analysis of the dystrophin protein by immunoblotting or of the dystrophin gene.[53,54]

2.8. Unclassified cardiomyopathies
2.8.1. Stress cardiomyopathy
Stress cardiomyopathy, also known as apical ballooning syndrome or takotsubo cardiomyopathy (after the Japanese

octopus pots which imitate the typical LV appearances in this condition), is a recently described condition.[56] More common in middle-aged, postmenopausal women, presentation typically follows an acutely stressful incident with clinical features suggestive of an acute coronary syndrome, including chest pain, acute injury pattern on electrocardiogram, and raised myocardial injury markers. These findings are associated with typical echocardiographic appearance of hypokinesis, akinesis, or dyskinesis involving the LV mid and apical segments in a pattern that involves more than a single coronary artery vascular distribution (Fig. 33.2). However, at angiography there is no evidence of obstructive epicardial coronary disease or acute plaque rupture. To confirm the diagnosis, pheochromocytoma and myocarditis must be excluded.

LV dysfunction and ECG changes are usually transient, resolving within 6 weeks. Mortality rates in-hospital are low (1% to 2%), but heart failure and ventricular arrhythmia due to QT interval prolongation are more common. Recurrent episodes have been reported in 10% of cases. The pathophysiology of stress cardiomyopathy is incompletely understood, but spasm of more than one epicardial coronary artery, microvascular impairment, direct catecholamine toxicity due to increased circulating catecholamines, or neurogenically mediated myocardial sympathetic activation may all play a role.[57,58] There are no established treatment guidelines, but supportive treatment for shock or heart failure is recommended. Combined α- and β-blockade may be preferred to isolated β-blockade.

LV appearance on contrast left ventriculography, echocardiography, or MR imaging is typical, with akinesis of the mid segments and ballooning or dyskinesis of the apical LV segments.[57,58] Apical segments of the right ventricle may also be involved. In the acute setting, perfusion defects may be demonstrated in the apical segments with myocardial contrast echocardiography.[57] Unlike ischemic cardiomyopathy with apical scarring, in stress cardiomyopathy there is no late gadolinium enhancement (LGE) on MR. MRI may, therefore, be helpful in differentiating myocarditis or prior myocardial infarction from stress cardiomyopathy.[59,60]

2.8.2. Noncompaction of the left ventricle

Isolated noncompaction of ventricular myocardium is a rare form of unclassified cardiomyopathy that results from interrupted cardiac embryogenesis.[61] Early in development, the embryonic heart consists of a spongiform mass of trabeculated muscle fibers interspersed with deep recesses that form sinuses communicating with the LV cavity.[62] Resorption of these sinuses produces the capillary network that communicates with the developing coronary circulation and the surrounding trabeculated myocardial fibers compact to produce normal myocardium. Interruption of this process results in persistence of the hyper trabeculated appearance. The cause for noncompaction is not clear, but gene association studies have identified familial and sporadic forms with novel mutations in sarcomeric proteins and in the α-dystrobrevin genes.[62,63] Prevalence is reported at <0.02% of the general population, and diagnosis is usually made in childhood although not uncommonly, the first presentation may occur in adult life.[62]

Noncompaction presents clinically with heart failure, arrhythmias, or systemic thromboembolism.[64] LV systolic and diastolic function are usually impaired at the time of first diagnosis or develop during follow-up in a nearly all subjects. Survival without transplant is ~50% at 5 years from the time of diagnosis with higher event rates in subjects with more advanced symptoms, higher LV end-diastolic pressures, conduction delay, or atrial fibrillation.[61,64] Treatment includes guideline-based medical therapy for systolic heart failure, anticoagulation, with consideration of ICD implant and cardiac transplantation in high-risk subjects with advanced symptoms.

Appearances on 2D echocardiography and color Doppler are characteristic (Fig. 33.3) with prominent trabeculation and deep recesses in the myocardium, usually affecting the apex and inferior wall.[65] In nearly half of the cases, the RV apex may be involved. Differentiation from DCM with prominent trabeculation may

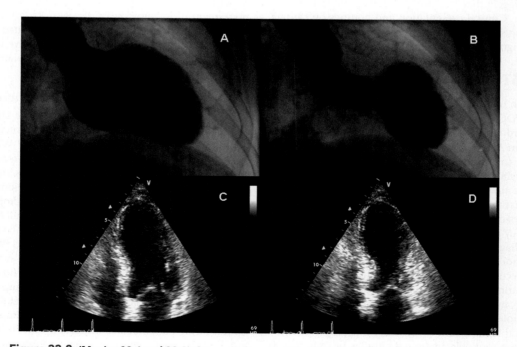

Figure 33.2 (Movies 33.1 and 33.2). Stress cardiomyopathy: Diastolic **(A,C)** and systolic **(B,D)** images from ventriculography and 2D echocardiography demonstrating typical "apical ballooning" appearance related to akinesis of left ventricular mid and apical segments in a 50-year-old female subject with acute stress cardiomyopathy.

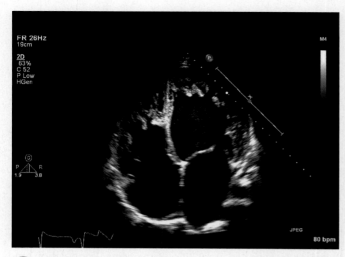

Figure 33.3 (Movie 33.3). 2D echocardiographic image demonstrating deep trabeculation of the left and right ventricular apexes in a 28-year-old man with isolated noncompaction and systolic heart failure. (Courtesy of Paul Bridgman.)

be difficult, but a ratio of 2:1 for thickness of trabeculation compared to compacted myocardial thickness at end systole provides good discrimination. LV systolic impairment is present in 60% and restrictive filling in one third of subjects at presentation. MRI provides excellent visualization of the trabeculated ventricular appearance.

2.8.3. Idiopathic dilated cardiomyopathy

In up to half of the cases of DCM, no underlying cause is found. In many of these, prior injury due to infectious myocarditis is suspected. Persistence of viral genome can be identified in myocardial biopsies from up to 70% of idiopathic DCM patients.[19,20] Genetic predisposition is also important but the interactions with environmental triggers that lead to cardiomyopathy are poorly defined at present. Clinical presentation and findings on cardiac imaging are nonspecific. The natural history of idiopathic DCM may be more benign than other forms.[7]

3. DIAGNOSTIC EVALUATION

Careful evaluation of patient history is important in the evaluation of suspected DCM. A history of antecedent infectious illness, malignancy treated with doxorubicin therapy, recent pregnancy, time spent in Latin America, or excess alcohol consumption may all provide clues to the underlying etiology. Family history of cardiomyopathy should be carefully documented, particularly in subjects where no other etiology is evident. Risk factors for coronary artery disease or history of myocardial infarction should be identified. Physical examination may demonstrate features of heart failure and LV dysfunction.

Appropriate diagnostic investigations should be targeted at identifying the underlying etiology of cardiomyopathy and severity of disease.[12] Electrocardiography and chest radiography should be performed routinely. B-type natriuretic peptide levels may be elevated and indicate symptomatic status and prognosis.[66]

Because the etiology of DCM can frequently be determined on the basis of clinical features and noninvasive imaging, endomyocardial biopsy is not routinely advocated but may be indicated in specific circumstances. These include new onset heart failure <2 weeks with hemodynamic compromise, or heart failure of 2 weeks

to 3 months duration or longer with failure to respond to therapy or with new ventricular arrhythmias or conduction block, or DCM associated with suspected allergic reaction or eosinophilia.[67]

Cardiac imaging is key to the investigation of DCM and should be directed at accurately quantifying the severity of cardiac dysfunction and identifying the underlying etiology.[34,68–70] Echocardiographic evaluation should include comprehensive 2D imaging of cardiac structure with 3D imaging for quantification of LV volumes and EF where possible.[71] Comprehensive hemodynamic assessment and evaluation of valves should be undertaken with color, pulsed, and continuous wave Doppler and tissue Doppler imaging. Newer indices such as 2D speckle tracking and tissue velocity imaging may allow more sophisticated assessment of ventricular function and synchrony.[44,68]

CMR imaging should include assessment of structure with fast spin-echo black blood sequences with and without fat suppression, and of function with cine steady-state free precession (SSFP) sequences. Phase contrast sequences allow assessment of filling patterns and hemodynamic status. Early and late enhancement T1 weighted inversion recovery sequences should be obtained after administration of gadolinium contrast for assessment of myocardial inflammation, fibrosis, and scar.[72]

Multidetector computed tomography (MDCT) allows visualization of the cardiac chambers, of the coronary arterial and venous anatomy, and of the pulmonary veins in subjects with sinus rhythm and controlled heart rate (70 to 80/min).[73] Prospective ECG gating may reduce contrast requirements and allow imaging in subjects with mild or moderate renal impairment.[74] Accurate assessment of LV volumes, mass, and EF is possible, and MDCT may also allow characterization of myocardial scar.[74] The main value of MDCT is the exclusion of significant epicardial coronary artery disease as the cause of LV dysfunction.

Nuclear imaging techniques allow characterization of coronary artery disease and ventricular function in appropriate patients. ECG-gated single photon emission computed tomography (SPECT) perfusion imaging and positron emission tomography (PET), particularly when used with hybrid MDCT imaging, allow for accurate assessment of ischemic heart disease.[70] Radionuclide ventriculography with gated pooled blood imaging or gated SPECT allows for assessment of LV volumes and EF. The relative utility of different imaging modalities for assessment of key variables in dilated cardiomyopathy is presented in table 33.2.

3.1. Evaluation of ventricular function

Accurate quantification of LV morphology, size, and function is vital in DCM as it provides more accurate functional assessment, risk stratification, and guides therapy decisions.[68] Where possible, 3D imaging by echocardiography, MRI, or MDCT, is preferable as it provides more accurate estimation of LV volumes, mass, and EF, while avoiding the pitfalls of accurate image acquisition and reproducibility that can occur with 2D imaging.[75] Echocardiography is the most commonly used modality and is recommended in guidelines as initial test of choice.[44,76] CMR and MDCT may be the first choice for accurate assessment of LV volumes, mass, and EF in some settings or where the acoustic window is inadequate even with the use of echocardiographic contrast agents.[74] Radionuclide ventriculography may be useful when more sophisticated imaging is not available.

Doppler echocardiography allows for careful assessment of LV filling patterns and diastolic function (see Chapter 16).[68,77] Transmitral filling patterns have important functional and prognostic implications, with pseudonormal or restrictive filling patterns indicating greater symptomatic limitation and increased risk of heart failure events or mortality.[77] Tissue Doppler or 2D strain imaging allows quantification of LV myocardial velocities.[78] In addition, Doppler indices allow accurate estimation of filling pressures. In this regard, a shortened early transmitral deceleration time (DT) with the ratio of early transmitral to either early mitral annular velocity (E/E') or the velocity of propagation of LV filling (E/V_p) in particular provides accurate estimates of LV filling pressure.[77]

Measurement of interventricular and intraventricular synchrony should be assessed in subjects with conduction delay, particularly when the QRS duration is between 120 and 150 ms (see Chapter 44). A range of indices should be assessed including septal posterior wall mechanical delay from parasternal M-mode, left and right ventricular pre-ejection times from pulsed wave Doppler outflow spectra.[79] Regional delay in longitudinal or radial peak systolic myocardial velocity or deformation in multiple segments can be measured from color-encoded tissue velocity imaging or 2D speckle tracking.[79] Variation in regional volume changes can be measured using real-time 3D volume.[71]

Important complications such as LV thrombus formation may be seen especially in Chagas disease or PPCM. MRI has greater sensitivity for detection of LV thrombus, while use of contrast agents may improve the accuracy of echocardiography.[80]

Right ventricular size and function are closely related to symptoms and outcome in DCM and should be assessed on each occasion the heart is imaged. Accurate volumetric quantification of the right ventricle is difficult due to chamber geometry and may be better facilitated by MRI or even MDCT techniques.[72,81] Quantification by echocardiography is more challenging, but availability of 3D echocardiography may allow greater accuracy.[82] Myocardial systolic velocities from the tricuspid lateral annulus provide quantification of RV systolic function that is less dependent on geometric assumptions.[81] Peak tricuspid regurgitation (TR) jet velocities allow accurate estimation of peak RV systolic pressures as an indication of pulmonary artery pressures.

Left atrial (LA) volume and mechanical function should also be assessed.[83] Higher LA volumes indicate greater severity of cardiac dysfunction and may act as a barometer of long-term LV filling pressures. Atrial transmitral or pulmonary vein reversal peak velocities and duration reflect atrial mechanical function and pressure, while mitral annular late diastolic tissue Doppler velocities are a marker of atrial mechanical function and stunning that may predict atrial fibrillation.

The appropriate frequency of serial imaging in heart failure is the subject of debate, but repeat imaging should be performed when there is a significant change in clinical status to guide important therapy decisions and to assess response to therapy.[76] 3D imaging by MRI or echocardiography provides greatest reproducibility and less technique-related variability on serial measurements of LV volumes and mass.[75] LV filling patterns and diastolic function, MR severity, RV function, and RV systolic pressure should also be undertaken at each assessment. In subjects with cardiac resynchronization therapy (CRT) or conduction delay indices of synchrony should also be assessed and pacing intervals may be optimized in the former.[79]

Changes in LVEF are dependent on loading and may also occur later in the pathophysiology of DCM. Newer imaging indices that allow characterization of regional and global myocardial functions may identify more subtle abnormality of LV function at an earlier stage. Tagged MRI imaging allows accurate characterization of longitudinal and radial myocardial deformation and can identify early LV dysfunction in high-risk subjects.[34] Early changes in regional or global myocardial velocities or strain may be detected by echocardiography using tissue velocity imaging or speckle tracking.[45] Similarly, abnormalities of radial deformation, torsion, or synchrony may be identified using echocardiographic 2D speckle tracking imaging.[84] And this modality has also demonstrated longitudinal rotation of the heart as a feature of subjects with DCM when there is QRS prolongation.[85]

3.2. Mitral valve assessment

Mitral regurgitation (MR) is seen frequently in DCM and is an important determinant of symptoms and outcome as well contributing to progressive ventricular remodeling.[86] Careful assessment of mitral valve structure and function is therefore paramount, and specific attention should be directed at confirming the mechanism of MR and accurately quantifying MR severity (see Chapter 30).[87,88]

The usual mechanism of MR in DCM is failure of coaptation due to tethering of otherwise normal leaflets as a consequence of LV dilatation and displacement of the papillary muscles.[89] The extent of annular dilatation and leaflet tenting can be measured by 3D echocardiography. Abnormality of either mitral leaflets or subvalvular apparatus or the presence of complex MR should alert the clinician to consider a primary valvular abnormality as the cause for LV dysfunction.

Qualitative and semiquantitative assessment of MR severity by echocardiography should include evaluation of MR jet size, continuous wave Doppler spectra intensity, pulmonary vein systolic flow blunting or reversal and the presence and size of vena contracta, and proximal convergence.[87,88] More importantly, mitral regurgitant volume and regurgitant fraction should be quantified by echocardiography or MRI. Echocardiography allows calculation of regurgitant volume from pulsed wave Doppler-derived measurements of aortic and mitral stroke volume. The proximal isovelocity surface area (PISA) method described elsewhere allows calculation of effective regurgitant orifice area and regurgitant volume.[88] The PISA method should be corrected if the hemisphere of proximal convergence is constrained or its radius varies through systole. MRI can accurately calculate MR regurgitant volume or fraction based on the difference between LV diastolic and systolic volumes measured from cine short-axis images and the aortic stroke volume measured from phase contrast sequences.[72] A regurgitant volume of <30 mL per beat or fraction <30% by either technique indicates mild MR, whereas a regurgitant volume >60 mL or a fraction >50% indicates severe MR.[87]

3.3. Establishing etiology

Cardiovascular imaging plays a critical role in establishing the etiology of DCM. Because of the important prognostic and therapeutic implications, coronary artery disease should be excluded, first by documenting the presence and extent of scarring from prior myocardial infarction and secondly by confirming the presence of coronary artery stenoses and the extent of viable myocardium.[90] LV wall thinning or regional wall motion abnormality on echocardiography or CMR are clues to an ischemic etiology, but lack sensitivity and specificity.[90] CMR imaging for LGE is the test of choice for identification of myocardial scar (Fig. 33.4).[91,92] Regional subendocardial or transmural LGE is pathognomonic for scar due to prior infarction, and this technique allows accurate assessment of the absolute amount of myocardial scar as well as the relative transmural extent of scarring. Transmural scar involving >50% of wall thickness indicates a low probability of functional recovery after revascularization, whereas scar involving <25% myocardial wall thickness has a high likelihood of functional recovery even

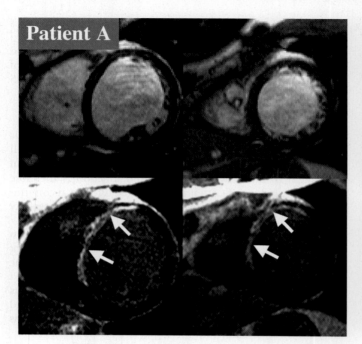

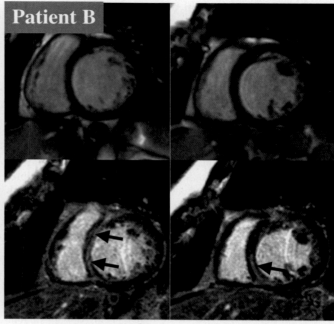

Figure 33.4 Short-axis images in two patients presenting with heart failure, enlarged left ventricle, and systolic dysfunction. The corresponding contrast cardiac magnetic resonance images demonstrate nearly transmural late gadolinium enhancement (LGE) in the anteroseptal wall consistent with a prior myocardial infarction in the patient with ischemic heart disease (**patient A**), whereas typical midwall stria-type LGE is present in the patient with nonischemic cardiomyopathy (**patient B**). (Adapted from Sechtem U, et al. Heart. 2007;93:1520–1527.)

when there is myocardial thinning. When ischemic cardiomyopathy is suspected from the clinical context or CMR appearances, selective coronary angiography is generally the test of choice to define the extent of coronary stenoses. In selected lower probability cases where coronary artery disease needs to be excluded, MDCT with (64-slice or greater) may be appropriate to exclude coronary stenosis with >50% diameter loss.

CMR provides accurate characterization of a number of specific cardiomyopathies. In Chagas disease, SSFP imaging by CMR provides excellent visualization of localized aneurysm formation, typically at the apex or basal inferolateral wall, frequently with associated mural thrombus formation and with subendocardial LGE consistent with scar in terminal vascular distributions.[34]

In cardiac sarcoidosis, LGE due to interstitial noncaseating granuloma formation is seen typically in a transmural pattern involving the septum, basal, and lateral segments (Fig. 33.5).[72] Early detection of this pattern prior to onset of LV dilatation and systolic impairment may facilitate early intervention. In acute myocarditis, CMR again is the test of choice. T2 weighting demonstrates edema in the lateral wall that typically correlates with multiple foci of late enhancement in the lateral LV often in the mid ventricular wall or toward the epicardium.[30] In the later phase, resolution of these changes may be seen or the development of LGE in the mid wall consistent with fibrosis (Fig. 33.6).[72]

Several cardiomyopathies have a distinctive appearance that allows diagnosis by echocardiography or CMR, including isolated noncompaction of the left ventricle (Fig. 33.3). The distinctive appearance of apical ballooning seen in stress or takotsubo cardiomyopathy may be pathognomonic (Fig. 33.2), but still requires correlation with clinical features and exclusion of acute coronary occlusion to confirm the diagnosis.

4. PROGNOSIS AND THERAPY GUIDANCE

A range of clinical, functional, biochemical, and haematological indices predict mortality and rehospitalization in DCM and heart failure. Clinical indicators include age, increasing symptomatic class, presence of a third heart sound or persistent JVP elevation, reduced peak oxygen consumption during exercise and conduction delay, ventricular ectopy or nonsustained ventricular tachycardia on electrocardiography.[12] Hematologic markers of anemia and biochemical indicators of renal dysfunction or neurohormonal activation including the B-type natriuretic peptides or norephinephrine are important markers of heart failure events.[66]

Cardiac imaging provides powerful risk stratification in DCM. Regardless of imaging modality, larger LV mass or volumes (particularly systolic) or reduced EF all predict increased mortality, as does RV enlargement or systolic dysfunction.[75]

Echocardiographic prognostic markers include the severity of diastolic dysfunction; progressively worse outcomes are seen for pseudonormal and restrictive filling patterns.[68,75,77] Doppler indices of LV compliance—especially early transmitral DT—and filling pressure—especially E/E'—provide incremental risk stratification.[78] Tissue velocity-based indices of LV synchrony are also associated with mortality.[78]

Specific findings on MRI also provide independent risk stratification. The extent of intramural late enhancement reflects the degree of fibrosis and is associated with increased mortality and tachyarrhythmias.[93,94] The presence of subendocardial late enhancement in patients without obstructive CAD is associated with increased risk of cardiac events.[93]

4.1. Medical therapy

While nonpharmacological interventions such as weight monitoring, salt restriction, and exercise play an important role, drug

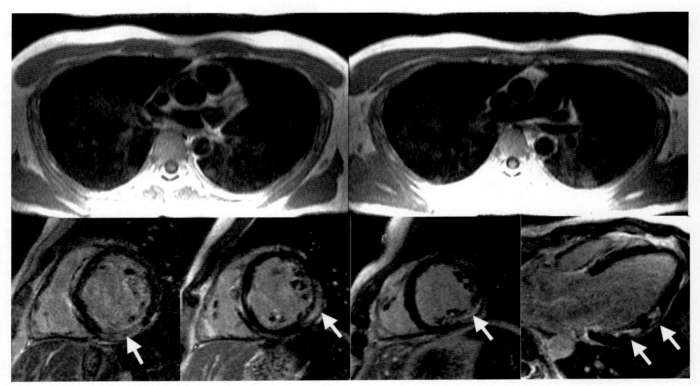

Figure 33.5 Spin-echo **(upper panel)** and late gadolinium enhancement-cardiac magnetic resonance (LGE-CMR; **lower panel)** images in a patient with biopsy proven with pulmonary sarcoidosis. A diffuse signal is seen in both lungs on spin-echo images. LGE short-axis images (three images from the left in the lower panel from base to apex) demonstrate inferior and lateral enhancement not dissimilar to that seen in myocarditis. (Adapted from Sechtem U, et al. *Heart.* 2007;93:1520–1527.)

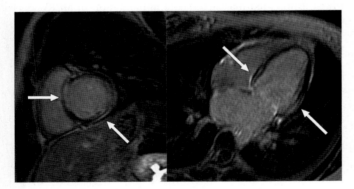

Figure 33.6 Cardiac MRI from a 19-year-old woman with a history of myocarditis when aged 10 years. Late-enhancement short-axis **(left panel)** and four-chamber long-axis **(right panel)** images showing meso-cardial striae of hyperenhancement located in the basal interventricular septum and posteroinferior and lateral LV walls (*arrows*). (Adapted from Belloni E, et al. *Am J Roentgenol.* 2008;191:1702–1710.)

therapy is the cornerstone of heart failure treatment.[76] Diuretic therapy is useful for managing volume overload and congestion, while the appropriate use of ACE inhibitors, ARBs, β-adrenergic receptor blockers (BB) and aldosterone receptor blockade has led to reductions in mortality and heart failure hospitalization in symptomatic systolic heart failure.[12] In asymptomatic patients with reduced EF, use of ACE inhibitors is associated with reduced mortality and ARB (in ACE intolerant subjects) and BB are also recommended in this setting.[12]

Cardiac imaging is vital for guiding implementation and assessing the response to appropriate medical therapy. Accurate assessment of systolic dysfunction in symptomatic patients is important to guide the implementation of the proven neurohormonal antagonists mentioned earlier. Serial measurement of volumes and EF allows monitoring of ventricular remodeling, which is attenuated by effective therapy. The presence of myocardial contractile reserve on stress echocardiography predicts a greater likelihood of symptomatic response and reverse remodeling with BB therapy, as does a lesser extent of myocardial scar on CMR late enhancement imaging.[95] Improvements in diastolic filling patterns are more readily measured by echocardiography and are associated with improvements in symptomatic status and outcome.[77]

4.2. Cardiac resynchronization and implantable cardioverter devices

Nearly half of all subjects with DCM die suddenly. Use of an ICD in symptomatic subjects with a reduced LVEF is associated with a mortality reduction of ~10% per annum.[12,14] ICD therapy is currently recommended for primary prevention in subjects with LVEF < 30% and NYHA class II–III symptoms receiving optimal medical therapy and may be considered in subjects with LVEF between 30% to 35%.[76] Cardiac imaging therefore plays a vital role in defining patients who are eligible for ICD therapy (Fig. 33.7), and accurate measurement of LVEF is pivotal. Specific imaging may also identify subjects at higher risk for arrhythmic events. Greater extent of gadolinium late enhancement on MRI identifies increased fibrosis or scar and greater substrate for arrhythmias and predicts a higher likelihood of sudden death.[96]

Up to 30% of subjects with DCM and systolic heart failure have left bundle branch block associated with mechanical LV dyssynchrony. In this context, CRT is associated with significant

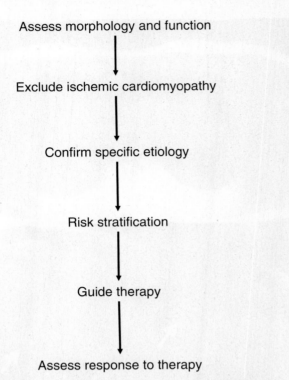

Assess morphology and function

↓

Exclude ischemic cardiomyopathy

↓

Confirm specific etiology

↓

Risk stratification

↓

Guide therapy

↓

Assess response to therapy

Figure 33.7 Aims of cardiovascular imaging in dilated cardiomyopathy.

reductions in mortality and rehospitalization and with reverse LV remodeling.[97,98] CRT with or without an ICD is currently recommended for symptomatic subjects receiving optimal medical therapy who have an LVEF < 35%, sinus rhythm, and cardiac dyssynchrony defined by QRS >120 ms on surface electrocardiogram.[76] Accurate measurement of LV volumes and EF is therefore essential to identify subjects who are eligible for CRT. Although multiple echocardiographic indices may indicate the degree of interventricular or LV intraventricular mechanical dyssynchrony, no single index can reliably predict the response to CRT.[75,99] Although echocardiographic indices may be helpful in confirming the presence of mechanical dyssynchrony in subjects with lesser degrees of QRS prolongation (120 to 150 ms), use of these indices to select eligible subjects for CRT is not currently advocated in guidelines.[76,99]

Cardiac imaging may provide helpful adjunctive information around the time of CRT implantation. Tissue velocity or 2D speckle tracking imaging may identify the point of latest mechanical LV activation.[100,101] Pacing at the site of greatest delay is associated with greater response to CRT.[100] Use of MDCT to define coronary venous anatomy in combination with tissue velocity or speckle tracking based measurements of regional mechanical delay may therefore be invaluable for facilitating implant planning. The presence of extensive scarring defined by reduced deformation on echocardiographic speckle tracking or tissue velocity imaging or by LGE on MRI, particularly involving the lateral wall, are associated with a reduced response to CRT.[75]

Following CRT, echocardiography can document reverse LV remodeling. Optimization of atrioventricular and ventriculoventricular pacing intervals guided by echocardiography is associated with improvements in LV contractility, EF, and diastolic filling profiles.

4.3. Mitral valve repair

In DCM, mitral regurgitation may occur secondary to displacement of papillary muscles and tethering of the MV leaflets. Although

MR severity may be reduced by effective medical therapy and CRT, in a proportion of subjects persisting MR contributes to progression of symptoms and ventricular remodeling.[86] Whether MV repair reduces mortality compared to optimal medical therapy has not been formally tested in a randomized clinical trial.[102,103] In selected surgical series mitral valve repair, with or without Alfieri stitch or plasty of the papillary muscles, has been performed in carefully chosen patients with relatively low perioperative mortality rates and sustained reduction of MR.[86] Careful case selection is important to avoid patients with greater LV dilatation, systemic hypotension, and advanced symptomatic limitation for whom mortality rates may be prohibitively high. For selected patients in whom mitral repair is indicated, cardiac imaging provides vital information for surgical planning and risk stratification. MR severity can be accurately quantified by MRI or echocardiography, while transesophageal echocardiography (TEE) can characterize leaflet morphology and confirm the mechanism for MR. Intraoperative TEE is imperative to ensure successful repair.

Postoperatively, echocardiography or MRI can be used to assess LV volumes and EF as well as residual MR. Use of a very small rigid annuloplasty ring may be associated with functional mitral stenosis, particularly on exertion, that can be detected by Doppler echocardiography at rest and after stress.

4.4. Support devices

Ventricular assist devices (VADs) can be used as a bridge to transplant in subjects with advanced stage D heart failure.[76] There is increasing interest in their role as a destination therapy for advanced heart failure or as a bridge to recovery.[104,105]

Cardiac imaging plays a vital role in assessing patients before and after implantation of a VAD. LV volumes and systolic function should be carefully characterized, as should RV function, which if impaired may necessitate implantation of an RV assist device. The presence of LV thrombus, atheroma or calcification, and aortic regurgitation should also be carefully noted as these may exclude implantation of an LVAD.

Although LVAD therapy is associated with improved survival in advanced heart failure compared to optimal medical therapy, there are significant complication rates due to bleeding, infection, and systemic thromboembolism.[104] With newer nonpulsatile devices, assessment of flow is more difficult, however, echocardiography may help identify thrombus or infection related to the aortic or LV cannula.[106] Echocardiography is also the test of choice to identify recovery of function during LVAD therapy and can guide weaning of the device.[105,107]

4.5. Heart transplantation

Worldwide there has been a gradual fall in the numbers of cardiac transplants performed due to a decline in donor hearts combined with improved survival in end-stage heart failure resulting from advances in drug and device therapy.[108] However, cardiac transplantation remains the treatment of choice for selected subjects with advanced heart failure that is refractory to medical and device therapy.[76]

Echocardiography allows comprehensive evaluation of LV systolic and diastolic function and of valvular function after transplant. Changes in tissue Doppler velocities may identify early rejection but do not replace the need for endomyocardial biopsy. Echocardiography can be used to guide endomyocardial biopsy in settings where fluoroscopic guidance is not available.[109]

Cardiac allograft vasculopathy occurs in up to 50% of recipients by 5 years after transplant and can be identified by selective coronary angiography, although MDCT may also be useful in this setting. Early detection is best achieved with intravascular ultrasound. A range of echocardiographic techniques including stress echo with strain imaging may allow for noninvasive detection of CAV in selected patients.[110]

5. FUTURE DIRECTIONS

Recent developments in imaging have led to improved diagnosis of cardiomyopathy and the ability to more accurately characterise cardiac function. These advances hold the promise that they may improve patient care and outcomes.

Newer echocardiographic modalities including 2D speckle tracking allow more sophisticated assessment of LV function including measurement of indices such as torsion and longitudinal rocking that cannot be assessed by conventional imaging.[85,101] Cardiac MRI also facilitates more comprehensive assessment of regional and global LV function through the use of tagged imaging.[72] The role of these newer modalities in assessment of DCM warrants further study, but early indications suggest they may facilitate earlier diagnosis of subclinical LV dysfunction and identify response to specific therapies such as CRT.

New developments in molecular imaging using CMR and nuclear imaging could have direct application in DCM.[111,112] Use of specific tracers now allows targeted imaging of molecules that may play an important role in the development or progression of the DCM phenotype. Molecules such as collagen have been targeted with cardiac MRI, to allow more accurate assessment of fibrosis. Similar techniques allow labeling of angiotensin or β-adrenergic receptors for detection by SPECT or PET imaging. Similar experimental techniques allow imaging of key processes such as apoptosis, angiogenesis, or vascular remodeling.[112] Development of these imaging modalities could potentially play a major role in enhancing our understanding the pathogenesis of DCM and in developing specific targeted therapies. These techniques could also guide the assessment of new cell-based therapies that are under investigation.[75]

Our understanding of the genetic basis for DCM has grown exponentially in recent times.[113] Already, many hundreds of mutations have been identified in a wide range of sarcomeric or nuclear proteins that can lead to cardiomyopathy. This number is likely to grow as will the need to better understand phenotype–genotype correlations. Cardiovascular imaging, especially newer modalities that allow assessment of torsion, regional deformation, or molecular imaging, is likely to play a critical role in early identification of structural or functional abnormality.[85] Equally, these forms of imaging will be important in assessing the efficacy of new gene transfer technologies or therapies.[75,111,112]

More immediately, integrated use of imaging modalities may provide more accurate assessment of cardiac dysfunction and may guide therapy. Hybrid imaging with MDCT and PET or SPECT modalities has already enhanced the assessment of ischemic cardiomyopathy.[70] Similarly, hybrid imaging such as MDCT of coronary venous anatomy combined with echocardiographic assessment of regional synchrony could result in more optimal planning and implantation of CRT in subjects with DCM.[75]

There is increasing interest in device-based therapy for advanced heart failure.[113] Percutaneous mitral valve repair, device-based monitoring of heart failure, and use of devices such as the CorCap device designed to attenuate remodeling are all the focus of intense investigation currently.[114,115] In the same way, LV assist devices are likely to play an increasing role as bridge to transplant or even as destination therapy.[113] Each of these new treatment approaches requires high-quality modern imaging to identify suitable candidates, guide implementation, and assess response to therapy.[75]

Each of the specific modalities faces technical challenges to enable application more broadly. Development of algorithms to allow imaging in subjects with common arrhythmias such as AF will be important for both CMR and MDCT. The ability to minimize radiation exposure and contrast dose will be critical for MDCT, whereas the development of pacing technologies that are compatible with CMR will be vital to allow imaging of the increasing number of DCM subjects with devices.[116]

REFERENCES

1. Maron BJ, Towbin JA, Thiene, G, et al. Contemporary definitions and classification of the cardiomyopathies: An American Heart Association Scientific Statement From the Council on Clinical Cardiology, Heart Failure and Transplantation Committee; Quality of Care and Outcomes Research and Functional Genomics and Translational Biology Interdisciplinary Working Groups; and Council on Epidemiology and Prevention. *Circulation.* 2006;113(14):1807–1816.
2. Elliott P, Andersson B, Arbustini E, et al. Classification of the cardiomyopathies: A position statement from the European Society Of Cardiology Working Group on Myocardial and Pericardial Diseases. *Eur Heart J.* 2008;29(2):270–276.
3. Dec GW, Fuster V. Idiopathic dilated cardiomyopathy. *N Engl J Med.* 1994;331(23):1564–1575.
4. Franz WM, Muller OJ, Katus HA. Cardiomyopathies: From genetics to the prospect of treatment. *Lancet.* 2001;358(9293):1627–1637.
5. McDonagh TA, Morrison CE, Lawrence A, et al. Symptomatic and asymptomatic left-ventricular systolic dysfunction in an urban population. *Lancet.* 1997;350(9081):829–833.
6. Devereux RB, Roman MJ, Paranicas M, et al. A population-based assessment of left ventricular systolic dysfunction in middle-aged and older adults: The Strong Heart Study. *Am Heart J.* 2001;141(3):439–446.
7. Felker GM, Thompson RE, Hare JM, et al. Underlying causes and long-term survival in patients with initially unexplained cardiomyopathy. *N Engl J Med.* 2000;342(15):1077–1084.
8. Burkett EL, Hershberger RE. Clinical and genetic issues in familial dilated cardiomyopathy. *J Am Coll Cardiol.* 2005;45(7):969–981.
9. Ashrafian H, Watkins H. Reviews of translational medicine and genomics in cardiovascular disease: New disease taxonomy and therapeutic implications: Cardiomyopathies: Therapeutics based on molecular phenotype. *J Am Coll Cardiol.* 2007;49(12):1251–1264.
10. Sliwa K, Damasceno A, Mayosi BM. Epidemiology and etiology of cardiomyopathy in Africa. *Circulation.* 2005;112(23):3577–3583.
11. Yacoub S, Mocumbi AO, Yacoub MH. Neglected tropical cardiomyopathies: I. Chagas disease. *Heart.* 2008;194(2):244–248.
12. Jessup M, Brozena S. Heart failure. *N Engl J Med.* 2003;348(20):2007–2018.
13. Elkayam U, Akhter MW, Singh H, et al. Pregnancy-associated cardiomyopathy: Clinical characteristics and a comparison between early and late presentation. *Circulation.* 2005;111(16):2050–2055.
14. Bardy GH, Lee KL, Mark DB, et al. Amiodarone or an implantable cardioverter-defibrillator for congestive heart failure. *N Engl J Med.* 2005;352(3):225–237.
15. Pasotti M, Klersy C, Pilotto A, et al. Long-term outcome and risk stratification in dilated cardiolaminopathies. *J Am Coll Cardiol.* 2008;52(15):1250–1260.
16. Binkley PF, Lesinski A, Ferguson JP, et al. Recovery of normal ventricular function in patients with dilated cardiomyopathy: Predictors of an increasingly prevalent clinical event. *Am Heart J.* 2008;155(1):69–74.
17. Magnani JW, Dec GW. Myocarditis: Current trends in diagnosis and treatment. *Circulation.* 2006;113(6):876–890.
18. Kawai C. From myocarditis to cardiomyopathy: Mechanisms of inflammation and cell death: Learning from the past for the future. *Circulation.* 1999;99(8):1091–1100.
19. Kuhl U, Pauschinger M, Seeberg B, et al. Viral persistence in the myocardium is associated with progressive cardiac dysfunction. *Circulation.* 2005;112(13):1965–1970.
20. Mahrholdt H, Wagner A, Deluigi CC, et al. Presentation, patterns of myocardial damage, and clinical course of viral myocarditis. *Circulation.* 2006;114(15):1581–1590.
21. Xiong D, Yajima T, Lim BK, et al. Inducible cardiac-restricted expression of enteroviral protease 2A is sufficient to induce dilated cardiomyopathy. *Circulation.* 2007;115(1):94–102.
22. Badorff C, Lee GH, Lamphear BJ, et al. Enteroviral protease 2A cleaves dystrophin: Evidence of cytoskeletal disruption in an acquired cardiomyopathy. *Nat Med.* 1999;5(3):320–326.
23. Feldman AM, McNamara D. Myocarditis. *N Engl J Med.* 2000;343(19):1388–1398.
24. Caforio AL, Calabrese F, Angelini A, et al. A prospective study of biopsy-proven myocarditis: Prognostic relevance of clinical and aetiopathogenetic features at diagnosis. *Eur Heart J.* 2007;28(11):1326–1333.
25. Kindermann I, Kindermann M, Kandolf R, et al. Predictors of outcome in patients with suspected myocarditis. *Circulation.* 2008;118(6):639–648.
26. Grogan M, Redfield MM, Bailey KR, et al. Long-term outcome of patients with biopsy-proved myocarditis: Comparison with idiopathic dilated cardiomyopathy. *J Am Coll Cardiol.* 1995;26(1):80–84.
27. McCarthy RE III, Boehmer JP, Hruban RH, et al. Long-term outcome of fulminant myocarditis as compared with acute (nonfulminant) myocarditis. *N Engl J Med.* 2000;342(10):690–695.

28. Skouri HN, Dec GW, Friedrich MG, et al. Noninvasive imaging in myocarditis. *J Am Coll Cardiol.* 2006;48(10):2085–2093.

29. Friedrich MG, Strohm O, Schulz-Menger J, et al. Contrast media-enhanced magnetic resonance imaging visualizes myocardial changes in the course of viral myocarditis. *Circulation.* 1998;97(18):1802–1809.

30. Mahrholdt H, Goedecke C, Wagner A, et al. Cardiovascular magnetic resonance assessment of human myocarditis: A comparison to histology and molecular pathology. *Circulation.* 2004;109(10):1250–1258.

31. Selvanayagam JB, Hawkins PN, Paul B, et al. Evaluation and management of the cardiac amyloidosis. *J Am Coll Cardiol.* 2007;50(22):2101–2110.

32. Vogelsberg H, Mahrholdt H, Deluigi CC, et al. Cardiovascular magnetic resonance in clinically suspected cardiac amyloidosis: Noninvasive imaging compared to endomyocardial biopsy. *J Am Coll Cardiol.* 2008;51(10):1022–1030.

33. Maceira AM, Joshi J, Prasad SK, et al. Cardiovascular magnetic resonance in cardiac amyloidosis. *Circulation.* 2005;111(2):186–193.

34. Sechtem U, Mahrholdt H, Vogelsberg H. Cardiac magnetic resonance in myocardial disease. *Heart.* 2007;93(12):1520–1527.

35. Anderson LJ, Holden S, Davis B, et al. Cardiovascular T2-star (T2*) magnetic resonance for the early diagnosis of myocardial iron overload. *Eur Heart J.* 2001;22(23):2171–2179.

36. Mavrogeni SI, Markussis V, Kaklamanis L, et al. A comparison of magnetic resonance imaging and cardiac biopsy in the evaluation of heart iron overload in patients with beta-thalassemia major. *Eur J Haematol.* 2005;75(3):241–247.

37. Umezawa ES, Stolf AM, Corbett CE, et al. Chagas' disease. *Lancet.* 2001;357(9258): 797–799.

38. Sliwa K, Fett J, Elkayam U. Peripartum cardiomyopathy. *Lancet.* 2006;368(9536): 687–693.

39. Sliwa K, Skudicky D, Bergemann A, et al. Peripartum cardiomyopathy: Analysis of clinical outcome, left ventricular function, plasma levels of cytokines and Fas/APO-1. *J Am Coll Cardiol.* 2000;35(3):701–705.

40. Elkayam U, Tummala PP, Rao K, et al. Maternal and fetal outcomes of subsequent pregnancies in women with peripartum cardiomyopathy. *N Engl J Med.* 2001;344(21):1567–1571.

41. Lucas DL, Brown RA, Wassef M, et al. Alcohol and the cardiovascular system research challenges and opportunities. *J Am Coll Cardiol.* 2005;45(12):1916–1924.

42. Elliott P. Pathogenesis of cardiotoxicity induced by anthracyclines. *Semin Oncol.* 2006;33(3 Suppl. 8):S2–S7.

43. Swain SM, Whaley FS, Ewer MS. Congestive heart failure in patients treated with doxorubicin: A retrospective analysis of three trials. *Cancer.* 2003;97(11): 2869–2879.

44. Cheitlin MD, Armstrong WF, Aurigemma GP, et al. ACC/AHA/ASE 2003 guideline update for the clinical application of echocardiography: Summary article: A report of the American College of Cardiology/American Heart Association Task Force on Practice Guidelines (ACC/AHA/ASE Committee to Update the 1997 Guidelines for the Clinical Application of Echocardiography). *Circulation.* 2003;108(9):1146–1162.

45. Ruxandra J, Hans W, Javier G, et al. Strain rate imaging detects early cardiac effects of pegylated liposomal doxorubicin as adjuvant therapy in elderly patients with breast cancer. *J Am Soc Echocardiogr.* 2008;21(12):1283–1289.

46. Slamon DJ, Leyland-Jones B, Shak S, et al. Use of chemotherapy plus a monoclonal antibody against HER2 for metastatic breast cancer that overexpresses HER2. *N Engl J Med.* 2001;344(11):783–792.

47. Guglin M, Cutro R, Mishkin JD. Trastuzumab-induced cardiomyopathy. *J Card Fail.* 2008;14(5):437–444.

48. Kamisago M, Sharma SD, DePalma SR, et al. Mutations in sarcomere protein genes as a cause of dilated cardiomyopathy. *N Engl J Med.* 2000;343(23):1688–1696.

49. Olson TM, Michels VV, Thibodeau SN, et al. Actin mutations in dilated cardiomyopathy, a heritable form of heart failure. *Science.* 1998;280(5364):750–752.

50. Caforio AL, Mahon NG, Baig MK, et al. Prospective familial assessment in dilated cardiomyopathy: Cardiac autoantibodies predict disease development in asymptomatic relatives. *Circulation.* 2007;115(1):76–83.

51. Koikkalainen JR, Antila M, Lotjonen JM, et al. Early familial dilated cardiomyopathy: Identification with determination of disease state parameter from cine MR image data. *Radiology.* 2008;249(1):88–96.

52. Matsumura Y, Elliott PM, Mahon NG, et al. Familial dilated cardiomyopathy: Assessment of left ventricular systolic and diastolic function using Doppler tissue imaging in asymptomatic relatives with left ventricular enlargement. *Heart.* 2006;92(3):405–406.

53. Towbin JA, Hejtmancik JF, Brink P, et al. X-linked dilated cardiomyopathy. Molecular genetic evidence of linkage to the Duchenne muscular dystrophy (dystrophin) gene at the Xp21 locus. *Circulation.* 1993;87(6):1854–1865.

54. Muntoni F, Cau M, Ganau A, et al. Brief report: Deletion of the dystrophin muscle-promoter region associated with X-linked dilated cardiomyopathy. *N Engl J Med.* 1993;329(13):921–925.

55. Rapezzi C, Leone O, Biagini E, et al. Echocardiographic clues to diagnosis of dystrophin related dilated cardiomyopathy. *Heart.* 2007;93(1):10.

56. Tsuchihashi K, Ueshima K, Uchida T, et al. Transient left ventricular apical ballooning without coronary artery stenosis: A novel heart syndrome mimicking acute myocardial infarction. *J Am Coll Cardiol.* 2001;38(1):11–18.

57. Shah DP, Sugeng L, Goonewardena SN, et al. Takotsubo cardiomyopathy. *Circulation.* 2006;113(19): e762.

58. Bybee KA, Prasad A. Stress-related cardiomyopathy syndromes. *Circulation.* 2008;118(4):397–409.

59. Eitel I, Behrendt F, Schindler K, et al. Differential diagnosis of suspected apical ballooning syndrome using contrast-enhanced magnetic resonance imaging. *Eur Heart J.* 2008; 29(21):2651–2659.

60. Nef HM, Mollmann H, Elsasser A. Tako-tsubo cardiomyopathy (apical ballooning). *Heart.* 2007;93(10):1309–1315.

61. Chin TK, Perloff JK, Williams RG, et al. Isolated noncompaction of left ventricular myocardium. A study of eight cases. *Circulation.* 1990;82(2):507–513.

62. Weiford BC, Subbarao VD, Mulhern KM. Noncompaction of the ventricular myocardium. *Circulation.* 2004;109(24):2965–2971.

63. Klaassen S, Probst S, Oechslin E, et al. Mutations in sarcomere protein genes in left ventricular noncompaction. *Circulation.* 2008;117(22):2893–2901.

64. Ichida F, Hamamichi Y, Miyawaki T, et al. Clinical features of isolated noncompaction of the ventricular myocardium: Long-term clinical course, hemodynamic properties, and genetic background. *J Am Coll Cardiol.* 1999;34(1): 233–240.

65. Koo BK, Choi D, Ha JW, et al. Isolated noncompaction of the ventricular myocardium: Contrast echocardiographic findings and review of the literature. *Echocardiography.* 2002;19(2):153–156.

66. Daniels LB, Maisel AS. Natriuretic peptides. *J Am Coll Cardiol.* 2007;50(25): 2357–2368.

67. Cooper LT, Baughman KL, et al. The role of endomyocardial biopsy in the management of cardiovascular disease: A scientific statement from the American Heart Association, the American College of Cardiology, and the European Society of Cardiology. *Circulation.* 2007;116(19):2216–2233.

68. Kirkpatrick JN, Vannan MA, Narula J, et al. Echocardiography in heart failure: Applications, utility, and new horizons. *J Am Coll Cardiol.* 2007;50(5):381–396.

69. Germans T, van Rossum AC. The use of cardiac magnetic resonance imaging to determine the aetiology of left ventricular disease and cardiomyopathy. *Heart.* 2008;94(4):510–518.

70. Higuchi T, Bengel FM. Cardiovascular nuclear imaging: From perfusion to molecular function: Non-invasive imaging. *Heart.* 2008;94(6):809–816.

71. Monaghan MJ. Role of real time 3D echocardiography in evaluating the left ventricle. *Heart.* 2006;92(1):131–136.

72. Belloni E, De Cobelli F, Esposito A, et al. MRI of cardiomyopathy. *Am J Roentgenol.* 2008;191(6):1702–1710.

73. Roberts WT, Bax JJ, Davies LC. Cardiac CT and CT coronary angiography: Technology and application. *Heart.* 2008;94(6):781–792.

74. Tops LF, Krishnan SC, Schuijf JD, et al. Noncoronary applications of cardiac multidetector row computed tomography. *J Am Coll Cardiol.* 2008;1(1):94–106.

75. Marwick TH, Schwaiger M. The future of cardiovascular imaging in the diagnosis and management of heart failure, Part 2: Clinical applications. *Circulation.* 2008;1(2):162–170.

76. Hunt SA, Abraham WT, Chin MH, et al. ACC/AHA 2005 guideline update for the diagnosis and management of chronic heart failure in the adult: A report of the American College of Cardiology/American Heart Association Task Force on Practice Guidelines (Writing Committee to Update the 2001 Guidelines for the Evaluation and Management of Heart Failure): Developed in collaboration with the American College of Chest Physicians and the International Society for Heart and Lung Transplantation: Endorsed by the Heart Rhythm Society. *Circulation.* 2005;112(12):e154–e235.

77. Lester SJ, Tajik AJ, Nishimura RA, et al. Unlocking the mysteries of diastolic function: Deciphering the rosetta stone 10 years later. *J Am Coll Cardiol.* 2008;51(7):679–689.

78. Yu C-M, Sanderson JE, Marwick TH. Tissue Doppler imaging: A new prognosticator for cardiovascular diseases. *J Am Coll Cardiol.* 2007;49(19): 1903–1914.

79. Anderson LJ, Miyazaki C, Sutherland GR, et al. Patient selection and echocardiographic assessment of dyssynchrony in cardiac resynchronization therapy. *Circulation.* 2008;117(15):2009–2023.

80. Weinsaft JW, Kim HW, Shah DJ. Detection of left ventricular thrombus by delayed-enhancement cardiovascular magnetic resonance: Prevalence and markers in patients with systolic dysfunction. *J Am Coll Cardiol.* 2008;52(2):148–157.

81. Greil GF, Beerbaum P, Razavi R. Imaging the right ventricle: Non-invasive imaging. *Heart.* 2008;94(6):803–808.

82. Sheehan F, Redington A. The right ventricle: Anatomy, physiology and clinical imaging. *Heart.* 2008;94(11):1510–1515.

83. Anderson JL, Horne BD, Pennell DJ. Atrial dimensions in health and left ventricular disease using cardiovascular magnetic resonance. *J Cardiovasc Magn Reson.* 2005;7(4):671–675.

84. Saito M, Okayama H, Nishimura K, et al. Determinants of left ventricular untwisting behavior in patients with dilated cardiomyopathy: Analysis by two-dimensional speckle tracking. *Heart.* 2008.

85. Popovic ZB, Grimm RA, Ahmad A, et al. Longitudinal rotation: An unrecognised motion pattern in patients with dilated cardiomyopathy. *Heart.* 2008;94(3):e11.

86. Mehra MR, Reyes P, Benitez RM, et al. Surgery for severe mitral regurgitation and left ventricular failure: What do we really know? *J Card Fail.* 2008;14(2):145–150.

87. Zoghbi WA, Enriquez-Sarano M, Foster E, et al. Recommendations for evaluation of the severity of native valvular regurgitation with two-dimensional and Doppler echocardiography. *J Am Soc Echocardiogr.* 2003;16(7):777–802.

88. O'Gara P, Sugeng L, Lang R, et al. The role of imaging in chronic degenerative mitral regurgitation. *J Am Coll Cardiol.* 2008;1(2):221–237.

89. He S, Fontaine AA, Schwammenthal E, et al. Integrated mechanism for functional mitral regurgitation: Leaflet restriction versus coapting force: In vitro studies. *Circulation.* 1997;96(6):1826–1834.

90. Rahimtoola SH, Dilsizian V, Kramer CM, et al. Chronic ischemic left ventricular dysfunction: From pathophysiology to imaging and its integration into clinical practice. *JACC Cardio Vasc Imaging.* 2008;1(4):536–555.

91. McCrohon JA, Moon JCC, Prasad SK, et al. Differentiation of heart failure related to dilated cardiomyopathy and coronary artery disease using gadolinium-enhanced cardiovascular magnetic resonance. *Circulation.* 2003;108(1):54–59.

92. Wu E, Judd RM, Vargas JD, et al. Visualisation of presence, location, and transmural extent of healed Q-wave and non-Q-wave myocardial infarction. *Lancet.* 2001;357(9249):21–28.

93. Assomull RG, Pennell DJ, Prasad SK. Cardiovascular magnetic resonance in the evaluation of heart failure. *Heart.* 2007;93(8):985–992.

94. Wu KC, Weiss RG, Thiemann DR, et al. Late gadolinium enhancement by cardiovascular magnetic resonance heralds an adverse prognosis in nonischemic cardiomyopathy. *J Am Coll Cardiol.* 2008;51(25):2414–2421.

95. Bello D, Shah DJ, Farah GM, et al. Gadolinium cardiovascular magnetic resonance predicts reversible myocardial dysfunction and remodeling in patients with heart failure undergoing beta-blocker therapy. *Circulation.* 2003;108(16):1945–1953.

96. Nazarian S, Bluemke DA, Lardo AC, et al. Magnetic resonance assessment of the substrate for inducible ventricular tachycardia in nonischemic cardiomyopathy. *Circulation.* 2005;112(18):2821–2825.

97. Cleland JG, Daubert JC, Erdmann E, et al. The effect of cardiac resynchronization on morbidity and mortality in heart failure. *N Engl J Med.* 2005;352(15):1539–1549.

98. Bristow MR, Saxon LA, Boehmer J, et al. Cardiac-resynchronization therapy with or without an implantable defibrillator in advanced chronic heart failure. *N Engl J Med.* 2004;350(21):2140–2150.

99. Chung ES, Leon AR, Tavazzi L, et al. Results of the Predictors of Response to CRT (PROSPECT) trial. *Circulation.* 2008;117(20):2608–2616.

100. Ypenburg C, van Bommel RJ, Delgado V, et al. Optimal left ventricular lead position predicts reverse remodeling and survival after cardiac resynchronization therapy. *J Am Coll Cardiol.* 2008;52(17):1402–1409.

101. Thomas JD, Popovic ZB. Assessment of left ventricular function by cardiac ultrasound. *J Am Coll Cardiol.* 2006;48(10):2012–2025.

102. McGee EC Jr. Should moderate or greater mitral regurgitation be repaired in all patients with LVEF < 30%? *Circ Heart Fail.* 2008;1(4):285–289.

103. Acker MA. Should moderate or greater mitral regurgitation be repaired in all patients with LVEF < 30%? *Circ Heart Fail.* 2008;1(4):281–284.

104. Rose EA, Gelijns AC, Moskowitz AJ, et al. Long-term use of a left ventricular assist device for end-stage heart failure. *N Engl J Med.* 2001;345(20):1435–1443.

105. Birks EJ, Tansley PD, Hardy J, et al. Left ventricular assist device and drug therapy for the reversal of heart failure. *N Engl J Med.* 2006;355(18):1873–1884.

106. Miller LW, Pagani FD, Russell SD, et al. Use of a continuous-flow device in patients awaiting heart transplantation. *N Engl J Med.* 2007;357(9):885–896.

107. Dandel M, Weng Y, Siniawski H, et al. Prediction of cardiac stability after weaning from left ventricular assist devices in patients with idiopathic dilated cardiomyopathy. *Circulation.* 2008;118(14 Suppl.):S94–S105.

108. Lietz K, Miller LW. Improved survival of patients with end-stage heart failure listed for heart transplantation: Analysis of Organ Procurement and Transplantation Network/U.S. United Network of Organ Sharing Data, 1990 to 2005. *J Am Coll Cardiol.* 2007;50(13):1282–1290.

109. Thorn EM, de Filippi CR. Echocardiography in the cardiac transplant recipient. *Heart Fail Clin.* 2007;3(1):51–67.

110. Eroglu E, D'Hooge J, Sutherland GR, et al. Quantitative dobutamine stress echocardiography for the early detection of cardiac allograft vasculopathy in heart transplant recipients. *Heart.* 2008;94(2):e3.

111. Sinusas AJ, Bengel F, Nahrendorf M, et al. Multimodality cardiovascular molecular imaging, Part I. *Circulation.* 2008;1(3):244–256.

112. Nahrendorf M, Sosnovik DE, French BA. Multimodality cardiovascular molecular imaging, Part II. *Circulation.* 2009;2(1):56–70.

113. Braunwald E. The management of heart failure: The past, the present, and the future. *Circ Heart Fail.* 2008;1(1):58–62.

114. Mann DL, Acker MA, Jessup M, et al. Clinical evaluation of the CorCap cardiac support device in patients with dilated cardiomyopathy. *Ann Thorac Surg.* 2007;84(4):1226–1235.

115. Ritzema J, Melton IC, Richards, AM, et al. Direct left atrial pressure monitoring in ambulatory heart failure patients: Initial experience with a new permanent implantable device. *Circulation.* 2007;116(25):2952–2959.

116. Dill T. Contraindications to magnetic resonance imaging: Non-invasive imaging. *Heart.* 2008;94(7):943–948.

Restrictive Cardiomyopathies

34

Ronan J. Curtin
Allan L. Klein

1. INTRODUCTION

Restrictive cardiomyopathies (RCMs) constitute a group of diseases characterized by increased myocardial stiffness resulting in impaired ventricular filling and elevated ventricular pressure in diastole. Traditionally, RCMs have been differentiated from hypertrophic, dilated, and arrhythmogenic right ventricular cardiomyopathy and classified as primary RCM or secondary to other diseases such as storage or infiltrative disorders.[1] However, RCMs have always been difficult to define and classify because the diagnosis is a physiological one and frequently overlaps in clinical practice with the anatomically defined hypertrophic and dilated cardiomyopathies. Recognizing the deficiencies in the traditional classification system and recent scientific advances, the latest American Heart Association (AHA) scientific statement on definition and classification of the cardiomyopathies proposed a more simple classification, with all cardiomyopathies designated as either primary or secondary, based on principal organ involvement.[2] Primary cardiomyopathies are those that predominantly or exclusively affect the heart and are further classified as genetic, mixed (genetic or nongenetic), or acquired. Under this new AHA classification system, restrictive cardiomyopathy refers only to primary restrictive cardiomyopathy, and traditional secondary RCMs such as cardiac amyloid are separately classified according to the primary disorder. The European Society of Cardiology (ESC) recently published its own position paper on the classification of cardiomyopathies, which does not follow the new AHA classification system, but instead builds on the traditional WHO classification.[3] In the ESC classification system, RCMs are defined as "restrictive ventricular physiology in the presence of normal or reduced diastolic volumes (of one or both ventricles), normal or reduced systolic volumes, and normal ventricular wall thickness." RCM so defined still incorporates the traditional primary and secondary causes. For the purpose of this chapter, we have continued to rely on the traditional classification system of RCM and will describe both primary and secondary RCMs, with secondary RCMs further subclassified as infiltrative, noninfiltrative, and storage disorders (Table 34.1). RCMs are rare disorders and provide a major diagnostic challenge. The diagnosis may be initially overlooked and when suspected, requires multiple diagnostic tests. Echocardiography and other noninvasive imaging modalities are central to the diagnosis.

1.1. Epidemiology

RCMs are considered rare disorders. Primary RCM is particularly rare, described in both children and adults in case reports and small series.[4,5] The secondary RCMs are more frequently encountered in clinical practice and usually affect adults. Probably, the most common restrictive cardiomyopathy encountered in hospital practice in Western countries is amyloid cardiomyopathy. However, globally the most common RCM is endomyocardial fibrosis (EMF), which is endemic in parts of Africa, Asia, and South America, and has been estimated to affect 12 million people worldwide.[6]

1.2. Clinical presentation

1.2.1. Symptoms and signs

Patients with RCM usually present with heart failure symptoms such as dyspnea, peripheral edema, and fatigue. Anginal chest discomfort may occur in cardiac amyloidosis due to microvascular infiltration with amyloid.[7] Patients with cardiac amyloidosis may also have dizziness or syncope related to autonomic dysfunction or conduction system disease, again related to amyloid infiltration of autonomic nerves or cardiac conducting tissue, respectively. Although first-degree heart block and interventricular conduction delay are common in cardiac amyloidosis, second- or third-degree heart block is uncommon.[8] The presence of advanced conduction disease should raise suspicion for a primary RCM related to a mutation in the desmin gene, but is also common in patients with cardiomyopathy related to mutations in PRKAG2.[9,10] Atrial fibrillation is common in amyloidosis and other secondary RCMs. Expected findings on physical examination in patients with RCM include an elevated jugular venous pulsation, prominent apical impulse, third or fourth heart sound, pulmonary rales, ascites, and peripheral edema. Patients with secondary RCM may also have symptoms and signs related to the primary diagnosis. For example, in cardiac amyloidosis, patients may present with renal failure, proteinuria, hepatomegaly, autonomic dysfunction, neuropathy, and carpal tunnel syndrome.[11] Patients with Fabry disease characteristically have associated end-stage renal disease, peripheral neuropathy manifesting as severe neuropathic limb pain and characteristic skin lesions called angiokeratomas.[12] Abdominal pain and diarrhea are also common due to deposition of glycosphingolipids in the gastrointestinal tract. In another glycogen storage disorder, Danon disease, skeletal myopathy, and mental retardation are common.[13] Noncardiac manifestations of hemochromatosis include liver cirrhosis, diabetes, skin hyperpigmentation, arthropathy, and hypogonadism.[14] Patients with sarcoidosis can have involvement of any organ system, leading to a wide range of presentations, although lung and ocular involvement are most common, followed by cutaneous and constitutional manifestations. Patients with EMF typically have predominant right sided heart failure with ascites out of proportion to the amount of peripheral edema.[15] Dyspnea predominates in patients with left sided heart failure. Thromboembolic complications may occur in the thrombotic phase of the disease.

TABLE 34.1
CLASSIFICATION OF THE RESTRICTIVE CARDIOMYOPATHIES

Primary
Genetic (e.g., mutations in troponin I)
Acquired (e.g., endomyocardial fibrosis)
Secondary
Infiltrative
Amyloidosis
Sarcoidosis
Noninfiltrative
Drugs
Radiation
Storage
Glycogen storage disorders
Hemochromatosis

1.2.2. Outcome

Untreated, advanced RCMs have a generally poor outcome. Reported 5- and 10-year survival in patients with symptomatic primary RCM is around 64% and 37% respectively.[16] Patients with symptomatic cardiac amyloidosis have a particularly poor survival with a median survival of 10.5 months as reported in one recent study.[17] Male patients with Fabry disease have a median cumulative survival of 50 years, representing an approximately 20-year reduction in life span compared to the normal population. In most cases, death is due to renal failure or stroke.[18] In patients with symptomatic cardiac sarcoidosis, mortality was 20% at mean follow-up of 1.7 years.[19] Although little specific data exists, the prognosis of EMF is considered poor with a high incidence of sudden death from fatal arrhythmias and thromboembolism.

2. PATHOPHYSIOLOGY

Primary and secondary RCMs have in common increased myocardial stiffness resulting in steep increases in left ventricular (LV) pressure with small changes in LV volume. There is a resultant upward shift of the LV pressure–volume curve and a characteristic "dip and plateau" or "square root" hemodynamic pattern.[20] In primary RCM, LV wall thickness is normal or mildly increased. The ventricular cavities are normal or decreased in size. Although little is known about the cause of diastolic impairment in these patients, increased myofilament sensitivity to calcium as well as increased accumulation of desmin and collagen type III have been implicated.[21–24] The morphological and physiological findings are more heterogenous in the secondary RCMs. LV wall thickness is more frequently increased due to expansion of the interstitial space in infiltrative disorders such as cardiac amyloidosis, or increased cellular size in the storage disorders such as Anderson-Fabry disease. Milder, nonrestrictive patterns of diastolic impairment are common, particularly in the earlier stages of disease.[25] In both primary and secondary RCMs increased diastolic filling pressures typically result in significant biatrial dilation and peripheral and pulmonary edema.

2.1. Primary restrictive cardiomyopathies

2.1.1. Genetic restrictive cardiomyopathies

Primary genetic RCM is rare, with case reports and small series published in the literature.[4,5] Both familial and sporadic cases have been described.[26,27] Familial cases are usually characterized by autosomal dominant inheritance with incomplete penetrance. Patients typically present at a young age, frequently in childhood. Skeletal myopathy may also be present. Primary RCM has been associated with mutations in genes encoding the sarcomeric proteins, troponin I, troponin T, alpha cardiac actin and beta-myosin heavy chain, which are more characteristically associated with hypertrophic cardiomyopathy (HCM).[28,29] In fact, cases of RCM and HCM, both related to a single mutation in troponin I have been described in a single, large family.[30] The "restrictive phenotype" of HCM appears to be rare, observed in 1.5% of 1,226 HCM patients or family members in one recent study.[31] RCM has also been linked to mutations in the desmin gene, which was originally associated with dilated cardiomyopathy.[9,32,33] In patients with mutations in the desmin gene, conduction system disorders are also frequently present.

2.1.2. Endomyocardial disease

EMF, although rare in developed countries, is probably the most common cause of RCM, affecting an estimated 12 million people worldwide.[6] It is endemic in tropical and subtropical Africa, Asia, and South America, but is also occasionally encountered outside the tropics.[34–36] Prognosis is poor with reported mortality as high as 40% in 1 year in patients with advanced disease.[37] EMF predominantly affects children and adolescents from poor socioeconomic backgrounds. The etiology remains unknown. Hypereosinophilia, parasitic infection, autoimmunity, dietary factors, and genetic factors have all been proposed.[15] An initial, acute inflammatory phase with fever and pancarditis is frequently associated with eosinophilia, facial and periorbital swelling, and urticaria. An intermediate phase is associated with ventricular endocardial thrombus formation. The final stage is endocardial fibrosis causing restrictive left and right ventricular physiology. Fibrosis characteristically involves the apex of the right and left ventricles. Mitral and tricuspid regurgitation are common due to tethering of the leaflets. Patients may present with right heart failure, left heart failure, or both. There may be marked systemic venous hypertension in patients with dominant right ventricular EMF with associated proptosis, facial edema, ascites, and hepatosplenomegaly. A recent study of a rural population in Mozambique found echocardiographic evidence for EMF in 211 (19.8%) of 1,063 randomly selected subjects.[38] Biventricular EMF was most common (55%), followed by isolated right (28%) and left (17%) sided EMF. Most patients had mild to moderate structural abnormalities and only 22.7% of subjects were symptomatic at the time of screening.

Hypereosinophilic syndrome (HES) is characterized by persistent, severe eosinophilia in the absence of a primary cause, and evidence of eosinophil-mediated end-organ damage.[39] Cardiac involvement is estimated to occur in 40% to 50% of patients, and is a major source of morbidity and mortality.[40] Loeffler[41] initially described endocardial fibrosis in the setting of eosinophilia in 1936, giving rise to the term "Loeffler's endocarditis." Pathologically, the disease is indistinguishable from endomyocardial fibrosis, with eosinophilic myocarditis in the first few weeks, endocardial thrombosis at around 10 months, and endocardial fibrosis from around 2 years.[39] Patients may present with heart failure, arrhythmia, pericarditis, or thromboembolism.[42] Echocardiography may show typical features of cardiac involvement in HES, including endomyocardial thickening, ventricular apical obliteration, and involvement of the posterior mitral leaflet.[40] Cardiac MRI can potentially provide additional diagnostic information due to its greater field of view, ability to detect myocardial fibrosis, and greater sensitivity for ventricular thrombus detection.[43,44] However, endomyocardial biopsy remains the diagnostic gold standard.

2.2. Secondary restrictive cardiomyopathies

Secondary RCM are further subclassified as infiltrative, noninfiltrative, and storage disorders. In infiltrative disorders deposits occur in the interstitial space, whereas in storage disorders deposits occur within the cell.

2.2.1. Infiltrative disorders

Cardiac amyloidosis. Cardiac amyloidosis is an infiltrative cardiomyopathy caused by deposition of insoluble fibrillar protein in the tissue interstitial space, which classically stains pink with Congo red and displays apple-green birefringence under polarizing light microscopy.[11] It typically occurs as part of a multisystem disorder with infiltration also occurring in a variety of organs including the liver, kidney, heart, nerves, skin, and tongue. Over 20 different amyloid proteins have been described, which arise either due to genetic mutations or overproduction.[45] Five major clinical types of cardiac amyloidosis are recognized, each associated with a different precursor protein (Table 34.2). Primary or systemic AL amyloidosis is the most common form of amyloidosis in developed countries. Monoclonal gammopathy of undetermined significance (MGUS) or plasma cell dyscrasia such as multiple myeloma results in excess production of immunoglobulin light chains leading to widespread tissue deposition of AL amyloid fibrils. Cardiac involvement in AL amyloidosis is common with up to 60% of patients demonstrating electrocardiogram (ECG) or echocardiographic abnormalities, and 90% of patients showing evidence of involvement on histological analysis.[46] Up to 2,500 new cases of AL amyloidosis are diagnosed in the United States each year, typically in patients over 50 years of age, with equal incidence in men and women.[47] Cardiac involvement is associated with a poor prognosis, with

a median survival from diagnosis of 1.08 years, falling to 0.75 years with the onset of heart failure.[48]

Cardiac involvement is also common in senile systemic amyloidosis, which is due to interstitial deposition of normal, wild-type transthyretin (TTR). It predominantly affects males older than 70 years. Reported prevalence in patients greater than 80 years of age is 25% to 36%.[49,50] Extensive amyloid deposits result in heart failure, although with a median survival of 75 months, the prognosis is better than with primary amyloidosis.[51] Senile systemic amyloidosis predominantly affects the heart with carpal tunnel syndrome being the only common extracardiac manifestation. Cardiac involvement is rare in secondary or systemic amyloid A (AA) amyloidosis, in which chronic inflammatory conditions lead to markedly increased production of serum AA protein and predominant renal disease.[52] Hereditary systemic amyloidosis is an autosomal dominant disorder due to tissue deposition of variant forms of seven different proteins including TTR and the apolipoproteins A-I and A-II.[53] Variant TTR protein is the most frequently implicated, and over 100 different mutations in the TTR gene have been described.[54] Hereditary systemic amyloidosis is rare, although geographic hot spots occur in areas in Northern Portugal, Japan, Northern Sweden, Finland, and Iceland.[53] The predominant feature of TTR hereditary systemic amyloidosis is peripheral or autonomic neuropathy. Cardiac involvement leading to heart failure is common, but is less aggressive than in AL amyloidosis. Cardiac amyloid deposition also occurs in isolated atrial natriuretic peptide (ANP) and dialysis related (β_2 microglobulin) amyloidosis, although with these conditions the clinical significance appears to be minimal. Isolated atrial amyloidosis may be associated with development of atrial fibrillation.[55] A number of prognostic factors have been determined for cardiac amyloidosis, including the underlying type of amyloidosis and presence of heart failure. In addition, echocardiography and laboratory testing may provide prognostic information in patients with cardiac amyloid and are discussed below.

Cardiac sarcoidosis. Although clinically evident cardiac sarcoid is uncommon, affecting approximately 5% of patients with the disorder, occult involvement may be detected in up to 39% of

TABLE 34.2
CLASSIFICATION OF CARDIAC AMYLOIDOSIS

	Precursor protein	Cardiac involvement	Other organ involvement	Treatment
Primary (AL)	Immunoglobulin light chain	Common	Kidney, liver, PNS, GI	Chemotherapy
Senile systemic	Wild-type transthyretin	Common	Lungs, carpal tunnel syndrome	Supportive
Hereditary systemic	Mutant transthyretin, Apo A-I, Apo A-II, etc.	Common	PNS	Liver transplantation
Secondary (AA)	Serum amyloid A	Rare	Kidney	Treatment of underlying disease
Isolated atrial amyloidosis	Atrial natriuretic peptide (ANP)	Common	None	None required

PNS, peripheral nervous system; GI, gastrointestinal.

patients.[56] Sarcoidosis can involve any part of the heart, including myocardium, endocardium, and pericardium. Symptomatic cardiac sarcoidosis is associated with a poor prognosis, with 20% mortality and 47% requiring pacemaker or AICD after 1.7 years of follow-up.[19,56] Arrhythmias or conduction defects are the most common causes of death due to cardiac sarcoidosis. However, progressive heart failure due to massive granulomatous infiltration of the myocardium accounts for approximately 25% of deaths.[57] Cardiomyopathy is present in approximately 50% of patients with cardiac sarcoid, with dilated cardiomyopathy more common than the restrictive type.[58]

2.2.2. Noninfiltrative disorders
Noninfiltrative restrictive cardiomyopathies are rare and include cases due to drug therapy and radiation.[59,60]

2.2.3. Storage disorders
Although, traditionally, storage disorders have been classified under RCM, these conditions both morphologically and physiologically bear more resemblance to HCM. Storage disorders are characterized by intracellular accumulation of a variety of substances, usually related to a defect in a gene coding for a metabolic pathway. Glycogen storage disorders, including Anderson-Fabry (Fabry) disease, Pompe disease, Danon disease (LAMP2), and PRKAG2 deficient cardiomyopathy, are associated with variable degrees of cardiac involvement (Table 34.3). Recent studies have highlighted how these disorders may initially be misdiagnosed as HCM.[61,62] Although Fabry disease is rare, it is one of the more common glycogen storage disorders, affecting approximately 1 in 50,000. It is an X-linked recessive disorder. Mutations in the α-galactosidase A gene lead to reduced or no activity of this enzyme and progressive lysosomal accumulation of glycosphingolipids in most body tissues. Renal, neurological, and cardiac involvement cause significant morbidity and mortality. Classically, Fabry disease presents in men during childhood or adolescence. However, the disease may present later in life with unexplained cardiomegaly or proteinuria. One study showed that Fabry disease was a relatively common cause of unexplained LV hypertrophy (LVH) in men with late onset HCM.[62] Five (6.3%) of 79 male patients aged 40 years or older diagnosed with HCM had low α-galactosidase A levels and corresponding gene mutations consistent with Anderson-Fabry disease. Heterozygous females are also commonly affected, particularly over the age of 45 years.[63] Cardiac symptoms including dyspnea, angina, and palpitations are common and are related to the degree of LVH.[64]

Findings that should raise suspicion for a glycogen storage disorder in a patient presenting with LVH include early or late age of onset, ventricular pre-excitation, skeletal myopathy, and elevation of skeletal muscle enzymes.[61,62] Hemochromatosis, a condition of iron overload, results in increased iron deposition in the sarcoplasmic reticulum of cells in a variety of organs including the liver, pancreas, heart, gonads, and other organs. Primary or hereditary hemochromatosis is an autosomal recessive disorder in which mutations in the HFE gene result in increased intestinal absorption of iron. It is the most common autosomal recessive disorder in Caucasians, affecting up to 0.8% of people of Northern European descent.[14] Secondary hemochromatosis results from multiple blood transfusions, ineffective erythropoiesis in severe thalassemia, sickle cell or sideroblastic anemia, excessive intake of iron, or chronic liver disease. Approximately 15% of patients with hemochromatosis present with cardiac symptoms and about 30% of untreated patients later develop cardiac symptoms.[65] More patients may have subclinical cardiac involvement.[66] RCM patients with hemochromatosis may also present with dilated cardiomyopathy and supraventricular arrhythmias such as atrial fibrillation.[67]

3. DIAGNOSTIC EVALUATION
3.1. Echocardiography
Echocardiography is required to detect the physiological alterations that characterize RCM (Fig. 34.1). Advanced impairment of LV diastolic filling is detected as a short early mitral inflow (E wave) deceleration time. Early or less severe disease may have an impaired relaxation or pseudonormal mitral inflow pattern. Tissue Doppler imaging of the mitral annulus typically shows reduced early diastolic (E') velocities. Pulmonary vein systolic velocities may be blunted due to increased left atrial pressure, and the velocity of propagation (Vp) of mitral inflow on color M-mode is typically reduced (<45 cm/s). LV systolic function is usually preserved, but may be decreased in advanced stages. Left and right ventricular wall thickness is normal or mildly increased with primary restrictive RCMs, but more frequently increased with secondary forms. Severe biatrial enlargement is a classic, if nonspecific feature. Constrictive pericarditis is the classical differential diagnosis, also leading to restrictive physiology with preserved LV systolic function. Many distinguishing characteristics have been described (Table 34.4). The presence of normal LV wall thickness, high tissue Doppler mitral annular early diastolic (E') velocities, a high Vp of mitral inflow on color M-mode, and significant respiratory variation in mitral and tricuspid inflow

TABLE 34.3
GLYCOGEN STORAGE DISORDERS WITH PREDOMINANT CARDIAC INVOLVEMENT

	Protein	Inheritance	Cardiac phenotype	Systemic phenotype
Fabry disease	α-Galactosidase A	X-linked recessive	Hypertrophic cardiomyopathy	Renal disease, neuropathy, gastrointestinal infiltration
Pompe disease	Lysosomal α-1, 4-glucosidase (GAA)	Autosomal recessive	Hypertrophic cardiomyopathy in infantile form	Skeletal myopathy
Danon disease	LAMP2	X-linked dominant	Hypertrophic or dilated cardiomyopathy, Wolff–Parkinson–White syndrome	Skeletal myopathy, variable mental retardation
Deficient cardiomyopathy	PRKAG2	Autosomal Dominant	Hypertrophic cardiomyopathy, Wolff–Parkinson–White syndrome, heart block	None

LAMP2, lysosome-associated membrane protein 2; PRKAG2, adenosine monophosphate-activated protein kinase gamma 2.

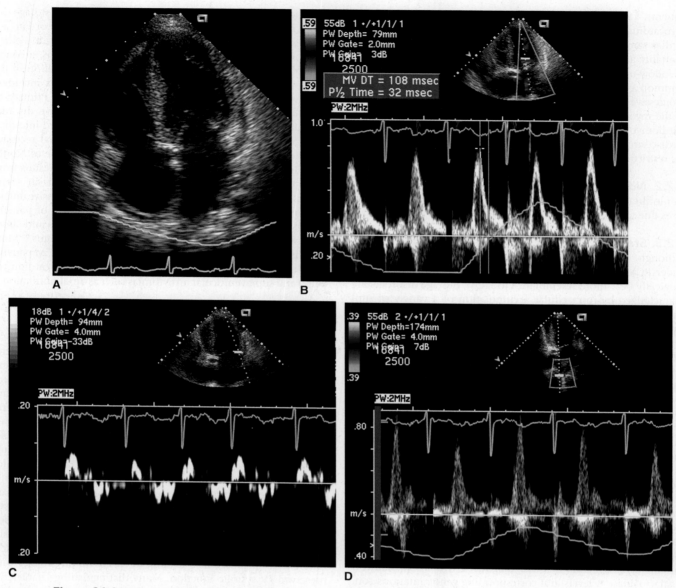

Figure 34.1 Patient with primary restrictive cardiomyopathy. **A:** Apical 4 chamber view shows normal LV and RV chamber sizes with normal wall thickness. **B:** Mitral inflow pulsed-wave Doppler demonstrates a restrictive filling pattern. **C:** Tissue Doppler imaging at the lateral mitral annulus demonstrates a low E' velocity. **D:** There is severe systolic blunting of pulmonary venous flow.

TABLE 34.4

DIFFERENTIATION OF RESTRICTIVE CARDIOMYOPATHY VERSUS CONSTRICTIVE PERICARDITIS

	Restrictive cardiomyopathy	Constrictive pericarditis
History	Amyloidosis, sarcoidosis	Pericarditis, open heart surgery, TB, connective tissue disease, radiation.
Labs	—	—
BNP	Elevated	Normal or mildly elevated
Echocardiography	—	—
Respiratory variation in mitral and tricuspid inflow	<10%	Mitral ≥25% Tricuspid ≥40%
Diastolic reversal of hepatic venous flow	Increased during inspiration	Increased during expiration
Mitral annular tissue Doppler velocity	Decreased (<8 cm/s)	Increased (>12 cm/s)
Cardiac catheterization		

(Continued)

TABLE 34.4

DIFFERENTIATION OF RESTRICTIVE CARDIOMYOPATHY VERSUS CONSTRICTIVE PERICARDITIS (Continued)

	Restrictive cardiomyopathy	Constrictive pericarditis
RV end diastolic/systolic pressure	<1/3	>1/3
Difference between LV and RV end diastolic pressures	>5 mm Hg	<5 mm Hg
Ventricular interdependence	Absent	Present
Cardiac CT or MRI		
Pericardium	Pericardium <2 mm	Pericardium >4 mm tethering
Myocardium	Myocardial scar or fibrosis	No myocardial scar

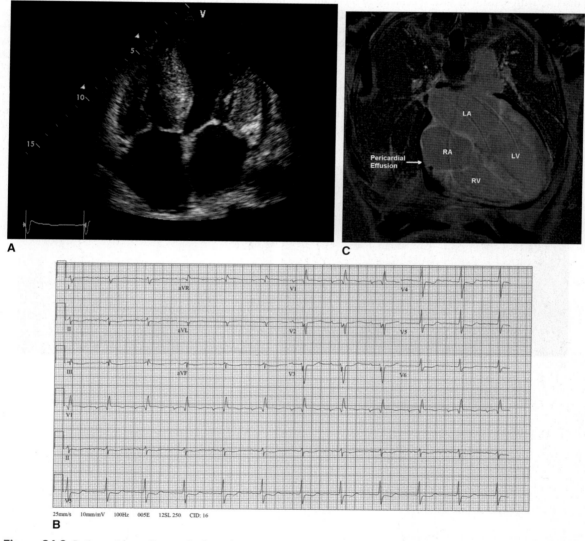

Figure 34.2 Patient with cardiac amyloidosis demonstrating (**A**) increased concentric, left ventricular wall thickness with a sparkling, granular appearance of the interventricular septum, (**B**) low voltage ECG pattern, and (**C**) a diffuse pattern of myocardial hyperenhancement after injection of gadolinium on cardiac MRI, which favors the subendocardial and midmyocardial layers. Also note delayed enhancement of the interatrial septum, atrial walls, and atrioventricular valves as well as a small circumferential pericardial effusion. LV, left ventricular; RV, right ventricular; LA, left atrium; RA, right atrium.

velocities point toward constrictive pericarditis. The pericardium is not easily assessed by echocardiography, although in some cases, particularly with TEE, pericardial thickening and pericardial tethering may be appreciated.[68]

The diagnosis of specific RCMs is sometimes possible by echocardiography. The myocardium in patients with amyloidosis is described as having a sparkling, granular appearance (Fig. 34.2A). Also seen are left and right ventricular wall thickening, thickening of the mitral and tricuspid leaflets and interatrial septum. Patients frequently have an associated small pericardial effusion. In the early stages of cardiac amyloidosis, diastolic function may be normal or mildly impaired, but progresses to restrictive physiology as the disease advances.[25] Restrictive filling on Doppler echocardiography, with an early mitral inflow (E) deceleration time of <150 ms has been associated with decreased 1 year survival (49% vs. 92%, p <0.001).[69] Other predictors of poor outcome include increased LV and RV wall thickness (≥15 mm and >7 mm, respectively), LV systolic dysfunction, and LV Tei index >0.77.[70,71] Echocardiographic measurement of cycle-dependent variation of myocardial integrated backscatter has been proposed to be a powerful prognostic indicator in cardiac amyloidosis, although its clinical utility remains limited.[72] The pattern of LVH in Fabry disease is frequently asymmetric and mimics HCM (Fig. 34.3A).[73] A binary appearance of the endocardium due to accumulation of glycosphingolipids in the endocardial and subendocardial layers has been described as characteristic of Fabry disease, with sensitivity and specificity of 94% and 100%, respectively.[74] However, these findings were not replicated in a later study, which demonstrated a much lower accuracy of a binary appearance of the endocardium for Fabry disease, with sensitivity and specificity of 35% and 79%, respectively.[75] Tissue Doppler imaging shows a decrease in systolic and diastolic mitral annular velocities, even before development of LVH.[76] This may facilitate earlier diagnosis in patients with a family history of Fabry disease or earlier institution of enzyme replacement therapy in patients who are known to be gene positive. LV Tei index

>0.60 and basal posterior wall thinning in Fabry disease have been associated with a worse prognosis.[77] Increased myocardial wall thickness is also present in other glycogen storage disorders; however, no specific identifying features have been described. In cardiac sarcoidosis echocardiography may reveal dilated cardiomyopathy, regional wall thinning, wall motion abnormalities, aneurysms, or restrictive physiology. However, cardiac MRI or nuclear myocardial perfusion imaging appears to be more sensitive for the detection of cardiac involvement in patients with sarcoidosis.[56] In hemochromatosis dilated cardiomyopathy is seen more commonly than RCM. In a review from Mayo Clinic seven (37%) of 19 patients with primary hemochromatosis had chamber dilation and systolic dysfunction.[66] Others have reported that the earliest finding is a restrictive filling pattern.[78] Doppler filling indices and tissue Doppler echocardiography may help to detect early involvement in patients with hereditary hemochromatosis.[79] In EMF the echocardiogram shows apical obliteration of the right, left, or both ventricular apices with small ventricular cavity size (Fig. 34.4A,B). Mitral and tricuspid regurgitations are common. Ventricular thrombus may also be detected.[35,80]

3.2. Electrocardiogram

The ECG has some utility in the diagnosis of RCMs. Low voltage and pseudoinfarct pattern are the most common ECG

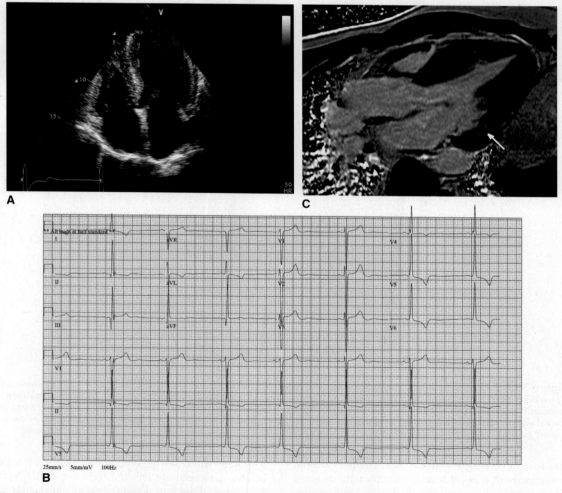

Figure 34.3 Patient with Anderson-Fabry disease demonstrating (**A**) a severe increase in left ventricular wall thickness, (**B**) relatively short PR interval on ECG with high voltage and secondary repolarization abnormalities and (**C**) small area of midmyocardial scar in the basal inferolateral wall, but otherwise normal (**dark**) myocardium on gadolinium delayed enhancement imaging with cardiac MRI.

abnormalities associated with amyloidosis, and in one study were detected in 46% and 47% of patients with biopsy proven cardiac involvement, whereas criteria for LVH were met in only 16% of patients (Fig. 34.2B).[8] A combination of low ECG voltage and interventricular septal thickness >1.98 cm by echocardiography has a sensitivity, specificity, positive and negative predictive values of 72%, 91%, 79% and 88%, respectively for the diagnosis of biopsy proven cardiac amyloidosis.[81]

ECG changes associated with Fabry disease include a short PR interval (<0.12 ms), widened QRS with right bundle branch block pattern, LVH, and giant negative T waves (Fig. 34.3B).[82,83] The short PR interval in Fabry disease is probably related to accumulation of glycosphingolipids in cardiac tissue, and has been reported to normalize after enzyme replacement therapy with recombinant human-galactosidase A.[84] Ventricular pre-excitation and Wolf Parkinson White syndrome are associated with the rarer inherited storage disorders, Danon disease and PRKAG2.[61]

3.3. Laboratory tests

Brain natriuretic peptide (BNP) is typically elevated in patients with heart failure secondary to RCM. By contrast, in patients with constrictive pericarditis the BNP is usually normal or mildly elevated.[85] Most patients with primary amyloidosis have a monoclonal gammopathy, more frequently due to a monoclonal gammopathy of uncertain significance (MGUS) than multiple myeloma. However, in approximately 10% of cases there is no monoclonal protein secreted (nonsecretory primary amyloidosis). Troponin may be increased in patients with amyloidosis, either due to myocyte necrosis from amyloid deposits or ischemia related to intramural vessel obstruction.[86] Not surprisingly, elevated serum levels of troponin and BNP suggest a worse prognosis.[87] Troponin T discriminates patients with AL amyloidosis who are at high risk for stem cell transplantation.[88] In a recent study, patients with troponin T levels of ≥0.06 ug/L before transplantation had a mortality rate of 28% at 100 days versus 7% in patients with troponin T levels <0.06 ug/L (p <0.001).

Fabry disease may be diagnosed on the basis of a low plasma α-galactosidase A concentration. In patients with Danon disease there are typically moderate elevations of creatine phosphokinase (CPK). In hemochromatosis there is increased serum ferritin, transferrin saturation, and increased ratio of plasma iron to total iron binding capacity. In EMF, the presence of hypereosinophilia is variable and more frequent early in the disease.

3.4. Cardiac magnetic resonance imaging

Cardiac amyloidosis is associated with short subendocardial T1 times and a distinctive pattern of diffuse, predominantly subendocardial and midmyocardial delayed gadolinium enhancement on cardiac MRI (Fig. 34.2C).[89] These findings reflect the tendency for amyloid fibrils to be deposited preferentially in the subendocardial layer. One recently published study showed that diffuse subendocardial delayed enhancement has a high degree of accuracy for the diagnosis of biopsy proven cardiac amyloidosis with a sensitivity and specificity of 80%, and 94%, and positive and negative predictive values of 92% and 85%, respectively.[90] Eosinophilic endocarditis also preferentially affects the subendocardium (Fig. 34.4D). Myocardial fibrosis may be detected by cardiac MRI in patients with Fabry disease. A midmyocardial pattern of hyperenhancement of the basal inferolateral wall appears to be typical, although the pattern of hyperenhancement may be more diffuse in patients with severe LVH (Fig. 34.3C).[91] Fabry disease has also been reported to be

associated with a prolonged myocardial T2 relaxation time.[92] However, the sensitivity and specificity of these findings is uncertain.

Cardiac MRI has high accuracy in the diagnosis of myocardial iron overload. Myocardial iron deposition results in lower T2 times with decreased myocardial signal on T2 weighted images (Fig. 34.5).[93] A T2* time of <20 ms has been associated with reduced LV function.[94] In addition, serial assessment of T2* times can allow monitoring of treatment for hemochromatosis.[95] Cardiac MRI appears to be more sensitive than standard assessment with ECG, echocardiography, and thallium scintigraphy in patients with sarcoidosis, detecting cardiac involvement in as many as 39% (Fig. 34.6).[56,96] The extent of scar correlates with the duration of disease, ventricular size and function, mitral regurgitation severity, and ventricular tachycardia, and hence may have prognostic significance.[97] Localized myocardial edema detected in T2-weighted sequences is usually indicative of active disease and may serve to guide clinical decisions regarding use of high-dose steroid therapy.

3.5. Cardiac catheterization

Echocardiography has largely supplanted cardiac catheterization for hemodynamic assessment in patients with RCM. However, invasive hemodynamic evaluation is still sometimes performed to demonstrate restrictive physiology. Patients have elevated left and right ventricular diastolic pressures with a characteristic "dip and plateau" pattern and an "M" or "W" venous tracing with steep X and Y descents. Although the hemodynamic profile is often similar in patients with constrictive pericarditis, patients with RCM tend to have higher pulmonary pressures (>50 mm Hg), a ratio of RV end diastolic to systolic pressure less than 1/3, a greater than 5 mm Hg difference between LV and RV end diastolic pressures, and absence of ventricular interdependence.[98]

3.6. Myocardial biopsy

Myocardial biopsy is the gold standard for diagnosis of many RCMs. In amyloidosis, Congo red staining results in amyloid fibrils displaying apple-green birefringence under a polarizing microscope. Alcian blue can also be used to stain for amyloid. Four endomyocardial biopsies are needed for 100% sensitivity for detecting the disease.[99] Diagnosis of systemic amyloidosis may be attempted with rectal submucosal or abdominal fat pad biopsy. However, these methods appear to have lower yield than myocardial biopsy with reported sensitivities of 75% to 85% and 84% to 88%, respectively.[100] Immunohistochemical staining using specific antibodies can discriminate between the different types of amyloidosis, although equivocal results may occur in some cases of primary or rare hereditary amyloidosis.[101] Endomyocardial biopsy in patients with Fabry disease reveals concentric lamellar bodies in the sarcoplasm of myocardial cells on electron microscopy.[102] Mutations in LAMP2 (Danon disease) and PRKAG2 show characteristic histological changes of myocyte enlargement with pronounced vacuole formation within the cells.[61,103] In hemochromatosis, light microscopy shows abnormal deposit of granular yellow–gray material within the sarcoplasm of the myocytes and Prussian blue stains positive for iron, which is diagnostic of iron overload.[104] Sarcoidosis is characterized histologically by noncaseating granulomas. In patients with suspected cardiac sarcoidosis the yield from myocardial biopsy appears to be low, particularly in patients with isolated conduction system disease, and a negative biopsy should not prevent treatment of patients with a high clinical suspicion for cardiac involvement.[105]

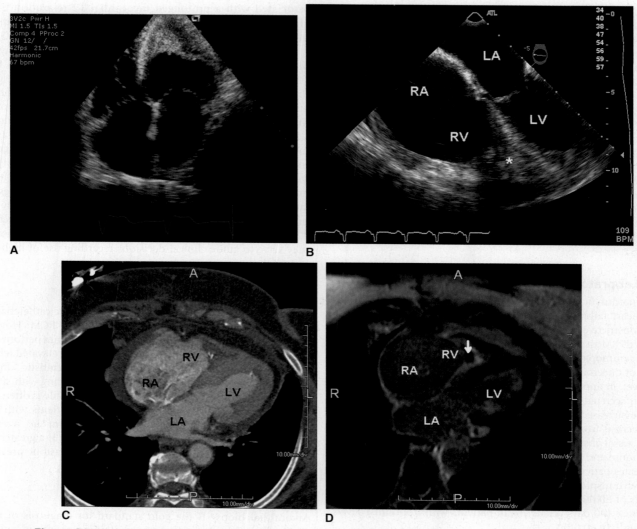

Figure 34.4 Two patients with Loeffler's endocarditis, predominantly involving the left ventricular apex (**A**) and right ventricular apex (**B**), respectively. In the second case, cardiac CT (**C**) demonstrates low attenuation filling defects with small areas of calcification in the right ventricular apex. Note also a small filling defect and calcification at the left ventricular apex. The tricuspid valve is tethered and nonfunctional. **D:** A cardiac MRI with gadolinium delayed enhancement shows diffuse endomyocardial fibrosis of the right and left ventricles, most prominent at the right ventricular apex. The area of decreased signal intensity at the right ventricular apex (*arrow*) is thrombus. LV, left ventricular; RV, right ventricular; LA, left atrium; RA, right atrium.

4. THERAPY

The primary goal of treatment in cardiac amyloidosis remains relief of symptoms. Diuretic therapy relieves congestion, but needs to be prescribed judiciously because of the tendency to orthostatic hypotension. Digoxin binds to amyloid fibrils potentially resulting in accumulation to toxic levels and should be avoided. Calcium channel blockers have also been associated with increased side effects in patients with cardiac amyloidosis.[106,107] Definitive therapy with chemotherapy and stem cell transplantation for AL have so far proved disappointing. Oral melphalan and prednisolone do not appear effective when there is cardiac or renal involvement. Stem cell transplantation has shown some promise for treatment of primary amyloidosis; however, compared to other hematological malignancies the early postprocedural mortality is significantly higher in patients with amyloidosis.[108,109]

Enzyme replacement therapy Agalsidase beta (Fabrazyme) in patients with Fabry disease reduces globotriaosylceramide levels

in infiltrated tissues throughout the body. In phase 3 studies, patients treated with agalsidase beta (1 mg/kg of body weight every 2 weeks) for 6 or 12 months had significant and sustained clearance of globotriaosylceramide from the vascular endothelium of the kidney, heart, and skin.[110] Enzyme replacement therapy with agalsidase beta has been reported to decrease LV wall thickness, decrease LV mass, and result in improvement in LV systolic and diastolic functions.[111-114] Studies have been underpowered to detect improvement in clinical endpoints and the cost effectiveness of therapy is uncertain.[115,116] Heart transplantation is an effective therapy for patients with end-stage primary RCM.[117,118] Pulmonary hypertension and high pulmonary vascular resistance are more common in restrictive than dilated cardiomyopathy and may preclude transplant in some patients. Close observation of pulmonary vascular resistance and prompt action when it increases is therefore recommended in these patients.[118] Heart transplantation is not generally considered a viable treatment option for patients with primary cardiac

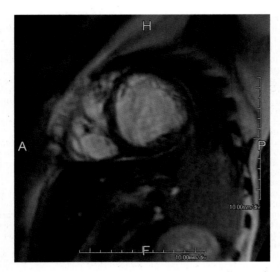

Figure 34.5 Cardiac MRI with T2-weighted gradient echo short-axis image of the heart shows decreased signal intensity of the myocardium and liver in a patient with hemochromatosis. Myocardial and liver T2* values of 9.1 and 5.5 ms, respectively, confirmed severe iron deposition in both organs. MRI, magnetic resonance imaging.

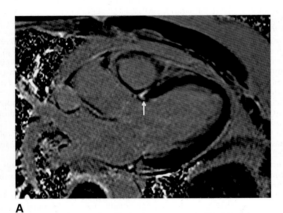

A

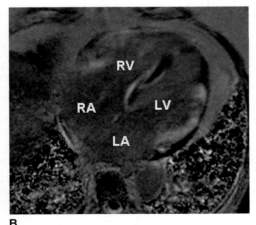

B

Figure 34.6 Cardiac MRI in two patients with cardiac sarcoidosis. **A:** Delayed enhancement imaging shows typical pattern of mid-myocardial scar involving the basal anteroseptum in a patient with palpitations. **B:** Extensive, patchy areas of transmural and epicardial scar in patient with severe cardiac sarcoidosis.

amyloidosis because of the tendency for disease recurrence in the allograft, despite adjuvant chemotherapy regimens.[119] In patients with hereditary amyloidosis, liver transplantation is the only known curative treatment and is associated with 5-year survival rates of 60% to 77%.[120,121] In patients with advanced cardiac disease, combined liver and cardiac transplantation has been successful.[122]

5. FUTURE DIRECTIONS

Greater understanding of the genetics and molecular mechanisms underlying RCMs may lead to earlier diagnosis and more specific treatments in the future. Newer imaging techniques such as cardiac MRI are likely to reduce the need for invasive testing such as myocardial biopsy. Enzyme replacement for Fabry disease is an example of how some of these conditions may be treatable or even curable with appropriate therapy. However, because of the rarity of many of these conditions, experience in their diagnosis and treatment is often limited among general cardiologists and management in specialist centers is generally recommended. This provides affected patients with appropriate expertise and the opportunity to participate in studies that may provide them with cutting edge treatments and improve our knowledge on how to best manage these conditions.

REFERENCES

1. Richardson P, McKenna W, Bristow M, et al. Report of the 1995 World Health Organization/International Society and Federation of Cardiology Task Force on the definition and classification of cardiomyopathies. *Circulation.* 1996;93(5):841–842.
2. Maron BJ, Towbin JA, Thiene G, et al. Contemporary definitions and classification of the cardiomyopathies: An American Heart Association Scientific Statement from the Council on Clinical Cardiology, Heart Failure and Transplantation Committee; Quality of Care and Outcomes Research and Functional Genomics and Translational Biology Interdisciplinary Working Groups; and Council on Epidemiology and Prevention. *Circulation.* 2006;113(14):1807–1816.
3. Elliott P, Andersson B, Arbustini E, et al. Classification of the cardiomyopathies: A position statement from the European Society Of Cardiology Working Group on myocardial and pericardial diseases. *Eur Heart J.* 2008;29(2):270–276.
4. Cetta F, O'Leary PW, Seward JB, et al. Idiopathic restrictive cardiomyopathy in childhood: Diagnostic features and clinical course. *Mayo Clin Proc.* 1995;70(7):634–640.
5. Siegel RJ, Shah PK, Fishbein MC. Idiopathic restrictive cardiomyopathy. *Circulation.* 1984;70(2):165–169.
6. Yacoub S, Kotit S, Mocumbi AO, et al. Neglected diseases in cardiology: A call for urgent action. *Nat Clin Pract Cardiovasc Med.* 2008;5(4):176–177.
7. Mueller PS, Edwards WD, Gertz MA. Symptomatic ischemic heart disease resulting from obstructive intramural coronary amyloidosis. *Am J Med.* 2000;109(3):181–188.
8. Murtagh B, Hammill SC, Gertz MA, et al. Electrocardiographic findings in primary systemic amyloidosis and biopsy-proven cardiac involvement. *Am J Cardiol.* 2005;95(4):535–537.
9. Arbustini E, Pasotti M, Pilotto A, et al. Desmin accumulation restrictive cardiomyopathy and atrioventricular block associated with desmin gene defects. *Eur J Heart Fail.* 2006;8(5):477–483.
10. Murphy RT, Mogensen J, McGarry K, et al. Adenosine monophosphate-activated protein kinase disease mimicks hypertrophic cardiomyopathy and Wolff-Parkinson-White syndrome: Natural history. *J Am Coll Cardiol.* 2005;45(6):922–930.
11. Selvanayagam JB, Hawkins PN, Paul B, et al. Evaluation and management of the cardiac amyloidosis. *J Am Coll Cardiol.* 2007;50(22):2101–2110.
12. Hauser AC, Lorenz M, Sunder-Plassmann G. The expanding clinical spectrum of Anderson-Fabry disease: A challenge to diagnosis in the novel era of enzyme replacement therapy. *J Intern Med.* 2004;255(6):629–636.
13. Sugie K, Yamamoto A, Murayama K, et al. Clinicopathological features of genetically confirmed Danon disease. *Neurology.* 2002;58(12):1773–1778.
14. McCarthy GM, Crowe J, McCarthy CJ, et al. Hereditary hemochromatosis: A common, often unrecognized, genetic disease. *Cleve Clin J Med.* 2002;69(3):224–226, 229–230, 232–233, 236–237.
15. Mocumbi AO, Yacoub S, Yacoub MH. Neglected tropical cardiomyopathies: II. Endomyocardial fibrosis: Myocardial disease. *Heart.* 2008;94(3):384–390.
16. Ammash NM, Seward JB, Bailey KR, et al. Clinical profile and outcome of idiopathic restrictive cardiomyopathy. *Circulation.* 2000;101(21):2490–2496.
17. Lebovic D, Hoffman J, Levine BM, et al. Predictors of survival in patients with systemic light-chain amyloidosis and cardiac involvement initially ineligible

for stem cell transplantation and treated with oral melphalan and dexamethasone. *Br J Haematol.* 2008;143(3):369–373.

18. MacDermot KD, Holmes A, Miners AH. Anderson-Fabry disease: Clinical manifestations and impact of disease in a cohort of 98 hemizygous males. *J Med Genet.* 2001;38(11):750–760.

19. Smedema JP, Snoep G, van Kroonenburgh MP, et al. Cardiac involvement in patients with pulmonary sarcoidosis assessed at two university medical centers in the Netherlands. *Chest.* 2005;128(1):30–35.

20. Abelmann WH, Lorell BH. The challenge of cardiomyopathy. *J Am Coll Cardiol.* 1989;13(6):1219–1239.

21. Zhang J, Kumar A, Stalker HJ, et al. Clinical and molecular studies of a large family with desmin-associated restrictive cardiomyopathy. *Clin Genet.* 2001;59(4):248–256.

22. Hayashi T, Shimomura H, Terasaki F, et al. Collagen subtypes and matrix metalloproteinase in idiopathic restrictive cardiomyopathy. *Int J Cardiol.* 1998;64(2):109–116.

23. Davis J, Wen H, Edwards T, et al. Allele and species dependent contractile defects by restrictive and hypertrophic cardiomyopathy-linked troponin I mutants. *J Mol Cell Cardiol.* 2008;44(5):891–904.

24. Yumoto F, Lu QW, Morimoto S, et al. Drastic Ca^{2+} sensitization of myofilament associated with a small structural change in troponin I in inherited restrictive cardiomyopathy. *Biochem Biophys Res Commun.* 2005;338(3):1519–1526.

25. Klein AL, Hatle LK, Taliercio CP, et al. Serial Doppler echocardiographic follow-up of left ventricular diastolic function in cardiac amyloidosis. *J Am Coll Cardiol.* 1990;16(5):1135–1141.

26. Angelini A, Calzolari V, Thiene G, et al. Morphologic spectrum of primary restrictive cardiomyopathy. *Am J Cardiol.* 1997;80(8):1046–1050.

27. Katritsis D, Wilmshurst PT, Wendon JA, et al. Primary restrictive cardiomyopathy: Clinical and pathologic characteristics. *J Am Coll Cardiol.* 1991;18(5):1230–1235.

28. Ware SM, Quinn ME, Ballard ET, et al. Pediatric restrictive cardiomyopathy associated with a mutation in beta-myosin heavy chain. *Clin Genet.* 2008;73(2):165–170.

29. Kaski JP, Syrris P, Burch M, et al. Idiopathic restrictive cardiomyopathy in children is caused by mutations in cardiac sarcomere protein genes. *Heart.* 2008;94(11):1478–1484.

30. Mogensen J, Kubo T, Duque M, et al. Idiopathic restrictive cardiomyopathy is part of the clinical expression of cardiac troponin I mutations. *J Clin Invest.* 2003;111(2):209–216.

31. Kubo T, Gimeno JR, Bahl A, et al. Prevalence, clinical significance, and genetic basis of hypertrophic cardiomyopathy with restrictive phenotype. *J Am Coll Cardiol.* 2007;49(25):2419–2426.

32. Pruszczyk P, Kostera-Pruszczyk A, Shatunov A, et al. Restrictive cardiomyopathy with atrioventricular conduction block resulting from a desmin mutation. *Int J Cardiol.* 2007;117(2):244–253.

33. Luethje LG, Boennemann C, Goldfarb L, et al. Prophylactic implantable cardioverter defibrillator placement in a sporadic desmin related myopathy and cardiomyopathy. *Pacing Clin Electrophysiol.* 2004;27(4):559–560.

34. Chew CY, Ziady GM, Raphael MJ, et al. Primary restrictive cardiomyopathy. Non-tropical endomyocardial fibrosis and hypereosinophilic heart disease. *Br Heart J.* 1977;39(4):399–413.

35. Hassan WM, Fawzy ME, Al Helaly S, et al. Pitfalls in diagnosis and clinical, echocardiographic, and hemodynamic findings in endomyocardial fibrosis: A 25-year experience. *Chest.* 2005;128(6):3985–3992.

36. Schneider U, Jenni R, Turina J, et al. Long-term follow up of patients with endomyocardial fibrosis: Effects of surgery. *Heart.* Apr 1998;79(4):362–367.

37. Barretto AC, Mady C, Nussbacher A, et al. Atrial fibrillation in endomyocardial fibrosis is a marker of worse prognosis. *Int J Cardiol.* 1998;67(1):19–25.

38. Mocumbi AO, Ferreira MB, Sidi D, et al. A population study of endomyocardial fibrosis in a rural area of Mozambique. *N Engl J Med.* 2008;359(1):43–49.

39. Ogbogu PU, Rosing DR, Horne MK III. Cardiovascular manifestations of hypereosinophilic syndromes. *Immunol Allergy Clin North Am.* 2007;27(3):457–475.

40. Ommen SR, Seward JB, Tajik AJ. Clinical and echocardiographic features of hypereosinophilic syndromes. *Am J Cardiol.* 2000;86(1):110–113.

41. Loeffler W. Endocarditis parietalis fibroplastica mit Bluteosinophilic. *Schweiz Me Wochenschr.* 1936;66:817.

42. Parrillo JE, Borer JS, Henry WL, et al. The cardiovascular manifestations of the hypereosinophilic syndrome. Prospective study of 26 patients, with review of the literature. *Am J Med.* 1979;67(4):572–582.

43. Srichai MB, Junor C, Rodriguez LL, et al. Clinical, imaging, and pathological characteristics of left ventricular thrombus: A comparison of contrast-enhanced magnetic resonance imaging, transthoracic echocardiography, and transesophageal echocardiography with surgical or pathological validation. *Am Heart J.* 2006;152(1):75–84.

44. Syed IS, Martinez MW, Feng DL, et al. Cardiac magnetic resonance imaging of eosinophilic endomyocardial disease. *Int J Cardiol.* 2008;126(3):e50–e52.

45. Westermark P, Benson MD, Buxbaum JN, et al. Amyloid fibril protein nomenclature – 2002. *Amyloid.* 2002;9(3):197–200.

46. Kyle RA, Gertz MA. Primary systemic amyloidosis: Clinical and laboratory features in 474 cases. *Semin Hematol.* 1995;32(1):45–59.

47. Gertz MA, Lacy MQ, Dispenzieri A. Amyloidosis. *Hematol Oncol Clin North Am.* 1999;13(6):1211–1233, ix.

48. Dubrey SW, Cha K, Anderson J, et al. The clinical features of immunoglobulin light-chain (AL) amyloidosis with heart involvement. *QJM.* 1998;91(2):141–157.

49. Cornwell GG III, Murdoch WL, Kyle RA, et al. Frequency and distribution of senile cardiovascular amyloid. A clinicopathologic correlation. *Am J Med.* 1983;75(4):618–623.

50. Tanskanen M, Kiuru-Enari S, Tienari P, et al. Senile systemic amyloidosis, cerebral amyloid angiopathy, and dementia in a very old Finnish population. *Amyloid.* 2006;13(3):164–169.

51. Ng B, Connors LH, Davidoff R, et al. Senile systemic amyloidosis presenting with heart failure: A comparison with light chain-associated amyloidosis. *Arch Intern Med.* 2005;165(12):1425–1429.

52. Dubrey SW, Cha K, Simms RW, et al. Electrocardiography and Doppler echocardiography in secondary (AA) amyloidosis. *Am J Cardiol.* 1996;77(4):313–315.

53. Saraiva MJ. Sporadic cases of hereditary systemic amyloidosis. *N Engl J Med.* 2002;346(23):1818–1819.

54. Connors LH, Lim A, Prokaeva T, et al. Tabulation of human transthyretin (TTR) variants, 2003. *Amyloid.* 2003;10(3):160–184.

55. Rocken C, Peters B, Juenemann G, et al. Atrial amyloidosis: An arrhythmogenic substrate for persistent atrial fibrillation. *Circulation.* 2002;106(16):2091–2097.

56. Mehta D, Lubitz SA, Frankel Z, et al. Cardiac involvement in patients with sarcoidosis: Diagnostic and prognostic value of outpatient testing. *Chest.* 2008;133(6):1426–1435.

57. Matsui Y, Iwai K, Tachibana T, et al. Clinicopathological study of fatal myocardial sarcoidosis. *Ann N Y Acad Sci.* 1976;278:455–469.

58. Johns CJ, Michele TM. The clinical management of sarcoidosis. A 50-year experience at the Johns Hopkins Hospital. *Medicine (Baltimore).* 1999;78(2):65–111.

59. Cotroneo J, Sleik KM, Rene Rodriguez E, et al. Hydroxychloroquine-induced restrictive cardiomyopathy. *Eur J Echocardiogr.* 2007;8(4):247–251.

60. Adams MJ, Lipsitz SR, Colan SD, et al. Cardiovascular status in long-term survivors of Hodgkin's disease treated with chest radiotherapy. *J Clin Oncol.* 2004;22(15):3139–3148.

61. Arad M, Maron BJ, Gorham JM, et al. Glycogen storage diseases presenting as hypertrophic cardiomyopathy. *N Engl J Med.* 2005;352(4):362–372.

62. Sachdev B, Takenaka T, Teraguchi H, et al. Prevalence of Anderson-Fabry disease in male patients with late onset hypertrophic cardiomyopathy. *Circulation.* 2002;105(12):1407–1411.

63. Kampmann C, Baehner F, Whybra C, et al. Cardiac manifestations of Anderson-Fabry disease in heterozygous females. *J Am Coll Cardiol.* 2002;40(9):1668–1674.

64. Linhart A, Kampmann C, Zamorano JL, et al. Cardiac manifestations of Anderson-Fabry disease: Results from the international Fabry outcome survey. *Eur Heart J.* 2007;28(10):1228–1235.

65. Cecchetti G, Binda A, Piperno A, et al. Cardiac alterations in 36 consecutive patients with idiopathic haemochromatosis: Polygraphic and echocardiographic evaluation. *Eur Heart J.* 1991;12(2):224–230.

66. Olson LJ, Baldus WP, Tajik AJ. Echocardiographic features of idiopathic hemochromatosis. *Am J Cardiol.* 1987;60(10):885–889.

67. Case records of the Massachusetts General Hospital. Weekly clinicopathological exercises. Case 31-1994. A 25-year-old man with the recent onset of diabetes mellitus and congestive heart failure. *N Engl J Med.* 1994;331(7):460–466.

68. Ling LH, Oh JK, Tei C, et al. Pericardial thickness measured with transesophageal echocardiography: Feasibility and potential clinical usefulness. *J Am Coll Cardiol.* 1997;29(6):1317–1323.

69. Klein AL, Hatle LK, Taliercio CP, et al. Prognostic significance of Doppler measures of diastolic function in cardiac amyloidosis. A Doppler echocardiography study. *Circulation.* 1991;83(3):808–816.

70. Tei C, Dujardin KS, Hodge DO, et al. Doppler index combining systolic and diastolic myocardial performance: clinical value in cardiac amyloidosis. *J Am Coll Cardiol.* 1996;28(3):658–664.

71. Cueto-Garcia L, Reeder GS, Kyle RA, et al. Echocardiographic findings in systemic amyloidosis: Spectrum of cardiac involvement and relation to survival. *J Am Coll Cardiol.* 1985;6(4):737–743.

72. Koyama J, Ray-Sequin PA, Falk RH. Prognostic significance of ultrasound myocardial tissue characterization in patients with cardiac amyloidosis. *Circulation.* 2002;106(5):556–561.

73. Tanaka H, Adachi K, Yamashita Y, et al. Four cases of Fabry's disease mimicking hypertrophic cardiomyopathy. *J Cardiol.* 1988;18(3):705–718.

74. Pieroni M, Chimenti C, De Cobelli F, et al. Fabry's disease cardiomyopathy: Echocardiographic detection of endomyocardial glycosphingolipid compartmentalization. *J Am Coll Cardiol.* 2006;47(8):1663–1671.

75. Kounas S, Demetrescu C, Pantazis AA, et al. The binary endocardial appearance is a poor discriminator of Anderson-Fabry disease from familial hypertrophic cardiomyopathy. *J Am Coll Cardiol.* 2008;51(21):2058–2061.

76. Pieroni M, Chimenti C, Ricci R, et al. Early detection of Fabry cardiomyopathy by tissue Doppler imaging. *Circulation.* 2003;107(15):1978–1984.

77. Kawano M, Takenaka T, Otsuji Y, et al. Significance of asymmetric basal posterior wall thinning in patients with cardiac Fabry's disease. *Am J Cardiol.* 2007;99(2):261–263.

78. Dabestani A, Child JS, Henze E, et al. Primary hemochromatosis: Anatomic and physiologic characteristics of the cardiac ventricles and their response to phlebotomy. *Am J Cardiol.* 1984;54(1):153–159.

79. Palka P, Macdonald G, Lange A, et al. The role of Doppler left ventricular filling indexes and Doppler tissue echocardiography in the assessment of cardiac involvement in hereditary hemochromatosis. *J Am Soc Echocardiogr.* 2002;15(9):884–890.

80. Acquatella H, Schiller NB. Echocardiographic recognition of Chagas' disease and endomyocardial fibrosis. *J Am Soc Echocardiogr.* 1988;1(1):60–68.

81. Rahman JE, Helou EF, Gelzer-Bell R, et al. Noninvasive diagnosis of biopsy-proven cardiac amyloidosis. *J Am Coll Cardiol.* 2004;43(3):410–415.

82. Yokoyama A, Yamazoe M, Shibata A. A case of heterozygous Fabry's disease with a short PR interval and giant negative T waves. *Br Heart J.* 1987;57(3):296–299.

83. Roudebush CP, Foerster JM, Bing OH. The abbreviated PR interval of Fabry's disease. *N Engl J Med.* 1973;289(7):357–358.

84. Waldek S. PR interval and the response to enzyme-replacement therapy for Fabry's disease. *N Engl J Med.* 2003;348(12):1186–1187.
85. Leya FS, Arab D, Joyal D, et al. The efficacy of brain natriuretic peptide levels in differentiating constrictive pericarditis from restrictive cardiomyopathy. *J Am Coll Cardiol.* 2005;45(11):1900–1902.
86. Miller WL, Wright RS, McGregor CG, et al. Troponin levels in patients with amyloid cardiomyopathy undergoing cardiac transplantation. *Am J Cardiol.* 2001;88(7):813–815.
87. Dispenzieri A, Gertz MA, Kyle RA, et al. Serum cardiac troponins and N-terminal pro-brain natriuretic peptide: A staging system for primary systemic amyloidosis. *J Clin Oncol.* 2004;22(18):3751–3757.
88. Gertz M, Lacy M, Dispenzieri A, et al. Troponin T level as an exclusion criterion for stem cell transplantation in light-chain amyloidosis. *Leuk Lymphoma.* 2008;49(1):36–41.
89. Maceira AM, Joshi J, Prasad SK, et al. Cardiovascular magnetic resonance in cardiac amyloidosis. *Circulation.* 2005;111(2):186–193.
90. Vogelsberg H, Mahrholdt H, Deluigi CC, et al. Cardiovascular magnetic resonance in clinically suspected cardiac amyloidosis: Noninvasive imaging compared to endomyocardial biopsy. *J Am Coll Cardiol.* 2008;51(10):1022–1030.
91. Moon JC, Sachdev B, Elkington AG, et al. Gadolinium enhanced cardiovascular magnetic resonance in Anderson-Fabry disease. Evidence for a disease specific abnormality of the myocardial interstitium. *Eur Heart J.* 2003;24(23):2151–2155.
92. Imbriaco M, Spinelli L, Cuocolo A, et al. MRI characterization of myocardial tissue in patients with Fabry's disease. *AJR Am J Roentgenol.* 2007;188(3):850–853.
93. Mavrogeni SI, Markussis V, Kaklamanis L, et al. A comparison of magnetic resonance imaging and cardiac biopsy in the evaluation of heart iron overload in patients with beta-thalassemia major. *Eur J Haematol.* 2005;75(3):241–247.
94. Anderson LJ, Holden S, Davis B, et al. Cardiovascular T2-star (T2*) magnetic resonance for the early diagnosis of myocardial iron overload. *Eur Heart J.* 2001;22(23):2171–2179.
95. Tanner MA, Galanello R, Dessi C, et al. A randomized, placebo-controlled, double-blind trial of the effect of combined therapy with deferoxamine and deferiprone on myocardial iron in thalassemia major using cardiovascular magnetic resonance. *Circulation.* 2007;115(14):1876–1884.
96. Smedema JP, Snoep G, van Kroonenburgh MP, et al. The additional value of gadolinium-enhanced MRI to standard assessment for cardiac involvement in patients with pulmonary sarcoidosis. *Chest.* 2005;128(3):1629–1637.
97. Schulz-Menger J, Wassmuth R, Abdel-Aty H, et al. Patterns of myocardial inflammation and scarring in sarcoidosis as assessed by cardiovascular magnetic resonance. *Heart.* 2006;92(3):399–400.
98. Talreja DR, Nishimura RA, Oh JK, et al. Constrictive pericarditis in the modern era: Novel criteria for diagnosis in the cardiac catheterization laboratory. *J Am Coll Cardiol.* 2008;51(3):315–319.
99. Pellikka PA, Holmes DR Jr, Edwards WD, et al. Endomyocardial biopsy in 30 patients with primary amyloidosis and suspected cardiac involvement. *Arch Intern Med.* 1988;148(3):662–666.
100. Shah KB, Inoue Y, Mehra MR. Amyloidosis and the heart: A comprehensive review. *Arch Intern Med.* 2006;166(17):1805–1813.
101. Kebbel A, Rocken C. Immunohistochemical classification of amyloid in surgical pathology revisited. *Am J Surg Pathol.* 2006;30(6):673–683.
102. Desnick RJ, Brady R, Barranger J, et al. Fabry disease, an under-recognized multisystemic disorder: Expert recommendations for diagnosis, management, and enzyme replacement therapy. *Ann Intern Med.* 2003;138(4):338–346.
103. Arad M, Benson DW, Perez-Atayde AR, et al. Constitutively active AMP kinase mutations cause glycogen storage disease mimicking hypertrophic cardiomyopathy. *J Clin Invest.* 2002;109(3):357–362.
104. Olson LJ, Edwards WD, Holmes DR Jr, et al. Endomyocardial biopsy in hemochromatosis: Clinicopathologic correlates in six cases. *J Am Coll Cardiol.* 1989;13(1):116–120.
105. Uemura A, Morimoto S, Hiramitsu S, et al. Histologic diagnostic rate of cardiac sarcoidosis: Evaluation of endomyocardial biopsies. *Am Heart J.* 1999;138(2 Pt 1):299–302.
106. Gertz MA, Falk RH, Skinner M, et al. Worsening of congestive heart failure in amyloid heart disease treated by calcium channel-blocking agents. *Am J Cardiol.* 1985;55(13 Pt 1):1645.
107. Griffiths BE, Hughes P, Dowdle R, et al. Cardiac amyloidosis with asymmetrical septal hypertrophy and deterioration after nifedipine. *Thorax.* 1982;37(9):711–712.
108. Moreau P, Leblond V, Bourquelot P, et al. Prognostic factors for survival and response after high-dose therapy and autologous stem cell transplantation in systemic AL amyloidosis: A report on 21 patients. *Br J Haematol.* 1998;101(4):766–769.
109. Comenzo RL, Vosburgh E, Simms RW, et al. Dose-intensive melphalan with blood stem cell support for the treatment of AL amyloidosis: One-year follow-up in five patients. *Blood.* 1996;88(7):2801–2806.
110. Eng CM, Guffon N, Wilcox WR, et al. Safety and efficacy of recombinant human alpha-galactosidase A–replacement therapy in Fabry's disease. *N Engl J Med.* 2001;345(1):9–16.
111. Hughes DA, Elliott PM, Shah J, et al. Effects of enzyme replacement therapy on the cardiomyopathy of Anderson-Fabry disease: A randomised, double-blind, placebo-controlled clinical trial of agalsidase alfa. *Heart.* 2008;94(2):153–158.
112. Beck M, Ricci R, Widmer U, et al. Fabry disease: Overall effects of agalsidase alfa treatment. *Eur J Clin Invest.* 2004;34(12):838–844.
113. Spinelli L, Pisani A, Sabbatini M, et al. Enzyme replacement therapy with agalsidase beta improves cardiac involvement in Fabry's disease. *Clin Genet.* 2004;66(2):158–165.
114. Weidemann F, Breunig F, Beer M, et al. Improvement of cardiac function during enzyme replacement therapy in patients with Fabry disease: A prospective strain rate imaging study. *Circulation.* 2003;108(11):1299–1301.
115. Banikazemi M, Bultas J, Waldek S, et al. Agalsidase-beta therapy for advanced Fabry disease: A randomized trial. *Ann Intern Med.* 2007;146(2):77–86.
116. Connock M, Juarez-Garcia A, Frew E, et al. A systematic review of the clinical effectiveness and cost-effectiveness of enzyme replacement therapies for Fabry's disease and mucopolysaccharidosis type 1. *Health Technol Assess.* 2006;10(20):iii–iv, ix–113.
117. Bograd AJ, Mital S, Schwarzenberger JC, et al. Twenty-year experience with heart transplantation for infants and children with restrictive cardiomyopathy: 1986–2006. *Am J Transplant.* 2008;8(1):201–207.
118. Weller RJ, Weintraub R, Addonizio LJ, et al. Outcome of idiopathic restrictive cardiomyopathy in children. *Am J Cardiol.* 2002;90(5):501–506.
119. Dubrey SW, Burke MM, Hawkins PN, et al. Cardiac transplantation for amyloid heart disease: The United Kingdom experience. *J Heart Lung Transplant.* 2004;23(10):1142–1153.
120. Herlenius G, Wilczek HE, Larsson M, et al. Ten years of international experience with liver transplantation for familial amyloidotic polyneuropathy: Results from the Familial Amyloidotic Polyneuropathy World Transplant Registry. *Transplantation.* 2004;77(1):64–71.
121. Parrilla P, Ramirez P, Andreu LF, et al. Long-term results of liver transplantation in familial amyloidotic polyneuropathy type I. *Transplantation.* 1997;64(4):646–649.
122. Nardo B, Beltempo P, Bertelli R, et al. Combined heart and liver transplantation in four adults with familial amyloidosis: Experience of a single center. *Transplant Proc.* 2004;36(3):645–647.

Hypertrophic Cardiomyopathy

35

Neal Lakdawala
Carolyn Ho

1. INTRODUCTION

Noninvasive cardiac imaging plays a paramount role in the diagnosis and management of hypertrophic cardiomyopathy (HCM). By characterizing anatomic changes and pathophysiology, assisting both in the determination of appropriate treatment and assessing therapeutic response, and aiding in stratifying risk for sudden death, cardiac imaging has facilitated the substantial evolution in the understanding and approach to this disease over the decades, since its modern characterization. What was once considered a rare disease with a uniformly poor prognosis has come to be appreciated as a relatively common condition which can be associated with normal longevity and manageable symptoms.[1] Advances in cardiac imaging technology have allowed for ever more refined understanding of the morphologic diversity, dynamic remodeling, and multifaceted perturbations of cardiac function associated with HCM. In this chapter we provide a brief overview of HCM, emphasizing how cardiac imaging can be integrated to optimize care of this complex and heterogeneous disease.

2. OVERVIEW

2.1. Epidemiology

HCM is defined by the presence of unexplained left ventricular hypertrophy (LVH) (Fig. 35.1), but demonstrates remarkable diversity with respect to disease course, age of onset, degree and pattern of LVH, severity of symptoms, hemodynamic perturbations, and risk for sudden cardiac death (SCD).[2] Echocardiographic screening studies of large cohorts across diverse ethnic backgrounds have estimated the prevalence of disease as approximately 1 in 500.[2-5] Reported annual mortality rates for HCM range from 4% to 6% in referral-based populations, to 1% to 2% in community-based studies.[1] Overall life expectancy is not dramatically impacted in the majority of patients with HCM. SCD (accounting for approximately half of HCM-related deaths), progressive heart failure, atrial fibrillation, and stroke are leading contributors to the morbidity and mortality associated with HCM.[2]

2.2. Histologic features

Myocyte hypertrophy with disarray and fibrosis are pathognomonic histologic features of HCM (Fig. 35.2), and have characterized the disease since the first modern description of HCM by British pathologist, Professor Donald Teare.[6] Disarray is often patchy with substantial regional variation, but more commonly seen in hypertrophied sections. Although mild degrees of disarray

have been reported in normal hearts (particularly at the right ventricular (RV) septal insertion point) and as a result of other diseases, the extent of disarray is unique to HCM and remains a defining feature of this disease; typically involving greater than 5% to 10% of the myocardium.[7]

2.3. Genetics

Although familial disease with autosomal dominant inheritance was recognized early in its description, the genetic etiology of HCM was identified in 1990 with the discovery of a mutation in the gene encoding β-cardiac myosin heavy chain (MYH7[8,9]). Follow-up studies established the paradigm that HCM is a disease of the sarcomere, caused by mutations in different components of the contractile apparatus (Fig. 35.3). To date over 800 mutations in ~12 sarcomere genes have been identified in patients and families with HCM[10] (updated genetic information is also available at http://cardiogenomics.med.harvard.edu). Most mutations do not tend to recur frequently in unrelated individuals, but rather are unique or private to individual families. Genetic studies in adult and pediatric populations have demonstrated that sarcomere mutations are a major cause of disease throughout life.[11-13] Despite differences in age of presentation, sarcomere mutations are identified in a similar percentage of adults and children with a clinical diagnosis of HCM; approximately 55% to 60%. Diagnostic yield is higher if a family history of disease is present (60% to 64%) than if absent (40% to 49%). The vast majority (>90%) of disease is accounted for by mutations in four sarcomere genes: MYH7 (encoding β-cardiac myosin heavy chain), MYBPC3 (cardiac myosin binding protein C), TNNT2 (cardiac troponin T), and TNNI3 (cardiac troponin I). It is important to note that sarcomere mutations are not identified in a proportion of patients with a clinical diagnosis of HCM, including individuals with a family history of disease. This indicates that other genetic and nongenetic etiologies importantly contribute to cardiac hypertrophy and await further characterization.

The substantial genetic heterogeneity of HCM has limited robust genotype–phenotype correlations, but some general trends have been identified. TNNT2 mutations may result in lesser degrees of hypertrophy but increased sudden death risk.[14] Elderly-onset disease has been associated with MYBPC3 mutations, but MYH7 mutations are notably absent in this cohort.[15] However, numerous exceptions to these associations have been described,[16-18] and rigorous prognostic information cannot typically be garnered solely from identifying the precise mutation responsible for causing the disease.

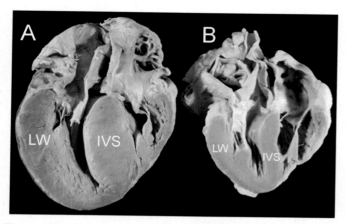

Figure 35.1 HCM: Gross pathology. The HCM heart (**A**) Demonstrates severe concentric left ventricular hypertrophy, most prominently in the interventricular septum (IVS) but also present in the free lateral wall (LW). This is in contrast to the normal heart (**B**) with normal wall thickness.

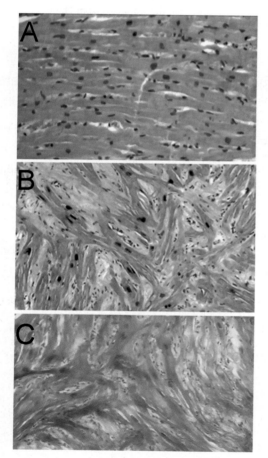

Figure 35.2 HCM: Microscopic pathology. Histologic examination of normal and HCM specimens. All images are at 10× magnification. **A:** Hematoxylin and eosin (H&E) stain of normal myocardium demonstrates the normal, orderly arrangement of myocytes and scant interstitial fibrosis. **B:** H&E stain of from a patient with HCM demonstrates myocyte hypertrophy and disarray with myocytes oriented at bizarre and varied angles. **C:** Masson trichrome staining of an HCM specimen demonstrates prominent fibrosis (*blue*). (Images courtesy of Robert Padera, MD, PhD. Brigham and Women's Hospital, Boston, MA.)

3. DIAGNOSTIC EVALUATION

3.1. Identification of left ventricular hypertrophy

The clinical diagnosis of HCM is based on the identification of unexplained LVH—increased LV wall thickness which occurs in the absence of other causes, such as pressure overload (systemic hypertension, aortic stenosis) or other relevant multisystem illness (e.g., storage diseases). Evaluation may be triggered in response to symptoms, or in asymptomatic individuals in the course of family screening or after detection of a systolic murmur or an abnormal EKG. Diagnosis is commonly made by transthoracic echocardiography, but is importantly facilitated by the use of complementary imaging techniques, including contrast echocardiography and cardiac magnetic resonance imaging (CMR). This is particularly critical if echocardiographic images are of suboptimal quality due to poor acoustic windows and inadequate endocardial definition. CMR allows true tomographic imaging and can provide accurate estimation of myocardial mass, superior visualization of the myocardium, and delineation of tissue borders, thereby improving the ability to diagnose HCM and to accurately quantify LV wall thickness. The LV apex and lateral free wall are particularly susceptible to beam spread artifact and diminished resolution on echocardiography. As demonstrated in Figure 35.4, CMR can often better visualize these regions as well as individual LV segments. Although several studies indicate that echo and CMR measured maximal LV wall thicknesses are highly correlated ($r^2 = 0.70$),[19,20] given the myriad of morphologic patterns seen in HCM, CMR may occasionally provide a diagnosis based on focal segmental hypertrophy that was unappreciated or underappreciated by echocardiography.[21] While the pattern of distribution of LVH probably does not substantially impact prognosis, accurate determination of LV wall thickness is clinically important because the extent of LVH is a risk predictor for SCD, with a higher risk associated with more extreme degrees of hypertrophy.[22,23]

Unexplained increased LV wall thickness in excess of 13 to 15 mm in adults or greater than two standard deviations above the normal population mean for age and body surface area in children[24] (z score >2) is considered diagnostic of disease. Diagnosis does not require the identification of increased LV mass. Approximately 21% of patients who meet diagnostic criteria for HCM based on increased wall thickness will have normal LV mass on CMR,[19] as focal or mild hypertrophy may not result in an abnormal increase in LV mass. Close relatives of patients with HCM are predicted to have a 50% likelihood of inheriting the disease-causing mutation and therefore, are at increased risk for disease development, relative to the general population. More subtle changes in LV wall thickness may indicate emerging or mild HCM in the context of familial disease. In recognition of this, modified echocardiographic and EKG criteria for the diagnosis of relatives of patients with HCM have been proposed,[25] as seen in Table 35.1. A diagnosis of familial HCM would be suggested by the presence of any of the following combinations: one major echocardiographic or EKG criterion, two minor echocardiographic criteria, or one minor echocardiographic plus 2 minor EKG criteria.

3.2. Evaluation of ventricular morphology

HCM exhibits a diverse morphologic spectrum, as illustrated in Figure 35.5. In addition to identifying and quantifying LVH, imaging studies allow description of LV morphology by characterizing the pattern and distribution of increased LV wall thickness. Hypertrophy can be focal or diffuse, and symmetric or asymmetric. Based

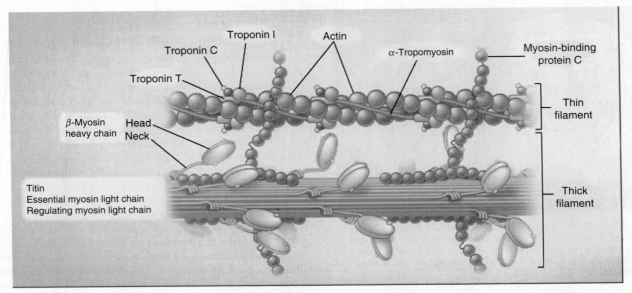

Figure 35.3 Hypertrophic cardiomyopathy is caused by mutations in sarcomere genes. Hypertrophic cardiomyopathy is a disease of the sarcomere, caused by dominantly acting mutations in contractile proteins. To date, over 800 mutations have been identified in all components of the sarcomere apparatus shown in this illustration. Mutations of β-myosin heavy chain, myosin binding protein C, troponin T, and troponin I are the most common. (Reproduced from Nabel E. *N Engl J Med.* 2003;349:60–72, with permission. Copyright © 2005 Massachusetts Medical Society. All rights reserved.)

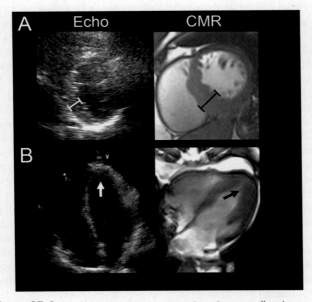

Figure 35.4 Cardiac magnetic resonance imaging may allow improved recognition and characterization of LV hypertrophy. Side by side comparisons of echocardiographic (**left**) and CMR images (**right**) where either inferoseptal hypertrophy (**A**) or apical hypertrophy (**B**) were not well visualized by echocardiography. **A:** Echocardiographic parasternal short axis at the level of the papillary muscles. Endocardial definition is suboptimal and maximal inferior septal thickness was 12 mm (*line*). CMR short-axis image allows precise quantification wall thickness (22 mm) at the inferior septum (*line*). **B:** Echocardiographic apical four-chamber image does not identify the apical hypertrophy that is clearly visible on the adjacent CMR image (*arrows*).

TABLE 35.1

DIAGNOSTIC CRITERIA FOR FAMILY MEMBERS OF PATIENTS WITH KNOWN HCM

Major criteria	Minor criteria
Echocardiography	
LV wall thickness ≥13 mm in anterior septum or posterior wall or ≥15 mm in the posterior septum or free wall Severe SAM	LV wall thickness 12 mm in anterior septum or posterior wall or 14 mm in the posterior septum or free wall ■ Moderate SAM ■ Redundant MV leaflets
Electrocardiography	
LVH ± repolarization changes T-wave inversion I and aVL (≥3 mm) discordant from QRS axis or Vr-V6 (≥3 mm) or II, III, and aVF (≥5 mm) Pathologic Q waves in at least two leads: II, III, aVF (in absence of L. anterior hemiblock) V1-V4; or I, aVl, V5, V6	■ Complete BBB or minor interventricular conduction defect ■ Minor repolarization changes in LV leads ■ Deep S V2 (≥25 mm)
—	Unexplained chest pain, dyspnea, or syncope.

LV, left ventricular; SAM, systolic anterior motion; MV, mitral valve; LVH, left ventricular hypertrophy.
Source: Adapted from McKenna WJ, Spirito P, Desnos M, et al. Experience from clinical genetics in hypertrophic cardiomyopathy: Proposal for new diagnostic criteria in adult members of affected families. *Heart.* 1997;77(2):130–132.

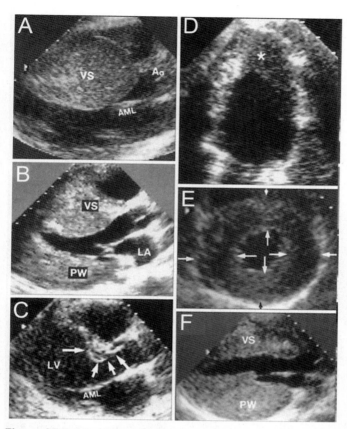

Figure 35.5 Diverse morphologic subtypes are seen in hypertrophic cardiomyopathy. Different patterns and distributions of wall thickening demonstrated in these diastolic still-frame images. **A:** Diffuse hypertrophy with massive hypertrophy of the anterior portion of the ventricular septum (50 mm), parasternal long-axis view. **B:** Prominent diffuse hypertrophy, parasternal long-axis view. **C:** Discrete upper septal hypertrophy (*arrows*) parasternal long-axis view. **D:** Apical hypertrophy (*), apical four-chamber view. **E:** Prominent diffuse hypertrophy, apical short-axis view. **F:** Hypertrophy predominantly of the posterior ventricular septum (PVS) and, to a lesser extent, the contiguous portion of the anterior septum, parasternal long-axis view. PW, posterior wall; AML, anterior mitral leaflet; VS, ventricular septum; LV, left ventricle; LA, left atrium. Calibration marks = 1 cm (Images courtesy of Barry J. Maron, MD. Minneapolis Heart Institute Foundation, Minneapolis, MN.)

on echo and CMR studies, site of LV involvement in descending order of prevalence is the septum (>80%), anterolateral free wall (~9%), apex (~4%), and midleft ventricle.[19] Typically, the pattern of LVH does not strongly influence prognosis.

Apical hypertrophy (Fig. 35.6) was first described in the Japanese medical literature, and is ~5 times more prevalent in Japanese than American populations.[26] The presence of apical hypertrophy is often accompanied by a distinctive EKG pattern with "giant" precordial T wave inversions (>10 mV), present in 30% to 60% of cases.[26] Favorable outcomes have been associated with apical HCM relative to more typical HCM with excellent long-term survival and lower symptom burden,[26,27] potentially because patients with apical HCM characteristically do not have concomitant hypertrophy beyond the midventricular level and therefore, do not develop outflow tract obstruction. However, the universality of this benign prognosis has recently been questioned as more varied outcomes have been observed.[28,29] Echocardiography is sufficient to make the diagnosis of apical HCM in ~ 90% cases,[27] nevertheless CMR or contrast echocardiography importantly improve diagnostic accuracy (Fig. 35.6).[30] Occasionally, LV noncompaction (LVNC) may mimic apical HCM and can be distinguished by using color flow

Doppler and/or echo contrast to visualize flow within the prominent LV trabeculations seen in LVNC,[31] or CMR to better visualize myocardial borders, as demonstrated in Figure 35.7.

Concentric, midventricular hypertrophy is an uncommon pattern of ventricular wall thickening in the context of HCM, but is of relevance because it may result in midventricular obstruction and apical aneurysm formation, as illustrated in Figure 35.8. This is a rare complication of disease, described in 2.2% of a cohort of over 1,300 patients.[32] In HCM, the development of apical aneurysms is not related to epicardial coronary artery disease, but rather appears to be associated with midcavitary obstruction, presumptively due to concentric hypertrophy that results in systolic apposition of the LV free wall and septum and formation of an intercavitary pressure gradient in the distal LV cavity and apex. These features were present in 68% of patients with LV aneurysm.[32] In this series, aneurysmal remodeling correlated with an unfavorable prognosis, including an increased risk for sudden death, progressive heart failure, and thromboembolic complications.

3.3. Family screening

HCM follows autosomal dominant inheritance, as such 50% of the offspring of an affected individual are predicted to inherit the mutation and be at risk for developing disease. Therefore, clinical screening of first degree relatives of patients with HCM is recommended, and it typically consists of history, physical examination, 12-lead EKG, and echocardiography to look for the presence of unexplained and asymptomatic LVH. The strategy outlined in Table 35.2 has been proposed for screening and following apparently healthy members of families with HCM.[33,34] Since the development of LVH is age-dependent, the absence of diagnostic clinical findings on initial assessment does not exclude the possibility of future disease development or the presence of an underlying sarcomere mutation, particularly in children. Serial follow-up is thus required, with the frequency of evaluation determined by the individual's age. Because most patients will develop LVH around the time of the adolescent growth spurt, the frequency of testing is greatest during that period. However, presentations in both early childhood and late adulthood are well described. As such, the presence of symptoms or abnormal exam findings should prompt testing regardless of age, and screening should continue at less frequent intervals throughout adulthood. As discussed above, modified diagnostic criteria have been proposed for the evaluation of familial disease (Table 35.1).[25] Genetic testing can potentially focus and clarify family management. In situations where a pathogenic sarcomere mutation is identified in an affected family member, mutation confirmation testing can then be performed on family members to determine which individuals who have inherited the disease-causing mutation are, therefore, definitively at risk for disease development. Longitudinal clinical screening can then be limited to just these individuals; family members who have not inherited the mutation can generally be reassured that neither they nor their offspring are at risk for developing disease.

3.4. Differential diagnosis

3.4.1. Athlete's heart

Intense athletic training can be accompanied by the development of physiologic hypertrophy and, if particularly pronounced, may raise concern for the possibility of underlying HCM. Most athletes have normal or only mildly increased LV wall thickness (6 to 12 mm), however ~2% of elite athletes, typically male, have LV wall thickness ≥13 mm and therefore, fall into an ambiguous "gray zone" between physiological hypertrophy and HCM.[35] Careful analysis of clinical features and noninvasive cardiac imaging

Figure 35.6 Apical hypertrophic cardiomyopathy. **A:** Typical EKG manifestations: Increased QRS amplitude and deep anterolateral T-wave inversions (*arrows*). **B:** Left ventriculogram, end-systolic still-frame image demonstrating apical chamber obliteration. **C:** Apical four-chamber echocardiogram with contrast demonstrating the "spade-shaped" LV cavity typical of apical HCM. **D:** Cardiac MRI: Prominent apical hypertrophy is seen in this diastolic still-frame image. LV, left ventricle.

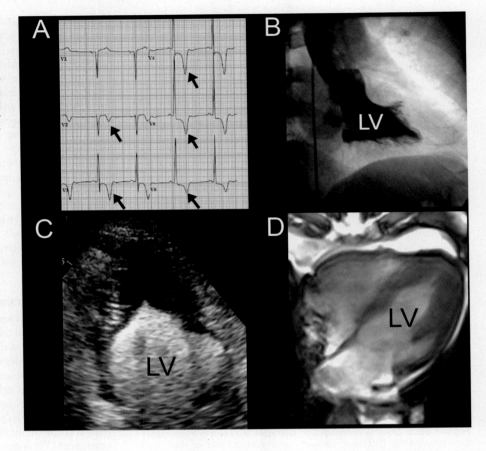

Figure 35.7 Color Doppler and CMR can distinguish left ventricular noncompaction from apical HCM. **A:** Noncompacted apical myocardium may have an appearance similar to apical hypertrophy on this grayscale apical four chamber diastolic still-frame image. **B:** Color Doppler demonstrates flow within apical trabeculations with color Doppler (*arrow*), identifying LVNC. **C:** CMR allows excellent myocardial visualization, demonstrating the prominent apical trabeculations of LVNC (*arrow*). LV, left ventricle; RV, right ventricle.

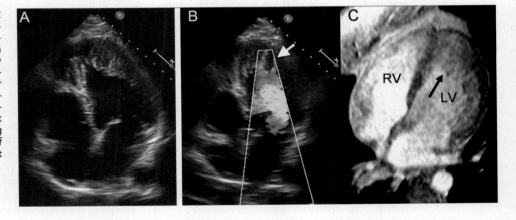

can assist in resolving this diagnostic dilemma summarized in Figure 35.9. In general, athletes will demonstrate other evidence of physiologic adaptations to intense training, including increased LV cavity size, uniform LV hypertrophy, and normal or supranormal indices of systolic and diastolic functions as well as peak oxygen consumption. By contrast, individuals with HCM, even if active and asymptomatic, tend to have more asymmetric LVH, small LV cavity size, markedly abnormal EKGs, and reduced systolic and diastolic myocardial velocities by tissue Doppler interrogation. In one study, S' velocity was 8.8 cm/s in HCM patients as compared to 10.6 cm/s in athletes; E' velocity was 11.7 cm/s as compared to 18.9 cm/s, in HCM patients and athletes, respectively.[36] Differentiating HCM from athlete's heart is important, since HCM is a lifelong genetic disease whose manifestations

could be adversely modified by continued involvement in competitive athletics. Moreover, there are significant familial implications associated with a diagnosis of HCM.

3.4.2. Phenocopies of hypertrophic cardiomyopathy: Metabolic and storage cardiomyopathies

Sarcomere mutations are not identified in ~30% to 50% of individuals with a clinical diagnosis of HCM. And the genetic basis of unexplained LVH in this context has not yet been fully elucidated. Such subjects tend to be slightly older at presentation and lack a clear family history of disease. Discrete upper septal hypertrophy seen in older patients, especially women with hypertension, is an example of a morphologic pattern of hypertrophy that is rarely associated with sarcomere mutations (<10%) and typically does

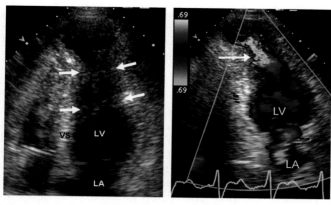

Figure 35.8 Apical aneurysm formation in HCM. Apical four-chamber still-frame systolic images, with and without color Doppler, showing a large LV apical aneurysm due to muscular mid-cavity narrowing and obstruction (*arrows*). LV, left ventricle; LA, left atrium; VS, ventricular septum. (Images courtesy of Barry J. Maron, MD. Minneapolis Heart Institute Foundation, Minneapolis, MN.)

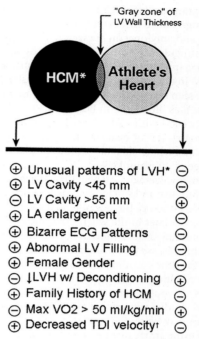

Figure 35.9 Athlete's heart versus HCM. About ~2% of elite athletes have an LV wall thickness ≥13mm and fall into a morphologic "gray zone" between physiological hypertrophy and HCM. Features on clinical examination and cardiac imaging can aid in distinguishing HCM from the benign, physiologic hypertrophy associated with intense athletic training. *LVH in which asymmetry is prominent, the anterior ventricular septum is spared, or the region of predominant thickening involves the posterior septum or LV free wall. †S' velocity and E' velocities are decreased in HCM and normal or supranormal in athletes. (Adapted from Barry J. Maron, MD. Distinguishing hypertrophic cardiomyopathy from athlete's heart: A clinical problem of increasing magnitude and significance. *Heart*. 2005;91(11):1380–1382, with permission. Copyright © 2008 BMJ Publishing Group. All rights reserved.)

not represent primary HCM,[11] but otherwise such individuals cannot be easily differentiated from those with underlying sarcomere mutations.

Genetic studies performed on families and sporadic cases of unexplained LVH with conduction abnormalities (progressive atrioventricular block, atrial fibrillation, ventricular pre-excitation) have led to the identification of a rare but distinct category of metabolic cardiomyopathies. In these situations, genetic cardiac hypertrophy is caused by mutations in the *PRKAG2* gene, encoding the γ2 regulatory subunit of adenosine monophosphate-activated protein kinase (AMPK), as well as mutations in the X-linked lysosome associated membrane protein (*LAMP2*) gene. Histopathologically, these metabolic cardiomyopathies do not display the prominent myocardial disarray or interstitial

---

TABLE 35.2

RECOMMENDED CLINICAL SCREENING OF FAMILY MEMBERS: PHYSICAL EXAMINATION, ECHOCARDIOGRAPHY, AND ELECTROCARDIOGRAM

The penetrance of LVH is age-dependent	
<12 years old	Optional unless: Severe family history of early HCM-related death, early development of LV hypertrophy, or other adverse complications Competitive athlete in intense training Suspected symptoms
12 to 22 years old	Repeat evaluation every 12 to 18 months
>23 years old	Repeat evaluation approximately every 5 years, or in response to symptoms.
If genetic results available:	Genotype (+) family members: Serial clinical evaluation, as above Genotype (−) family members: Reassurance; no need for further testing

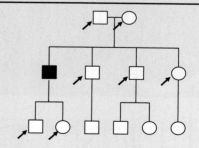

The proband is indicated by the solid square, indicating a male with a diagnosis of HCM.

Clinical evaluation is recommended for 1st degree relatives, indicated by the arrows.

Source: Adapted from Barry J. Maron, MD et al. Proposal for contemporary screening strategies in families with hypertrophic cardiomyopathy. *J Am Coll Cardiol.* 2004;44:2125–2132.

fibrosis pathognomonic for HCM. Instead, myocardial vacuolization with glycogen-filled myocytes (*PRKAG2*) or autophagic vacuoles (*LAMP2*) and amylopectin are seen.[37] These disorders cannot be reliably distinguished from HCM caused by sarcomere mutations by cardiac imaging, although massive concentric LVH with prominent RV involvement as well as ventricular pre-excitation are frequently seen in association with *LAMP2* mutations (cardiac Danon disease), as illustrated in Figure 35.10. *LAMP2* cardiomyopathy is associated with early onset LVH (often in childhood) with rapid progression of heart failure and poor prognosis, particularly in males, whose survival without cardiac transplantation beyond the age of 25 is unlikely.[37]

Multisystem involvement can help distinguish cardiac hypertrophy due to infiltrative and storage disorders, which can be familial, from HCM. Nevertheless, there is potential for ambiguity because HCM may present later in life when other medical comorbidities may be confounding factors. Moreover, cardiac-predominant phenotypes of Fabry disease (an X-linked recessive disorder caused by mutations in the gene encoding the lysosomal hydrolase α-galactosidase (GLA) resulting in glycosphyngolipid accumulation in the heart, kidneys, nervous system, and skin)[38-40] and amyloidosis[41] are well described. Studies suggest that at least 3% of unexplained LVH in adult males may be due to underlying Fabry disease.[42] Careful evaluation of extracardiac disease and review of family history can typically distinguish these conditions and are clinically relevant due to the availability of specific treatments for these disorders, including chemotherapy for amyloidosis due to plasma cell dyscrasias and enzyme replacement therapy for Fabry disease.[43] CMR may also help to identify characteristic patterns of delayed enhancement in these conditions. Preliminary reports suggest that focal midwall delayed gadolinium enhancement in the basal inferolateral LV is characteristic of Fabry associated cardiomyopathy.[44]

4. PATHOPHYSIOLOGY

The varied morphologic and functional changes associated with HCM may result in complex changes in cardiac physiology, leading to diastolic dysfunction, left ventricular outflow tract obstruction, mitral regurgitation, and overt systolic dysfunction. These pathophysiologic alterations relate to symptoms of effort intolerance, angina, fatigue, and syncope which commonly accompany HCM.

4.1. Diastolic dysfunction

Diastolic dysfunction is a consistent feature of disease and underlies central disease-related phenomena, including symptoms of dyspnea, exercise intolerance, and pulmonary congestion, as well as pathophysiologic changes of increased filling pressures and left atrial enlargement. A variety of imaging modalities (invasive hemodynamic measurements, radionuclide angiography, and echocardiography) have reliably identified diastolic abnormalities in HCM, manifested by increased LV diastolic pressures, prolonged isovolumic relaxation time, and impaired early diastolic filling.[45-47] These abnormalities stem from a multitude of factors affecting contraction and relaxation loads, myocardial calcium handling, and LV chamber stiffness that are perturbed in HCM.[48] Specifically, intracavitary obstruction may result in increased systolic load as well as delayed and impaired early relaxation. The prominent hypertrophy, increased myocardial mass, and myocardial fibrosis associated with the disease likely culminate in increased myocardial stiffness. Echocardiographic indices of diastolic function can identify patterns consistent with impaired relaxation or restrictive filling[49] and can assist in characterizing diastolic function and guiding treatment in patients with HCM (Fig. 35.11). However, direct clinical application and accurate quantification have been challenging in this disease. Diastolic filling parameters have not reliably predicted resting filling pressures or exercise capacity in patients with HCM. In patients studied simultaneously with cardiac catheterization and echocardiography, no relationship between transmitral indices of diastolic function and LV end-diastolic pressure was identified.[50-52] In addition, there has not been a consistent correlation with transmitral Doppler flow patterns and the extent of LVH, presence or absence of LVOT obstruction, symptoms, or exercise capacity.[50-53]

The use of newer indices of diastolic function derived from tissue Doppler interrogation (TDI) of myocardial velocity have improved detection and understanding of the pathophysiology of diastolic dysfunction in patients with HCM, but have not resolved all challenges. Measurement of early diastolic mitral

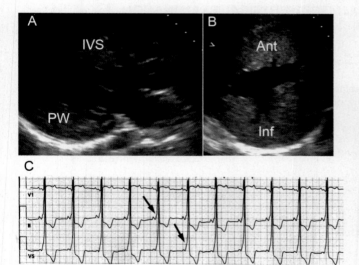

Figure 35.10 Phenocopies of HCM: Electrocardiogaphic and echocardiograhpic manifestations of LAMP2 mutations (cardiac Danon disease). **A:** Parasternal long axis and (**B**) short-axis images demonstrate severe, diffuse LV hypertrophy with a maximal LV septal wall thickness of 35 mm. **C:** Ventricular pre-excitation identifiable by the presence of delta waves (*arrows*). IVS, intraventricular septum; PW, posterior wall; Inf, inferior wall; Ant, anterior wall.

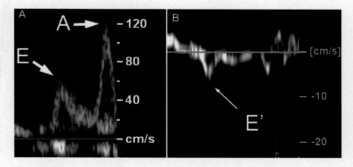

Figure 35.11 Impaired relaxation is a consistent feature of HCM and can be identified with Doppler techniques. Standard mitral inflow and tissue Doppler interrogation demonstrates diastolic dysfunction in a patient with HCM. **A:** Impaired relaxation demonstrated by pulse wave spectral Doppler assessment of mitral inflow. The peak velocity of early diastolic filling (E) is reduced compared to late diastolic filling (A), with an E/A wave ratio of 0.6. **B:** Impaired relaxation demonstrated by myocardial tissue velocity. The peak velocity of early diastolic mitral annular descent (E') is reduced (6 cm/s).

annular velocity (E') reflects LV relaxation and improves when outflow tract obstruction is mechanically relieved, either by surgical myectomy or alcohol septal ablation.[54,55] The ratio of early diastolic mitral inflow velocity (E) to early diastolic mitral annular velocity (E') has been proposed to estimate LV filling pressures in a variety of conditions, with an elevated E/E' ratio >15 suggesting increased left atrial pressure.[49,56] However, a recent validation study in patients with HCM found only a modest correlation ($r = 0.28$) between E/E' and invasively determined left atrial pressure, and found that E/E' had insufficient accuracy to predict increased wedge pressure (ROC c-statistic: $0.65 +/- 0.55$)[57] in this population. Although the integrated use of mitral inflow and TDI is currently the best approach to characterize diastolic function, the difficulties encountered in identifying an accurate, noninvasive, and quantitative method are indicative of the complex and heterogeneous nature of diastolic abnormalities in HCM.

There is compelling data from animal and human studies which indicate that diastolic dysfunction is an intrinsic manifestation of sarcomere mutations, detectable early in disease development *prior* to the development of LVH or even microscopic changes of disarray and fibrosis.[58,59] Tissue Doppler echocardiographic studies on genotyped human subjects have demonstrated that individuals with sarcomere gene mutations have impaired LV relaxation early in disease, prior to the development of LVH. Impaired relaxation was manifested by decreased E' velocity, compared to normal controls without sarcomere mutations (Fig. 35.12).[60–62] Owing to the substantial overlap in E' velocities from G + /LVH- subjects and normal controls, tissue Doppler indices alone are not sufficiently predictive of genetic status to replace genetic testing in families. However, these studies provide insights regarding the pathogenesis of HCM, suggesting that diastolic abnormalities are an early and direct manifestation of the underlying sarcomere mutation, rather than merely a secondary consequence of altered myocardial compliance characteristics due to the distinct changes in myocardial architecture that accompany overt disease.

4.2. Systolic dysfunction

Reduced systolic function may be a more prevalent feature of HCM than was previously suspected. Sophisticated measures of contractile function have shown evidence of diminished contractility in spite of a preserved or hyperdynamic LV ejection fraction (LVEF), the traditional metric of systolic function. This discrepancy may be partially explained by regional differences in contractile function that are not recognized with global tests such as the LVEF, but can be quantified with contemporary techniques. Moreover, LVEF does not reflect longitudinal systolic function and may not detect impaired long-axis performance.[63] Both CMR and echocardiographic strain imaging demonstrate abnormal contractility in HCM, particularly in hypertrophied segments and the interventricular septum.[64,65] The pathophysiologic basis and clinical implications of regional systolic dysfunction are not known at present.

4.3. Left ventricular outflow tract obstruction and systolic anterior motion of the mitral valve

Left ventricular outflow obstruction (LVOTO) was a defining physiologic feature of HCM when it was first described. It remains a highly visible feature of disease and a source of important morbidity and mortality. In addition to contributing to the symptoms, evidence from a large retrospective study suggests that obstruction is also an independent predictor of mortality. In a cohort of 1,101 patients followed for an average of 6.3 years, 25% of whom had a resting outflow tract gradient >30 mm Hg, the presence of

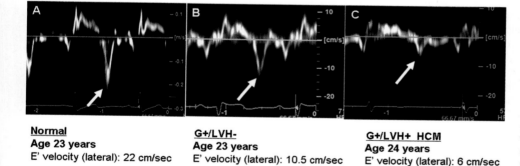

Normal
Age 23 years
E' velocity (lateral): 22 cm/sec

G+/LVH-
Age 23 years
E' velocity (lateral): 10.5 cm/sec

G+/LVH+ HCM
Age 24 years
E' velocity (lateral): 6 cm/sec

Figure 35.12 Impaired relaxation is present in carriers of sarcomere mutations prior to the development of LVH. Normal E' velocity of 22 cm/s is seen in a healthy relative who does not carry the sarcomere mutation that causes HCM in the family (**A**, normal control). By contrast, E' velocity is mildly reduced to 10.5 cm/s in an asymptomatic young family member who carries the sarcomere mutation but has not yet developed LVH (**B**, G+/LVH-). With the development of overt HCM (**C**, G+/LVH+), E' velocity is substantially reduced to 6 cm/s. There is substantial overlap in E' velocities between normal genotype (+) controls and G+/LVH- family members (**D**), limiting the diagnostic accuracy of using E' velocities alone to predict genotype status in families with HCM.

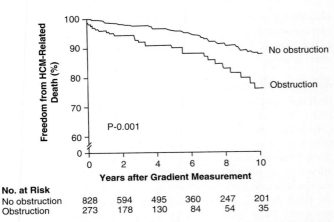

No. at Risk

No obstruction	828	594	495	360	247	201
Obstruction	273	178	130	84	54	35

Figure 35.13 Left ventricular obstruction is associated with decreased survival due to HCM-related death. The presence of a resting outflow tract gradient of 30 mm Hg or greater was associated with a significant reduction in survival. The magnitude of the gradient beyond 30 mm Hg did not add incremental risk. (Reproduced from Maron MS, Olivotto I, Betocchi S, et al. Effect of left ventricular outflow tract obstruction on clinical outcome in hypertrophic cardiomyopathy. *N Engl J Med.* 2003;348(4):295–303, with permission. Copyright © 2008 Massachusetts Medical Society. All rights reserved.)

obstruction predicted adverse outcomes.[66] Patients with obstruction were nearly 5 times more likely to progress to severe symptoms of heart failure and heart failure-related death, and after adjustment for potential confounding factors, the presence of obstruction was associated with a 60% increased risk of mortality (Fig. 35.13). Of note, there was no relationship between the severity of the obstruction and clinical outcomes in this study.

The causes of LVOTO in HCM are complex and multifactorial, relating to septal hypertrophy, redundant, elongated, and often anteriorly positioned mitral apparatus, altered ventricular loading conditions, and reduced ventricular chamber volume. These conditions lead to systolic anterior motion (SAM) of the mitral apparatus into the LV outflow tract which in turn obstructs the egress of blood from the heart and leads to the development of an outflow pressure gradient. Typically in younger patients, the mitral leaflets are elongated and flexible causing the tip of the anterior mitral leaflet to make localized septal contact, as illustrated in Figure 35.14. M-mode imaging can define the presence and duration of septal-leaflet contact (Fig. 35.14) and allowed development of a

grading system for SAM. Septal-leaflet contact for more than 30% of systole is considered severe SAM, lesser duration of contact is moderate, and if the leaflet is within 10 mm of the septum during systole without making contact, the SAM is graded as mild.[67] M-mode imaging can also detect systolic notching of the aortic valve (Fig. 35.15). This premature aortic valve closure occurs when LV outflow tract obstruction interrupts LV ejection.

There is a consensus that SAM of the mitral valve is the result of LV flow on the protruding mitral leaflet, however the precise mechanism is unclear. Initially, it was hypothesized that high velocity flow in the outflow tract created a local low-pressure region which lifts the mitral leaflet toward the septum (Venturi effect). More recent experimental and observational studies have found that the pushing force of flow (termed flow drag) is the dominant hemodynamic mechanism underlying SAM.[68] Blood flow is posteriorly and laterally reflected off the hypertrophied septum, generating a pressure gradient between the LV cavity and outflow tract which pushes the underside of the mitral leaflets toward the septum, creating a self-amplifying loop where longer durations of SAM-septal contact lead to further increases in the gradient.

Echocardiography plays a key role in characterizing the mechanism and quantifying the severity of obstruction. Careful evaluation is increasingly relevant and critical to management due to the variety of treatments now available to specifically target obstruction. The appropriate choice of therapy: medical and surgical myectomy or percutaneous alcohol septal ablation depends on accurate assessment of the specific morphologic and hemodynamic features present in each individual. For example, distinct from SAM, systolic cavity obliteration is also seen in HCM, owing to the small LV cavity, hypertrophied myocardium, and vigorous systolic function. Intraventricular pressure gradients can result which may respond to medical therapy, but invasive mechanical strategies (myectomy or alcohol ablation) designed to address obstruction related to SAM may not be appropriate.

Obstruction at rest occurs in approximately one third of the patients, but the propensity to develop obstruction is more common and may be missed without careful evaluation incorporating provocative maneuvers.[69] Obstruction can be provoked by increasing contractility and/or heart rate (exercise, postpremature ventricular contraction) or by altering the loading conditions of the heart through reducing either preload or afterload (standing, amyl nitrate or Valsalva maneuver), as illustrated in Figure 35.16. For the purposes of diagnosing latent obstruction, especially when

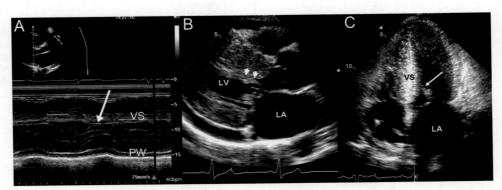

Figure 35.14 Systolic anterior motion (SAM) of the mitral valve. These still-frame images illustrate typical SAM which produces mechanical impedance to LV outflow and mitral regurgitation. **A:** M-mode representation of SAM: Arrows indicate anterior motion of the mitral valve and prolonged septal contact in midsystole. **B:** Parasternal long-axis view showing typical SAM in which the anterior mitral leaflet (*arrows*) bends acutely resulting in localized septal contact and obstruction to flow. **C:** Apical four-chamber view demonstrating the same acute-angled conformation of SAM. LV, left ventricle; LA, left atrium; VS, ventricular septum.

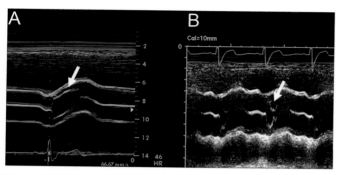

Figure 35.15 Premature closure of the aortic valve as a result of LV outflow tract obstruction. M-mode images of the base of the heart in a normal patient (**A**) and HCM (**B**). **A:** Normal: Wide separation of the aortic valve leaflets throughout systole (*arrow*). **B:** HCM: Midsystolic partial closure or notching of the aortic valve (*arrow*) secondary to LVOT obstruction interrupting ejection to the aorta.

4.4. Mitral valve anatomical and functional alterations

A number of anatomic and functional abnormalities of the mitral valve are seen in HCM and may be a manifestation of the underlying cardiomyopathy, related hemodynamic abnormalities, or may result from primary pathology unrelated to HCM such as rheumatic heart disease or myxomatous degeneration. Prominent developmental abnormalities of the mitral valve associated with HCM are increased leaflet area and abnormal origination and insertion of the papillary muscles.[70] The papillary muscle may insert directly into the anterior leaflet without intervening chordae tendinae in over 10% of patients with obstruction,[71] as seen in Figure 35.17. Echocardiographic features include exaggerated anterior displacement of the papillary muscles and decreased mobility of the mitral apparatus due to direct continuity of the anterolateral papillary muscle and anterior mitral leaflet. Recognition may require nontraditional transthoracic windows (slightly rotated parasternal long-axis view of the LV) but is critical for appropriate management. In patients undergoing myectomy, surgical approaches have been adapted for this setting and include creating a deeper myectomy trough and partial resection of papillary attachments to ensure adequate relief of obstruction postoperatively (Fig. 35.18).[72]

SAM of the mitral valve leads to diminished systolic coaptation of the mitral leaflets and creation of an "interleaflet gap" resulting in mitral regurgitation.[72] Because the leaflets, typically the anterior leaflets, are selectively pulled into the LVOT, the jet of mitral regurgitation due to SAM is characteristically eccentric and posteriorly directed, as illustrated in Figure 35.19A. The severity of the mitral regurgitation secondary to SAM is proportional to the severity of the outflow tract gradient.[73] Careful imaging is critical in guiding treatment decisions. If mitral regurgitation is *not* secondary to SAM, the management differs significantly and surgical treatment of primary mitral valve pathology may be required, whereas mitral regurgitation secondary to SAM resolves upon relieving obstruction and correcting the altered hemodynamics which lead to SAM; typically neither mitral valve repair nor

nonpharmacologic therapy is considered, exercise is the preferred method to quantify provokable and physiologically relevant obstruction. It is important to recognize that SAM of the mitral valve and dynamic LVOT obstruction may occur in patients without HCM. These abnormalities may occur in patients with small ventricular cavity size, such as elderly women, in the setting of acute hypovolemia, vasodilation, or increased inotropic state. Typical scenarios include induction of anesthesia after prolonged fasting, dobutamine stress testing, and postapical myocardial infarction.

Differentiation of the spectral Doppler signal of obstruction from that of mitral regurgitation requires careful attention to detail, and is complicated by the close anatomic proximity of these two phenomena. The spectral Doppler profile of obstruction typically has a "dagger appearance" that accelerates during mid to late systole, whereas MR begins at the onset of systole and has a smoother, more symmetric contour (Fig. 35.16). Moreover, MR typically generates a higher velocity signal that is usually in excess of 5 to 6 m/s.

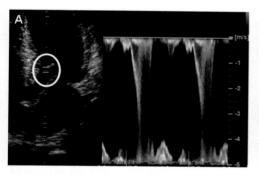
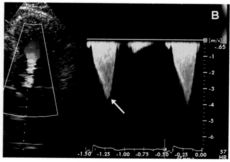
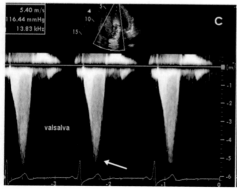
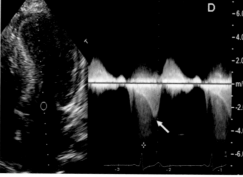

Figure 35.16 Spectral Doppler mapping of LV outflow tract gradient. **A:** Interrogation starts with pulse wave Doppler in the midLV cavity, advancing the sample volume (*circled*) to the outflow tract to identify the site of flow velocity acceleration; typically at the site of maximal SAM-septal contact. **B:** Continuous-wave Doppler identifies the peak instantaneous outflow gradient of 4.1 m/s (*arrow*), corresponding to a peak LVOT gradient of 68 mm Hg. **C:** With Valsalva maneuver the peak velocity (*arrow*) increases to 5.4 m/s (peak gradient 116 mm Hg). **D:** Distinguishing the Doppler signal from the LV outflow tract from the jet of mitral regurgitation (MR). The mitral regurgitant waveform has a more symmetric, parabolic shape and begins at the onset of systole with an abrupt increase in peak velocity (5.5 m/s; *asterisk*). The later-peaking, "dagger shaped," midsystolic signal from the LV outflow tract is embedded within the MR signal (3.1 m/s; *arrow*).

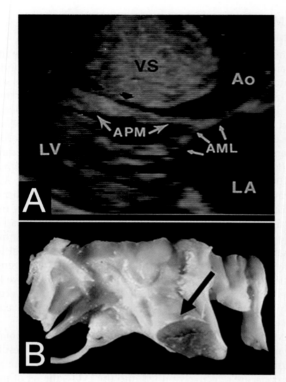

Figure 35.17 Abnormal mitral valve morphology is common in HCM. **A:** Parasternal long-axis image shows a hypertrophied APM which inserts directly into the AML. This produces midcavity obstruction (*arrowheads*) due to muscular apposition with the VS. **B:** Pathologic specimen: The excised mitral valve shows a massively hypertrophied and anomalous papillary muscle which inserts directly into the anterior mitral leaflet without the interposition of chordae tendineae (*arrow*). APM, anterolateral papillary muscle; AML, anterior mitral leaflet; VS, ventricular septum; LV, left ventricle; RV, right ventricle; Ao, aorta. (Images courtesy of Barry J. Maron, MD. Minneapolis Heart Institute Foundation, Minneapolis, MN.)

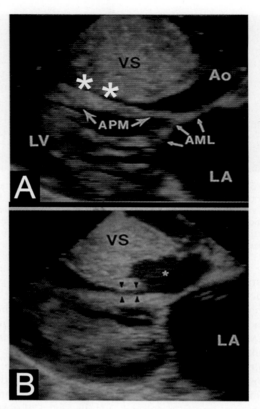

Figure 35.18 Anatomic variant of HCM amenable only to surgical myectomy. **A:** Preoperative echocardiogram: Parasternal long-axis image shows that the hypertrophied anterolateral papillary muscle (APM) inserts directly into the anterior mitral leaflet (AML) producing midcavity obstruction (*asterisks*) due to muscular apposition with the ventricular septum (VS). In the surgical treatment of obstruction, this anomalous papillary muscle must be addressed to fully attend to outflow obstruction. **B:** Postoperative echo: Parasternal long-axis image after standard surgical myectomy shows that the resection did not extend sufficiently distally or address the hypertrophied papillary muscle, allowing muscular obstruction due to anomalous papillary muscle to persist (*arrowheads*), despite enlargement of the proximal LV outflow tract (*asterisk*). LV, left ventricle; LA, left atrium; Ao, aorta; APM, anterolateral papillary muscle; AML, anterior mitral leaflet; VS, ventricular septum. (Images courtesy of Barry J. Maron, MD. Minneapolis Heart Institute Foundation, Minneapolis, MN.)

replacement is required. Intrinsic mitral valve disease should be excluded, including mitral valve prolapse, severe annular calcification, or valvular vegetations. It has been recognized that a significant proportion of patients with HCM and SAM have abnormally elongated posterior mitral valve leaflets and even overt prolapse. The direction of the regurgitant jet is a key component of the differentiation of primary mitral valve disease from MR secondary to SAM. Centrally or anteriorly directed MR strongly suggest that MR would not resolve with amelioration of obstruction and SAM (i.e., intrinsic mitral valve disease) (Fig. 35.19B&C). Moreover, patients with long standing SAM can develop traumatic fibrosis of the anterior mitral leaflet due to recurrent septal contact which can become a determinant of mitral regurgitation independent of obstruction severity.[48]

4.5. Myocardial perfusion and fibrosis

Myocardial ischemia is well described in HCM, contributes to symptoms of angina and dyspnea, and may play a role in the pathogenesis of heart failure, ventricular arrhythmia, and sudden death.[74] Ischemia in HCM is typically not the result of obstructive atherosclerotic plaque in the epicardial arteries, but rather a microvascular disease. Microvascular ischemia can be detected and quantified by single-photon computed tomography (SPECT), positron emission tomography (PET), and CMR as a blunted increase in myocardial flow after exercise (SPECT) or administration of a coronary vasodilator such as dipyridamole (PET,

SPECT, or CMR). Perfusion abnormalities can be identified both in symptomatic patients with invasive demonstration of ischemia as well as asymptomatic patients without other evidence of ischemia.[75] As such, SPECT and PET myocardial perfusion imaging can lead to the false impression of epicardial disease. Differentiation of microvascular abnormalities from epicardial stenosis may be facilitated by identifying nonanatomic perfusion abnormalities which do not follow typical coronary artery distribution. As shown in Figure 35.20, CMR may be more useful in this regard, given its superior spatial resolution.

The presence of myocardial perfusion abnormalities correlates with poor prognosis. A prospective, controlled study of 51 patients with HCM found that blunted vasodilator mediated flow, strongly predicted adverse events.[74] The hazard ratios of death from cardiovascular causes and a composite outcome of death, class III-IV HF or significant ventricular arrhythmia were 9.6 and 20.1, respectively, in patients in the tertile with the worst microvascular function ($p < 0.05$ for both comparisons). Ischemia-induced scarring and fibrosis have been the proposed mechanism by which microvascular ischemia is linked to adverse events.[74,75]

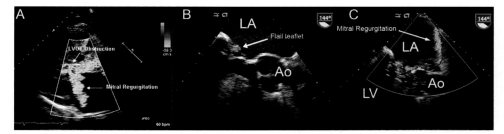

Figure 35.19 Characterizing abnormalities of mitral valve structure and function influence management decisions. Mitral regurgitation secondary to SAM and LVOTO can be expected to improve with amelioration of LVOTO, whereas MR secondary to intrinsic mitral valve disease requires definitive repair or replacement. **A:** Mitral regurgitation associated with SAM and LVOT obstruction is posteriorly directed (transthoracic echocardiography, parasternal long axis, midsystolic-still image). **B,C:** Transesophageal echocardiography of a patient with HCM demonstrates a partially flail segment of the posterior leaflet (**B**) which results in an anteriorly directed jet of mitral regurgitation (**C**) seen in these midesophageal, midsystolic still-frame images. LV, left ventricle; LA, left atrium; Ao, aorta.

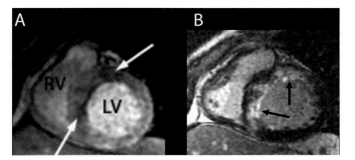

Figure 35.20 CMR can identify abnormal myocardial perfusion in HCM that is not typical of epicardial coronary disease. These basal short-axis images demonstrate a noncoronary distribution of abnormal first pass gadolinium perfusion and delayed enhancement, indicating impaired perfusion and fibrosis. The diffuse pattern of distribution does not correlate anatomically with epicardial coronary artery disease, but is more patchy and consistent with the underlying cardiomyopathic process. **A:** First pass perfusion images: Well-perfused myocardium enhances with gadolinium administration (*bright*) whereas the dark, poorly perfused segments do not (*arrows*). There is abnormal first pass perfusion with a subendocardial perfusion defect involving the basal and mid anterior, anteroseptal, and anterolateral segments. **B:** In the delayed images, bright gadolinium enhancement (*black arrows*) signifies myocardial scar tissue. There is extensive delayed hyperenhancement involving the basal to distal anterior wall and anterior septum and the RV aspect of the mid-to-distal inferior wall. This pattern is atypical of myocardial infarction and suggests scar or fibrosis of the LV myocardium unrelated to coronary artery disease. RV, right ventricle; LV, left ventricle. (Images courtesy of Shuaib Abdullah, MD, Brigham and Women's Hospital, Boston, MA.)

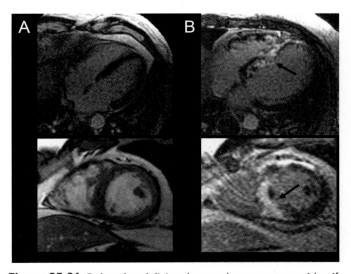

Figure 35.21 Delayed gadolinium hyperenhancement may identify areas of myocardial fibrosis. This patient with end-stage HCM underwent baseline and delayed T1-weighted MRI images, late gadolinium enhancement (*bright*) suggests underlying scar. Long-axis images are displayed above short-axis images. **A:** Baseline images demonstrate normal first pass perfusion. **B:** Imaging repeated 15 min after injection of gadolinium contrast demonstrates extensive delayed hyperenhancement throughout the septum. (Images courtesy of Raymond Kwong, MD, Brigham and Women's Hospital, Boston, MA.)

Interstitial fibrosis, identifiable by histologic examination (Fig. 35.2) affects the heart at several levels in HCM. There is a general increase in cardiac collagen content, which is more prominently present at sites of (presumed) prior ischemic injury (replacement fibrosis), myocyte disarray, and prominently in the region of RV insertion in the interventricular septum.[59] Interstitial fibrosis may be detected clinically by visualizing delayed gadolinium enhancement (DE) with CMR (Fig. 35.21).[59] Gadolinium is an extracellular tracer that has previously been validated to identify myocardial scar in patients suffering myocardial infarction[76] and with HCM.[77] It has been suggested that increased fibrosis may play a role in the pathogenesis of ventricular arrhythmias and sudden death, however direct studies are not yet available. Furthermore, the clinical relevance and functional consequences of DE remain incompletely characterized. Increased DE is commonly present in patients with end-stage HCM, a group with a recognized poor prognosis.[78,79]

Preliminary studies have found a modest correlation between the presence of DE and either sudden death risk factors[80] or ventricular ectopy.[81] However, the extent of DE has neither correlated with outcomes nor has it been found to be a significant predictor of adverse events.[79] DE at the site of septal RV insertion is relatively common and not associated with a profile of increased risk.[80] The accuracy and incremental value of including DE in sudden death prediction remains unknown and it is currently not included as a standard element of sudden death risk stratification.

5. CLINICAL FEATURES

In addition to diagnosing disease, screening family members, and characterizing pathophysiology and hemodynamic abnormalities, noninvasive cardiac imaging plays an important role in the management of HCM. Serial imaging studies are used in risk assessment for SCD, monitoring for complications of disease, determining treatment strategies, and assessing response to therapy.

5.1. Symptoms

As with other aspects of HCM, there is remarkable diversity in the severity of symptoms associated with disease.[2] Some individuals experience no or only minor symptoms, while others develop refractory symptoms or end-stage heart failure requiring cardiac transplantation. Exertional dyspnea is the most common symptom of HCM, occurring in up to 90% of patients. Other manifestations include chest pain, palpitations, atrial and ventricular arrhythmias, orthostatic lightheadedness, presyncope and syncope, volume overload, and fatigue.[82] The location or degree of LVH is not closely predictive of the severity of symptoms associated with HCM.[2]

5.2. Prognosis: Assessment of risk for sudden cardiac death

The risk for SCD is increased in HCM. This disorder is an important cause of sudden death in young people[83] and the leading cause of sudden death in competitive athletes, responsible for approximately a third of such cases.[84,85] Therefore, assessment of SCD risk and appropriate implementation of therapy are important, although challenging, components of clinical management. Predicting which patients are at increased risk of sudden death is imperfect and controversial. Currently employed clinical predictors of increased risk are summarized in Table 35.3 and include a family history of sudden death, unexplained syncope, hypotensive blood pressure response to exercise, nonsustained ventricular tachycardia on ambulatory Holter monitoring, and extreme LVH (wall thickness ≥30 mm by echocardiography). In this regard, cardiac imaging can assist in the identification of patients with extreme LVH who are at increased risk for SCD and may be eligible for implantable cardiovertor defibrillator (ICD) therapy for primary prevention of sudden death.[22,86] Importantly, the positive predictive accuracy for a wall thickness of ≥30 mm is <20%, suggesting that interpretation of this parameter must be in the context of a thorough clinical assessment. Making the decision to implant an ICD for primary prevention is, therefore, guided by the number and nature of predictors, as well as individualized clinical judgment and personal input from patients who have been well educated and informed. Patients who do not demonstrate any of the above risk factors are at low risk for SCD (<1% annual risk) and should have periodic re-evaluation of risk factors. Individuals who have survived cardiac arrest or sustained ventricular tachycardia are at high risk for recurrent events and should receive ICDs for secondary prevention.[87]

5.3. End-stage hypertrophic cardiomyopathy

Since the 1970s, it has been recognized that a small but important subset of patients with HCM will develop LV systolic dysfunction as their disease progresses.[88,89] Due to the heterogeneous pattern of cardiac remodeling associated with this phenotype, a variety of descriptive terms have been used in the literature, including end-stage HCM, burnt-out HCM, and dilated-hypokinetic evolution of HCM. End-stage HCM is most consistently characterized by the evolution from the typical hypertrophied, nondilated, and hyperdynamic state to one of systolic dysfunction (LV EF < 50%) as illustrated in Figure 35.22. Approximately 50% of patients also develop restrictive physiology, LV wall thinning, and LV cavity dilatation.[78] The etiology of this form of remodeling is not known, but when compared to classic HCM, patients with end-stage disease were more likely to have a family history of HCM, sudden death, or need for cardiac transplantation, suggesting that genetic factors may influence development.[78,90] Prevalence has been estimated at 3.5% to 4.9% with an incidence of 0.5 to 1.1 cases per 100 person-years,[77,90] and occurring 14 years after initial

TABLE 35.3

RISK PREDICTORS FOR SUDDEN DEATH IN HCM

	Criteria	Comments
History	Exertional or recurrent syncope	Risk is greatest in children
	Family history of sudden death or known malignant genotype	Risk is related to family size and number of affected family members with SCD
Diagnostic evaluation	Severe LVH (maximal wall thickness ≥30 mm)	Risk increases as wall thickness increases
	Nonsustained ventricular tachycardia (ambulatory Holter monitoring)	Higher predictive value in children and patients with history of syncope
	Abnormal hemodynamic response to exercise (failure to augment SBP by at least 20 mm Hg)	Less applicable to patients >40 years old

SCD, sudden cardiac death.

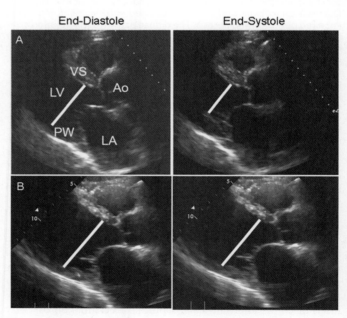

Figure 35.22 Development of end-stage HCM. These parasternal long-axis images at end-diastole (**left**) and end-systole (**right**) demonstrate the development of diminished LV ejection fraction, regression of LV hypertrophy, and LV cavity dilation associated with evolution to end-stage HCM. Baseline images (**A**) show mild LVH (septal thickness of 14 mm), normal LV cavity size (LV end-diastolic dimension of 5.2 cm, and LV end-systolic dimension of 3.5 cm), and normal LVEF of 55%. Five years later (**B**), there is LV wall thinning (septal thickness of 9 mm), LV enlargement (LV end-diastolic dimension of 6.2 cm, LV end-systolic dimension of 5.6 cm), and severely reduced LVEF of 18%. LV, left ventricle; LA, left atrium; Ao, aorta, PW, posterior wall; VS, ventricular septum.

diagnosis of HCM. End-stage HCM has been reported to develop at any age, but usually presents prior to the age of 40 and is relatively more common when HCM was diagnosed in childhood or adolescence.

Compared to patients with classic HCM, outcomes with end-stage HCM are less favorable.[91] Once features develops, average transplantation-free survival is short (2.7 years), moderate-to-severe heart failure is common (>75%), and arrhythmias (AF and VT) are substantially more common that in classic HCM.[78,90] The suggested medical therapy for end-stage HCM is the same regimen that is used in systolic heart failure; involving conversion to agents such as ACE inhibitors or angiotensin-II receptor blockers, diuretics, digitalis, β-blockers, and spironolactone.[2]

6. MANAGEMENT OF DISEASE

Comprehensive cardiac imaging is essential to determine appropriate treatment strategies and to monitor response to therapy. As described above, imaging can define altered hemodynamics, systolic and diastolic functions, obstructive physiology, and valvular dysfunction; factors which importantly contribute to the symptoms related to HCM and influence therapeutic approach. Serial imaging, typically echocardiography with Doppler interrogation, is a critical component of optimal medical therapy to guide the choice of therapy and assess response to treatment by assessing changes in obstructive physiology (as indicated by decrease in LVOT gradients/ velocity, decreased SAM and related mitral regurgitation) and improvement in diastolic function (as indicated by increased early diastolic filling, more rapid time to peak filling).

6.1. Medical management

The general goals of medical management are to mitigate symptoms by decreasing obstruction (if present), lowering heart rate to enhance diastolic filling time, and to reduce volume overload. First line agents are either β-adrenergic blockers (BB) or L-type calcium channel blockers (CCB, verapamil or diltiazem). Both of these classes of medication can decrease LV gradients and mitral regurgitation due to SAM, improve exercise tolerance, and increase NYHA functional class. Patients who remain symptomatic on recommended doses of CCB or BB may have further relief of symptoms with the addition of disopyramide, a class IA antiarrhythmic agent that is utilized in the management of HCM because its negative inotropic properties may decrease intracavitary obstruction. If volume overload is prominent, diuretic therapy may be judiciously used, recognizing that volume depletion may exacerbate obstructive physiology and compromise stroke volume. Symptomatic patients who do not exhibit obstructive physiology, even after careful assessment including provocative maneuvers, should be treated with standard medical therapy. Echocardiography may also be useful to evaluate changes in diastolic function following specific medical interventions.

Patients who remain significantly symptomatic secondary to severe outflow tract obstruction (NYHA Class III-IV, Gradient >50 mm Hg at rest or with exercise provocation) despite maximal medical therapy are candidates for nonpharmacologic approaches to relieve outflow tract obstruction: surgical myectomy or alcohol septal ablation. The role of imaging prior to either procedure is to identify the presence of sufficient obstruction, characterize key anatomic and functional features (e.g., site of maximal gradient and mechanism of obstruction), and to prospectively identify the presence of other abnormalities which would favor surgical therapy (e.g., intrinsic mitral valve disease or severe coronary artery disease).[92] Because exercise testing recapitulates the conditions in

which patients become symptomatic, it is the preferred method used to identify dynamic obstruction in patients with gradients < 30 mm Hg at rest. Alternate methods such as dobutamine infusion may provoke gradients that would not be present under normal physiological conditions and may dictate a management course which may not improve symptoms. The choice between these two options is dictated by the severity of concomitant medical comorbidities (favors septal ablation), need for non-HCM related surgery (coronary artery bypass, valve surgery) and well-informed patient preference.[93] A general approach to managing symptomatic patients with obstruction is summarized in Fig. 35.23.

6.2. Surgical myectomy

Surgical myectomy was first developed at the National Institutes of Health but the initial Morrow procedure has been refined and has been performed successfully in thousands of patients over several decades. In the current era, operative mortality in experienced centers is less than 1%,[93] symptomatic benefit is prompt and durable,[94] and need for permanent pacemaker is minimal. Beyond its obvious value in helping identify severe obstruction, preoperative echocardiography should identify unusual patterns of obstruction of mitral valve morphology that could influence the nature of the operative repair, concomitant RVOT obstruction and to delineate the thickness of the interventricular septum. Intraoperative transesophageal echocardiography (TEE) has assumed a central role in the guidance of surgical myectomy by localizing the site of obstruction and identifying the optimal location for the myectomy. Moreover, it can immediately identify residual obstruction or mitral regurgitation that requires reintervention.[95] Surgical myectomy relieves obstruction by debulking the septum (Fig. 35.24) and can, therefore, be expected to produce immediate improvement of gradients which are sustained with time. Moreover, long-term outcomes following myectomy are excellent with improvement of symptoms, exercise capacity, and overall prognosis, including survival, as compared to nonoperated patients with obstruction.[96]

6.3. Alcohol septal ablation

Alcohol septal ablation is the intentional and controlled creation of a septal myocardial infarction, demonstrated in Figure 35.25. Dehydrated (100%) ethanol is selectively injected into the septal perforator coronary artery which subtends the septal bulge and site of maximal SAM-septal contact. This results in transmural scar formation and thinning of the proximal septum as the ventricle remodels, thereby decreasing SAM, outflow tract obstruction, and related mitral regurgitation. While alcohol ablation has been shown to improve symptoms, exercise capacity, and oxygen consumption, long-term follow-up comparable to the surgical myectomy experience is not currently available. Furthermore, the impact of the resultant myocardial scar on SCD risk in HCM is currently unresolved. About 1% to 2% mortality rates have generally been reported with this procedure.[97] The most common complication is complete heart block requiring permanent pacemaker implantation, occurring at an incidence of ~5% to 30%. Because of the small risk of septal rupture, it is recommended that septal ablation be avoided in patients with septal thickness less than 15 mm.[97]

As with surgical myectomy, echocardiography plays a key role in the planning, performance, and postprocedural follow-up of alcohol septal ablation (Table 35.4). Before and during the procedure, echocardiographic guidance, including the use of contrast, plays an important role (Fig. 35.24). Imaging is used to verify

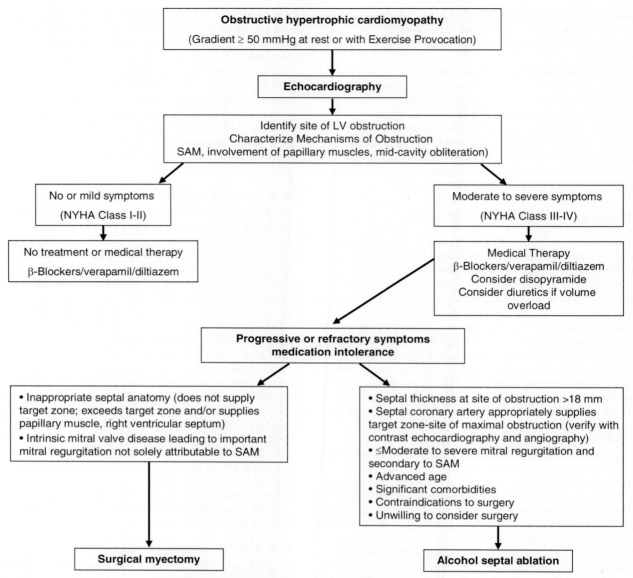

Figure 35.23 Algorithm for the diagnosis and treatment of obstructive HCM.

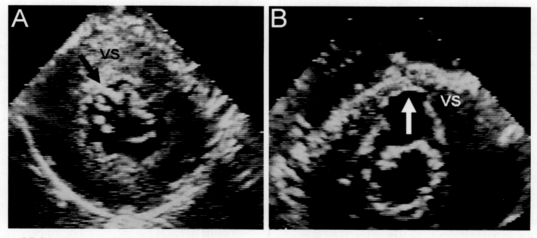

Figure 35.24 Surgical myectomy results in enlargement of the LVOT with resolution of SAM and LVOT obstruction. **A:** Preoperative parasternal short-axis view shows severe septal hypertrophy (VS) with systolic anterior motion of the anterior mitral leaflet (*black arrow*). **B:** Postmyectomy parasternal short-axis view shows a myectomy "notch" (*white arrow*) representing the portion of the upper septum that was resected. (Images courtesy of Maron BJ, MD. Minneapolis Heart Institute Foundation, Minneapolis, MN.)

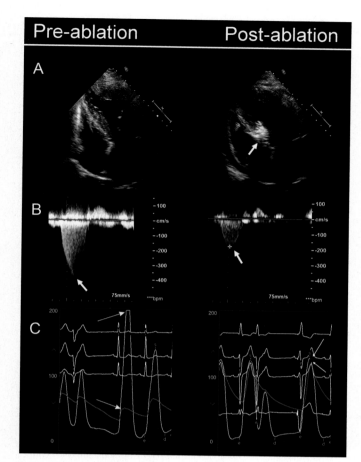

Pre-ablation Post-ablation

Figure 35.25 Alcohol septal ablation: Echocardiographic appearance and hemodynamic response. Preprocedure (**left**) and postprocedure (**right**) images from a patient who has undergone alcohol septal ablation. **A:** Apical four-chamber view demonstrates the echo-bright appearance of the basal septum (*arrow*) after alcohol ablation (alcohol depot). **B:** Spectral Doppler (CW) of the LVOT demonstrates a reduction in the estimated resting gradient from 64 mm Hg to 16 mm Hg (*arrows*). **C:** Invasive hemodynamic measurements confirm the reduction in outflow tract gradient. The post-PVC difference between the LV (*yellow*) and aortic (*magenta*) pressures (*arrows*) has decreased dramatically (160 mm Hg to 16 mm Hg). (Images courtesy of Pinak Shah, MD, Brigham and Women's Hospital, Boston, MA.)

TABLE 35.4

ECHOCARDIOGRAPHIC GUIDANCE FOR ALCOHOL SEPTAL ABLATION

Baseline	Intraprocedural	Postprocedural
• Measure gradient • Visualize and localize SAM-septal contact • Assess mitral valve pathology Identify suboptimal candidates for septal ablation: • Atypical location of obstruction • Primary mitral valve disease (MVP, central or anteriorly directed severe MR) • Septum <15 mm	Pre-EtOH ablation • Verify appropriate location with myocardial contrast injection • Site of maximal SAM-septal contact and flow acceleration • Avoidance of RV, papillary muscles, nonseptal LV Post-EtOH ablation • Verify location of EtOH depot • Identify proximal septal stunning • Reassess gradients	Predischarge and after 3 months • Repeat assessment of gradients • Check location and extent of septal thinning and wall motion involvement

RV, right ventricle; MR, mitral regurgitation.

7. FUTURE DIRECTIONS

Noninvasive cardiac imaging has provided key insights into natural history and has refined management of this diverse and complex disease. In the future, evolution of CMR technology will improve our ability to visualize and understand the clinical significance and functional consequences of prototypic histologic features of HCM—myocardial fibrosis and disarray. Integration of genetic testing with comprehensive imaging will allow better characterization of the early consequences of gene mutations, prior to the development of overt disease. This will facilitate the identification of surrogate outcomes to study disease pathogenesis and monitor response to novel treatment strategies, which target preclinical gene mutation carriers to prevent or modify disease development. Further advances in echocardiographic strain imaging and CMR will help to better define the mechanical perturbations of HCM through more sophisticated characterization of systolic and diastolic functions, looking not only at two-dimensional motion and deformation, but the more complex actions of rotation, torsion, and twist. In this ongoing manner, advances in imaging technology will continue to drive advances in our understanding of the pathogenesis and management of HCM.

that anatomy is appropriate for ablation, exclude the presence of important mitral regurgitation from primary (not related to SAM) mitral valve disease that would require surgical intervention, target the appropriate septal perforator branch for injection (the branch that perfuses the segment adjacent to maximal flow acceleration and the site of SAM-septal contact should be selected[98]), and reduce the likelihood of potential complications. Moreover, contrast echocardiography has been shown to improve procedural success, reduce procedural time and infarct size, and minimize the occurrence of heart block.[99] The echocardiographic features of a successful septal ablation include regional, septal hypokinesis and a reduction in the outflow tract gradient. Immediate reductions of 40 mm Hg can be expected, but in the acute setting a significant number of patients will have a substantial provokable gradient. Because remodeling of the infarcted segment will take days to weeks, the maximal procedural benefit is delayed during which there are further reductions in both the resting a provokable gradients.[100]

REFERENCES

1. Maron BJ, Casey SA, Hauser RG, et al. Clinical course of hypertrophic cardiomyopathy with survival to advanced age. *J Am Coll Cardiol.* 2003;42(5):882–888.
2. Maron BJ, McKenna WJ, Danielson GK, et al. American College of Cardiology/European Society of Cardiology Clinical Expert Consensus Document on Hypertrophic Cardiomyopathy: A report of the American College of Cardiology Foundation Task Force on Clinical Expert Consensus Documents and the European Society of Cardiology Committee for Practice Guidelines. *J Am Coll Cardiol.* 2003;42(9):1687–1713.

3. Maron BJ, Gardin JM, Flack JM, et al. Prevalence of hypertrophic cardiomyopathy in a general population of young adults: Echocardiographic analysis of 4111 subjects in the CARDIA Study. *Circulation*. 1995;92(4):785–789.

4. Maron BJ, Peterson EE, Maron MS, et al. Prevalence of hypertrophic cardiomyopathy in an outpatient population referred for echocardiographic study. *Am J Cardiol*. 1994;73(8):577–580.

5. Zou Y, Song L, Wang Z, et al. Prevalence of idiopathic hypertrophic cardiomyopathy in China: A population-based echocardiographic analysis of 8080 adults. *Am J Med*. 2004;116(1):14–18.

6. Teare D. Aasymmetrical hypertrophy of the heart in young adults. *Br Heart J*. 1958;20(1):1–8.

7. Davies MJ. The current status of myocardial disarray in hypertrophic cardiomyopathy. *Br Heart J*. 1984;51(4):361–363.

8. Geisterfer-Lowrance AA, Kass S, Tanigawa G, et al. A molecular basis for familial hypertrophic cardiomyopathy: A beta cardiac myosin heavy chain gene missense mutation. *Cell*. 1990;62(5):999–1006.

9. Jarcho JA, McKenna W, Pare JA, et al. Mapping a gene for familial hypertrophic cardiomyopathy to chromosome 14q1. *N Engl J Med*. 1989;321(20):1372–1378.

10. Keren A, Syrris P, McKenna WJ. Hypertrophic cardiomyopathy: The genetic determinants of clinical disease expression. *Nat Clin Pract Cardiovasc Med*. 2008;5(3):158–168.

11. Binder J, Ommen SR, Gersh BJ, et al. Echocardiography-guided genetic testing in hypertrophic cardiomyopathy: Septal morphological features predict the presence of myofilament mutations. *Mayo Clin Proc*. 2006;81(4):459–467.

12. Morita H, Rehm HL, Menesses A, et al. Shared genetic causes of cardiac hypertrophy in children and adults. *N Engl J Med*. 2008;358(18):1899–1908.

13. Richard P, Charron P, Carrier L, et al. For the EUROGENE Heart Failure Project. Hypertrophic cardiomyopathy: Distribution of disease genes, spectrum of mutations, and implications for a molecular diagnosis strategy. *Circulation*. 2003;107(17):2227–2232.

14. Watkins H, McKenna WJ, Thierfelder L, et al. Mutations in the genes for cardiac troponin T and {alpha}-tropomyosin in hypertrophic cardiomyopathy. *N Engl J Med*. 1995;332(16):1058–1065.

15. Niimura H, Bachinski LL, Sangwatanaroj S, et al. Mutations in the gene for cardiac myosin-binding protein C and late-onset familial hypertrophic cardiomyopathy. *N Engl J Med*. 1998;338(18):1248–1257.

16. Ackerman MJ, Van Driest SL, Bos M. Are longitudinal, natural history studies the next step in genotype-phenotype translational genomics in hypertrophic cardiomyopathy? *J Am Coll Cardiol*. 2005;46(9):1744–1746.

17. Kubo T, Kitaoka H, Okawa M, et al. Lifelong left ventricular remodeling of hypertrophic cardiomyopathy caused by a funder frameshift deletion mutation in the cardiac myosin-binding protein C gene among Japanese. *J Am Coll Cardiol*. 2005;46(9):1737–1743.

18. Van Driest SL, Vasile VC, Ommen SR, et al. Myosin binding protein C mutations and compound heterozygosity in hypertrophic cardiomyopathy. *J Am Coll Cardiol*. 2004;44(9):1903–1910.

19. Olivotto I, Maron MS, Autore C, et al. Assessment and significance of left ventricular mass by cardiovascular magnetic resonance in hypertrophic cardiomyopathy. *J Am Coll Cardiol*. 2008;52(7):559–566.

20. Romano R, Losi MA, Migliore T, et al. Evaluation of the left ventricular anatomy in hypertrophic cardiomyopathy: Comparison between echocardiography and cardiac magnetic resonance imaging. *Minerva Cardioangiol*. 2008;56(2):181–187.

21. Rickers C, Wilke NM, Jerosch-Herold M, et al. Utility of cardiac magnetic resonance imaging in the diagnosis of hypertrophic cardiomyopathy. *Circulation*. 2005;112(6):855–861.

22. Spirito P, Bellone P, Harris KM, et al. Magnitude of left ventricular hypertrophy and risk of sudden death in hypertrophic cardiomyopathy. *N Engl J Med*. 2000;342(24):1778–1785.

23. Elliott PM, Gimeno Blanes JR, Mahon NG, et al. Relation between severity of left-ventricular hypertrophy and prognosis in patients with hypertrophic cardiomyopathy. *The Lancet*. 2001;357(9254):420–424.

24. Colan SD, Lipshultz SE, Lowe AM, et al. Epidemiology and cause-specific outcome of hypertrophic cardiomyopathy in children: Findings from the pediatric cardiomyopathy registry. *Circulation*. 2007;115(6):773–781.

25. McKenna WJ, Spirito P, Desnos M, et al. Experience from clinical genetics in hypertrophic cardiomyopathy: Proposal for new diagnostic criteria in adult members of affected families. *Heart*. 1997;77(2):130–132.

26. Hiroaki K, Yoshinori D, Susan AC, et al. Comparison of prevalence of apical hypertrophic cardiomyopathy in Japan and the United States. *Am J Cardiol*. 2003;92(10):1183–1186.

27. Eriksson MJ, Sonnenberg B, Woo A, et al. Long-term outcome in patients with apical hypertrophic cardiomyopathy. *J Am Coll Cardiol*. 2002;39(4):638–645.

28. Refaat M. Prognosis of apical hypertrophic cardiomyopathy. *JAMA*. 2007;298(17):2006–.

29. Abinader EG. Long-term outcome in patients with apical hypertrophic cardiomyopathy. *J Am Coll Cardiol*. 2002;40(4):837–838.

30. Moon JCC, Fisher NG, McKenna WJ, et al. Detection of apical hypertrophic cardiomyopathy by cardiovascular magnetic resonance in patients with nondiagnostic echocardiography. *Heart*. 2004;90(6):645–649.

31. Spirito P, Autore C. Apical hypertrophic cardiomyopathy or left ventricular noncompaction? A difficult differential diagnosis. *Eur Heart J*. 2007;28(16):1923–1924.

32. Maron MS, Finley JJ, Bos JM, et al. Prevalence, clinical significance, and natural history of left ventricular apical aneurysms in hypertrophic cardiomyopathy. *Circulation*. 2008;118(15):1541–1549.

33. Maron BJ, Seidman JG, Seidman CE. Proposal for contemporary screening strategies in families with hypertrophic cardiomyopathy. *J Am Coll Cardiol*. 2004;44(11):2125–2132.

34. Ho CY, Seidman CE. A contemporary approach to hypertrophic cardiomyopathy. *Circulation*. 2006;113(24):e858–e862.

35. Maron BJ. Distinguishing hypertrophic cardiomyopathy from athlete's heart: A clinical problem of increasing magnitude and significance. *Heart*. 2005;91(11):1380–1382.

36. Cardim N, Oliveira AG, Longo S, et al. Doppler tissue imaging: Regional myocardial function in hypertrophic cardiomyopathy and in athlete's heart. *J Am Soc Echocardiogr*. 2003;16(3):223–232.

37. Arad M, Maron BJ, Gorham JM, et al. Glycogen storage diseases presenting as hypertrophic cardiomyopathy. *N Engl J Med*. 2005;352(4):362–372.

38. von Scheidt W, Eng CM, Fitzmaurice TF, et al. An atypical variant of Fabry's disease with manifestations confined to the myocardium. *N Engl J Med*. 1991;324(6):395–399.

39. Linhart A, Elliott PM. The heart in Anderson-Fabry disease and other lysosomal storage disorders. *Heart*. 2007;93(4):528–535.

40. Chimenti C, Pieroni M, Morgante E, et al. Prevalence of Fabry disease in female patients With late-onset hypertrophic cardiomyopathy. *Circulation*. 2004;110(9):1047–1053.

41. Falk RH. Diagnosis and management of the cardiac amyloidoses. *Circulation*. 2005;112(13):2047–2060.

42. Sachdev B, Takenaka T, Teraguchi H, et al. Prevalence of Anderson-Fabry disease in male patients with late onset hypertrophic cardiomyopathy. *Circulation*. 2002;105(12):1407–1411.

43. Gahl WA. New therapies for Fabry's disease. *N Engl J Med*. 2001;345(1):55–57.

44. De Cobelli F, Esposito A, Belloni E, et al. Delayed–enhanced cardiac MRI for differentiation of Fabry's disease from symmetric hypertropic cardiomyopathy. *Am J. Roentgenol*. 2009;192:W97–102.

45. Stewart S, Mason DT, Braunwald E. Impaired rate of left ventricular filling in idiopathic hypertrophic subaortic stenosis and valvular aortic stenosis. *Circulation*. 1968;37(1):8–14.

46. Maron BJ, Spirito P, Green KJ, et al. Noninvasive assessment of left ventricular diastolic function by pulsed Doppler echocardiography in patients with hypertrophic cardiomyopathy. *J Am Coll Cardiol*. 1987;10(4):733–742.

47. Stewart RA, McKenna WJ. Assessment of diastolic filling indexes obtained by radionuclide ventriculography. *Am J Cardiol*. 1990;65(3):226–230.

48. Wigle ED, Sasson Z, Henderson MA, et al. Hypertrophic cardiomyopathy. The importance of the site and the extent of hypertrophy. A review. *Prog Cardiovasc Dis*. 1985;28(1):1–83.

49. Ommen SR, Nishimura RA, Appleton CP, et al. Clinical utility of Doppler echocardiography and tissue Doppler imaging in the estimation of left ventricular filling pressures: A comparative simultaneous Doppler-catheterization study. *Circulation*. 2000;102(15):1788–1794.

50. Nihoyannopoulos P, Karatasakis G, Frenneaux M, et al. Diastolic function in hypertrophic cardiomyopathy: Relation to exercise capacity. *J Am Coll Cardiol*. 1992;19(3):536–540.

51. Nishimura RA, Appleton CP, Redfield MM, et al. Noninvasive doppler echocardiographic evaluation of left ventricular filling pressures in patients with cardiomyopathies: A simultaneous Doppler echocardiographic and cardiac catheterization study. *J Am Coll Cardiol*. 1996;28(5):1226–1233.

52. Briguori C, Betocchi S, Losi MA, et al. Noninvasive evaluation of left ventricular diastolic function in hypertrophic cardiomyopathy. *Am J Cardiol*. 1998;81(2):180–187.

53. Spirito P, Maron BJ. Relation between extent of left ventricular hypertrophy and diastolic filling abnormalities in hypertrophic cardiomyopathy. *J Am Coll Cardiol*. 1990;15(4):808–813.

54. Nagueh SF, Lakkis NM, Middleton KJ, et al. Changes in left ventricular diastolic function 6 months after nonsurgical septal reduction therapy for hypertrophic obstructive cardiomyopathy. *Circulation*. 1999;99(3):344–347.

55. Menon SC, Ackerman MJ, Ommen SR, et al. Impact of septal myectomy on left atrial volume and left ventricular diastolic filling patterns: An echocardiographic study of young patients with obstructive hypertrophic cardiomyopathy. *J Am Soc Echocardiogr*. 2008;21(6):684–688.

56. Nagueh SF, Lakkis NM, Middleton KJ, et al. Doppler estimation of left ventricular filling pressures in patients with hypertrophic cardiomyopathy. *Circulation*. 1999;99(2):254–261.

57. Geske JB, Sorajja P, Nishimura RA, et al. Evaluation of left ventricular filling pressures by Doppler echocardiography in patients with hypertrophic cardiomyopathy: Correlation with direct left atrial pressure measurement at cardiac catheterization. *Circulation*. 2007;116(23):2702–2708.

58. Geisterfer-Lowrance AA, Christe M, Conner DA, et al. A mouse model of familial hypertrophic cardiomyopathy. *Science*. 1996;272(5262):731–734.

59. Georgakopoulos D, Christe ME, Giewat M, et al. The pathogenesis of familial hypertrophic cardiomyopathy: Early and evolving effects from an alpha-cardiac myosin heavy chain missense mutation. *Nat Med*. 1999;5(3):327–330.

60. Ho CY, Sweitzer NK, McDonough B, et al. Assessment of diastolic function with Doppler tissue imaging to predict genotype in preclinical hypertrophic cardiomyopathy. *Circulation*. 2002;105(2):2992–2997.

61. Nagueh SF, Bachinski LL, Meyer D, et al. Tissue Doppler imaging consistently detects myocardial abnormalities in patients with hypertrophic cardiomyopathy and provides a novel means for an early diagnosis before and independently of hypertrophy. *Circulation*. 2001;104(2):128–130.

62. Nagueh SF, McFalls J, Meyer D, et al. Tissue Doppler imaging predicts the development of hypertrophic cardiomyopathy in subjects with subclinical disease. *Circulation*. 2003;108(4):395–398.

63. Vinereanu D, Khokhar A, Fraser AG. Reproducibility of pulsed wave tissue Doppler echocardiography. *J Am Soc Echocardiogr.* 1999;12(6):492–499.
64. Kato TS, Izawa H, Komamura K, et al. Heterogeneity of regional systolic function detected by tissue Doppler imaging is linked to impaired global left ventricular relaxation in hypertrophic cardiomyopathy. *Heart.* 2008;94(10):1302–1306.
65. Yang H, Sun JP, Lever HM, et al. Use of strain imaging in detecting segmental dysfunction in patients with hypertrophic cardiomyopathy. *J Am Soc Echocardiogr.* 2003;16(3):233–239.
66. Maron MS, Olivotto I, Betocchi S, et al. Effect of left ventricular outflow tract obstruction on clinical outcome in hypertrophic cardiomyopathy. *N Engl J Med.* 2003;348(4):295–303.
67. Gilbert BW, Pollick C, Adelman AG, et al. Hypertrophic cardiomyopathy: Subclassification by M mode echocardiography. *Am J Cardiol.* 1980;45(4):861–872.
68. Sherrid MV, Gunsburg DZ, Moldenhauer S, et al. Systolic anterior motion begins at low left ventricular outflow tract velocity in obstructive hypertrophic cardiomyopathy. *J Am Coll Cardiol.* 2000;36(4):1344–1354.
69. Maron MS, Olivotto I, Zenovich AG, et al. Hypertrophic cardiomyopathy is predominantly a disease of left ventricular outflow tract obstruction. *Circulation.* 2006;114(21):2232–2239.
70. Klues HG, Maron BJ, Dollar AL, et al. Diversity of structural mitral valve alterations in hypertrophic cardiomyopathy. *Circulation.* 1992;85(5):1651–1660.
71. Klues HG, Roberts WC, Maron BJ. Anomalous insertion of papillary muscle directly into anterior mitral leaflet in hypertrophic cardiomyopathy. Significance in producing left ventricular outflow obstruction. *Circulation.* 1991;84(3):1188–1197.
72. Maron BJ, Nishimura RA, Danielson GK. Pitfalls in clinical recognition and a novel operative approach for hypertrophic cardiomyopathy with severe outflow obstruction due to anomalous papillary muscle. *Circulation.* 1998;98(23):2505–2508.
73. Yu EHC, Omran AS, Wigle ED, et al. Mitral regurgitation in hypertrophic obstructive cardiomyopathy: Relationship to obstruction and relief with myectomy. *J Am Coll Cardiol.* 2000;36(7):2219–2225.
74. Cecchi F, Olivotto I, Gistri R, et al. Coronary microvascular dysfunction and prognosis in hypertrophic cardiomyopathy. *N Engl J Med.* 2003;349(11):1027–1035.
75. Cannon RO III, Dilsizian V, O'Gara PT, et al. Myocardial metabolic, hemodynamic, and electrocardiographic significance of reversible thallium-201 abnormalities in hypertrophic cardiomyopathy. *Circulation.* 1991;83(5):1660–1667.
76. Kim RJ, Wu E, Rafael A, et al. The use of contrast-enhanced magnetic resonance imaging to identify reversible myocardial dysfunction. *N Engl J Med.* 2000;343(20):1445–1453.
77. Moon JC, Reed E, Sheppard MN, et al. The histologic basis of late gadolinium enhancement cardiovascular magnetic resonance in hypertrophic cardiomyopathy. *J Am Coll Cardiol.* 2004;43(12):2260–2264.
78. Harris KM, Spirito P, Maron MS, et al. Prevalence, clinical profile, and significance of left ventricular remodeling in the end-stage phase of hypertrophic cardiomyopathy. *Circulation.* 2006;114(3):216–225.
79. Maron MS, Appelbaum E, Harrigan CJ, et al. Clinical profile and significance of delayed enhancement in hypertrophic cardiomyopathy. *Circ Heart Fail.* 2008;1(3):184–191.
80. Moon JC, McKenna WJ, McCrohon JA, et al. Toward clinical risk assessment in hypertrophic cardiomyopathy with gadolinium cardiovascular magnetic resonance. *J Am Coll Cardiol.* 2003;41(9):1561–1567.
81. Nazarian S, Lima JA. Cardiovascular magnetic resonance for risk stratification of arrhythmia in hypertrophic cardiomyopathy. *J Am Coll Cardiol.* 2008;51(14):1375–1376.
82. Nishimura RA, Holmes DR Jr. Clinical practice. Hypertrophic obstructive cardiomyopathy. *N Engl J Med.* 2004;350(13):1320–1327.
83. Spirito P, Autore C. Management of hypertrophic cardiomyopathy. *BMJ.* 2006;332(7552):1251–1255.
84. Maron BJ, Shirani J, Poliac LC, et al. Sudden death in young competitive athletes. Clinical, demographic, and pathological profiles. *JAMA.* 1996;276(3):199–204.
85. Drezner JA, Khan K. Sudden cardiac death in young athletes. *BMJ.* 2008;337:a309.
86. McKenna WJ, Behr ER. Hypertrophic cardiomyopathy: Management, risk stratification, and prevention of sudden death. *Heart.* 2002;87(2):169–176.
87. Zipes DP, Camm AJ, Borggrefe M, et al. ACC/AHA/ESC 2006 Guidelines for Management of Patients With Ventricular Arrhythmias and the Prevention of Sudden Cardiac Death: a report of the American College of Cardiology/American Heart Association Task Force and the European Society of Cardiology Committee for Practice Guidelines (writing committee to develop Guidelines for Management of Patients With Ventricular Arrhythmias and the Prevention of Sudden Cardiac Death): Developed in collaboration with the European Heart Rhythm Association and the Heart Rhythm Society. *Circulation.* 2006;114(10):e385–e484.
88. ten Cate FJ, Roelandt J. Progression to left ventricular dilatation in patients with hypertrophic obstructive cardiomyopathy. *Am Heart J.* 1979;97(6):762–765.
89. Spirito P, Maron BJ, Bonow RO, et al. Occurrence and significance of progressive left ventricular wall thinning and relative cavity dilatation in hypertrophic cardiomyopathy. *Am J Cardiol.* 1987;60(1):123–129.
90. Biagini E, Coccolo F, Ferlito M, et al. Dilated-Hypokinetic evolution of hypertrophic cardiomyopathy: Prevalence, incidence, risk factors, and prognostic implications in pediatric and adult patients. *J Am Coll Cardiol.* 2005;46(8):1543–1550.
91. Shirani J, Maron BJ, Cannon RO, et al. Clinicopathologic features of hypertrophic cardiomyopathy managed by cardiac transplantation. *Am J Cardiol.* 1993;72(5):434–440.
92. Nagueh SF, Mahmarian JJ. Noninvasive Cardiac imaging in patients with hypertrophic cardiomyopathy. *J Am Coll Cardiol.* 2006;48(12):2410–2422.
93. Maron BJ. Surgical myectomy remains the primary treatment option for severely symptomatic patients with obstructive hypertrophic cardiomyopathy. *Circulation.* 2007;116(2):196–206.
94. Woo A, Williams WG, Choi R, et al. Clinical and echocardiographic determinants of long-term survival after surgical myectomy in obstructive hypertrophic cardiomyopathy. *Circulation.* 2005;111(16):2033–2041.
95. Ommen SR, Park SH, Click RL, et al. Impact of intraoperative transesophageal echocardiography in the surgical management of hypertrophic cardiomyopathy. *Am J Cardiol.* 2002;90(9):1022–1024.
96. Ommen SR, Maron BJ, Olivotto I, et al. Long-term effects of surgical septal myectomy on survival in patients with obstructive hypertrophic cardiomyopathy. *J Am Coll Cardiol.* 2005;46(3):470–476.
97. Fifer MA. Most fully informed patients choose septal ablation over septal myectomy. *Circulation.* 2007;116(2):207–216.
98. Lakkis NM, Nagueh SF, Kleiman NS, et al. Echocardiography-guided ethanol septal reduction for hypertrophic obstructive cardiomyopathy. *Circulation.* 1998;98(17):1750–1755.
99. Faber L, Seggewiss H, Gleichmann U. Percutaneous transluminal septal myocardial ablation in hypertrophic obstructive cardiomyopathy: Results with respect to intraprocedural myocardial contrast echocardiography. *Circulation.* 1998;98(22):2415–2421.
100. Faber L, Seggewiss H, Gietzen FH, et al. Catheter-based septal ablation for symptomatic hypertrophic obstructive cardiomyopathy: Follow-up results of the TASH-registry of the German Cardiac Society. *Z Kardiol.* 2005;94(8):516–523.

Acute and Chronic Pericardial Disease

36

Craig R. Asher
Gian M. Novaro
Jacobo Kirsch

1. INTRODUCTION

Diseases of the pericardium encompass a broad spectrum of acute and chronic conditions that are encountered by physicians in multiple specialties and clinical settings. Generations ago, prior to the advent of multimodality imaging and invasive cardiac hemodynamics, these disorders where astutely recognized by physicians based on pathognomonic physical examination findings. Contemporary evaluation of pericardial disease is largely reliant on echocardiography, cardiac computed tomography (CT), and magnetic resonance imaging (MRI). These tests are widely available and can be performed safely, rapidly, and repeatedly to make diagnoses and guide therapy. Most anatomic and hemodynamic features of pericardial disease can be assessed noninvasively. Recognizing the utility and limitations of each of the available technologies to assess pericardial disease is essential to cardiologists, radiologists, emergency room and critical care physicians.

This chapter will review the structure and function of the pericardium, the presentation, etiology, pathophysiology, diagnosis, and management of both uncommon and common pericardial disorders, focusing on the role of noninvasive cardiac imaging.

2. PATHOPHYSIOLOGY

2.1. Pericardial structure

The pericardium is a fibroserous sac located in the middle mediastinum posterior to the sternum and costal cartilages and anterior to the vertebrae. The sac encases the heart and the proximal portion of the great vessels and pulmonary veins (Fig. 36.1). The pericardium has ligamentous attachments to the sternum, vertebral bodies, pleura, and the central tendon of the diaphragm.

The pericardium has two layers: an external fibrous layer and an internal serous layer (further separated into inner visceral and outer parietal layers). The inner portion of the serous layer (visceral pericardium or epicardium) is invaginated by the heart and is contiguous with the outer portion of the serous layer (parietal pericardium), creating a potential space. The serous layer contains mesothelial cells with microvilli for fluid secretion, and the fibrous layer is composed of collagen and elastin fibers that are responsible for the elasticity of the pericardium.[1,2] There are three major regions of the heart called sinuses that are not covered by parietal pericardium. The transverse sinus is posterior to the proximal ascending aorta and main pulmonary artery between the left atrium, pulmonary veins, and superior vena cava (SVC); the oblique sinus is posterior between the left atrium and

pulmonary veins, and the superior sinus is at the level of the tracheal bifurcation in the region of the ascending aorta.[3]

The pericardial thickness is normally <4 mm consisting primarily of the parietal pericardium. Between both pericardial layers and in the pericardial sinuses, there is a small amount of pericardial fluid that is normally <40 mL of transudative fluid. The left internal mammary artery and other intrathoracic arteries provide blood supply to the pericardium. The phrenic nerve provides the primary innervation, and venous drainage occurs through the azygous veins. Pericardial fluid is drained through the lymphatic system of the thorax ending in the thoracic duct or pleural space.

2.2. Pericardial function

The pericardium is a dynamic structure that has multiple physiologic and protective roles including (i) preventing excessive motion and providing lubrication of the heart during movement; (ii) inhibiting acute distension of the heart; (iii) contributing to "diastolic coupling" or even filling of the cardiac chambers; (iv) preventing the spread of infection, malignancy, inflammation or hematoma between surrounding organs and the heart; (v) producing substances within pericardial fluid including prostaglandins that aid in regulation of sympathetic and coronary tone and cardiac contractility; (vi) providing afferent and efferent cardiac feedback regulation responsive to neuroreceptors, chemoreceptors, and mechanoreceptors; (vii) directing lymphatic fluid for drainage.[4]

The pericardium is a tense, elastic membrane that regulates cardiac filling based on an exponential stress–strain relationship (Fig. 36.2). There is little effect of the pericardium on cardiac filling under normal conditions (flat portion of the curve). But, with an acute increase in intracardiac volume, the pericardial pressure rises rapidly, thus restricting acute distension (exponential portion of the curve).[5]

In the normal state in the right heart, a negative intrathoracic pressure with inspiration is transmitted directly to reduce intrapericardial pressure, thus creating a transmural myocardial filling pressure. A normal pericardial pressure is near (−) 5 mm Hg (with inspiration) that, given a right ventricular diastolic pressure of 5 mm Hg, would result in a 10 mm Hg transmural myocardial pressure to promote right ventricular filling.[4,6] In the normal state in the left heart, a similar negative intrathoracic pressure during inspiration results in increased pulmonary compliance and therefore, a decreased filling gradient between the pulmonary veins and left ventricle. Hence, with inspiration, right heart filling is greater than left heart filling and reciprocal changes occur with expiration. When intrathoracic pressure is dissociated from

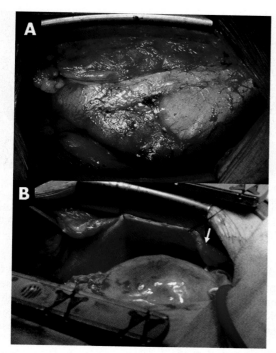

Figure 36.1 Anatomic picture of pericardium. **A:** Surgical view of the heart with a closed pericardium. The head is to the left and feet toward the right. **B:** Surgical view after the pericardium has been opened. The arrow points to the pericardium.

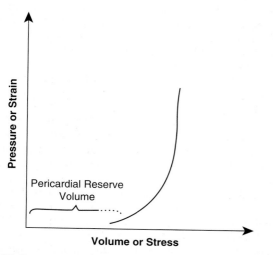

Figure 36.2 Stress–strain relationship. After the relatively small pericardial reserve volume is exhausted by filling of the pericardial sinuses and recesses, the curve at first rises gently; with continued filling at some point more acutely, the time scale and exact proportions are variable depending on the rate of filling of the intact pericardial sac. (From Spodick DH, *The Pericardium: A Comprehensive Textbook.* Ed. Marcel Dekker Inc., Figure 3.1, Schema of stress–strain and pressure–volume curves of the normal pericardium, with permission.)

intrapericardial or intracardiac pressure (e.g., constrictive pericarditis), see Figure 36.3, or when intrapericardial pressure is greater or equal to intracardiac pressure (e.g., cardiac tamponade) the normal physiologic state is markedly exaggerated resulting in interventricular dependence. Cardiac volume is fixed, and any filling of one side of the heart results in a reciprocal decrease in filling of the other side due to ventricular septal shift.

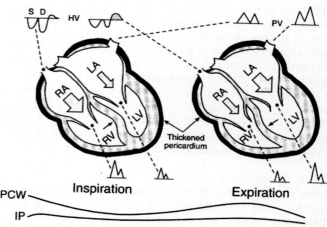

Figure 36.3 Physiology of interventricular dependence. Diagram of the heart with a thickened pericardium to illustrate the respiratory variation in ventricular filling and the corresponding Doppler features of the mitral valve, tricuspid valve, pulmonary vein (PV), and hepatic vein (HV). These changes are related to discordant pressure changes in the vessels in the thorax such as the pulmonary capillary wedge pressure (PCW) and intrapericardial (IP) and intracardiac pressures. Hatched area under curve indicates the reversal of flow. *Thicker arrows* indicate greater filling. D, diastolic flow; S, systolic flow; LA, left atrium; LV, left ventricle; RA, right atrium; RV, right ventricle. (From Oh JK. *The Echo Manual*, Chapter 14. Lippincott Williams & Wilkins, with permission.)

3. DIAGNOSTIC IMAGING

The role of an imaging test is to demonstrate the anatomical characteristics and to assess the hemodynamic alterations that characterize different diseases of the pericardium, serving as a guide to specific therapeutic interventions.

3.1. Congenital absence of the pericardium

This is a rare condition characterized as either partial or complete absence of the pericardium. An iatrogenic form of absence of the pericardium is created in patients who have complete pericardial stripping due to chronic pericarditis or constrictive pericarditis.

Although mostly recognized incidentally during cardiac or thoracic imaging or direct surgical inspection and autopsy, symptomatic presentation may occur. Characteristic findings suggestive of congenital absence of the pericardium include laterally displaced and migratory apical pulsations on examination, and sharp, stabbing, nonexertional chest pains, most often positional and worsened lying on the left side.[7,8] A study of a series of 10 patients from Toronto found that 70% of patients were female with a mean age of 21 years, while other studies have identified predominantly males.[8] Associated congenital cardiac defects include atrial and ventricular septal defects, bicuspid aortic valves, Tetralogy of Fallot, and patent ductus arteriosus.[7] Pleural and musculoskeletal defects may also be present, including pectus excavatum. On electrocardiography, a late transition point in the precordial leads, right axis deviation, right bundle branch block, bradycardia, and peaked precordial P waves may be seen.[9]

Most congenital absence of the pericardium is partial, usually involving the left side of the heart along the base of the heart with inferior left-sided and isolated right-sided defects less common.[3]

Herniation or compression of a cardiac segment or chamber usually involves the left atrial appendage or left atrium, though right-sided chambers, great vessels, and coronary arteries may be involved. Rarely, this has been described as the cause of arrhythmias or sudden cardiac death due to strangulation of the coronary vessels. Patients with complete absence of the pericardium are usually asymptomatic and may present during the workup of right ventricular dilation or tricuspid regurgitation.[10]

The embryologic basis for this congenital anomaly is related to failure of growth or fusion of the pleural–pericardial membrane during early development.[11] The absent pericardial segments include the fibrous and the parietal portion of the serous pericardium and not the visceral pericardium.

3.1.1. Chest X-ray

When the pericardial absence is complete, the right ventricle appears shifted to the left chest, in a position horizontal to the chest wall. Despite this shift in cardiac position, the trachea remains midline suggesting the absence of a contralateral hyperexpanded hemithorax (such as in tension pneumothorax) or compressive mass, as well as no ipsilateral volume loss (i.e., atelectasis or postsurgical change). The obscuration of the right cardiac contour as it superimposes over the thoracic spine becomes easier to detect. A characteristic appearance of lung tissue interposed between the aorta and main pulmonary artery has been described as a diagnostic feature for congenital absence of the pericardium. Partial absence of the pericardium is less evident on chest X-ray, with only a nonspecific bulge in the expected location of the main pulmonary artery or left atrial appendage.[12]

3.1.2. Echocardiography

Complete or significant regions of partial absence of the pericardium allows for excessive motion of the heart, abnormal septal motion in systole and diastole, and an abnormal twisting appearance.[13] The right ventricle, which is a volume-adapted chamber, has increased compliance without the restraint of the pericardium and therefore appears enlarged by conventional imaging views with a shift of the left ventricle laterally in the thorax.[14] Many patients are detected with an echocardiographic appearance of right ventricular dilation of unknown etiology. Severe tricuspid regurgitation may occur due to enhanced distensibility in the right ventricle. A bulging motion of the inferior wall has been described that occurs in diastole, distinguishing it from a ventricular aneurysm.[15]

3.1.3. Cardiac computed tomography and magnetic resonance imaging

These modalities best diagnose absence of the pericardium and can distinguish partial and complete defects. Detection of a pericardial defect relies on the absence of visualization of the fibrous layer of the pericardium and associated epicardial fat.[11,16–18] Other findings on cross-sectional imaging include the presence of lung tissue interposed between the aorta and pulmonary artery, and less commonly between the inferior wall of the heart and diaphragm (this appearance is impossible with an intact pericardium) (Fig. 36.4). An alteration in the main axis of the pulmonary artery may also be seen.[19,20]

3.1.4. Management

Follow-up is indicated even in asymptomatic patients with partial defects, since the size of the defect may change and herniation may be anticipated. Indications for repair are based on symptoms or complications related to herniation of partial defects. Various surgical procedures including pericardiectomy either partial or complete, patch repair or extension of the defect, and left atrial

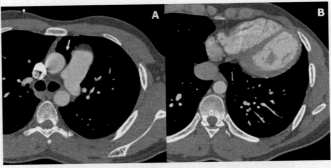

Figure 36.4 Congenital absence of pericardium. Two contrast-enhanced CT axial images through the chest in a patient with complete absence of the pericardium. In (**A**) note the interposed lung between the aorta and main pulmonary artery (*arrow*). (**B**) Mediastinal shift to the left is noticeable with mild clockwise rotation of the heart.

appendage excision to reduce complications, have been described.[3] Tricuspid repair may be required in some patients due to secondary annular distortion and significant tricuspid regurgitation. Complete absence of the pericardium less often requires surgical intervention, though remains at risk for exercise related torsion.

3.2. Pericardial cysts

Although rare, mediastinal cysts including pericardial cysts are readily visualized by multiple cardiac imaging modalities. The most common primary mass in the pericardium is a cyst. These are saccular structures generally with one lobe, a smooth surface, and no stalk.[3,21] On average, pericardial cysts are up to 3 cm in size though very large cysts have been described.[22] They do not communicate with the pericardial cavity, a distinction from pericardial diverticuli. They are filled with a clear plasma fluid transudate often with hyaluronic acid present.

Most often pericardial cysts are incidental findings on chest X-ray or CT, though less often they are detected during an evaluation of chest pain or dyspnea.[21] They are benign cysts of variable size most frequently found in the right costophrenic angle. Other sites include the left costophrenic angle, the hilum, and anterior mediastinum. Cysts in these unusual locations can make them difficult to distinguish from other mediastinal cysts, such as a bronchogenic or thymic cysts.[19,23]

Pericardial cysts are congenital in origin. It is thought that they occur during pericardial development when a portion of the embryonic pericardium is redundant and pinched off from the cavity. Pseudocysts may also occur due to inflammatory, infectious, or traumatic etiologies. The differential diagnosis includes a pericardial or pleural effusion or other forms of mediastinal cysts or masses.

3.2.1. Chest X-ray

Pericardial cysts have a radio-opacity similar to water/soft tissue. Although they are most commonly found in the right cardiophrenic angle, in approximately 20% of patients they are located on the left heart border where they can mimic a prominent left atrial appendage or a left ventricular aneurysm (Fig. 36.5).[18,24] On the lateral chest radiograph, pericardial cysts usually extend to the angle formed by the junction of the anterior hemidiaphragm and chest wall.

3.2.2. Echocardiography

Pericardial cysts, particularly small cysts or those outside the confines of the cardiac chambers may not be detected by

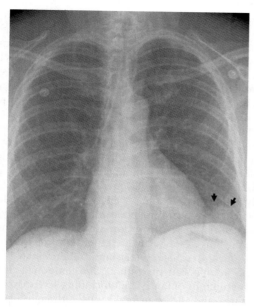

Figure 36.5 Pericardial cyst. PA view of the chest shows a rounded opacity located at the left cardiophrenic angle (*arrowheads*).

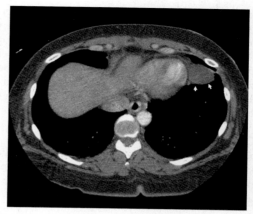

Figure 36.6 Pericardial cyst. Axial image of a contrast-enhanced CT of the chest (same patient as in Fig. 36.5) shows a well-defined rounded lesion at the left cardiophrenic angle (*arrowheads*) in continuity with the pericardium. Its attenuation is homogeneous and in keeping with simple fluid.

echocardiography. Modified views such as a right parasternal long-axis or subcostal views may best visualize cysts in the right costophrenic angle.[25] It is important that they are not misinterpreted as a right pleural effusion.

3.2.3. Computed tomography

This is the modality of choice to evaluate a suspicious finding on chest X-ray. Standard protocols without ECG gating can be utilized for the assessment of paracardiac masses. With CT, pericardial cysts usually have an attenuation coefficient in the range of simple fluid (mean HU between 0 and 10), although cases of high attenuation cysts have been reported and are thought to represent complicated cysts (with secondary infection or hemorrhage).[26] They are usually spherical or oval structures contiguous with the pericardium, have imperceptible walls without internal septa, and do not enhance after contrast material administration (Fig. 36.6).[19,27,28] Rarely, the capsule of a pericardial cyst may calcify, which CT can demonstrate better than other modalities.[29] A discriminatory feature of pericardial cysts is that they commonly change in size and shape with respiration or change in position.[30]

3.2.4. Magnetic resonance imaging

As with other fluid collections in the body, MRI has the best capacity for characterization. With MRI, pericardial cysts will show low or intermediate signal intensity on T1-weighted images and homogeneous high intensity on T2-weighted images, and will not enhance after the administration of gadolinium chelates. A cyst may contain proteinaceous fluid or blood by-products, which may show high signal intensity on T1-weighted images. As with other modalities, no communication with the pericardial space can be demonstrated.[24,27,31]

3.2.5. Management

Asymptomatic cysts require no treatment, though large cysts may cause symptoms or compression of cardiac structures and potentially cyst rupture. Approximately, one third of pericardial cysts may progress to symptoms. One mechanism by which cyst

expansion occurs is by intracavitary hemorrhage. Until recently, thoracotomy with resection and aspiration was the standard procedure for pericardial cyst removal. Percutaneous video-assisted robotic aspiration of pericardial cysts can now be performed.[32,33] Of note, recurrence of pericardial cysts following drainage has been reported. Spontaneous resolution does not occur unless there is rupture.

3.3. Pericardial tumors

Primary pericardial tumors are exceedingly rare so that most neoplastic pericardial diseases are related to an extracardiac metastatic malignancy or less often a primary benign or malignant cardiac tumor. The reported prevalence of pericardial tumors is approximately 3% of all primary cardiac tumors.

Malignant pericardial disease may present with chest pain, dyspnea, palpitations, arrhythmias, or sudden cardiac death, or may manifest as pericarditis, cardiac tamponade, or an incidental pericardial effusion.[34,35] Other presentations include infectious and vasculitic manifestations particularly in immunocompromised patients. Malignant pericardial effusions tend to be large and hemorrhagic.

The presence of pericardial involvement with a neoplasm is usually associated with a poor prognosis. There are four pathways for tumors to involve the pericardium: retrograde lymphatic extension, hematogenous spread, direct contiguous extension, or transvenous extension.[36]

In adults, the most common benign tumors to involve the pericardium are fibromas and lipomas.[3] They may be very large and invade the pericardium and myocardium. Sarcomas (angio- and fibro-) and mesotheliomas are the primary malignant cardiac tumors that most frequently involve the pericardium.[37,38] Pericardial mesotheliomas have an association with asbestosis similar to with pleural disease. Lung, breast, esophagus, lymphoma, leukemia, and melanoma are the most common secondary malignancies that involve the pericardium.

In autopsy series, metastatic involvement of the pericardium is relatively frequent, however, by imaging it has been difficult to demonstrate. The most common and usually first imaging manifestation of pericardial primary or metastatic disease is a pericardial effusion.[17,20] When an unexplained pericardial effusion is suspected, age-appropriate cancer testing should be undertaken to determine if a primary cancer can be detected. If testing is unrevealing, particularly if a large effusion is present, pericardiocentesis should be performed for diagnostic purposes. General laboratory testing should include specific gravity, protein, glucose, LDH, cell counts, bacterial cultures, and cytology.[39] The sensitivity of fluid cytology for a malignant etiology is reported to be high.[39] Tumor markers including CEA, AFP, and CA-125 should only be obtained if suspicion is high. If the diagnosis remains elusive, a biopsy should be considered.

3.3.1. Chest X-ray
Other than identifying a pericardial effusion, plain radiography plays no significant role in assessing for pericardial neoplastic or metastatic detection. In some cases, an irregular cardiac contour or mediastinal enlargement may be noted.

3.3.2. Echocardiography
The role of echocardiography is usually limited to the detection and follow-up of a pericardial effusion. Often the recognition of a pericardial effusion by echocardiography may be the first sign of a neoplasm. Extracardiac masses cannot generally be seen by echocardiography. The presence of suspected tumor metastatic foci or seeding in the pericardial space can sometimes be suggestive of a metastatic effusion.

3.3.3. Cardiac computed tomography and magnetic resonance imaging
In addition to the role these modalities play in detecting and characterizing pericardial effusions, direct extension of tumor from an adjacent lung or mediastinal structures can be detected by both CT and MRI, by observing the obliteration of the normal pericardial line and intervening fat plane.[17] Pericardial nodularity, in the presence or absence of an effusion, should be viewed with a high degree of suspicion in patients with known primary tumors.[20] On MRI, most neoplasms will demonstrate a low-signal intensity on T1-weighted images and high-signal intensity on T2-weighted images. Metastatic melanoma is an exception due to its T1 shortening effect.

3.3.4. Management
Benign pericardial tumors are amenable to resection if associated with symptoms or complications.[40] The prognosis for sarcomas is poor despite attempts at resection, mediastinal irradiation, and chemotherapy.[3] Malignant pericardial effusions are managed by treating the underlying primary neoplasm. Specific management of malignant pericardial effusions is still controversial with several options.[41] For recurrent malignant effusions a pleural–pericardial window is often performed. Subxiphoid balloon pericardiotomy can also be undertaken with low risk. Sclerosing agents are less often utilized to prevent recurrence.[42]

3.4. Pericardial effusion and cardiac tamponade
Pericardial effusions are commonly seen on routine transthoracic echocardiography.[43,44] Typically, effusions are trivial or small and are generally considered physiologic with no associated symptomatology. However, pathologic effusions may be small and acute development of a pericardial effusion can lead to cardiac tamponade. By contrast, large pericardial effusions may develop over time without symptoms. Therefore, clinicians following patients with known chronic pericardial effusions must consider the etiology and follow-up to avoid progression to symptoms or cardiac tamponade.

Cardiac tamponade is a medical emergency resulting in a marked impediment to cardiac filling with a subsequent reduction in cardiac output and eventually, shock and pulseless electrical

alternans. It may be an unexpected complication of a cardiac procedure or the initial presentation of a patient with symptoms or hemodynamic deterioration. All critical care physicians caring for patients with acute, hemodynamically unstable illnesses (ER, ICU, CCU, catheterization laboratory, OR) must be aware of the clinical settings and diagnostic clues that suggest cardiac tamponade.

Detection of a pericardial effusion may occur in asymptomatic patients undergoing cardiac or thoracic imaging, without the suspicion of pericardial disease. Symptomatic presentation typically occurs in the setting of acute pericarditis as a result of myriad etiologies (Table 36.1). Iatrogenic etiologies related to intracardiac perforation during catheterization, electrophysiology procedures, or following cardiac surgery may present with acute symptoms or primarily hemodynamic collapse and cardiac tamponade.

Unrelated to pericarditis, pericardial effusions may present with nonspecific chest discomfort or noncardiac compressive effects on the lungs, esophagus, abdomen, or phrenic nerve resulting in dyspnea, dysphagia, hoarseness, abdominal discomfort, nausea, or hiccups. Patients with cardiac tamponade experience signs and symptoms of low output including severe dyspnea, dizziness, fatigue, and altered mental status. Although there may be an initial compensatory phase with sustained or elevated blood pressure, hemodynamic instability with tachycardia and hypotension subsequently occurs.

On cardiac examination when tamponade is present, Beck triad's may occur (hypotension, raised jugular venous pressure, and decreased heart sounds). Elevated jugular venous pressure with a prominent "x" descent and loss of "y" descent, dull heart tones, Ewart's sign (due to compression of the left bronchus), and rales due to atelectasis are associated findings.[45] A pulsus paradoxus in the setting of a known pericardial effusion has a sensitivity of 82% for cardiac tamponade. A pooled review by Roy et al.[46] of clinical findings most consistent with cardiac tamponade found that dyspnea, tachycardia, pulsus paradoxus, elevated

TABLE 36.1
ETIOLOGIES OF PERICARDITIS

- **Idiopathic**
- **Infectious**
  Viral, bacterial (purulent), tuberculous, fungal
- **Isolated condition**
- **After injury**
  Acute myocardial infarction (acute, Dressler syndrome), postpericardiotomy syndrome, postpercutaneous interventions, trauma, chest radiation therapy
- **Related to local structure**
  Neoplasm, aortic dissection, pneumonia, esophageal perforation
- **Systemic conditions**
- **Autoimmune diseases**
  Systemic lupus erythematosus, rheumatoid arthritis, scleroderma, sarcoidosis, Sjögren syndrome, rheumatic fever, Behcet syndrome, reactive arthritis, ankylosing spondylitis, familial Mediterranean fever, vasculitis
- **Metabolic disorders**
  Hypothyroidism, renal failure (uremic, dialysis associated), cholesterol
- **Drug induced**
  Hydralazine, procainamide, isoniazid, minoxidil, doxorubicin, phenytoin, methyldopa, mesalazine, dantrolene, cromolyn sodium, methysergide

jugular venous pressure, and cardiomegaly on chest X-ray were most common. Pulsus paradoxus may not occur despite cardiac tamponade in cardiac conditions, where right or left ventricular diastolic pressures are chronically elevated or with large shunts such as an atrial septal defect.[3] In addition, pulsus paradoxus is present in many conditions unrelated to cardiac tamponade such as obesity, chronic obstructive lung disease, pregnancy, pneumothorax, and pulmonary embolism, where there are large swings in intrathoracic pressures. An electrocardiogram during cardiac tamponade may show electrical alternans and low voltage.

If hemodynamic monitoring is performed, the classic features of cardiac tamponade include elevated central venous, right and left atrial pressure with waveforms similar to those seen on the jugular venous waveforms (described earlier). There is near equalization of the right atrial, right ventricular end-diastolic, pulmonary capillary wedge pressure and left ventricular end-diastolic pressure. The cardiac output will be decreased (Fig. 36.7).

There are several atypical presentations with cardiac tamponade (Table 36.2). Low-pressure tamponade is a milder form of tamponade which occurs when intrapericardial pressure is greater than right atrial and right ventricular diastolic pressures with clinical features of classic tamponade in only 24% of patients.[47] This occurs mostly in the setting of severe hypovolemia, and hemodynamics and symptoms may improve with pericardiocentesis. Hypertensive cardiac tamponade is unusual, occurring with elevated blood pressure but otherwise typical findings of hemodynamic impairment.[48] Localized forms of cardiac tamponade usually occur in the postoperative setting or after iatrogenic cardiac perforation. Often this is due to loculated fluid or hematoma compressing a cardiac chamber. This form may be more difficult to identify by transthoracic echocardiography. Effusive-constrictive pericarditis manifests as cardiac tamponade with limited pericardial fluid volume and a rigid pericardium and then subsequently as persistent constrictive physiology when fluid is removed.[49] Most of these patients eventually require pericardiectomy. Cardiac tamponade with left ventricular diastolic collapse has been described without a pericardial effusion associated with a large left pleural effusion.[50,51]

Understanding the physiology and pathophysiologic abnormalities leading to pericardial fluid accumulation is useful in considering the etiologies. Normal pericardial fluid is a filtrate of plasma with a low protein concentration (of which most is albumin). Drainage of pericardial fluid is through the lymphatic system. Therefore, the mechanisms leading to pericardial fluid accumulation include (i) lymphatic obstruction (e.g., prior chest radiation, cancer); (ii) elevated venous pressure; (iii) low oncotic

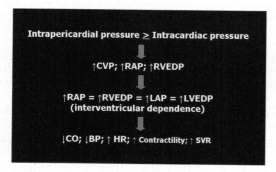

Figure 36.7 Sequential hemodynamic abnormalities that lead to cardiac tamponade. CVP, central venous pressure; RVEDP, right ventricular end diastolic pressure; LAP, left atrial pressure; LVEDP, left ventricular end diastolic pressure; CO, cardiac output; BP, blood pressure; HR, heart rate; RAP, right atrial pressure; SVR, systemic vascular resistance.

TABLE 36.2
CLINICAL VARIANT PRESENTATIONS OF CARDIAC TAMPONADE

- "Classical"
- Low pressure
- Hypertensive
- Effusive-constrictive
- Right-sided (early)
- Localized
- Associated with ↑ LV/RV/PA pressures
- Without pericardial effusion (left pleural effusion)

LV, left ventricle; RV, right ventricle; PA, pulmonary artery.

pressure; (iv) inflammation (e.g., direct extension or generalized serositis); and (v) hemorrhage (e.g., cardiac rupture or systemic coagulopathy).[3]

The determinants of hemodynamic effect/risk of cardiac tamponade due to a pericardial effusion are related to the (i) volume of pericardial effusion; (ii) rate of accumulation; (iii) intracardiac pressures; and (iv) etiology. When a critical volume is reached on the stress–strain curve, the intrapericardial pressure rises rapidly and the sequence of hemodynamic alterations results in a decreased cardiac output.[52]

The diagnosis of a probable pericardial effusion can be made on chest X-ray, scintigraphic myocardial perfusion imaging, and ventriculography, though most often is confirmed by echocardiography, CT, and cardiac MRI. CT and MRI are usually used in patients with limited echocardiographic windows, inconclusive findings, when loculated effusions or pericardial thickening is suspected, or those when there is a discrepancy between the echocardiogram and the clinical data.

3.4.1. Chest X-ray

Unsuspected pericardial disease may first be suggested by an unexplained increased cardiac silhouette on routine chest X-ray. With a large pericardial effusion the heart appears enlarged and globular in shape, the so-called "water-bottle" or "flask-shape" without significant pulmonary venous congestion. The absence of interstitial fluid may aid to differentiate pericardial effusion from multichamber cardiac enlargement. Small effusions are usually not discernable on a chest X-ray. Approximately 250 mL of pericardial fluid is expected before enlargement of the cardiac silouette is evident.[16,18] The separation of the epicardial fat layer and parietal pericardium by more than a 2 mm is consistent with a pericardial effusion. This is best seen along the anterior aspect of the heart in the lateral view as the pericardial "fat-pad" or "sandwich" sign.[18]

Although there are no specific findings on the chest X-ray to suggest cardiac tamponade, a rapid development of a pericardial effusion (or rapid progressive cardiomegaly) on serial chest X-rays should raise consideration. When the pericardial effusion results in hemodynamic compromise, pulmonary venous congestion may be seen.

3.4.2. Cardiac SPECT

Patients with chest pain referred for nuclear perfusion imaging may have an unrecognized pericardial effusion that can be detected by cardiac SPECT imaging. A circumferential region around the heart that is count poor as seen on raw projection images is suggestive of a pericardial effusion (Fig. 36.8).[53]

Figure 36.8 Pericardial effusion during nuclear SPECT imaging. Left-sided panel shows raw projection image at rest and with stress. There is a count poor region (*arrow point*) that surrounds the left and right ventricles that is consistent with a pericardial effusion. Right-sided panel shows SPECT images at rest and stress with similar count poor region surrounding the heart (*arrow point*). The study was done in a patient with chest pain of unknown etiology subsequently demonstrated on echocardiogram to be a pericardial effusion (From Austin DA, Kwon DH, Jaber WA. Pericardial effusion on Tc-99m SPECT perfusion study. J *Nucl Cardiol* 2008;15(6):e35–6, with permission.).

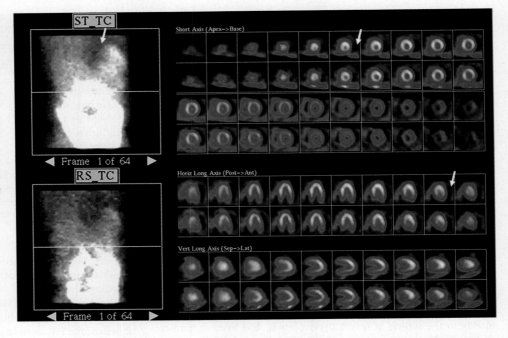

3.4.3. Echocardiography

The gold standard test for detection and follow-up of pericardial effusions providing both diagnostic and physiologic information is echocardiography. By two-dimensional imaging, pericardial effusion is identified as an echolucent space surrounding the heart and representing fluid in the pericardial cavity. Pleural effusions can be distinguished in the parasternal and apical views from pericardial effusions. Left pleural effusions are seen extending posterior to the descending aorta in the parasternal view and laterally in the apical view. Left pleural effusions can also be distinguished by imaging from the left back. Pericardial effusion may often be misdiagnosed when localized epicardial fat is present anterior to the right ventricle or adjacent to the right atrium. Epicardial fat can be distinguished as having a fine, linear bright stippling appearance not seen with pericardial effusions. Although not as effective as CT, the character of a pericardial effusion can sometimes be determined (i.e., hematoma versus free-flowing fluid). In addition, the chronicity of an effusion can be inferred by fibrous strands and loculation. The distribution of pericardial fluid should be described as circumferential, loculated, or adjacent to a cardiac chamber, anterior or posterior. The size of a pericardial effusion is generally regarded as small (<1 cm), medium (1 to 2 cm), and large (>2 cm) as measured in systole and diastole.[54] Small effusions usually appear first posterior to the heart around the atrioventricular groove, though may appear anteriorly, particularly if there are posterior adhesions.

Transthoracic echocardiography is the test of choice for the diagnosis of cardiac tamponade, since it is portable and can be performed rapidly. In most cases, imaging windows are adequate but in some patients particularly on life-support systems, transesophageal echocardiography (TEE) is necessary. Echocardiography also allows for the detection of alternative diagnoses in unstable or critically ill patients.

The echocardiographic evaluation for cardiac tamponade is well described, including two-dimensional imaging, M-mode and Doppler examinations (Fig. 36.9). The sensitivity and specificity of echocardiographic criteria for tamponade are variably reported (Table 36.3).[55–59] Right atrial collapse is a highly sensitive (>90%) finding and easy to assess.[55] However, this finding is not specific particularly when there is a brief inversion of the right atrial wall.

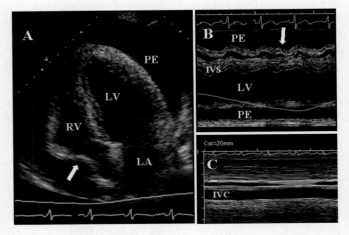

Figure 36.9 Echocardiographic images of a large pericardial effusion with cardiac tamponade. **A:** Apical four-chamber view of LV, LA, and RV that shows large PE with diastolic right atrial collapse (*arrow*). **B:** M-mode image with cursor placed through RV, IVS, and LV in parasternal long axis. The view shows circumferential PE with diastolic collapse of RV free wall (*arrow*) during expiration. **C:** M-mode image from subcostal window in the same patient that shows IVC plethora without inspiratory collapse. PE, pericardial effusion; LV, left ventricle; RV, right ventricle; LA, left atrium; IVS, interventricular septum; IVC, inferior vena cava. (From Troughton RW, *Lancet.* 2004;363:717–727, with permission.)

Specificity is enhanced by chamber collapse greater that one third of the cardiac cycle and inferior vena cava (IVC) plethora (dilated IVC with no collapse during inspiration). Right ventricular diastolic collapse is specific, especially if it is greater that one-third of the cardiac cycle, but may not be as sensitive (approximately 80%).[58] Conditions with high pulmonary and right ventricular pressures will prevent the manifestation of right ventricular collapse with tamponade. Left atrial collapse is uncommon but specific and generally occurs postoperatively or in conditions where right-sided pressures are very high (e.g., chronic pulmonary hypertension). Left ventricular diastolic collapse may occur with cardiac rupture or hemorrhage in the pericardial cavity.

M-mode echocardiography is useful to confirm the duration, timing, and presence of chamber collapse. Pulsed Doppler flow

TABLE 36.3

ECHOCARDIOGRAPHIC PARAMETERS TO ASSESS CARDIAC TAMPONADE

	Sensitivity	Specificity	Obtainable
RA diastolic collapse	++++	+++	++++
RV diastolic collapse	+++	++++	++++
LA diastolic collapse	++	++++	+++++
LV diastolic collapse	+	+++++	+++++
Mitral/ tricuspid inflow	+++++	+++	++++
Hepatic vein flow	++++	++++	++
IVC size/ collapse	++++	++	++++

RA, right atrium; RV, right ventricle; LA, left atrium; LV, left ventricle; IVC, inferior vena cava.

with abnormal respiratory variation in mitral and tricuspid inflow is the most sensitive indicator for cardiac tamponade, occurring before definite right heart collapse. However, the specificity of this finding is reduced in the presence of other conditions such as chronic lung disease.[60] Criteria for cardiac tamponade are a mitral E wave inspiratory fall >25% and tricuspid E wave inspiratory increase >40% (Fig. 36.10). A hepatic vein Doppler profile with absence of diastolic filling (D wave) is a specific feature of cardiac tamponade concordant with the loss of the "Y" descend on the venous waveform.

3.4.4. Computed tomography

Relative to echocardiography, localized pericardial fluid may be better visualized and other pericardial characteristics such as the thickness and presence of calcification or masses can be assessed. As with MRI, the use of ECG gating results in the best quality images. In the supine patient, small effusions will collect posterior to the left atrium and ventricle, while large effusions surround the heart (Fig. 36.11).[61] The size of a pericardial effusion as seen on CT often appears greater relative to echocardiography.

The CT attenuation values (Hounsfield units) of pericardial fluid can allow for distinction of the contents of pericardial fluid (e.g., blood, transudates or exudates, and chyle). A fluid collection with attenuation close to that of water (0 to 10 HU) is consistent with a simple effusion, while attenuation coefficient values greater than that of water will suggest malignancy, hemopericardium (the denser of the effusions), purulent exudate, or effusion associated with hypothyroidism.[19] Hemopericardium may be difficult to detect in the absence of epicardial fat or intravenous contrast, since blood will have an attenuation coefficient very similar to that of the adjacent myocardium.[16] In cases of chylopericardium, lower than water attenuation effusions have been reported.[19] Small pericardial effusions may be misinterpreted on CT in view of its similar appearance to pericardial thickening, especially when the image acquisition is done without ECG gating.

The role of CT to diagnose cardiac tamponade is limited. In both CT and MR imaging, the presence of a pericardial effusion with loss of definition of the subepicardial fat and compression of the right atria and ventricle will suggest tamponade. The use of ECG-gated EBCT or MDCT to construct cine images improves accuracy. Few findings on static images of the chest will be suggestive of tamponade in the appropriate clinical setting. Bowing of the interventricular septum is equivalent to the paradoxical motion of the septum seen on cine images. Compression of low-pressure intrapericardial structures like the coronary sinus, the pericardial trunk, or the intrapericardial segment of the IVC should raise the concern of tamponade.

One advantage of CT over echocardiography and to some degree over MRI is its capacity to include the entire chest in the examination, rather than being an organ focused exam. Therefore, ancillary findings associated with tamponade pathophysiology can be detected, such as enlargement of the SVC and IVC, periportal edema, and reflux of the contrast bolus into the hepatic or azygous veins.

3.4.5. Magnetic resonance imaging

Cardiac MRI has many of the same advantages as CT. Additionally, MRI is superior in differentiating fluid from a thickened pericardium, and may be superior to echocardiography in defining

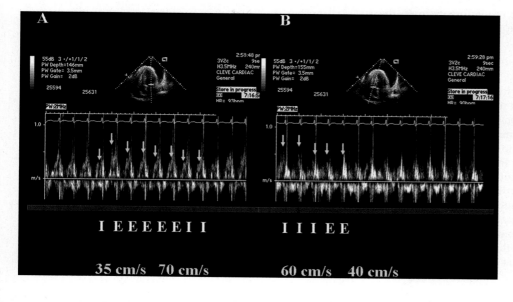

Figure 36.10 Mitral and tricuspid inflow respiratory variation in cardiac tamponade. **A:** Mitral inflow pulsed Doppler. *Yellow arrows* point to peak E wave velocity in inspiration and expiration. Respiratory variation calculated as *E − I/E* × 100% (70 − 35/70 × 100% = 50%). **B:** Tricuspid inflow pulsed Doppler. Respiratory variation calculated as *I − E/I* × 100% (60 − 40/60 × 100% = 33%). I, inspiration; E, expiration.

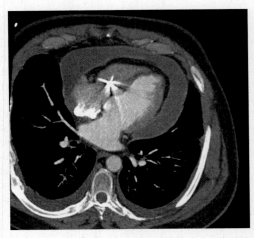

Figure 36.11 Computed tomography with large pericardial effusion. Axial image of a contrast-enhanced CT of the chest shows a moderate to large pericardial effusion. The effusion is homogeneous and with an attenuation coefficient in keeping with simple fluid representing a trasudative type of effusion.

the nature and assessing the extent of the effusion.[24,31] MRI is also especially useful in identifying localized or loculated effusions. A simple effusion will demonstrate low intensity on T1-weighted spin echo images and high intensity on T2-weighted spin echo and gradient echo images. Complex pericardial effusions, due to their high protein content, will typically exhibit greater signal intensity on T1-weighted images. Conversely, hemorrhagic effusions and hemopericardium will have high signal intensity on spin echo images and low intensity on GRE sequences, secondary to the presence of paramagnetic blood byproducts. However, these hemorrhagic effusions can show areas of both medium and high signal intensities, reflecting the variable age of the blood.[27,31] Spin echo images, either T1 or T2 weighted, may have an important amount of motion artifact. Newer, faster cine sequences, such as fast gradient echo or balanced steady-state free precession gradient echo, can be very useful to show the moving heart within the pericardial space and the pericardial fluid that can be characterized by its T1/T2 ratio.[18,24]

Similar to echocardiography, MRI using ECG-gated cine sequences may be able to demonstrate right-sided chamber collapse in diastole. However, one advantage of echocardiography over MRI is the possibility of following specific breathing instructions during real-time scanning, since the degree of chamber collapse can vary during the respiratory cycle. In the emergent setting of cardiac tamponade, MRI is of limited clinical assistance.

3.4.6. Management

Medical treatment of asymptomatic pericardial effusions without hemodynamic significance is generally not required. Diagnostic consideration should be given for cardiac, systemic, inflammatory, infectious, metabolic, malignant, traumatic, or drug etiologies, and appropriate testing performed. If no leading systemic symptoms or signs are present, basic testing including an appropriate malignancy evaluation particularly for lung and breast cancer and limited laboratory testing should be carried out (see Section 3.5). While pericardiocentesis is generally undertaken for therapeutic reasons or hemodynamic deterioration, it may also be required if there is concern for malignancy or purulent infectious etiologies. Depending on the etiology, other therapeutic measures that are disease specific may reduce effusions size (e.g., more intense

dialysis for end-stage renal disease). Steroids, nonsteroidal anti-inflammatory agents, or colchicine are not recommended for asymptomatic effusions. Anticoagulation or antiplatelet agents are also avoided if possible.

There is a small subset of patients (2% of patients with pericardial disease) with large chronic idiopathic pericardial effusions.[62,63] In one relatively large series of 28 patients who fulfilled this criteria and were followed for a median of 7 years, cardiac tamponade occurred in 29% of patients.[63] Since close follow-up is required for patients with large pericardial effusions, it is reasonable to consider elective pericardiocentesis.

When cardiac tamponade is identified, rapid drainage is required, which can usually be done by percutaneous pericardiocentesis. Temporary stabilization of some patients with mild hypotension by volume expansion may be effective.[64] In few circumstances such as following trauma, cardiac rupture, or acute aortic dissection, open surgical drainage is preferred.[65] This option can only be considered if immediate surgical support is available and the patient is stable enough to allow for transfer to the operating room. Echocardiography is important to mark the entry site for pericardiocentesis, allowing identification of a region with >1 cm of free-flowing pericardial fluid during diastole. The subxiphoid and apical approaches are most commonly utilized and the procedure can be performed with low procedural risk. For recurrent effusions especially of malignant etiology, a pericardial window should be performed.

3.5. Acute and chronic pericarditis

Pericardial inflammation can present in a variety of clinical scenarios, and may occur as either an isolated pericardial condition or as a manifestation of a systemic disease. Characterized by chest pain and sequential electrocardiographic changes, it is an entity more common in men and in adults. Pericarditis accounts for 1 in every 1,000 hospitalized patients and is diagnosed in 5% of patients presenting to emergency departments, with chest pain unrelated to myocardial infarction.[66,67] Although mortality is very low with an often self-limiting course, morbidity related to pericarditis depends on the underlying etiology and the development of potential complications, which include pericardial effusion, relapsing pericarditis, and constrictive pericarditis.

Although typically presenting in the acute phase, pericarditis can present in subacute and chronic recurrent forms. Acute pericarditis presents with severe retrosternal chest pain, often sharp, pleuritic, and sudden during onset. The pain can radiate to the neck, arms, and classically to the trapezius muscle ridge (related to phrenic nerve irritation).[68] It is aggravated when lying supine or with excess body motion, coughing, or deep inspiration and alleviated by sitting upright. Fever is a common associated symptom.

Chronic or relapsing pericarditis can be of the incessant or intermittent type. The presenting features during relapses of the intermittent type are similar to the initial episode but become progressively milder.[69,70] In some cases, exercise may precipitate a recurrent attack. While the frequency of relapses is unpredictable, the majority of patients have few episodes and these tend to disappear in the long term. Despite the recurrent nature, the risk of developing constrictive pericarditis in idiopathic relapsing pericarditis is very low (<1%). The incessant type of chronic pericarditis is more frequent in patients treated with steroids during their initial attack.

The hallmark finding of pericarditis is the pericardial friction rub. A friction rub is heard in most patients during the disease course. It is a high-pitched scratchy or creaking sound, most audible in end-expiration when the patient is leaning forward. The sound is typically triphasic (three components corresponding to ventricular ejection, rapid diastolic filling, and atrial contraction), but can be biphasic or monophasic in half the cases.[68] It can be differentiated from a pleural rub that corresponds to the respiratory cycle, and ceases with breath holding and may be heard even when a pericardial effusion is present.

For most presentations of acute pericarditis, extensive laboratory testing is not required, since the etiology is most often viral or idiopathic. If systemic, neoplastic, or purulent related pericarditis is not suspected, a CBC, CMP, Troponin, CPK, CRP, and ESR are sufficient initial tests. Blood cultures and viral serologies are generally not recommended. Acute and convalescent levels of viral serologies are time consuming and costly, and require a knowledge of the endemic strains in the region. Tuberculosis and HIV testing should be considered when exposures or risk factors are present.

Viral or idiopathic etiologies account for up to 90% of causes of pericarditis. The remaining 10% of etiologies comprise an extensive list.[71-73] Etiologies most commonly related to the chronic recurrent forms of pericarditis are also idiopathic and viral pericarditis. Postmyocardial infarction and postpericardiotomy syndromes are conditions recognized to cause relapsing pericarditis, thought to be related to an immune-mediated process.

The diagnosis of pericarditis is based on the clinical history, examination, and electrocardiographic findings. The most widely used diagnostic tool for acute pericarditis is the electrocardiogram, which classically shows diffuse concave ST-segment elevation along with PR-segment depression. The typical electrocardiographic abnormalities evolve through four stages: Stage I, ST-segment elevation and upright T waves; stage II, normalization of ST-segments and T-wave flattening; stage III, diffuse T-wave inversions; and stage IV, resolution of T-wave inversions and return to baseline state.[74,75] The differential diagnosis includes myocardial infarction and early repolarization. Complimentary diagnostic modalities such as chest X-ray, echocardiography, CT, and cardiac MRI can be used when the simple diagnostic tools are inconclusive and for the detection of complications related to pericarditis.

3.5.1. Chest X-ray
In acute pericarditis, the chest X-ray is often normal, but should be obtained to exclude mediastinal or pulmonary pathologies. The cardiac silhouette can enlarge to take on the "water bottle" shape in the presence of a large pericardial effusion.

3.5.2. Echocardiography
Usually recommended in acute pericarditis, echocardiography is often the initial imaging modality used in suspected pericardial inflammation. It can be normal or may show a small pericardial effusion, which helps to confirm the diagnosis. Echocardiography will define the size and physiologic effects of the effusion, and help determine if evidence for cardiac tamponade or constriction is present. It may also uncover other underlying primary disease processes like myocarditis that require an entirely different treatment approach. TEE is useful when a transthoracic study is suboptimal or in the postoperative period when loculated pericardial effusions or pericardial hematomas are suspected.

3.5.3. Computed tomography
As compared to echocardiography, CT provides higher spatial resolution imaging of the heart, pericardial space, and entire chest. When pericarditis is present, a small amount of pericardial effusion or mild amount of pericardial thickening may be present, though they are often times indistinguishable from one another. When acute pericarditis is present, early contrast enhancement of a thickened pericardium (≥ 4 mm) may be identified.[19] The presence of significant and irregular pericardial thickening generally implies chronicity.[20,76] The presence of a normal thickness pericardium makes the diagnosis of chronic pericarditis unlikely.

3.5.4. Magnetic resonance imaging
When the diagnosis of pericarditis is suspected, MRI can easily identify pericardial thickening and associated effusions with fluid characterization. It can also help visualize the inflammatory involvement of the pericardium and adjacent structures (Fig. 36.12). The signal intensity of the thickened pericardium can be variable depending on the amount of inflammatory and granulation tissue seen in acute pericarditis (mildly elevated signal on spin echo sequences) and the fibrous tissue or calcification that is usually present in the more chronic cases (lower signal intensity on spin echo sequences).[19,24] As on CT, enhancement of the inflamed pericardium can be seen after the administration of contrast, which can also further assist in separating the pericardial layers from the fluid between them and reveal septations that may be present in cases of loculated effusions.[19,77] Recently, the use of late enhancement sequences to detect myocardial infarction has been proposed as a method of identifying active inflammation of the pericardial layers, differentiating inflammatory from fibrosing forms of pericarditis.[77]

Although not generally the first line of imaging for the diagnosis of pericarditis, MRI can be of value to the clinician in monitoring for the resolution. For cases of chronic relapsing pericarditis related to postpericardiotomy syndrome, imaging may show the potential evolution to pericardial constriction.

3.5.5. Management
Because of its self-limited nature, the treatment of acute pericarditis is supportive, largely aimed at relief of chest pain (Fig. 36.13). Poor prognostic variables necessitating hospital admission identified from a prospective study of 453 patients include fever >38°C, subacute course, large pericardial effusion, and ASA or nonsteroidal anti-inflammatory drug (NSAID) failure.[78] Other variables that predict adverse outcomes include left ventricular

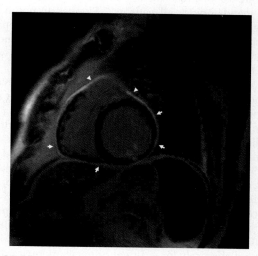

Figure 36.12 Magnetic resonance imaging in a patient with acute pericarditis. Delayed enhancement MRI sequence in the short axis demonstrates persistent enhancement of the pericardium circumferentially (*arrowheads*), suggesting an inflammatory process.

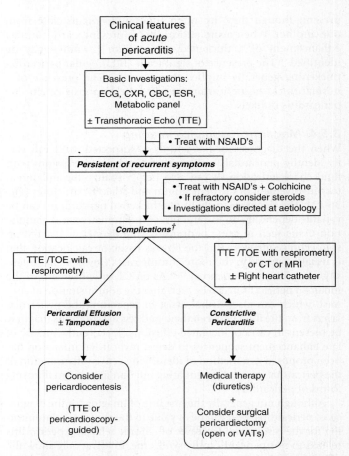

Figure 36.13 Suggested approach to investigation and management of pericarditis and its complications. TTE, transthoracic echocardiogram; TOE, transesophageal echocardiogram; †Defined as hemodynamic instability, right heart failure, volume overload, or both, or unexplained cardiovascular symptoms. (From Troughton RW, *Lancet.* 2004;363: 717–727, with permission.)

regional or global dysfunction (i.e., myopericarditis), anticoagulation therapy, immunosuppression, or trauma. Admission for a brief hospital observation period is reasonable to assure that patients are responsive to therapy and have no high risk features, but not mandatory for all patients.[79] Elevated troponin I levels have been reported in 32% to 49% of patients with idiopathic or viral pericarditis and correlate with younger age, male gender, and a pericardial effusion.[80,81] However, in this setting they were not found to be a negative prognostic factor.[80]

If an underlying etiology of acute pericarditis is known, treatment should be targeted at the primary cause. For most cases of idiopathic or viral pericarditis, the mainstay of therapy is a NSAID. Multiple regimens including aspirin, NSAIDs and colchicines have been utilized and tested as first line therapy.[82–85] Nonsteroidal anti-inflammatory agents (e.g., ibuprofen 400 to 800 mg tid or ASA 650 to 975 mg tid) are preferred agents for 2 to 4 weeks with a tapering course and consideration for gastrointestinal prophylaxis. Colchicine can be given along with NSAIDs or ASA for 3 months to reduce recurrence. Aspirin is the preferred agent for postmyocardial infarction pericarditis. For patients who may be intolerant to NSAIDs, a colchicine-only regimen can be utilized. Colchicine can be used effectively for recurrent or refractory pericarditis, and has been used in combination with ASA for a first episode of acute pericarditis (2 mg daily for 1 to 2 days, then 0.5 mg to 1 mg daily for 3 months).[84] The threshold to initiate corticosteroids should

be very high due to the high likelihood of relapse with tapering. If corticosteroids are absolutely required, underdosing should be avoided (1 to 1.5 mg/kg for at least 1 month before tapering over 3 months, with NSAIDs or colchicine).[83,86,87]

3.6. Constrictive pericarditis

A long-term sequela of most etiologies of acute and chronic pericarditis and constrictive pericarditis has been well recognized for centuries. Many of the classic physical examination findings including Broadbent (systolic apical retraction), Friedreich (rapid y descent of the jugular venous pulse), and Kussmaul sign (rise or failure of the jugular venous pulse to fall with inspiration), described before modern imaging, have corresponding diagnostic findings on echocardiography and hemodynamic waveforms. Despite extensive research to understand its pathophysiology, the diagnosis of constrictive pericarditis continues to elude even modern day specialists. Multiple diagnostic imaging modalities to assess anatomic and pathophysiologic features of constrictive pericarditis are often required. Differentiation from restrictive cardiomyopathy still remains difficult. However, detection of constrictive pericarditis continues to be vital, since often pericardiectomy can be done with low risk and result in substantial functional improvement.[88]

The clinical presentation of constrictive pericarditis ranges from exertional dyspnea and fatigue, to symptoms of longstanding right and left heart failure.[89] Patients may present with lower extremity swelling or abdominal distension as a sole manifestation. Many patients are first seen and evaluated by a gastroenterologist for liver disease or ascites of unknown etiology. Angina due to pericardial restriction of coronary artery compression is uncommon. Atrial arrhythmias may be a presenting sign of constriction.

Similarly, the signs may be variable including manifestations of predominantly right heart failure with elevated jugular venous distension and a prominent "x" and rapid "y" descent, Kussmaul sign, hepatosplenomegaly with a pulsatile liver, ascites, and edema.[90] The heart sounds may be reduced with a pericardial knock occurring at the trough of the y descent in early diastole (similar in timing to an S3).[91] There may be systolic retraction of the apical impulse. Left heart failure signs may also be present but generally are not advanced. Pulsus paradoxus does not occur unless there is effusive-constrictive pericarditis.

There are no specific features on electrocardiography. A low voltage QRS complex, nonspecific ST changes, biatrial enlargement, and atrial fibrillation may be present. Brain natriuretic peptide levels in patients with isolated constriction are not elevated in contrast to a marked elevation in patients with restrictive cardiomyopathy.[92]

The cause of constrictive pericarditis has changed in the past several decades. Contemporary identifiable etiologies include viral, cardiac surgery, and radiation in that order, though still a large proportion of cases are idiopathic.[88] In all cases, inflammation leads to a combination of thickening, fibrosis, and calcification that contribute to diastolic dysfunction. The exception is neoplastic processes that may cause constrictive physiology through direct seeding of the pericardium and compression.

As a result of pericardial encasement, two fundamental pathophysiologic changes occur that lead to the hemodynamic abnormalities found in constrictive pericarditis: (i) exaggerated interventricular dependence (filling of one side of the heart directly affects the volume and pressure of filling of the other side of the heart)—interventricular dependence is manifested as reciprocal changes occurring with respiration—and (ii) dissociation between intracardiac and intrathoracic pressures (the decrease in intrathoracic pressures due to inspiration is not transmitted to result in an enhanced filling pressure) (Fig. 36.3).[93] These pathophysiologic changes can be assessed by echocardiography and direct hemodynamic assessment in the catheterization laboratory.[94-96] With inspiration, left ventricular transmyocardial filling pressure is not enhanced due to the dissociation from intrathoracic pressure, though the lungs and pulmonary veins (not encased by the pericardium) become more compliant. This results in a lower driving pressure from the pulmonary veins to the left ventricle in diastole and thus, a lower diastolic volume and stroke volume. Concomitantly, with interventricular dependence, a lower left ventricular diastolic volume allows for a greater right ventricular diastolic volume with inspiration, with reciprocal changes occurring in expiration.

Restrictive cardiomyopathy can be distinguished from constrictive pericarditis by the absence of interventricular dependence and dissociation of intracardiac and intrathoracic pressures.[97] Isolated constrictive pericarditis is a disorder of compliance, while restrictive cardiomyopathy effects both relaxation and compliance.[98-100] These properties are the basis for many techniques that aid in differentiating these two disease processes. In addition, isolated constrictive pericarditis affects diastolic function and not systolic function, whereas restrictive cardiomyopathies ultimately lead to systolic impairment. There is an extensive body of literature comparing diagnostic testing to distinguish constrictive pericarditis from restrictive cardiomyopathy (see Chapter 34 on Restrictive cardiomyopathy).

3.6.1. Chest X-ray
Pericardial calcifications are strongly suggestive of constrictive pericarditis (Fig. 36.14). These are usually best seen in the lateral view. However, the pericardium calcifies only in 20% to 40% of constrictive cases.[101,102] Secondary findings, such as an enlarged left atrium or pulmonary redistribution, may be seen.

It is important to distinguish pericardial and myocardial calcifications. Pericardial calcification is usually thin and linear and can extend over the atrial contours. However, it serves only as a diagnostic test and may not correlate with functional class and

hemodynamic effect. Additional findings on chest X-ray such as biatrial enlargement, pleural effusions, and volume overload would be consistent with high filling pressures.

3.6.2. Echocardiography
Transthoracic echocardiography is often the first line test used in patients with suspected constrictive pericarditis or symptoms and signs of right and left heart failure. Although the anatomic evaluation of the pericardium may be limited with transthoracic echocardiography, even technically limited studies may allow for the detection of structural and hemodynamic features that are consistent with the disease. When evaluating the possibility of constrictive pericarditis on echocardiography, the sonographer and interpreting physician must do a careful and comprehensive examination that requires additional time and detail compared to a conventional study.

Two-dimensional images: Direct evaluation of the pericardium should be performed for the presence of a pericardial effusion, calcification, and thickening, and specific anatomic variants of constriction can be identified. The measurement of pericardial thickness and calcification by transthoracic echocardiography is usually limited, and 18% of cases of constrictive pericarditis occur with normal pericardial wall thickness.[103] Signs of focal atrial or ventricular tethering and reduced motion of the atrioventricular groove or annulus may be seen, though require experience and heightened awareness.[104] The presence of atrial dilation with normal ventricular chambers and a dilated IVC or hepatic veins is also suggestive of constriction particularly when atrial fibrillation is not present. The most specific sign for constrictive pericarditis by two-dimensional imaging is a "septal bounce" (sensitivity: 62%, specificity: 93%).[104] This diastolic motion of the septum represents rapid early filling of a noncompliant ventricle with exaggerated interventricular dependence.

M-mode: Direct pericardial visualization can also be done with M-mode to assess for similar findings of an effusion, calcification, and thickening. M-mode of the left and right ventricular cavities can show the reciprocal changes in cavity size related to respiration and early diastolic flattening of the left ventricular posterior wall (Fig. 36.15).[105] Less commonly sought findings of

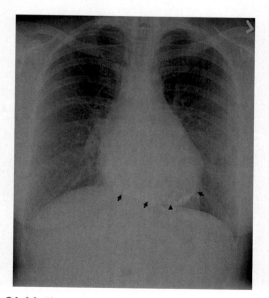

Figure 36.14 Chest X-ray with constrictive pericarditis. PA view of the chest shows dense, linear coarse calcifications following the contour of the heart in keeping with pericardial calcification. Note that it involves the periphery of both left and right cardiac structures making myocardial calcification a very unlikely possibility.

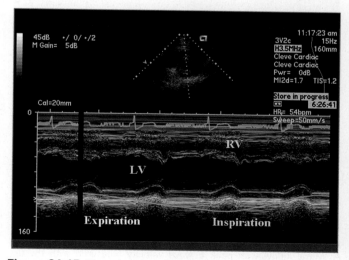

Figure 36.15 M-mode echocardiogram in constrictive pericarditis. Parasternal short-axis view. Respiratory variation in septal motion seen with a smaller LV cavity size with inspiration and larger cavity size with expiration. Flattening of the posterior wall is also seen. LV, left ventricle; RV, right ventricle.

constrictive physiology by M-mode include premature diastolic opening of the pulmonary valve and an early posterior motion of the aortic root in diastole.[106,107]

Diastology and Doppler: The Doppler examination, utilizing mitral and tricuspid inflow and pulmonary and hepatic vein flows, is the most fundamental part of a constriction evaluation.[93,95,108,109] Technical aspects of performing this evaluation are essential. A high quality ECG tracing and appropriate Doppler alignment, sweep speed, filter, gain, sample placement, and size are required (1 to 2 mm for mitral and tricuspid, and 3 to 4 mm for pulmonary and hepatic). A nasal respirometer is preferred to determine timing of inspiration and expiration, and the first beat convention is used to minimize the effect due to respiratory effort. Figure 36.16 shows typical Doppler profiles of constrictive pericarditis and calculation of respiratory variation of mitral and tricuspid inflow. Other disorders such as pulmonary embolism, right ventricular infarction, severe tricuspid regurgitation, large pleural effusions, chronic obstructive lung disease, and atrial fibrillation may also cause right or left ventricular inflow respiratory variation. In both constrictive pericarditis and restrictive cardiomyopathy, the deceleration time is short consistent with a restrictive filling pattern. However, significant respiratory variation of mitral, tricuspid, pulmonary, and hepatic flows occurs only with constriction. Additionally, with constriction inspiration results in a decreased mitral deceleration time and an increased isovolumic relaxation time relative to expiration.

Pulmonary and hepatic vein flows provide ancillary information to the mitral and tricuspid inflow patterns.[108] Respiratory variation in the pulmonary vein diastolic flow (D wave) mirrors the mitral inflow E wave variation with reduced systolic and diastolic flows (S and D waves) during inspiration that are increased with expiration. Hepatic vein flow provides very specific evidence for constrictive physiology. The hepatic vein (D wave) mirrors the tricuspid inflow E wave and along with the S wave increases with

inspiration. With expiration the S and D waves are reduced and there may be a prominent reversed atrial reversal (AR) and ventricular reversal (VR) flows (Fig. 36.17). Significant blunting of the S wave of pulmonary or hepatic veins is more consistent with restrictive physiology.

SVC flow can be obtained by imaging below the right clavicle. The pattern of flow is similar to hepatic vein flow with a systolic and diastolic flow and VR and AR. Boonyaratavej et al.[110] demonstrated the utility of SVC flow to differentiate right-sided respiratory variation due to chronic obstructive lung disease and constrictive pericarditis. In patients with constrictive pericarditis, SVC flows demonstrate less respiratory variation, whereas there is a marked respiratory variation with chronic obstructive lung disease (Fig. 36.18).

Doppler tissue imaging (DTI) and color M-mode (CMM) patterns in constriction have been well studied and are useful to distinguish from restrictive physiology. A normal DTI E' velocity >8 cm/s and CMM propagation slope >90 cm/s represent normal relaxation and rapid early filling. With restrictive physiology, relaxation and compliance are abnormal and therefore, E' velocity is <8 cm/s and

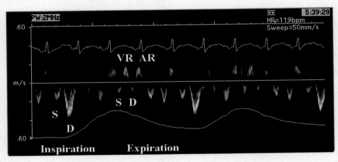

Figure 36.17 Hepatic vein flow with constrictive pericarditis. Hepatic vein forward D flow is increased with inspiration. In expiration, forward D flow is decreased with more prominent VR and AR. D, diastolic; VR, ventricular reversal; AR, atrial reversal.

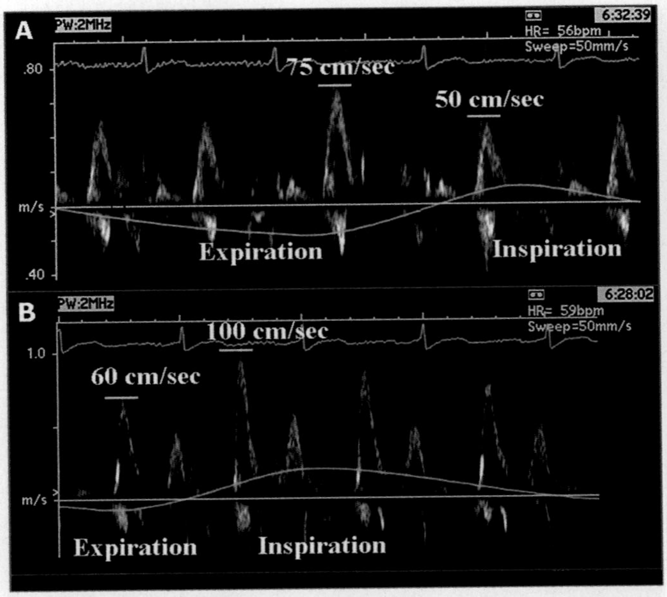

Figure 36.16 Pulsed Doppler inflows in constrictive pericarditis. **A:** Mitral inflow with peak E wave velocity measured with the first beat of inspiration and expiration. Respiratory variation calculated as $E - I/E \times 100\% = (75 - 50)/75 \times 100\% = 33\%$. **B:** Tricuspid inflow with peak E wave velocity measured with the first beat of inspiration and expiration. Respiratory variation calculated as $I - E/I \times 100\% = (100 - 60/100 \times 100\%) = 40\%$.

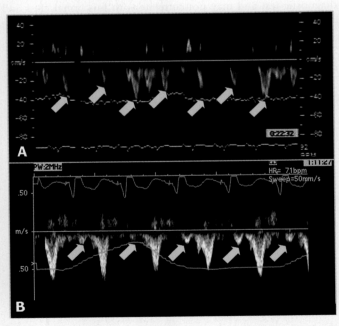

Figure 36.18 Superior vena cava pulsed Doppler flow with chronic obstructive lung disease and constrictive pericarditis. **A:** Chronic obstructive lung disease. *Arrows* demonstrate respiratory variation in systolic forward flow. **B:** Constrictive pericarditis. *Arrows* demonstrate lack of respiratory variation in systolic forward flow.

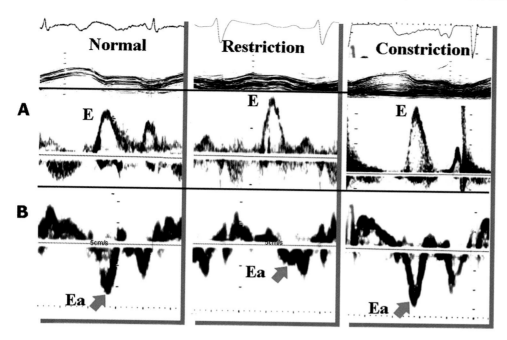

Figure 36.19 Tissue Doppler imaging to distinguish constrictive pericarditis and restrictive cardiomyopathy. Annular M-mode, pulsed Doppler E wave mitral inflow (E) and tissue Doppler mitral annulus (Ea) are shown for normal individual and patients with restrictive cardiomyopathy and constrictive pericarditis. The mitral E wave in constriction and restriction cannot distinguish the disorders, though the Ea velocities identify a markedly reduced velocity with restriction and preserved velocity with constriction. (From Garcia MJ, *JACC* 1996;27:108, with permission.)

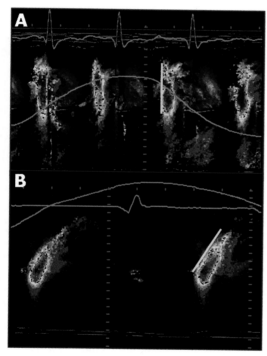

Figure 36.20 Color M-mode to distinguish constrictive pericarditis and restrictive cardiomyopathy. Color M-mode propagation into the left ventricle. **A:** Constrictive pericarditis with rapid propagation velocity. **B:** Restrictive cardiomyopathy with slow propagation velocity. *Yellow lines* show color M-mode propagation slope.

CMM propagation slope is generally <50 cm/s (Figs. 36.19 and 36.20).[98,100] Although an elevated E/E_{ann} ratio is associated with an elevated pulmonary capillary wedge pressure among patients with restrictive cardiomyopathy, an inverse relation occurs with constrictive pericarditis ("annulus paradoxus").[111] The use of DTI of the mitral annulus for the diagnosis of constrictive pericarditis in the presence of significant mitral annular calcification is less accurate.

Additional echocardiographic techniques: Approximately, 20% of patients with constrictive pericarditis may not have respiratory

variation of Doppler flow profiles. This may occur because filling pressures are too low or too high. Therefore, if constriction is suspected but not readily apparent, maneuvers to reduce preload including Valsalva, sitting up, or diuretics can be used, and to increase preload leg lifts or fluid loading can be performed.[112–114] The tricuspid regurgitant jet can be interrogated as an additional manifestation of interventricular dependence. With constrictive pericarditis, the maximum velocity of tricuspid regurgitation, the width of the regurgitant jet profile, and velocity-time integral (VTI) increase relative to normal controls.[115]

If transthoracic echocardiography is suboptimal for assessing patients with suspected constrictive pericarditis, TEE can be utilized.[108] Studies comparing TEE to CT for determining pericardial thickness have shown a good correlation.[116]

Invasive hemodynamic evaluation of patients with suspected constrictive pericarditis and inconclusive noninvasive testing may be required in a small proportion of patients (Fig. 36.21). Criteria for the diagnosis of constriction and differentiation from

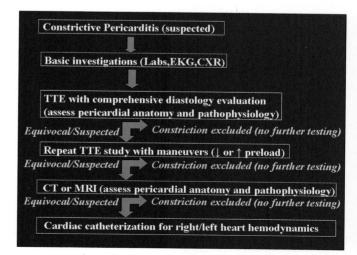

Figure 36.21 Algorithm for suggested workup of patients with suspected constrictive pericarditis. EKG, electrocardiogram; CXR, chest X-ray; TTE, transthoracic echocardiogram; CT, computed tomography; MRI, magnetic resonance imaging.

restriction have been established.[97] Classic echocardiographic criteria consistent with constrictive pericarditis are summarized in Table 36.4. Anatomic variants of constrictive pericarditis have also been described with implications regarding likelihood of postsurgical improvement (Fig. 36.22).[117]

3.6.3. Computed tomography

The diagnostic hallmark of constrictive pericarditis is pericardial thickening with or without calcifications in the appropriate clinical scenario (Fig. 36.23). An advantage of CT over other modalities is its capacity to detect minute amounts of pericardial calcium. It is also a useful tool for defining the location and extent of the focal thickening and pericardial calcification in the presurgical

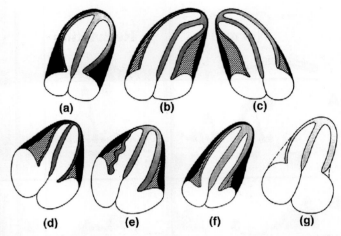

Figure 36.22 Pathoanatomic forms of constrictive pericarditis versus restrictive cardiomyopathy. **A**: Annular form constriction; **B**: Left-sided form constriction; **C**: Right-sided form constriction; **D**: Myocardial atrophy and global form of constriction; **E**: Perimyocardial fibrosis and global form of constriction; **F**: Global form of constriction; and **G**: Restrictive cardiomyopathy. (From *Eur Heart J.* 2004;25:587. European Society of Cardiology: Guidelines on the diagnosis and management of pericardial diseases, Executive Summary, with permission.)

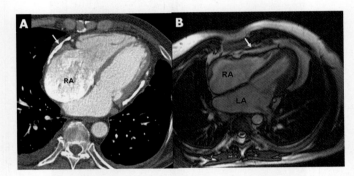

Figure 36.23 Computed tomography and magnetic resonance imaging with constrictive pericarditis. **A**: Axial image of a contrast-enhanced CT of the chest shows dense pericardial calcification (*arrowheads*) and atrial enlargement (only the RA is well seen at this level). Note the small pleural effusion posteriorly. **B**: Balanced steady-state free precession image in the four-chamber view in a patient with pericardial constriction. The atria are enlarged (RA and LA), while the ventricles show a tubular appearance with some bowing of the interatrial septum. There is some focal pericardial thickening (*arrowheads*).

TABLE 36.4

SUMMARY OF "CLASSIC" ECHOCARDIOGRAPHIC FEATURES OF CONSTRICTIVE PERICARDITIS

Two-dimensional

- Pericardial thickening, calcification, effusion
- LA/RA cavity dilation
- LV/RV function preserved
- Chamber/AV groove tethering
- Diastolic "septal" bounce
- Dilated IVC/hepatic veins
- Atrial septum bows to LA with inspiration

M-mode

- Reciprocal respiratory variation in LV/RV cavity size
- LV posterior wall flattening in early diastole
- Aortic abrupt posterior motion in early diastole
- Premature opening of pulmonary valve
- Color M-mode mitral inflow, rapid propagation slope >90 cm/s

Doppler

Inspiration

- ↓ Mitral E and A wave (>25% respiratory variation considered abnormal)
- ↓ pulmonary vein S and D wave
- ↓ Mitral E wave deceleration time
- ↑ LV IVRT
- ↑ Tricuspid E and A wave (>40% respiratory variation considered abnormal)
- ↓ Tricuspid E wave deceleration time
- ↑ Hepatic vein diastolic forward flow
- ↓ Hepatic vein diastolic flow reversal
- ↑ Superior vena cava diastolic forward flow
- ↑ V_{max} tricuspid regurgitant velocity and TDI

Reciprocal changes with expiration

- TDI E annular >8 cm/s

LA, left atrium; RA, right atrium; LV, left ventricle; RV, right ventricle; AV, atrioventricular; IVC, inferior vena cava; IVRT, isovolumic relaxation time; TDI, tissue Doppler imaging.

planning stages. The calcification is commonly located along the regions of the atrioventricular grooves, and extends over both the atria and ventricles. When the calcifications are myocardial, as in cases of remote infarctions, they are exclusive to the left side of the heart.[61] In the absence of calcifications, in the appropriate clinical settings, pericardial thickening and a normal appearing myocardium can be helpful for the diagnosis of constriction. However, altered physiology should be demonstrated. With the advent of EBCT and MDCT with increased temporal resolution, ECG-gated cine images can be constructed and abnormal interventricular dependence caused by the lack of pericardial distensibility can be seen.[20,118] Additional findings seen with constriction include distorted contours of the ventricles, tubular-shaped ventricles (sometimes with enlarged atria, the so-called "acorn-shaped" heart), dilatation of the intrahepatic IVC, or coronary sinus. There may be other extracardiac findings like dilatation of the hepatic

TABLE 36.5

ADVANTAGES AND DISADVANTAGES OF COMPUTED TOMOGRAPHY VERSUS MAGNETIC RESONANCE IMAGING FOR EVALUATION OF CONSTRICTIVE PERICARDITIS

Findings	Modality	
	CT	MRI
Morphologic		
Pericardial thickening	+++	+++
Mild thickening vs. small effusion	+	+++
Significant thickening vs. large effusion	++	+++
Pericardial calcifications	+++	+
Tubelike configuration of the ventricles	+++	+++
Sigmoid-shaped interventricular septum	+++	+++
Atrial enlargement	+++	+++
Dilated inflow veins (IVC, SVC, or CS)	+++	++
Functional		
Delayed of contrast bolus in vascular system	+++	+
Paradoxical motion of the IVC	++	+++
Regurgitant flow in the PV or HV	−	+++

CT, computed tomography; MRI, magnetic resonance imaging; IVC, inferior vena cava; SVC, superior vena cava; CS, coronary sinus; PV, pulmonary veins; HV, hepatic veins.

veins, hepatic venous congestion, ascites or mesenteric soft tissue stranding, and pleural effusions.[17,61,119] Reflux of contrast material into the coronary sinus or IVC can sometimes be seen following the bolus administration of intravenous contrast.[26] The absence of thickened pericardium argues against the diagnosis of constriction, but does not rule it out.

3.6.4. Magnetic resonance imaging

In contrast to CT, even significant foci of calcification can be missed on MR. However, constriction can occur without calcification, and MRI has the better ability to differentiate between small pericardial effusions and pericardial thickening.[20] Table 36.5 shows the contrast between CT and MRI for assessment of constrictive pericarditis. Pericardial thickening can be quite variable and as in CT, a thickness of 4 mm or more is considered abnormal. MRI is a valuable tool in assessing the pericardial thickening and the characteristic sequelae of constrictive pathophysiology (ancillary findings described earlier). With the use of spin echo sequences, a thickened pericardium can be demonstrated in most patients. However, newer sequences with cine acquisition capabilities, such as cine fast gradient echo and balanced steady-state fast precession gradient echo are as good, or even better, to visualize small amounts of pericardial fluid and functional information.[24] These cine-MR images often prove useful in assessing the reduced diastolic capacity of the left ventricle and, as with CT, the paradoxical motion of the interventricular septum. Real-time low resolution cine-imaging during free breathing may also be performed to demonstrate reciprocal changes in left and right ventricular volumes during inspiration and expiration. The use of velocity-encoded sequences is being investigated for the measurement and analysis of transmitral velocities that could expand the role of MRI.[23]

3.6.5. Management

The treatment of constrictive pericarditis is dependent on the severity of heart failure, the etiology, and risk of pericardiectomy. Initial treatment with salt and fluid restriction and diuretics

(including loop diuretics and aldosterone) should be given to all patients.[120] There are reported cases of constrictive pericarditis due to infectious or inflammatory causes that are responsive to targeted medical therapy. Surgery should only be considered in patients considered refractory to medical therapy and balanced against the risk of pericardiectomy.[87,121–124] The surgical mortality of pericardiectomy in high volume centers depends on the etiology with an overall mortality of 6%. In a large series from the Cleveland Clinic, the 30-day mortality was 2.7% for idiopathic constriction, 8.3% for postsurgical constriction, and 21.4% for postradiation induced constriction (Fig. 36.24).[88] Predictors of increased surgical mortality included prior radiation, increased creatinine, increased pulmonary artery systolic pressure, decreased serum sodium, left ventricular dysfunction, and advanced age. Following pericardiectomy, significant tricuspid regurgitation may develop due to re-expansion of the right ventricle.

Two subgroups, transient constrictive pericarditis and effusive-constrictive pericarditis, should be identified due to differing presentations and prognosis relative to chronic constrictive pericarditis. Transient constrictive pericarditis presents within weeks after an episode of pericarditis with mild manifestations of constrictive physiology.[125] This form of constriction resolves with medical therapy for pericarditis due to infectious or inflammatory etiologies. Effusive-constrictive pericarditis presents with clinical features and hemodynamics most consistent with cardiac tamponade.[49] Following pericardial fluid drainage, a transition to clinical and hemodynamic features consistent with constrictive pericarditis occurs. Most patients in this subgroup ultimately require pericardiectomy.

4. FUTURE DIRECTIONS

Diagnostic cardiac imaging continues to evolve as a vital tool for the diagnosis and management of pericardial disease. Echocardiography remains the foundation for the detection, confirmation, and follow-up of most pericardial diseases, allowing for both structural and functional information. Defining the distinct roles

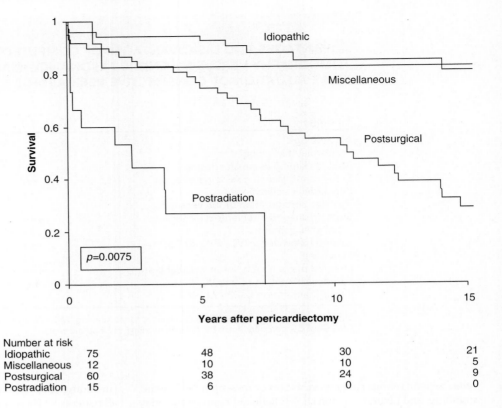

Figure 36.24 Kaplan–Meier plots showing survival postpericardiectomy for constrictive pericarditis based on etiology. There is a statistically significant difference in survival based on a cause of constrictive pericarditis. (From Bertog SC, JACC 2004;43:1445, with permission.)

Number at risk				
Idiopathic	75	48	30	21
Miscellaneous	12	10	10	5
Postsurgical	60	38	24	9
Postradiation	15	6	0	0

and selection of CT and MRI to assess pericardial disease require further refinement. Although currently diagnostic imaging of the pericardium is aimed at the management of pericardial diseases, ultimately the pericardial space may be utilized as a window for therapeutic cardiac interventions.

REFERENCES

1. Spodick DH. Macrophysiology, microphysiology, and anatomy of the pericardium: A synopsis. *Am Heart J.* 1992;124(4):1046–1051.
2. Manner J, Perez-Pomares JM, Macias D, et al. The origin, formation and developmental significance of the epicardium: A review. *Cells Tissues Organs.* 2001;169(2):89–103.
3. Spodick DH. *The Pericardium: A Comprehensive Textbook.* Editor Marcel Dekker, Inc. 1997.
4. Spodick D. Role of the pericardium in diastolic dysfunction and diastolic heart failure. In Klein AL and Garcia MJ, Diatology: Clinical approach to diastolic heart failure. Philadelphia, Elsevier; 2008:28–31.
5. Spodick DH. Threshold of pericardial constraint: The pericardial reserve volume and auxiliary pericardial functions. *J Am Coll Cardiol.* 1985;6(2):296–297.
6. Boltwood CM, Jr. Ventricular performance related to transmural filling pressure in clinical cardiac tamponade. *Circulation.* 1987;75(5):941–955.
7. Abbas AE, Appleton CP, Liu PT, et al. Congenital absence of the pericardium: Case presentation and review of literature. *Int J Cardiol.* 2005;98(1):21–25.
8. Gatzoulis MA, Munk MD, Merchant N, et al. Isolated congenital absence of the pericardium: Clinical presentation, diagnosis, and management. *Ann Thorac Surg.* 2000;69(4):1209–1215.
9. Nasser WK, Helmen C, Tavel ME, et al. Congenital absence of the left pericardium. Clinical, electrocardiographic, radiographic, hemodynamic, and angiographic findings in six cases. *Circulation.* 1970;41(3):469–478.
10. Rashid A, Ahluwalia G, Griselli M, et al. Congenital partial absence of the left pericardium associated with tricuspid regurgitation. *Ann Thorac Surg.* 2008;85(2):645–647.
11. Montaudon M, Roubertie F, Bire F, et al. Congenital pericardial defect: Report of two cases and literature review. *Surg Radiol Anat.* 2007;29(3):195–200.
12. White CS. MR evaluation of the pericardium. *Top Magn Reson Imaging.* 1995;7(4):258–266.
13. Oki T, Tabata T, Yamada H, et al. Cross sectional echocardiographic demonstration of the mechanisms of abnormal interventricular septal motion in congenital total absence of the left pericardium. *Heart.* 1997;77(3):247–251.
14. Abbas A, Awan S. Rhabdomyosarcoma of the middle ear and mastoid: A case report and review of the literature. *Ear Nose Throat J.* 2005;84(12):780, 782, 784.
15. Candan I, Erol C, Sonel A. Cross sectional echocardiographic appearance in presumed congenital absence of the left pericardium. *Br Heart J.* 1986;55(4):405–407.
16. Hoit BD. Imaging the pericardium. *Cardiol Clin.* 1990;8(4):587–600.
17. Breen JF. Imaging of the pericardium. *J Thorac Imaging.* 2001;16(1):47–54.
18. Axel L. Assessment of pericardial disease by magnetic resonance and computed tomography. *J Magn Reson Imaging.* 2004;19(6):816–826.
19. Kim JS, Kim HH, Yoon Y. Imaging of pericardial diseases. *Clin Radiol.* 2007;62(7):626–631.
20. Grizzard JD, Ang GB. Magnetic resonance imaging of pericardial disease and cardiac masses. *Cardiol Clin.* 2007;25(1):111–140.
21. Feigin DS, Fenoglio JJ, McAllister HA, et al. Pericardial cysts. A radiologic-pathologic correlation and review. *Radiology.* 1977;125(1):15–20.
22. Satur CM, Hsin MK, Dussek JE. Giant pericardial cysts. *Ann Thorac Surg.* 1996;61(1):208–210.
23. Francone M, Dymarkowski S, Kalantzi M, et al. Magnetic resonance imaging in the evaluation of the pericardium. A pictorial essay. *Radiol Med (Torino).* 2005;109(1–2):64–74; quiz 75–76.
24. Maksimovic R, Dill T, Seferovic PM, et al. Magnetic resonance imaging in pericardial diseases. Indications and diagnostic value. *Herz.* 2006;31(7):708–714.
25. Hynes JK, Tajik AJ, Osborn MJ, et al. Two-dimensional echocardiographic diagnosis of pericardial cyst. *Mayo Clin Proc.* 1983;58(1):60–63.
26. Olson MC, Posniak HV, McDonald V, et al. Computed tomography and magnetic resonance imaging of the pericardium. *Radiographics.* 1989;9(4):633–649.
27. Wang ZJ, Reddy GP, Gotway MB, et al. CT and MR imaging of pericardial disease. *Radiographics.* 2003;23 Spec No:S167–S180.
28. Karia DH, Xing YQ, Kuvin JT, et al. Recent role of imaging in the diagnosis of pericardial disease. *Curr Cardiol Rep.* 2002;4(1):33–40.
29. Smith WH, Beacock DJ, Goddard AJ, et al. Magnetic resonance evaluation of the pericardium. *Br J Radiol.* 2001;74(880):384–392.
30. Oyama N, Oyama N, Komuro K, et al. Computed tomography and magnetic resonance imaging of the pericardium: Anatomy and pathology. *Magn Reson Med Sci.* 2004;3(3):145–152.
31. Frank H, Globits S. Magnetic resonance imaging evaluation of myocardial and pericardial disease. *J Magn Reson Imaging.* 1999;10(5):617–626.
32. Sharma R, Harden S, Peebles C, et al. Percutaneous aspiration of a pericardial cyst: An acceptable treatment for a rare disorder. *Heart.* 2007;93(1):22.
33. Bacchetta MD, Korst RJ, Altorki NK, et al. Resection of a symptomatic pericardial cyst using the computer-enhanced da Vinci Surgical System. *Ann Thorac Surg.* 2003;75(6):1953–1955.
34. Yoo SY, Park CB, Cheong SS. Primary pericardial malignant fibrosarcoma presenting as sudden onset of substernal pain. *Heart.* 2008;94(3):265.
35. Imazio M, Demichelis B, Parrini I, et al. Relation of acute pericardial disease to malignancy. *Am J Cardiol.* 2005;95(11):1393–1394.
36. Chiles C, Woodard PK, Gutierrez FR, et al. Metastatic involvement of the heart and pericardium: CT and MR imaging. *Radiographics.* 2001;21(2):439–449.
37. Montalescot G, Chapelon C, Drobinski G, et al. Diagnosis of primary cardiac sarcoma. Report of 4 cases and review of the literature. *Int J Cardiol.* 1988;20(2):209–219.

38. Thomason R, Schlegel W, Lucca M, et al. Primary malignant mesothelioma of the pericardium. Case report and literature review. *Tex Heart Inst J.* 1994;21(2):170–174.
39. Meyers DG, Meyers RE, Prendergast TW. The usefulness of diagnostic tests on pericardial fluid. *Chest.* 1997;111(5):1213–1221.
40. Segawa D, Yoshizu H, Haga Y, et al. Successful operation for solitary fibrous tumor of the epicardium. *J Thorac Cardiovasc Surg.* 1995;109(6):1246–1248.
41. Vaitkus PT, Herrmann HC, LeWinter MM. Treatment of malignant pericardial effusion. *JAMA.* 1994;272(1):59–64.
42. Maher EA, Shepherd FA, Todd TJ. Pericardial sclerosis as the primary management of malignant pericardial effusion and cardiac tamponade. *J Thorac Cardiovasc Surg.* 1996;112(3):637–643.
43. Berger M, Bobak L, Jelveh M, et al. Pericardial effusion diagnosed by echocardiography. Clinical and electrocardiographic findings in 171 patients. *Chest.* 1978;74(2):174–179.
44. Riba AL, Morganroth J. Unsuspected substantial pericardial effusions detected by echocardiography. *JAMA.* 1976;236(23):2623–2625.
45. Shabetai R. Symposium: Pericardial disease. Introduction. *Am J Cardiol.* 1970;26(5):445–446.
46. Roy CL, Minor MA, Brookhart MA, et al. Does this patient with a pericardial effusion have cardiac tamponade? *JAMA.* 2007;297(16):1810–1818.
47. Sagrista-Sauleda J, Angel J, Sambola A, et al. Low-pressure cardiac tamponade: Clinical and hemodynamic profile. *Circulation.* 2006;114(9):945–9452.
48. Brown J, MacKinnon D, King A, et al. Elevated arterial blood pressure in cardiac tamponade. *N Engl J Med.* 1992;327(7):463–466.
49. Sagrista-Sauleda J, Angel J, Sanchez A, et al. Effusive-constrictive pericarditis. *N Engl J Med.* 2004;350(5):469–475.
50. Kopterides P, Lignos M, Papanikolaou S, et al. Pleural effusion causing cardiac tamponade: Report of two cases and review of the literature. *Heart Lung.* 2006;35(1):66–67.
51. Bilku RS, Bilku DK, Rosin MD, et al. Left ventricular diastolic collapse and late regional cardiac tamponade postcardiac surgery caused by large left pleural effusion. *J Am Soc Echocardiogr.* 2008;21(8):978 e9–e11.
52. Freeman GL, LeWinter MM. Pericardial adaptations during chronic cardiac dilation in dogs. *Circ Res.* 1984;54(3):294–300.
53. Austin DA, Kwon DH, Jaber WA. Pericardial effusion on Tc-99m SPECT perfusion study. *J Nucl Cardiol.* 2008;15(6):e35–36.
54. Spodick DH. Pericarditis, pericardial effusion, cardiac tamponade, and constriction. *Crit Care Clin.* 1989;5(3):455–476.
55. Gillam LD, Guyer DE, Gibson TC, et al. Hydrodynamic compression of the right atrium: A new echocardiographic sign of cardiac tamponade. *Circulation.* 1983;68(2):294–301.
56. Kronzon I, Cohen ML, Winer HE. Diastolic atrial compression: A sensitive echocardiographic sign of cardiac tamponade. *J Am Coll Cardiol.* 1983;2(4):770–775.
57. Armstrong WF, Schilt BF, Helper DJ, et al. Diastolic collapse of the right ventricle with cardiac tamponade: An echocardiographic study. *Circulation.* 1982;65(7):1491–1496.
58. Singh S, Wann LS, Klopfenstein HS, et al. Usefulness of right ventricular diastolic collapse in diagnosing cardiac tamponade and comparison to pulsus paradoxus. *Am J Cardiol.* 1986;57(8):652–656.
59. Appleton CP, Hatle LK, Popp RL. Cardiac tamponade and pericardial effusion: Respiratory variation in transvalvular flow velocities studied by Doppler echocardiography. *J Am Coll Cardiol.* 1988;11(5):1020–1030.
60. Gonzalez MS, Basnight MA, Appleton CP. Experimental pericardial effusion: Relation of abnormal respiratory variation in mitral flow velocity to hemodynamics and diastolic right heart collapse. *J Am Coll Cardiol.* 1991;17(1):239–248.
61. Boxt LM, Lipton MJ, Kwong RY, et al. Computed tomography for assessment of cardiac chambers, valves, myocardium and pericardium. *Cardiol Clin.* 2003;21(4):561–585.
62. Merce J, Sagrista Sauleda J, Permanyer Miralda G, et al. Pericardial effusion in the elderly: A different disease? *Rev Esp Cardiol.* 2000;53(11):1432–1436.
63. Sagrista-Sauleda J, Angel J, Permanyer-Miralda G, et al. Long-term follow-up of idiopathic chronic pericardial effusion. *N Engl J Med.* 1999;341(27):2054–2059.
64. Sagrista-Sauleda J, Angel J, Sambola A, et al. Hemodynamic effects of volume expansion in patients with cardiac tamponade. *Circulation.* 2008;117(12):1545–1549.
65. Isselbacher EM, Cigarroa JE, Eagle KA. Cardiac tamponade complicating proximal aortic dissection. Is pericardiocentesis harmful? *Circulation.* 1994;90(5):2375–2378.
66. Launbjerg J, Fruergaard P, Hesse B, et al. Long-term risk of death, cardiac events and recurrent chest pain in patients with acute chest pain of different origin. *Cardiology.* 1996;87(1):60–66.
67. Friman G, Fohlman J. The epidemiology of viral heart disease. *Scand J Infect Dis Suppl.* 1993;88:7–10.
68. Spodick DH. Acute pericarditis: Current concepts and practice. *JAMA.* 2003;289(9):1150–1153.
69. Fowler NO, Harbin AD III. Recurrent acute pericarditis: Follow-up study of 31 patients. *J Am Coll Cardiol.* 1986;7(2):300–305.
70. Guindo J, Rodriguez de la Serna A, Ramio J, et al. Recurrent pericarditis. Relief with colchicine. *Circulation.* 1990;82(4):1117–1120.
71. Permanyer-Miralda G, Sagrista-Sauleda J, Soler-Soler J. Primary acute pericardial disease: A prospective series of 231 consecutive patients. *Am J Cardiol.* 1985;56(10):623–630.
72. Maisch B, Ristic AD. The classification of pericardial disease in the age of modern medicine. *Curr Cardiol Rep.* 2002;4(1):13–21.
73. Zayas R, Anguita M, Torres F, et al. Incidence of specific etiology and role of methods for specific etiologic diagnosis of primary acute pericarditis. *Am J Cardiol.* 1995;75(5):378–382.
74. Spodick DH. Diagnostic electrocardiographic sequences in acute pericarditis. Significance of PR segment and PR vector changes. *Circulation.* 1973;48(3):575–580.
75. Spodick DH. Differential characteristics of the electrocardiogram in early repolarization and acute pericarditis. *N Engl J Med.* 1976;295(10):523–526.
76. Sechtem U, Tscholakoff D, Higgins CB. MRI of the abnormal pericardium. *Am J Roentgenol.* 1986;147(2):245–252.
77. Taylor AM, Dymarkowski S, Verbeken EK, et al. Detection of pericardial inflammation with late-enhancement cardiac magnetic resonance imaging: Initial results. *Eur Radiol.* 2006;16(3):569–574.
78. Imazio M, Cecchi E, Demichelis B, et al. Indicators of poor prognosis of acute pericarditis. *Circulation.* 2007;115(21):2739–2744.
79. Little WC, Freeman GL. Pericardial disease. *Circulation.* 2006;113(12):1622–1632.
80. Imazio M, Demichelis B, Cecchi E, et al. Cardiac troponin I in acute pericarditis. *J Am Coll Cardiol.* 2003;42(12):2144–2148.
81. Bonnefoy E, Godon P, Kirkorian G, et al. Serum cardiac troponin I and ST-segment elevation in patients with acute pericarditis. *Eur Heart J.* 2000;21(10):832–836.
82. Arunasalam S, Siegel RJ. Rapid resolution of symptomatic acute pericarditis with ketorolac tromethamine: A parenteral nonsteroidal antiinflammatory agent. *Am Heart J.* 1993;125(5 Pt 1):1455–1458.
83. Artom G, Koren-Morag N, Spodick DH, et al. Pretreatment with corticosteroids attenuates the efficacy of colchicine in preventing recurrent pericarditis: A multi-centre all-case analysis. *Eur Heart J.* 2005;26(7):723–727.
84. Imazio M, Bobbio M, Cecchi E, et al. Colchicine in addition to conventional therapy for acute pericarditis: Results of the COlchicine for acute PEricarditis (COPE) trial. *Circulation.* 2005;112(13):2012–2016.
85. Imazio M, Bobbio M, Cecchi E, et al. Colchicine as first-choice therapy for recurrent pericarditis: Results of the CORE (COlchicine for REcurrent pericarditis) trial. *Arch Intern Med.* 2005;165(17):1987–1991.
86. Imazio M, Brucato A, Trinchero R, et al. Corticosteroid therapy for pericarditis: A double-edged sword. *Nat Clin Pract Cardiovasc Med.* 2008;5(3):118–119.
87. Guidelines on the diagnosis and management of pericardial diseases executive summary: The task force on the diagnosis and management of pericardial diseases of the European Society of Cardiology. *Eur Heart J.* 2004;25:587–610.
88. Bertog SC, Thambidorai SK, Parakh K, et al. Constrictive pericarditis: Etiology and cause-specific survival after pericardiectomy. *J Am Coll Cardiol.* 2004;43(8):1445–1452.
89. Myers RB, Spodick DH. Constrictive pericarditis: Clinical and pathophysiologic characteristics. *Am Heart J.* 1999;138(2 Pt 1):219–232.
90. Manga P, Vythilingum S, Mitha AS. Pulsatile hepatomegaly in constrictive pericarditis. *Br Heart J.* 1984;52(4):465–467.
91. Nicholson WJ, Cobbs BW Jr, Franch RH, et al. Early diastolic sound of constrictive pericarditis. *Am J Cardiol.* 1980;45(2):378–382.
92. Leya FS, Arab D, Joyal D, et al. The efficacy of brain natriuretic peptide levels in differentiating constrictive pericarditis from restrictive cardiomyopathy. *J Am Coll Cardiol.* 2005;45(11):1900–1902.
93. Hatle LK, Appleton CP, Popp RL. Differentiation of constrictive pericarditis and restrictive cardiomyopathy by Doppler echocardiography. *Circulation.* 1989;79(2):357–370.
94. Hurrell DG, Nishimura RA, Higano ST, et al. Value of dynamic respiratory changes in left and right ventricular pressures for the diagnosis of constrictive pericarditis. *Circulation.* 1996;93(11):2007–1013.
95. Oh JK, Hatle LK, Seward JB, et al. Diagnostic role of Doppler echocardiography in constrictive pericarditis. *J Am Coll Cardiol.* 1994;23(1):154–162.
96. Santamore WP, Bartlett R, Van Buren SJ, et al. Ventricular coupling in constrictive pericarditis. *Circulation.* 1986;74(3):597–602.
97. Vaitkus PT, Kussmaul WG. Constrictive pericarditis versus restrictive cardiomyopathy: A reappraisal and update of diagnostic criteria. *Am Heart J.* 1991;122(5):1431–1441.
98. Rajagopalan N, Garcia MJ, Rodriguez L, et al. Comparison of new Doppler echocardiographic methods to differentiate constrictive pericardial heart disease and restrictive cardiomyopathy. *Am J Cardiol.* 2001;87(1):86–94.
99. Palka P, Lange A, Donnelly JE, et al. Differentiation between restrictive cardiomyopathy and constrictive pericarditis by early diastolic doppler myocardial velocity gradient at the posterior wall. *Circulation.* 2000;102(6):655–662.
100. Garcia MJ, Rodriguez L, Ares M, et al. Differentiation of constrictive pericarditis from restrictive cardiomyopathy: Assessment of left ventricular diastolic velocities in longitudinal axis by Doppler tissue imaging. *J Am Coll Cardiol.* 1996;27(1):108–114.
101. Suh SY, Rha SW, Kim JW, et al. The usefulness of three-dimensional multidetector computed tomography to delineate pericardial calcification in constrictive pericarditis. *Int J Cardiol.* 2006;113(3):414–416.
102. Chen SJ, Li YW, Wu MH, et al. CT and MRI findings in a child with constrictive pericarditis. *Pediatr Cardiol.* 1998;19(3):259–262.
103. Talreja DR, Edwards WD, Danielson GK, et al. Constrictive pericarditis in 26 patients with histologically normal pericardial thickness. *Circulation.* 2003;108(15):1852–1857.
104. Himelman RB, Lee E, Schiller NB. Septal bounce, vena cava plethora, and pericardial adhesion: Informative two-dimensional echocardiographic signs in the diagnosis of pericardial constriction. *J Am Soc Echocardiogr.* 1988;1(5):333–340.

105. Voelkel AG, Pietro DA, Folland ED, et al. Echocardiographic features of constrictive pericarditis. *Circulation.* 1978;58(5):871–875.

106. Engel PJ, Fowler NO, Tei CW, et al. M-mode echocardiography in constrictive pericarditis. *J Am Coll Cardiol.* 1985;6(2):471–474.

107. D'Cruz IA, Dick A, Gross CM, et al. Abnormal left ventricular-left atrial posterior wall contour: A new two-dimensional echocardiographic sign in constrictive pericarditis. *Am Heart J.* 1989;118(1):128–132.

108. Klein AL, Cohen GI, Pietrolungo JF, et al. Differentiation of constrictive pericarditis from restrictive cardiomyopathy by Doppler transesophageal echocardiographic measurements of respiratory variations in pulmonary venous flow. *J Am Coll Cardiol.* 1993;22(7):1935–1943.

109. Klein AL, Cohen GI. Doppler echocardiographic assessment of constrictive pericarditis, cardiac amyloidosis, and cardiac tamponade. *Cleve Clin J Med.* 1992;59(3):278–290.

110. Boonyaratavej S, Oh JK, Tajik AJ, et al. Comparison of mitral inflow and superior vena cava Doppler velocities in chronic obstructive pulmonary disease and constrictive pericarditis. *J Am Coll Cardiol.* 1998;32(7): 2043–2048.

111. Ha JW, Oh JK, Ling LH, et al. Annulus paradoxus: Transmitral flow velocity to mitral annular velocity ratio is inversely proportional to pulmonary capillary wedge pressure in patients with constrictive pericarditis. *Circulation.* 2001;104(9):976–978.

112. Oh JK, Tajik AJ, Appleton CP, et al. Preload reduction to unmask the characteristic Doppler features of constrictive pericarditis. A new observation. *Circulation.* 1997;95(4):796–799.

113. Bush CA, Stang JM, Wooley CF, et al. Occult constrictive pericardial disease. Diagnosis by rapid volume expansion and correction by pericardiectomy. *Circulation.* 1977;56(6):924–930.

114. Abdalla IA, Murray RD, Lee JC, et al. Does rapid volume loading during transesophageal echocardiography differentiate constrictive pericarditis from restrictive cardiomyopathy? *Echocardiography.* 2002;19(2):125–134.

115. Klodas E, Nishimura RA, Appleton CP, et al. Doppler evaluation of patients with constrictive pericarditis: Use of tricuspid regurgitation velocity curves to determine enhanced ventricular interaction. *J Am Coll Cardiol.* 1996;28(3):652–657.

116. Ling LH, Oh JK, Tei C, et al. Pericardial thickness measured with transesophageal echocardiography: Feasibility and potential clinical usefulness. *J Am Coll Cardiol.* 1997;29(6):1317–1323.

117. Reinmuller R, Gurgan M, Erdmann E, et al. CT and MR evaluation of pericardial constriction: A new diagnostic and therapeutic concept. *J Thorac Imaging.* 1993;8(2):108–121.

118. Ghersin E, Lessick J, Litmanovich D, et al. Septal bounce in constrictive pericarditis. Diagnosis and dynamic evaluation with multidetector CT. *J Comput Assist Tomogr.* 2004;28(5):676–678.

119. Johnson KT, Julsrud PR, Johnson CD. Constrictive pericarditis at abdominal CT: A commonly overlooked diagnosis. *Abdom Imaging.* 2008;33(3):349–352.

120. Anand IS, Ferrari R, Kalra GS, et al. Pathogenesis of edema in constrictive pericarditis. Studies of body water and sodium, renal function, hemodynamics, and plasma hormones before and after pericardiectomy. *Circulation.* 1991;83(6):1880–1887.

121. Senni M, Redfield MM, Ling LH, et al. Left ventricular systolic and diastolic function after pericardiectomy in patients with constrictive pericarditis: Doppler echocardiographic findings and correlation with clinical status. *J Am Coll Cardiol.* 1999;33(5):1182–1188.

122. Ling LH, Oh JK, Schaff HV, et al. Constrictive pericarditis in the modern era: Evolving clinical spectrum and impact on outcome after pericardiectomy. *Circulation.* 1999;100(13):1380–1386.

123. Uchida T, Bando K, Minatoya K, et al. Pericardiectomy for constrictive pericarditis using the harmonic scalpel. *Ann Thorac Surg.* 2001;72(3):924–925.

124. DeValeria PA, Baumgartner WA, Casale AS, et al. Current indications, risks, and outcome after pericardiectomy. *Ann Thorac Surg.* 1991;52(2):219–224.

125. Haley JH, Tajik AJ, Danielson GK, et al. Transient constrictive pericarditis: Causes and natural history. *J Am Coll Cardiol.* 2004;43(2):271–275.

Benign Cardiac Tumors

37

Lori B. Croft

1. INTRODUCTION

Benign primary cardiac masses and tumors have the potential to cause significant morbidity and mortality, but are possibly curable if accurately diagnosed. They may be identified by different imaging techniques including echocardiography (transthoracic echo and transesophageal echo), computer tomography (CT) or magnetic resonance imaging (MRI). With an incidence of 0.002% to 0.3 % in autopsy series,[1–3] primary tumors of the heart are rare. Benign cardiac tumors are more frequent than malignant ones, but far less common than metastatic tumors to the heart.[4] Seventy-five percent of primary tumors are benign, with myomas comprising about 50%. The majority of the rest are papillary fibroelastomas, lipomas, and rhabdomyomas.[5] Fibromas and hemangiomas are less frequent, and paragangliomas are very rare.[2,6,5]

Other cardiac masses that are incidentally found include benign cysts and intracardiac thrombi. Cardiac cysts are found within the heart and pericardium. The most common cysts include pericardial cysts, echinococcal (hydatid) cysts, and blood cysts. Pericardial cysts are uncommon intrathoracic developmental abnormalities, occurring in 1/100,000 persons.[7] Cardiac hydatid cysts are intracardiac cysts that arise from the larval stage of the echinococcus parasite and account for less than 2% of all hydatid disease.[8] Blood cysts, though common findings at infant autopsy, are extremely rare in adults.[9] Intracardiac thrombi are associated with a variety of diseases. Left ventricular thrombus formation is a complication after acute myocardial infarction, occurring in at least 5% of patients.[10,11] The prevalence of thrombi of the left atrium or left atrial appendage in patients with atrial fibrillation is 7% to 21%.[12–16] Finally, deep vein thrombosis leading to right heart thrombi occur in 7% to 18% of patients.[17,18]

Normal anatomic variants exist that can be confused with cardiac masses and tumors. Mitral annular calcification is observed at autopsy in 3% to 8% of the population,[19] and rarely (0.6%) has a large calcified burden with central "caseous" necrosis resembling a tumor. The incidence of this finding is 0.6% in patients with mitral annular calcification.[20] Chiari network, remnants of the Eustachian valve, false tendons, and prominent pectinate muscles are occasionally misdiagnosed as tumors or thrombi and lead to unnecessary diagnostic workup and even surgical removal. Thus, the cardiac imaging specialist needs to familiarize with the typical appearance of these findings.

2. GENERAL PRINCIPLES OF DIAGNOSTIC EVALUATION

Transthoracic echocardiography (TTE) is the primary diagnostic modality for imaging cardiac tumors and masses. Because

of harmonic imaging, advances in three-dimensional echo and contrast agents, TTE provides high resolution real-time images of diagnostic quality in most cases. Additionally, it is widely available, portable, and fairly inexpensive. It is capable of detecting a cardiac mass and defining its location, extent, and relationship to adjacent structures. However, the technique is operator-dependant and imaging may be suboptimal because of an inadequate acoustic window. Echo is also limited by its inability to discriminate among various masses because of its lack of tissue characterization. Transesophageal echo (TEE) provides further information in cases with a suboptimal TTE, in particular, small masses and lesions located in the left atrium. Although TEE is widely available and portable, it requires special skills for proper performance and interpretation. In addition, TEE is a semi-invasive test, usually performed with the use of conscious sedation.

Cardiac CT and MR are complementary methods in the diagnostic workup of cardiac masses and tumors. Both modalities image the entire mediastinum, evaluate the extent of extracardiac disease, and do not depend on acoustic windows. Multidetector CT provides high-quality noninvasive images of the heart, great vessels, and coronary vasculature. The current scanners allow rapid scanning of the cardiac anatomy, requiring a shorter breath hold, and have improved image quality (better spatial and temporal resolution). Cardiac CT is capable of characterizing and quantifying calcification, which is an important feature in the differential diagnosis of cardiac tumors. Iodine contrast administration helps differentiate vascular tumors from avascular thrombi. Additionally, CT can characterize tissues better than TEE or TTE, based on X-ray attenuation. CT however, requires a single breath hold, which is sometimes difficult for patients. Additionally, it exposes the patient to radiation and iodine contrast.

MR images can be acquired in any desired plane. MR provides excellent tissue characterization of intracardiac lesions. Its high soft-tissue contrast using different T1 and T2 weighted sequences provides a more distinct tissue characterization of the mass. It affords detailed morphological information by providing simultaneous assessment of all cardiac chambers, the pericardium, and surrounding structures. It also evaluates cardiac function and tumor mobility. It has the capability to evaluate flowing blood and the effect of tumor mass on blood flow. Contrast enhancement with gadolinium provides information on the vascularity of the mass and assists in the differentiation of thrombus from tumor. Suppression of fat signal is useful in the detection of lipid containing masses such as lipomas. The advantages of cardiac MRI, compared with cardiac CT, are the absence of radiation exposure and the avoidance of iodinated contrast media. It also has greater tissue characterization. However, cardiac MRI also has several disadvantages compared with CT. Cardiac MR examination time is much longer, it is more expensive, it cannot demonstrate calcium, and it cannot be performed in patients with implanted metallic devices.

3. SPECIFIC CARDIAC TUMORS AND MASSES

Although benign primary cardiac tumors are rare, it is extremely important to diagnosis their presence early and accurately. Additionally, it is equally important to distinguish these tumors from other masses and normal variants in the heart. By identifying the location of the tumor or mass within the heart (Fig. 37.1) and by classifying the features of the tumor or mass on different imaging modalities (Table 37.1), an expedient diagnosis can be made and appropriate treatment begun.

3.1. Myxomas

3.1.1. Clinical features

Myxomas are the most common primary cardiac tumors.[21] They may occur in all age groups but are particularly frequent between the third and sixth decades of life and are predominate in women.[2] They can be sporadic, familial, or complex (syndrome myxoma). Cardiac myxomas usually develop in the atria. Up to 80% of myxomas are localized in the left atrium, of which 75% involve the interatrial septum; 7% to 20% are found in the right atrium; the rest of up to 10% each are either biatrial, in the right ventricle, or in the left ventricle.[22] Myxomas emerging from valve tissue are extraordinarily rare.[23] Most myxomas arise from the interatrial septum at the border of the fossa ovalis, but can also originate from the posterior atrial wall, anterior atrial wall, and atrial appendage.[24]

Myxomas are tumors of endocardial origin arising from a multipotential mesenchymal cell.[25] Myomas are gelatinous, smooth, and round, or they can be friable and either polypoid or irregular.

They can be pedunculated, with a stalk that may be narrow or broad base, or they can be sessile. Clinical features of myxomas vary depending on the size and location of the tumor. Patients with myxoma often present with the triad of constitutional signs, embolization, and intracardiac obstruction. Myxomas can present with signs and symptoms similar to those of collagen vascular diseases, rheumatic heart disease, malignant disease, and infective endocarditis.[26-30] Embolization can occur in 30% to 40% of patients, most commonly systemic, since most myxomas are located in the left atrium.[31,23,32] Obstructive valvular dysfunction can occur leading to dyspnea, recurrent pulmonary edema, and right heart failure. With left ventricular outflow obstruction, patients are at increased risk for acute cardiogenic shock or sudden cardiac death.[33,34]

3.1.2. Diagnostic imaging

TTE can be used to determine the location, size, shape, attachment, and mobility of the myxoma.[35] TTE has high sensitivity and specificity for the diagnosis of cardiac myxoma, and is therefore the imaging modality of choice (Fig. 37.2). The usual finding on TTE or TEE is a spherical mobile tumor connected to the interatrial septum by a narrow stalk.[36] Tumors are heterogeneous with occasional internal hypoechoic areas, speckled echogenic foci, and frondlike surface projections (Fig. 37.3). Prolapse across the atrioventricular valve during diastole can also be seen (Fig. 37.4). The most important characteristic to determine the diagnosis of myxoma by TEE or TEE is the location in the left atrium and origin from the midportion of the atrial septum.[37] TTE is usually sufficient to make the diagnosis, but if the results are suboptimal or the tumors are small, TEE should be employed to visualize the extent of the mass and exclude the presences of additional tumors.

Contrast-enhanced CT can usually identify myxomas as spherical or oval, well-defined intracavitary masses. CT may not be able to identify the thin stalk of a myxoma, but can visualize a

Figure 37.1 Common location of cardiac tumors, masses, and tumorlike structures.

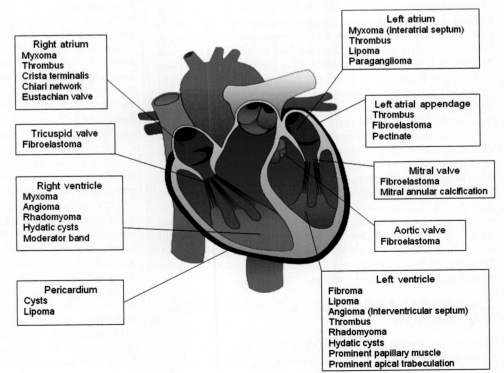

Right atrium
Myxoma
Thrombus
Crista terminalis
Chiari network
Eustachian valve

Tricuspid valve
Fibroelastoma

Right ventricle
Myxoma
Angioma
Rhadomyoma
Hydatic cysts
Moderator band

Pericardium
Cysts
Lipoma

Left atrium
Myxoma (interatrial septum)
Thrombus
Lipoma
Paraganglioma

Left atrial appendage
Thrombus
Fibroelastoma
Pectinate

Mitral valve
Fibroelastoma
Mitral annular calcification

Aortic valve
Fibroelastoma

Left ventricle
Fibroma
Lipoma
Angioma (Interventricular septum)
Thrombus
Rhadomyoma
Hydatic cysts
Prominent papillary muscle
Prominent apical trabeculation

TABLE 37.1
IMAGING FEATURES OF BENIGN CARDIAC TUMORS

Type of tumor	Echocardiographic features	CT features	MR features[a]
Myxoma	Mobile tumor connected by a narrow stalk	Heterogenous low attenuation	T1-low signal intensity T2-high signal intensity
Papillary fibroelastoma	Multiple fronds attached by small pedicle	Usually not seen	Usually not seen
Lipoma	Homogeneous, broad base, nonmobile	Homogeneous fat attenuation (low attenuation)	Homogeneous mass with T1-increased signal intensity; no enhancement
Rhadomyoma	Solid, hyperechoic mass, diffuse myocardial thickening	Hypodense on contrast CT	T1-isointense signal, similar to adjacent myocardium T2-hyperintense
Fibroma	Intramural, hetergeneous echogenic mass, calcified	Low attenuation, calcified	T1-isointense to hyperintense T2-homogeneous and hypointense
Angioma	No uniform echo features; echodense bulge of interventricular septum, multilobulated mass or unilocular mass with a cystic structure	Heterogeneous lesions on unenhanced CT, intensely enhanced with contrast	Increased vascularity with rapid enhancement during first pass gadolinium
			T1-intermdeiate signal intensity T2-hyperintense
Paraganglioma	Broad-based, ovoid, well circumscribed	Markedly enhanced on contrast enhanced CT, low attenuation	T1-hypoisotense T2-very hyperintense
Cysts	Pericardial cyst-cystic mass in pericardium Hydatid cyst- Spheroid mass with liquid content	Pericardial cyst-failure to enhance with contrast	Simple fluid with no enhancement after contrast T1-hypoisotense T2-hyperintense

[a]T1-, T1-weighted image; T2-, T2-weighted image.

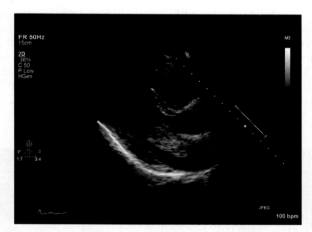

Figure 37.2 TTE long-axis view of myxoma prolapsing from the left atrium into the left ventricle.

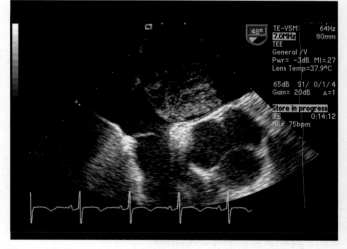

Figure 37.3 TEE short-axis view of a myxoma attached to the interatrial septum in the left ventricle.

narrow base attachment. Myxomas usually have heterogeneous low attenuation at CT. Heterogeneity is thought to reflect hemorrhage, necrosis, cyst formation, fibrosis, calcification, or ossification.[38] CT may occasionally show myxomas prolapsing through cardiac valves.

Cardiac-gated MRI demonstrates myxomas as spherical or ovoid, lobular masses of heterogeneous enhancement with intravenous gadolinium contrast. Myxomatous components appear low in signal intensity on T1-weighted images and high intensity

on T2-weighted images (Fig. 37.5, Movies 37.1 and 37.2). Cine images can demonstrate tumor motion and prolapse across the atrioventricular valve.

3.1.3. Therapeutic options
The treatment for myxoma is surgical resection. Once the diagnosis is made, surgery should be performed because of the possibility of obstructive complications, risk of sudden death and embolic

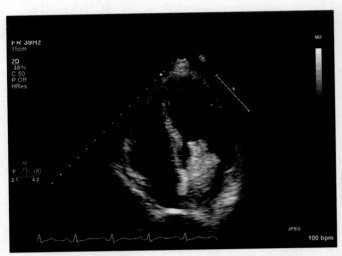

Figure 37.4 TTE apical four-chamber view of a myxoma attached to the interatrial septum. The myxoma is seen prolapsing into the left ventricle.

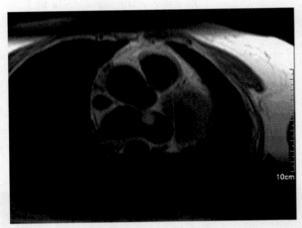

Figure 37.5 MRI T2-weighted image of a myxoma along intra-atrial septum; **Movie 37.1**: SSFP cine sequence; **Movie 37.2**: First pass gadolinium perfusion.

complications.[39] Surgical access and technique vary depending on the location of the myxoma. The operative mortality has been reported between 3% and 4%.[40,41] The long-term prognosis for patients with myxoma is excellent. Late reoccurrences have been reported in 0.4% to 5% of surgically treated patients up to 22 years after the initial operation.[31] Careful follow-up is indicated in patients with familial or syndrome myxoma, as the tumor reoccurrence may be as high as 21%.[42]

3.2. Papillary fibroelastomas

3.2.1. Clinical features

Cardiac papillary fibroelastomas (CPF) are benign tumors comprising 10% of all primary cardiac tumors.[43] They are usually found incidentally at autopsy, during heart surgery or echocardiography. CPF affect men and women equally, in patients with a mean age of 60 years.[44–46] About 80% to 90% of CPFs are found on valvular endocardium, most commonly the aortic and mitral valves.[47] A comprehensive analysis of 661 patients with CPF revealed that in 44% of cases the tumor was located on the aortic valve, followed by the mitral valve in 35%, the tricuspid valve in 15%, and the pulmonary valve in 8%.[48] CPFs

are usually found on the atrial side on the atrioventricular valve and can be found on either side on semilunar valves. CPFs can be located on various parts of the cusps including the free edge, closing margin, or on the body of the cusps. CPFs have been reported to originate from a variety of locations within the heart including the left ventricle,[49–51] the ostium of the right coronary artery,[52,53] the ostium of the left coronary artery,[54] the left atrial appendage,[55,54] atrial septum,[56,57] ventricular septum,[58,59,46] right atrium,[60,61] right ventricle,[62] left ventricular outflow tract,[63] Eustachian valve and Chiari network,[64] right atrial appendage,[65] and right ventricular outflow tract.[66]

CPF have a characteristic frondlike appearance and resemble a sea anemone, especially when placed in saline. They are avascular papillomas. Most CPFs are less than 20 mm in diameter.[67] Though most CPFs are asymptomatic, neurological events,[68–71] sudden death,[49,72] angina,[73] acute myocardial infarction,[74–76] pulmonary emboli,[77] and retinal artery embolism[78] related to CPF have been reported.

3.2.2. Diagnostic imaging

Most CPFs are usually discovered by echocardiography. Tumors appear round, oval, or irregular, but are well demarcated and homogenous in appearance (Figs. 37.6 and 37.7, Movie 37.3). They are mobile, pedunculated masses with small stalks that flutter or prolapse with cardiac motion. There may be stippling around the perimeter that correlates with papillary surface projections.[46] Because of their small size and high mobility, small CPFs are not usually seen on CT but larger CPFs may be visualized (Fig. 37.8). MRI can demonstrate a mass on the endocardial surface or a valve leaflet. Valvular CPFs can result in turbulence of blood flow which can be seen with cine MR.[79]

3.2.3. Therapeutic options

There is controversy about the management of CPFs. Some suggest that CPFs should be resected even in asymptomatic patients[80] while others recommend that small asymptomatic left-sided tumors should be observed, whereas larger mobile tumors are excised especially in young patients with low cardiovascular surgical risk and high risk of embolization.[67] For right-sided tumors, only symptomatic tumors should be excised.[81]

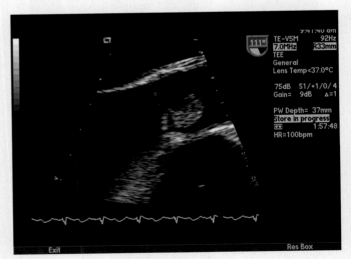

Figure 37.6 Movie 37.3. TEE long-axis view demonstrating a fibroelastoma on the aortic valve.

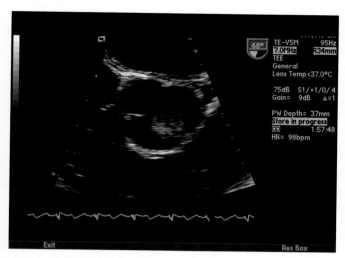

Figure 37.7 TEE short-axis of the aortic valve demonstrating a fibroelastoma on the left coronary cusp.

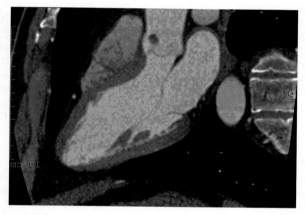

Figure 37.8 Contrast-enhanced CT demonstrating a fibroelastoma on the aortic valve.

3.3. Lipomas

3.3.1. Clinical features

Cardiac lipomas are rare, benign neoplasms composed of adipose tissue. They account for only 10% of all primary cardiac tumors and 14% of benign cardiac tumors.[82] Lipomas occur with equal frequency in both sexes and occur at all ages. Lipomas are more common in obese persons and often increase in size during a period of rapid weight gain.[83] They are thought to originate either from the subendocardium, subpericardium, or from the myocardium. Cardiac lipomas have been divided into lipomatous hypertrophy in the atrial septum and true lipomas. True lipomas are less frequent and can occur anywhere in the heart including the pericardial space. The left ventricle and left atrium are the most commonly involved chambers.[84] Half of the lipomas arise subendocardially, one-quarter arise subepicardially and the rest are intramyocardial.[85]

Lipomas are polypoid or sessile masses. Lipomatous hypertrophy in the atrial septum is continuous with the epicardial fat and consists of a noncapsulated mass of adipose tissue. True lipomas are encapsulated adipose tissue. In true lipomas, myocytes are not seen throughout the tumor, as they are in lipomatous hypertrophy of the intra-atrial septum. Lipomas are mostly asymptomatic. When lipomas are subpericardial, the location allows some to reach an enormous size altering ventricular function and causing

symptoms such as angina and dsypnea on exertion.[86] Intramyocardially located lipomas can interfere with the conduction system and may cause arrhythmias.

3.3.2. Diagnostic imaging

TTE, TEE, CT, and MR are all helpful in identifying true cardiac lipomas. TTE and TEE typically demonstrate an echogenic, nonmobile mass.[87] The TTE/TEE appearance of a lipoma varies with location. Lipomas in the pericardial space vary in echogenicity from hypoechoic to hyperechoic.[87-89] Intracavitary lipomas are usually homogeneous and hyperechoic.[90] The affected myocardium is usually hypokinetic.[91]

Both CT and MR are accurate in the diagnosis of cardiac lipoma.[92] CT and MR can exactly predict the intramyocardial extent and the relationship to other cardiac structures.[93] Additionally, both can identify fat with a high degree of specificity and therefore, accurately establish the diagnosis of a lipoma. In cardiac CT lipomas appear as low attenuation (−100 Hounsfield unit) homogenous masses.[90] They can demonstrate interposed soft tissue septa or scattered strands of higher attenuation tissue.[94,95] MRI shows lipomas as homogenous masses with increased signal intensity on T1-weighted images (Fig. 37.9). Cardiac lipomas do not enhance with contrast material.

3.3.3. Therapeutic options

Cardiac lipomas are generally incidental findings and in most cases, require no treatment or surgical intervention. However,

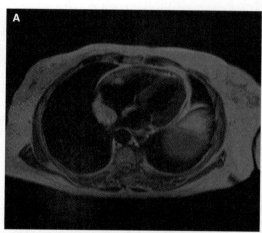

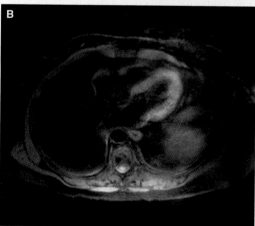

Figure 37.9 A: MR T1-weighted image of a subpericardial lipoma. **B:** Triple inversion recovery image (fat suppression).

when they cause symptoms surgical resection is recommended. Patients undergoing surgical resection generally have an excellent outcome.[96]

3.4. Rhabdomyomas

3.4.1. Clinical features

Cardiac rhabdomyoma is the most common benign cardiac tumor in infants, but in adults it is very rare. Rhabdomyomas represent up to 90% of cardiac tumors in infants and children, and are usually discovered in patients less than 1 year of age.[97] They are benign myocardial hamartomas, and in about 50% are associated with tuberous sclerosis.[98]

Rhabdomyomas show pathological features of cardiac striated muscle tumors.

They are firm, white, well-circumscribed, lobulated nodules that occur in any location in the heart, but are more common in the ventricles. The tumors usually invade the ventricular myocardium or ventricular septum but occasionally protrude into the left ventricular space or freely moving mass.[99] The tumors may be multiple (rhabdomyomatosis), measuring less than 1 mm in diameter. Single tumors may also measure up to 10 cm, with an average size of 3 to 4 cm.[3]

Although the tumor is benign, rhabdomyoma can present as right ventricular outflow tract obstruction, congestive heart failure, murmur, tachyarrhythmia, or sudden death. In addition, it can also cause pre-excitation syndrome.[100,101] Only a few adult cases with cardiac rhabdomyoma have been reported in the literature.[102,103]

3.4.2. Diagnostic imaging

Rhabdomyomas appear as solid hyperechoic masses on echo. Diffuse myocardial thickening with small, multiple lesions are also seen.[104] Echo can demonstrate small (<0.5 cm) or entirely intramural lesions.[105] MRI assessment of these tumors can be extremely helpful. MR may allow better definition of tumor margins and may help demonstrate individual lesions. The tumors appear as isointense on T1-weighted images, which is similar to adjacent myocardium, and hyperintense on T2-weighted images.[106] CT with contrast can demonstrate tumors attached to the interventricular septum.

3.4.3. Therapeutic options

Because majority of cardiac rhabdomyomas regress spontaneously, surgery is not necessary. When they are associated with life-threatening symptoms, surgery is often necessary. The biologic behavior of adult cardiac rhabdomyoma is clearly not known. For this reason, long-term prognosis is uncertain and these patients should be followed up.[107]

3.5. Fibromas

3.5.1. Clinical features

Cardiac fibroma is a congenital neoplasm, and is the second most common benign cardiac tumor in infants and children.[97] However, approximately 15% of cardiac fibromas occur in adolescents and adults.[45,91,108] The mean age of affected patients is 13 years, with an age range of 0 to 56 years.[91] There is an increased risk of cardiac fibromas in patients with Gorlin (basal cell nevus) syndrome, which is characterized by multiple nevoid basal cell carcinomas of the skin, jaw cysts, and bifid ribs. About 14% of these patients have cardiac fibromas.[109]

Cardiac fibromas are typically solitary, intramural tumors with a predilection for the left ventricular free wall or interventricular septum. The tumors range in size from 2 to 10 cm. They are round, bulging, well-circumscribed tumors that can extend into or obliterate the chamber. Calcification is common.[91] Fibromas tend to grow rapidly.

One-third of patients with cardiac fibromas are asymptomatic, and their tumors are discovered because of a cardiac murmur detected during physical examination or chest radiography.[110,91] Depending on the size and location, cardiac fibomas may be symptomatic and can possibly result in heart failure, arrhythmias, or sudden death. Invasion or compression of the cardiac conduction system resulting in arrhythmia is considered to be the cause of death in most patients who die with this tumor. It is the second most common primary cardiac tumor associated with sudden death.[111]

3.5.2. Diagnostic imaging

TTE and TEE can reveal a heterogeneous echogenic mass with possible calcifications. The affected myocardium is usually hypocontractile.[112,91] The fibroma can appear as a solid mass in a ventricular wall or may mimic focal hypertrophic cardiomyopathy[113,110] or hypertrophy of the ventricular septum.[114] CT of these tumors demonstrate a mural mass. The fibroma may appear homogeneous with soft-tissue attenuation that may be sharply marginated or infiltrative.[115] CT is highly sensitivity for the detection of tumor calcification (Fig. 37.10).[91] MRI demonstrate a discrete mural mass or focal myocardial thickening. Because of the fibrous composition of the tumor, it is usually homogeneous and hypointense on T2-weighted images and isointense to hyperintense relative to the myocardium on T1-weighted images (Fig. 37.11, Movies 37.4 and 37.5).[116,117,91]

3.5.3. Therapeutic options

Surgery is the optimal treatment in patients with symptomatic, resectable tumors. The prognosis after complete resection is excellent. However, depending on the size and location of the tumor, incomplete resection or single-ventricle palliation as a bridge to heart transplantation may be necessary.[118] Partial resection can result in long-term relief of symptoms. The surgical outcome is less favorable in patients with large masses, severe heart failure at initial presentation, or recurrent arrhythmias.[108] Unresectable cardiac fibromas have been successfully treated by transplantation.

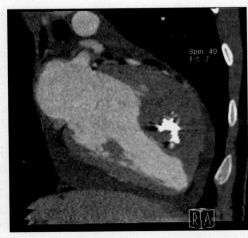

Figure 37.10 CT scan showing a fibroma with central calcification.

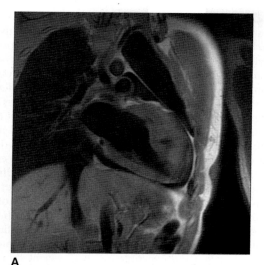

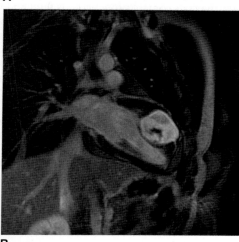

Figure 37.11 A: MR T1-weighted image of a fibroma. **B**: Delayed gadolinium enhancement; **Movie 37.4**: Cine SSFP long-axis image; **Movie 37.5**: First-pass gadolinium perfusion sequence.

3.6. Angiomas

3.6.1. Clinical features

Composed of benigned proliferation of endothelial cells, lymphangiomas and hemangiomas are rare tumors of the heart. Cardiac lymphangioma is an extremely rare tumor mainly discovered during childhood. They can occur anywhere in the heart or in the pericardium. Presenting symptoms include congestive heart failure, syncope, arrhythmia, palpitations, or cardiac tamponade.[119,120]

Hemangiomas of the heart account for only 2% to 3% of all benign primary cardiac tumors.[121] Cardiac hemangiomas (including capillary, venous, racemose, and cavernous histological subtypes) occur in persons of all ages, with a mean presenting age of 43 years with a slight male predominance.[122] Hemangiomas are red, hemorrhagic, generally sessile or polypoid subendocardial nodules, ranging from 2 to 4 cm in diameter. They can be pericardial, intramyocardial, or subendocardial in location.[123]

Within the heart they may occur in any part, but more commonly are found in the lateral wall of the left ventricle (21%), the anterior wall of the right ventricle (21%), or the interventricular septum (17%).[124] Hemangiomas are usually intramural, but they may also protrude intraluminally.

Although cardiac hemangiomas are often asymptomatic, the main symptoms include dyspnea, palpitation, atypical chest pain, and arrhythmia. When intramural they are often in the interventricular septum or AV node. where they can cause complete heart block and sudden death. Other symptoms may result from compression of surrounding structures, obstruction of the outflow tracts, pericardial effusion (which may be hemorrhagic), or embolization.[125] Cardiac hemangiomas can occur in the clinical setting of Kasabach–Merritt syndrome, which is characterized by multiple systemic hemangiomas associated with recurrent thrombocytopenia and consumptive coagulopathy.[124]

3.6.2. Diagnostic imaging

The diagnosis of cardiac angiomas can be made by TTE, TEE, CT, or MR. TTE is an accurate and reliable tool for visualization of angiomas. Cardiac hemangioma was visualized with TTE in 81% of cases in a review of 23 cases reported in the literature.[124] Angiomas appear as hyperechoic lesions on TTE. Because they are vascular tumors, myocardial contrast echocardiography has been particularly helpful in identifying their vascular nature.[126,127] CT and MR can evaluate the dimensions and invasiveness of the tumor. Cardiac hemangiomas appear as heterogeneous lesions on unenhanced CT and, in most cases, intensely enhance on CT performed after contrast administration. Cardiac hemangiomas typically demonstrate intermediate signal intensity on T1-weighted images and become hyperintense on T2-weighted images.[128] Finally, it should be mentioned that coronary angiography is sometimes useful in revealing how the tumor is fed and its characteristic tumor blush.[124]

3.6.3. Therapeutic options

Angiomas can be successfully excised. Surgery is the optimal treatment in patients with symptomatic tumors. The long-term prognosis after resection in patients with symptomatic tumors is excellent.[124] Spontaneous regression of a cardiac hemangioma has been reported.[129] Therefore, surgery may not always be necessary particular in patients with extensive and difficult to resect tumors who are asymptomatic.

3.7. Paragangliomas

3.7.1. Clinical features

Cardiac paragangliomas are extremely rare neoplasms with fewer than 50 cases reported in the medical literature.[130] They arise from intrinsic cardiac paraganglial (chromaffin) cells that lie adjacent to sympathetic fibers innervating the heart or ectopic chromaffin cells.[131] Patients range in age from 18 to 85 years, but are typically younger adults with a mean age of 40 years.[132] Cardiac paragangliomas are large, poorly circumscribed masses that typically measure 2 to 14 cm in their greatest dimension. They are most commonly located on the epicardial surface of the roof of the left atrium, with less common locations including the right atrium, interatrial septum, and rarely, the ventricles.[3] It is referred to as pheochromocytoma or chemodectoma when the tumor is functionally active.

Although hypertension represents the most common clinical presentation, functional tumors may also cause symptoms related to catecholamine excess, including palpitations, headache, sweating, and flushing.[133,132] Constitutional symptoms, chest pain, heart failure, mitral insufficiency, embolic phenomenon, hypertensive crisis, and compressive or obstructive symptoms have also been reported.[134,132] The biochemical laboratory abnormalities that lead to the diagnosis of a paraganglioma include elevated levels of urinary norepinephrine, vanelylmandelic acid, and total metanephrine or elevated levels of plasma norepinephrine and epinephrine.[133]

3.7.2. Diagnostic imaging

Once excess plasma or urinary catecholamines or their metabolites are demonstrated, TTE, TEE, CT, and MR have been used to successfully localize the tumor. At TTE/TEE, a paraganglioma can appear as large echogenic mass usually in the left atrium and rarely in the interatrial septum. It is usually broad based and firm appearing.[135] At CT, paragangliomas appear as well circumscribed, heterogeneous masses with low attenuation.[115] On contrast-enhanced CT the mass is markedly enhanced and likely seen adherent to or involving the left atrium.[136,133] Some of these lesions have central areas of low attenuation likely representing areas of necrosis. MRI typically demonstrates a mass that is hypointense on T1-weighted images and very hyperintense on T2-weighted images.[137] MR easily demonstrates the relationship of paraganglioma to cardiovascular structures.[138]

3.7.3. Therapeutic options

Treatment consists of complete surgical resection of the paraganglioma. Since most tumors are benign, most patients with complete resection have a good long-term prognosis.[132] However, because these tumors are highly vascular and frequently supplied by the coronary arteries, complete resection is often technically difficult. Patients may require extensive cardiac reconstruction, cardiac autotransplantation, or orthotopic cardiac transplantation.[139,140]

3.8. Cysts

3.8.1. Clinical features

Cysts are occasionally found within the heart and pericardium. The most common cysts are pericardial cysts, echinococcal (hydatid) cysts, and blood cysts.

Pericardial cysts are uncommon intrathoracic developmental abnormalities, occurring in 1/100,000 persons.[7] Cysts are more common in men than women (61.5% vs. 38.5%).[141] Cysts are unilocular, round, or ellipsoid. The fluid is transudate. Blood supply comes from the pericardium. The size of the cyst varies from 2 to 3 cm to as large as 28 cm.[142] Pericardial cysts are typically extremely slow growing.[143] Pericardial cysts are usually found at the right costophrenic angle, although they may occur anywhere in the mediastinum. The most common symptoms that patients present with are chest pain dyspnea and coughing in approximately one-third of the patients.[144] Other signs and symptoms include atelectasis, venous obstruction, retrosternal pain, pulse alterations, palpitations, and pain at the cardiac apex, fullness, and difficulty eating.[7]

Cardiac hydatid cysts are intracardiac cysts that arise from the larval stage of the echinococcus parasite. Intracardiac cysts account for less than 2% of all hydatid disease, and invade the myocardium by the coronary circulation. During the early stages, the disease is asymptomatic and may be discovered accidentally. Hydatid cysts grow slowly but continuously and increase in volume. The most common presenting symptoms include chest pain and dyspnea on exertion. Cysts size ranges from 1.8 to 11 cm in diameter, and are found in the left ventricular free wall, the interventricular septum, the right ventricle, and the pericardium. Intracardiac rupture, dysrhythmia, and emboli are common and can result in death.[8]

Blood cysts though common findings at infant autopsy are extremely rare in adults and only a few prospective series are available. Blood cysts are presumed congenital cysts typically found on the lines of closure of the valvular endocardium.[145,9]

3.8.2. Diagnostic imaging

TTE is an excellent noninvasive modality to delineate the exact location of a pericardial cyst and to differentiate a cyst from other potential diagnoses such as a prominent fat pad, left ventricular aneurysm, prominent left atrial appendage, aortic aneurysm, and solid tumors. Color and spectral Doppler can help in differentiating a pericardial cyst from other vascular structures such as a coronary aneurysm.[146] A common TTE appearance is that of a cystic mass behind the right atrium. Cysts may also be located in other locations within the pericadium (Fig. 37.12). Characteristic CT findings of the pericardial cyst are failure of the lesion to enhance with intravenous contrast and attenuation value compatible with a cystic lesion.[147] However, some pericardial cysts may not appear cystic on a CT scan when the attenuation exceeds that of water, and confirmation by percutaneous cyst aspiration may be necessary.[143] MRI demonstrates the characteristics of simple fluid and no enhancement after contrast. The cysts are usually hypotense on T1-weighted images and hyperintense on T2-weighted images.[148] Occasionally, the cysts contain proteinaceous fluid and therefore, have high signal intensity on both T1- and T2-weighted images.[149]

Cardiac hydatid cysts on TTE appear as spheroid masses of liquid content with a well-contrasted capsule. TTE is able to identify the location of the cyst, extension into other cavities, any obstruction to flow, and any deformation of valves. Additionally, echo can demonstrate honeycomb appearance of multiple hydatid cysts. CT can demonstrate cardiopericarial hydatid cysts, but generally adds little to the overall diagnosis value than echocardiography. MRI is helpful in determining extracardiac extension of the cysts. It is more reliable than CT in the diagnosis.[8,150]

Blood cysts on TTE appear as well-circumscribed masses with thin walls and an echolucent core. TTE and TEE are excellent modalities for anatomic definition (Fig. 37.13, Movies 37.6 and 37.7).[145,151,9] MRI can assess the contents of cyst and differentiate it from myxoma, other neoplasms, or thrombus.

3.8.3. Therapeutic options

Pericardial cysts are usually associated with an excellent long-term prognosis.[144] Surgical excision of pericardial cysts is recommended in symptomatic patients, while asymptomatic cases are managed conservatively with a close follow-up.[152] Minimally invasive thoracoscopic resection of a pericardial cyst is a good alternative option to open surgical resection because it minimizes surgical trauma and postoperative pain, has a shorter recovery period and a better

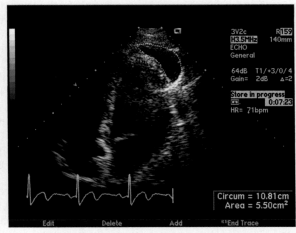

Figure 37.12 A pericardial cyst measuring 5.5 cm² is seen at the lateral apex of the left ventricle.

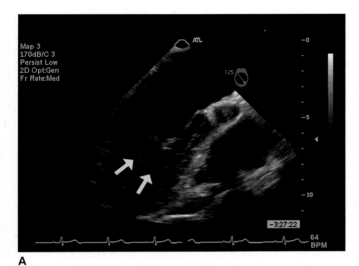

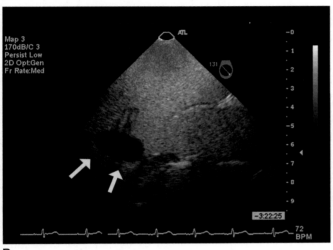

Figure 37.13 Blood cyst. **A**: TEE 2-chamber view demonstrating a blood cyst attached to the mitral valve chordae (**Movie 37.6**). **B**: Echo contrast is given to establish absent blood flow within the cyst (**Movie 37.7**).

cosmetic outcome.[153] Percutaneous aspiration of cyst contents is another alternative to surgical resection in symptomatic patients. A 3-year follow-up study of post percutaneous resection showed no recurrence in four out of six patients.[143] Spontaneous resolution of a pericardial cyst has been reported in few cases managed conservatively, the probable mechanism being cyst rupture.[154,155]

Surgical resection should be considered in every diagnosed case of cardiac hydatid cyst. Surgeons should proceed in cyst sterilization before removal. Medical treatment with albendazole or mebendazol alone or in combination with surgery should be always considered in an effort to prevent recurrences as well as accidental contamination during surgery.[156]

Because blood cysts are so rare, consensus is also lacking concerning appropriate treatment. Careful echocardiographic monitoring of the cysts for change in size and for the assessment of change in cardiac function may be appropriate. Removal may be indicated when the cysts are noted to cause cardiac dysfunction.[157,9]

3.9. Thrombi

3.9.1. Clinical features

Intracardiac thrombi are associated with a variety of diseases. Functional disorders such as myocardial infarction or atrial

fibrillation are a common cause of cardiac thrombi.[158,159] Most thrombi develop within the first week after the infarction, and are most often noted at the apex of the left ventricle in patients who have had an anterior myocardial infarction.[158] In atrial fibrillation the thrombus is usually located in the left atrial appendage. Deep vein thrombosis or the use of central venous catheters may lead to the development of thrombi in the right heart.[160,161] Several disorders and diseases such as Behçet syndrome, coagulopathies, Löffler endocarditis, and Churg–Strauss syndrome are also potential causes of intracardiac thrombi.[162,163,164]

3.9.2. Diagnostic imaging

TEE/TEE is an excellent diagnostic imaging modality for the detection of cardiac thrombus. With the addition of echo contrast, most thrombi can be identified within the cardiac chambers (Fig. 37.14). TEE is considered the reference standard modality for detecting left atrial appendage thrombi (Fig. 37.15). TEE offers high-resolution images of the left atrium and its appendage. Additionally, TEE can visualize thrombi on catheters and pacemakers within the heart that may not be seen by transthoracic echo. Multidetector CT has high spatial resolution, and is therefore, another tool for detecting intracardiac thrombus (Fig. 37.16). However, presence of slow flow may be often misdiagnosed as LA appendage thrombi

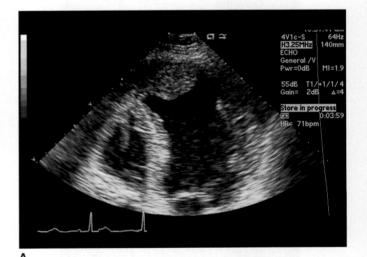

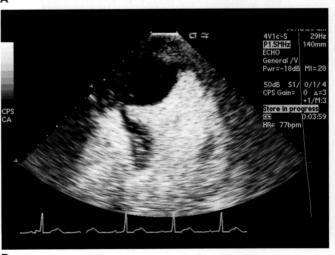

Figure 37.14 **A**: Apical four-chamber view with apical thrombus. **B**: After echo contrast.

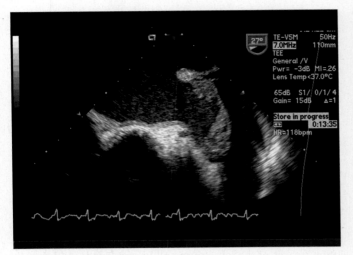

Figure 37.15 TEE of left atrial appendage. Thrombi are seen adherent to appendage wall.

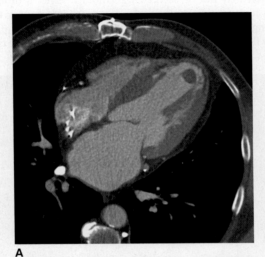

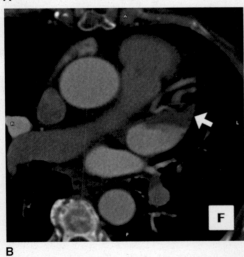

Figure 37.16 Thrombi detected by CT. **A:** Left ventricular thrombus. **B:** Left atrial appendage thrombus.

on contrast-enhanced CT studies. Additonally, a small intracardiac thrombus may be difficult to diagnose by CT because of motion artifacts. MRI can accurately image cardiac thrombi in all the chambers of the heart. MR appears to have greater sensitivity than echocardiography and similarly high specificity for the detection

of intracardiac thrombus in the left ventricle.[165,166] The signal intensity characteristics of the thrombus vary at MRI depending on the age of the thrombus. Acute thrombus will appear bright on both T1- and T2-weighted images. Subacute thrombus will appear bright on T1-weighted images with low-signal-intensity areas on T2-weighted images. Chronic organized thrombus will have low-signal-intensity areas on both T1- and T2-weighted images. With gadolinium contrast the thrombus should not enhance as compared to a tumor.[167]

3.9.3. Therapeutic options

Anticoagulation therapy is the usual treatment for intracardiac thrombi to prevent systemic embolization. Surgical resection can be performed in highly mobile thrombi that have an extremely high risk of systemic embolization.[168]

4. NORMAL ANATOMICAL VARIANTS

Numerous normal anatomical variants exist that can be confused with cardiac masses and tumors. In the left ventricle, prominent or calcified papillary muscles and dense mitral annular calcification can mimic abnormal pathology (Fig. 37.17). Mitral annular calcification is a common echocardiographic finding (Fig. 37.18). Caseous calcification is a rare variant seen as a large mass with echolucencies that resembles a tumor.[20] Additionally, prominent apical trabeculations can also be confused with tumors. Though both apical hypertrophic cardiomyopathy and left ventricular noncompaction are diseases and not normal variants, they should be mentioned in the context of findings in the left ventricle that may appear as an apical mass. A dilated coronary sinus can mimic a left atrial mass. Occasionally, multiple lobes of the left atrial appendage can be confused with mass lesions in the main pulmonary artery. Pectinate muscles in the appendage can mimic thrombus (Fig. 37.19).[169] The prominent moderator band in the right ventricle can appear as a right ventricular mass. Crista terminalis is a fibromuscular ridge that extends between the right sides of the superior and inferior caval orifices. It can mimic a right atrial mass.[170] Other normal structures in the right atrium that can mimic cardiac masses include remnants of the Chiari network and Eustachian valve (Fig. 37.20).

5. FUTURE DIRECTIONS

Benign primary cardiac tumors are rare but are extremely important to diagnosis. It is important to integrate all the clinical information provided including age, past medical history, and presenting symptoms. Using TTE and TEE, CT, or MR alone or in combination can accurately characterize larger masses, but TEE

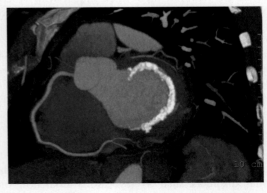

Figure 37.17 CT image of severe mitral annular calcification.

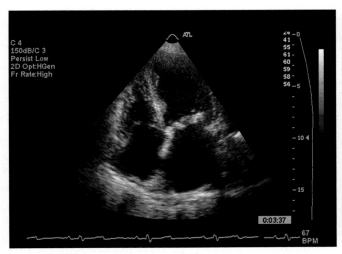 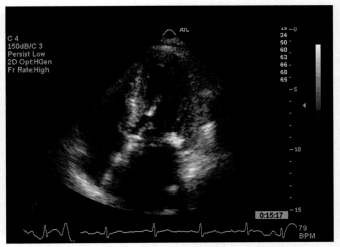

Figure 37.18 TTE apical four-chamber view of mitral annular calcification shown in systole (left panel) and diastole (right panel).

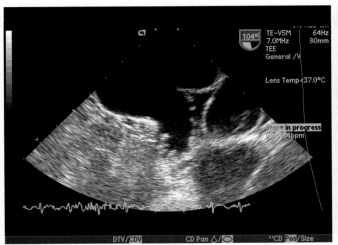 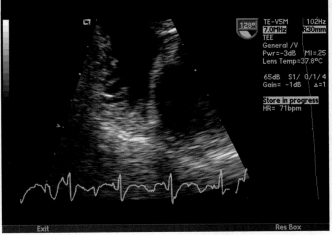

Figure 37.19 TEE images of the left atrial appendage. Prominent pectinate muscles in the appendage can mimic thrombus.

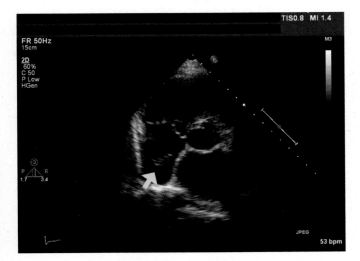

Figure 37.20 TTE parasternal short-axis image of a prominent Chiari network in the right atrium, which can mimic a cardiac mass.

and TEE are superior in detecting smaller mobile masses due their greater spatial and temporal resolution. With the advent of real-time 3D echocardiography, the ability to detect characterize benign tumors may increase in the future. It is important to be familiar with the strengths and limitations of all these imaging modalities as well as the clinical features of these tumors and masses. This knowledge will provide an accurate and expedient diagnosis leading to appropriate treatment if necessary.

REFERENCES

1. McAllister HA, Fenoglio JJ. Tumors of the cardiovascular system. In: Hartman WH, Cowan WR, eds. *Atlas of Tumor Pathology*. 2nd series, Fasc 15. Washington, D.C.: Armed Forces Institute of Pathology; 1978:1–3.
2. Reynen K. Frequency of primary tumors of the heart. *Am J Cardiol*. 1996;77:107.
3. Burke A, Virmani R. Tumors of the heart and great vessels. *Atlas of Tumor Pathology*. 3rd series. Armed Forces Institute of Pathology; 1996.
4. Hanson EC. Cardiac tumors: A current perspective perspective. *NY State Med*. 1992;92:41.
5. Silverman NA. Primary cardiac tumors. *Ann Surg*. 1980;191:127–138.
6. McAllister HA, Fenoglio JJ. Tumors of the cardiovascular system. In: Hartman WH, Cowan WR, eds. *Atlas of Tumor Pathology*. Second Series, Fascicle 15. Washington, DC: Armed Forces Institute of Pathology; 1978:1–3.
7. Roover PD, Maisin J, Lacquet A. Congenital pleural pericardial cysts. *Thorax*. 1963;18:146–150.

8. Ben-Hamda K, Maatouk F, Ben-Farhat M, et al. Eighteen year experience with Echinococcosus of the heart clinical and echocardiographic features in 14 patients. *Int J Cardiol.* 2003;91:145–151.
9. Sim EKW, Wong ML, Tan TK, et al. Blood cyst of the tricuspid valve. *Ann Thorac Surg.* 1996;61:1012–1013.
10. Asinger R, Mikell R, Elsperger J, et al. Incidence of left ventricular thrombosis after acute transmural myocardial infarction. *N Engl J Med.* 1981;305:297–302.
11. Chiarella F, Santoro E, Domenicucci S, et al. Predischarge two-dimensional echocardiographic evaluation of left ventricular thrombosis after acute myocardial infarction in the GISSI-3 study. *Am J Cardiol.* 1998;81:822–877.
12. Leung DY, Black IW, Cranney GB, et al. Prognostic implications of left atrial spontaneous echo contrast in nonvalvular atrial fibrillation. *J Am Coll Cardiol.* 1994;24:755–762.
13. Black IW, Chesterman CN, Hopkins AP, et al. Hematologic correlates of left atrial spontaneous echo contrast and thromboembolism in nonvalvular atrial fibrillation. *J Am Coll Cardiol.* 1993;21:451–457.
14. Fatkin D, Kelly RP, Feneley MP. Relations between left atrial appendage blood flow velocity, spontaneous echocardiographic contrast and thromboembolic risk in vivo. *J Am Coll Cardiol.* 1994;23:961–969.
15. Manning WJ, Silverman DI, Keighley CS, et al. Transesophageal echocardiographically facilitated early cardioversion from atrial fibrillation using short-term anticoagulation: Final results of a prospective 4.5-year study. *J Am Coll Cardiol.* 1995;25:1354–1361.
16. Stoddard MF, Dawkins PR, Prince CR, et al. Left atrial appendage thrombus is not uncommon in patients with acute atrial fibrillation and a recent embolic event: A transesophageal echocardiographic study. *J Am Coll Cardiol.* 1995;25:452–459.
17. Chapoutot L, Nazeyrollas P, Metz D, et al. Floating right heart thrombi and pulmonary embolism: Diagnosis, outcome and therapeutic management. *Cardiology.* 1996;87:169–174.
18. Casazza F, Bongarzoni A, Centonze F, et al. Prevalence and prognostic significance of right-sided cardiac mobile thrombi in acute massive pulmonary embolism. *Am J Cardiol.* 1997;79:1433–1435.
19. Pomerance A. Pathological and clinical study of calcification of the mitral valve ring. *J Clin Pathol.* 1970;23:354–361.
20. Harpaz D, Auerbach I, Vered Z, et al. Caseous calcification of the mitral annulus: A neglected, unrecognised diagnosis. *J Am Soc Echocardiogr.* 2001;14:825–831.
21. Sabatine MS, Colucci WS, Schoen FJ. Primary tumors of the heart. In: Zipes DP, Libby P, Bonow RO, et al, eds. *Braunwald's Heart Disease.* 7th Ed. Philadelphia, PA: Elsevier; 2041–755.
22. Keeling IM, Oberwalder P, Anelli-Monti M, et al. Cardiac myxomas: 24 years of experience in 49 patients. *Eur J Cardiothorac Surg.* 2002;22:971–977.
23. Chakfe N, Kretz JG, Valentin P, et al. Clinical presentation and treatment options for mitral valve myxoma. *Ann Thorac Surg.* 1997;64:872–877.
24. Reynen K. Cardiac myxomas. *N Engl J Med.* 1996;333:1610–1617.
25. Johansson L. Histogenesis of cardiac myxomas. An immunohistochemical study of 19 cases including some with glandular structures and review of the literature. *Arch Pathol Lab Med.* 1989;113(7):735–741.
26. Peters MN, Hall RJ, Cooley DA, et al. The clinical syndrome of atrial myxoma. *JAMA.* 1974;230:695–701.
27. Kaminsky ME, Ehlers KH, Engle MA, et al. Atrial myxoma mimicking a collagen disorder. *Chest.* 1979;75:93–95.
28. Cohen AI, McIntosh HD, Orgain ES. The mimetic nature of left atrial myxomas: Report of a case presenting as a severe systemic illness and simulating massive mitral insufficiency at cardiac catheterization. *Am J Cardiol.* 1963;11:802–807.
29. Huston KA, Combs JJ Jr, Lie JT, et al. Left atrial myxoma simulating peripheral vasculitis. *Mayo Clin Proc.* 1978;53:752–756.
30. Thomas MH. Myxoma masquerading as polyarteritis nodosa. *J Rheumatol.* 1981;8:133–137.
31. Castells E, Ferran V, Octavio de Toledo MC, et al. Cardiac myxomas: Surgical treatment, long-term results and recurrence. *J Cardiovasc Surg Torino.* 1993;34:49–53.
32. Chakfe N, Kretz JG, Valentin P, et al. Clinical presentation and treatment options for mitral valve myxoma. *Ann Thorac Surg.* 1997;64:872–877.
33. Vassiliadis N, Vassiliadis K, Karkavelas G. Sudden death due to cardiac myxoma. *Med Sci Law.* 1997;37:76–78.
34. Cilliers AM, van Unen H, Lala S, et al. Massive biatrial myxomas in a child. *Pediatr Cardiol.* 1999;20:150–151.
35. DePace NL, Soulen RL, Kotler MN, et al. Two dimensional echocardiographic detection of intraatrial masses. *Am J Cardiol.* 1981;48:954–960.
36. Braunwald E. *Heart Disease: A Textbook of Cardiovascular Medicine.* 6th Ed. Philadelphia, PA: WB Saunders Co.; 2001.
37. Masses, tumors, and source of embolus. In: Feigenbaum H, Armstrong WF, Ryan T, eds. *Feigenbaum's Echocardiography.* 6th Ed. Philadelphia, PA: Lippincott Williams & Wilkins; 2005:701–733.
38. Tsuchiya F, Kohno A, Saitoh R, et al. CT findings of atrial myxoma. *Radiology.* 1984;151:139–143.
39. Livi U, Bortolotti U. Milano A, et al. Cardiac myxomas: Results of 14 years' experience. *Thorac Cardiovasc Surg.* 1984;32:143–147.
40. Lad VS, Jain J, Agarwala S, et al. Right atrial trans-septal approach for left atrial myxomas – nine-year experience. *Heart Lung Circ.* 2006;15:38–43.
41. Ipek G, Erentug V, Bozbuga N, et al. Surgical management of cardiac myxoma. *J Card Surg.* 2005;20:300–304.
42. Van Gelder M, O'Brien DJ, Staples ED, et al. Familial cardiac myxoma. *Ann Thorac Surg.* 1992;552:419–424.
43. Sastre-Garriga J, Molina C, Montaner J, et al. Mitral papillary fibroelastoma as a cause of cardiogenic embolic stroke: Report of two cases and review of the literature. *Eur J Neurol.* 2000;7(4):449–453.
44. Edwards FH, Hale D, Cohen A, et al. Primary cardiac valve tumors. *Ann Thorac Surg.* 1991;52:1127–1131.
45. Tazelaar HD, Locke TJ, McGregor CG. Pathology of surgically excised primary cardiac tumors. *Mayo Clin Proc.* 1992;67:957–965.
46. Klarich KW, Enriquez-Sarano M, Gura GM, et al. Papillary fibroelastoma: Echocardiographic characteristics for the diagnosis and pathologic correlation. *J Am Coll Cardiol.* 1997;30:784–790.
47. Koji T, Fujioka M, Imai H, et al. Infected papillary fibroelastoma attached to the atrial septum. *Circ J.* 2002;66(3):305–307.
48. Gowda RM, Khan IA, Nair CK, et al. Cardiac papillary fibroelastoma: A comprehensive analysis of 725 cases. *Am Heart J.* 2003;146:404–410.
49. Cha SD, Incarvito J, Fernandez J, et al. Giant Lambl's excrescences of papillary muscle and aortic valve: Echocardiographic, angiographic, and pathologic findings. *Clin Cardiol.* 1981;4:51–54.
50. de Menezes IC, Fragata J, Martins FM. Papillary fibroelastoma of the mitral valve in a 3-year-old child: Case report. *Pediatr Cardiol.* 1996;17:194–195.
51. Espada R, Talwalker NG, Wilcox G, et al. Visualization of ventricular fibroelastoma with a video-assisted thoracoscope. *Ann Thorac Surg.* 1997;63:221–223.
52. Rona G, Feeney N, Kahn DS. Fibroelastic hamartoma of the aortic valve producing ischemic heart disease. Associated pulmonary glomus bodies. *Am J Cardiol.* 1963;12:869–874.
53. Prahlow JA, Barnard JJ. Sudden death due to obstruction of coronary artery ostium by aortic valve papillary fibroelastoma. *Am J Forensic Med Pathol.* 1998;19:162–165.
54. Howard RA, Aldea GS, Shapira OM, et al. Papillary fibroelastoma: Increasing recognition of a surgical disease. *Ann Thorac Surg.* 1999;68:1881–1885.
55. Tsukube T, Ataka K, Taniguchi T, et al. Papillary fibroelastoma of the left atrial appendage: Echocardiographic findings. *Ann Thorac Surg.* 2000;70:1416–1417.
56. Nakao T, Hollinger I, Attai L, et al. Incidental finding of papillary fibroelastoma on the atrial septum. *Cardiovasc Surg.* 1994;2:423–424.
57. Watchell M, Heritage DW, Pastore L, et al. Cytogenetic study of cardiac papillary fibroelastoma. *Cancer Genet Cytogenet.* 2000;120:174–175.
58. Schuetz WH, Welz A, Heymer B. A symptomatic papillary fibroelastoma of the left ventricle removed with the aid of transesophageal echocardiography. *Thorac Cardiovasc Surg.* 1993;41:258–260.
59. Lee KS, Topol EJ, Stewart WJ. Atypical presentation of papillary fibroelastoma mimicking multiple vegetations in suspected subacute bacterial endocarditis. *Am Heart J.* 1993;125:1443–1445.
60. Schiller AL, Schantz A. Papillary endocardial excrescence of the right atrium: Report of two cases. *Am J Clin Pathol.* 1970;53:617–621.
61. Gallas MT, Reardon MJ, Reardon PR, et al. Papillary fibroelastoma. A right atrial presentation. *Tex Heart Inst J.* 1993;20:293–295.
62. Bapat VN, Varma GG, Hordikar AA, et al. Right-ventricular fibroma presenting as tricuspid stenosis - A case report. *Thorac Cardiovasc Surg.* 1996;44:152–154.
63. Uchida S, Obayashi N, Yamanari H, et al. Papillary fibroelastoma in the left ventricular outflow tract. *Heart Vessels.* 1992;7:164–167.
64. Wasdahl DA, Wasdahl WA, Edwards WD. Fibroelastic papilloma arising in a Chiari network. *Clin Cardiol.* 1992;15:45–47.
65. Schwinger ME, Katz E, Rotterdam H, et al. Right atrial papillary fibroelastoma: Diagnosis by transthoracic and transesophageal echocardiography and percutaneous transvenous biopsy. *Am Heart J.* 1989;118:1047–1050.
66. Anderson KR, Fiddler GI, Lie JT. Congenital papillary tumor of the tricuspid valve. An unusual cause of right ventricular outflow obstruction in a neonate with trisomy E. *Mayo Clin Proc.* 1997;52:665–669.
67. Sun JP, Asher CR, Yang XS, et al. Clinical and echocardiographic characteristics of papillary fibroelastomas: A retrospective and prospective study in 162 patients. *Circulation.* 2001;103(22):2687–2693.
68. McFadden PM, Lacy JR. Intracardiac papillary fibroelastoma: An occult cause of embolic neurologic deficit. *Ann Thorac Surg.* 1987;43:667–669.
69. Mann J. Papillary fibroelastoma of the mitral valve: A rare cause of transient neurological deficits. *Br Heart J.* 1994;71:6.
70. Kasarskis EJ, O'Connor W, Earle G. Embolic stroke from cardiac papillary fibroelastomas. *Stroke.* 1988;19:1171–1173.
71. Topol EJ, Biern RO, Reitz BA. Cardiac papillary fibroelastoma and stroke: Echocardiographic diagnosis and guide excision. *Am J Cardiol.* 1986;80:129–132.
72. Fine G, Pai SR. Cardiac papillary fibroelastoma: A source of coronary artery emboli and myocardial infarction. *Henry Ford Hosp Med J.* 1984;32:204–208.
73. Israel DH, Sherman W, Ambrose JA, et al. Dynamic coronary ostial obstruction due to papillary fibroelastoma leading to myocardial ischemia and infarction. *Am J Cardiol.* 1991;67:104–105.
74. Grote J, Mugge A, Schafers HJ, et al. Multiplane transesophageal echocardiography detection of a papillary fibroelastoma of the aortic valve causing myocardial infarction. *Eur Heart J.* 1995;16:426–429.
75. Etienne Y, Jobic Y, Houel JF, et al. Papillary fibroelastoma of the aortic valve with myocardial infarction: Echocardiographic diagnosis and surgical excision. *Am Heart J.* 1994;127:443–445.
76. Richard J, Castello R, Dressller FA, et al. Diagnosis of papillary fibroelastoma of the mitral valve complicated by non-q-wave infarction with apical thrombus: Transesophageal and transthoracic echocardiographic study. *Am Heart J.* 1993;126:710–712.
77. Waltenberger J, Thelin S. Papillary fibroelastoma as an unusual source of repeated pulmonary embolism. *Circulation.* 1994;89:24–33.

78. Zamora RL, Adelberg DA, Berger AS, et al. Branch retinal artery occlusion caused by a mitral valve papillary fibroelastoma. *Ophthalmology.* 1995;119:325–329.

79. Al-Mohammad A, Pambakian H, Young C. Fibroelastoma: Case report and review of the literature. *Heart.* 1998;79:301–304.

80. Minatoya K, Okabayashi H, Yokota T, et al. Cardiac papillary fibroelastomas: Rationale for excision. *Ann Thorac Surg.* 1996;62(5):1519–1521.

81. Yee HC, Nwosu JE, Lii AD, et al. Echocardiographic features of papillary fibroelastomas and their consequences and management. *Am J Cardiol.* 1997;80(6):811–814.

82. McAllister HA. Primary tumours and cysts of the heart and pericardium. *Curr Probl Cardiol.* 1979;4:1–51.

83. Weiss SW, Goldblum JR. *Enzinger and Weiss's Soft Tissue Tumors.* St Louis, MO: Mosby; 2001:571–639.

84. Roberts WC, Spray TL. Pericardial heart disease: A study of its causes, consequences and morphologic features. *Cardiovasc Clin.* 1976;7:11–65.

85. Grande AM, Minzioni G, Pederzolli C, et al. Cardiac lipomas. Description of 3 cases. *J Cardiovasc Surg.* 1998;39:813–815.

86. Grande AM, Minzioni G, Pederzolli C, et al. Cardiac lipomas: Description of 3 cases. *J Cardiovasc Surg.* 1998;39:813–815.

87. Conces DJ Jr, Vix VA, Tarver RD. Diagnosis of a myocardial lipoma by using CT. *Am J Roentgenol.* 1989;153:725–726.

88. Doshi S, Halim M, Sing H, et al. Massive intrapericardial lipoma, a rare cause of breathlessness: Investigations and management. *Int J Cardiol.* 1998;66:211–215.

89. Mullen JC, Schipper SA, Sett SS, et al. Right atrial lipoma. *Ann Thorac Surg.* 1995;59:1239–1241.

90. Kamiya H, Ohno M, Iwata H, et al. Cardiac lipoma in the interventricular septum: Evaluation by computed tomography and magnetic resonance imaging. *Am Heart J.* 1990;119:1215–1217.

91. Burke AP, Rosado-de-Christenson M, Templeton PA, et al. Cardiac fibroma: Clinicopathologic correlates and surgical treatment. *J Thorac Cardiovasc Surg.* 1994;108:862–870.

92. Murugasu P, Edwards James RM, Bastian Bruce C, et al. Pericardial lipoma: Ultrasound, computed tomography and magnetic resonance imaging findings. *Aust Radiol.* 2000;44:321–324.

93. Lang-Lazdunski L, Oroudjii M, Pansard Y, et al. Successful resecton of giant intrapericaridal lipoma. *Ann Thorac Surg.* 1994;58:238–241.

94. Zingas AP, Carrera JD, Murray CA, III, et al. Lipoma of the myocardium. *J Comput Assist Tomogr.* 1983;7:1098–1100.

95. Hananouchi GI, Goff WB. Cardiac lipoma: Six-year follow-up with MRI characteristics and a review of the literature. *Magn Reson Imaging.* 1990;8:825–828.

96. Sankar NM, Thiruchelvam T, Thirunavukkaarasu K, et al. Symptomatic lipoma in the right atrial free wall. *Tex Heart Inst J.* 1998;25:152–154.

97. Beghetti M, Gow RM, Haney I, et al. Pediatric primary benign cardiac tumors: A 15-year review. *Am Heart J.* 1997;134:1107–1114.

98. Harding CO, Pagon RA. Incidence of tuberous sclerosis in patients with cardiac rhabdomyoma. *Am J Med Genet.* 1990;37:443–446.

99. Verhaaren HA, Vanakker O, De Wolf D, et al. Left ventricular outflow obstruction in rhabdomyoma of infancy: Meta-analysis of the literature. *J Pediatr.* 2003;143:258–263.

100. Mehta AV. Rhabdomyoma and ventricular preexitation syndrome. A report of two cases and review of literature. *Am J Dis Child.* 1993;147:669–671.

101. Grebene ML, Rosado de Christenson ML, Burke AP, et al. Primary cardiac and pericardial neoplasms: Radiologic–pathologic correlation. *Radiographics.* 2000;20:1073–1103.

102. Hirsch JL, Chays A, Jouven JC, et al. Cardiac rhabdomyoma in the adult. Echocardiographic diagnosis and successful surgical treatment. *Arch Mal Coeur Vaiss.* 1987;80:1189–1192.

103. Burke AP, Gato-Weis C, Griego JE, et al. Adult cellular rhabdomyoma of the heart: A report of 3 cases. *Hum Pathol.* 2002;33:1092–1097.

104. Coates TL, McGahan JP. Fetal cardiac rhabdomyomas presenting as diffuse myocardial thickening. *J Ultrasound Med.* 1994;13:813–816.

105. Rienmüller R, Lloret JL, Tiling R, et al. MR imaging of pediatric cardiac tumors previously diagnosed by echocardiography. *J Comput Assist Tomogr.* 1989;13:621–626.

106. Kiaffas MG, Powell AJ, Geva T. Magnet resonance imaging evaluation of cardiac tumor characteristics in infants and children. *Am J Cardiol.* 2002;89:1229–1233.

107. Aktoz M, Tatli E, Ege T, et al. Cardiac rhabdomyoma in an adult patient presenting with right ventricular outflow tract obstruction. *Int J Cardiol.* 2007.

108. Yamaguchi M, Hosokawa Y, Ohashi H, et al. Cardiac fibroma: Long-term fate after excision. *J Thorac Cardiovasc Surg.* 1992;103:140–145.

109. Vidaillet HJ. Cardiac tumors associated with hereditary syndromes. *Am J Cardiol.* 1988;61:1355.

110. Parmley LF, Salley RK, Williams JP, et al. The clinical spectrum of cardiac fibroma with diagnostic and surgical considerations: Noninvasive imaging enhances management. *Ann Thorac Surg.* 1988;45:455–465.

111. Cina SJ, Smialek JE, Burke AP, et al. Primary cardiac tumors causing sudden death: A review of the literature. *Am J Forensic Med Pathol.* 1996;17:271–281.

112. Blanchard DG, DeMaria AN. Cardiac and extracardiac masses: Echocardiographic evaluation. In: Skorton DJ, ed. *Marcus Cardiac Imaging: A Companion to Braunwald's Heart Disease.* 2nd Ed. Philadelphia, Pa: Saunders; 1996:452–480.

113. Grinda JM, Mace L, Dervanian P, et al. Obstructive right ventricular cardiac fibroma in an adult. *Eur J Cardiothorac Surg.* 1998;13:319–321.

114. Veinot JP, O'Murchu B, Tazelaar HD, et al. Cardiac fibroma mimicking apical hypertrophic cardiomyopathy: A case report and differential diagnosis. *J Am Soc Echocardiogr.* 1996;9:94–99.

115. Araoz PA, Mulvagh SL, Tazelaar HD, et al. CT and MR imaging of benign primary cardiac neoplasms with echocardiographic correlation. *Radiographics.* 2000;20(5):1303–1319.

116. Winkler M, Higgins CB. Suspected intracardiac masses: Evaluation with MR imaging. *Radiology.* 1987;165:117–122.

117. Amparo EG, Higgins CB, Farmer D, et al. Gated MRI of cardiac and paracardiac masses: Initial experience. *Am J Roentgenol.* 1984;143:1151–1156.

118. Waller BR, Bradley SM, Crumbley AJ III, et al. Cardiac fibroma in an infant: Single ventricle palliation as a bridge to heart transplantation. *Ann Thorac Surg.* 2003;75:1306–1308.

119. Kaji T, Takamatsu H, Noguchi H, et al. Cardiac lymphangioma: Case report and review of the literature. *J Pediatr Surg.* 2002;37(10):E32.

120. Kim SJ, Shin ES, Kim SW, et al. Lee SGA case of cardiac lymphangioma presenting as a cystic mass in the right atrium. *Yonsei Med J.* 2007;48(6):1043–1047.

121. Thomas JE, Eror AT, Kenney M, et al. Asymptomatic right atrial cavernous hemangioma: A case report and review of the literature. *Cardiovasc Pathol.* 2004;341–344.

122. Tabry IF, Nassar VH, Rizk G, et al. Cavernous hemangioma of the heart: Case report and review of the literature. *J Thorac Cardiovasc Surg.* 1975;69:415–420.

123. Tanrikulu MA, Ozben B, Cincin AA, et al. A pedunculated left ventricular hemangioma initially misdiagnosed as thrombus in a woman with atypical chest pain. *J Thromb Thrombolysis.* 2008;27:227–232.

124. Brizard C, Latremouille C, Jebara VA et al. Cardiac hemangiomas. *Ann Thorac Surg.* 1993;56:390–394.

125. Cunningham T, Lawrie GM, Stavinoha J Jr, et al. Cavernous hemangioma of the right ventricle: Echocardiographic-pathologic correlates. *J Am Soc Echocardiogr.* 1993;6:335–340.

126. Kirkpatrick JN, Wong T, Bednarz JE, et al. Differential diagnosis of cardiac masses using contrast echocardiographic perfusion imaging. *J Am Coll Cardiol.* 2004;43:1412–1419.

127. Lepper W, Shivalkar B, Rinkevich D, et al. Assessment of the vascularity of a left ventricular mass using myocardial contrast echocardiography. *J Am Soc Echocardiogr.* 2002;15:1419–1422.

128. Emami B, Antoniades J. *Heart and Blood Vessels: Principles and Practice of Radiation Oncology.* 2nd Ed. Philadelphia, Pa: JB Lippincott; 1994:871–876.

129. Palmer TE, Tresch DD, Bonchek LI. Spontaneous resolution of a large cavernous hemangioma of the heart. *Am J Cardiol.* 1986;58:184–185.

130. Okum EJ, Henry D, Kasirajan V, et al. Cardiac pheochromocytoma. *J Thorac Cardiovasc Surg.* 2005;129:674–675.

131. David TE, Lenkei SC, Marquez-Julio A, et al. Pheochromocytoma of the heart. *Ann Thorac Surg.* 1986;41:98–100.

132. Jebara VA, Uva MS, Farge A, et al. Cardiac pheochromocytomas. *Ann Thorac Surg.* 1992;53:356–361.

133. Heufelder AE, Hofbauer LC. Greetings from below the aortic arch! The paradigm of cardiac paraganglioma. *J Clin Endocrinol Metab.* 1996;81:891–895.

134. Turley AJ, Hunter S Stewart MJ. A cardiac paraganglioma presenting with atypical chest pain. *Eur J Cardiothorac Surg.* 2005;28:352–354.

135. Cane ME, Berrizbeitia LD, Yang SS, et al. Paraganglioma of the interatrial septum. *Ann Thorac Surg.* 1996;61:1845–1847.

136. Fisher MR, Higgins CB, Andereck W. MR imaging of an intrapericardial pheochromocytoma. *J Comput Assist Tomogr.* 1985;9:1103–1105.

137. Hamilton BH, Francis IR, Gross BH, et al. Intrapericardial paragangliomas (pheochromocytomas): Imaging features. *Am J Roentgenol.* 1997;168:109–113.

138. Conti VR, Saydjari R, Amparo EG. Paraganglioma of the heart. *Chest.* 1986;90:604–606.

139. Jeevanandam V, Oz MC, Shapiro B, et al. Surgical management of cardiac pheochromocytoma Resection versus transplantation. *Ann Thorac Surg.* 1995;221:415–419.

140. Reardon MJ, Malaisrie SC, Walkes J et al. Cardiac autotransplantation for primary cardiac tumors. *Ann Thorac Surg.* 2006;82:645–650.

141. Grundmann G, Fischer R, Griesser G. Congenital pericardial cysts. *Thoraxchirurgie.* 1955;2(6):492–504.

142. Braude PD, falk G, McCaughan BC et al. Giant pericardial cyst. *Aust N Z J Surg.* 1996;60(8):640–641.

143. Stoller JK, Shaw C, Mattay RA. Enlarging, atypically located pericardial cyst: Recent experience and literature review. *Chest.* 1986;3:402–406.

144. Feigin DS, Fenoglio JJ, Mc Allister HA, et al. Pericardial cysts: A radiologic-pathologic correlation and review. *Radiology.* 1977;125:15–20.

145. Pelikan HMP, Tsang TSM, Seward JB. Giant blood cyst of the mitral valve. *J Am Soc Echocardiogr.* 1999;13:1005–1007.

146. Patel J, Park C, Michaels J, et al. Pericardial cyst case reports and a literature review. *Echocardiography.* 2004;21:269–272.

147. Kaimal KP. Computed tomography in the diagnosis of pericardial cyst. *Am Heart J.* 1982;103:566–567.

148. Syed IS, Feng D, Harris SR, et al. MR imaging of cardiac masses. *Magn Reson Imaging Clin N Am.* 2008;16(2):137–164.

149. White CS. MR evaluation of the pericardium. *Top Magn Reson Imaging.* 1995;7:258–266.

150. Atilgan D, Kudar H, Tukek T, et al. Role of transesophageal echocardiography in diagnosis and management of cardiac hydatid cyst report of three cases and review of the literature. *J Am Soc Echocardiogr.* 2002;15:271–274.

151. Nkomo V, Miller FA. Eustachian valve cyst. *J Am Soc Echocardiogr.* 2001;14:1224–1226.

152. Abad C, Rey A, Feijoo J, et al. Pericardial cyst: Surgical resection in two symptomatic cases. *J Cardiovasc Surg.* 1996;37(2):199–202.

153. Szinicz G, Taxer F, Riedlinger J, et al. Thoracosocopic resection of a pericardial cyst. *Thorac Cardiovasc Surg.* 1992;40(4):190–191.

154. Kruger SR, Michaud J, Canrom DS. Spontaneous resolution of a pericardial cyst. *Am Heart J.* 1985;109(6):1390–1391.
155. Ambalavanan SK, Mehta JB, Tayor RA, et al. Spontaneous resolution of a large pericardial cyst. *Tenn Med.* 1997;90(3):97–98.
156. Niarchos C, Kounis GN, Frangides CR, et al. Large hydatid cyst of the left ventricle associated with syncopal attacks. *Int J Cardiol.* 2007;118(1):e24–6.
157. Pelikan HMP, Tsang TSM, Seward JB. Giant blood cyst of the mitral valve. *J Am Soc Echocardiogr.* 1999;13:1005–1007.
158. van Dantzig JM, Delemarre BJ, Bot H, et al. Left ventricular thrombus in acute myocardial infarction. *Eur Heart J.* 1996;17:1640–1645.
159. Giardina EG. Atrial fibrillation and stroke: Elucidating a newly discovered risk factor. *Am J Cardiol.* 1997;80:11D–18D.
160. Chartier L, Bera J, Delomez M, et al. Free-floating thrombi in the right heart: Diagnosis, management, and prognostic indexes in 38 consecutive patients. *Circulation.* 1999;99:2779–2783.
161. Shapiro MA, Johnson M, Feinstein SB. A retrospective experience of right atrial and superior vena caval thrombi diagnosed by transesophageal echocardiography. *J Am Soc Echocardiogr.* 2002;15:76–79.
162. Mogulkoc N, Burgess MI, Bishop PW. Intracardiac thrombus in Behçet's disease: A systematic review. *Chest.* 2000;118:479–487.
163. Yamamoto H, Nakatani S, Hashimura K. Löffler's endomyocarditis. *Heart.* 2005;91(2):135.
164. Schwab J, Schwab M, Manger K, et al. Churg-Strauss syndrome with right ventricular tumor. *Dtsch Med Wochenschr.* 1998;123:487–492.
165. Mollet NR, Dymarkowski S, Volders W, et al. Visualization of ventricular thrombi with contrast-enhanced magnetic resonance imaging in patients with ischemic heart disease. *Circulation.* 2002;106(23):2873–2876.
166. Srichai MB, Junor C, Rodriguez LL, et al. Clinical, imaging, and pathological characteristics of left ventricular thrombus: A comparison of contrast-enhanced magnetic resonance imaging, transthoracic echocardiography, and transesophageal echocardiography with surgical or pathological validation. *Am Heart J.* 2006;152(1):75–84.
167. Sparrow PJ, Kurian JB, Jones TR, et al. MR imaging of cardiac tumors. *Radiographics.* 2005;25(5):1255–1276.
168. Nili M, Deviri E, Jortner R, et al. Surgical removal of a mobile, pedunculated left ventricular thrombus: Report of 4 cases. *Ann Thorac Surg.* 1988;46:396–400.
169. Peters PJ, Reinhardt S. The echocardiographic evaluation of intracardiac masses: A review. *J Am Soc Echocardiogr.* 2006;19(2):230–240.
170. Pharr JR, West M, Kusomoto F, et al. Prominent crista terminalis appearing as a right atrial mass on transthoracic echocardiogram. *J Am Soc Echocardiogr.* 2002;15:753–755.

Malignant Cardiac Masses and Tumors

38

Raymond Wong
Milind Y. Desai

1. INTRODUCTION

1.1. Epidemiology

Primary cardiac tumors are rare entities with an autopsy frequency of 0.19% to 0.56%.[1-3] Only a quarter of these tumors are malignant; 95% of these are sarcomas.[4] Undifferentiated soft tissue sarcomas are the commonest, followed by angiosarcomas, leiomyosarcomas, rhabdomyosarcomas, malignant mesotheliomas, and fibrosarcomas.[5,6] Primary cardiac sarcomas typically affect adults (mean age 41 years) and are rare in children. Angiosarcoma and osteosarcoma are approximately twice as common in men.[7,8] By contrast, metastases to the heart and pericardium are more common than primary cardiac tumors by a more than a 100-fold,[9] with an incidence of 1.23%[3] (Figs. 38.1 and 38.2). In a single-center report, carcinoma of all types accounted for 76% of metastases. Others included lymphoma (13.6%), leukemia (3.2%), melanoma, and sarcoma (2.6% each). A review of 12,485 autopsies revealed only 7 cases of primary neoplasm of the heart compared to 154 cases of metastatic heart tumors.[3]

1.2. Clinical presentation

1.2.1. Symptoms

Up to 12% of primary cardiac tumors are asymptomatic and are detected during incidental cardiac evaluation or at autopsy.[10] Most patients have disseminated metastases, yet producing clinical signs and symptoms in only a tenth of afflicted patients.[11] The classic triad of clinical manifestation of these tumors include signs and symptoms resulting from intracardiac/intracavitary obstruction[12]; signs of arterial/systemic embolization; and systemic or constitutional symptoms.[10,11] Piazza et al.[13] described the commonest symptoms in adult patients included dyspnea (38%) or central nervous system embolic events (24%), whereas in the pediatric group, the most frequent presenting symptom was hypoxia (50%) (Table 38.1).

2. PATHOPHYSIOLOGY

2.1. Primary malignant cardiac tumors

2.1.1. Primary sarcomas

Primary sarcomas comprise the largest group in adult malignant primary cardiac tumors and second most common primary cardiac tumors.[14] In one series of pathological and surgical specimens sarcomas represented 35% of tumors.[7] The pluripotent mesenchymal cell is likely the cell of origin. These tumors can present as virtually any type of soft tissue sarcoma, located anywhere systemically and in any part of the heart.[15] The pathologic features of cardiac sarcoma vary widely, ranging from endocardial-based lesions similar to benign myxoma to large, infiltrative tumors. Cut sections of cardiac sarcomas are typically firm and heterogeneous, but the myofibroblastic tumors may be homogenous (Table 38.2).[7,14]

2.1.2. Rhabdomyosarcomas

These rare invasive sarcomas have a male preponderance and mean age of presentation of 15 years (Fig. 38.3).[4,7] Rhabdomyosarcoma is the commonest cardiac tumor in children and adolescents. Frequently multicentric and bulky, these may arise from either ventricles or atria. Gross specimens may be gelatinous and friable,[16] firm and fleshy,[17] or cystlike.[18] Large areas of central necrosis may be seen at gross examination.[19] The tumor grows rapidly and may have invaded cardiac valves and pericardium at the time of diagnosis.[17,20] They have a tendency to metastasize and recur.[21] Surgical excision of small tumors may be possible, but local and distant metastasis coupled with a poor response to radiation or chemotherapy limit survival to less than a year.[17,20,22]

2.1.3. Liposarcomas

Liposarcomas are very rare, comprising only of 1% of primary malignant cardiac tumors.[23] Grossly, they are bulky tumors as large as 10 cm, often arising from the right heart, and are soft and bosselated.

2.1.4. Fibrosarcomas

Primary sarcoma of the pulmonary vein, most of them leiomyosarcomas,[24,25] appear to be in the smallest subgroup of rare cases of primary sarcomas of the great vessels (Fig. 38.4).[26] There is strong female preponderance. The mean age of presentation is 50 years, with a range of 23 to 74 years.[27] At gross examination, fibrosarcomas have been described as soft, lobulated, gelatinous masses.[7,28] Fibrosarcomas contain areas of hemorrhage and necrosis and frequently involve multiple heart chambers.[3,13] Like all sarcomas of the great vessels and the heart, the prognosis of pulmonary vein sarcoma is poor, with a 3-year survival rate of about 5%.[25,29]

2.1.5. Malignant histiocytomas

Malignant fibrous histiocytoma (MFH) is the second or third most common cardiac sarcoma,[7] originating from fibroblasts or histioblasts.[14] The mean age at diagnosis is 44 years with no sexual predilection. Grossly these tumors are generally lobulated,[30] soft or even creamy in texture.[31] Valvular involvement has been reported in as many as half of lesions. Patients often die of local cardiac disease before the development of metastasis.

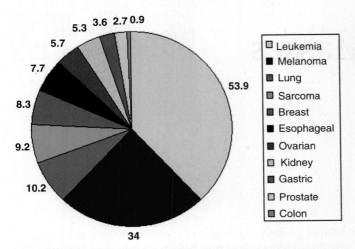

Figure 38.1 Sources of cardiac metastases. Numbers shown are indicative of percentages of cases. (Adapted from Neragi-Miandoab S, Gangadharan SP, Sugarbaker DJ. Cardiac sarcoma 14 years after treatment for pleural mesothelioma. *N Engl J Med.* 2005;352(18):1929–1930.)

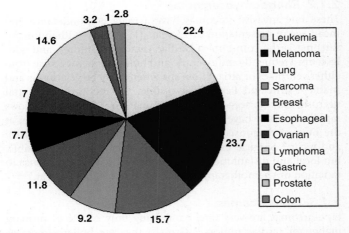

Figure 38.2 Sources of pericardial metastases. Numbers shown are indicative of percentages of cases. (Adapted from Neragi-Miandoab S, Gangadharan SP, Sugarbaker DJ. Cardiac sarcoma 14 years after treatment for pleural mesothelioma. *N Engl J Med.* 2005;352(18): 1929–1930.)

2.1.6. Angiosarcomas

Angiosarcoma is the most frequent malignant tumor of the heart[32] with 75% occurring in the right heart, especially in the right atrium, and 40% extending into the pericardium (Fig. 38.5). It presents between the third and fifth decades of life, with a male-to-female ratio of 2:1.[33] Metastases develop in 47% to 89% of patients, mostly in the lungs, but also in the brain, bone, and colon.[34] Gross angiosarcomas are usually large and multilobular, completely replace the atrial wall and often fill the entire cardiac chambers, and may invade adjacent structures, including great veins.[35,36] They are usually hemorrhagic. Without resection, 90% of patients die within 9 to 12 months after diagnosis.

2.1.7. Mesotheliomas/pericardial tumors

Primary malignant pericardial mesothelioma is a very rare tumor of the heart and pericardium with an incidence of 0.0022%.[22,37] Metastatic tumors from the lung, breast, melanomas, lymphoma, or leukemia are much more common.[38] The mean age at diagnosis is 51 years with a male-to-female ratio of 2:1.[7] There may be a

TABLE 38.1
CLINICAL MANIFESTATION OF MALIGNANT TUMORS

Sarcoma
Cardiopulmonary symptoms at 5 months mean duration.[7] Dyspnea is the commonest presenting complaint. Other symptoms/signs include cardiac tamponade, embolic phenomena, chest pain, syncope, pneumonia, fever, arrhythmias, peripheral edema, and sudden death.[8,14,60,109] Primary cardiac sarcomas most commonly metastasize to the lungs but also to lymph nodes, bone, liver, skin, and other organs.[7,8,14]

Angiosarcoma
Nonspecific chest pain (46% of patients in a recent review[34]), dyspnea, malaise, and fever. Symptoms from right-sided heart inflow obstruction or cardiac tamponade are common due to right atrial and pericardial involvement.[7] If metastatic lung lesions are present, dyspnea can also occur.[34] Diagnosis are often based on biopsy of metastases, which are found in 66%–89% of patients at the time of presentation.[7,92]

Osteosarcoma
Congestive heart failure. Respiratory symptoms if atria are involved; recurrent ventricular tachyarrhythmia if ventricles are involved.

Leiomyosarcoma
Patients generally present 5–10 years earlier than other cardiac sarcomas. Pulmonary lesions present with dyspnea, chest pain, and dry cough; cardiac lesions present with right heart failure, valve stenosis, dysrhythmias, hemopericardium, and sudden death.

Rhabdomyosarcoma
Nonspecific symptoms, sometimes pleuropericardial symptoms and distal embolization, arrhythmias, and obstructive symptoms.

Cardiac Lymphoma
Cardiac tamponade, heart failure, exertional dyspnea, atrial fibrillation, and features of right-sided heart obstruction.[110]

Malignant Histiocytoma
Symptoms related to pulmonary congestion since the tumor usually arises from the posterior wall of the left atrium causing extrinsic compression of the pulmonary veins.

Pericardial mesothelioma
Patients present with a mean age of 46 years and a 2:1 male-to-female ratio. Clinical symptoms include chest pain, cough, dyspnea, and palpitations. Diffuse pericardial involvement may cause pericarditis or cardiac tamponade. Widespread metastases may occur. Causal effect of asbestos exposure has been suspected but a definite association is difficult to establish.

Metastatic cardiac tumor
Tachycardia, arrhythmias, cardiomegaly, or heart failure in patient with carcinoma may indicate cardiac involvement. Majority are clinically silent.

Source: Adapted from Butany J, Nair V, Naseemuddin A, et al. Cardiac tumours: Diagnosis and management. *Lancet Oncol.* 2005;6(4):219–228.

causal link between asbestos exposure and pleural mesothelioma, though this has not been conclusively proven.[7] Malignant mesotheliomas form bulky nodules that fill the pericardial cavity, often encircling the heart. Other rare malignant primary tumors of the pericardium include sarcoma and yolk sac tumor.[7]

TABLE 38.2

INCIDENCE, SITES, CLINICAL PRESENTATION, PERICARDIAL, AND VALVE INVOLVEMENT OF PRIMARY CARDIAC SARCOMAS

Type of sarcoma	Incidence	Site	Most common clinical presentation	Pericardial involvement	Valve involvement
Angiosarcoma	37%; M > F	RA, RV	Right heart failure or tamponade	+ + + +, hemopericardium, tamponade	Occasional
Undifferentiated sarcoma	0%–24%	LA	Pulmonary congestion	+ +, hemopericardium	Occasional
Rhabdomyo-sarcoma	4%–7%; common in infants and children	Myocardium	Variable	Frequent, nodular masses	Likely to involve valves
Osteosarcoma	3%–9%	LA	Pulmonary congestion	—	Occasional
Fibrosarcoma	5%	LA, multiple sites	Pulmonary congestion	Direct invasion, deposition of tumor nodules	Occasional
Leiomyosarcoma	8%–9%	Pulmonary vessels, LA, aorta, cavae	Pulmonary congestion	Effusion, nodules or irregular masses	Extension to pulmonary veins
Liposarcoma	2/145; 18 cases	RA, RV	Pulmonary congestion	Effusion, nodules or irregular masses	Occasional
Mesothelioma	50% primary pericardial tumors; M > F	Extends into myocardium and lung	Pericardial constriction, pericarditis	Pericarditis, tamponade	Unusual

Source: Adapted from Shanmugam G. Primary cardiac sarcoma. *Eur J Cardiothorac Surg.* 2006;29(6):925–932 and Araoz PA, Eklund HE, Welch TJ, et al. CT and MR imaging of primary cardiac malignancies. *Radiographics.* 1999;9(6):1421–1434.

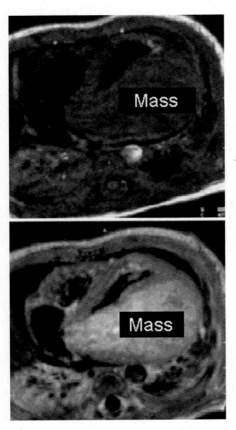

Figure 38.3 Rhabdomyosarcoma on MRI. A large malignant mass involves the free wall of the left ventricle and fills the left ventricular cavity, as seen on T1-weighted (**top**) and postcontrast T1-weighted axial images (**bottom**).

2.1.8. Leiomyosarcoma

These are rare, highly aggressive, and locally invasive tumors with a frequency of 0.25%.[39] Right heart failure, valve stenosis, arrhythmias, hemopericardium, and sudden death have been reported.[40] Generally seen in the fourth to fifth decade of life, they are usually located in the posterior left atrium and present as sessile masses. Pulmonary veins or the mitral valve is involved in about 10% of cases. Leiomyosarcomas usually appear as gelatinous, sessile masses at gross examination and may be multiple in 30% of cases.[7]

2.1.9. Osteosarcoma

These rare tumors account for 3% to 9% of primary cardiac sarcomas.[7] They usually arise from the left atrium leading to

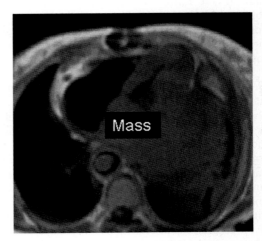

Figure 38.4 Fibrosarcoma involving the left atrial cavity, with extension into the pericardial space on T1-weighted imaging, seen on MRI.

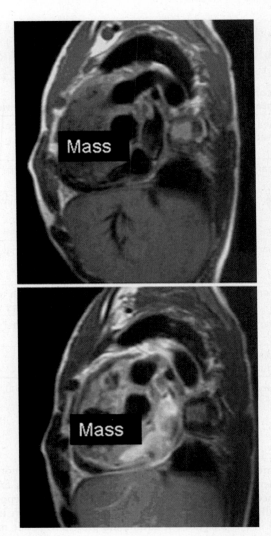

Figure 38.5 Angiosarcoma, as seen on sagittal MRI. Precontrast **(top)** and postcontrast T1-weighted imaging **(bottom)** reveals a large mass of the right atrioventricular groove with peripheral enhancement reflecting its hypervascular nature with central necrosis.

respiratory complaints. They typically present as large sessile tissue masses, ranging from 4 to 10 cm in diameter. Invasion of the atrial wall and mitral valve is seen. The surface may have a mucoid or gelatinous appearance, while sections through it demonstrate a gritty consistency and areas of calcification. Amplifications at 1q21–23 and at 17p are frequent in conventional osteosarcoma.

2.1.10. Undifferentiated sarcoma/other primary cardiac tumors

Undifferentiated or unclassifiable sarcomas are defined as without specific histological, ultrastructural, or specific immunohistochemical characteristics and constitute 0% to 24% of sarcomas.[7] In the most recent AFIP series,[7] 81% of unclassified sarcomas arose in the left atrium. The tumors may take the form of discrete or polypoid myocardial masses.[41] Genomic imbalances as detected by comparative genomic hybridization frequently include loss of 2p24-pter and 2q32-qter, as well as gain of 7p 15-pter, 7q32, and 1p31.[42] Myosarcoma, chondromyxosarcoma, and plasmacytoma of the heart have also been reported.[43,44]

2.2. Metastatic cardiac tumors

Secondary malignancies involving the heart are 20 to 40 times more frequent than primary cardiac neoplasms (Fig. 38.6). In autopsy studies, patients with known malignant neoplasms will have cardiac metastatic involvement in 10% to 12% of cases.[45,46] This assumes a variety of ways that include contiguous extension, hematogenous or lymphatic spread, or entry via the inferior vena cava. Pericardium is the commonest site of involvement, nearly 2/3 of the time; in many cases metastatic spread involves multiple sites.[3] Rarely, the coronary arteries can be implicated, or intracavitary obstruction may occur by direct neoplastic growth through the inferior vena cava.[47] The highest rate of metastases to the heart occurs with malignant melanoma.[7,48] In males, the most common tumor metastatic to the heart was lung carcinoma (32%), followed by esophageal carcinoma (29%) and lymphoma (12%). In females, carcinoma of the lung was also most common at 36%, followed by lymphoma (17%) and breast cancer (8%).[3] Metastatic lesions from carcinoma of the cervix have also been reported.[49]

2.2.1. Lymphomas

Primary cardiac lymphoma, which by definition is localized to the heart and pericardium with no evidence of lymphoma elsewhere in the body,[7] is an uncommon malignancy, accounting for 1.3% of primary cardiac tumors and 0.5% of extranodal lymphomas.[50] They are usually part of disseminated disease; up to 20% of patients with disseminated non-Hodgkin lymphoma will have evidence of cardiac involvement at autopsy. The mean

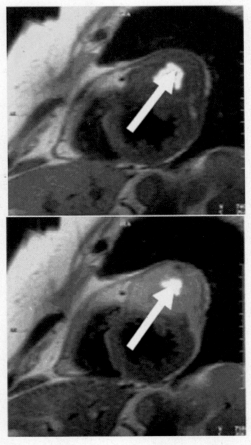

Figure 38.6 Metastatic gastric carcinoma on MRI, within the pericardial sac, with invasive characteristics. Compared to T1-weighted imaging **(top)**, the mass appears to be bright on the more edema-weighted T2-weighted imaging **(bottom)**.

age at presentation for cardiac lymphoma is 38 years with a slight predominance in men.[51] More than one cardiac chamber is involved in over 75% of cases, and contiguous invasion of the pericardium is typical.[7] The heart is typically enlarged and the weight is a reflection of the size of the tumor. Grossly, lymphomas manifest as an ill-defined, multiple, firm, whitish-yellow infiltrative mass, in which case they are typically best depicted with cardiac magnetic resonance (CMR) because of its superior soft tissue contrast.[52] Atrial location is typical, with infiltration of atrial or ventricular walls.

2.2.2. Hepatoma

Extension of hepatocellular carcinoma (HCC) to the inferior vena cava and right atrium is very uncommon, with a 1% to 4% prevalence[53] and a male-to-female ratio of 3:1.[54] In advanced HCC, tumor thrombi into the IVC or right atrium are usually associated with extremely poor outcome, including fatality.[55] Transthoracic echocardiogram (TTE) and transesophageal echocardiogram (TEE) are the noninvasive diagnostic methods of choice followed by CT, CMR, and cavography.[56] The high prevalence of subclinical cardiac metastasis in HCC mandates the use of TEE in all patients with HCC prior to surgical intervention.[57]

2.2.3. Hypernephroma

Quarter patients with renal cell carcinoma have evidence of metastatic disease at the time of diagnosis.[58] In autopsy series, cardiac metastases occur in 10% to 20% of patients dying of malignancy, and 8.2% of renal cell carcinoma.

3. DIAGNOSTIC EVALUATION

3.1. Electrocardiogram and chest X-ray

Infiltration of a cardiac fibroma within the myocardium, may lead to an ECG that suggests a previous myocardial infarction with no clinical history of the event.[59] In patients with cardiac myxoma, chest X-ray is nonspecific, demonstrating left atrial enlargement and signs characteristic of pulmonary hypertension. Calcification of the tumor may rarely be seen.[11,47] A chest X-ray may be abnormal and even show a mass lesion in the form of enlargement of the cardiac silhouette or mediastinal widening. Tumors such as fibromas might show calcifications on X-ray.[14,60]

3.2. Echocardiography

TTE is the initial diagnostic test of choice for cardiac tumors. It is noninvasive and allows for real time analysis of the tumor shape, size, location, and mobility within the heart and the assessment of hemodynamic consequences with Doppler.[52] TEE improves visualization of the right and left atria, especially the appendages.[61]

The potential advantages of TEE include improved resolution of the tumor and its attachment, the ability to detect some masses not visualized by TTE, and improved visualization of right atrial tumors.[62] Both TEE and TTE are equally effective in visualizing tumors originating from the heart. However, when comparing TTE with TEE in patients with mediastinal tumors, marked differences were seen. Tumors originating from the mediastinum were 2.9 times less likely to be detected by TTE than TEE, and TEE was also superior in diagnosing tumor infiltration and invasion of the heart and the great vessels.[62]

Echocardiography is the optimal imaging modality for imaging small masses (<1 cm) or masses arising from valves. The diagnostic sensitivity of TTE and TEE has been reported to be 93% and 97% respectively.[63] Echocardiography can also identify involvement of the valves and their competency, ventricular function, irregular

pericardial thickening, and intracavity masses interfering with blood flow.[14,60] TEE in particular guides transvenous tumor biopsy especially with right atrial masses.[64] The three-dimensional echocardiography has advantages with respect to quantitative precision in unusually shaped ventricles and in accurate anatomical description of complex anatomy of the heart.[65,66] Echocardiography in general has limitations for tissue characterization and requires advanced research techniques (ultrasonic backscatter, tissue Doppler imaging with strain rate analysis, or contrast perfusion imaging).

3.2.1. Contrast echo

Microbubble contrast agents have been used with two-dimensional echocardiography to delineate the myocardium-blood interface, to define intracavitary structures, and to evaluate myocardial perfusion.[67,68] One study found qualitative and quantitative differences in the gray scale between the levels of perfusion in various types of cardiac masses and sections of adjacent myocardium using power modulation and dedicated video-intensity detection software. Malignant or highly vascular tumors demonstrated greater enhancement than the adjacent myocardium.[69]

3.3. Computerized axial tomography and cardiac magnetic resonance

Cardiac CT and CMR do not unequivocally differentiate benign from malignant tumors; however, there are certain findings that suggest malignancy. Involvement of the right side of the heart, masses in the ventricles that infiltrate the myocardium, and associated hemopericardium support the diagnosis of malignant tumors. This is invaluable in detecting metastases and determining the resectablity of the tumor.[42,70] CMR and CT are capable of differentiating between adipose tissue, soft tissue, and cystic fluid collection.[71]

CT scanners have spatial resolution superior to MRI and echocardiography. CT has better soft tissue contrast than echocardiography and can be used to definitively characterize fatty content and calcifications.[52] However, the overall soft tissue contrast and ability to characterize tumor infiltration and tumor type is less than that of MRI.[72] Due to the highest soft tissue contrast, MRI is the imaging modality of choice for structural myocardial pathology and juxta-cardiac anatomy. It is the most sensitive modality for detection of tumor infiltration.[73] Furthermore, T2 weighted fast spin echo sequence distinguishes tumors with high water content, such as hemangioma, from tumors with low water content, such as fibroma. MRI can characterize tumor vascularity with intravenous contrast and allows for wall motion evaluation, characterization of ventricular function, inflow or outflow obstruction, and valve regurgitation. MRI can also differentiate tumor from myocardium, thrombus, vegetation, and blood flow artifact. MRI, however, is not capable of differentiating between benign and malignant tumors.

CMR is also useful in evaluation of other cardiac masses. CMR can be used to verify intracardiac masses found on echocardiography and to exclude a mass when the echocardiogram is equivocal.[74] The primary contribution of CMR is not the ability to obtain tissue diagnosis, but rather its ability to delineate the anatomic extent and to aid in treatment planning.[75] Accurate and fast detection of cardiac masses is also obtained by real-time CMR, which delineates all functional impediments.[76,77] The wide field of view, high-contrast and spatial resolution, and multiplanar imaging capabilities allow precise demonstration and localization of a mass, including its anatomic relationship to the cardiac chambers and any involvement of the myocardium, pericardium, or contiguous structures. T1-weighted, T2-weighted, and gadolinium-enhanced sequences are used for anatomic definition and tissue characterization, whereas cine gradient-echo imaging is used to assess functional consequences. Differences in characteristic locations and features by CMR imaging allow confident differentiation between benign and malignant tumors. Indicators of malignancy at CMR imaging are invasive behavior, involvement of the right side of the heart or the pericardium, tissue inhomogeneity, diameter greater than 5 cm, and enhancement after administration of gadolinium contrast material (as a result of higher tissue vascularity). Concomitant pericardial or pleural effusions are rare in benign processes but occur in about 50% of cases of malignant tumors. An important diagnostic limitation of cardiac MR imaging is an inability to demonstrate calcium.[78] Most of the CMR protocols are based on breath-held imaging. Another limitation of CMR is the requirement of synchronizing data acquisition to the cardiac cycle, commonly done via ECG gating. Perhaps the biggest limitation to CMR is that the technique carries a relative contraindication for pacemakers, intracardiac defibrillators, and certain surgical devices such as cerebral aneurysm clips.[79]

3.3.1. Technical considerations of CMR

Black-blood imaging sequences permit accurate depictions of the heart anatomy.[80] The various endogenous contrast responses to T1-weighted, T2-weighted, proton-density, and other specialized sequences help characterize masses by detecting fat, fluid, or blood products. A detailed description of physical principles, instrumentation, and protocols is provided in chapters 5 and 6. Bright-blood imaging methods, based on steady-state free precession methods (SSFP), yield images with excellent contrast between blood and myocardium and high spatial and moderate temporal resolutions. These improve evaluation of effect of the mass on global and regional cardiac function.[81] Tissue plane delineation is superior with CMR than 2D echo and the exact attachment and extent of the mass is more likely determined. A promising CMR technique is MR spectroscopy. With spectroscopy, the spectral signatures of metabolites and tissue components can be isolated.[79] Table 38.3 demonstrates a typical recommended MRI approach for evaluation of cardiac masses. Table 38.4 demonstrates the typical appearance of malignant cardiac tumors on various MRI sequences.

3.4. Nuclear scintigraphy

Positron emission tomography (PET) has been useful in identifying cardiac involvement in patients with metastatic tumors,[82,83] atrial myxoma,[84] or lipomatous septal hypertrophy. The major utilization of PET consists of imaging the distribution of fluorine 18 fluorodeoxy-glucose (FDG), where the transport and phosphorylation of 18F-FDG to 18F-FDG-6-phosphate occur at a higher rate in cancer cells than in normal, hence 18F-FDG will preferentially accumulate in tumor cells and be used as a radioactive marker of neoplastic activity, both diagnostically[85] and for tracking disease progression or recurrence. PET can elucidate the functional and metabolic activities of tumors which modalities like CT is unable to differentiate. The Society of Nuclear Medicine approves PET for detecting and localizing unknown primary tumors, differentiating malignant from benign tissues, staging and evaluating recurrences, differentiating recurrence from postsurgical changes, and monitoring the treatment response.[86] In particular, PET can identify malignant pleural mesothelioma and appears to be a useful noninvasive staging modality for patients being considered for aggressive combined modality therapy.[87]

3.5. Angiography

In patients with cardiac neoplasms, angiography is particularly useful in detecting compression or displacement of cardiac cavities or large masses and determining the magnitude of the intracavitary filling defects.[88] The most frequent angiographic findings are intracavitary filling defects, which may be fixed or mobile, lobulated or smooth and attached over a broad base or by a narrow stalk.[89] Coronary angiography is sometimes helpful in visualizing the vascular supply of the neoplasm and the relation of the neoplasm to the coronary arteries. The angiographic sign of "tumor vascularity" was found to be present in some patients with highly vascularized atrial myxomas.[90] The vascular pattern is not helpful, however, in differentiating benign from malignant tumors. Cardiac catheterization and selective angiography are no longer necessary in all patients with cardiac neoplasm because adequate preoperative information can usually be obtained by echocardiography, CT or CMR.[89] Table 38.5 summarizes the relative value and limitation of different imaging modalities used for diagnostic evaluation of cardiac masses.

A diagnostic algorithm for cardiac tumors is shown in Figure 38.7.

4. PROGNOSIS AND THERAPY GUIDANCE

4.1. Prognosis and outcome

Nearly all malignant cardiac tumors are rapidly fatal, with death reportedly occurring within 6 months postsurgery regardless of histology.[91] Cardiac sarcomas may have a better prognosis if they arise in the left atrium, have a low mitotic count, no necrotic regions, and have not metastasized at the time of diagnosis,[92] whereas age, gender, the presence of differentiation, and histologic type had no impact on prognosis.[14] Achieving full remission is unusual except in cases of chemotherapy with lymphomas. Recurrence of primary cardiac sarcomas is relatively common, whereby adjuvant chemotherapy and radiation should be considered.[15] Angiosarcomas are associated with poor outcomes, and surgery, with chemotherapy and radiotherapy, results in survival of only 6 to 9 months.[33] Prognosis of mesothelioma is poor with approximately 50% survival at 6 months. Pericardial resection or attempted sclerosis of the pericardium to prevent pericardial effusion can be performed to attempt symptomatic improvement.[7] Treatment of all other malignant cardiac tumors provides mainly palliation. Mean survival of affected patients is 3 months to 1 year for sarcomas in general.[23] Lymphoma patients can live up to 5 years if adequately treated.[93] In patients undergoing cardiac transplantations for tumors, outcome depends on the success of the transplant procedure and has been limited.[50,94]

Table 38.5 addresses the various strengths and limitations of different imaging modalities in diagnosis of malignant cardiac tumors.

4.2. Therapy

4.2.1. Surgery

Surgery may be performed for prognostic or symptomatic reasons. Complete surgical resection of malignant cardiac tumors is only possible in less than half of cases, rarely curative, and carries high perioperative risks. In a series of 33 patients with malignant cardiac tumors who underwent radical surgical resection, extensive procedures such as resection and repair of the interatrial septum and atrial walls and valve replacement did not improve survival.[32] Cardiac autotransplantation[95] (cardiac explantation, ex vivo tumor resection with cardiac reconstruction, and cardiac reimplantation) has been described but more data is needed regarding durability and applicability of this technique. The dominant role of surgery is to provide palliation of symptoms.[7] Patients may undergo palliative debulking for rapidly progressive obstructive symptoms. Surgery is indicated urgently when there is potential for catastrophic embolization or occlusion of a valve orifice. Creation of a

TABLE 38.3

PROPOSED MR IMAGING SEQUENCE FOR EVALUATION OF CARDIAC MASSES

1. LV structure and function	
A. Scout imaging—transaxial, coronal, sagittal	
B. Transaxial (8–10 mm) set of steady state free precession (SSFP) or fast spin echo images through the chest.	
C. Scout to line up short axis cine images	a. Vertical long axis prescribed orthogonal to transaxial scouts aligned through the apex and center of the mitral valve
	b. Horizontal long axis aligned orthogonal to the vertical long axis, passing through the apex and center of the mitral valve
D. SSFP short axis cine images, from the mitral valve plane through the apex	a. Slice thickness 6–8 mm, with two to four interslice gaps to equal 10 mm
E. SSFP long axis cine images	a. The four-chamber long axis is prescribed from the vertical long axis through the apex and center of the mitral and tricuspid valves. This can be cross-checked on basal short axis cines, using the costophrenic angle (margin) of the RV free wall.
	b. Vertical long axis, prescribed from the scout already acquired
	c. LV outflow tract (LVOT) long axis, passing through the apex, the center of the mitral valve and aligned with the center of LVOT to aortic valve, as seen on a basal short axis cine.
2. T1-weighted fast spin echo—slices through the mass and surrounding structures (number of slices depends on size of the mass)	
3. T2-weighted fast spin echo with fat suppression (optional without fat suppression)—through the mass and surrounding structures as above. See nonischemic cardiomyopathies for sequence details.	
4. First-pass perfusion module with slices through mass	
5. Repeat T1-weighted turbo spin echo with fat suppression	
7. Late gadolinium enhancement	
A. Need at least 10 min wait after gadolinium injection (0.1–0.2 mmol/kg)	
B. 2D segmented inversion recovery GRE imaging during diastolic standstill	a. segmented inversion recovery GRE imaging during diastolic standstill
	b. Same views as for cine imaging (short- and long-axis views)
	c. Same views as for cine imaging (short- and long-axis views)
	d. Slice thickness, same as for cine imaging
	e. In-plane resolution, ~1.4–1.8 mm
	f. Inversion time set to null normal myocardium. Alternative is to use fixed TI with a phase-sensitive sequence

Source: Adapted from a Society of CMR consensus statement by Kramer CM, Barkhausen J, Flamm SD, Kim, R and Nagel E.

pericardial window or percutaneous drainage and sclerosis of the pericardium may alleviate symptoms of pericardial effusions.[96]

4.2.2. Radiotherapy and chemotherapy

Patients with systemic metastases, cardiac metastases from a peripheral sarcoma, or an unresectable tumor are incurable and should be offered palliative therapy. Preoperative or postoperative radiotherapy is an effective adjuvant to complete excision for sarcomas arising at other sites.[97] Low-dose radiotherapy might have a role as an adjuvant to complete surgery for cardiac sarcomas. Patients with localized disease of borderline resectability

should be considered for cytoreductive chemotherapy with the aim of proceeding to complete resection if sufficient regression is obtained, especially in the postoperative setting.

No conclusive evidence exists to support routine use of chemotherapy as an adjuvant to complete surgery for cardiac sarcoma,[98] although application of chemotherapy to cytoreduce a tumor prior to surgery or for palliation of unresectable disease might be of value.[99] Chemotherapy has been used alone or combined with radiotherapy. In cardiac lymphoma, treatment primarily includes anthracycline-based chemotherapy and anti-CD20 treatment (rituximab).[100]

TABLE 38.4
MRI FEATURES OF SELECTED COMMON PRIMARY MALIGNANT CARDIAC TUMORS

	T1-weighted	T2-weighted	Postcontrast	Cine-MRI	Other data
Angiosarcoma	Isointense, with hyperintense areas	Isointense, heterogeneous	Strong	Hypointense foci	Hemorrhage, possible pericardial origin
Undifferentiated sarcoma	Isointense	Isointense	Nonspecific		Possible pericardial origin, infiltrative or masslike appearance
Rhabdomyosarcoma	Isointense	Isointense, heterogeneous	Central non-enhancing areas		Necrosis
Osteosarcoma	Hyperintense	Hyperintense	Nonspecific		Calcifications
MFH	Isointense	Hyperintense, heterogeneous	Nonspecific		Pulmonary veins involvement
Leiomyosarcoma	Isointense	Hyperintense	Nonspecific		Pulmonary veins and mitral valve involvement
Fibrosarcoma	Isointense, heterogeneous	Hyperintense	Central non-enhancing areas	Possible pericardial origin	Necrosis
Liposarcoma	Non published	Not published	Non published		Possible pericardial origin, little intratumoral macroscopic fat
Lymphoma	Hypo- or isointense	Hyperintense	Variable		No necrosis, possible pericardial origin, rare intracavitary

Source: Adapted from Luna A, et al. *Eur Radiol.* 2005;15:1446–1455.

TABLE 38.5
COMPARISONS OF MODALITIES: ECHO, CT, AND MRI

	Echocardiogram	CT	MRI
Availability	Excellent	Limited	Limited
Applicability	Excellent	Good	Fair
Cost	Low	Intermediate	High
Contrast use	None	Yes	Yes
Tissue resolution	Fair, limited by acoustic windows	Fair	Excellent, good visualization of myocardial infiltration, multiplanar imaging, and quantitates tumor volume
Tissue characterization	Poor	Excellent, especially calcification and fats	Excellent, the best soft tissue characterization
Functional data	Excellent	Poor	Some information such as flow direction and velocity in large vessels
Blood flow			
Valve	Excellent	Good	Good
Pericardium visualization	Fair	Excellent	Excellent
Extracardiac extension	Poor	Excellent	Excellent

4.2.3. Orthotropic heart transplantation
Orthotropic heart transplantation (OHT) after neoadjuvant chemoradiation is a rarely explored but reasonable option for patients with extensive local disease without distant metastases.[5,12,60] Patients most likely to benefit from OHT are those with low grade neoplasm and metastatic tendencies.[101]

A treatment algorithm for cardiac tumors is shown in Figure 38.8.

5. FUTURE DIRECTIONS

Research into different apoptotic pathways in the heart can contribute to improved and safer anticancer therapies for the heart.[102] Cytogenic and molecular genetic studies of sarcomas have elucidated a reproducible chromosomal translocation causing the production of chimeric genes, which may code for fusion proteins causing malignant changes in cells and resistance to apoptosis.[103]

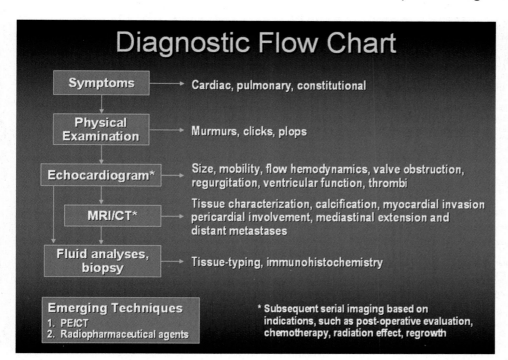

Figure 38.7 Diagnostic algorithm of cardiac masses.

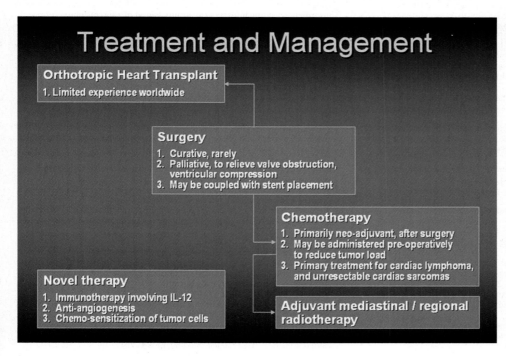

Figure 38.8 Treatment algorithm of cardiac tumors.

This translocation occurs in chromosomes 12 and 15, which results in a fusion protein and a tyrosine kinase that has oncogenic potential.[104] The new tyrosine kinase inhibitors might have beneficial effect in mitigating the disease progression. Targeting mRNA with antisense oligonucleotide and downregulation of protein expression can also induce apoptosis and render these tumors chemosensitive.[105] The fusion proteins increase the production of the antiapoptotic protein bcl-xl. Antisense oligonucleotides directed at this oncoprotein mRNA have led to apoptosis in rhabdomyosarcoma cells.[106]

Despite the seemingly normal expression of p53, the mdm-2 gene is often overexpressed in many sarcomas, including angiosarcoma. mdm-2 binds to and inhibits p53 activity, potentially inducing cellular transformation. The overexpression of mdm-2

has also been implicated in vascular endothelial growth factor overproduction and angiogenesis.[107] Angiosarcoma is an obvious target for therapies based on antiangiogenesis.[108]

REFERENCES

1. Reynen K. Frequency of primary tumors of the heart. *Am J Cardiol.* 1996;77(1):107.
2. Centofanti P, Di Rosa E, Deorsola L, et al. Primary cardiac tumors: Early and late results of surgical treatment in 91 patients. *Ann Thorac Surg.* 1999;68(4):1236–1241.
3. Lam KY, Dickens P, Chan AC. Tumors of the heart. A 20-year experience with a review of 12,485 consecutive autopsies. *Arch Pathol Lab Med.* 1993;117(10):1027–1031.
4. Shapiro LM. Cardiac tumours: Diagnosis and management. *Heart.* 2001;85(2):218–222.
5. Vander Salm TJ. Unusual primary tumors of the heart. *Semin Thorac Cardiovasc Surg.* 2000;12(2):89–100.

6. Grandmougin D, Fayad G, Decoene C, et al. Total orthotopic heart transplantation for primary cardiac rhabdomyosarcoma: Factors influencing long-term survival. *Ann Thorac Surg.* 2001;71(5):1438–1441.
7. Burke A, Virmani R. Tumors of the heart and great vessels. In: *Atlas of tumor pathology.* 3rd series, fasc 16. Washington, DC: Armed Forces Institute of Pathology; 1996.
8. Burke AP, Virmani R. Osteosarcomas of the heart. *Am J Surg Pathol.* 1991;15(3):289–295.
9. Chiles C, Woodard PK, Gutierrez FR, et al. Metastatic involvement of the heart and pericardium: CT and MR imaging. *Radiographics.* 2001;21(2):439–449.
10. Pinede L, Duhaut P, Loire R. Clinical presentation of left atrial cardiac myxoma. A series of 112 consecutive cases. *Medicine.* 2001;80(3):159–172.
11. Reynen K. Cardiac myxomas. *N Engl J Med.* 1995;333(24):1610–1617.
12. Molina JE, Edwards JE, Ward HB. Primary cardiac tumors: Experience at the University of Minnesota. *Thorac Cardiovasc Surg.* 1990;38(Suppl. 2):183–191.
13. Piazza N, Chughtai T, Toledano K, et al. Primary cardiac tumours: Eighteen years of surgical experience on 21 patients. *Can J Cardiol.* 2004;20(14):1443–1448.
14. Burke AP, Cowan D, Virmani R. Primary sarcomas of the heart. *Cancer.* 1992;69(2):387–395.
15. Donsbeck AV, Ranchere D, Coindre JM, et al. Primary cardiac sarcomas: An immunohistochemical and grading study with long-term follow-up of 24 cases. *Histopathology.* 1999;34(4):295–304.
16. Sholler GF, Hawker RE, Nunn GR, et al. Primary left ventricular rhabdomyosarcoma in a child: Noninvasive assessment and successful resection of a rare tumor. *J Thorac Cardiovasc Surg.* 1987;93(3):465–468.
17. Poole GV Jr, Breyer RH, Holliday RH, et al. Tumors of the heart: Surgical considerations. *J Cardiovasc Surg.* 1984;25(1):5–11.
18. Awad M, Dunn B, al Halees Z, et al. Intracardiac rhabdomyosarcoma: Transesophageal echocardiographic findings and diagnosis. *J Am Soc Echocardiogr.* 1992;5(2):199–202.
19. Rheeder P, Simson IW, Mentis H, et al. Cardiac rhabdomyosarcoma in a renal transplant patient. *Transplantation.* 1995;60(2):204–205.
20. Thomas CR Jr, Johnson GW Jr, Stoddard MF, et al. Primary malignant cardiac tumors: Update 1992. *Med Pediatr Oncol.* 1992;20(6):519–531.
21. Nagatani M, Ikeda T, Otsuki H, et al. Sellar fibrosarcoma following radiotherapy for prolactinoma. *No shinkei geka.* 1984;12(Suppl. 3):339–346.
22. Miralles A, Bracamonte L, Soncul H, et al. Cardiac tumors: Clinical experience and surgical results in 74 patients. *Ann Thorac Surg.* 1991;52(4):886–895.
23. Grebenc ML, Rosado de Christenson ML, Burke AP, et al. Primary cardiac and pericardial neoplasms: Radiologic-pathologic correlation. *Radiographics.* 2000;20(4):1073–1103,quiz 110–111,112.
24. Laroia ST, Potti A, Rabbani M, et al. Unusual pulmonary lesions: Case 3. Pulmonary vein leiomyosarcoma presenting as a left atrial mass. *J Clin Oncol.* 2002;20(11):2749–2751.
25. Oliai BR, Tazelaar HD, Lloyd RV, et al. Leiomyosarcoma of the pulmonary veins. *Am J Surg Pathol.* 1999;23(9):1082–1088.
26. Burke AP, Virmani R. Sarcomas of the great vessels. A clinicopathologic study. *Cancer.* 1993;71(5):1761–1773.
27. Burke A, Jeudy J Jr, Virmani R. Cardiac tumours: An update: Cardiac tumours. *Heart(British Cardiac Society).* 2008;94(1):117–123.
28. Shrivastava S, Chopra P, Kumar AS. Fibrosarcoma of the right ventricle–a case report. *Int J Cardiol.* 1985;9(2):234–238.
29. Okuno T, Matsuda K, Ueyama K, et al. Leiomyosarcoma of the pulmonary vein. *Pathol Int.* 2000;50(10):839–846.
30. Herrmann MA, Shankerman RA, Edwards WD, et al. Primary cardiac angiosarcoma: A clinicopathologic study of six cases. *J Thorac Cardiovasc Surg.* 1992;103(4):655–664.
31. Nowrangi SK, Ammash NM, Edwards WD, et al. Calcified left ventricular mass: Unusual clinical, echocardiographic, and computed tomographic findings of primary cardiac osteosarcoma. *Mayo Clin Proc.* 2000;75(7):743–747.
32. Vitovskii RM. Efficacy of the surgical treatment for malignant heart tumors. *Klinichna khirurhiia/Ministerstvo okhorony zdorov'ia Ukrainy, Naukove tovarystvo khirurhiv Ukrainy.* 2005;(1):35–38.
33. Corso RB, Kraychete N, Nardeli S, et al. Spontaneous rupture of a right atrial angiosarcoma and cardiac tamponade. *Arquivos brasileiros de cardiologia.* 2003;81(6):611–613,8–10.
34. Butany J, Yu W. Cardiac angiosarcoma: Two cases and a review of the literature. *Can J Cardiol.* 2000;16(2):197–205.
35. Rettmar K, Stierle U, Sheikhzadeh A, et al. Primary angiosarcoma of the heart. Report of a case and review of the literature. *Jpn Heart J.* 1993;34(5):667–683.
36. Bear PA, Moodie DS. Malignant primary cardiac tumors. The Cleveland Clinic experience, 1956 to 1986. *Chest.* 1987;92(5):860–862.
37. Tse GM, Tsang AK, Putti TC, et al. Stromal CD10 expression in mammary fibroadenomas and phyllodes tumours. *J Clin Pathol.* 2005;58(2):185–189.
38. Suman S, Schofield P, Large S. Primary pericardial mesothelioma presenting as pericardial constriction: A case report. *Heart (British Cardiac Society).* 2004;90(1):e4.
39. Evans BJ, Haw MP. Surgical clearance of invasive cardiac leiomyosarcoma with concomitant pneumonectomy. *Eur J Cardiothorac Surg.* 2003;24(5):843–846.
40. Willaert W, Claessens P, Vanderheyden M. Leiomyosarcoma of the right ventricle extending into the pulmonary trunk. *Heart (British Cardiac Society).* 2001;86(1):e2.
41. Lazoglu AH, Da Silva MM, Iwahara M, et al. Primary pericardial sarcoma. *Am Heart J.* 1994;127(2):453–458.
42. Butany J, Nair V, Naseemuddin A, et al. Cardiac tumours: Diagnosis and management. *Lancet oncol.* 2005;6(4):219–228.
43. Winer HE, Kronzon I, Fox A, et al. Primary cardiac chondromyxosarcoma–clinical and echocardiographic manifestations. A case report. *J Thorac Cardiovasc Surg.* 1977;74(4):567–570.
44. Orban M, Tousek P, Becker I, et al. Cardiac malignant tumor as a rare cause of acute myocardial infarction. *Int J Cardiovasc Imaging.* 2004;20(1):47–51.
45. Abraham KP, Reddy V, Gattuso P. Neoplasms metastatic to the heart: Review of 3314 consecutive autopsies. *Am J Cardiovasc Pathol.* 1990;3(3):195–198.
46. Klatt EC, Heitz DR. Cardiac metastases. *Cancer.* 1990;65(6):1456–1459.
47. Hall R, Cooley D, McAllister H, et al. Neoplastic heart disease. In: Fuster V, Alexander RW, O'Rourke RA, eds. *Hurst's the Heart.* 10th Ed. USA: McGraw-Hill; 2001:2179–2195.
48. Gibbs P, Cebon JS, Calafiore P, et al. Cardiac metastases from malignant melanoma. *Cancer.* 1999;85(1):78–84.
49. Batchelor WB, Butany J, Liu P, et al. Cardiac metastasis from primary cervical squamous cell carcinoma: Three case reports and a review of the literature. *Can J Cardiol.* 1997;13(8):767–770.
50. Gowda RM, Khan IA. Clinical perspectives of primary cardiac lymphoma. *Angiology.* 2003;54(5):599–604.
51. Sarjeant JM, Butany J, Cusimano RJ. Cancer of the heart: Epidemiology and management of primary tumors and metastases. *Am J Cardiovasc Drugs.* 2003;3(6):407–421.
52. Araoz PA, Eklund HE, Welch TJ, et al. CT and MR imaging of primary cardiac malignancies. *Radiographics.* 1999;19(6):1421–1434.
53. Miller DL, Katz NM, Pallas RS. Hepatoma presenting as a right atrial mass. *Am Heart J.* 1987;114(4 Pt 1):906–908.
54. El-Serag HB, Mason AC. Rising incidence of hepatocellular carcinoma in the United States. *N Engl J Med.* 1999;340(10):745–750.
55. Uemura M, Sasaki Y, Yamada T, et al. Surgery for hepatocellular carcinoma with tumor thrombus extending into the right atrium: Report of a successful resection without the use of cardiopulmonary bypass. *Hepato-gastroenterology.* 2004;51(59):1259–1262.
56. Fujisaki M, Kurihara E, Kikuchi K, et al. Hepatocellular carcinoma with tumor thrombus extending into the right atrium: Report of a successful resection with the use of cardiopulmonary bypass. *Surgery.* 1991;109(2):214–219.
57. Tse HF, Lau CP, Lau YK, et al. Transesophageal echocardiography in the detection of inferior vena cava and cardiac metastasis in hepatocellular carcinoma. *Clin Cardiol.* 1996;19(3):211–213.
58. Janzen NK, Kim HL, Figlin RA, et al. Surveillance after radical or partial nephrectomy for localized renal cell carcinoma and management of recurrent disease. *Urol Clin North Am.* 2003;30(4):843–852.
59. Kanemoto N, Usui K, Fusegawa Y. An adult case of cardiac fibroma. *Intern Med (Tokyo, Japan).* 1994;33(1):10–12.
60. Putnam JB Jr, Sweeney MS, Colon R, et al. Primary cardiac sarcomas. *Ann Thorac Surg.* 1991;51(6):906–910.
61. Reeder GS, Khandheria BK, Seward JB, et al. Transesophageal echocardiography and cardiac masses. *Mayo Clin Proc.* 1991;66(11):1101–1109.
62. Geibel A, Kasper W, Keck A, et al. Diagnosis, localization and evaluation of malignancy of heart and mediastinal tumors by conventional and transesophageal echocardiography. *Acta Cardiologica.* 1996;51(5):395–408.
63. Meng Q, Lai H, Lima J, et al. Echocardiographic and pathologic characteristics of primary cardiac tumors: A study of 149 cases. *Int J Cardiol.* 2002;84(1):69–75.
64. Burling F, Devlin G, Heald S. Primary cardiac lymphoma diagnosed with transesophageal echocardiography-guided endomyocardial biopsy. *Circulation.* 2000;101(17):e179–e181.
65. Vieira ML, Ianni BM, Mady C, et al. Left atrial myxoma: Three-dimensional echocardiographic assessment. *Arquivos brasileiros de cardiologia.* 2004;82(3):281–283.
66. Harada T, Ohtaki E, Sumiyoshi T, et al. Successful three-dimensional reconstruction using transesophageal echocardiography in a patient with a left atrial myxoma. *Jpn Heart J.* 2001;42(6):789–792.
67. Lindner JR. Assessment of myocardial viability with myocardial contrast echocardiography. *Echocardiography.* 2002;19(5):417–425.
68. Mengozzi G, Rossini R, Palagi C, et al. Usefulness of intravenous myocardial contrast echoardiography in the early left ventricular remodeling in acute myocardial infarction. *Am J Cardiol.* 2002;90(7):713–719.
69. Kirkpatrick JN, Wong T, Bednarz JE, et al. Differential diagnosis of cardiac masses using contrast echocardiographic perfusion imaging. *J Am Coll Cardiol.* 2004;43(8):1412–1419.
70. Debourdeau P, Gligorov J, Teixeira L, et al. Malignant cardiac tumors. *Bulletin du cancer.* 2004;91(Suppl. 3):136–146.
71. Schvartzman PR, White RD. Imaging of cardiac and paracardiac masses. *J Thorac Imaging.* 2000;15(4):265–273.
72. Tatli S, Lipton MJ. CT for intracardiac thrombi and tumors. *Int J Cardiovasc Imaging.* 2005;21(1):115–131.
73. Siripornpitak S, Higgins CB. MRI of primary malignant cardiovascular tumors. *J Comput Assist Tomogr.* 1997;21(3):462–466.
74. Winkler M, Higgins CB. Suspected intracardiac masses: Evaluation with MR imaging. *Radiology.* 1987;165(1):117–122.
75. Lund JT, Ehman RL, Julsrud PR, et al. Cardiac masses: Assessment by MR imaging. *AJR.* 1989;152(3):469–473.
76. Spuentrup E, Kuehl HP, Wall A, et al. Visualization of cardiac myxoma mobility with real-time spiral magnetic resonance imaging. *Circulation.* 2001;104(19):E101.

77. Spuentrup E, Mahnken AH, Kuhl HP, et al. Fast interactive real-time magnetic resonance imaging of cardiac masses using spiral gradient echo and radial steady-state free precession sequences. *Invest Radiol.* 2003;38(5):288–292.

78. Sparrow PJ, Kurian JB, Jones TR, et al. MR imaging of cardiac tumors. *Radiographics.* 2005;25(5):1255–1276.

79. Altbach MI, Squire SW, Kudithipudi V, et al. Cardiac MRI is complementary to echocardiography in the assessment of cardiac masses. *Echocardiography.* 2007;24(3):286–300.

80. Simonetti OP, Finn JP, White RD, et al. "Black blood" T2-weighted inversion-recovery MR imaging of the heart. *Radiology.* 1996;199(1):49–57.

81. Barkhausen J, Ruehm SG, Goyen M, et al. MR evaluation of ventricular function: True fast imaging with steady-state precession versus fast low-angle shot cine MR imaging: Feasibility study. *Radiology.* 2001;219(1):264–269.

82. Garcia JR, Simo M, Huguet M, et al. Usefulness of 18-fluorodeoxyglucose positron emission tomography in the evaluation of tumor cardiac thrombus from renal cell carcinoma. *Clin Transl Oncol.* 2006;8(2):124–128.

83. Buchmann I, Wandt H, Wahl A, et al. FDG PET for imaging pericardial manifestations of Hodgkin lymphoma. *Clin Nucl Med.* 2003;28(9):760–761.

84. Agostini D, Babatasi G, Galateau F, et al. Detection of cardiac myxoma by F-18 FDG PET. *Clin Nucl Med.* 1999;24(3):159–160.

85. Duhaylongsod FG, Lowe VJ, Patz EF Jr, et al. Detection of primary and recurrent lung cancer by means of F-18 fluorodeoxyglucose positron emission tomography (FDG PET). *J Thorac Cardiovasc Surg.* 1995;110(1):130–139.

86. Delbeke D, Coleman RE, Guiberteau MJ, et al. Procedure Guideline for SPECT/CT Imaging 1.0. *J Nucl Med.* 2006;47(7):1227–1234.

87. Schneider DB, Clary-Macy C, Challa S, et al. Positron emission tomography with f18-fluorodeoxyglucose in the staging and preoperative evaluation of malignant pleural mesothelioma. *J Thorac Cardiovasc Surg.* 2000;120(1):128–133.

88. Ekmektzoglou KA, Samelis GF, Xanthos T. Heart and tumors: Location, metastasis, clinical manifestations, diagnostic approaches and therapeutic considerations. *J Cardiovasc Med.* 2008;9(8):769–777.

89. Roberts WC. Neoplasms involving the heart, their simulators, and adverse consequences of their therapy *Burnc. Proceedings.* 2001;14(4):358–376.

90. Chow WH, Chow TC, Tai YT, et al. Angiographic visualization of 'tumour vascularity' in atrial myxoma. *Eur Heart J.* 1991;12(1):79–82.

91. Poole GV Jr, Meredith JW, Breyer RH, et al. Surgical implications in malignant cardiac disease. *Ann Thorac Surg.* 1983;36(4):484–491.

92. Tazelaar HD, Locke TJ, McGregor CG. Pathology of surgically excised primary cardiac tumors. *Mayo Clin Proc.* 1992;67(10):957–965.

93. Goldstein DJ, Oz MC, Rose EA, et al. Experience with heart transplantation for cardiac tumors. *J Heart Lung Transplant.* 1995;14(2):382–386.

94. Anghel G, Zoli V, Petti N, et al. Primary cardiac lymphoma: Report of two cases occurring in immunocompetent subjects. *Leuk Lymphoma.* 2004;45(4):781–788.

95. Reardon MJ, Malaisrie SC, Walkes JC, et al. Cardiac autotransplantation for primary cardiac tumors. *Ann Thorac Surg.* 2006;82(2):645–50.

96. Anderson TM, Ray CW, Nwogu CE, et al. Pericardial catheter sclerosis versus surgical procedures for pericardial effusions in cancer patients. *J Cardiovasc Surg.* 2001;42(3):415–419.

97. O'Sullivan B, Davis AM, Turcotte R, et al. Preoperative versus postoperative radiotherapy in soft-tissue sarcoma of the limbs: A randomised trial. *Lancet.* 2002;359(9325):2235–2241.

98. Llombart-Cussac A, Pivot X, Contesso G, et al. Adjuvant chemotherapy for primary cardiac sarcomas: The IGR experience. *Br J Cancer.* 1998;78(12):1624–1628.

99. Reardon MJ, Walkes JC, Benjamin R. Therapy insight: Malignant primary cardiac tumors. *Nat Clin Pract.* 2006;3(10):548–553.

100. Nakagawa Y, Ikeda U, Hirose M, et al. Successful treatment of primary cardiac lymphoma with monoclonal CD20 antibody (rituximab). *Circ J.* 2004;68(2):172–173.

101. Catton C. The management of malignant cardiac tumors: Clinical considerations. *Semin Diagn Pathol.* 2008;25(1):69–75.

102. Perik PJ, de Vries EG, Gietema JA, et al. The dilemma of the strive for apoptosis in oncology: Mind the heart. *Crit Rev Oncol Hematol.* 2005;53(2):101–113.

103. Tomescu O, Barr FG. Chromosomal translocations in sarcomas: Prospects for therapy. *Trends Mol Med.* 2001;7(12):554–559.

104. Graadt van Roggen JF, Bovee JV, Morreau J, et al. Diagnostic and prognostic implications of the unfolding molecular biology of bone and soft tissue tumours. *J Clin Pathol.* 1999;52(7):481–489.

105. Smythe WR, Mohuiddin I, Ozveran M, et al. Antisense therapy for malignant mesothelioma with oligonucleotides targeting the bcl-xl gene product. *J Thorac Cardiovasc Surg.* 2002;123(6):1191–1198.

106. Bernasconi M, Remppis A, Fredericks WJ,. Induction of apoptosis in rhabdomyosarcoma cells through down-regulation of PAX proteins. *Proc Natl Acad Sci USA.* 1996;93(23):13164–13169.

107. Milas M, Yu D, Lang A, et al. Adenovirus-mediated p53 gene therapy inhibits human sarcoma tumorigenicity. *Cancer Gene Ther.* 2000;7(3):422–429.

108. Momand J, Zambetti GP. Mdm-2: "big brother" of p53. *J Cell Biochem.* 1997;64(3):343–352.

109. Kim EE, Wallace S, Abello R, et al. Malignant cardiac fibrous histiocytomas and angiosarcomas: MR features. *J Comput Assist Tomogr.* 1989;13(4):627–632.

110. Burke A, Virmani R. Tumours and tumour-like conditions of the heart. In: Silver MD, Gotleib AG, Schoen FJ, eds. *Cardiovascular Pathology.* New york, NY: Churchill Livingstone; 2001:583–605.

111. Neragi-Miandoab S, Gangadharan SP, Sugarbaker DJ. Cardiac sarcoma 14 years after treatment for pleural mesothelioma. *N Engl J Med.* 2005;352(18):1929–1930.

Prosthetic Valves and Devices

39

Jennifer A. Dickerson
Subha V. Raman

1. INTRODUCTION

Contemporary management of patients with valvular heart disease (VHD) includes a vast array of percutaneous and surgical options. Replacement includes both biological and mechanical prostheses. Increasing emphasis on repair over replacement has resulted in increased use of annuloplasty and clip devices to address regurgitant valvular lesions. In addition to the valvular lesion, VHD patients often require implantation of pacemaker and cardiac defibrillator devices. And in patients with advanced heart failure refractory to medical management alone, ventricular assist and resynchronization devices are ever increasing in frequency. Over the last 10 years the number of valve repairs and replacements has increased due to both aging of the population as well as improvement in surgical techniques that allow for intervention in higher-risk patients. In addition, the cost-effectiveness of aortic valve procedures in octogenarians and nonagenarians has been demonstrated.[1,2] In 2006, over 56,000 valvular procedures were performed in the United States alone.[3]

With implantation of devices comes a challenge in adequate diagnostic imaging of both implanted devices as well as native cardiovascular structures. In an era of multiple modalities and an array of clinical queries requiring diagnostic imaging, this chapter provides the cardiovascular clinician with algorithms for efficient and accurate evaluation of prosthetic valves and devices.

1.1. Clinical presentation

Clinical presentation of patients with VHD varies, particularly in the setting of prosthetic valve dysfunction. Typical symptoms include signs and symptoms of systolic heart failure such as dyspnea, orthopnea, and lower extremity edema. In addition, patients may have symptoms of low cardiac output such as fatigue or malaise. An attentive patient history is especially important in the setting of subtherapeutic anticoagulation for mechanical valve prostheses or in patients with signs and symptoms of endocarditis. Prosthetic valve dysfunction can occur as a result of primary structural degeneration or as a secondary phenomenon from pannus development, thrombus formation, or infective masses. The clinical presentation may be acute, subacute, or chronic. The clinician's first sign of prosthetic valve dysfunction may be detected with auscultation revealing a change in the quality or crispness of valve sounds, muffled valve sounds, or development of a new or worsening murmur of insufficiency. Any clinical suspicion of prosthetic valve dysfunction warrants further evaluation given the significant morbidity and mortality if left untreated.

2. PATHOPHYSIOLOGY

2.1. Normal prosthetic valve morphology and function

Starting from the first generation Starr–Edwards valve implanted in the 1960s to present-day stentless tissue valves, mechanical and bioprosthetic valves have evolved to provide increasing durability in a variety of clinical applications. The traditional modality for evaluating prosthetic valve morphology and function is echocardiography. As a Class I indication in the most current societal guidelines, patients with a newly-implanted prosthetic valve (both bioprosthetic and mechanical) should undergo baseline echocardiography within 2 to 4 weeks after hospital discharge or more acutely if clinically indicated.[4] In addition to visualization of the prosthesis location, excursion, and associated stenosis or insufficiency, echocardiography can provide information regarding ventricular size and function. Estimated pulmonary artery systolic pressure and visualization of the pericardial space for effusion are of specific interest in the assessment of the patient who is recently status-post cardiac valve surgery. Documentation of baseline transvalvular pressure gradients is helpful for subsequent comparison when there is suspected prosthetic valve obstruction. In addition, many prosthetic valves have a wide range of "normal" gradients, making it essential to establish what is "normal" in an individual patient with a specific valve type.[4]

For routine surveillance, transthoracic echocardiography (TTE) of a biologic valve can be considered 5 years after implantation. Routine, annual echocardiography is not warranted unless there is concern regarding change in ventricular function, clinical status, or auscultatory findings.[4]

A complete TTE or transesophageal echocardiogram (TEE) in a patient with a prosthetic cardiac valve consists of two-dimensional imaging and Doppler interrogation to evaluate valvular and cardiac structure and function. Complete assessment includes identifying the type and location of prosthetic valves in addition to morphology, gradients, and regurgitation. The complete valve annulus and sewing ring deserve close scrutiny; opening and closing motion of the valve should also be queried.[5] Rocking motion of the valve may suggest valvular dehiscence, especially if accompanied by perivalvular leaks. Abnormal motion of the valve leaflets or discs may suggest concomitant abnormalities such as vegetation, thrombus, or pannus.

Both TTE and TEE are used to evaluate prosthetic heart valves, and the two tests can be complementary to one another. The greatest limitation to ultrasound evaluation of prosthetic heart valves remains acoustic shadowing from the prosthesis. This is especially difficult when two or more prosthetic valves are present. TTE can identify the type of mechanical prosthesis; for example, most prostheses are low profile valves with tilting-disc or bileaflet structure, while one occasionally comes across the high profile ball-cage valve. TTE of bioprosthetic valves are adequate to evaluate general leaflet mobility as well as sewing ring stability. Stentless valves may be difficult to distinguish from native valves and save greater echogenicity at the valve annulus. Table 39.1 categorizes the various types of prosthetic valves according to their material and design.

Doppler evaluation forms an essential component of echocardiographic assessment of prosthetic valves; in general, transvalvular velocities are higher across prosthetic valves than across native valves. Bioprosthetic valves also produce greater resistance to blood flow, causing flow acceleration compared to velocities obtained in normal native valves. Average prosthetic velocities are widely available for specific valve types; however, defining an individual patient's prosthetic valve velocities at baseline postoperatively is most useful to serve as a "normal" reference.[6] The continuity equation is used to calculate the peak and mean pressure gradients from Doppler velocities, as is done for native valves. The same limitations to Doppler echocardiography apply, in that transducer angulation relative to jet direction introduces errors in estimations of valve areas. Doppler-derived measurements of prosthetic valve area, which corresponds to the vena contracta of the valve orifice, are typically smaller than that of the expected area reported by the manufacturer.[7] Doppler-derived velocity index (DVI) is a simple alternative for the evaluation of prosthetic valve stenosis.[5] This dimensionless index is calculated as a ratio of the outflow tract velocity to the velocity across the prosthesis. DVI for a normally functioning prosthesis is typically between 0.35 and 0.5. The DVI removes the error introduced into the continuity equation by manual measurement of the left ventricular outflow tract (LVOT) diameter. Causes of increasing velocity across a prosthetic valve with decreasing effective orifice area can include pannus, thrombosis, and endocarditis, which will be discussed separately in the next section of this chapter. Color Doppler is another tool for prosthetic valve evaluation. The amount of regurgitation can be qualitatively evaluated with color Doppler; however, technical limitations must be appreciated. Acoustic shadowing can lead to an underestimation of regurgitation due to reduced size of the visualized regurgitant jet. TTE is generally superior for the evaluation of

TABLE 39.1
TYPES OF PROSTHETIC CARDIAC VALVES

Mechanical

Single tilting disc	Björk-Shiley (600 reported cases of strut fractures)
	Medtronic hall (low thrombogenicity and good mechanical performance)
	Omniscience/Omnicarbon
	Monostrut valve (struts are machines connected to housing to reduce the chance of strut fracture)
	Ultracor valve (used outside the United States)
	Lillihei-Kaster
Bileaflet disc	St Jude's
	St Jude regent valve (supra-annular cuff to provide a greater orifice area for given annular diameter, resulting in lower transvalvular gradients)
	Carbomedics
	Sorin biocarbon
	Edwards-Duramedics
	Medtronic advantage

Bioprosthetic

Stented porcine	Carpentier-Edwards
	Hancock standard mitral
	Hancock modified aortic
	Hancock II aortic and mitral
	Hancock modified orifice II aortic
	Mosaic aortic and mitral (anticalcification treatment)
	Bicor/St Jude Medical
	Epic
Stentless porcine	Medtronic freestyle
	St Jude Toronto SPV
	Biocor stentless
	CryoLife-O'Brien valve (low pressure gluteraldehyde fixation)
	CryoLife-Ross valve
Bovine pericardial	Carpentier-Edwards perimount pericardial valve
	Carbomedics mitroflow synergy stented pericardial
	Ionescu-Shiley
Homograft	Pulmonary and aortic valves explanted from human hearts, sterilized and cryopreserved
Pulmonary autograft	(Ross procedure)

aortic prosthetic regurgitation, and TEE is preferred for mitral prosthesis insufficiency due to the relative positions of the probe to the valve in question. However, overall, TEE performs better than TTE for the evaluation of severity of prosthetic valve regurgitation.[8] In addition, continuous wave Doppler is more sensitive than pulsed wave Doppler for identifying regurgitant jets.

While TTE is typically used in the initial evaluation of prosthetic valves, TEE may be the first-line test in the setting of high suspicion for prosthetic valve dysfunction where an unrevealing TTE would be inadequate. In direct comparisons, TEE has demonstrated increased sensitivity and specificity (86% and 88%, respectively) compared to TTE (57% and 63%, respectively) for diagnosis of prosthetic valve dysfunction.[8]

While echocardiography remains the workhorse for imaging of prosthetic valves, other modalities are proving their merit for visualization and assessment of prosthetic valves. Multidetector row computed tomography (MDCT) is particularly well suited to visualization of prosthetic valves with minimal artifact. MDCT gives information regarding calcification of bioprosthetic valves and mechanical leaflets. Its volumetric nature and submillimeter isotropic spatial resolution allow for visualization in any plane or volume to evaluate for restricted leaflet motion. MDCT not only gives the interpreter unrestricted planes of interrogation for the valve, but also information regarding adjacent structures such as the aorta and coronary arteries. While not limited by acoustic windowlike echocardiography, image quality still suffers in case of obese patients due to attenuation of X-rays. MDCT also affords visualization of complications secondary to endocarditis such as perivalvular abscesses, fistulae, or pseudoaneurysms.[9]

Clinical use of cardiac magnetic resonance (CMR) imaging for prosthetic valve assessment is also emerging at many centers. It is worthy to note that all prosthetic heart valves—mechanical valves, biologic valves, and repair hardware such as annuloplasty rings—can be safely imaged with magnetic resonance.[10]

CMR is a powerful tool to evaluate cardiac morphology, function, and hemodynamics. The prosthetic material of valves provides minimal signal due to low proton density. Furthermore, there may be local susceptibility artifact that can be minimized using spin echo versus gradient echo imaging and other acquisition parameter optimization.[11] Based on CMR appropriateness criteria, CMR is considered appropriate in the evaluation of prosthetic heart valves for investigation of stenosis or regurgitation, especially in those patients with technically inadequate echocardiographic studies.[12] This is especially useful in patients with concomitant aortic disease, where CMR provides a comprehensive cardiovascular evaluation for not only valvular disease but also cardiac function, aortic morphology, and aortic compliance. Given the vast array of acquisition techniques, a typical CMR examination is designed using those techniques required for the diagnostic needs of the individual patient and referring physician. A comprehensive CMR evaluation includes assessment of left ventricular (LV) structure and function, velocity-encoded sequences for assessment of valvular function, and delayed postgadolinium imaging for myocardial evaluation. Aortic imaging often utilizes precontrast dark blood imaging and contrast-enhanced magnetic resonance angiography (MRA).[13] Comprehensive CMR evaluation is most beneficial and economical for patients with multiple cardiovascular issues that require serial assessment. These include patients with aortopathies or congenital heart disease that may have prosthetic valves and valved conduits, patients who are status-post Ross procedures and whenever evaluation of right heart function is required.[14,15] Figure 39.1 and Movie 39.1 show a bioprosthetic aortic valve on CMR.

2.2. Prosthetic valve dysfunction

Familiarity with the normal function of prosthetic valves across varying modalities facilitates identification of prosthetic valve dysfunction. The overall incidence of complications in appropriately managed patients with prosthetic valves is 3% per year.[16-19] In this section, we will discuss the issues of structural deterioration, thrombosis, and pannus formation as well as valve thrombosis, dehiscence, and endocarditis.

2.2.1. Structural deterioration

Structural deterioration is a problem most specific to bioprosthetic valves. In the Veterans Affairs Cooperative Study on VHD, the 11-year failure rate for bioprosthetic valves due to structural deterioration was 15% in the aortic position and 36% for mitral bioprostheses. No valve failures occurred in mechanical valves over the same 11-year period.[16] The mechanism of failure in bioprosthetic dysfunction due to structural degeneration is the development of severe regurgitation due to tearing of calcified valve leaflets. Calcification and stiffening can lead to significant stenosis. Structural deterioration of a bioprosthetic valve should be suspected whenever increased valvular regurgitation or stenosis develops. This is evaluated most commonly with TTE or TEE, though CMR is increasingly used especially in the setting of congenital heart disease or aortopathy.

Figure 39.1 Bioprosthetic aortic valve seen on CMR SSFP imaging in LVOT (**left**) and three-chamber (**right**) orientations. **Movie 39.1**: Three-chamber cine CMR shows a bioprosthetic aortic valve.

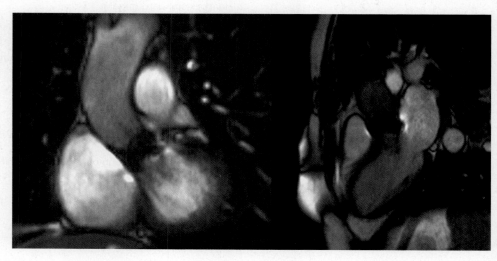

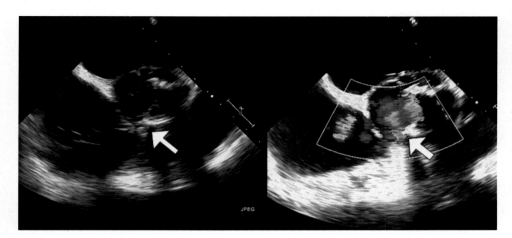

Figure 39.2 TEE of a bioprosthetic aortic valve with a perivalvular leak; the defect is suspected on two-dimensional imaging (**left**) and confirmed with color Doppler (**right**).

2.2.2. Valvular dehiscence

A perivalvular leak can signify prosthetic valvular dehiscence; however, one must exert caution in evaluating signs of periprosthetic regurgitation. Small jets of regurgitation between the annulus and the sewing ring are not uncommon and do not necessarily indicate dehiscence. In one series, the frequency of this finding was as high as 10% for aortic and 15% for mitral prostheses.[20] Risk factors for pathologic perivalvular leaks include smaller body habitus, bioprosthetic valves, supra-annular position, and Marfan syndrome.[21] Also, presence of moderate or severe regurgitation or progressive worsening of small jets of perivalvular regurgitation should augment one's concern for valvular dehiscence. A rocking motion or movement of the prosthetic valve that exceeds 15 degree in one direction is an indication of dehiscence.[22] Overt valvular dehiscence can result from a variety of mechanisms. The integrity of the suture line could have been compromised by usual wear or age-related deterioration of the valve, the valve may have been poorly seated at the time of the surgery or a secondary process such as endocarditis may have produced disruption of the suture line. Figure 39.2 illustrates a bioprosthetic valve with evidence of a perivalvular leak with abnormal color Doppler extending outside the suture line. Figure 39.3 and Movie 39.2 show a similar perivalvular leak in the setting of a St. Jude aortic valve.

2.2.3. Prosthetic valve endocarditis

Mechanical valves carry a lifelong risk of endocarditis of about 0.4% per year.[19] TTE is complementary to TEE in the diagnosis of prosthetic valve endocarditis, especially with limitations imposed by the significant acoustic shadowing produced by mechanical prostheses. In several case series comparing sensitivity of the two modalities, TEE performed much better in detecting prosthetic valve endocarditis with a sensitivity of 82% to 96% versus TTE sensitivity of 17% to 36%.[8,23,24] One study of patients with suspected endocarditis, 30% of whom had prosthetic valves, evaluated the potential diagnostic impact of TEE versus TTE. They found that TEE improved the sensitivity of the Duke criteria, especially with prosthetic valves, with TEE reclassifying 34% of patients with prosthetic valves and 11% of patients with suspected native valve endocarditis.[25] The ability of TTE and TEE to diagnose prosthetic valve endocarditis based on valve type and location may be limited by the adequacy of the images (Table 39.2).[26] Figure 39.4 and Movie 39.3 illustrate a patient with extensive prosthetic valve endocarditis with a large mobile mass affixed to the St. Jude aortic valve with extensive perivalvular abscess formation.

While echocardiography remains the mainstay for detecting prosthetic valve endocarditis, other imaging modalities may offer useful information particularly in conjunction with myocardial or coronary assessment. Current generation MDCT technology has sufficient spatial resolution to visualize valvular structures with multiphase reconstruction of ECG-gated acquisitions; demonstration of vegetations should improve with ongoing technological advances in MDCT's temporal resolution. Computed tomography (CT) has shown ability to detect vegetations on both

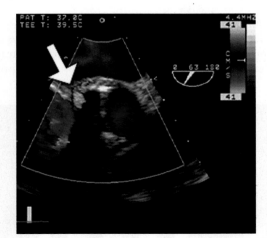

Figure 39.3 TEE demonstrates a St. Jude prosthetic aortic valve with perivalvular leak (*arrow*). **Movie 39.2**: TEE shows perivalvular leak around a bileaflet tilting-disc aortic valve prosthesis.

TABLE 39.2

ADEQUACY OF TTE AND TEE IN DIAGNOSING PROSTHETIC VALVE ENDOCARDITIS

Prosthesis type and position	Nondiagnostic TTE (%)	Nondiagnostic TEE (%)
Aortic position	47	15
Bioprosthesis	50	8
Mechanical valve	45	18
Mitral position	86	11
Bioprosthesis	75	20
Mechanical valve	89	7

Source: Karchmer AW, Longworth DL. Infections of intracardiac devices. *Cardiol Clin.* 2003;21(2):253–271, vii.

Figure 39.4 TEE shows a St Jude aortic valve with endocarditis; note the large vegetation seen with magnification *(arrow)*. **Movie 39.3:** Prosthetic aortic valve endocarditis. Note the large, mobile vegatation as well as excessive thickening around the aortic root indicating abscess.

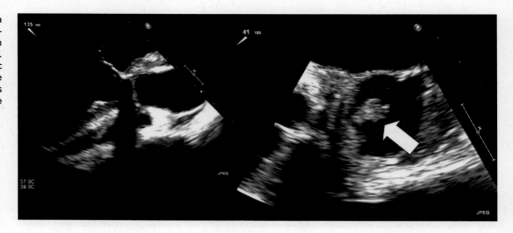

mechanical and bioprosthetic valves with 64-slice platforms.[9] Both MDCT and CMR have been shown to demonstrate complications of endocarditis such as fistulae or pseudoaneurysms.

2.2.4. Thrombosis and pannus formation

The diagnostic tests of choice for prosthetic valve thrombosis have traditionally been TEE or cinefluoroscopy. These tests can provide information regarding leaflet mobility and clot burden; additionally, echo Doppler can provide information regarding hemodynamic significance. When prosthetic valve thrombosis is suspected, the guidelines support either TTE or TEE as the initial imaging investigation.[4,27] Montorsi et al.[28] compared the diagnostic accuracy of cinefluoroscopy, TTE, and TEE in a series of 82 patients with suspected prosthetic valve thrombosis. The specific diagnostic criteria used were restricted leaflet motion with fluoroscopy, increased Doppler gradients with TTE, and visualization of thrombi with TEE. Cinefluoroscopy alone had 87% sensitivity and 78% specificity in detecting prosthetic valve thrombosis, while TTE alone had 75% sensitivity and 64% specificity; together, the two modalities had 85% accuracy. TEE was felt to be required in only 15% of cases, including (i) single tilting-disc valves where cinefluoroscopy is abnormal and (ii) clinical situations where a high index of suspicion exists for nonobstructive prosthetic valve thrombus such as mitral prostheses, atrial fibrillation, and systemic embolism. In patients with diagnosed prosthetic valve thrombosis receiving thrombolytic therapy, thrombus area >0.8 cm² by TEE predicts higher risk of complications such as stroke, peripheral embolic events, and death.[29] Figure 39.5 and Movie 39.4 illustrate a case with extensive thrombus on a mechanical mitral valve; note the increased gradient across the valve and the large thrombus burden.

Pannus formation due to fibrotic tissue overgrowth of the valve is less common than prosthetic valve thrombosis, but making the correct diagnosis is essential for accurate treatment selection.[30] Distinction of pannus from thrombi can be difficult with echocardiography, though pannus tends to be smaller and fixed to valve apparatus versus thrombi that are larger and more mobile. In addition, pannus is typically highly echogenic.[31] Coupled with imaging characteristics, clinical data such as the adequacy of anticoagulation and duration of symptoms help establish the correct diagnosis.[30,32] More recently, MDCT has shown promise in evaluating prosthetic valve thrombosis through visualization of the mechanical valve leaflets with ECG-gated, two-dimensional and three-dimensional renderings in any plane or volume. One series using MDCT in 16 patients with St. Jude valves in the aortic position demonstrated pannus extending from the interventricular septum to the pivot guard of the valve leaflets. Even with minor streak artifact from the metallic leaflets, the attenuation of pannus could be measured and was found to be similar to that of myocardium.[33,34] Thus, MDCT can be used not only to visualize the restricted movement of the leaflets but also to characterize perivalvular tissue. Movie 39.5 shows a MDCT of a patient with abnormal mechanical valve leaflet movement, suggestive of pannus formation. Figure 39.6 provides a basic algorithm for multimodality evaluation of prosthetic dysfunction. Table 39.3 compares the multiple imaging modalities for prosthetic cardiac valves.

2.3. Arterial grafts
2.3.1. Normal morphology

Evaluation of the thoracic aorta in patients who have undergone aortic root and/or arch replacement is a common request to the cardiovascular imaging specialist. An underappreciated

Figure 39.5 Left: TEE shows a mechanical mitral valve with extensive thrombus *(arrow)*. **Right:** Continuous wave Doppler across this valve indicates elevated transmitral velocities. **Movie 39.4:** TEE color Doppler in a patient with a thrombosed St. Jude mitral valve. **Movie 39.5:** Multiphase cine-MDCT images show a fixed posterior leaflet in a patient with prosthetic mitral valve dysfunction.

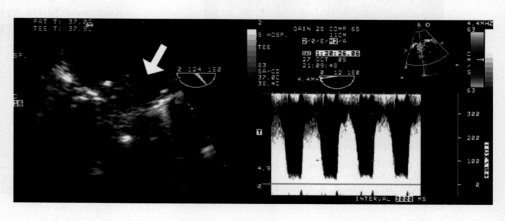

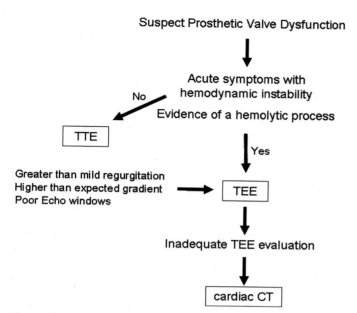

Suspect Prosthetic Valve Dysfunction

Acute symptoms with hemodynamic instability
Evidence of a hemolytic process

No → TTE

Greater than mild regurgitation
Higher than expected gradient
Poor Echo windows → TEE

Yes → TEE

Inadequate TEE evaluation

cardiac CT

Figure 39.6 Suggested algorithm for evaluation of prosthetic valve dysfunction includes TTE as the first-line modality unless there are features that warrant TEE. Inadequate TEE should prompt considerate of CT imaging.

extension of the heart, the postsurgical aorta can be evaluated with multiple imaging modalities each with distinct advantages and disadvantages.[35] The clinical use of echocardiography to evaluate the postsurgical aorta is most common intraoperatively. Given the availability of other imaging techniques and the limited extent of aortic coverage with TEE, it is not the imaging modality of first choice for chronic evaluation of patients with aortic repair.[36]

Comprehensive postoperative imaging evaluation of aortic grafts with or without prosthetic aortic valves ideally utilizes MDCT or CMR. When selecting and imaging modality and evaluating the study of a patient who has undergone an aortic surgical procedure, it is paramount that the interpreter understands the extent of the surgery to help guide the noninvasive evaluation. Items for consideration include the extent and location of the aortic graft material, the need to reimplant coronaries, the presence of a prosthetic aortic valve, and of course the indication for the imaging procedure at the present time.

Patients who have had surgery for aortic pathology will typically be subject to a lifetime of surveillance aortic imaging. A significant number of patients may require reoperations for complications or progressive aortic disease. Recognizing the lifetime risk, limiting exposure to ionizing radiation is an important consideration. Magnetic resonance imaging (MRI) is often a suitable alternative to CT, and both offer significant advantages over biplane invasive angiography. A comprehensive cardiovascular magnetic resonance (CMR) protocol in patients with a postsurgical aorta may include aortic bright blood and dark blood anatomy, assessment of the aortic valve, first-pass perfusion in cases of suspected leaks, plaque imaging, and quantification of ventricular function.[35] Cine imaging of the aorta offers direct assessment of vessel wall compliance and may be useful in evaluating vessel wall in regions without grafts.

CMR imaging techniques to generate this spectrum of information are numerous. Traditional techniques include three-dimensional contrast-enhanced MRA. However, imagers should also be aware of noncontrast three-dimensional steady-state free precession (SSFP) MRA that can be done without breath hold using respiratory navigator techniques. Noncontrast, dark blood, ECG-gated T2-weighted turbo spin echo (TSE) sequences provide high-resolution anatomy and vessel wall characterization.[37,38] Velocity-encoded sequences are available to assist in the hemodynamic evaluation of aortic dissection, coarctation,

TABLE 39.3
OVERVIEW OF MODALITIES AVAILABLE FOR IMAGING PROSTHETIC CARDIAC VALVES

Modality	Pros	Cons
TTE	Widely available Good patient tolerance Gross assessment of the prosthetic valve and hemodynamics Lower cost	Limited by acoustic window—obesity, kyphoscoliosis, pulmonary disease, chest wall thickness Acoustic shadowing by prosthetic material Error introduced by Doppler angle of interrogation
TEE	Better assessment of sewing ring and valve leaflets Hemodynamics Superior visualization of small, highly mobile masses	Invasive Lower patient tolerance Acoustic shadowing by prosthetic material Difficult when multiple prosthetic valves/devices are present Blind spot at the level of the carina
MDCT	Three-dimensional data set Not severely limited by body habitus or chest wall deformities Evaluation of aortic pathology Good patient tolerance High sensitivity for detection of calcification	Ionizing radiation exposure Nephrotoxic contrast Streak artifact with metallic objects Allergic risk with iodinated contrast
CMR	Three-dimensional data set Hemodynamic assessment Evaluation of aortic pathology No ionizing radiation Noncontrast three-dimensional aortic imaging feasible	Gadolinum-based contrast risk in patients with end-stage renal disease Claustrophobia MRI safety contraindications

and the aortic valve. Postoperatively, residual dissection can be identified with T1-weighted gradient echo sequences or with three-dimensional noncontrast or contrast-enhanced MRA as described earlier. Wall thickening around the graft may indicate perigraft fibrosis; asymmetric thickening with appropriate signal characteristics and localization should raise concern for hematoma or anastomotic leak.[39,40] Thickening of the vessel wall ≤10 mm postoperatively is considered normal; ≥15 mm may be considered high risk for anastomotic leak that can be confirmed with contrast imaging.[40]

Aortic grafts can be made of biologic tissue as in porcine grafts or, more typically, man-made material such as Dacron or Gortex. Synthetic material has higher attenuation on noncontrast CT. ECG-gated contrast-enhanced computed tomographic angiography (CTA) can define the anatomy of the aortic root and any coronary ostial changes in cases of coronary reimplantation. If an aortic valve prosthesis is present, its function can be evaluated with either CMR or MDCT as described in the valve section. In situations where the aortic arch was involved, different surgical techniques for the head vessels may have been employed. The great vessels may be carried as a single "island" and anastomosed into the graft material or the graft itself may be fashioned with head vessels. Thus, in cases of aortic arch disease the great vessels require close interrogation as part of the aortic imaging protocol. Tables 39.4 and 39.5 provide protocols for comprehensive cardiac and aortic evaluation using CMR.[13]

2.3.2. Dehiscence, infection, and late complications of arterial grafts

Graft anastomotic dehiscence and graft infection are rare complications of aortic surgery, with a rate <2%.[41] The majority of graft infections develop within the first month after surgery, but occurrences have been reported years later as well.[42] Anastomotic dehiscence typically results from graft infection. On MDCT, recognition of an area of low attenuation around the site of surgical anastomosis, especially if enlarging on serial scans, should prompt consideration of infection or dehiscence with or without hematoma.[43] Perivascular extravasation at the site of dehiscence can be appreciated on postcontrast imaging. Rarely, pseudoaneurysm of the composite graft material may occur.[44] Figure 39.7 and Movie 39.6 demonstrate a complex aortic pseudoaneurysm in a patient with a prior Bentall procedure. Both the MDCT and the CMR evaluation are used together to clearly define the extent of aortic disease prior to surgical intervention.

In addition to traditional surgical repairs of aortic disease, there is an increasing interest in percutaneous repair techniques. Endovascular stent graft procedures may be considered in lieu of traditional surgery for descending aortic dissections, aneurysms, ulcerations, and posttraumatic ruptures. MDCT has been established as the preferred imaging modality for serial postprocedure evaluations of these patients. The protocol typically involves a noncontrast scan to identify calcification followed by a contrast-enhanced helical acquisition triggered by bolus tracking at the onset of contrast opacification in the appropriate aortic segment. Imaging evaluation includes identification of residual aortic disease, new disease or dissection postprocedure, patency of graft, and evaluation for endograft leaks or signs of infection. Graft thrombosis can be either concentric or eccentric and can occur in up to 19% of cases. It may appear as a nonenhancing region within the lumen of the graft. Regional stent graft collapse or angulation is a frequent mechanism of thrombus formation. Stent graft fractures can also be identified. Position of the stent should be noted, as stent migration can occur. This is particularly important in the aortic arch where migration may compromise great vessel ostia. Endovascular leaks are not infrequent complications after stent graft placement. They appear as high attenuation areas outside the boundary of the graft material. The leak can be contained within the aneurismal wall of the vessel. Endovascular leaks are classified based on the integrity of the graft and native aorta; location, and morphology drive subsequent leak repair.[45]

TABLE 39.4

COMPREHENSIVE CMR PROTOCOL FOR IMAGING THE THORACIC AORTA

Localizers: Axial, sagittal, coronal

Axial stack of single-shot turbo spin echo (TSE) and/or SSFP images

Breath-hold T1-weighted TSE for high-resolution imaging of dissection and hematoma

Oblique sagittal (candy-cane) cine of the aorta

Contrast-enhanced MRA with 0.1–0.2 mol/kg gadolinium-based contrast, oblique sagittal orientation

Repeat at least two acquisitions after contrast injection

Optional postcontrast axial T1-weighted gradient echo imaging in aortitis evaluation

Include the following in the setting of aortopathy or connective tissue disease:

– multiplane cardiac cine imaging (Table 39.5)

– axial cine 3 cm above aortic valve for aortic distensibility

---

TABLE 39.5

COMPREHENSIVE CMR PROTOCOL FOR CARDIAC FUNCTION AND VALVES

Localizers: Axial, sagittal, coronal

Multiplane cine imaging: horizontal long axis, vertical long axis, multiplane short axis, three-chamber and LVOT views

Additional cine views of the right ventricular outflow tract or right ventricular inflow as needed

Flow velocity measurements perpendicular to the vessel distal to valve leaflet tips

– adjust velocity encoding to anticipated peak velocity, using the lowest velocity without aliasing

Late gadolinium enhancement for myocardial fibrosis (optional)

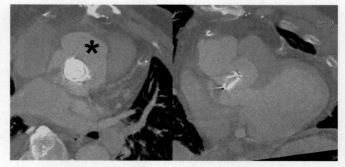

Figure 39.7 MDCT in a patient with a history of Bentall procedure with a St. Jude aortic valve. Complex pseudoaneurysm is seen at the aortic root (*asterisk*). **Movie 39.6:** First-pass dynamic MRA in a patient with a history of a Bentall procedure shows a complex pseudoaneurysm at the aortic root.

2.4. Ventricular assist devices

2.4.1. Normal morphology and function

The cardiovascular community is seeing an increase in ventricular assist device (VAD) utilization, both as a destination therapy and as a bridge to cardiac transplantation. The cardiac imager of present day needs to have a working knowledge of normal VAD morphology and function and a firm grasp on potential causes of mechanical failure and how to utilize imaging modalities to most effectively assist surgical colleagues in trouble shooting the device.

Echocardiographic assessment is typically employed before, during, and after VAD implantation. Typically, a TEE is the test of choice for this patient population. Prior to VAD implantation, echocardiography is used to identify intracardiac shunting, either via a patent foramen ovale or an atrial septal defect. A priori knowledge of this is fundamental, due to the fact that presence of a shunt can compromise LV emptying or lead to systemic destaturation or paradoxical emboli. Echocardiography is also used to diagnosis mitral valve disease that may restrict VAD flows. Significant mitral valve stenosis can limit LV filling. The ascending aorta anatomy also needs to be clearly delineated, as it is frequently a site for outflow cannula implantation. And the left ventricle should be interrogated for apical thrombi, given that it is the typical site for inflow cannula implantation. Right ventricular function is evaluated to ensure functional pulmonary blood flow if only a left ventricular assist device (LVAD) is implanted. There are certain morphologic signs of correct cannulae position that the echocardiographer must be familiar with. These are outlined as follows:

1. Neutral interventricular septal position. This demonstrates adequate ventricular filling.
2. Inflow cannula positioned toward the mitral valve. The cannula should not be directed toward an adjacent myocardial wall. Low flow or high resistance states can occur with the ventricular free wall or septum being sucked into the inflow cannula or with a leaflet of the mitral valve obstructing.
3. Minimal mitral regurgitation. With a correctly positioned LVAD only minimal mitral regurgitation is expected.
4. Aortic valve remains closed or opens intermittently, without significant regurgitation.
5. Left ventricle appears decompressed. The overall cavity dimension is smaller relative to that in the preoperative state.
6. Unidirectional VAD flow. This is indicated by low-velocity flow with color and continuous wave Doppler; minimal pulsatility is seen by pulsed wave Doppler at the location of the entrance of the cannulae.[46]

Figures 39.8 and 39.9 are images of normal LVAD anatomy, one via TEE and one with MDCT.

2.4.2. Mechanical failure of ventricular assist devices

In the echocardiographic assessment of LVAD malfunction, first-line imaging evaluation often involves TEE. Certain features identified with imaging suggest VAD malfunction:

1. Poor LV decompression and/or a rightward shift of the interventricular septum;
2. Significant mitral valve regurgitation;
3. Excessive aortic valve opening during systole;

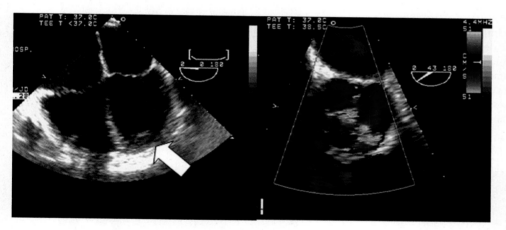

Figure 39.8 TEE in a patient with an LVAD shows the inflow cannula in the LV apex *(arrow)*. There is moderately severe aortic insufficiency on color Doppler **(right)** suggesting LVAD dysfunction.

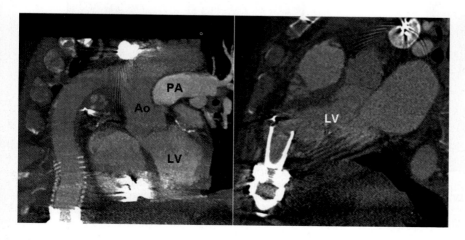

Figure 39.9 MDCT in a patient with an LVAD shows normal position of both outflow **(left)** and inflow **(right)** cannulae. The LV cavity is decompressed and the cannulae appear unobstructed. Ao, aorta; PA, pulmonary artery; LV, left ventricle.

4. Spontaneous contrast in the left ventricle or left atrium;
5. Extrinsic compression of the heart from a pericardial effusion or hematoma;
6. Cannulae appearing kinked or obstructed from thrombus or ventricular wall;
7. Right ventricular dysfunction; and
8. Excess LV cavity decompression precluding adequate LVAD filling.

The typical TEE examination allows assessment of the outflow cannula via a midesophageal view at 100 degree to 120 degree. This shows the cannula and the ascending aorta; color Doppler should show unidirectional flow, and peak velocity by pulsed wave Doppler should be 1.0 to 2.0 m/s. Obstruction may increase velocities or decrease the size of flow by color Doppler.

Inflow cannula assessment with TEE is best visualized with a four-chamber midesophageal view by looking at the cannula through the apex of the left ventricle. This too is best evaluated with color Doppler and pulsed wave Doppler, with high-velocity flow aliasing suggestive of obstruction.[46,47]

While TEE remains the most widely reported method for LVAD imaging, MDCT is rapidly emerging as a useful modality for detailed imaging of VAD placement and performance. With contrast enhancement, MDCT can provide a three-dimensional data set for limitless planes of evaluating cannulae and associated structures.[48] This modality provides excellent visualization of both inflow and outflow cannulae. Cardiac function and valve movement can be delineated with standard ECG-gating for pulsatile VADs. Figure 39.10 is a MDCT evaluation of a patient with LVAD dysfunction, demonstrating the abnormal position of the inflow cannula.

2.5. Catheters, pacemakers, and other devices
2.5.1. Overview (normal morphology)
With ever-growing inclusion criteria for implantable devices such as pacemakers and implantable cardiac defibrillators (ICD), the number of patients requiring cardiac imaging with such devices continues to escalate. Overall, there are almost 4.5 million people worldwide with an intracardiac device.[49,50] The role of cardiac imaging in these patients include assessment of cardiac function, device infection, malfunction, and other postprocedure complications.

A cornucopia of cardiac devices exist, ranging from pacemakers and ICDs to closure devices for atrial septal defects/patent foramen ovale and devices placed around the heart to influence remodeling. Echocardiography holds the advantage of being "compatible" with all the devices mentioned above though acoustic shadowing may limit direct visualization postimplantation. Echocardiography is heavily used prior to placement of septal occluder devices, both preprocedure and intraoperatively with TEE and/or intracardiac echocardiography. Postprocedure evaluation serves not only to evaluate for complications from the procedure but also to evaluate procedural efficacy. Figure 39.11 is a MDCT of a septal occluder device. Figure 39.12 is a MDCT of a patient who had previously undergone apical myectomy for hypertrophic obstructive cardiomyopathy.

The presence of a cardiac device does not necessarily preclude cardiac examination via magnetic resonance. Septal occluder devices are MRI compatible and so are most cardiac remodeling devices. These are typically made of materials like nitinol or MP35N that do not possess ferromagnetic properties. An ongoing source of debate is whether or not MRI can be safely performed in patients with active implants, such as pacemakers and ICDs. Overall, MRI is still considered relatively contraindicated in

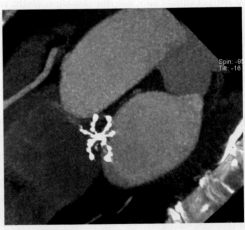

Figure 39.11 MDCT shows a CardioSEAL atrial septal defect closure device.

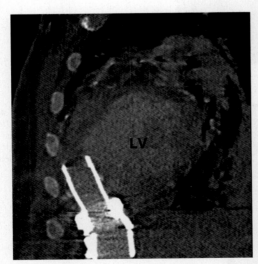

Figure 39.10 MDCT in a patient with LVAD dysfunction shows a smaller region for inflow with the left ventricular (LV) inflow cannula nearly flushed against the interventricular septum.

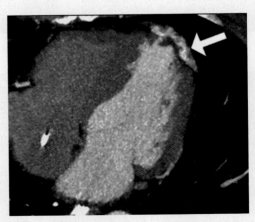

Figure 39.12 MDCT in a patient who underwent prior apical myectomy with placement of an apical patch. Synthetic material placed over the apex (arrow) at the time of the myectomy is seen. Part of a defibrillator lead is seen in the right atrium.

patients with active electronic cardiac implants due to concerns of tissue heating due to current induction at lead tips, programming changes, and mode switching. One formal investigation that included meticulous device interrogation before and after MRI[51] evaluated 54 nonpacemaker-dependent patients undergoing multiple types of MRI and MRA procedures in a 1.5 Tesla scanner. There were no adverse clinical consequences to patients or devices. These authors contended that MRI could be considered in individuals with pacemakers if adhering to the following safety guidelines: (i) the patient understands the risks and benefits for undergoing the imaging procedure; (ii) appropriately trained medical personnel are available, including physicians adept at making programming changes with devices; (iii) interrogation of the device immediately before and after the MRI procedure is done; (iv) when applicable, minute ventilation features on devices are disabled; and (v) continuous cardiac monitoring is done throughout the MRI.[51] There have been other protocols proposed for patients with pacemaker dependence that minimized gradient amplitude and specific absorption rate (SAR) during scanning.[52] The current clinical standard of care is that MRI in patients with pacemakers or ICDs should be done only under the auspices of a research protocol. In general, questions concerning the MRI safety and compatibility of any device are best answered by consulting the manufacturer's guidelines specific to the device, and reference sites such as that maintained by the U.S. Food and Drug Administration for medical device safety (http://www.fda.gov/cdrh/safety/mrisafety.html) or www.mrisafety.com should be consulted. Ultimately, these authors anticipate that incorporation of lead systems specifically designed for MR compatibility, such as those that use fiber optics, represents the safest approach to MRI in patients with active implants.

2.5.2. Migration, infection, lead fracture, and other complications

Cardiovascular imaging can provide insight into complications related to implanted pacemakers and ICDs. This section highlights where cardiac imaging is most commonly used and where there is the greatest evidence to support its use for this application.

The most common complications of pacemaker and ICD devices are: cardiac tamponade, right ventricular perforation, lead infection, lead fracture, migration of lead or lead misplacement, and vascular complications. Figure 39.13 is taken from a patient

where the ICD lead crossed to the left heart via a patent foramen ovale (PFO). The lead appears to cross the mitral valve and is affixed in the LV apex. In settings where one is clinically suspicious of pacemaker lead infection, TEE is the test of choice. Sensitivity to detect vegetations with TEE ranges from 91% to 96%, whereas TTE sensitivity is 23% to 30%.[53] Vegetations can be visualized on the lead, tricuspid valve complex, or right atrium particularly at the ostium of the coronary sinus or the superior vena cava–right atrial junction. Vegetations can be single or multiple, lobular and highly mobile. They can have variable echogenicity due to varying age and extent of superimposed thrombus.[54]

Thrombi can form on pacemaker leads and cause not only regional problems such as an obstructed superior vena cava, but events due to distal embolization such as pulmonary artery occlusion. TEE is the most clinically utilized modality to evaluate for intracardiac thrombi related to device leads.[55]

Other devices that may require serial imaging are septal occluders. Concerns for device migration, coronary sinus obstruction, strut fractures, or residual shunts can be answered with MDCT.[56,57] MDCT is an ideal modality to evaluate septal occluder devices, in that it provides three-dimensional views of the device and surrounding structures. Erosion and perforation rates with septal occluder devices have been reported to be as high as 0.3%. MDCT can visualize the device in association with the adjacent aortic structures and demonstrate formation of aortoatrial fistulas. There is no consensus statement regarding standardization of device surveillance; prospective trials incorporating MDCT in patient evaluation and management may be forthcoming.[58]

3. FUTURE DIRECTIONS

Advances in cardiovascular imaging technology often bring questions regarding utilization. Cost containment measures set forth by government agencies and insurers are designed to prevent unchecked utilization of diagnostic imaging. Cardiac imaging technologies provide detailed device visualization and functional assessment, thus complementing thoughtful bedside decision making. These may lead to improved patient outcomes when the information provided impacts patient management. The appropriateness criteria set forth by professional societies will help the clinician make an educated, informed decision; however, that may not be all there is to the art of clinical care. All cardiovascular physicians need to maintain an understanding of diagnostic modalities including strengths and weaknesses of each test. Anticipating a future that may reimburse for limited number of tests, it is imperative for the patient and physician alike to choose the test most suitable to address each individual patient's clinical needs with the highest accuracy.

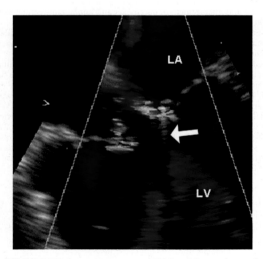

Figure 39.13 TEE demonstrates an ICD lead (arrow) crossing a patent foramen ovale and entering the left ventricle (LV). LA, left atrium.

REFERENCES

1. Wu Y, Grunkemeier GL, Starr A. The value of aortic valve replacement in elderly patients: An economic analysis. *J Thorac Cardiovasc Surg.* 2007;133(3):603–607.
2. Wu Y, Jin R, Gao G, et al. Cost-effectiveness of aortic valve replacement in the elderly: an introductory study. *J Thorac Cardiovasc Surg.* 2007;133(3):608–613.
3. STS Executive Summary. Available at: http://www.sts.org/documents/pdf/ndb/Fall_2007_Executive_Summary.pdf, 2007.
4. Bonow RO, Carabello BA, Kanu C, et al. ACC/AHA 2006 guidelines for the management of patients with valvular heart disease: A report of the American College of Cardiology/American Heart Association Task Force on Practice Guidelines (writing committee to revise the 1998 Guidelines for the Management of Patients With Valvular Heart Disease): developed in collaboration with the Society of Cardiovascular Anesthesiologists: Endorsed by the Society for Cardiovascular Angiography and Interventions and the Society of Thoracic Surgeons. *Circulation.* 2006;114(5):e84–e231.
5. Feigenbaum H, Armstrong W, Ryan T. *Feigenbaum's Echocardiography.* 6th Ed. Philadelphia, PA: Lippincott Williams & Wilkins; 2005.

6. Rosenhek R, Binder T, Maurer G, et al. Normal values for Doppler echocardiographic assessment of heart valve prostheses. *J Am Soc Echocardiogr.* 2003;16(11):1116–1127.

7. Bech-Hanssen O, Wallentin I, Larsson S, et al. Reference Doppler echocardiographic values for St. Jude Medical, Omnicarbon, and Biocor prosthetic valves in the aortic position. *J Am Soc Echocardiogr.* 1998;11(5):466–477.

8. Daniel WG, Mugge A, Grote J, et al. Comparison of transthoracic and transesophageal echocardiography for detection of abnormalities of prosthetic and bioprosthetic valves in the mitral and aortic positions. *Am J Cardiol.* 1993;71(2):210–215.

9. Kim RJ, Weinsaft JW, Callister TQ, et al. Evaluation of prosthetic valve endocarditis by 64-row multidetector computed tomography. *Int J Cardiol.* 2007;120(2):e27–29.

10. Prasad SK, Pennell DJ. Safety of cardiovascular magnetic resonance in patients with cardiovascular implants and devices. *Heart.* 2004;90(11):1241–1244.

11. Cook SC, Shull J, Pickworth-Pierce K, et al. An unusual cause of susceptibility artifact in magnetic resonance imaging. *J Magn Reson Imaging.* 2006;24(5):1148–1150.

12. Hendel RC, Patel MR, Kramer CM, et al. ACCF/ACR/SCCT/SCMR/ASNC/NASCI/SCAI/SIR 2006 appropriateness criteria for cardiac computed tomography and cardiac magnetic resonance imaging: A report of the American College of Cardiology Foundation Quality Strategic Directions Committee Appropriateness Criteria Working Group, American College of Radiology, Society of Cardiovascular Computed Tomography, Society for Cardiovascular Magnetic Resonance, American Society of Nuclear Cardiology, North American Society for Cardiac Imaging, Society for Cardiovascular Angiography and Interventions, and Society of Interventional Radiology. *J Am Coll Cardiol.* 2006;48(7):1475–1497.

13. Society of Cardiac Magnetic Resonance CMR Protocols. Available at: http://www.scmr.org/documents/SCMR_protocols_2007.pdf. Accessed May, 2008.

14. Kawamoto S, Bluemke DA, Traill TA, et al. Thoracoabdominal aorta in Marfan syndrome: MR imaging findings of progression of vasculopathy after surgical repair. *Radiology.* 1997;203(3):727–732.

15. Grotenhuis HB, de Roos A, Ottenkamp J, et al. MR imaging of right ventricular function after the Ross procedure for aortic valve replacement: Initial experience. *Radiology.* 2008;246(2):394–400.

16. Hammermeister KE, Sethi GK, Henderson WG, et al. Comparison of outcomes in men 11 years after heart-valve replacement with a mechanical valve or bioprosthesis. Veterans affairs cooperative study on valvular heart disease. *N Engl J Med.* 1993;328(18):1289–1296.

17. O'Brien MF, Stafford EG, Gardner MA, et al. Allograft aortic valve replacement: Long-term follow-up. *Ann Thorac Surg.* 1995;60(Suppl. 2):S65–70.

18. Vongpatanasin W, Hillis LD, Lange RA. Prosthetic heart valves. *N Engl J Med.* 1996;335(6):407–416.

19. Aslam AK, Aslam AF, Vasavada BC, et al. Prosthetic heart valves: Types and echocardiographic evaluation. *Int J Cardiol.* 2007;122(2):99–110.

20. Ionescu A, Fraser AG, Butchart EG. Prevalence and clinical significance of incidental paraprosthetic valvar regurgitation: A prospective study using transoesophageal echocardiography. *Heart.* 2003;89(11):1316–1321.

21. Rallidis LS, Moyssakis IE, Ikonomidis I, et al. Natural history of early aortic paraprosthetic regurgitation: A five-year follow-up. *Am Heart J.* 1999;138 (2 Pt 1):351–357.

22. Sachdev M, Peterson GE, Jollis JG. Imaging techniques for diagnosis of infective endocarditis. *Cardiol Clin.* 2003;21(2):185–195.

23. Morguet AJ, Werner GS, Andreas S, et al. Diagnostic value of transesophageal compared with transthoracic echocardiography in suspected prosthetic valve endocarditis. *Herz.* 1995;20(6):390–398.

24. Vered Z, Mossinson D, Peleg E, et al. Echocardiographic assessment of prosthetic valve endocarditis. *Eur Heart J.* 1995;16(Suppl. B):63–67.

25. Roe MT, Abramson MA, Li J, et al. Clinical information determines the impact of transesophageal echocardiography on the diagnosis of infective endocarditis by the duke criteria. *Am Heart J.* 2000;139(6):945–951.

26. Karchmer AW, Longworth DL. Infections of intracardiac devices. *Cardiol Clin.* 2003;21(2):253–271, vii.

27. Alpert JS. The thrombosed prosthetic valve: current recommendations based on evidence from the literature. *J Am Coll Cardiol.* 2003;41(4):659–660.

28. Montorsi P, De Bernardi F, Muratori M, et al. Role of cine-fluoroscopy, transthoracic, and transesophageal echocardiography in patients with suspected prosthetic heart valve thrombosis. *Am J Cardiol.* 2000;85(1):58–64.

29. Tong AT, Roudaut R, Ozkan M, et al. Transesophageal echocardiography improves risk assessment of thrombolysis of prosthetic valve thrombosis: Results of the international PRO-TEE registry. *J Am Coll Cardiol.* 2004;43(1):77–84.

30. Barbetseas J, Nagueh SF, Pitsavos C, et al. Differentiating thrombus from pannus formation in obstructed mechanical prosthetic valves: An evaluation of clinical, transthoracic and transesophageal echocardiographic parameters. *J Am Coll Cardiol.* 1998;32(5):1410–1417.

31. Lin SS, Tiong IY, Asher CR, et al. Prediction of thrombus-related mechanical prosthetic valve dysfunction using transesophageal echocardiography. *Am J Cardiol.* 2000;86(10):1097–1101.

32. Girard SE, Miller FA, Jr, Orszulak TA, et al. Reoperation for prosthetic aortic valve obstruction in the era of echocardiography: Trends in diagnostic testing and comparison with surgical findings. *J Am Coll Cardiol.* 2001;37(2):579–584.

33. Teshima H, Hayashida N, Enomoto N, et al. Detection of pannus by multidetector-row computed tomography. *Ann Thorac Surg.* 2003;75(5):1631–1633.

34. Teshima H, Hayashida N, Fukunaga S, et al. Usefulness of a multidetector-row computed tomography scanner for detecting pannus formation. *Ann Thorac Surg.* 2004;77(2):523–526.

35. Raman SV, Cook SC. Cardiovascular computed tomography and MRI in clinical practice: Aortopathy. *J Cardiovasc Med (Hagerstown).* 2007;8(7):535–540.

36. Morocutti G, Gelsomino S, Spedicato L, et al. Transesophageal echocardiography follow-up of patients undergoing replacement of the ascending aorta and aortic valve with a Cabrol procedure for chronic aneurysm and dissection. *J Am Soc Echocardiogr.* 2003;16(4):360–366.

37. Francois CJ, Tuite D, Deshpande V, et al. Unenhanced MR angiography of the thoracic aorta: Initial clinical evaluation. *AJR Am J Roentgenol.* 2008;190(4):902–906.

38. Koktzoglou I, Chung YC, Carroll TJ, et al. Three-dimensional black-blood MR imaging of carotid arteries with segmented steady-state free precession: initial experience. *Radiology.* 2007;243(1):220–228.

39. Nienaber CA, Fattori R. Aortic diseases—do we need MR techniques? *Herz.* 2000;25(4):331–341.

40. Fattori R, Descovich B, Bertaccini P, et al. Composite graft replacement of the ascending aorta: leakage detection with gadolinium-enhanced MR imaging. *Radiology.* 1999;212(2):573–577.

41. Sundaram B, Quint LE, Patel S, et al. CT appearance of thoracic aortic graft complications. *AJR Am J Roentgenol.* 2007;188(5):1273–1277.

42. Coselli JS, Koksoy C, LeMaire SA. Management of thoracic aortic graft infections. *Ann Thorac Surg.* 1999;67(6):1990–1993.

43. Sundaram B, Quint LE, Patel HJ, et al. CT findings following thoracic aortic surgery. *Radiographics.* 2007;27(6):1583–1594.

44. Mesana TG, Caus T, Gaubert J, et al. Late complications after prosthetic replacement of the ascending aorta: What did we learn from routine magnetic resonance imaging follow-up? *Eur J Cardiothorac Surg.* 2000;18(3):313–320.

45. Iezzi R, Cotroneo AR, Marano R, et al. Endovascular treatment of thoracic aortic diseases: Follow-up and complications with multi-detector computed tomography angiography. *Eur J Radiol.* 2008;65(3):365–376.

46. Catena E, Milazzo F, Montorsi E, et al. Left ventricular support by axial flow pump: the echocardiographic approach to device malfunction. *J Am Soc Echocardiogr.* 2005;18(12):1422.

47. Horton SC, Khodaverdian R, Powers A, et al. Left ventricular assist device malfunction: a systematic approach to diagnosis. *J Am Coll Cardiol.* 2004;43(9):1574–1583.

48. von Smekal A, Lachat ML, Willmann JK, et al. Multislice spiral CT follow-up of a patient with implanted debakey ventricular assist device. *Circulation.* 2000;102(15):1871–1872.

49. Josephson M, Wellens HJ. Implantable defibrillators and sudden cardiac death. *Circulation.* 2004;109(2 2):2685–2691.

50. Hauser RG. The growing mismatch between patient longevity and the service life of implantable cardioverter-defibrillators. *J Am Coll Cardiol.* 2005;45(12):2022–2025.

51. Martin ET, Coman JA, Shellock FG, et al. Magnetic resonance imaging and cardiac pacemaker safety at 1.5-Tesla. *J Am Coll Cardiol.* 2004;43(7):1315–1324.

52. Nazarian S, Roguin A, Zviman MM, et al. Clinical utility and safety of a protocol for noncardiac and cardiac magnetic resonance imaging of patients with permanent pacemakers and implantable-cardioverter defibrillators at 1.5 tesla. *Circulation.* 2006;114(12):1277–1284.

53. Kerut EK, Hanawalt C, Everson CT. Role of the echocardiography laboratory in diagnosis and management of pacemaker and implantable cardiac defibrillator infection. *Echocardiography.* 2007;24(9):1008–1012.

54. Dumont E, Camus C, Victor F, et al. Suspected pacemaker or defibrillator transvenous lead infection. Prospective assessment of a TEE-guided therapeutic strategy. *Eur Heart J.* 2003;24(19):1779–1787.

55. Korkeila PJ, Saraste MK, Nyman KM, et al. Transesophageal echocardiography in the diagnosis of thrombosis associated with permanent transvenous pacemaker electrodes. *Pacing Clin Electrophysiol.* 2006;29(11):1245–1250.

56. Lee T, Tsai IC, Fu YC, et al. MDCT evaluation after closure of atrial septal defect with an Amplatzer septal occluder. *AJR Am J Roentgenol.* 2007;188(5):W431–439.

57. Wheatley GH III, Opie SR, Maas D, et al. Atrial septal occluder device surveillance using 64 multi-slice computed tomography. *J Card Surg.* 2007;22(6):537.

58. Delaney JW, Li JS, Rhodes JF. Major complications associated with transcatheter atrial septal occluder implantation: A review of the medical literature and the manufacturer and user facility device experience (MAUDE) database. *Congenit Heart Dis.* 2007;2(4):256–264.

Acyanotic Congenital Lesions

40

Bruce F. Landeck II
Brian Fonseca
Adel Younoszai

1. INTRODUCTION

In the past, patients born with congenital heart lesions were almost exclusively managed by the pediatric cardiologist. However, with the advent of cardiopulmonary bypass, continual improvements in surgical technique and the development of catheter-based interventions, survival and quality of life have both improved dramatically for these patients. In fact, there are now more adults with congenital heart disease than children, and this growth of the adult population with congenital heart disease is only going to expand.[1] This chapter is designed to provide the reader with a basic understanding of acyanotic congenital heart lesions, including their epidemiology, pathophysiology, clinical presentation, imaging modalities, surgical repair, and prognosis.

2. EPIDEMIOLOGY

Approximately 8 in 1,000 live-born infants in the United States have a congenital heart defect.[2] These defects range from simple to very complex. For example, a child may be born with a small muscular ventricular septal defect (VSD), which closes spontaneously in the first months of life, having no impact on the quality or duration of life. Another child may have a severe complex lesion such as hypoplastic left heart syndrome, which will require a lifetime of specialized medical care at significant cost and stress to the family.

Most cases of congenital heart disease are sporadic and their cause is unknown. However, there are many known factors, which if present can predispose a particular infant to congenital heart disease. This is important when counseling prospective parents with certain of these factors. Perhaps, the most well-known is the association between advanced maternal age and the increased risk of infants with Down syndrome, which carries a 40% to 50% risk of congenital heart lesions.

The most comprehensive study involving the epidemiology of congenital heart defects was the Baltimore–Washington Infant Study, conducted from 1981 to 1989.[3] Among other things, this study showed a variation in gender distribution based on a specific lesion, with males predominating in conotruncal defects, branchial arch defects, and left-sided heart defects. All other lesions had an equal or slight female preponderance. Ethnic differences were less clear; however, in general there was no difference in race between cases and controls. Of note, there is a clearly higher incidence of conotruncal defects in Japan than the United States, while left-sided outflow obstructive defects are lower in Japan.[4]

Other factors that increase a child's risk of congenital heart disease include maternal diabetes, maternal exposure to alcohol, diazepam, cocaine, maternal phenylketonuria, and smoking (mother or father). Conversely, folate supplementation during the periconceptual period has been shown to reduce the risk for conotruncal defects.[5]

2.1. Clinical presentation

While the clinical presentation of each acyanotic congenital heart lesion is unique, there are some common themes. Lesions with shunting of blood from the left to the right side of the heart typically present clinically with signs and symptoms of *congestive heart failure* (CHF), while those with significant obstruction to flow along the left side of the heart present with signs and symptoms of *shock*. Other lesions with right to left shunting (sometimes with obstruction along the right side of the heart) or transposition syndromes present with *cyanosis* and will be discussed in Chapter 41.

2.2. Symptoms

Many acyanotic heart lesions present clinically with CHF as a result of systemic-to-pulmonary (left-to-right) shunting of blood (Table 40.1). The basic mechanism behind the direction of shunting is that blood flows to the path of least resistance. Normal cardiopulmonary physiology dictates that pulmonary vascular resistance (PVR) is lower than systemic vascular resistance (SVR); therefore, blood will follow the path of least resistance to the lungs. The degree of shunting depends on the relative resistances of the vascular beds, and the size and location of the shunting defect(s). The relative amount of flow to the pulmonary circulation (Qp) versus the systemic circulation (Qs), known as the Qp/Qs ratio, helps define the degree of pulmonary overcirculation caused by the lesion.

Symptoms of CHF depend on the age of the patient. In infants and small children, these include tachypnea, feeding difficulties, slower-than-expected growth (especially weight), sweating (owing to increased sympathetic tone), and frequent respiratory infections. In older children and adults, CHF can present as dyspnea with exertion, orthopnea, and fatigue. Signs of CHF include tachycardia, tachypnea, hepatomegaly and/or splenomegaly, pulmonary edema on chest X-ray, and S3 or S4 heart sounds on auscultation.

Other acyanotic heart lesions present with shock (Table 40.1). These lesions cause obstruction to blood flow at some point through the left side of the heart or systemic circulation. The level of the obstruction(s) determines the signs and symptoms. For example, a patient with aortic valve stenosis might have globally decreased systemic perfusion, poor pulses, and signs of impaired coronary artery flow. Alternatively, a patient with coarctation of

TABLE 40.1

CLINICAL PRESENTATION OF SELECTED ACYANOTIC CONGENITAL HEART LESIONS

Congenital heart lesions presenting with CHF

Lesion	Percent of all CHD (%)	Percent male (%)
ASD	16	40
VSD	50	slightly <50
AVSD	5	approximately 50
PDA	4	35
Anomalous pulmonary venous return (total or partial)	1	84

Congenital heart lesions presenting with decreased systemic perfusion

Lesion	Incidence (%)	Percent male (%)
Coarctation of the aorta	5	slightly >50
AS	3	66
Mitral stenosis	<1	unknown

the aorta will typically present with normal or bounding pulses in the upper extremities (proximal to the coarctation site) and poor perfusion and pulses in the lower extremities (distal to the coarctation site).

Symptoms of shock also depend on the age of the patient. Infants can present with lethargy, poor urine output, poor skin color, vomiting and/or diarrhea, and tachypnea. Older children and adults present similarly but may also describe nausea, confusion, agitation, and fatigue. Signs of shock include poor pulses, delayed capillary refill, oliguria, tachycardia, tachypnea, hypotension, mottling or cyanosis, cold extremities, and anemia. With coarctation of the aorta in particular it is important to observe for differences in pulse and blood pressure between upper and lower extremities.

2.3. Outcome

In the presurgical era, only about one in three children born with congenital heart disease survived to his or her tenth birthday.[6] The first surgery for congenital heart disease was performed by Drs. Blalock and Taussig at Johns Hopkins in 1944 and described in 1945.[7] Improvements in early diagnosis (including fetal diagnosis), medical management, surgical technique, postoperative care, and longitudinal monitoring with noninvasive imaging have helped improve survival to adulthood to approximately 80% to 85% of all children born with congenital heart disease.[8]

3. PATHOPHYSIOLOGY

The following acyanotic congenital lesions encompass a wide range of severity in pathophysiology. Each lesion has its own unique factors, which determine its natural history, therapeutic options, and both short- and long-term prognosis. Given the scope of this text, only a basic overview of more commonly encountered lesions will be discussed. For detail beyond what is described in this chapter, it is suggested the reader consult a textbook devoted to congenital heart disease.

3.1. Atrial septal defect

Atrial septal defect (ASD) makes up 16% of all congenital heart lesions, and is more common in females than males with an approximate ratio of 1.5:1.[2] Most occur sporadically, but ASDs have occurred in multiple family members. Of note, the term patent foramen ovale (PFO) is used to denote persistence of a normal fetal and infantile structure which represents a potential interatrial communication. A PFO is a persistent communication between the left and right atria through an opening between the septum secundum and the septum primum, whereas ASD is an actual defect in either the septum secundum or primum. Finding a PFO is very common in the adult population, with approximately one in four people with normal hearts being found to have a PFO in a large autopsy series.[9] There is an increased incidence of a PFO in patients with migraine headaches, and percutaneous closure has been proposed as a potential treatment for migraines.[10] The presence of a PFO creates the potential for a paradoxical embolus, possibly causing stroke, and this has led to the practice of percutaneous device closure in patients who have had embolic stroke and are found to have PFO.[11]

A defect of the atrial septum, is categorized by its location into the secundum (most common), primum, sinus venosus, and coronary sinus types (Fig. 40.1). A communication at the atrial level will result in left-to-right shunting of blood due to increased compliance of the right ventricle as compared to the left. In significantly large defects, this increased volume load will lead to right atrial and ventricular enlargement. Patients are typically asymptomatic and present most commonly for evaluation of their murmur caused by increased flow across the pulmonary valve. Less commonly, a large defect can cause symptoms of pulmonary overcirculation, including poor growth, tachypnea and tachycardia in young children, and mild fatigue and dyspnea in older children and adults. The physical exam is normal for small defects. In defects with a significant volume load classic findings include fixed, wide splitting of the second heart sound, a pronounced cardiac impulse, a systolic ejection murmur (as described above) and a middiastolic flow rumble due to increased flow across the tricuspid valve. If left untreated, ASDs can cause irreversible pulmonary hypertension and eventual cyanosis (Eisenmenger

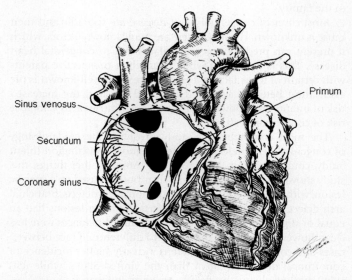

Figure 40.1 Drawing of the four types of ASDs, viewed from the right atrium. Secundum ASD is the most common form, and is usually amenable to catheter-based device closure. (Illustration by Steven Goldberg, MD.)

syndrome), although the onset of pulmonary vascular disease is typically later in life. It has been suggested in natural history studies that the life span of an adult with an untreated ASD is shorter than normal adults.[12]

Treatment options for an ASD include medical management, percutaneous device closure, or surgical closure. In most, congenital heart disease centers the standard therapy for a secundum ASD requiring closure is by percutaneous device. Multiple types of devices are commercially available. The device is placed transvenously by catheter, usually with echo guidance (either transesophageal echo or intracardiac echo). Considerations to be made while attempting device closure are presence of adequate rims of tissue to prevent dislodging and embolization of the device, avoidance of disruption of the mitral valve, tricuspid valve, or aorta (causing valvar insufficiency), and avoidance of causing obstruction to the right pulmonary veins. Those ASDs not amenable to catheter-based closure (including primum, coronary sinus, or sinus venosus defects) can be safely closed surgically.

3.2. Ventricular septal defects

VSD is the most common congenital heart lesion, making up 50% of all congenital heart lesions, with a slight female preponderance. A VSD can occur in relation with many genetic disorders including chromosomal abnormalities (most notably Trisomy 21), but are usually isolated. Many of these defects close spontaneously in the first 3 years of life. Defects that require closure are typically repaired in early childhood.

Defects of the ventricular septum are categorized by location into membranous, muscular, inlet, and outlet/supracristal types (Fig. 40.2).[13] Membranous VSDs made up 80% of all defects in one autopsy series,[13] but a recent echocardiographic study shows a higher prevalence of muscular VSDs in neonates, many of which spontaneously close.[14] Muscular defects can involve more than one area of the ventricular septum and can be multiple.

A communication at the ventricular level will result in left-to-right shunting, and, if significant, will cause left atrial and left ventricular enlargement. A VSD will almost always present initially

in childhood with a systolic (typically holosystolic) murmur. Other findings of a hemodynamically significant VSD include a diastolic rumble and hepatomegaly. Infants present with failure to thrive, tachypnea, tachycardia, and diaphoresis. Older children and adults can be asymptomatic or can have dyspnea. An unrepaired large VSD can lead to fixed pulmonary vascular disease with resultant right-to-left flow across the defect causing cyanosis (Eisenmenger syndrome).

Treatment of a significant VSD is surgical closure at an early age to prevent the advent of pulmonary vascular disease. Percutaneous device closure has been performed and is evolving as an option in some types of VSD.

3.3. Atrioventricular septal defects (AVSDs)

An AVSD, also known as an atrioventricular canal or endocardial cushion defect, makes up approximately 5% of all congenital heart lesions.[2] It has a fairly equal gender distribution, and is often associated with Trisomy 21 (Down syndrome) but can be seen in isolation.

An AVSD occurs due to inadequate development of the atrioventricular septum which is responsible for dividing the common atrioventricular valve into the tricuspid and mitral valves during fetal heart development. Maldevelopment of the atrioventricular septum also is typically associated with an inlet VSD and primum ASD.[15] A complete AVSD includes the above features (Fig. 40.3), while a partial AVSD will typically include just the primum ASD and a cleft in the mitral valve. Typically, a complete AVSD is associated with normal or "balanced" development of both ventricles, however, in some cases preferential flow into one ventricle is associated with concomitant growth failure of the other; this is termed an unbalanced AVSD.

An AVSD causes left-to-right shunting at both the atrial and ventricular levels, and can cause enlargement of all cardiac chambers. This marked pulmonary overcirculation is often complicated by insufficiency of the common atrioventricular valve. Children with an AVSD typically present in infancy with a systolic murmur, failure to thrive, tachypnea, and tachycardia. Similar to a large VSD,

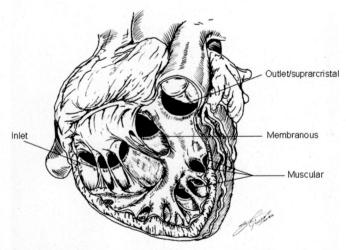

Figure 40.2 Drawing of the four types of VSDs, viewed from the right ventricle. A membranous VSD, the most common, occurs in the membranous septum between the inlet and outlet portions of the ventricular septum, and often extends into any combination of the inlet, outlet, or muscular septum. An inlet VSD occurs underneath the atrioventricular valve apparatus, while an outlet/supracristal VSD occurs in the outflow tract just beneath the pulmonary valve. A muscular VSD occurs in the muscular portion of the septum, often behind the right ventricular trabeculations. (Illustration by Steven Goldberg, MD.)

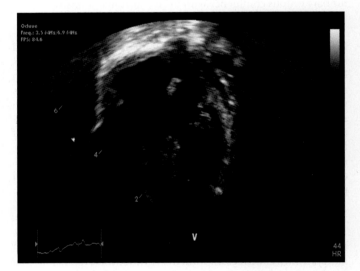

Figure 40.3 AVSD shown by transthoracic echocardiography. In this apical four-chamber view the crux of the heart is absent, resulting in absence of the bottom portion of the atrial septum (primum ASD), inlet portion of the ventricular septum (inlet VSD), and resulting in a common atrioventricular valve (shown open during diastole in this image). A secundum ASD is shown higher in the atrial septum in this image.

the risk of pulmonary hypertension and development of Eisenmenger syndrome typically leads to surgical repair during the first 6 months of life. Postoperative considerations include routine evaluation for residual shunting defects, left- or right-sided atrioventricular valve stenosis or regurgitation, and subaortic obstruction. Approximately 10% of patients with a repaired AVSD will need reoperation, with the most common indication being significant residual left atrioventricular valve regurgitation.[16]

3.4. Anomalous pulmonary venous return

Anomalous pulmonary venous drainage is defined by pulmonary veins which drain into a vessel or chamber other than the left atrium. If one or several veins drain anomalously, it is termed partial anomalous pulmonary venous return (PAPVR), however, if none of the veins return to the left atrium, it is called total anomalous pulmonary venous return (TAPVR). Anomalous drainage of the pulmonary veins comprises around 1% of all congenital heart lesions and has a significant male preponderance (more than 4:1 male to female ratio).[2] It is thought to be a result of failure of the fetal pulmonary veins, which have their embryonic origins in the lung buds to form a confluence and connect appropriately with the left atrium during fetal development.[15] Both TAPVR and PAPVR typically occur as isolated lesions, but can occur in combination with other syndromes including abnormalities of atrial and abdominal situs, Tetralogy of Fallot, and AVSD. In the case of TAPVR, a shunting defect (typically an ASD) is critical for survival in order to provide left ventricular preload.

In the most common form of TAPVR, the pulmonary veins form a confluence, which then communicates with a vertical vein to drain pulmonary venous return up into the innominate vein. This is known as the supracardiac form of TAPVR. Less commonly, the pulmonary venous confluence communicates with a vessel that drains blood through the liver and the ductus venosus (infracardiac TAPVR), or directly into the coronary sinus to the right atrium (cardiac TAPVR). In some cases the pulmonary veins drain into a variety of areas in which case it is referred to as mixed TAPVR.

Anomalous drainage of the pulmonary veins is distinct from cor triatriatum in which there is normal connection of the pulmonary venous confluence with the left atrium but obstruction of flow within the left atrium due to an anomalous membrane.

In PAPVR if only a single pulmonary vein drains anomalously to the superior vena cava or right atrium, the volume load is inconsequential and the patient is clinically asymptomatic. Unobstructed TAPVR can be clinically silent and often mimics an ASD in clinical presentation (right heart enlargement, dyspnea with or without exertion, pulmonary flow murmur). Similar to an ASD, TAPVR is a left-to-right shunt with the potential to eventually cause pulmonary vascular disease (Eisenmenger syndrome) if untreated. Obstructed TAPVR presents in infancy with pulmonary edema and low systemic cardiac output. Treatment is surgical, and postoperative considerations typically are related to residual pulmonary venous obstruction.[17]

3.5. Patent ductus arteriosus

The ductus arteriosus is a normal fetal structure connecting the main pulmonary artery to the proximal descending aorta to facilitate systemic venous return from the right ventricle to the placenta for oxygenation. The ductus arteriosus typically closes within the first hours to days of life. If it does not close in that time frame, it is considered a pathologic patent ductus arteriosus (PDA). Normal transition of the open ductus arteriosus to a closed ligamentum arteriosum is facilitated by an increase in PO_2 as well as other vasoactive substances (vascular endothelial growth factor,

TGF-β).[18] A PDA can be seen in isolation, but has greatly increased the incidence in premature infants and can be seen in conjunction with other forms of congenital heart disease.

A PDA results in left-to-right shunting of blood, with the amount of shunting depending on the relative resistances of the pulmonary and systemic vascular beds. A significant shunt from a PDA will result in left atrial and left ventricular enlargement. If left untreated, a PDA may increase the lifetime risk of bacterial endocarditis or pulmonary vascular disease and cyanosis (Eisenmenger syndrome). Treatment in premature infants consists of either indomethacin administration to stimulate closure or surgical ligation. Percutaneous closure with coil or occlusion device can usually be safely performed in children more than a few months of age.[19] In the absence of significant pulmonary vascular disease, closure of the PDA is curative and long-term residual problems are rare.

3.6. Coarctation of the aorta

Coarctation of the aorta is a fairly common defect, making up approximately 5% of all congenital heart lesions.[2] It has a slight male preponderance and typically occurs sporadically, however, more recent data suggest a hereditary component in some cases, with an increased occurrence in twins, siblings, and first degree relatives.[20] About 35% of individuals with Turner (XO) syndrome have a coarctation of the aorta. In addition, a possible environmental influence is seen with an increased incidence of coarctation in the late fall and winter months.[21]

Coarctation of the aorta usually implies a discrete stenosis of the proximal descending thoracic aorta (Fig. 40.4); however, the lesion can appear as a longer segment stenosis or with considerable arch hypoplasia. It can present in the newborn period with shock during ductal closure (critical coarctation), or can present later in childhood or even in adulthood. Of note, a berry aneurysm in the circle of Willis occurs in 3% to 5% of people with coarctation, and can even be a presenting in rare cases.[22]

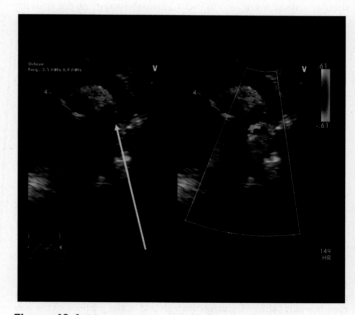

Figure 40.4 Discrete coarctation of the aorta shown by transthoracic echocardiography (suprasternal view) with 2D and color Doppler images displayed side by side. The yellow arrow points to the posterior shelf which causes a discrete narrowing in the proximal descending aorta. Aliasing of color Doppler flow in the picture on the right shows the origin of accelerated blood flow.

There is a wide spectrum of severity of disease depending on the degree of stenosis. Physical examination will reveal diminished and delayed pulses in the legs compared to the right upper extremity (left upper extremity findings vary depending on location of the coarctation in relation to the left subclavian artery). The hallmark of the physical examination is a systolic blood pressure gradient between the right arm (which is typically hypertensive) and either legs, and this gradient may be amplified with exercise. A systolic murmur can be heard in the midscapular area of the back. Additionally, a systolic ejection murmur is often heard over the right upper sternal border caused by a bicuspid aortic valve which is commonly found in patients with arch obstruction.

The natural history of untreated coarctation of the aorta is poor, with a mean age at death of 34 years,[23] therefore treatment of coarctation is warranted. Repair of coarctation depends on age at presentation. Neonates and infants more commonly undergo surgical repair, whereas older children and adults can often be adequately treated with percutaneous balloon angioplasty and often placement of aortic stent.[24]

Coarctation deserves lifetime monitoring for residual effects. These include residual coarctation, aneurysmal dilation of repair site, pseudoaneurysm, endocarditis, and the development of systemic hypertension at both rest and exercise over time.[25]

3.7. Ebstein anomaly of the tricuspid valve

Ebstein anomaly of the tricuspid valve is a rare defect (<1% of all congenital heart lesions[2]), and consists of a spectrum of pathologic findings involving not only the tricuspid valve but also the right atrium and right ventricle. Embryologically, the tricuspid valve leaflets and tensile apparatus are derived from detachment of the inner layers of the inlet zone of the right ventricle, a process called delamination. Incomplete delamination may account for the inferior displacement of the leaflets that is the essence of this congenital cardiac malformation. In Ebstein anomaly, the septal and posterior/inferior mural leaflets do not attach normally to the valve annulus and are displaced apically, thereby causing the effective orifice of the tricuspid valve to be displaced into the right ventricular cavity at the junction of the inlet and trabecular portions of the right ventricle.[26] An echocardiographic example of significant apical displacement of the tricuspid valve is shown in Figure 40.5. The anterior leaflet is large and redundant, often

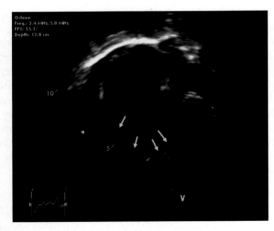

Figure 40.5 Ebstein anomaly of the tricuspid valve shown by transthoracic echocardiography. This apical four-chamber view shows severe apical displacement of the tricuspid valve (*yellow arrows*), resulting in "atrialization" of the inlet and trabecular portions of the right ventricle.

described as "sail like" and may contain fenestrations, contributing to tricuspid regurgitation which is frequently severe. The right ventricle is divided into two components by these displaced leaflets: the proximal atrialized portion and the distal functional right ventricle, which in severe Ebstein malformations can be prohibitively small for normal repair of the tricuspid valve. In the case of severe right ventricular hypoplasia, single ventricle palliation with surgical exclusion of the right ventricle is required for survival. Abnormalities in the conduction system exist in Ebstein anomaly which predispose these patients to Wolff-Parkinson-White syndrome (ventricular pre-excitation due to accessory conduction pathway) and possible supraventricular tachycardia.[27] An atrial level communication (ASD or PFO) is present in most patients with Ebstein malformation.[26]

The severity of Ebstein anomaly typically varies inversely with age with patients presenting in infancy, having more severe displacement of the tricuspid valve toward the right ventricular apex and more significant tricuspid insufficiency. These children present with cyanosis due to reduced forward flow through the right heart into the pulmonary arteries, with increased flow from right-to-left through the atrial communication. By contrast, milder forms of Ebstein's present later in life and may be clinically silent. Indeed, it is not uncommon for mild Ebstein anomaly to be an incidental finding at autopsy.[15] Older children and adults with unrepaired Ebstein's may have a prominent jugular venous distention and a systolic murmur at the left lower sternal border related to tricuspid regurgitation. Symptoms in adulthood can include dyspnea on exertion, fatigue, palpitations, and cyanosis, and depend on the severity of the lesion as well as on whether an atrial communication exists.

Repair for severe Ebstein malformation in infancy often involves, as previously mentioned, exclusion of the right ventricle via the Starnes procedure. This surgery includes placing a patch, often fenestrated, over the tricuspid valve annulus effectively excluding the right ventricle, an atrial septectomy, and insertion of a Blalock–Taussig shunt to provide blood flow from the subclavian artery to the pulmonary circulation.[28] Later in childhood, these children will need to undergo rerouting of the systemic venous return to the pulmonary arteries via a bidirectional Glenn shunt (superior vena cava) at 6 months of age followed by a Fontan operation (inferior vena cava) at approximately 3 years of age.

Milder cases of Ebstein's can have surgery delayed into childhood or adulthood. Surgical repair later in life usually includes tricuspid valvuloplasty or replacement with plication of the enlarged right atrium and atrialized portion of the right ventricle. These patients have done quite well, with a relatively low risk of reoperation.[29] Longer term complications of Ebstein anomaly are often related to the development of supraventricular tachycardia.

3.8. Left ventricular inflow obstruction

Obstruction to left ventricular inflow can be at the pulmonary venous, left atrial, or mitral valve level. Isolated left ventricular inflow is a rare congenital defect, since intrauterine restriction to left ventricular inflow will usually cause downstream maldevelopment resulting in hypoplastic left heart syndrome with aortic valve and arch hypoplasia.[30]

Lesions that cause obstruction to flow at the left atrial level include cor triatriatum (incomplete fusion of the pulmonary venous confluence with the left atrial wall) and a supramitral ring. These abnormal tissue collections within the left atrium prevent diastolic filling of the left ventricle and result in elevated pulmonary venous pressure and pulmonary edema.

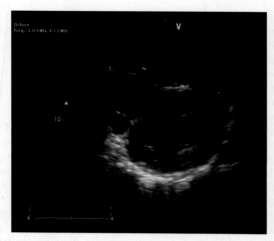

Figure 40.6 Double orifice mitral valve (DOMV) shown by transthoracic echocardiography. This parasternal short-axis view shows an accessory bridge of tissue dividing the mitral valve into two orifices, which then empty into the left ventricle during diastole. Although in this example the openings are relatively balanced in size, more commonly they are unequal with a dominant primary orifice and much smaller secondary one.

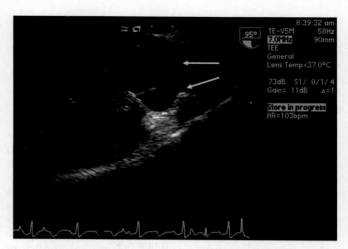

Figure 40.7 Supravalvar AS shown by TEE. This TEE image shows the aortic valve opening during systole (left ventricle is leftward in this picture). Just distal to the aortic valve is a discrete stenosis at the sinotubular junction (*yellow arrows*). This condition is often associated with Williams syndrome.

Congenital mitral valve stenosis can be related to hypoplasia of the annulus, commissural fusion, or excessive or abnormal chordal tissue and attachments. Abnormal chordal apparatus can manifest as double-orifice mitral valve (DOMV), where accessory bridging of tissue divides the mitral valve into two openings into the left ventricle (Fig. 40.6). A mitral valve arcade occurs when the mitral valve leaflets are thickened and chordal attachments are shortened or absent. A parachute mitral valve is defined as having all of the chordal attachments to the mitral valve connect to a single papillary muscle.

The clinical presentation of left ventricular inflow obstruction depends on the severity. Signs and symptoms include growth failure, tachypnea, cough, fatigue, dyspnea on exertion, and low cardiac output. More severe obstruction causes pulmonary hypertension. The physical examination can be remarkable for diminished peripheral perfusion and pulses and for a low-frequency diastolic murmur at the apex (during mitral inflow). A systolic murmur at the apex may indicate mitral regurgitation.

Treatment for left ventricular inflow obstruction depends on the mechanism of obstruction. Historically, surgery has been the preferred repair for all causes of inflow obstruction, however, balloon angioplasty has been shown to have a place in the treatment of isolated stenosis of the mitral valve.[31] The prognosis depends on adequacy of surgical repair or catheter-based treatment, and on whether the mitral valve needs to be replaced.

3.9. Left ventricular outflow obstruction

Obstruction to left ventricular outflow can occur at multiple places in relation to the aortic valve, including the subvalvar, valvar, and supravalvar levels. The most common of these is valvar aortic stenosis (AS), which occurs in approximately 3% to 6% of all congenital heart lesions.[15] This incidence does not include bicuspid aortic valve, a more common finding which often is clinically silent in childhood but can cause stenosis later in adulthood. There is a male preponderance of valvar AS, approximately 2:1.[2]

Congenital valvar AS has an aortic valve with thickened leaflets which are rigid and dome during systole. It often has partial fusion of the leaflets, causing a functionally bicuspid or even unicuspid valve. Stenotic aortic valves often calcify later in life.

Hemodynamically significant obstruction can lead to left ventricular hypertrophy and poststenotic dilation of the ascending aorta. Subaortic obstruction can be caused by a discrete fibrous membrane below the aortic valve or a longer fibromuscular narrowing of the left ventricular outflow tract. Supravalvar AS can be a localized or diffuse narrowing of the ascending aorta, usually originating at the superior edge of the sinus of Valsalva (Fig. 40.7), and is commonly associated with Williams syndrome.[32]

Clinical presentation of left ventricular outflow obstruction varies depending on the severity of the obstruction. Most children with AS are asymptomatic, and the lesion is detected by auscultation of a systolic ejection murmur at routine examination. However, patients with AS can present with fatigue, exertional dyspnea, angina pectoris, and syncope. Physical examination reveals an ejection click from aortic valve opening as well as a systolic ejection murmur best heard at the base of the heart.

Natural history studies suggest progression of AS from childhood to adulthood.[33] Definitive treatment of valvar AS usually begins with balloon valvuloplasty in the catheterization laboratory, often with good relief of the gradient. However, an expected complication is the development of aortic insufficiency, and if significant insufficiency exists before treatment, surgery is the preferred method of repair. If the valve cannot be primarily repaired it will need to be replaced. The native aortic valve can be replaced with a mechanical prosthesis, bioprosthesis or translocation of the pulmonary valve to the aortic position with the insertion of a conduit from the right ventricle to the pulmonary artery (Ross operation). Results from surgical repair of valvar AS have generally been very good.[34,35] Subaortic and supravalvar AS are not amenable to percutaneous balloon procedures and require surgical repair.

3.10. Right ventricular inflow obstruction

Isolated obstruction of right ventricular inflow is very rare and more commonly presents in combination with other obstructive lesions of the right heart (pulmonary stenosis [PS] or atresia) at the tricuspid valve. Tricuspid stenosis is typically associated with a hypoplastic right ventricle and may lead to single ventricle palliation if severe.

Patients presenting with tricuspid stenosis are similar to those with tricuspid atresia. In infancy right-to-left shunting of blood is seen across the foramen ovale causing cyanosis. Later in life if the foramen ovale closes, the right atrium is under high pressure and patients show jugular venous distention and hepatomegaly on physical examination. In addition, a diastolic murmur of tricuspid inflow is present at the left lower sternal border. Patients with tricuspid stenosis who have adequate right ventricular size are repaired with commissurotomy or valve replacement.

3.11. Right ventricular outflow obstruction

Obstruction to the right ventricular outflow can occur at multiple sites, including within the right ventricle, at the pulmonary valve, at the supravalvar level, and at the branch pulmonary arteries. The most common of these is valvar PS, which comprises approximately 7% of all congenital heart lesions[2] and makes up 80% to 90% of all right ventricular outflow obstructive lesions.[15] Valvar PS usually is due to fusion of a valve of normal thickness and appearance, but PS with dysplasia of the pulmonary valve is found in patients with Noonan syndrome.

Obstruction of the right ventricular outflow tract, if hemodynamically significant, can cause right ventricular hypertrophy. Patients are often asymptomatic in all but the most severe cases, with the diagnosis made by auscultation of a murmur during routine examination. Patients with clinical symptoms may show exercise intolerance, fatigue, and in severe cases without therapy, right ventricular failure.

Consensus recommendations for valvar PS suggest observation only in patients with mild gradients, with intervention being suggested in those with peak-to-peak gradients in the catheterization laboratory of at least 40 mm Hg or at least 30 mm Hg if symptomatic.[36] Intervention in the absence of significant pulmonary insufficiency is almost always performed in the catheterization laboratory with balloon valvuloplasty, usually with significant relief of the stenosis.[37] If severe pulmonary insufficiency is present, treatment is surgical, often with replacement of the pulmonary valve with a valved conduit.

Subvalvar PS is typically seen with malalignment of the infundibular septum and excessive right ventricular outflow tract muscle bundles in Tetralogy of Fallot. In this case, surgical incision and resection of the anomalous muscle bundles (typically performed as part of the overall repair for Tetralogy of Fallot) is the treatment of choice. Supravalvar stenosis, either at the main pulmonary artery level or in the branches, may be treated with balloon dilation and/or stent placement. Results depend on the severity of the stenosis compared to adjacent vessel size. Typically, patients with isolated right ventricular outflow obstruction have a good long-term prognosis.[38]

3.12. Coronary anomalies

Congenital abnormalities of the coronary arteries are relatively rare, and can present in isolation or as part of more complex congenital heart disease. Coronary artery formation has been shown to start in the myocardium, with vessels coalescing and then penetrating the aorta in the appropriate sinus.[39] Abnormalities of this process lead to coronary anomalies. Isolated coronary artery lesions can include single coronary artery, anomalous origin of the right coronary artery from the left sinus of Valsalva, anomalous origin of the left coronary artery from the right sinus of Valsalva, and anomalous left coronary artery from the pulmonary artery (ALCAPA) (Fig. 40.8).

ALCAPA is a rare but well-known abnormality of the left coronary artery which presents in infancy. It is usually clinically silent

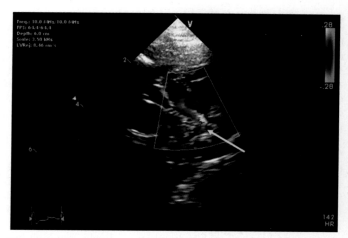

Figure 40.8 ALCAPA is shown in this transthoracic echocardiogram. This modified high parasternal short-axis view shows diastolic flow from the left main coronary artery (*yellow arrow*) into the pulmonary artery, confirming the diagnosis.

in the neonatal period, and manifests when PVR falls over the first weeks to months of life. The decrease in pulmonary artery pressure causes diastolic steal from the left coronary artery into the pulmonary artery, leading to ischemia of the left ventricle in the distribution of the left main coronary artery and the appearance of a dilated cardiomyopathy. If children present at a later age, there is often formation of coronary collateral vessels from the right coronary artery to the left ventricle. The classic presentation for ALCAPA is initially discomfort with exertion (feeding or crying), with eventual progression to infarction and CHF. Significant mitral regurgitation is typically seen due to infarction of the papillary muscles of the mitral valve. There is dilation and failure of the left ventricle, and if undetected this will lead to death. Of interest, some patients with ALCAPA that was not corrected in infancy can show recovery of left ventricular function presumably due to extensive collateralization. Unfortunately, ALCAPA has presented in older children and even adults with sudden death after exertion.

The treatment of ALCAPA is surgical. Multiple surgical approaches have been performed, with the current standard being direct reimplantation of the left coronary artery into the aorta.[40] Prognosis depends on the amount of ischemia suffered by the myocardium, with some children experiencing recovery of function and others progressing to cardiac transplantation or death.

Other congenital abnormalities of the coronary arteries are typically clinically silent. The anomalous origin of one coronary from the opposite sinus of Valsalva is often an incidental finding on echocardiography. Some patients may present in childhood (especially adolescence) with chest pain with or without exertion, ventricular arrhythmias, or sudden death. It is not known why patients with similar anomalies have such a wide spectrum of presentation. Often at surgery or autopsy, coronaries arising from the opposite sinus of Valsalva are found to have a slitlike orifice with an intramural course, which is postulated to cause ischemia, during times of increased cardiac output and myocardial oxygen consumption (i.e., exercise). Treatment of an anomalous left coronary artery from the right sinus is surgical, usually with widening of the opening of the orifice with unroofing of the transmural portion. Whether to intervene surgically for asymptomatic anomalous right coronary artery arising from the left sinus is controversial.

4. DIAGNOSTIC EVALUATION

Evaluation of patients with acyanotic congenital heart lesions requires careful imaging due to the complexity of their anatomy. Techniques used by pediatric cardiologists to image these patients are both invasive and noninvasive, however, with the expansion of technology in the past two decades, noninvasive imaging, especially echocardiography, has become the standard for initial diagnostic evaluation and serial clinical monitoring.

4.1. Fetal imaging

Current ultrasound systems and transducers have very high spatial and temporal resolution, which has vastly expanded the role of fetal echocardiography in detecting congenital heart lesions and fetal arrhythmias. Fetal echocardiograms are performed for several reasons, including abnormal screening ultrasound,[41] abnormal chromosomal analysis, polyhydramnios or oligohydramnios, history of maternal or paternal congenital heart disease or other certain genetic disorders, mothers with prior children with congenital heart lesions, and in the increasingly high number of women with maternal diabetes (existing before or acquired during pregnancy). Benefits of fetal diagnosis include providing counseling of parents to provide choices for location of delivery (i.e., tertiary care center) and options for termination of pregnancy for those who choose to do so. In addition, fetal intervention has become a new therapeutic option for some diseases, with imaging being critical in deciding the best candidates.

The fetal echocardiographic examination can be performed in most patients as early as 16 weeks gestation with the best imaging obtained between 18 and 24 weeks.[42] Many imaging planes are used during the examination. The quality of the examination is dependent on the expertise of the sonographer performing and echocardiographer interpreting the exam. In addition, the examination can be limited by fetal movement or positioning in the uterus. Careful and detailed examination can allow for the detection of most congenital heart lesions.

Fetal arrhythmias can also be detected by fetal echocardiography. Rhythm abnormalities are typically detected by simultaneous M-mode recording of the atrium and ventricle, with abnormal atrioventricular contraction patterns being indicative of arrhythmias such as complete heart block, atrial flutter, and atrial or ventricular extrasystoles. Figure 40.9 shows an example of complete heart block diagnosed in a fetus by fetal M-mode echocardiography. Detection of tachyarrhythmias with transplacental treatment with high maternal doses of antiarrhythmic medications has been shown to improve or arrest the development of hydrops fetalis, a life-threatening complication of many fetal arrhythmias.[43]

Fetal cardiac intervention is an emerging field, in which an appropriately timed intervention for a carefully selected patient with congenital heart disease may lead to improved prenatal cardiac development in an effort to decrease the severity of postnatal disease and eventual outcome. Most attempts have been made in limited centers in the setting of aortic valvar stenosis in order to provide for the growth of the left heart and aorta.[44] Fetal echocardiography is essential in detecting these abnormalities and other factors, which determine if a particular fetus is a good candidate for this high-risk procedure.[45]

4.2. Transthoracic echocardiography

The transthoracic echocardiogram remains the centerpiece of diagnostic imaging for all congenital heart lesions. Current technology allows for easily available high resolution, high framerate images of most infants and children with congenital heart

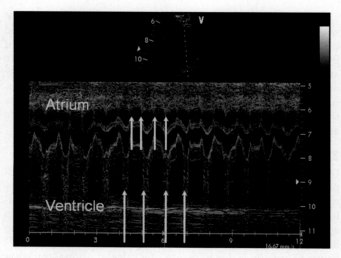

Figure 40.9 Fetal M-mode echocardiogram of fetus with congenital complete heart block. In this ice pick view of the heart, the atrium is on the top of the image while the ventricle is on the bottom. The *arrows* indicate the contractile pattern of each chamber, which is faster in the atrium than the ventricle and completely dissociated from one another.

disease. In the repaired adult the echocardiographic examination is often more difficult due to body habitus and other factors such as lung disease. In these patients transesophageal echocardiography (TEE) may be helpful in situations where the demand for information exceeds the relatively low risk of the procedure.

Standard imaging planes have been used to assess acyanotic congenital heart disease, and guidelines for the complete pediatric echocardiogram exist.[46] The standard echocardiogram for congenital heart disease follows a similar protocol as most adult studies, however, more emphasis is placed on subcostal and suprasternal notch imaging. In addition, the majority of echocardiography laboratories that primarily image congenital heart disease will invert the image on the ultrasound machine in the apical and subcostal windows to provide a more anatomically correct presentation of the cardiac structures. In general, defects of the atrial or ventricular septae should be imaged from a plane perpendicular to the septum to minimize axial drop-out artifact. This approach also will typically present a good angle for Doppler interrogation of flow across the defect. Valvar abnormalities should evaluated by two-dimensional imaging separate from color Doppler analysis to help describe the valve anatomy. Color Doppler analysis is then used to evaluate regurgitation and help determine the optimal angle of interrogation for spectral analysis of flow patterns. Table 40.2 provides useful echocardiographic imaging planes for evaluation of selected acyanotic congenital heart lesions.

4.2.1. Parasternal window

The parasternal window provides a good angle to evaluate VSDs, tricuspid and mitral valve abnormalities, and pulmonary valve abnormalities. The long-axis plane is used to evaluate the morphology of the aortic, mitral, and pulmonary valves. A significant portion of the ventricular septum is well seen, although some perimembranous defects may be out of plane somewhat behind the tricuspid valve. The left anterior descending coronary artery is well seen traversing along the anterior surface of the ventricular septum just right of the pulmonary valve. The short-axis view allows for easy evaluation of all types of VSDs, as you scan the septum from the base to the apex, and is the view of choice to

TABLE 40.2

OPTIMAL ECHOCARDIOGRAPHIC IMAGING PLANES FOR ACYANOTIC CONGENITAL HEART LESIONS

	Parasternal long axis	Parasternal short axis	Apical four-chamber	Subcostal long axis	Subcostal short axis	Suprasternal long axis	Suprasternal short axis
ASD		✓		✓	✓		
VSD	✓	✓			✓		
AVSD	✓	✓	✓	✓	✓		
Anomalous pulmonary venous return		✓	✓			✓	✓
PDA	✓	✓				✓	
Coarctation of the aorta					✓	✓	✓
Ebstein anomaly	✓	✓	✓	✓			
Left ventricular inflow obstruction	✓	✓	✓	✓	✓		
Left ventricular outflow obstruction	✓		✓	✓		✓	
Right ventricular inflow obstruction	✓	✓	✓	✓			
Right ventricular outflow obstruction		✓		✓	✓		✓
Coronary anomalies		✓					

evaluate perimembranous defects. From this plane the pulmonary valve and branch pulmonary arteries, and proximal coronary artery anatomy are also well seen. Doppler interrogation is optimal along the right ventricular outflow tract, pulmonary valve and proximal left pulmonary artery.

4.2.2. Apical window

The apical window, mainly in the four chamber view, allows for examination of mitral and tricuspid valve abnormalities (including estimation of right ventricular and pulmonary artery pressure from tricuspid regurgitant flow). This window allows for optimal evaluation of tricuspid and mitral inflow as well as aortic outflow. The degree of apical displacement of the tricuspid valve in Ebstein anomaly is well seen in the four chamber view. Some of the pulmonary veins can be seen entering the left atrium and may be evaluated by Doppler. The left ventricular outflow tract also can be well seen.

4.2.3. Subcostal window

The subcostal window with the transducer aimed directly at the spine and mark toward the left helps determine situs--that is the relationship of the aorta and inferior vena cava to the spine and each other. Normal situs reveals the aorta leftward of the spine and posterior to a rightward inferior vena cava. In cases of complex congenital anatomic defects, the subcostal views in the coronal and sagittal planes are often times the most useful to the echocardiographer as all of the intracardiac and most of the vascular anatomy can be well seen and identified in relationship to the planes of the body. This window is especially helpful in evaluating the atrial septum for defects, and the sagittal plane is essential for diagnosing a sinus venosus type ASD.

4.2.4. Suprasternal and high parasternal windows

The suprasternal notch view is an essential component of the pediatric echocardiogram, and is used to detect abnormalities in upper-body systemic venous return, pulmonary venous return, and aortic arch abnormalities including coarctation of the aorta. With the probe in the suprasternal notch the entire aortic arch may be imaged in the sagittal plane. Further definition of the

head and neck vessels including their branching patterns can be shown by sweeping upward in the coronal plane. From a high left parasternal window in the sagittal plane the branch pulmonary artery bifurcation can be well seen and evaluated by Doppler (pant-leg view). With counterclockwise rotation into a left anterior oblique plane, the left pulmonary artery can be well seen. Returning to the sagittal plane and tipping the transducer inferiorly, all of the pulmonary veins can be identified entering the left atrium and evaluated with Doppler (crab view). The high right parasternal window, optimally with the patient placed in the right lateral decubitus position, in the sagittal plane is used to identify the entry of the superior vena cava to the right atrium where superior sinus venosus defects are found often. In addition, with angulation to the left the ascending aorta can be well seen in length. This view is often the best for Doppler interrogation of the flow across the aortic valve in the setting of valvar or supra valvar AS.

4.3. Transesophageal echocardiography

TEE is not routinely used in infants and children for the diagnosis of congenital heart lesions as the transthoracic imaging windows are very clear and allow for definition of all cardiac structures. In children, TEE is more commonly used in the setting of preoperative and postoperative evaluation of patients in the operating room, or to provide assistance in the catheterization laboratory for interventional procedures. TEE can usually be performed in infants as small as 3 kg using a specialized pediatric probe. Less common uses of TEE in the setting of congenital heart lesions include determining whether adequate rims of tissue exist for large secundum ASDs to be closed by device, or in evaluating for thrombus, or vegetation in patients with poor transthoracic imaging windows.

4.4. Three-dimensional echocardiography (3DE)

3DE is a rapidly evolving technology working its way into the assessment of patients with acyanotic congenital heart lesions. Current technology allows for either live 3D imaging or capture of full volume datasets, which then can be analyzed on a desktop computer using commercially available software programs. Certain anomalies such as cor triatriatum or aortopulmonary window can be better appreciated using 3DE.[47,48] In addition, the right and left ventricles can both be assessed for volumes and systolic function using semiautomatic border tracking algorithms applied to 3D datasets, creating computer models of the ventricular chambers.[49–51] Figures 40.10 and 40.11 provide examples of computer models of the left and right ventricles, respectively. In addition, 3DE can be used to help clarify anatomic abnormalities such as showing an ASD or VSD en face. Through postprocessing software it is possible to determine the precise location and mechanism of mitral valve regurgitation. Potential applications for 3DE in imaging of patients with congenital heart disease are rapidly expanding.

4.5. Magnetic resonance imaging

When considering the appropriateness of cardiac magnetic resonance (CMR) imaging in a patient with congenital heart disease, it is best to think in terms of the strengths and limitations of CMR as a modality. CMR has unique advantages in imaging extra cardiac anatomy, quantifying ventricular volumes without geometric assumptions, quantifying flow in through valves and vessels, cardiac tissue characterization. As a second line imaging technique, CMR is most frequently used when other techniques prove insufficient and therefore, is most often used in older children and adults as acoustic windows deteriorate and sequelae from surgical palliation become apparent. In younger children (<8 years of age) cooperation with the scan becomes an issue and many centers routinely use general anesthesia for this age group.

4.5.1. Extracardiac anatomy

Using a contrast agent (gadolinium) a magnetic resonance angiogram of the chest can be produced. The resulting angiogram is a 3D representation of the vessels of the chest which can be reformatted into any two-dimensional plane and volume rendered 3D models of the vasculature. This technique is most useful for complicated 3D relationships of vessels and for measuring vessels in the chest. Clinically, this technique is used for accurate and reproducible measurement of the ascending aorta and aortic arch (bicuspid aortic valves, Marfan syndrome, Loeys–Dietz syndrome, D-transposition after arterial switch, and coarctation of the aorta), accurate and reproducible measurement of the pulmonary arteries (branch PS, supravalvar PS), and for delineation of the pulmonary venous anatomy (PAPVR, complex TAPVR and pulmonary vein stenosis). Figure 40.12 provides an example of a patient with severe coarctation of the aorta with evidence of extensive collateral flow. Figure 40.13 shows another patient with recoarctation of the aorta.

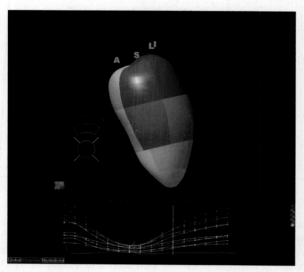

Figure 40.10 3D computer model of the left ventricle, created using QLAB 3DQ ADV Release 6.0 software (Philips Ultrasound, Bothell, WA). The ventricle is displayed with apex at the bottom. Anterior (A), septal (S), lateral (L), and inferior (I) portions of the mitral valve annulus are shown at the top of the ventricle. The ventricular chamber is divided into 17 segments, which are represented in the time (x-axis)–volume (y-axis) curves on the bottom of this image of a normal heart.

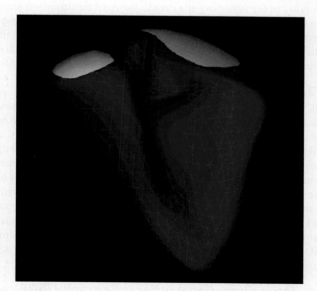

Figure 40.11 3D model of the right ventricle, created using 4D RV-Function© version 1.1 software (TomTec Imaging Systems, GmbH, Unterschleissheim, Germany). The right ventricle chamber is viewed from the left ventricular side, with the broader tricuspid valve shown in white on the right side of the image and the narrower outflow tract leading to the pulmonary valve (shown in white on the left side of the image). The left ventricle would fit into the "pocket" shown in the middle of the model in this image of a normal heart.

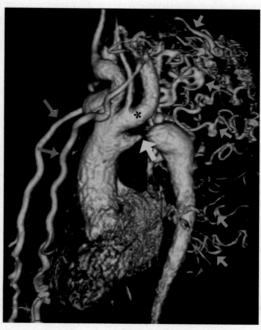

Figure 40.12 Severe coarctation of the aorta (*yellow arrow*) shown by 3D contrast MRA. Dilated internal thoracic (*red arrows*) vertebral and intercostals arteries (*green arrows*) with collateral flow.

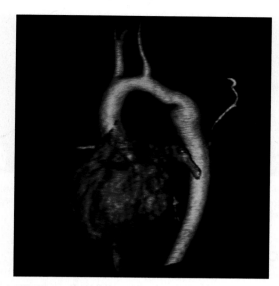

Figure 40.13 Recoarctation of the aorta shown in this 3D MRI reconstruction. This patient with discrete recoarctation of the proximal descending aorta originally had a subclavian flap repair. A small collateral artery is shown just distal to the recoarctation.

4.5.2. Quantifying ventricular volumes

CMR is an inherently volumetric modality in that 2D images are acquired at a slice thickness giving each pixel in the image an associated volume. Therefore, a stack of short-axis images that covers the heart can be used to determine the volumes of both ventricles, without using geometric assumptions. By calculating the volume of a ventricle in diastole and systole, both stroke volume and ejection fraction can be determined. In the normal left ventricle this technique is both accurate and reproducible. The technique is particularly advantageous in right ventricles, systemic right ventricles, and single ventricles where no presumptive geometric model exists. Clinically, this technique is used to quantify ventricular volumes and function for nearly all patients who undergo CMR for congenital heart disease. In patients with systemic right ventricles (D-transposition after atrial switch [Senning, Mustard], congenitally corrected transposition), and in patients with poor acoustic windows CMR is often the only way to determine ventricular function (muscular dystrophy). Quantifying ventricular volumes is also useful in gauging the severity and progression of aortic and pulmonic regurgitation. Figure 40.14 shows dilated pulmonary artery (A) and right ventricle (Movie 40.1) in a patient with a large secundum ASD.

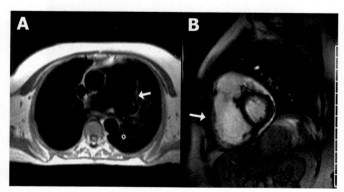
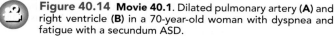

Figure 40.14 Movie 40.1. Dilated pulmonary artery (A) and right ventricle (B) in a 70-year-old woman with dyspnea and fatigue with a secundum ASD.

4.5.3. Quantification of flow

Phase contrast imaging can determine the flow through a designated plane. This can be used to quantitative aortic, pulmonic, and to a lesser extent, tricuspid regurgitant fractions where through plane motion complicates analysis. By comparing the flow in the main pulmonary artery (Qp) and aorta (Qs), a Qp:Qs ratio can be calculated in a variety of lesions (ASD, VSD, PDA, and anomalous pulmonary venous return), with good correlation to values obtained invasively by oximetry.[52,53] Flow quantification can also be used to measure the proportion of blood flow to each lung in the setting of branch pulmonary artery stenosis. Figure 40.15, (Movies 40.2 and 40.3) show a secundum ASD imaged in a cross-sectional SSFP cine image before (A) and after placement of a saturation band (B). The saturation band nulls the signal from the blood in the left atrium. The blood entering the right atrium through the ASD then appears black. Figure 40.16 (Movies 40.4 and 40.5) demonstrate the visualization of the size and location of the ASD using phase contrast imaging. Figure 40.17 illustrates the method to quantify shunt flow (Qp:Qs).

4.5.4. Tissue characterization

Myocardial delayed enhancement is a technique used to diagnose myocardial fibrosis. It is routinely used in any patient who has undergone surgical correction of congenital heart disease to screen for the sequelae of cardiopulmonary bypass or surgery. As in the patient without congenital heart disease, myocardial first-past perfusion with or without adenosine or dobutamine stress can be used to diagnosis myocardial ischemia or delayed perfusion.[54] This technique is most often used in patients with congenital coronary anomalies or Kawasaki syndrome with coronary aneurysms. A combination of first-pass perfusion, myocardial delayed enhancement imaging, T1/T2 weighted black blood imaging can be used to help characterize intracardiac tumor types, myocarditis, arrhythmogenic right ventricular cardiomyopathy, and pericardial disease.[55]

4.5.5. Coronary imaging

3D steady-state free precession imaging is routinely used to evaluate anomalous coronary origins and proximal coronary artery

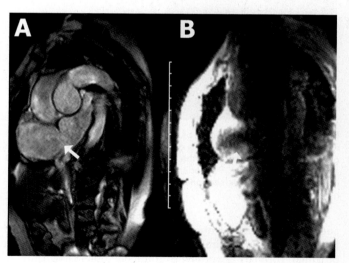
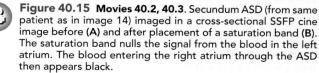

Figure 40.15 Movies 40.2, 40.3. Secundum ASD (from same patient as in image 14) imaged in a cross-sectional SSFP cine image before (A) and after placement of a saturation band (B). The saturation band nulls the signal from the blood in the left atrium. The blood entering the right atrium through the ASD then appears black.

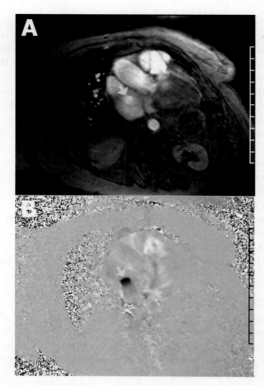

Figure 40.16 (**Movies 40.4, 40.5**). In the same patient as in Figures 40.14 and 40.15, the size and location of the ASD are shown using through-plane phase contrast imaging. **A:** Localizer image. **B:** Phase-encoded image.

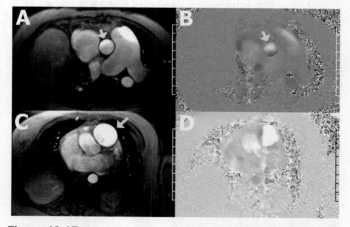

Figure 40.17 Quantification of shunt (Qp:Qs) in the previous patient with ASD. Systemic flow (Qs) is quantified as the product of the area of the ascending aorta (**A**) by the integrated flow velocity in the same area (**B**) during systole. Pulmonary flow (Qs) is quantified in the same manner from the cross-sectional image of the proximal main pulmonary artery (**C,D**).

aneurysms in patients with congenital heart disease and acquired heart disease. Due to limitations of resolution and signal level, proximal coronary anatomy is routinely obtainable only in patient with heart rates <110 beats per min and weighting over 15 kg. This technique can be used to cover the entire heart for patients with very complex anatomic relationships. Figure 40.18 shows an example of anomalous origin of the circumflex coronary artery shown by MRI.

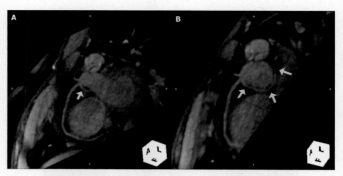

Figure 40.18 Anomalous origin of the left circumflex (*arrows*) from the right sinus of Valsalva (**A**). The retroaortic course is best depicted in **panel B**.

4.6. Computed tomography

Patients with congenital heart disease often require a lifetime of serial noninvasive imaging studies. Therefore, techniques using ionizing radiation are used as judiciously as possible. Multidetector computed tomography (MDCT), however, has some unique advantages which make it useful for imaging in congenital heart disease.[56,57] Cardiac CT is used when detailed, noninvasive images of the entire coronary artery system is required. In the setting of patients with pacemakers, or significant metal artifact on CMR, gated MDCT can be used to obtain quantitative ventricular volumes and function. Similar to magnetic resonance angiographic techniques, MDCT can produce high resolution 3D imaging of extracardiac anatomy. When detailed imaging of the cardiac anatomy in relation to airway anomalies is required, MDCT is the imaging modality of choice. Using prospective ECG gating and low kVp settings, adequate images of the coronaries can be obtained with reduced radiation doses between 1 and 3 mSv. Figures 40.19–40.21 (Movies 40.6–40.8) show examples of anomalous coronary artery origin by MDCT. Figure 40.22 shows an example of a patient with a congenital circumflex to coronary sinus fistula.

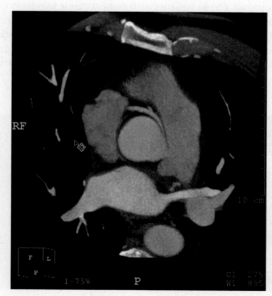

Figure 40.19 (**Movie 40.6**). Anomalous origin of the right coronary artery from the left sinus of Valsalva. Notice in this case the narrow, slitlike origin.

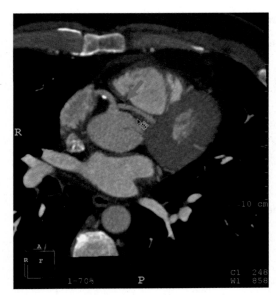

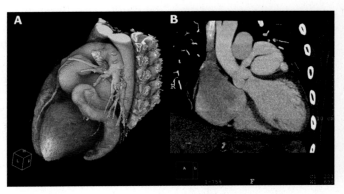

Figure 40.22 MDCT images of a large left circumflex-coronary sinus fistula shown in volume-rendered (**A**) and oblique coronal maximum intensity (**B**) projections.

imaging is in the evaluation of patients with abnormal coronary artery anatomy, especially after repair to evaluate for functional abnormalities. One potential application may be determining whether coronaries arising from the wrong sinus and traversing between the great arteries are at risk for ischemia,[59] however, further study of this patient population is required before functional testing becomes part of the standard evaluation.

5. SELECTING AND GUIDING THERAPY

Treatment options for patients with acyanotic congenital heart lesions range from careful observation to complex surgical repair or even heart transplantation.

An ongoing challenge to specialists in congenital heart disease is the diversity of congenital heart lesions and their relatively low incidence limiting the ability to perform well-powered prospective studies. Compared to disorders such as adult onset coronary artery disease in which a study with thousands of participants can be performed in months, most institutions see well under 100 patients in a year with any single lesion and may see less than 10 patients a year that require therapy for more complex disorders.

This fact combined with the rapid evolution of a variety of surgical and catheter-based interventions for these lesions has led to significant differences in treatment algorithms, varying by institution and even between well-experienced physicians within institutions. With this in mind, the following section will attempt to address therapeutic considerations for the previously described acyanotic congenital heart lesions. Reasonable therapeutic algorithms for diagnosis and management of ASD (Fig. 40.23) and coarctation of the aorta (Fig. 40.24) appear at in this section.

5.1. Medical therapy

Most significant congenital heart lesions require surgical repair as definitive therapy. However, it is often necessary to medically manage these patients prior to surgery to allow for growth and for maturity of the pulmonary vasculature. In addition, medications are commonly used postoperatively as the heart recovers from surgery and the body adjusts to new circulatory patterns. Diuretics such as furosemide, spironolactone, and chlorothiazide reduce preload, and are commonly used for patients with significant left-to-right shunt lesions to treat symptoms of CHF and pulmonary edema. Angiotensin converting enzyme (ACE) inhibitors such as captopril and enalapril are used to reduce afterload in patients with significant left-sided valvar regurgitation. Positive inotropic agents (dopamine, dobutamine, epinephrine, norepinephrine are examples) are often needed after surgery to augment cardiac

Figure 40.20 (Movie 40.7). Anomalous origin of the left coronary artery from the right sinus of Valsalva, with intramyocardial (between aorta and right ventricular outflow tract) course.

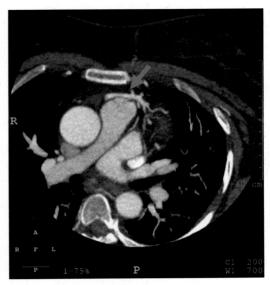

Figure 40.21 (Movie 40.8). Anomalous origin of the left coronary artery from the right sinus of Valsalva, with anterior (over right ventricular outflow tract) course. This patient has also a persistent left-sided superior vena cava draining in the coronary sinus.

4.7. Nuclear scintigraphy

Nuclear medicine, while common in adults with acquired heart disease, has a more limited role in acyanotic congenital heart lesions. As with MDCT the use of ionizing radiation in this technique limits its use to patients who have contraindications for other noninvasive measures of the above parameters. Cardiac nuclear scintigraphy can be used to assess the physiologic consequences of acyanotic congenital heart lesions, such as quantitating shunts, myocardial perfusion, and differential branch pulmonary artery blood flow.[58] One particularly useful indication for nuclear

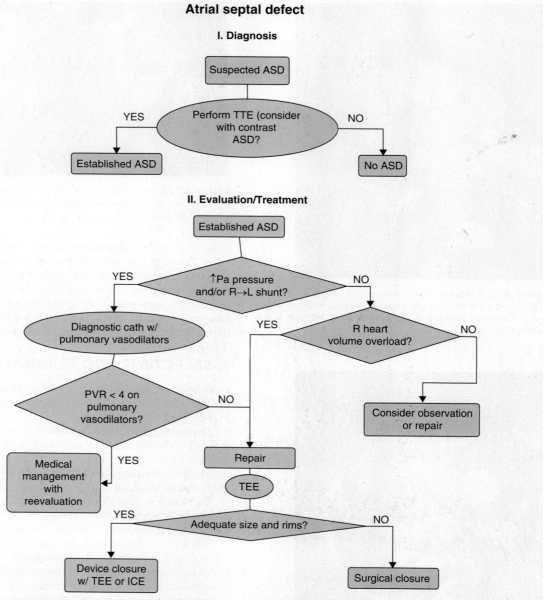

Figure 40.23 Flow diagram for diagnosis and management of ASD suspected in the adult. *Note:* Any ASD which is not secundum is not likely amenable to catheter-based device closure.

output in the recovering heart. The phosphodiesterase inhibitor milrinone has gained widespread acceptance in the postoperative setting as well as in patients with a dilated cardiomyopathy. Pulmonary vasodilators such as oxygen, nitric oxide, and sildenafil are used in the treatment of pulmonary hypertension due to congenital heart lesions. Antihypertensives such as nitroprusside, esmolol, and ACE inhibitors are used postoperatively to treat systemic hypertension following coarctation repair.

5.2. Percutaneous interventions

Catheter-based interventions are becoming increasingly common in the treatment of several acyanotic congenital heart lesions. ASDs are commonly closed with growing number of percutaneously placed devices. Select VSDs are now able to be closed with percutaneous devices as well. A PDA or other collateral vessels can be successfully closed by coil (if small) or vascular plug (if large). Balloon valvuloplasty is used as a treatment for pulmonary valve or aortic valve stenosis. Balloons or stents can be used

to treat branch pulmonary artery stenosis and coarctation of the aorta. This approach, as opposed to surgery, is usually reserved for older children or after the initial surgical repair to address a recoarctation.

The benefits of percutaneous intervention are generally centered around reduced morbidity of the patient. Patients undergoing a catheterization with intervention can often go home from the hospital after overnight observation or even the same day, without any scars or disfiguration of the chest. Recovery is much faster as the patient only has skin entry at the point of vascular access (groin, neck, liver, etc.) avoiding both sternotomy and cardiotomy. These devices permanently remain in the heart or great vessels, and the long-term sequelae of many of the newer devices are not yet known. Consideration for percutaneous intervention versus surgical repair depends on institutional preference and experience, but also must weigh the risks and benefits of each approach. Preprocedural and intraprocedural imaging is important to determine feasibility, provide guidance, and evaluate

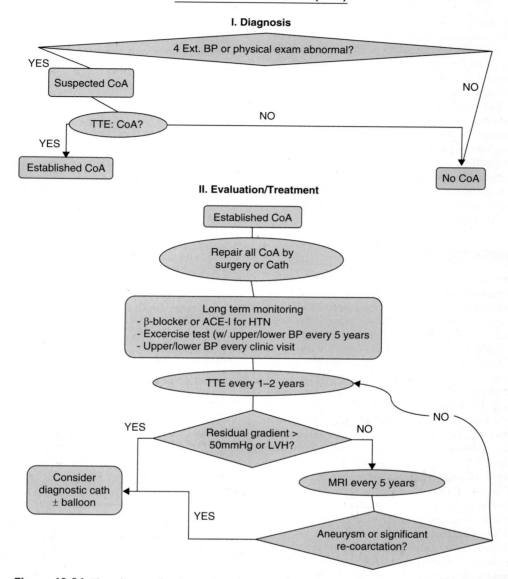

Coarctation of the aorta (CoA)

I. Diagnosis

4 Ext. BP or physical exam abnormal?

YES → Suspected CoA

NO → No CoA

TTE: CoA?

NO → No CoA

YES → Established CoA

II. Evaluation/Treatment

Established CoA

Repair all CoA by surgery or Cath

Long term monitoring
- β-blocker or ACE-I for HTN
- Excercise test (w/ upper/lower BP every 5 years
- Upper/lower BP every clinic visit

TTE every 1–2 years

Residual gradient > 50mmHg or LVH?

YES → Consider diagnostic cath ± balloon

NO → MRI every 5 years

Aneurysm or significant re-coarctation?

YES → Consider diagnostic cath ± balloon

NO → TTE every 1–2 years

Figure 40.24 Flow diagram for diagnosis and management of coarctation of the aorta in an adult.

outcome. Preprocedural imaging with echocardiography, MRI and/or CT permits to evaluate the anatomy in order to select appropriate devices, identify associated lesions, and evaluate systemic and pulmonary circulation. Intraprocedural guidance is most often performed with TEE, including real-time 3D imaging (see Chapter 11). A few centers in the United States are using MRI guidance for selected procedures. Special MRI compatible catheters are designed to perform these procedures. Advantages include reduction of ionizing radiation and better 3D visualization.

5.3. Surgical repair

For the majority of significant acyanotic congenital heart lesions surgical repair remains the most definitive therapy. Ideally, these operations should be performed by a team of professionals who are specifically trained and experienced in the management of congenital heart disease. Details of surgical technique can be found in a number of cardiac surgical textbooks.

Intracardiac cardiac lesions including septal defects and most outflow and valvar abnormalities, require cardiopulmonary

bypass and often circulatory arrest in order to perform the repair. Use of cardiopulmonary bypass will lead to predictable postoperative considerations such as transiently diminished cardiac function and peripheral edema, which usually require an initial period of inotropic support followed by aggressive diuresis.[60]

Extracardiac lesions can often be repaired without cardiopulmonary bypass. Thoracic repairs such as ligation of PDA or resection of coarctation of the aorta with extended end-to-end anastomosis can be performed via thoracotomy. Others, such as pulmonary artery augmentation for branch pulmonary artery stenosis, must be done via median sternotomy.

Outcomes for surgical repair are dependent of many variables, including individual patient comorbidities, timing of surgical referral, surgeon and surgical team experience, and postoperative management. The range from simple to complex lesions and surgical approaches make it somewhat difficult to predict outcomes for an individual patient, however, attempts have been made to create a scoring system to evaluate surgical results, such as the Aristotle score.[61]

6. IMAGING AND PROGNOSIS

Imaging plays a very important role in determining the prognosis of patients affected by congenital heart lesions. Echocardiography is routinely used to assess the severity of AS or PS and to monitor for progression.[36] As in adults with acquired heart disease, strain and strain rate measured by echocardiography can provide valuable information on regional wall mechanics and synchrony in patients who have had surgically repaired acyanotic congenital heart lesions.[62] Assessment of atrial and ventricular chambers by echo or CMR is important in determining hemodynamic effect of left-to-right shunting lesions (such as ASD or VSD) and tricuspid or mitral valve regurgitation, and degree of enlargement seen by echo can assist the cardiologist in determining whether to surgically intervene and if so the correct timing. CMR can also be used to assess myocardial viability in patients with congenital heart disease who have events resulting in myocardial damage.[63]

7. FUTURE DIRECTIONS

Noninvasive cardiac imaging, and especially echocardiography, remains the core diagnostic approach for defining and following patients with acyanotic congenital heart lesions. Improvements on existing modalities and the introduction of newer technologies both add to the understanding of these sometimes very complex anatomic abnormalities. 3DE has existed for some time, but often has been inefficient in clinical application due to the huge computing demands necessary for image processing and manipulation. Great strides in both transducer and 3D software technology have been made in the last several years, improving the workflow and allowing the gradual introduction of 3D echo into many pediatric laboratories. This will only increase as more physicians are trained in 3D imaging techniques and industry brings higher frequency, higher frame-rate transducers to the market, all of which are essential in 3D evaluation of young children with acyanotic congenital heart lesions.

Catheter-based interventions have reduced the morbidity and mortality in several types of congenital heart disease. Device closure of straightforward secundum ASD in the catheterization laboratory is now the standard of care. Cooperation between surgeons and interventional cardiologists has led to innovative, new hybrid approaches to the treatment of some congenital heart lesions. Many exciting new interventions are now undergoing trials, including percutaneous pulmonary valve replacement, mitral valve clip to reduce mitral regurgitation, and left atrial plug to reduce thrombus formation. Other devices are in development, such as biodegradable stents and closure devices. All of these new techniques bring the hope of improving both quality and duration of life for individuals afflicted with congenital heart disease. However, these innovations do not yet have long-term follow-up data, and these patients must be followed during adulthood to monitor for any unexpected late complications.

The advances made in the diagnosis and management of acyanotic congenital heart disease in the last several decades are truly remarkable. There is every reason to expect continued improvement in diagnostic, medical, catheter-based, and operative techniques in the coming years.

ACKNOWLEDGMENTS

The authors would like to thank Dr. Steven Goldberg for his original drawings shown in Figures 40.1 and 40.2. The authors would also like to thank Dr Karrie Villavicencio for her contributions and consultation for this chapter.

REFERENCES

1. Williams RG, Pearson GD, Barst RJ, et al. Report of the National Heart, Lung, and Blood Institute Working Group on Research in adult congenital heart disease. *J Am Coll Cardiol.* 2006;47:701–707.
2. Reller MD, Strickland MJ, Riehle-Colarusso T, et al. Prevalence of congenital heart defects in metropolitan Atlanta, 1998–2005. *J Pediatr.* 2008;153(6):807–813.
3. Ferencz C, Rubin J, Loffredo C, eds. *Epidemiology of Congenital Heart Disease: The Baltimore-Washington Infant Heart Study 1981–1989.* Mount Kisco, NY: Futura; 1993.
4. Nakazawa M, Seguchi M, Takao A. Prevalence of congenital heart disease in Japan. In: Clark E, Takao A, eds. *Developmental Cardiology: Morphogenesis and Function.* Mount Kisco, NY: Futura; 1990:541–548.
5. Scanlon KS, Ferencz C, Loffredo CA, et al. Preconceptional folate intake and malformations of the cardiac outflow tract. *Epidemiology.* 1998;9:95–98.
6. Macmahon B, McKeown T, Record RG. The incidence and life expectation of children with congenital heart disease. *Br Heart J.* 1953;15:121–129.
7. Baker C, Brock R, Campbell M, et al. Morbus coeruleus: A study of 50 cases after the blalock-taussig operation. *Br Heart J.* 1949;11:170–200.
8. Borghi A, Ciuffreda M, Quattrociocchi M, et al. The grown-up congenital cardiac patient. *J Cardiovasc Med.* 2007;8:78–82.
9. Hagen P, Scholz D, Edwards W. Incidence and size of patent foramen ovale during the first 10 decades of life: An autopsy study of 965 normal hearts. *Mayo Clin Proc.* 1984;59:17–20.
10. Post MC, Luermans JGLM, Plokker HWM, et al. Patent foramen ovale and migraine. *Catheter Cardiovasc Interv.* 2007;69:9–14.
11. Holmes DR, Cohen H, Katz WE, et al. Patent foramen ovale, systemic embolization and closure. *Curr Probl Cardiol.* 2004;29:56–94.
12. Campbell M. Natural history of atrial septal defect. *Br Heart J.* 1970;32:820–826.
13. Soto B, Becker AE, Moulaert AJ, et al. Classification of ventricular septal defects. *Br Heart J.* 1980;43:332–343.
14. Roguin N, Du Z-D, Barak M, et al. High prevalence of muscular ventricular septal defect in neonates. *J Am Coll Cardiol.* 1995;26:1545–1548.
15. Allen HD, Gutgesell HP, Clark EB, et al., eds. *Moss and Adams' Heart Disease in Infants, Children, and Adolescents - Including the Fetus and Young Adult.* 6th Ed. Philadelphia, PA: Lippincott Williams & Wilkins; 2001.
16. Suzuki T, Bove EL, Devaney EJ, et al. Results of definitive repair of complete atrioventricular septal defect in neonates and infants. *Ann Thorac Surg.* 2008;86:596–602.
17. Kanter KR. Surgical repair of total anomalous pulmonary venous connection. *Semin Thorac Cardiovasc Surg Pediatr Card Surg Annu.* 2006;9:40–44.
18. Hermes-DeSantis E, Clyman R. Patent ductus arteriosus: Pathophysiology and management. *J Perinatol.* 2006;26:S14–S18.
19. Bilkis AA, Alwi M, Hasri S, et al. The amplatzer duct occluder: Experience in 209 patients. *J Am Coll Cardiol.* 2001;37:258–261.
20. Beekman RH, Robinow M. Coarctation of the aorta inherited as an autosomal dominant trait. *Am J Cardiol.* 1985;56:818–819.
21. Miettinen OS, Reiner ML, Nadas AS. Seasonal incidence of coarctation of the aorta. *Br Heart J.* 1970;32:103–107.
22. Aris A, Bonnin O, Sole O, et al. Surgical management of aortic Coarctation associated with ruptured cerebral artery aneurysm. *Tex Heart Inst J.* 1986;13:313–319.
23. Campbell M. Natural history of coarctation of the aorta. *Br Heart J.* 1970;32:633–640.
24. Rodés-Cabau J, Miró J, Dancea A, et al. Comparison of surgical and transcatheter treatment for native coarctation of the aorta in patients ≥1 year old. The Quebec native coarctation of the aorta study. *Am Heart J.* 2007;154:186–192.
25. Maron B, Humphries J, Rowe R, et al. Prognosis of surgically corrected coarctation of the aorta. A 20-year postoperative appraisal. *Circulation.* 1973;47:119–126.
26. Frescura C, Angelini A, Daliento L, et al. Morphological aspects of Ebstein's anomaly in adults. *Thorac Cardiovasc Surg.* 2000;203–208.
27. Ho SY, Goltz D, McCarthy K, et al. The atrioventricular junctions in Ebstein malformation. *Heart.* 2000;83:444–449.
28. Reemtsen BL, Polimenakos AC, Fagan BT, et al. Fate of the right ventricle after fenestrated right ventricular exclusion for severe neonatal Ebstein anomaly. *J Thorac Cardiovasc Surg.* 2007;134:1406–1412.
29. Vargas FJ, Mengo G, Granja MA, et al. Tricuspid annuloplasty and ventricular plication for Ebstein's malformation. *Ann Thorac Surg.* 1998;65:1755–1757.
30. Rudolph A, Heymann M, Spitznas U. Hemodynamic considerations in the development of narrowing of the aorta. *Am J Cardiol.* 1972;30:514–525.
31. McElhinney DB, Sherwood MC, Keane JF, et al. Current management of severe congenital mitral stenosis: Outcomes of transcatheter and surgical therapy in 108 infants and children. *Circulation.* 2005;112:707–714.
32. Williams J, Barratt-Boyes B, Lowe J. Supravalvular aortic stenosis. *Circulation.* 1961;24:1311–1318.
33. Keane J, Driscoll D, Gersony W, et al. Second natural history study of congenital heart defects. Results of treatment of patients with aortic valvar stenosis. *Circulation.* 1993;87:I16–I27.
34. HL Walters I, Lobdell K, Tantengco V, et al. The ross procedure in children and young adults with congenital aortic valve disease. *J Heart Valve Dis.* 1997;6:335–342.
35. Elkins RC, Thompson DM, Lane MM, et al. Ross operation: 16-year experience. *J Thorac Cardiovasc Surg.* 2008;136:623–630,e625
36. Bonow RO, Carabello BA, Kanu C, et al. ACC/AHA 2006 guidelines for the management of patients with valvular heart disease: A report of the American College of Cardiology/American Heart Association Task Force on practice guidelines (writing committee to revise the 1998 guidelines for the management of patients with valvular heart disease): Developed in collaboration with the Society of Cardiovascular Anesthesiologists: Endorsed by the Society for

Cardiovascular Angiography and Interventions and the Society of Thoracic Surgeons. *Circulation.* 2006;114:e84–e231.

37. McCrindle B. Independent predictors of long-term results after balloon pulmonary valvuloplasty. Valvuloplasty and angioplasty of congenital anomalies (VACA) registry investigators. *Circulation.* 1994;89:1751–1759.

38. Hayes C, Gersony W, Driscoll D, et al. Second natural history study of congenital heart defects. Results of treatment of patients with pulmonary valvar stenosis. *Circulation.* 1993;87:I28–I37.

39. Tomanek RJ. Formation of the coronary vasculature: A brief review. *Cardiovasc Res.* 1996;31:E46–E51.

40. Grace R, Angelini P, Cooley D. Aortic implantation of anomalous left coronary artery arising from pulmonary artery. *Am J Cardiol.* 1977;39:609–613.

41. Lee W, Carvalho J, Chaoui R, et al. Cardiac screening examination of the fetus: Guidelines for performing the "basic" and "extended basic" cardiac scan. *Ultrasound Obstet Gynecol.* 2006;27:107–113.

42. Rychik J, Ayres N, Cuneo B, et al. American Society of Echocardiography guidelines and standards for performance of the fetal echocardiogram. *J Am Soc Echocardiogr.* 2004;17:803–810.

43. Gembruch U, Redel DA, Bald R, et al. Longitudinal study in 18 cases of fetal supraventricular tachycardia: Doppler echocardiographic findings and pathophysiologic implications. *Am Heart J.* 1993;125:1290–1301.

44. Tworetzky W, Marshall A. Balloon valvuloplasty for congenital heart disease in the fetus. *Clin Perinatol.* 2003;30:541–550.

45. Makikallio K, McElhinney DB, Levine JC, et al. Fetal aortic valve stenosis and the evolution of hypoplastic left heart syndrome: Patient selection for fetal intervention. *Circulation.* 2006;113:1401–1405.

46. Lai WW, Geva T, Shirali GS, et al. Guidelines and standards for performance of a pediatric echocardiogram: A report from the task force of the pediatric council of the American Society of Echocardiography. *J Am Soc Echocardiogr.* 2006;19:1413–1430.

47. Vogel M, Simpson JM, Anderson D. Live three-dimensional echocardiography of cor triatriatum in a child. *Heart.* 2008;94:794.

48. Singh A, Mehmood F, Romp RL, et al. Live/real time three-dimensional transthoracic echocardiographic assessment of aortopulmonary window. *Echocardiography.* 2008;25:96–99.

49. Grison A, Maschietto N, Reffo E, et al. Three-dimensional echocardiographic evaluation of right ventricular volume and function in pediatric patients: Validation of the technique. *J Am Soc Echocardiogr.* 2007;20:921–929.

50. Jenkins C, Bricknell K, Hanekom L, et al. Reproducibility and accuracy of echocardiographic measurements of left ventricular parameters using real-time three-dimensional echocardiography. *J Am Coll Cardiol.* 2004;44:878–886.

51. Jenkins C, Chan J, Bricknell K, et al. Reproducibility of right ventricular volumes and ejection fraction using real-time three-dimensional echocardiography: Comparison with cardiac MRI. *Chest.* 2007;131:1844–1851.

52. Powell AJ, Geva T. Blood flow measurement by magnetic resonance imaging in congenital heart disease. *Pediatr Cardiol.* 2000;21:47–58.

53. Powell AJ, Tsai-Goodman B, Prakash A, et al. Comparison between phase-velocity cine magnetic resonance imaging and invasive oximetry for quantification of atrial shunts. *Am J Cardiol.* 2003;91:1523–1525.

54. Prakash A, Powell AJ, Krishnamurthy R, et al. Magnetic resonance imaging evaluation of myocardial perfusion and viability in congenital and acquired pediatric heart disease. *Am J Cardiol.* 2004;93:657–661.

55. Kiaffas MG, Powell AJ, Geva T. Magnetic resonance imaging evaluation of cardiac tumor characteristics in infants and children. *Am J Cardiol.* 2002;89:1229–1233.

56. Goo HW, Park I-S, Ko JK, et al. Computed tomography for the diagnosis of congenital heart disease in pediatric and adult patients. *Int J Cardiovasc Imaging.* 2005;21:347–365.

57. Ou P, Celermajer DS, Calcagni G, et al. Three-dimensional CT scanning: A new diagnostic modality in congenital heart disease. *Heart.* 2007;93:908–913.

58. Dae MW. Pediatric nuclear cardiology. *Semin Nucl Med.* 2007;37:382–390.

59. De Luca L, Bovenzi F, Rubini D, et al. Stress-rest myocardial perfusion SPECT for functional assessment of coronary arteries with anomalous origin or course. *J Nucl Med.* 2004;45:532–536.

60. Wernovsky G, Wypij D, Jonas RA, et al. Postoperative course and hemodynamic profile after the arterial switch operation in neonates and infants: A comparison of low-flow cardiopulmonary bypass and circulatory arrest. *Circulation.* 1995;92:2226–2235.

61. Lacour-Gayet F, Clarke D, Jacobs J, et al. The aristotle score: A complexity-adjusted method to evaluate surgical results. *Eur J Cardiothorac Surg.* 2004;25:911–924.

62. Voigt JU, Flachskampf FA. Strain and strain rate. New and clinically relevant echo parameters of regional myocardial function. *Z Kardiol.* 2004;93:249–258.

63. Whitham J, Hasan B, Schamberger M, et al. Use of cardiac magnetic resonance imaging to determine myocardial viability in an infant with in utero septal myocardial infarction and ventricular noncompaction. *Pediatr Cardiol.* 2008;29:950–953.

Cyanotic Congenital Lesions

41

Wyman W. Lai

1. INTRODUCTION

Based on an analysis of multiple studies in various populations, the incidence of moderate or severe congenital heart disease (CHD) has been stable at 6/1,000 live births over the past 50 years. The median incidence of cyanotic CHD was reported at 1.3/1,000 live births, with an upper quartile value of 1.5/1,000 live births indicating consistency among the studies.[1] With advances in fetal echocardiography, approximately 25% to 35% of congenital heart lesions are now detected *in utero*, and routine prenatal screening has lowered the prevalence of the more severe forms of CHD in some regions.[2,3]

At the 32nd Bethesda Conference, a panel of experts estimated that, due to advances in care, there were approximately 787,000 adults with CHD in the United States in the year 2000: 117,000 adults with complex heart disease, 302,000 with moderate heart disease, and 368,000 with simple heart disease.[4] A rapid increase in the prevalence of adult CHD has also occurred in Canada and Europe. The categories of complex, moderate, and simple were based on the health care resources needed to care for this growing population of patients.

The term *cyanosis* is defined as a blue discoloration of the skin (Gr. kyanos = blue, osis = condition). Central cyanosis—cyanosis of the skin, lips, and mucous membranes—occurs with an absolute concentration of 3 to 5 g/dL of reduced (deoxygenated) hemoglobin in the capillaries which generally occurs with an arterial oxygen saturation of 75% to 85%.[5,6] Almost any form of CHD can present with cyanosis, depending on the pathophysiology at the time of evaluation, but certain types of CHD predominate. Cyanosis occurs in the newborn and young child due to right-to-left shunting found in complex CHD such as conotruncal abnormalities and single ventricles. In uncorrected simple CHD, cyanosis can occur in late childhood and adulthood with the development of pulmonary vascular obstructive disease, as seen in Eisenmenger syndrome. Other relatively common causes of cyanosis include lung disease, abnormally elevated hemoglobin levels, heart failure, and liver disease.

2. CLINICAL PRESENTATION

The clinical presentation of cyanotic CHD depends on the age of the patient and the underlying diagnosis. The newborn often presents with a murmur, but may present with cyanosis alone. The older child may present with lightheadedness, fatigue, or a history of squatting for relief of dyspnea. The physical appearance of patients with cyanotic CHD may be dominated by an underlying genetic diagnosis and/or syndrome, such as Down syndrome

or velocardiofacial syndrome. Digital clubbing is associated with chronic cyanosis in older children and adults; this finding may resolve following relief of cyanosis.

The importance of rapid and accurate diagnosis is greatest in the newborn with complex CHD. In many forms of complex-CHD, the systemic or pulmonary circulation is dependent on the patency of the ductus arteriosus. A prompt diagnosis allows the initiation of treatment with a prostaglandin infusion before the development of circulatory or pulmonary collapse, resulting in improved survival. Although the advances in medical and surgical treatments for cyanotic CHD have resulted in significantly more patients surviving into adulthood, many have sequelae requiring ongoing clinical care and monitoring.[4]

3. PATHOPHYSIOLOGY

For the purposes of discussion in this chapter, congenital cyanotic lesions are divided into the following categories: (i) simple CHD with right-to-left shunting, (ii) conotruncal abnormalities, and (iii) single ventricles.

3.1. Simple CHD with right-to-left shunting

The anatomy of simple CHD, such as septal defects and patent ductus arteriosus, is discussed in the previous chapter on Acyanotic Congenital Lesions. These lesions present with left-to-right shunting in early childhood, beginning with the fall in pulmonary vascular resistance seen normally in the first few days of life. Cyanosis occurs as the result of reversal of shunting across the cardiac lesion.

The pathophysiology of cyanosis due to right-to-left shunting across a large ventricular septal defect was called Eisenmenger complex by Maude Abbot in 1932 and popularized as Eisenmenger syndrome by Paul Wood in a landmark paper published in 1958.[7,8] The term *Eisenmenger syndrome* is now frequently used to refer to simple CHD associated with pulmonary hypertension, defined as a mean pulmonary artery (PA) pressure of 25 mm Hg at rest and 30 mm Hg with exercise, and cyanosis. The cyanosis is due to bidirectional or strictly right-to-left shunting of poorly oxygenated blood into the systemic arterial circulation. In order of occurrence, the most common forms of CHD involved are ventricular septal defect, atrial septal defect, and complete common atrioventricular canal (also called atrioventricular septal defect).[9] In patients with a ventricular septal defect or complete common atrioventricular canal, the presence of increased pulmonary pressures in addition to increased pulmonary blood flow leads to pulmonary vascular obstructive disease in the first decade of life (Fig. 41.1). In patients with atrial septal defect, the onset of

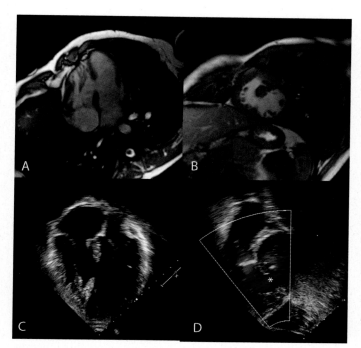

Figure 41.1 Magnetic resonance imaging and echocardiogram on a 30-year-old man with a ventricular septal defect and Eisenmenger syndrome. The pulmonary-to-systemic blood flow ratio (Q_P/Q_S) was 0.84:1 on room air. Magnetic resonance ECG-triggered steady-state free precession (SSFP) four-chamber (**A**) and short-axis (**B**) images demonstrating a large, mid muscular ventricular septal defect and RV hypertrophy. **C**: Echocardiographic apical four-chamber view of the defect. **D**: Subxiphoid short-axis color Doppler imaging of the right-to-left systolic shunt (*asterisk*).

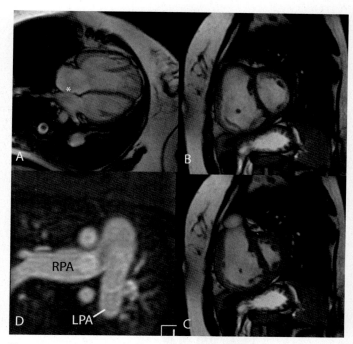

Figure 41.2 Magnetic resonance imaging on a 26-year-old woman with an atrial septal defect and Eisenmenger syndrome. The Q_P/Q_S was 1.1:1 on supplemental oxygen by nasal cannula. **A**: ECG-triggered SSFP cine four-chamber image of a moderate-to-large secundum atrial septal defect (*asterisk*) and dilated RV. **B**: SSFP cine short-axis image at end-diastole. **C**: SSFP cine short-axis at end-systole demonstrating ventricular septal flattening secondary to pulmonary hypertension. **D**: Gadolinium-enhanced MRA (subvolume maximal intensity projection) showing dilated right and left pulmonary arteries (RPA and LPA).

pulmonary hypertension and pulmonary vascular obstructive disease is delayed until the second or third decade of life (Fig. 41.2). Pulmonary hypertension also occurs with more complex forms of CHD, such as truncus arteriosus or single ventricle.

In simple CHD, Eisenmenger syndrome can almost always be prevented with early transcatheter or surgical closure of the cardiac lesion. Pulmonary vascular obstructive disease, however, can progress in a small minority of patients even after correction of the cardiac lesion. With increased right-to-left shunting and worsening cyanosis, the associated problems of erythrocytosis, hemoptysis, and right heart failure become the dominant features of Eisenmenger syndrome. Treatment consists of oxygen, pulmonary vasodilator therapy, anticoagulation, and prevention of dehydration and endocarditis.[10] Phlebotomy should be used cautiously because of the potential to cause microcytosis and exacerbate hyperviscosity.[11] Patients with Eisenmenger syndrome are at particular risk for heart failure and sudden death during pregnancy.

3.2. Conotruncal abnormalities

Conotruncal lesions involve abnormalities at the junction of the ventricular infundibulum, or conus, with the proximal great arteries, or—embryologically—the truncus arteriosus. Conotruncal abnormalities can be classified based on the ventriculoarterial alignments (i.e., concordant, discordant, or double outlet). For an understanding of the pathophysiology, it is also important to note the atrioventricular alignment, the status of the ventricular septum (number, size, and location of ventricular septal defects), the presence of subvalvular or valvular stenosis, and the position

of the great arteries. In addition, abnormalities of the great arteries are common, with the potential occurrence of stenosis or atresia either proximally or distally. As with simple right-to-left shunts, the hemodynamic component of the examination (assessment of pressure and flow) is essential for clinical decision making.

3.2.1. Tetralogy of Fallot

The most common conotruncal abnormality is tetralogy of Fallot, which consists of a ventricular septal defect (in the outlet region), pulmonary stenosis (generally subvalvular), overriding of the aorta, and right ventricular (RV) hypertrophy. Cyanosis results from right-to-left shunting across the ventricular septal defect. The amount of shunting and the level of cyanosis are directly proportional to the degree of pulmonary stenosis. In cases with pulmonary atresia, blood flow to the lungs is through a patent ductus arteriosus and/or major aortopulmonary collaterals. Another important—but rarer—morphological variant is tetralogy of Fallot with absent pulmonary valve syndrome, which is associated with severe pulmonary regurgitation and enlarged pulmonary arteries that may cause airway obstruction (Fig. 41.3).

The treatment for tetralogy of Fallot and its variants consists of ventricular septal defect closure and relief of RV outflow tract obstruction. Classically, a systemic-to-PA shunt was used to provide adequate pulmonary blood flow until the time a complete repair could be performed.[12] At the time of corrective surgery, a RV outflow tract patch may be utilized to widen the subpulmonary infundibulum, often crossing the pulmonary annulus. As a result, significant pulmonary regurgitation is a common sequela of repair.

In patients with absent or severely hypoplastic branch pulmonary arteries, the initial palliative procedure may be to bring together, or "unifocalize," the aortopulmonary collaterals to create a central pulmonary arterial tree.[13] Multiple interventional catheterizations are often required for balloon dilation of stenosis of the distal pulmonary arteries, intravascular stent placement, and coil embolization of collaterals[14] prior to or after corrective surgery. In cases with pulmonary atresia, a conduit is frequently necessary to connect the RV to the native or unifocalized pulmonary arteries.

Whether performed in one or multiple stages, the postoperative RV pressure is dependent on the status of the pulmonary arterial tree (number of pulmonary segments perfused, relief of proximal and distal stenoses, and intravascular pressures). The ultimate goal of surgery and catheterization is to bring the RV systolic pressure to less than or equal to one half of systemic level systolic pressure.[15] In patients with absent pulmonary valve syndrome, plication of the branch pulmonary arteries is often necessary at the time of surgical correction.

Following successful tetralogy of Fallot surgery, patients must be monitored for residual RV outflow tract or PA obstruction; the effects of pulmonary regurgitation; worsening ventricular function; and arrhythmia. Late reoperation for subsequent native or conduit pulmonary stenosis and/or pulmonary regurgitation is common. Based on two large series, the average conduit longevity was approximately 5 to 10 years for infants and young children and approximately 10 to 15 years for older children and young adults.[16,17] The surgical mortality for conduit replacement is low.[18] Percutaneous pulmonary valve implantation is now a viable alternative to surgery in selected patients.[19]

3.2.2. Truncus arteriosus

Truncus arteriosus is defined as a single arterial trunk arising from the heart due to failure of septation of the truncus arteriosus into the aorta and main PA during development. The conotruncal anatomy in truncus arteriosus is similar to tetralogy of Fallot with pulmonary atresia, except that the pulmonary arteries arise—together or separately—from the proximal arterial trunk (Fig. 41.4). Cyanosis results

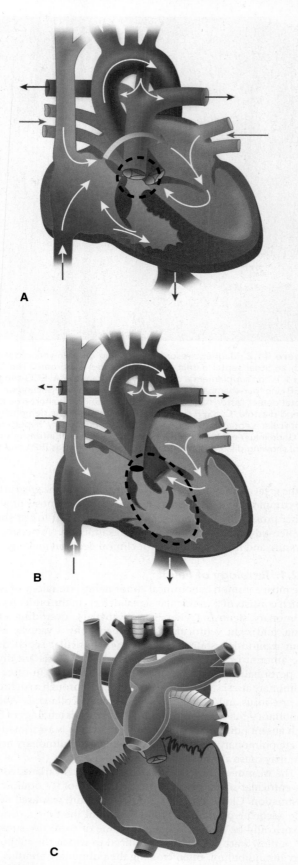

Figure 41.3 Drawings of tetralogy of Fallot (**A**), tetralogy of Fallot with pulmonary atresia (**B**), and tetralogy of Fallot with absent pulmonary valve syndrome (**C**). In this example with pulmonary atresia, confluent pulmonary arteries are supplied by a patent ductus arteriosus.

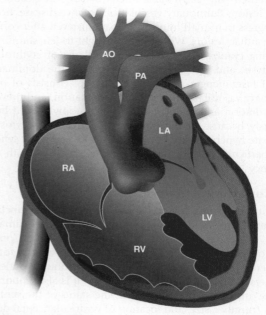

Figure 41.4 Drawing of truncus arteriosus with branch pulmonary arteries arising together from a main pulmonary artery segment off the common arterial trunk.

from right-to-left shunting across the ventricular septal defect, but symptoms of congestive heart failure frequently occur, due to excessive pulmonary blood flow, with a fall in pulmonary vascular resistance. The truncal valve generally overrides a large conoventricular septal defect. Most truncal valves have three leaflets, but valves with two or four leaflets are also common.[20,21] In a series of 205 patients, moderate or severe truncal valve stenosis was reported in 13% and moderate or severe regurgitation in 11%[22]; but the prevalence of truncal valve dysfunction may be significantly greater in the subset of patients with pulmonary hypertension.[23] Interrupted aortic arch has been reported in approximately 11% of patients.[24]

Surgical correction of truncus arteriosus consists of ventricular septal defect closure and placement of a conduit from the RV to the pulmonary arteries. As seen in other lesions, conduit stenosis develops with progressive size mismatch due to somatic growth and also intimal proliferation, frequently necessitating conduit replacement. Long-term monitoring of truncal valve function is required.

3.2.3. Transposition of the great arteries

In transposition of the great arteries, the aorta arises from the RV and the PA from the left ventricle (LV), a condition also known as ventriculoarterial discordance (Fig. 41.5). With normal atrial and ventricular anatomy (atrial situs solitus and D-ventricular looping), the deoxygenated systemic venous return is pumped back into the systemic arterial system, resulting in profound cyanosis. Postnatal survival is dependent upon the presence of atrial, ventricular, and/or ductal level shunting. Under echocardiographic guidance, a balloon atrial septostomy can be performed at the bedside to increase atrial level shunting.[25] Patency of the ductus arteriosus improves mixing and may be required in some patients even after an atrial septostomy.

Surgery for D-loop transposition of the great arteries transitioned from a Mustard or Senning procedure ("atrial switch") in the 1960 to 1970s to an arterial switch operation (Jatene) in the 1980 to 1990s (Fig. 41.6).[26] In the Mustard and Senning procedures, the systemic venous blood is baffled to the LV and the pulmonary venous blood to the RV. The LV pumps to the pulmonary

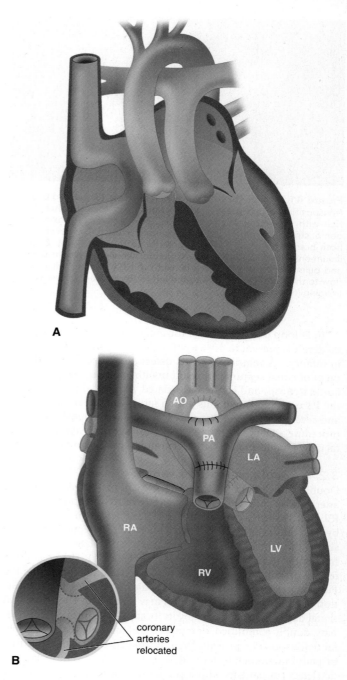

A

B

coronary arteries relocated

Figure 41.6 Drawings of transposition of the great arteries following Mustard procedure (**A**) and arterial switch operation with LeCompte maneuver, resulting in the right pulmonary artery coursing anterior to the ascending aorta (**B**).

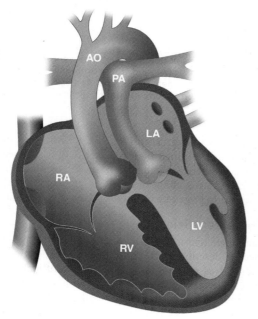

Figure 41.5 Drawing of transposition of the great arteries with a ventricular septal defect. Ao, aorta; PA, pulmonary artery; RA, right atrium; LA, left atrium; RV, right ventricle; LV, left ventricle.

circulation, while the RV functions as the systemic ventricle. Many adult patients with these atrial switch procedures are alive but suffer from arrhythmia, systemic atrioventricular valve (tricuspid) regurgitation, RV failure, and pulmonary hypertension.[27] In the arterial switch operation, the aorta and PA are surgically transposed, and the coronary arteries are reimplanted onto the neoaorta. The LV is thus transformed into the systemic ventricle. An accompanying LeCompte maneuver results in both proximal branch pulmonary arteries crossing anterior to the ascending aorta (Fig. 41.7). Midterm results of the neonatal arterial switch operation have been promising, but patients must be monitored regularly for neoaortic valve function, neoaortic root dilation, and coronary function.[28-30]

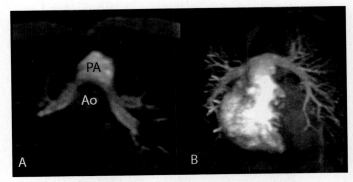

Figure 41.7 Magnetic resonance imaging on a 13-year-old boy with transposition of the great arteries, status post arterial switch operation with LeCompte maneuver. **A:** ECG-triggered SSFP axial image demonstrating an anterior main pulmonary artery (PA) bifurcating with both branch pulmonary arteries anterior to the aorta (Ao). **B:** Gadolinium-enhanced MRA (3D reconstruction) showing the right ventricle and pulmonary arteries. There is mild right PA stenosis with 43% of flow to the right PA and 57% to the left PA by phase-contrast velocity imaging (not shown).

In D-loop transposition of the great arteries, a ventricular septal defect is present in 40% to 45% of cases, some of which close in infancy.[31] A ventricular septal defect associated with malalignment of conal septum can result in either subpulmonary or subaortic stenosis, and is often associated with distal obstruction of the PA or aorta. In patients with a large ventricular septal defect and severe subvalvular or valvular pulmonary stenosis, a Rastelli procedure—LV-to-aortic valve baffle through the ventricular septal defect baffle and a RV-to-PA conduit—may be indicated.[32]

3.2.4. Double outlet right ventricle

Double outlet right ventricle (DORV) occurs when both great arteries arise entirely or predominantly from the morphologically RV. DORVs form a complex group of anomalies which are defined by the features of the great arteries, ventricular septal defect, and size of the ventricles. DORV can occur as an isolated anomaly or, frequently, in the setting of more complex CHD. The great arteries are described by the position of the aorta relative to the PA. Pulmonary stenosis is present in a majority of cases, but obstruction of either or both great arteries may be present. The ventricular septal defect is characterized by its location (subaortic, subpulmonary, doubly committed, or remote), and multiple ventricular septal defects may be present. Even in isolated DORV, the spectrum of pathophysiology varies widely. It may mimic ventricular septal defect (in patients with a subaortic ventricular septal defect), tetralogy of Fallot (subaortic ventricular septal defect with pulmonary stenosis), transposition of the great arteries (subpulmonary ventricular septal defect), or single ventricle pathophysiology (Fig. 41.8).[33] In complex DORV, the associated findings include complete common atrioventricular canal, straddling atrioventricular valve(s), superoinferior ventricles, and/or heterotaxy syndrome.[34] Hypoplasia of either the RV or LV may be present.

In patients with two relatively normal ventricles, the surgical procedure is selected to separate the two ventricles, to direct the pulmonary venous blood to the aorta, and to relieve ventricular outflow tract obstruction. If possible, the surgery will result in the morphologically LV functioning as the systemic ventricle. In one large series, the patients were grouped as having had one of five types of repair: "intraventricular tunnel repair, arterial switch with ventricular septal defect-to-PA baffle, Rastelli-type extracardiac conduit repair, Damus–Kaye–Stansel repair, and atrial inversion

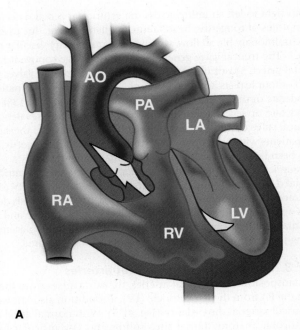

A

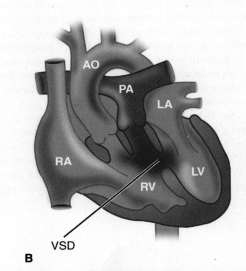

B

Figure 41.8 Drawings of double outlet right ventricle with tetralogy of Fallot-like conotruncus (**A**): and transposition-like conotruncus (**B**). VSD, ventricular septal defect. PA, pulmonary artery; Ao, aorta; RA, right atrium; LA, left atrium; RV, right ventricle; LV, left ventricle.

with ventricular septal defect-to-PA baffle.[35]" The timing of the surgery was often determined by the presence of associated cardiac anomalies. As evidenced by the list of surgical techniques utilized, the preoperative assessment of DORV is challenging and postoperative monitoring must be tailored to the individual patient.

3.3. Single ventricles

The terms *single ventricle* and *univentricular heart* have classically been used to describe a doublet inlet ventricle, with two atrioventricular valves entering a single, large ventricular chamber. The use of these terms to describe cases with an additional rudimentary chamber has been debated without resolution.[36,37] The morphology of the large ventricular chamber can usually be recognized by its shape, the presence of basal septal trabeculations, and the location of an accessory chamber (if present). The single, morphologically LV is often a prolate ellipsoid with fine or inapparent trabeculations and is usually associated with an anterior outlet chamber from which the aorta often arises. The single, morphologically RV is generally pyramidal in shape with prominent trabeculations, may have a bisecting midline posterior muscle band, and may be associated with a posterior accessory chamber at the posterior atrioventricular groove that represents a rudimentary LV. A caveat in the imaging of single ventricles is that a ventricle of either morphology may assume a more spherical shape with thinning out of trabeculations, especially in the setting of dilation and systolic dysfunction. The term *single ventricle* has also been used to describe any form of CHD with single ventricle pathophysiology.

3.3.1. Single or dominant left ventricle
The most common form of double inlet ventricle is a morphologically LV with L-loop and transposition of the great arteries (aorta arising from an anterior and leftward outlet chamber).[38] The eponym *Holmes heart* describes a double inlet LV with normally related great arteries.

Tricuspid atresia is characterized by absence of the tricuspid valve and RV hypoplasia. Patient with tricuspid atresia can be classified by the ventriculoarterial alignment (i.e., normally related great arteries versus transposition of the great arteries) and restrictiveness of the ventricular septal defect.[39]

Patients with pulmonary atresia with intact ventricular septum are categorized by tricuspid annular size, RV size, and RV morphology (bipartite vs. tripartite).[40,41] These morphologic features, plus the presence or absence of severe coronary artery abnormalities, allow for planning of surgery (single ventricle palliation vs. staged biventricular repair).[42,43]

3.3.2. Single or dominant right ventricle
Relatively rare forms of single right ventricles with a single or double inlet exist, often with other associated anomalies. Double outlet ventriculo-arterial connections are generally present. Some CHD with two ventricles but severe LV hypoplasia will also be considered as part of the hypoplastic left heart syndrome, for example, the more severe forms of RV-dominant complete common atrioventricular canal and critical aortic stenosis.

In the usual form of hypoplastic left heart syndrome, the aortic valve is atretic. Mitral valve stenosis or atresia is also seen, as is hypoplasia of the ascending aorta and aortic coarctation.[44,45]

3.3.3. Single ventricle pathophysiology
The pathophysiology of single ventricles share some common features, but are also specific to the group of anatomical abnormalities present. In most patients, there is complete mixing of the systemic and pulmonary venous blood return, resulting in identical oxygen saturations in the aorta and pulmonary arteries regardless of the position of the great arteries. In a small minority of patients with single ventricles, streaming may occur; the presence of incomplete mixing, in turn, could result in either ventricular septal defect or transposition physiology.

In both double inlet LV and tricuspid atresia, obstruction of the bulboventricular foramen—the communication between the ventricular chambers—is common and is frequently associated with narrowing of the aorta or PA. With normally related great arteries, the size of the bulboventricular foramen determines the degree of subpulmonary stenosis. In transposition of the great arteries, a restrictive bulboventricular foramen results in subaortic stenosis and is frequently associated with coarctation of the aorta.

With pulmonary atresia and intact ventricular septum, the pulmonary circulation is dependent on left-to-right flow across a patent ductus arteriosus. A hypoplastic and often hypertensive ("suprasystemic") RV is present. The patent foramen ovale in both tricuspid atresia and pulmonary atresia with intact ventricular septum is rarely restrictive.

With hypoplastic left heart syndrome, the systemic circulation—including the coronary circulation—is dependent on right-to-left flow across a patent ductus arteriosus. The interatrial communication in hypoplastic left heart syndrome may be severely restrictive, thereby increasing pulmonary venous pressures and limiting pulmonary blood flow.[46] With a nonrestrictive or mildly restrictive interatrial communication and a widely patent ductus arteriosus, or surgical shunt, the pulmonary-to-systemic circulation ratio will depend on the relative vascular resistances in those circulations; an optimal pulmonary-to-systolic blood flow ratio (Q_p/Q_s) is approximately 1:1, which would yield a systemic arterial oxygen saturation of approximately 75% to 80%.[47,48]

3.3.4. Single ventricle palliation
The initial goal of single ventricle palliation is to establish a stable systemic circulation (adequate systemic blood flow with an oxygen saturation ≥70%) and a stable pulmonary circulation (Fig. 41.1). In patients with critical obstruction to the pulmonary circulation, a systemic-to-PA shunt is generally indicated to provide a stable source of pulmonary blood flow. A biventricular repair may be considered in some cases with favorable RV and coronary artery anatomy.

For patients with aortic atresia, the most common surgical approach is the Norwood procedure,[49] which consists of an anastomosis of the ascending aorta to the transected main PA with aortic arch augmentation, atrial septectomy, and a systemic-to-PA, usually in the form of a modified Blalock–Taussig shunt (a conduit from the right subclavian artery to right PA).[50] The Sano modification to the Norwood procedure which utilizes a right ventricle-to-PA conduit in place of the Blalock–Taussig shunt[51] has been reported to improve survival,[52] and a multicenter randomized clinical trial comparing the classic Norwood procedure and the Sano modification is ongoing. Yet another initial palliative procedure for aortic atresia is termed the "hybrid" approach, which consists of surgical banding the branch pulmonary arteries and transcatheter stenting the patent ductus arteriosus.[53] Using this approach, the more involved surgical reconstruction of the aorta and branch pulmonary arteries is deferred until the second stage procedure.

In single ventricle patients with primarily subvalvular obstruction to the systemic circulation, an anastomosis of the ascending aorta and main PA with transection of the main PA (Damus–Kaye–Stansel procedure) is performed.[54] A systemic-to-PA shunt is required.

In single ventricle patients without ventricular outflow obstruction, banding of the main PA is performed to prevent pulmonary overcirculation and to guard against pulmonary hypertension. The protection of the pulmonary vasculature is critical, as a low pulmonary vascular resistance is necessary for subsequent single ventricle palliative procedures. Some single ventricle patients are born with a "well-balanced" circulation, which can be defined as an unobstructed systemic circulation and just the right amount of pulmonary stenosis to be free of pulmonary overcirculation (which would result in congestive heart failure), pulmonary undercirculation (severe cyanosis), and pulmonary hypertension.

The second stage for most single ventricle patients is a bidirectional Glenn anastomosis (also called a bidirectional cavopulmonary anastomosis) or a variant of this procedure (e.g., the hemi-Fontan procedure). With the bidirectional Glenn anastomosis, the superior vena cava is connected directly into the pulmonary circulation with an end-to-side anastomosis to the right PA. With the hemi-Fontan procedure, a dividing patch is placed within the right atrium and the superior portion of the right atrium is anastomosed to the main PA. The physiology following the bidirectional Glenn and hemi-Fontan procedures is the same. Some centers choose to leave an additional source of pulmonary blood flow, which may obviate the need for a Fontan procedure in certain patients.[55]

The final step in palliative surgery for most single ventricle patients is the Fontan procedure.[56] Most commonly, the systemic venous blood is directed to the pulmonary arteries by way of a right atrium-to-PA anastomosis (Fig. 41.9); a noncircumferential conduit, or "lateral tunnel," of the inferior vena cava to the right PA; or an extracardiac conduit from the inferior vena cava to the right PA (Fig. 41.10). The risk factors for morbidity and mortality in the Fontan procedure include high pulmonary arterial pressures and elevated pulmonary vascular resistance; poor ventricular function; significant atrioventricular valvular regurgitation; and pulmonary venous obstruction. In at least one study, the performance of a bidirectional Glenn anastomosis as a second stage appeared to confer survival benefit in the period before the Fontan

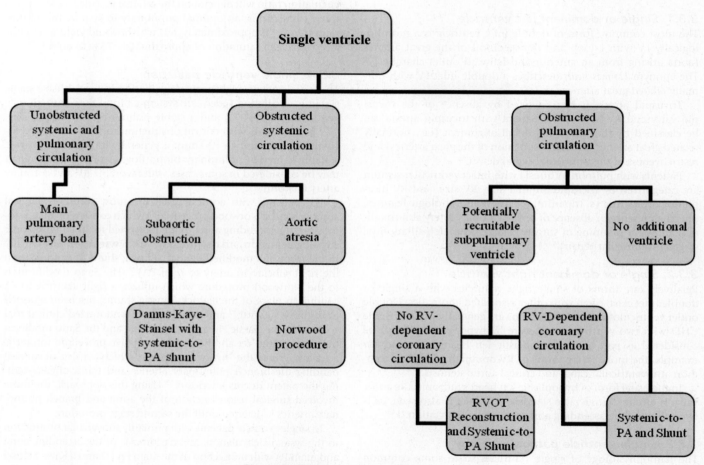

Figure 41.9 Initial single ventricle palliation.

Figure 41.10 Gadolinium-enhanced MRA with 3D reconstruction on a 37-year-old man with double inlet left ventricle, status post right atrial-to-pulmonary artery Fontan procedure. **A:** Initial phase of demonstrating the dilated right atrium, right atrial-to-pulmonary artery anastomosis, and branch pulmonary arteries. **B:** Second phase showing the venae cavae, heart, and aorta.

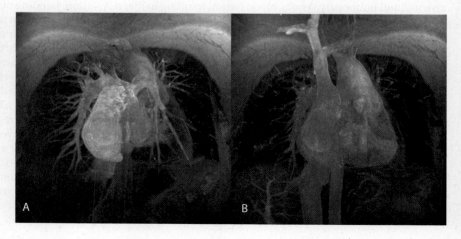

procedure, rather than at the time of the Fontan.[57] The incorporation of a fenestration between the pulmonary and systemic circulations, which acts to maintain cardiac output in the setting of elevated pulmonary vascular resistance, improves perioperative hemodynamics. Its long-term benefits are still debated,[58,59] and subsequent transcatheter closure of the fenestration may be necessary for significant cyanosis in some patients.

The Fontan procedure is a palliative rather than a corrective procedure. Despite many advances in surgical technique and perioperative management, patients with a Fontan circulation remain at high risk for early ventricular failure, arrhythmia, thromboembolic events, and protein losing enteropathy.[60] Exercise testing reveals subnormal performance as a rule.[61] The occurrence of sudden death is presumed to be secondary to arrhythmia. In the Fontan circulation, the long-term myocardial function of the single right ventricle is poorer than the single LV and overall prognosis is generally worse for the patient with a single, or dominant, right ventricle.[62,63] Patients following a Fontan procedure for single ventricle anatomy require monitoring at frequent intervals.

4. DIAGNOSTIC EVALUATION

Irrespective of the method of diagnosis, the evaluation of a patient with cyanotic CHD requires a systematic approach based on the knowledge of the cardiac segments and their connections or alignments. In the commonly used segmental classification systems, the heart may be described as formed of three major cardiac segments (atria, ventricles, and great arteries) joined together by two interconnecting segments (atrioventricular canal and conus or infundibulum).[64,65] Detailed examination of the systemic and pulmonary venous connections is especially important in the patient with cyanosis. A key concept of the segmental approach is that the cardiac segments may develop independent of one another.

One approach to the diagnosis of complex CHD is to define each segment separately. After the determination of visceral situs, or sidedness, the veins and atria are identified. Ventricular morphology and looping are determined, and the identity and location of the great arteries are established. Finally, the atrioventricular and ventriculoarterial connections are carefully evaluated. Knowledge of the common associations among lesions is helpful. Another approach is to follow the blood flow: from the systemic

venous return into and out of the heart, and similarly with the pulmonary venous return. The use of a common nomenclature facilities communication between specialties and aids in the analysis of outcomes.[66,67]

The goals of any diagnostic test will vary with the specific diagnosis and the stage at which the patient with CHD is being evaluated (i.e., hypoplastic left heart syndrome status post Norwood procedure vs. status post bidirectional Glenn anastomosis, etc.). The relative strengths of each of the commonly utilized noninvasive diagnostic[66,67] tests are provided in Table 41.1. The selection of an appropriate test is dependent on the age or size of the patient, the clinical question being asked, and the expertise available at the institutions involved.

4.1. Fetal echocardiography

The fetal echocardiogram is a unique test for the assessment of the fetal cardiovascular system with ultrasound.[68] Although technically more challenging than the echocardiogram in a young child, the fetal echocardiogram provides diagnostic information that allows for appropriate counseling, monitoring of the growth of cardiovascular structures, assessment of hemodynamic status, and determination of the optimal timing and method of delivery. Identification of patients with a ductal-dependent systemic or pulmonary circulation is particularly important for perinatal management.[69]

As it is currently practiced, fetal cardiac screening with a four-chamber view allows for the detection of 16% to 35% of all cases of CHD before birth.[70,71] Universal screening with a more detailed fetal echocardiogram could improve the detection rate of CHD to as high as 80% to 85% (Fig. 41.11).[72,73] The cost-to-benefit ratio of universal screening does not currently support this approach,[70] but survival in some studies of transposition of the great arteries[74] and hypoplastic left heart syndrome[75] has been improved with prenatal detection.

4.2. Echocardiography

Echocardiography is the primary imaging tool for the diagnosis and management of cyanotic CHD in children.[76] Its major advantages are high-resolution images in real time, the ability to assess cardiac function, and the availability of hemodynamic information with Doppler and color Doppler. With good two-dimensional (2D) imaging, the practitioner is able to create a

TABLE 41.1
RELATIVE STRENGTHS OF COMMONLY UTILIZED NONINVASIVE DIAGNOSTIC TESTS

	Echocardiography in the young child	Echocardiography in the older child/adult	Cardiac MRI in the young child	Cardiac MRI in the older child/young adult	CT scan
Shunt lesions	2D/3D anatomy +++ Output/flow ++ Pressure ++	2D/3D anatomy ++ Output/flow ++ Pressure +	2D/3D anatomy ++ Output/flow +++ Pressure +	2D/3D anatomy ++ Output/flow +++ Pressure +	2D/3D anatomy ++ Output/flow + Pressure −
Conotruncal abnormalities	2D/3D anatomy +++ Output/flow ++ Pressure ++	2D/3D anatomy ++ Output/flow ++ Pressure ++	2D/3D anatomy ++ Output/flow ++ Pressure +	2D/3D anatomy +++ Output/flow +++ Pressure +	2D/3D anatomy +++ Output/flow + Pressure −
Single ventricles	2D/3D anatomy +++ Output/flow ++ Pressure ++	2D/3D anatomy + Output/flow ++ Pressure +	2D/3D anatomy ++ Output/flow ++ Pressure +	2D/3D anatomy +++ Output/flow +++ Pressure +	2D/3D anatomy ++ Output/flow + Pressure −

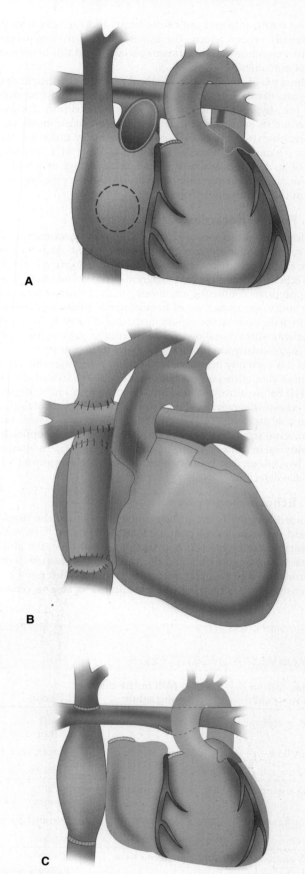

Figure 41.11 Drawings of the three more common types of Fontan procedure: atriopulmonary anastomosis (**A**), lateral tunnel (**B**), and extracardiac conduit (**C**).

3D image of the heart mentally. The greatest contributions of 3D echocardiography in the management of CHD have been in the description of relationships between intracardiac structures, which is important for the planning of interventional catheterization or surgery and in the quantification of ventricular function. Recent advances in the echocardiographic assessment of myocardial performance with tissue Doppler and speckle tracking for systolic function, diastolic function, synchronicity, and torsion, have also been applied to patients with cyanotic CHD.[77-79]

As the patient transitions into adulthood, the diagnostic capabilities of both 2D and 3D transthoracic echocardiographies lessen due to technical limitations. Transesophageal echocardiography (TEE) is a useful technique for imaging CHD in patients of all ages, particularly in patients with a nondiagnostic transthoracic echocardiogram, in the intraoperative setting, and for echocardiographic guidance of interventions (Fig. 41.12).[80] While the issue of safety can be reasonably addressed in most patients, the requirement for anesthesia in younger patients limits the utility of TEE in the outpatient setting. The common indications for TEE in patients with CHD are listed in Table 41.2.[80]

In patients with Eisenmenger syndrome, the focus of the echocardiogram is directed toward determination of the etiology, assessment of the degree of pulmonary hypertension, and evaluation of RV function. The noninvasive assessment of RV function is covered in Chapter 16.

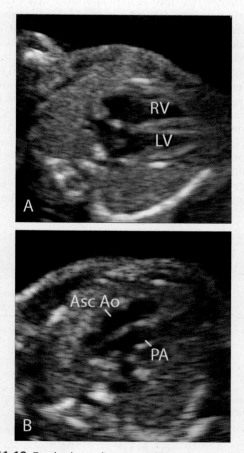

Figure 41.12 Fetal echocardiogram at 22 weeks gestation of transposition of the great arteries. **A:** A normal four-chamber view is present (LV, left ventricle; RV, right ventricle). **B:** The outflow tracts and proximal great arteries are parallel instead of crossing, with a rightward/anterior ascending aorta (Asc Ao) and leftward/posterior pulmonary artery (PA).

TABLE 41.2

COMMON INDICATIONS FOR TRANSESOPHAGEAL ECHOCARDIOGRAPHY IN CONGENITAL HEART DISEASE PATIENTS

Diagnostic indications

Patient with suspected CHD and nondiagnostic transthoracic echocardiogram

Presence of patent foramen ovale and direction of shunting

Evaluation of intra- or extra-cardiac baffles for stenosis or leaks following surgery (e.g., Mustard or Senning procedure for transposition of the great arteries or Fontan procedure)

Aortic dissection (Marfan syndrome)

Evaluation for intracardiac vegetation or periaortic abscess

Evaluation for pericardial effusion or cardiac function in postoperative patients with poor transthoracic windows

Evaluation for intracardiac thrombus prior to cardioversion for atrial flutter/fibrillation

Evaluation of prosthetic valve

Perioperative indications

Immediate preoperative definition of cardiac anatomy and function

Intravascular or intracardiac line or catheter location

Postoperative surgical results and function

Indications and guidelines for performance of transesophageal echocardiography in the patient with pediatric acquired or congenital heart disease: Report from the task force of the Pediatric Council of the American Society of Echocardiography.

CHD, congenital heart disease.

Source: Adapted from Ayres NA, Miller-Hance W, Fyfe DA, et al. Indications and guidelines for performance of transesophageal echocardiography in the patient with pediatric acquired or congenital heart disease: Report from the task force of the Pediatric Council of the American Society of Echocardiography. *J Am Soc Echocardiogr.* 2005;18(1):91–98.

Echocardiographic diagnosis alone permits the planning of surgery for most patients undergoing primary repair of CHD,[81] a group that includes many of the conotruncal anomalies. Single ventricle patients, however, often require additional testing in order to fully assess PA structure and pressures prior to the second and third stages of palliative surgery (the bidirectional Glenn anastomosis and Fontan procedure, respectively), which are dependent on a low pulmonary vascular resistance for success.

In all preoperative cyanotic CHD patients, a thorough transthoracic echocardiogram should address the potential risks and roadblocks for each surgical alternative. Standard imaging windows usually suffice for simple lesions,[76] but unconventional views are often required for complex abnormalities. The ability of 3D echocardiography to demonstrate complex anatomy in CHD has increased significantly (Fig. 41.13).[82] Preoperative information gathered by TEE is often complimentary to information from a less invasive transthoracic echocardiogram; therefore, a recent complete transthoracic examination is indicated prior to TEE.

The limitations of echocardiography are primarily due to the inability of ultrasound to penetrate through air or bone. In larger patients, image quality is worse because imaging at higher ultrasound frequencies, which provides the best resolution, is encumbered by poorer penetration due to energy loss. There is also a trade-off between spatial and temporal resolution that becomes more pronounced as the focal depth increases. The limited availability of adequate ultrasound windows also affects the accuracy of Doppler interrogation which is dependent on the angle of insonation. Because of these reasons, the echocardiogram in an older child or adult provides poorer anatomical and hemodynamic information than in a young child.

4.3. Magnetic resonance imaging

The main indications for cardiovascular magnetic resonance (CMR) imaging in patients with CHD are the delineation of cardiovascular anatomy, assessment of ventricular function, and measurement of blood flow.[83] As with other cardiac conditions, CMR can also aid in the assessment of myocardial perfusion, ischemia, and viability, as well as assist in the detection of tumor and thrombus. Unlike echocardiography, CMR is not limited by the availability of acoustic windows and provides better 3D spatial information on the relative positions of cardiac and extracardiac structures. The clinical data obtained on CMR are often complimentary to that by echocardiography and may allow avoidance of cardiac catheterization in selected patients (see next description).

In patients with cyanotic CHD, phase-contrast velocity imaging sequences provide important information on the cardiac output, pulmonary-to-systemic flow ratio, valvular regurgitation, and right-to-left lung perfusion ratio. In Eisenmenger syndrome, an advantage of CMR over echocardiography is in the assessment of RV size and function. In conotruncal abnormalities and single ventricles, CMR is able to reliably visualize the pulmonary vasculature, including aortopulmonary and veno-venous collaterals (Fig. 41.14).[84,85] Quantification of ventricular size, function, and mass is also achievable by CMR in patients with a systemic RV or a single ventricle.

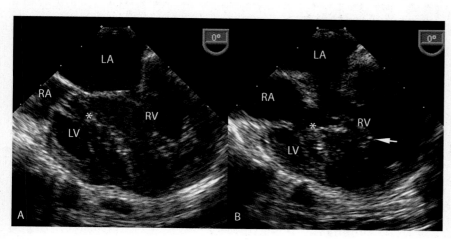

Figure 41.13 Tranesophageal echocardiogram on a 7-year-old boy with double outlet right ventricle, L-ventricular loop, and ventricular septal defect. **A:** In a mid esophageal four-chamber image, the mitral valve is aligned with the LV, to the right of the ventricular septal crest (*) (atrioventricular valves closed). **B:** More anteriorly, overriding and straddling of the MV are seen across an outlet ventricular septal defect (atrioventricular valves open). A prominent muscle band/papillary muscle is present (*arrow*) in the right ventricle (RV). LA, left atrium; LV, left ventricle; RA, right atrium.

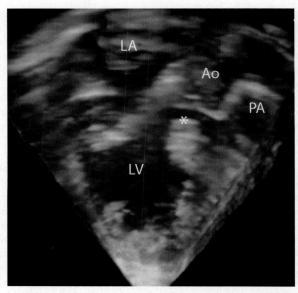

Figure 41.14 Three-dimensional echocardiogram on a 2-month-old boy with tetralogy of Fallot demonstrating the relationship of the aorta (Ao) and pulmonary artery (PA) to the ventricular septal defect (*, crest of ventricular septum). LA, left atrium; LV, left ventricle.

In contrast to echocardiography, the quality of images by CMR in younger children is worse than in adults due to lower signal strength and the limitations in image resolution. Children are also usually unable to cooperate sufficiently with CMR protocols until the age of 6 to 8 years, even with the aid of distraction tools. Although standardized protocols may be applicable for routine congenital CMR cases (e.g., assessment of RV size/function and pulmonary regurgitation in postoperative tetralogy of Fallot), the examination often must be tailored to the clinical indication(s) specified. Direct physician involvement in image acquisition is usually required for patients with cyanotic CHD to ensure that all pertinent clinical questions have been addressed.

4.4. Computed tomography

Cardiovascular imaging by multidetector computed tomography (MDCT) provides high spatial resolution images with a short examination time.[86] In younger children, the requirement for sedation can be significantly shortened or eliminated. MDCT data can be optimized for 3D reconstruction, and visualization algorithms allow for the extraction of surrounding tissues. In patients with Eisenmenger syndrome, pulmonary emboli can be detected[87] and the lung parynchema evaluated.[88] In conotruncal abnormalities, the pulmonary vasculature can be visualized by MDCT with adequate detail to detect stenosis and plan surgery.[89] Cardiac CT has also been utilized to detect coronary abnormalities following the arterial switch operation for transposition of the great arteries.[90,91]

The injection of an iodinated contrast medium is required for cardiac CT and CT angiography. High-resolution cardiac or coronary imaging also requires ECG triggering, which further increases the radiation exposure. Therefore, the benefits of CT imaging must be weighed against the increased risk of cancer associated with radiation exposure, especially in children.[92]

CT scanning has been developed into a complimentary imaging modality that is useful for patients with CHD in whom other imaging modalities are inadequate or contraindicated (e.g., CMR on patients with a susceptibility imaging artifact (Fig. 41.15) or a pacemaker, respectively).[93] Developments to reduce radiation dosages will further enhance its utility in the care for children with cyanotic CHD who require serial follow-up through adulthood.

5. SELECTING AND GUIDING THERAPY

The treatment decision making for cyanotic CHD is complex. In the cyanotic newborn, a rapid and accurate diagnosis is necessary to determine if a ductal-dependent systemic or pulmonary circulation is present. Ideally, this determination is made prenatally by fetal echocardiography. Because of its portability and high image resolution in young children, echocardiography is the ideal initial test for the cyanotic newborn. Once the cyanotic patient is stabilized, the decision-making process turns to identifying those patients who are candidates for primary or staged biventricular repair versus those who will require single ventricle palliation.

In the older patient, the emphasis shifts to the monitoring of residual lesions, assessment of ventricular function, and determination of the need and timing for reintervention. The typical treatment decisions for some of the more common cyanotic CHD lesions are outlined below, with emphasis on the potential role of noninvasive imaging in the guidance of treatment. A detailed description of the clinical imaging protocols for each cyanotic congenital lesion is beyond the scope of this textbook, but the interested reader is referred to other references for additional information.[83,94,95]

Figure 41.15 Gadolinium-enhanced MRA (subvolume maximal intensity projections) on a 36-year-old man with double inlet left ventricle with L-transposition of the great arteries, status post (s/p) lateral tunnel Fontan procedure. **A:** Bidirectional Glenn anastomosis of the superior vena cava (SVC) to the right pulmonary artery (RPA). A dilated ascending aorta (Ao) is present. **B:** Coronal oblique image of the lateral tunnel connection (*double asterisk*) of the inferior vena cava to the RPA with image plane selected to show the ligated main PA (*arrow*) and left pulmonary artery (LPA).

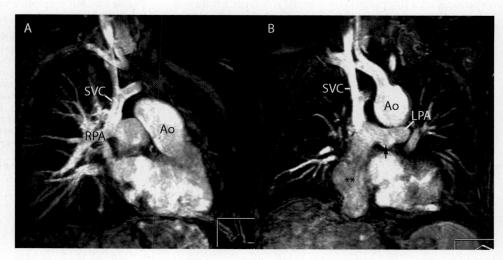

5.1. Eisenmenger syndrome

The combination of noninvasive diagnostic information and cardiac catheterization data can be used to guide treatment decisions in Eisenmenger syndrome (Fig. 41.2). The complexity of the underlying cardiac malformation affects prognosis.[23] The transthoracic echocardiogram is the initial screening test of choice, with the capability to define cardiac anatomy, determine the direction of shunting, and assess ventricular function.[96] Ventricular septal position at end-systole and Doppler echocardiography also provide a means of estimating pulmonary pressures.

With Doppler interrogation of flow velocity (V), pressures can be calculated using the simplified Bernoulli equation (ΔPressure = $4V^2$). The PA systolic pressure is equivalent to RV systolic pressure in the absence of pulmonary stenosis. Using the peak tricuspid regurgitation jet velocity (V_{TR}), RV systolic pressure can be calculated as $4V_{TR}^2$ plus the estimated right atrial pressure (RAP). The peak pulmonary regurgitation jet velocity (V_{PR}) is used to estimate the mean PA pressure ($4V_{PR}^2$ plus the estimated RAP), and the end-diastolic pulmonary regurgitation velocity (V_{EDPR}) is used to estimate the end-diastolic PA pressure ($4V_{EDPR}^2$ plus the estimated RAP) (Fig. 41.16).[97]

Magnetic resonance can be used to confirm the intracardiac anatomy; measure cardiac output and Q_P/Q_S; evaluate the pulmonary and systemic vasculatures; and provide a more detailed assessment of RV function.[98] As noted above, high-resolution CT scan is especially useful to assess pulmonary arterial thrombi and the pulmonary parenchyma.[88]

5.2. Conotruncal abnomalities

Some of the following discussion on tetralogy of Fallot can be generalized to patients with truncus arteriosus and certain forms of DORV—those with ventricular septal defect or tetralogy of Fallotlike physiology. DORV patients with transpositionlike physiology, on the other hand, generally require more complex decision making regarding potential interventricular baffling procedures and their complications. Many patients with complex DORVs may go down the path of single ventricle palliation. The monitoring of patients with transposition of the great arteries is divided by surgical era—atrial versus arterial switch procedure—and their follow-up is quite disparate.

5.2.1. Tetralogy of Fallot

The diagnosis of tetralogy of Fallot can be made reliably on fetal and newborn echocardiography. Examination of the RV outflow and pulmonary arteries are essential components of the preoperative assessment (Fig. 41.3). In addition, the presence of associated lesions such as additional ventricular septal defects, aortic arch anomalies, and anomalous origin of the left coronary artery must be determined. The intraoperative TEE and later postoperative evaluations place emphasis on the assessment of residual lesions and ventricular function (Fig. 41.4).

The echocardiogram generally provides an adequate screening evaluation for a residual ventricular septal defect, tricuspid regurgitation, residual RV outflow tract obstruction, and pulmonary regurgitation. Further assessment of a residual ventricular septal defect by CMR or cardiac catheterization may be needed for quantification of the residual shunt. If indicated, an interventional catheterization for device occlusion of the residual ventricular septal defect would likely require TEE guidance. Additional imaging of residual RV outflow tract obstruction and the pulmonary arteries is possible by CMR (Figs. 41.17 and 41.18), CT scanning, and cardiac catheterization. If transcatheter dilation of a residual obstruction is likely indicated, then X-ray angiography at the time of catheterization would be the imaging technique of choice.

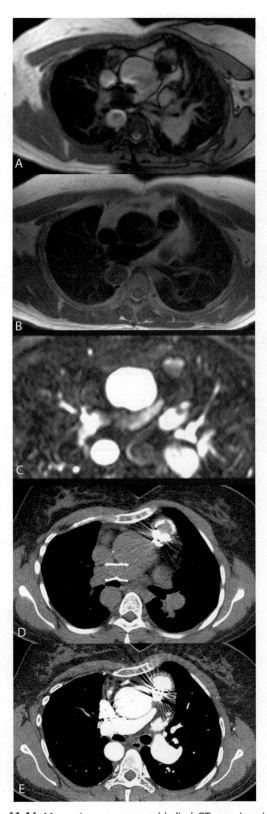

Figure 41.16 Magnetic resonance and helical CT scan imaging on a 40-year-old woman with repaired tetralogy of Fallot and subsequent RPA stent placement. **A:** Nongated SSFP axial image demonstrating a susceptibility imaging artifact due to a metallic stent in the mid RPA. **B:** Fast spin echo with double inversion recovery sequence showing a reduction in the artifact. **C:** Gadolinium-enhanced magnetic resonance angiography. The right-to-left lung perfusion ratio was 40%:60% by phase-contrast velocity imaging (not shown). Helical CT axial images without **D:** and with **E:** contrast better demonstrating the stented RPA anatomy.

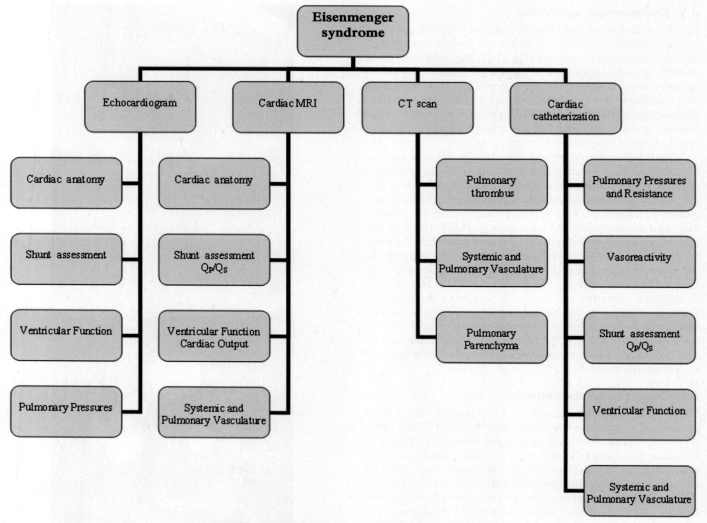

Figure 41.17 Eisenmenger syndrome—diagnostic tests.

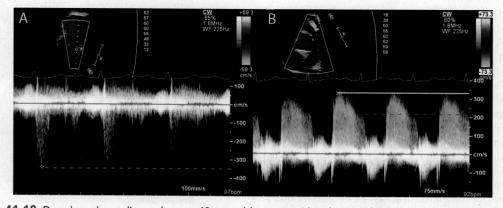

Figure 41.18 Doppler echocardiography on a 48-year-old woman with pulmonary hypertension. **A:** Technically limited Doppler assessment of a trivial-to-mild tricuspid regurgitation jet yielded an estimated RV/pulmonary artery (PA) systolic pressure of $4 \times (3.5)^2$ + right atrial pressure (RAP). RAP was estimated in this patient at 10 mm Hg by imaging of the inferior vena cava (not shown). Therefore, the estimated RV/PA systolic pressure was 59 mm Hg (*dashed green line*) with technically limited tricuspid regurgitation assessment. **B:** Better Doppler interrogation of a mild pulmonary regurgitation jet yielded a more reliable estimated PA mean pressure of $4 \times (3.3)^2$ + RAP = 54 mm Hg (*yellow line*). Estimated PA diastolic pressure was $4 \times (2.2)^2$ + RAP = 29 mm Hg (*dashed red line*). A cardiac catheterization 5 days later showed a mean RAP of 6 mm Hg, systolic PA pressure of 95 mm Hg, mean PA pressure of 63 mm Hg, and diastolic PA pressure of 36 mm Hg on room air.

The optimum timing of pulmonary valve replacement for pulmonary regurgitation following tetralogy of Fallot repair has been a topic of considerable interest.[99–101] A delay in pulmonary valve replacement places the patient at increased risk of exercise intolerance, RV failure, ventricular arrhythmia, syncope, and sudden death. Early pulmonary valve replacement will subject the patient to unnecessary risks and an increased total number of reinterventions. While other clinical criteria must also be factored in, there is now a consensus that the asymptomatic patient with severe pulmonary regurgitation, severe RV dilation (RV end-diastolic volume ≥160 to 170 mL/m^2), and/or poor RV systolic function (RV ejection fraction ≤45%) benefits from pulmonary valve replacement. CMR is ideally suited for the serial assessment of the postoperative tetralogy of Fallot patient because of its ability to assess the pulmonary vasculature, determine the degree of pulmonary regurgitation, and quantify RV size and function. A sample CMR imaging protocol for the postoperative patient with tetralogy of Fallot is provided in Table 41.3.

5.2.2. Transposition of the great arteries

Despite a positive survival benefit, the current fetal detection rate of D-loop transposition of the great arteries has remained low at 25% in one population-based study, with improvement to 40% when transposition of the great arteries was associated with a ventricular septal defect.[102] The prenatal diagnosis of transposition of the great arteries allows for a planned birth at a tertiary medical center where medical and surgical care are available. Prostaglandin therapy is promptly initiated to maintain patency of the ductus arteriosus. Prenatal detection of a restrictive interatrial communication allows for planning of an emergency balloon atrial septostomy procedure immediately after birth.[74]

The newborn echocardiogram focuses on coronary artery imaging and the identification of associated lesions for surgical planning.[103,104] In patients either with an intact ventricular septum or a ventricular septal defect, the arterial switch operation is the preferred surgical option (Fig. 41.5). The presence of significant LV outflow tract obstruction (i.e., subvalvular or valvular pulmonary stenosis), as determined primarily by imaging, in association with a ventricular septal defect, may dictate consideration of a Rastelli repair.

The postoperative evaluation of an adult patient with transposition of the great arteries following a Mustard or Senning procedure involves assessment of the systemic and pulmonary venous pathways for a leak or obstruction, valvular function, and ventricular function (Fig. 41.6). The most common site of systemic venous pathway narrowing or obstruction is the superior vena caval baffle near its entrance into the right atrium (Fig. 41.19). TEE is well suited for visualization of the systemic venous pathways and guidance of transcatheter intervention.[105] Tissue Doppler echocardiography provides a method for evaluating global and regional myocardial function of the systemic right ventricle in patients following an atrial switch procedure.[106,107]

CMR is a useful tool for the assessment of venous pathways[108] as well systemic RV function at rest and with exercise (Table 41.4).[109] CT scan is valuable in demonstrating the site of baffle obstruction following stent implantation,[110] and in the significant number of patients who are not candidates for CMR due to pacemaker implantation (Figs. 41.20–41.25).

Following an arterial switch operation, the goals of echocardiography and CMR (Fig. 41.7 and Table 41.5) on routine assessment are the evaluation for stenosis at the arterial anastomoses, monitoring for neoaortic dilation, assessment of branch PA stenosis, and assessment of global and regional ventricular function. Coronary stenosis or occlusion following reimplantation occurs in approximately 7% to 8% of patients after arterial switch operation.[111,112] These postoperative coronary abnormalities are difficult to detect by routine echocardiography,[113] but stress echocardiography[114] and recently, CT scan[90,91] have been shown to be useful in this patient group. Surgical revascularization following an arterial switch operation is possible (Fig. 41.26).[115]

5.3. Single ventricles
5.3.1. Single or dominant left ventricles

As noted above, the different forms of CHD with a single, or dominant, LV can share a similar pathophysiology. The initial decision making revolves around ensuring an adequate systemic arterial oxygen saturation while protecting the pulmonary vasculature from high pressure and flow. Obstruction to pulmonary blood flow can occur from atresia of the tricuspid or pulmonary valve. Obstruction at the level of the bulboventricular foramen or ventricular septal defect can result in either subpulmonary or subaortic narrowing, depending on the ventriculoarterial connections. The imager must be aware of the lesions commonly associated with each form of single LV and the information required for surgical planning.

In patients with transposition of the great arteries and either double inlet LV or tricuspid atresia, subaortic stenosis is poorly tolerated in the Fontan circulation.[116] The future restrictiveness of the bulboventricular foramen or ventricular septal defect is sometimes difficult to predict. A group of 28 infants with double inlet LV or tricuspid atresia, an initial indexed bulboventricular foramen area of <2 cm^2/m^2 defined by 2D echocardiography, who did not undergo early bulboventricular foramen bypass, developed late obstruction.[117]

In a patient with pulmonary atresia and intact ventricular septum with suprasystemic RV pressures, a RV outflow tract patch plasty may be indicated. Before doing so, it is important to exclude a RV-dependent coronary circulation in the setting of

---

TABLE 41.3
CARDIAC MAGNETIC RESONANCE IMAGING PROTOCOL FOR POSTOPERATIVE TETRALOGY OF FALLOT

Three-plane localizing images

Axial stack of ECG-gated double inversion recovery ("black blood") or ECG-gated cine steady-state free precession (SSFP) sequences to assess morphology of the pulmonary arteries and ascending aorta

ECG-gated cine SSFP sequences in the four-chamber, two-chamber, and short-axis planes, including a short-axis stack from base to apex for quantification of LV and RV size, mass, and ejection fraction

ECG-gated cine SSFP sequences parallel to the left and right ventricular outflow tracts to rule out obstruction or aneurysmal dilation

ECG-gated phase-contrast velocity imaging sequences perpendicular to the ascending aorta and main pulmonary artery (to measure cardiac output, Q_p/Q_s); also to the branch pulmonary arteries (for $Q_pR{:}Q_pL$) and atrioventricular valves (for MR, TR) if indicated

Gadolinium-enhanced 3D magnetic resonance angiography

Myocardial delayed enhancement imaging if indicated

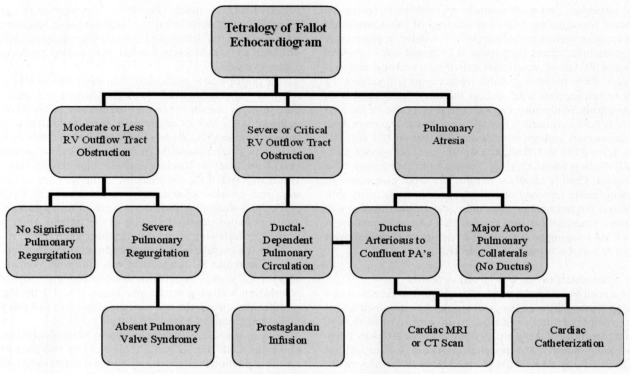

Figure 41.19 Tetralogy of Fallot—fetal and newborn diagnosis.

TABLE 41.4

CARDIAC MAGNETIC RESONANCE IMAGING PROTOCOL FOR TRANSPOSITION OF THE GREAT ARTERIES STATUS POST MUSTARD OR SENNING PROCEDURE

Three-plane localizing images

ECG-gated double inversion recovery ("black blood") or ECG-gated cine steady-state free precession (SSFP) axial stack and oblique coronal sequences to assess the systemic and venous pathways for obstruction or leak

ECG-gated cine SSFP sequences in the four-chamber, two-chamber, and short-axis planes, including a short-axis stack from base to apex for quantification of subpulmonary LV and systemic RV size, mass, and ejection fraction

ECG-gated cine SSFP sequences parallel to the left and right ventricular outflow tracts to rule out obstruction

ECG-gated phase-contrast velocity imaging sequences perpendicular to the ascending aorta and main pulmonary artery (to measure cardiac output, Q_p/Q_s), and atrioventricular valves (for MR, TR) if indicated

Gadolinium-enhanced 3D magnetic resonance angiography

Myocardial delayed enhancement imaging

coronary fistulous communications.[43] Some patients with pulmonary atresia and intact ventricular septum may be candidates for biventricular repair. In a large, multi-institutional study, the most important variable for predicting biventricular repair was the size of the tricuspid valve annulus.[42]

5.3.2. Single or dominant right ventricles

Many lesions are associated with significant LV hypoplasia, including some that are primarily acyanotic lesions. Knowledge of the various approaches to surgical palliation for LV hypoplasia is required for guiding therapy and assessing its outcome. Not all patients with LV hypoplasia require single ventricle palliation, and the adequacy of the LV for biventricular repair can usually be determined based on morphologic and hemodynamic factors assessed noninvasively by echocardiography.[118,119] For example, in RV dominant common atrioventricular canal, investigators have proposed a minimum LV volume of 15 mL/m² [120] or atrioventricular valve index of 0.67 (the area of the common atrioventricular valve apportioned to the LV vs. the right ventricle)[121] as predictive of a successful biventricular repair. In critical aortic stenosis, two popular scoring systems have been developed that assess the separate components of the LV (e.g., mitral valve annulus diameter, LV length, etc.) in order to determine the likelihood of survival using a biventricular approach.[122,123] At least in the short term, a disproportionate pursuit of biventricular repair in borderline candidates can result in an increased number of deaths.[124]

In the usual form of hypoplastic left heart syndrome associated with aortic atresia, the fetal and newborn echocardiograms focus on the assessment of LV hypoplasia; restrictiveness of the interatrial communication; diameter of the ascending aorta and aortic arch; tricuspid regurgitation; and RV function. The presence of severe interatrial restriction identifies a group of patients with a very high risk of mortality after birth, even with immediate surgical intervention.[125,126] The impact of prenatal intervention to create an atrial septal defect in this small cohort of patients is currently under investigation.[127]

Each of the initial palliative procedures for hypoplastic left heart syndrome, described above, leaves the patient with all of the

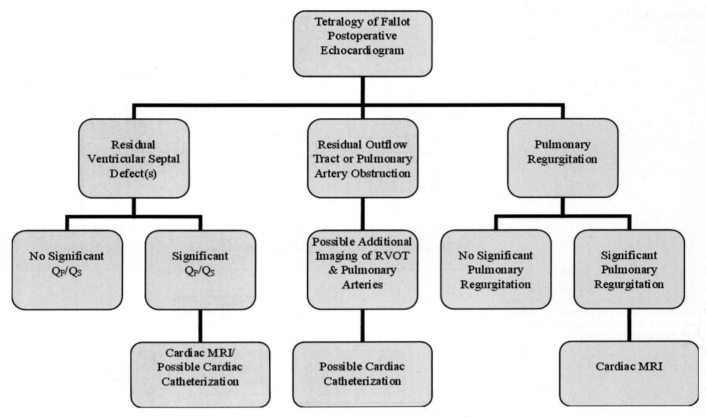

Figure 41.20 Tetralogy of Fallot—postoperative evaluation.

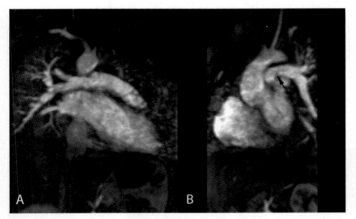

Figure 41.21 Gadolinium-enhanced magnetic resonance angiography (MRA) on an 18-year-old man with repaired tetralogy of Fallot demonstrating the RPA and LPA. There is mild proximal LPA stenosis (*arrow*) with 65% of flow to the right pulmonary artery and 35% to the left pulmonary artery by phase-contrast velocity imaging (not shown). (**A**) coronal; (**B**) sagital images to caption.

systemic and pulmonary venous blood mixing in the right ventricle and a controlled portion of the cardiac output directed toward the lungs. The imager should specifically examine for the different complications seen with each procedure, such as left PA stenosis beneath the neoascending aorta in the Norwood procedure, right ventricle-to-PA conduit stenosis with the Sano modification, and proximal aortic arch obstruction with the hybrid procedure. The presence of any complication in a patient with hypoplastic left syndrome is potentially serious and may affect the planning and timing of the second stage procedure.

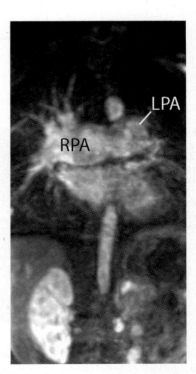

Figure 41.22 Magnetic resonance imaging on a 9-year-old boy with tetralogy of Fallot with absent pulmonary valve syndrome, s/p repair. Gadolinium-enhanced MRA (subvolume maximal intensity projection) demonstrating severely dilated right and left pulmonary arteries (RPA and LPA) which were not plicated at the time of repair.

Figure 41.23 D-loop transposition of the great arteries—fetal and newborn diagnosis.

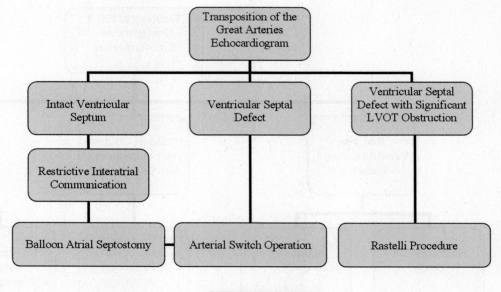

Figure 41.24 Transposition of the great arteries (TGA)—postoperative evaluation status post (s/p) Mustard or Senning ("Atrial Switch") procedure.

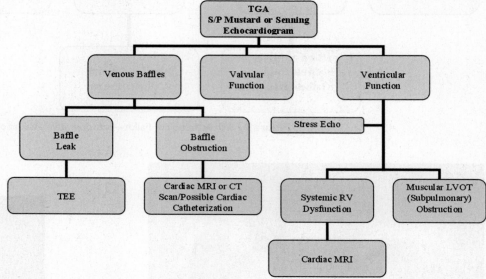

Figure 41.25 Gadolinium-enhanced MRA (subvolume maximal intensity projections) on a 33-year-old man with transposition of the great arteries, s/p Mustard procedure. There is complete obstruction of the superior vena caval baffle pathway (**A**, *arrow*) with decompression through the azygos (**AZ**) and hemiazygos (**HZ**) veins on parasagittal (**B**), and coronal (**C**) images.

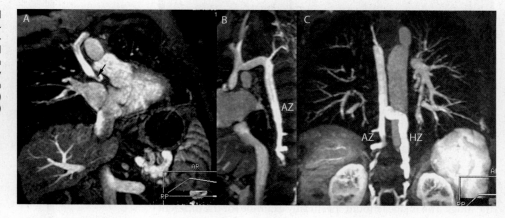

5.3.3. Single ventricles following initial palliation

In preparation for a bidirectional Glenn anastomosis, a single ventricle patient usually undergoes a cardiac catheterization to assess PA anatomy and pulmonary vascular resistance. In a randomized, single-center clinical trial of 92 patients, CMR was demonstrated to be a safe and less costly alternative to routine catheterization prior to a bidirectional Glenn anastomosis.[128] Of the patients who underwent catheterization, 41% received some form of intervention, with the most common ones being coil occlusion of an aortopulmonary collateral in 19%, balloon dilation of coarctation in 7%, and balloon dilation of the RV-to-PA conduit in 7%. There was no difference in perioperative morbidity or mortality

TABLE 41.5

CARDIAC MAGNETIC RESONANCE IMAGING PROTOCOL FOR TRANSPOSITION OF THE GREAT ARTERIES STATUS POST ARTERIAL SWITCH OPERATION

Three-plane localizing images

ECG-gated double inversion recovery ("black blood") or ECG-gated cine steady-state free precession (SSFP) axial stack and oblique sequences to assess morphology of the outflow tracts and great arteries

ECG-gated cine SSFP sequence in the four-chamber, two-chamber, and short-axis planes, including a short-axis stack from base to apex for quantification of LV and RV size, mass, and ejection fraction

ECG-gated cine SSFP sequences parallel to the left and right ventricular outflow tracts to rule out anastomotic obstruction and neoaortic dilation

ECG-gated phase-contrast velocity imaging sequences perpendicular to the ascending aorta and main pulmonary artery (to measure cardiac output); if indicated, also the branch pulmonary arteries (for $Q_pR{:}Q_pL$) and atrioventricular valves (for MR, TR)

Consider Gadolinium-enhanced myocardial perfusion imaging

Gadolinium-enhanced 3D magnetic resonance angiography

Myocardial delayed enhancement imaging

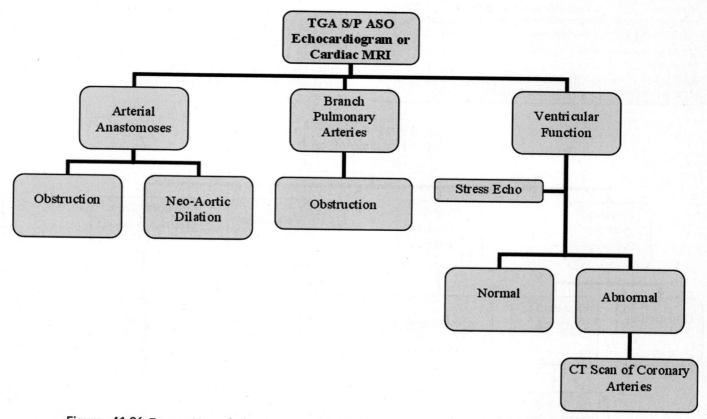

Figure 41.26 Transposition of the great arteries (TGA)—Postoperative evaluation status postarterial switch operation (s/p ASO).

between the CMR and catheterization groups, but further study was recommended to determine the long-term benefits of the interventional procedures.

CMR has also proven to be a valuable noninvasive imaging technique prior to and after the Fontan procedure for patients with any form of single ventricle.[85,129] CMR has the capability to assess the systemic venous pathways, pulmonary arteries, and ventricle in patients with poor acoustic windows. It can also detect systemic arterial obstruction; pulmonary venous obstruction; Q_p/Q_s in patients with a fenestration or baffle leak; aortopulmonary, systemic venous, or systemic-to-pulmonary venous collateral vessels;

and thrombus (Fig. 41.8).[83] A sample CMR imaging protocol for a single ventricle patient before or after Fontan procedure is provided in Table 41.6. TEE is a useful tool for the detection of baffle leaks and obstruction, and for the guidance of transcather interventions in these patients.

The evaluation of myocardial performance in patients with a single ventricle is particularly challenging. CMR provides a mechanism for accurately assessing global ventricular function without the need for geometric assumptions, and 3D echocardiography has shown the ability to do so in young patients.[130] Tissue Doppler echocardiography allows for a

TABLE 41.6

CARDIAC MAGNETIC RESONANCE IMAGING PROTOCOL FOR SINGLE VENTRICLE PATIENTS BEFORE OR AFTER FONTAN PROCEDURE

Three-plane localizing images

ECG-gated double inversion recovery ("black blood") or ECG-gated cine steady-state free precession (SSFP) axial stack and oblique sequences to assess the systemic venous pathways and pulmonary arteries for obstruction, leak, or thrombus

ECG-gated cine SSFP sequences in the long-axis and short-axis planes, including a short-axis stack from base to apex for quantification of ventricular size, mass, and ejection fraction

ECG-gated cine SSFP sequences parallel to the outflow tract(s) to assess morphology

ECG-gated phase-contrast velocity imaging sequences perpendicular to the ascending aorta (to measure cardiac output) and atrioventricular valve(s) (for cardiac output and regurgitation); if indicated, also across selected points in the systemic venous pathways and/or branch pulmonary arteries (for Q_p/Q_s and/or differential flow assessment, including $Q_pR{:}Q_pL$)

Consider myocardial tagging and/or first-pass perfusion sequences

Gadolinium-enhanced 3D magnetic resonance angiography
Myocardial delayed enhancement imaging

more quantitative approach in the serial assessment of single ventricular function.[131,132] Echocardiography with speckle tracking has recently been used to demonstrate mechanical dyssynchrony in the RV of patients with hypoplastic left heart syndrome.[133]

6. FUTURE DIRECTIONS

Over the past four decades, the field of congenital cardiac noninvasive imaging has steadily improved in diagnostic accuracy for the planning of surgery and/or interventional catheterization. As the tools for noninvasive congenital cardiac imaging have expanded, so too have the requirements for advanced training in imaging.[80,134–136] Congenital cardiac noninvasive imaging is now a more quantitative and analytical discipline, but the relatively small number of patients with cyanotic CHD still limits the ability to predict outcomes for many lesions.

Quantitative measures of systolic and diastolic function in cyanotic CHD have improved our understanding of the underlying pathology. The utility of speckle tracking and other noninvasive imaging techniques, such as myocardial tagging with CMR and stress imaging, to assess the myocardial function of patients with a systemic RV, the RV in Eisenmenger syndrome, or a single ventricle, is an exciting area for future investigation (Fig. 41.27).

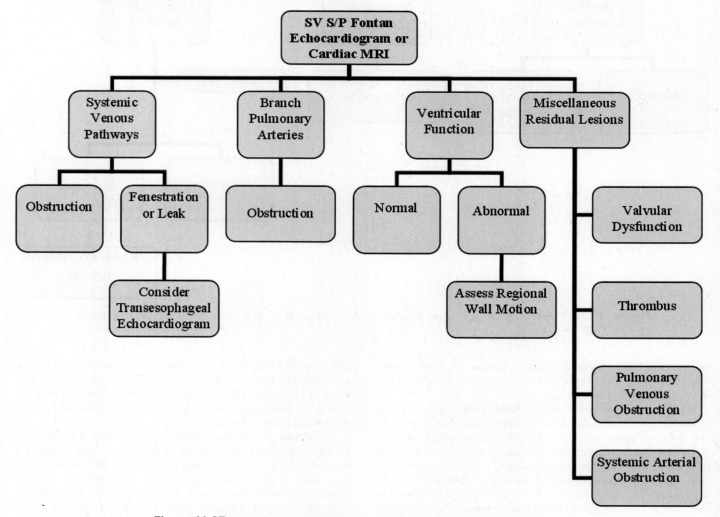

Figure 41.27 Single ventricle (SV)—postoperative evaluation s/p Fontan procedure.

Additional improvements in the quality of 3D images and methods of display for all noninvasive imaging modalities will continue to facilitate communication between the imager and the surgeon. Real-time MRI with diagnostic-level resolution will be a major advancement for the imaging of complex congenital CHD in young children as well as adults. The availability of lower-dose radiation CT scanning will increase its acceptance for serial imaging in patients with CHD.

REFERENCES

1. Hoffman JI, Kaplan S. The incidence of congenital heart disease. *J Am Coll Cardiol.* 2002;39(12):1890–1900.
2. Friedman AH, Kleinman CS, Copel JA. Diagnosis of cardiac defects: Where we've been, where we are and where we're going. *Prenat Diagn.* 2002;22(4):280–284.
3. Allan L. Prenatal diagnosis of structural cardiac defects. *Am J Med Genet C Semin Med Genet.* 2007;145C(1):73–76.
4. Warnes CA, Liberthson R, Danielson GK, et al. Task force 1: The changing profile of congenital heart disease in adult life. *J Am Coll Cardiol.* 2001;37(5):1170–1175.
5. Martin L, Khalil H. How much reduced hemoglobin is necessary to generate central cyanosis? *Chest.* 1990;97(1):182–185.
6. Lees MH, King DH. Cyanosis in the newborn. *Pediatr Rev.* 1987;9(2):36–42.
7. Perloff JK. *The Clinical Recognition of Congenital Heart Disease.* 3rd Ed. Philadelphia, PA: WB Saunders Company; 1987.
8. Wood P. The Eisenmenger syndrome or pulmonary hypertension with reversed central shunt. *Br Med J.* 1958;2(5099):755–762.
9. Duffels MG, Engelfriet PM, Berger RM, et al. Pulmonary arterial hypertension in congenital heart disease: An epidemiologic perspective from a Dutch registry. *Int J Cardiol.* 2007;120(2):198–204.
10. Berman Rosenzweig E, Barst RJ. Pulmonary arterial hypertension: A comprehensive review of pharmacological treatment. *Treat Respir Med.* 2006;5(2):117–127.
11. Vongpatanasin W, Brickner ME, Hillis LD, et al. The Eisenmenger syndrome in adults. *Ann Intern Med.* 1998;128(9):745–755.
12. Perloff JK, Friedman WF, Laks H, et al. From cyanotic infant to acyanotic adult—the odyssey of blue babies. *West J Med.* 1983;139(5):673–687.
13. Duncan BW, Mee RB, Prieto LR, et al. Staged repair of tetralogy of Fallot with pulmonary atresia and major aortopulmonary collateral arteries. *J Thorac Cardiovasc Surg.* 2003;126(3):694–702.
14. Pagani FD, Cheatham JP, Beekman RH III, et al. The management of tetralogy of Fallot with pulmonary atresia and diminutive pulmonary arteries. *J Thorac Cardiovasc Surg.* 1995;110(5):1521–1532.
15. Murphy JG, Gersh BJ, Mair DD, et al. Long-term outcome in patients undergoing surgical repair of tetralogy of Fallot. *N Engl J Med.* 1993;329(9):593–599.
16. Niemantsverdriet MB, Ottenkamp J, Gauvreau K, et al. Determinants of right ventricular outflow tract conduit longevity: A multinational analysis. *Congenit Heart Dis.* 2008;3(3):176–184.
17. Dearani JA, Danielson GK, Puga FJ, et al. Late follow-up of 1095 patients undergoing operation for complex congenital heart disease utilizing pulmonary ventricle to pulmonary artery conduits. *Ann Thorac Surg.* 2003;75(2):399–410.
18. Rodefeld MD, Ruzmetov M, Turrentine MW, et al. Reoperative right ventricular outflow tract conduit reconstruction: Risk analyses at follow up. *J Heart Valve Dis.* 2008;17(1):119–126.
19. Lurz P, Coats L, Khambadkone S, et al. Percutaneous pulmonary valve implantation: Impact of evolving technology and learning curve on clinical outcome. *Circulation.* 2008;117(15):1964–1972.
20. Butto F, Lucas RV Jr, Edwards JE. Persistent truncus arteriosus: Pathologic anatomy in 54 cases. *Pediatr Cardiol.* 1986;7(2):95–101.
21. Fuglestad SJ, Puga FJ, Danielson GK, et al. Surgical pathology of the truncal valve: A study of 12 cases. *Am J Cardiovasc Pathol.* 1988;2(1):39–47.
22. Williams JM, de Leeuw M, Black MD, et al. Factors associated with outcomes of persistent truncus arteriosus. *J Am Coll Cardiol.* 1999;34(2):545–553.
23. Niwa K, Perloff JK, Kaplan S, *et al.* Eisenmenger syndrome in adults: Ventricular septal defect, truncus arteriosus, univentricular heart. *J Am Coll Cardiol.* 1999;34(1):223–232.
24. Konstantinov IE, Karamlou T, Blackstone EH, et al. Truncus arteriosus associated with interrupted aortic arch in 50 neonates: A Congenital Heart Surgeons Society study. *Ann Thorac Surg.* 2006;81(1):214–222.
25. Martin AC, Rigby ML, Penny DJ, et al. Bedside balloon atrial septostomy on neonatal units. *Arch Dis Child Fetal Neonatal Ed.* 2003;88(4):F339–F340.
26. Freedom RM, Lock J, Bricker JT. Pediatric cardiology and cardiovascular surgery: 1950–2000. *Circulation.* 2000;102(20 Suppl. 4):IV58–IV68.
27. Love BA, Mehta D, Fuster VF. Medscape. Evaluation and management of the adult patient with transposition of the great arteries following atrial-level (Senning or Mustard) repair. *Nat Clin Pract Cardiovasc Med.* 2008;5(8):454–467.
28. Wernovsky G, Hougen TJ, Walsh EP, et al. Midterm results after the arterial switch operation for transposition of the great arteries with intact ventricular septum: Clinical, hemodynamic, echocardiographic, and electrophysiologic data. *Circulation.* 1988;77(6), 1333–1344.
29. Bove T, De Meulder F, Vandenplas G, et al. Midterm assessment of the reconstructed arteries after the arterial switch operation. *Ann Thorac Surg.* 2008;85(3):823–830.
30. Losay J, Touchot A, Serraf A, et al. Late outcome after arterial switch operation for transposition of the great arteries. *Circulation.* 2001;104(12 Suppl. 1):I121–I126.
31. Kirklin JW, Barrat Boyes B, eds. *Complete Transposition of the Great Arteries.* New York, NY: Churchill Livingston; 1993.
32. Dearani JA, Danielson GK, Puga FJ, et al. Late results of the Rastelli operation for transposition of the great arteries. *Semin Thorac Cardiovasc Surg Pediatr Card Surg Annu.* 2001;4:3–15.
33. Keane JF, Fyler DC. Double-outlet right ventricle. In: Keane JF, Lock JE, Fyler DC, eds. Nadas' Pediatric Cardiology, 2nd Ed. Philadelphia, PA: Saunders Elsevier; 2006:735–741.
34. Van Praagh S, Davidoff R, Chin A, et al. Double outlet right ventricle: Anatomic types and developmental implications based on a study of 101 autopsied cases. *Coeur.* 1982;XIII:389–440.
35. Aoki M, Forbess JM, Jonas RA, et al. Result of biventricular repair for double-outlet right ventricle. *J Thorac Cardiovasc Surg.* 1994;107(2):338–349.
36. Van Praagh R, Leidenfrost RD, Lee SK, et al. The morphologic method applied to the problem of "single" right ventricle. *Am J Cardiol.* 1982;50(4):929–932.
37. Anderson RH, Macartney FJ, Tynan M, et al. Univentricular atrioventricular connection: The single ventricle trap unsprung. *Pediatr Cardiol.* 1983;4(4):273–280.
38. Bevilacqua M, Sanders SP, Van Praagh S, et al. Double-inlet single left ventricle: Echocardiographic anatomy with emphasis on the morphology of the atrioventricular valves and ventricular septal defect. *J Am Coll Cardiol.* 1991;18(2):559–568.
39. Rao PS. A unified classification for tricuspid atresia. *Am Heart J.* 1980;99(6):799–804.
40. Daubeney PE, Delany DJ, Anderson RH, et al. Pulmonary atresia with intact ventricular septum: Range of morphology in a population-based study. *J Am Coll Cardiol.* 2002;39(10):1670–1679.
41. de Leval M, Bull C, Stark J, et al. Pulmonary atresia and intact ventricular septum: Surgical management based on a revised classification. *Circulation.* 1982;66(2):272–280.
42. Hanley FL, Sade RM, Blackstone EH, et al. Outcomes in neonatal pulmonary atresia with intact ventricular septum. A multiinstitutional study. *J Thorac Cardiovasc Surg.* 1993; 105(3):406–423, 424–427.
43. Satou GM, Perry SB, Gauvreau K, et al. Echocardiographic predictors of coronary artery pathology in pulmonary atresia with intact ventricular septum. *Am J Cardiol.* 2000;85(11):1319–1324.
44. Noonan JA, Nadas AS. The hypoplastic left heart syndrome; an analysis of 101 cases. *Pediatr Clin North Am.* 1958;5(4):1029–1056.
45. Von Rueden TJ, Knight L, Moller JH, et al. Coarctation of the aorta associated with aortic valvular atresia. *Circulation.* 1975;52(5):951–954.
46. Vida VL, Bacha EA, Larrazabal A, et al. Hypoplastic left heart syndrome with intact or highly restrictive atrial septum: Surgical experience from a single center. *Ann Thorac Surg.* 2007;84(2):581–585.
47. Sommer RJ, Rossi AF, Griepp RB. Computer-simulated and clinical models agree on optimal postoperative management for hypoplastic left heart syndrome. *J Am Coll Cardiol.* 1995;25(7):1740–1741.
48. Migliavacca F, Pennati G, Dubini G, et al. Modeling of the Norwood circulation: Effects of shunt size, vascular resistances, and heart rate. *Am J Physiol Heart Circ Physiol.* 2001; 280(5):H2076–H2086.
49. Pigott JD, Murphy JD, Barber G, et al. Palliative reconstructive surgery for hypoplastic left heart syndrome. *Ann Thorac Surg.* 1988;45(2):122–128.
50. Norwood WI, Lang P, Hansen DD. Physiologic repair of aortic atresia-hypoplastic left heart syndrome. *N Engl J Med.* 1983;308(1):23–26.
51. Sano S, Ishino K, Kawada M, et al. Right ventricle-pulmonary artery shunt in first-stage palliation of hypoplastic left heart syndrome. *J Thorac Cardiovasc Surg.* 2003;126(2): 504–509.
52. Sano S, Ishino K, Kado H, et al. Outcome of right ventricle-to-pulmonary artery shunt in first-stage palliation of hypoplastic left heart syndrome: A multi-institutional study. *Ann Thorac Surg.* 2004;78(6):1951–1957.
53. Galantowicz M, Cheatham JP. Lessons learned from the development of a new hybrid strategy for the management of hypoplastic left heart syndrome. *Pediatr Cardiol.* 2005;26(3):190–199.
54. Carter TL, Mainwaring RD, Lamberti JJ. Damus-Kaye-Stansel procedure: Midterm follow-up and technical considerations. *Ann Thorac Surg.* 1994;58(6):1603–1608.
55. Day RW, Etheridge SP, Veasy LG, et al. Single ventricle palliation: Greater risk of complications with the Fontan procedure than with the bidirectional Glenn procedure alone. *Int J Cardiol.* 2006;106(2):201–210.
56. Tweddell JS, Litwin SB, Thomas JP Jr, et al. Recent advances in the surgical management of the single ventricle pediatric patient. *Pediatr Clin North Am.* 1999;46(2):465–480,xii.
57. Lee JR, Choi JS, Kang CH, et al. Surgical results of patients with a functional single ventricle. *Eur J Cardiothorac Surg.* 2003;24(5):716–722.
58. Ono M, Boethig D, Goerler H, et al. Clinical outcome of patients 20 years after Fontan operation—effect of fenestration on late morbidity. *Eur J Cardiothorac Surg.* 2006; 30(6):923–929.
59. Thompson LD, Petrossian E, McElhinney DB, et al. Is it necessary to routinely fenestrate an extracardiac fontan? *J Am Coll Cardiol.* 1999;34(2):539–544.
60. Khairy P, Fernandes SM, Mayer JE Jr, et al. Long-term survival, modes of death, and predictors of mortality in patients with Fontan surgery. *Circulation.* 2008;117(1):85–92.
61. Driscoll DJ, Durongpisitkul K. Exercise testing after the Fontan operation. *Pediatr Cardiol.* 1999;20(1):57–59.

62. Anderson PA, Sleeper LA, Mahony L, et al. Contemporary outcomes after the Fontan procedure: A Pediatric Heart Network multicenter study. *J Am Coll Cardiol.* 2008; 52(2):85–98.

63. McGuirk SP, Winlaw DS, Langley SM, et al. The impact of ventricular morphology on midterm outcome following completion total cavopulmonary connection. *Eur J Cardiothorac Surg.* 2003;24(1):37–46.

64. Van Praagh R. The segmental approach clarified. *Cardiovasc Intervent Radiol.* 1984;7(6): 320–325.

65. Anderson RH, Becker AE, Freedom RM, et al. Sequential segmental analysis of congenital heart disease. *Pediatr Cardiol.* 1984;5(4):281–287.

66. Jacobs JP, Mavroudis C, Jacobs ML, et al. Nomenclature and databases – the past, the present, and the future: A primer for the congenital heart surgeon. *Pediatr Cardiol.* 2007;28(2):105–115.

67. Rocchini AP. Congenital Heart Surgery Nomenclature and Database Project: Therapeutic cardiac catheter interventions. *Ann Thorac Surg.* 2000;69(4 Suppl.):S332–S342.

68. Rychik J, Ayres N, Cuneo B, et al. American Society of Echocardiography guidelines and standards for performance of the fetal echocardiogram. *J Am Soc Echocardiogr.* 2004;17(7):803–810.

69. Mellander M. Perinatal management, counselling and outcome of fetuses with congenital heart disease. *Semin Fetal Neonatal Med.* 2005;10(6):586–593.

70. Bahtiyar MO, Copel JA. Improving detection of fetal cardiac anomalies: A fetal echocardiogram for every fetus? *J Ultrasound Med.* 2007;26(12):1639–1641.

71. Todros T, Faggiano F, Chiappa E, et al. Accuracy of routine ultrasonography in screening heart disease prenatally. Gruppo Piemontese for Prenatal Screening of Congenital Heart Disease. *Prenat Diagn.* 1997;17(10):901–906.

72. Yagel S, Weissman A, Rotstein Z, et al. Congenital heart defects: Natural course and in utero development. *Circulation.* 1997;96(2):550–555.

73. Stumpflen I, Stumpflen A, Wimmer M, et al. Effect of detailed fetal echocardiography as part of routine prenatal ultrasonographic screening on detection of congenital heart disease. *Lancet.* 1996;348(9031):854–857.

74. Bonnet D, Coltri A, Butera G, et al. Detection of transposition of the great arteries in fetuses reduces neonatal morbidity and mortality. *Circulation.* 1999;99(7):916–918.

75. Tworetzky W, McElhinney DB, Reddy VM, et al. Improved surgical outcome after fetal diagnosis of hypoplastic left heart syndrome. *Circulation.* 2001;103(9):1269–1273.

76. Lai WW, Geva T, Shirali GS, et al. Guidelines and standards for performance of a pediatric echocardiogram: A report from the Task Force of the Pediatric Council of the American Society of Echocardiography. *J Am Soc Echocardiogr.* 2006;19(12):1413–1430.

77. Chow PC, Liang XC, Lam WW, et al. Mechanical right ventricular dyssynchrony in patients after atrial switch operation for transposition of the great arteries. *Am J Cardiol.* 2008;101(6):874–881.

78. Abd El Rahman MY, Hui W, Yigitbasi M, et al. Detection of left ventricular asynchrony in patients with right bundle branch block after repair of tetralogy of Fallot using tissue-Doppler imaging-derived strain. *J Am Coll Cardiol.* 2005;45(6):915–921.

79. Friedberg MK, Rosenthal DN. New developments in echocardiographic methods to assess right ventricular function in congenital heart disease. *Curr Opin Cardiol.* 2005;20(2): 84–88.

80. Ayres NA, Miller-Hance W, Fyfe DA, et al. Indications and guidelines for performance of transesophageal echocardiography in the patient with pediatric acquired or congenital heart disease: Report from the task force of the Pediatric Council of the American Society of Echocardiography. *J Am Soc Echocardiogr.* 2005;18(1):91–98.

81. Tworetzky W, McElhinney DB, Brook MM, et al. Echocardiographic diagnosis alone for the complete repair of major congenital heart defects. *J Am Coll Cardiol.* 1999;33(1): 228–233.

82. Bharucha T, Roman KS, Anderson RH, et al. Impact of multiplanar review of three-dimensional echocardiographic data on management of congenital heart disease. *Ann Thorac Surg.* 2008;86(3):875–881.

83. Geva T, Powell AJ. Pediatric heart disease. In: Edelman RR, Hesselink JR, Zlatkin MB, et al., eds. *Clinical Magnetic Resonance Imaging.* 3rd Ed. Philadephia, PA: Saunders Elsevier; 2006:1041–1069.

84. Dorfman AL, Geva T. Magnetic resonance imaging evaluation of congenital heart disease: Conotruncal anomalies. *J Cardiovasc Magn Reson.* 2006;8(4):645–659.

85. Fogel MA. Cardiac magnetic resonance of single ventricles. *J Cardiovasc Magn Reson.* 2006;8(4):661–670.

86. Crean A. Cardiovascular MR and CT in congenital heart disease. *Heart (British Cardiac Society).* 2007;93(12):1637–1647.

87. Silversides CK, Granton JT, Konen E, et al. Pulmonary thrombosis in adults with Eisenmenger syndrome. *J Am Coll Cardiol.* 2003;42(11):1982–1987.

88. Sheehan R, Perloff JK, Fishbein MC, et al. Pulmonary neovascularity: A distinctive radiographic finding in Eisenmenger syndrome. *Circulation.* 2005;112(18):2778–2785.

89. Wang XM, Wu LB, Sun C, et al. Clinical application of 64-slice spiral CT in the diagnosis of the Tetralogy of Fallot. *Eur J Radiol.* 2007;64(2):296–301.

90. Oztunc F, Baris S, Adaletli I, et al. Coronary events and anatomy after arterial switch operation for transposition of the great arteries: Detection by 16-row multislice computed tomography angiography in pediatric patients. *Cardiovasc Intervent Radiol.* 2009;32(2):206–212.

91. Ou P, Mousseaux E, Azarine A, et al. Detection of coronary complications after the arterial switch operation for transposition of the great arteries: First experience with multislice computed tomography in children. *J Thorac Cardiovasc Surg.* 2006;131(3):639–643.

92. Hall EJ, Brenner DJ. Cancer risks from diagnostic radiology. *Br J Radiol.* 2008;81(965):362–378.

93. Leschka S, Oechslin E, Husmann L, et al. Pre- and postoperative evaluation of congenital heart disease in children and adults with 64-section CT. *Radiographics.* 2007;27(3):829–846.

94. Snider AR, Serwer GA, Ritter SB. *Echocardiography in Pediatric Heart Disease.* 2nd Ed. St Louis, MO: Mosby; 1997.

95. Silverman NH. *Pediatric Echocardiography.* Baltimore, MD: Williams & Wilkins; 1993.

96. Diller GP, Gatzoulis MA. Pulmonary vascular disease in adults with congenital heart disease. *Circulation.* 2007;115(8):1039–1050.

97. Lee KS, Abbas AE, Khandheria BK, et al. Echocardiographic assessment of right heart hemodynamic parameters. *J Am Soc Echocardiogr.* 2007;20(6):773–782.

98. McLure LE, Peacock AJ. Imaging of the heart in pulmonary hypertension. *Int J Clin Pract Suppl.* 2007;(156):15–26.

99. Ammash NM, Dearani JA, Burkhart HM, et al. Pulmonary regurgitation after tetralogy of Fallot repair: Clinical features, sequelae, and timing of pulmonary valve replacement. *Congenit Heart Dis.* 2007;2(6):386–403.

100. Geva T. Indications and timing of pulmonary valve replacement after tetralogy of Fallot repair. *Semin Thorac Cardiovasc Surg Pediatr Card Surg Annu.* 2006;9(1): 11–22.

101. Therrien J, Provost Y, Merchant N, et al. Optimal timing for pulmonary valve replacement in adults after tetralogy of Fallot repair. *Am J Cardiol.* 2005 Mar 15;95(6):779–782.

102. Blyth M, Howe D, Gnanapragasam J, et al. The hidden mortality of transposition of the great arteries and survival advantage provided by prenatal diagnosis. *BJOG.* 2008;115(9):1096–1100.

103. Pasquini L, Sanders SP, Parness IA, et al. Coronary echocardiography in 406 patients with d-loop transposition of the great arteries. *J Am Coll Cardiol.* 1994;24(3):763–768.

104. Skinner J, Hornung T, Rumball E. Transposition of the great arteries: From fetus to adult. *Heart (British Cardiac Society).* 2008;94(9):1227–1235.

105. Hashmi A, Hosking M, Teixeira O, et al. Transoesophageal echocardiographic assessment of obstruction to the pulmonary venous pathway in children with Mustard or Senning repair. *Cardiol Young.* 1998;8(1):79–85.

106. Bos JM, Hagler DJ, Silvilairat S, et al. Right ventricular function in asymptomatic individuals with a systemic right ventricle. *J Am Soc Echocardiogr.* 2006;19(8):1033–1037.

107. Rentzsch A, Abd El Rahman MY, Hui W, et al. Assessment of myocardial function of the systemic right ventricle in patients with D-transposition of the great arteries after atrial switch operation by tissue Doppler echocardiography. *Z Kardiol.* 2005;94(8):524–531.

108. Fogel MA, Hubbard A, Weinberg PM. A simplified approach for assessment of intracardiac baffles and extracardiac conduits in congenital heart surgery with two- and three-dimensional magnetic resonance imaging. *Am Heart J.* 2001;142(6):1028–1036.

109. Tops LF, Roest AA, Lamb HJ, et al. Intraatrial repair of transposition of the great arteries: Use of MR imaging after exercise to evaluate regional systemic right ventricular function. *Radiology.* 2005;(3):861–867.

110. Cook SC, McCarthy M, Daniels CJ, et al. Usefulness of multislice computed tomography angiography to evaluate intravascular stents and transcatheter occlusion devices in patients with d-transposition of the great arteries after mustard repair. *Am J Cardiol.* 2004; 94(7):967–969.

111. Hutter PA, Bennink GB, Ay L, et al. Influence of coronary anatomy and reimplantation on the long-term outcome of the arterial switch. *Eur J Cardiothorac Surg.* 2000;18(2):207–213.

112. Bonnet D, Bonhoeffer P, Piechaud JF, et al. Long-term fate of the coronary arteries after the arterial switch operation in newborns with transposition of the great arteries. *Heart (British Cardiac Society).* 1996;76(3):274–279.

113. Legendre A, Losay J, Touchot-Kone A, et al. Coronary events after arterial switch operation for transposition of the great arteries. *Circulation.* 2003;108(Suppl. 1):II186–II190.

114. Kimball TR. Pediatric stress echocardiography. *Pediatr Cardiol.* 2002;23(3): 347–357.

115. Raisky O, Bergoend E, Agnoletti G et al. Late coronary artery lesions after neonatal arterial switch operation: Results of surgical coronary revascularization. *Eur J Cardiothorac Surg.* 2007 May;31(5):894–898.

116. Rothman A, Lang P, Lock JE, et al. Surgical management of subaortic obstruction in single left ventricle and tricuspid atresia. *J Am Coll Cardiol.* 1987;10(2):421–426.

117. Matitiau A, Geva T, Colan SD, et al. Bulboventricular foramen size in infants with double-inlet left ventricle or tricuspid atresia with transposed great arteries: Influence on initial palliative operation and rate of growth. *J Am Coll Cardiol.* 1992;19(1):142–148.

118. Corno AF. Borderline left ventricle. *Eur J Cardiothorac Surg.* 2005;27(1):67–73.

119. Phoon CK, Silverman NH. Conditions with right ventricular pressure and volume overload, and a small left ventricle: "hypoplastic" left ventricle or simply a squashed ventricle? *J Am Coll Cardiol.* 1997;30(6):1547–1553.

120. van Son JA, Phoon CK, Silverman NH et al. Predicting feasibility of biventricular repair of right-dominant unbalanced atrioventricular canal. *Ann Thorac Surg.* 1997;63(6):1657–1663.

121. Cohen MS, Jacobs ML, Weinberg PM, et al. Morphometric analysis of unbalanced common atrioventricular canal using two-dimensional echocardiography. *J Am Coll Cardiol.* 1996;28(4):1017–1023.

122. Rhodes LA, Colan SD, Perry SB, et al. Predictors of survival in neonates with critical aortic stenosis. *Circulation.* 1991;84(6):2325–2335.

123. Lofland GK, McCrindle BW, Williams WG, et al. Critical aortic stenosis in the neonate: A multi-institutional study of management, outcomes, and risk factors. Congenital Heart Surgeons Society. *J Thorac Cardiovasc Surg.* 2001;121(1):10–27.

124. Hickey EJ, Caldarone CA, Blackstone EH, et al. Critical left ventricular outflow tract obstruction: The disproportionate impact of biventricular repair in borderline cases. *J Thorac Cardiovasc Surg.* 2007;134(6):1429–1436.

125. Rychik J. Hypoplastic left heart syndrome: From in-utero diagnosis to school age. *Semin Fetal Neonatal Med.* 2005;10(6):553–566.

126. Glatz JA, Tabbutt S, Gaynor JW, et al. Hypoplastic left heart syndrome with atrial level restriction in the era of prenatal diagnosis. *Ann Thorac Surg.* 2007;84(5):1633–1638.

127. Marshall AC, Levine J, Morash D, et al. Results of in utero atrial septoplasty in fetuses with hypoplastic left heart syndrome. *Prenat Diagn.* 2008;28(11):1023–1028.

128. Brown DW, Gauvreau K, Powell AJ, et al. Cardiac magnetic resonance versus routine cardiac catheterization before bidirectional glenn anastomosis in infants with functional single ventricle: A prospective randomized trial. *Circulation.* 2007;116(23):2718–2725.

129. Festa P, Ait Ali L, Bernabei M, et al. The role of magnetic resonance imaging in the evaluation of the functionally single ventricle before and after conversion to the Fontan circulation. *Cardiol Young.* 2005;15(Suppl. 3):51–56.

130. Soriano BD, Hoch M, Ithuralde A, et al. Matrix-array 3-dimensional echocardiographic assessment of volumes, mass, and ejection fraction in young pediatric patients with a functional single ventricle: A comparison study with cardiac magnetic resonance. *Circulation.* 2008;117(14):1842–1848.

131. Lunze FI, Hui W, Abd El Rahman MY, et al. Preserved regional atrial contractile function following extra-atrial rather than intra-atrial type Fontan operation: A tissue Doppler imaging study. *Clin Res Cardiol.* 2007;96(5):264–271.

132. Vitarelli A, Conde Y, Cimino E, et al. Quantitative assessment of systolic and diastolic ventricular function with tissue Doppler imaging after Fontan type of operation. *Int J Cardiol.* 2005;102(1):61–69.

133. Friedberg MK, Silverman NH, Dubin AM, et al. Right ventricular mechanical dyssynchrony in children with hypoplastic left heart syndrome. *J Am Soc Echocardiogr.* 2007 Sep;20(9):1073–1079.

134. Sanders SP, Colan SD, Cordes TM, et al. ACCF/AHA/AAP recommendations for training in pediatric cardiology. Task force 2: Pediatric training guidelines for noninvasive cardiac imaging endorsed by the American Society of Echocardiography and the Society of Pediatric Echocardiography. *J Am Coll Cardiol.* 2005;46(7):1384–1388.

135. Helbing WA, Mertens L, Sieverding L. Recommendations from the Association for European Paediatric Cardiology for training in congenital cardiovascular magnetic resonance imaging. *Cardiol Young.* 2006;16(4):410–412.

136. Child JS, Freed MD, Mavroudis C, et al. Task force 9: Training in the care of adult patients with congenital heart disease. *J Am Coll Cardiol.* 2008;51(3):389–393.

Cardiovascular Imaging in Atrial Fibrillation

42

Sabe De
Richard A. Grimm

1. INTRODUCTION

Atrial fibrillation (AF) is a supraventricular arrhythmia characterized by chaotic irregular atrial activation that leads to reduced atrial mechanical function adversely affecting cardiac function and associated with an increased risk of cardioembolic stroke. It is the most common of all cardiac arrhythmias occurring in 0.4% to 1% of the general population, and an estimated 2.2 million Americans per year with this number expected to rise to 5.6 million by 2050.[1-4] The incidence increases with age affecting at least 10% of the population above the age of 80.[3,5,6] AF is associated with increased morbidity and increased mortality.[7,8] AF is the most common cause of embolic strokes with an annual stroke rate between 4.2% and 4.5% per year.[9,10]

Advances in cardiovascular imaging modalities, including echocardiography, computed tomography (CT), and magnetic resonance imaging (MRI) are playing important roles in understanding the structural and clinical consequences and management of this arrhythmia as well as serving as an important guide to therapeutic interventions.

2. PATHOPHYSIOLOGY

2.1. Structural and functional alterations

AF may occur in the absence of any identifiable structural heart disease (Lone AF). The absence of structural heart disease or significant left atrial (LA) dilatation may suggest a favorable candidate for radiofrequency ablation (RFA). Conversely, the presence of structural heart disease or left ventricular (LV) dysfunction may help guide medical antiarrhythmic therapy (Fig. 42.1).

Sustained AF results in a progressive enlargement of the atrium, termed atrial remodeling.[11] This may be reversed or prevented with cardioversion to normal sinus rhythm.[12] LA enlargement may provide an indirect marker of the duration of AF or the likelihood of success from cardioversion particularly in rheumatic disease. Increased LA size is related to increased wall tension reflecting elevated filling pressures.[13,14] Increased LA size may serve as an important marker of diastolic dysfunction.[15] Patients with AF may have an increased LA size as a consequence of LV dysfunction, hypertension (HTN), or mitral valve disease. LA size is important prognostically in patients with AF, as enlargement decreases the likelihood of successful maintenance of normal sinus rhythm (NSR) following cardioversion. For patients with rheumatic mitral stenosis, LA diameter is a predictor of developing AF and the recovery of atrial function following cardioversion. This is recognized by current guidelines for which a class IIb recommendation is that patients with mitral stenosis and a LA dimension >5.5 cm in sinus rhythm should be considered for anticoagulation.[16]

Systolic and diastolic heart failure often manifests with the development of AF. Conversely, simply eliminating the atrial contribution to filling will predictably adversely impact LV systolic function.[17] Furthermore, AF can directly cause reductions in global systolic function with prolonged uncontrolled ventricular rates resulting in a dilated cardiomyopathy (tachycardia-mediated cardiomyopathy).[18] LV dysfunction is a major predictor of cerebrovascular events in patients with nonvalvular AF.[19,20] Pooled analysis from three AF anticoagulation trials (BAATAF, SPINAF, and SPAF) showed that stroke risk increases with worsening LV dysfunction.[21] The relative risk of stroke was 9.3% per year for patients with moderate to severe LV dysfunction compared to 4.4% per year for patients with normal or mild-LV dysfunction. The degree of LV dysfunction has been shown to interact with clinical features in assessing stroke risk, as patients deemed low risk by clinical features with moderate to severe LV dysfunction have a significantly higher annual risk than those with high-risk clinical features but with normal or mild LV dysfunction (9.3% vs. 4.4%). In the same pooled analysis, among all patients in a clinically low-risk group, 38% were felt to be high risk (annual stroke risk >5% per year) when LV function data was added.[21] LV dysfunction and associated congestive heart failure has been incorporated into many models assessing stroke risk including the CHADS2 score (Table 42.1) which has been validated in several population cohorts.[19,20]

Diastolic dysfunction has several important considerations with respect to AF. Not only does it directly lead to an increased likelihood of developing AF, but when it occurs, it is often poorly tolerated. The contribution of the atrial kick to LV filling has been shown to be ~20% to 30%, with a reduction in stroke volume and cardiac output of similar magnitude seen in AF from a loss of atrial systole. Patients with diastolic dysfunction have a loss of LV compliance that shifts diastolic filling toward the latter part of diastole when atrial contraction occurs. This accounts for the hemodynamic instability and significant symptoms that may occur in a patient with diastolic dysfunction and AF. In addition, there are significant beat-to-beat variations in atrial pressure (preload) and myocardial contractility that may contribute to unfavorable hemodynamics.[22]

2.2. Spontaneous echocardiographic contrast and thrombus formation

The left atrial appendage (LAA) is characterized as a multilobed, long, and sharply pointed recess with a relatively narrow point of origin from the body of the LA. The LAA acts as a decompression chamber during LV systole and periods of LA pressure

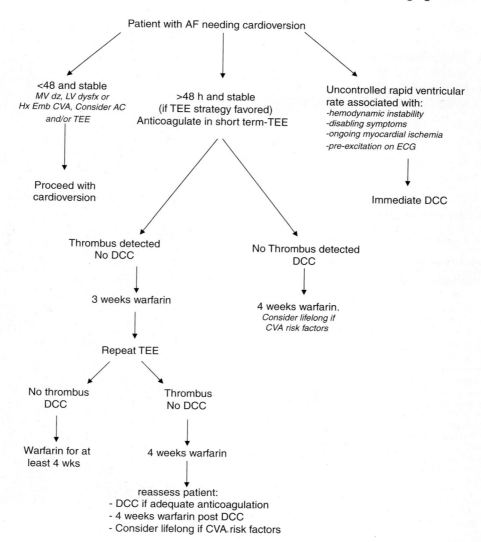

Figure 42.1 Recommended antiarrhythmic drug therapy for maintenance of normal sinus rhythm for patients with AF, based on ACC 2006 guidelines.

elevations.[23] AF results in thrombus formation with a predilection for the LAA in part due to its shape and its trabeculated nature, in addition to the reduction in atrial function and appendage emptying ability associated with the arrhythmia.[24] Direct visualization of a thrombus is seen in up to 13% of patients with nonrheumatic AF, particularly if in AF for >3 days duration.[25,26] The risk of thrombus development increases in the presence of mitral stenosis, LV dysfunction, LA enlargement, or recent embolic event. Evidence of thrombus carries a poor prognosis with an annual risk of embolus as high as 10.4% per year.[27]

It is hypothesized that the low flow state associated loss of atrial function in AF results in low shear forces and increased erythrocyte aggregation and red cell Rouleaux formation.[24,28–31] Spontaneous echocardiographic contrast (SEC) may be detected by transesophageal echocardiography (TEE) in over 70% of patients with AF and associated with increased risk of thrombus formation and thromboembolic events. Severe SEC or sludge refers to a prethrombotic milieu or thrombus in situ. It signifies the presence of a viscid, gelatinous echodensity in either the left atrium or appendage with no clear, organized mass present. It is more dense and layered than smoke, and is usually visible throughout the

cardiac cycle (Fig. 42.2). SEC is associated with increased blood viscosity and diminished atrial emptying velocities.[32,33] SEC is not reversed by anticoagulation.

3. TREATMENT OF ATRIAL FIBRILLATION

Cardioversion to normal sinus rhythm for AF provides synchronized atrial activity and improves atrial function before improvements in LV function and peak oxygen consumption are observed.[34] Current guidelines suggest RFA for patients who poorly tolerate AF that is refractory to antiarrhythmic therapy.[16] AF often results from ectopic beats arising from fascicles in the LA extending to the pulmonary veins (PVs). Techniques directed at focal RFA in the PVs have associated difficulties with accurate localization of ablation site and in eliciting ectopic beats during electrophysiology studies. This approach has also been associated with increased risk of PV stenosis. Several newer techniques have evolved that include pulmonary vein isolation (PVI) or circumferential LA ablation. Segmental ostial ablation removes the conductive pathways between the ostia of the PVs and LA, resulting in electrical dissociation between the two sites. Circumferential LA ablation results in preferential ablation of the

TABLE 42.1

CHADS2 SCORE, THROMBOEMBOLIC RISK, AND EFFECT OF WARFARIN IN 11,526 PATIENTS WITH NONVALVULAR ATRIAL FIBRILLATION AND NO CONTRAINDICATIONS TO WARFARIN THERAPY

Clinical parameter	Points
Congestive heart failure (any history)	1
Hypertension (prior history)	1
Age ≥75	1
Diabetes mellitus	1
Secondary prevention in patients with a prior ischemic stroke or a TIA; most experts also include patients with a systemic embolic event	2

CHADS2 score	Events per 100 person-years[a]	
	Warfarin	No warfarin
0	0.25	0.49
1	0.72	1.52
2	1.27	2.50
3	2.20	5.27
4	2.35	6.02
5 or 6	4.60	6.88

[a]The CHADS2 score estimates the risk of stroke, which is defined as focal neurologic signs or symptoms that persist for >24 h and that cannot be explained by hemorrhage, trauma, or other factors, or peripheral embolization, which is much less common. TIAs are not included. All differences between warfarin and nonwarfarin groups are statistically significant except for a trend with a CHADS2 score of 0. Patients are considered to be at low risk with a score of 0, at intermediate risk with a score of 1 or 2, and at high risk with a score ≥3. One exception is that most experts would consider patients with a prior ischemic stroke, TIA, or systemic embolic event to be at high risk even if they had no other risk factors and therefore, a score of 2. However, the great majority of these patients have some other risk factor and a score of at least 3. *Source:* Data from Go AS, Hylek EM, Chang Y, et al, *JAMA.* 2003;290:2685 and CHADS2 score from Gage BF, Waterman AD, Shannon W, *JAMA.* 2001;285:2864.

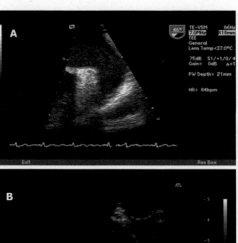
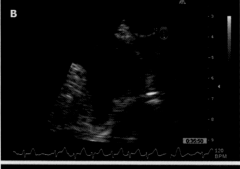
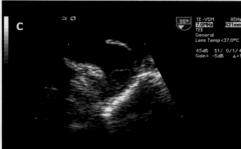

Figure 42.2 TEE appearance of (**A**) SEC, (**B**) sludge, and (**C**) thrombus.

region encircling the PVs. The superiority of segmental versus circumferential techniques is still subject to debate. Both techniques may be complimentary and both are associated with complications in ~6% of cases.[35] These may include thromboembolism, atrioesophageal fistula, LA flutter, and PV stenosis. PV stenosis may present with exertional dyspnea, chest pain, increased cough, or frank hemoptysis. There may be chest X-ray evidence of pleural effusion. Given the technical complexity of RFA techniques and the complications noted, successful and safe procedures rely on preprocedural imaging and knowledge of PV and LA anatomy. The PVs can have several anatomic variations. These include common ostia of the PVs, more frequently involving the left PV. There may be additional PVs or anomalous insertion of the PVs. Both preprocedural CT and MRI help identify such anomalies so as to enable lessened procedural time and technical complexity.

4. ROLE OF IMAGING IN DIAGNOSTIC EVALUATION AND THERAPEUTIC GUIDANCE

4.1. Echocardiography

Echocardiography remains the most important imaging modality in the diagnosis and management of AF. There are multiple indications for transthoracic echocardiography (TTE) or TEE in patients with AF (Table 42.2). Echocardiography allows for identification

of structural heart disease along with underlying cardiac causes of AF. It is most commonly employed as a diagnostic modality that provides information salient in the risk stratification for thromboembolic events (Table 42.3).

4.1.1. Transthoracic echocardiography

TTE provides important information on cardiac structure, function, and anatomy and identifies patients that may be at risk of developing AF. All newly diagnosed patients with AF will benefit from TTE evaluation. Current guidelines advocate the use of TTE to assess for valvular heart disease, LA size and volume, left ventricular hypertrophy (LVH), LV function, peak right ventricular (RV) pressure, and pericardial disease. TTE provides important information that may guide therapies for AF.[16]

The LA size is well assessed by TTE. The left atrium is tapered and pillow shaped, and may be imaged from numerous echocardiographic windows. 2D measurements are typically taken from the parasternal long axis either directly or by M-mode imaging. In this view the anterior to posterior dimension is measured. The normal anteroposterior LA dimension is <4 cm. Given the irregular shape of the LA and the asymmetric remodeling that occurs, diameter measurements may not be accurate and LA volume is felt to be superior in accurately quantifying true LA enlargement.[36] LA volume has been shown to more strongly correlate with cardiovascular disease compared to linear measurements.[15,37] Echocardiographic derived measurements may be calculated using an

TABLE 42.2
INDICATIONS FOR ECHOCARDIOGRAPHY IN AF

Assessment of cardiac structure and function
Assessment of etiology of AF
Assessment of thromboembolic risk
TEE guided DC cardioversion/stratification for anticoagulation
TEE guidance of percutaneous or surgical LAA closure
RF ablation procedures

TABLE 42.3
ECHO PREDICTORS OF THROMBOEMBOLISM IN AF

Valve disease
LV systolic dysfunction
LA dilatation
*Complex aortic atheroma
*LAA thrombus > sludge > smoke
*Reduced LAA velocities (<20 cm/s)

*Detectable on TEE

ellipsoid model or Simpson rule using a method of disks, with good agreement noted when compared to values derived from CT and MRI.[38] Although highly specific, TTE is not sensitive for determining the presence of thrombus in the left atrium or LAA, for which detection by TEE is superior.[39,40]

TTE is an excellent modality to also interrogate for LV dysfunction that may contribute to AF. Imaging with TTE provides valuable information on the presence of diastolic dysfunction as well as potential causes that have lead to AF. These include LVH, which may be associated with hypertension or other causes of diastolic heart failure including hypertrophic cardiomyopathy, aortic stenosis, or restrictive cardiomyopathies.

TTE assesses diastolic function based on several parameters obtained from transmitral Doppler inflow velocities, tissue Doppler, and PV velocities. Patients with AF lack an A wave (second wave of diastolic filling from atrial contraction) when sampling mitral and PV flow velocities. As a result, the ratio of peak early transmitral velocity (E) to peak late transmitral velocity (A) cannot be measured. Additionally, the atrial filling fraction of the PV retrograde A velocity may also not be used in the assessment of LV filling pressures in patients with AF. The PV velocity profile often shows a blunted systolic wave regardless of mean atrial pressure, and is often reduced irrespective of the mean atrial pressure.[41]Tissue Doppler-derived early transmitral annular velocities (Ea) may vary in AF and are characteristically reduced, however, E/Ea has been shown to correlate with pulmonary capillary wedge pressures in patients with AF.[42] The deceleration time (DT) of the early transmitral filling curve is relatively easy to measure, yet may be falsely shortened when measured from an interval with a very short diastolic filling period as occurs with rapid AF. Technically, one should measure peak E velocities and DT from cardiac cycles with clear completion of LV diastolic filling before QRS onset. When measured correctly, a DT <130 ms suggests an increased LA pressure and restrictive filling.[43]

Atrial mechanical function and changes that occur with cardioversion are challenging to assess with TTE. Cardioversion allows reassessment of velocity amplitude and duration of transmitral A wave and PV atrial reversal. However, in the immediate postcardioversion period for up to 4 weeks, atrial stunning may occur, evidenced by a reduction in peak A wave velocity.[44] During this time period, it is important to recognize that a "pseudorestrictive pattern" of diastolic filling by mitral inflow interrogation may temporarily exist due to a lower than normal A wave amplitude as result of atrial stunning and not ventricular diastolic dysfunction.[45] For this reason, anticoagulation is suggested during the 4-week period following cardioversion in most guidelines.[16,45] A similar reduction occurs in atrial mechanical function as evidenced by a reduction in tissue Doppler-derived peak velocity in late diastole due to atrial contraction (A') in patients undergoing RFA and PVI for chronic AF.[46]

4.1.2. Transesophageal echocardiography

TEE involves placing a high-frequency ultrasound transducer into the esophagus, posterior to the heart, providing high quality images of major cardiac structures.[47,48] TEE has the major advantage over TTE in providing direct visualization of the LAA, enabling detection of thrombi with a sensitivity of 93% and a specificity of 100%.[40] By contrast, TTE is considered a poor imaging modality for the detection of LAA thrombi with sensitivity in one study of only 53%.[40] The higher resolution of TEE allows superior visualization of the appendage. Despite a high sensitivity, TEE may miss thrombi <2 mm given the complex anatomy of the LAA. Pectinate muscles extend from the lateral to medial walls of the LAA, and may appear as indentation of similar reflectance to the LAA wall. They are typically nonmobile and linear in nature, and may be mistaken for thrombi. For a patient with known thrombus, TEE should be performed prior to cardioversion to ensure appropriate resolution.

As a clot forms, there are different stages and echocardiographic findings that occur, ranging from SEC to severe SEC or sludge (Fig. 42.2). SEC develops as echodensities that are swirling and "smoke" like in appearance, typically arising in the left atrium or the LAA.

The mechanical function of the LAA is best assessed using pulsed wave Doppler on TEE. The pulsed Doppler, when sampled from the mouth of LAA in patients who are in normal sinus rhythm, demonstrates a regular filling pattern with atrial emptying waves that are timed with atrial contraction.[49] Normal filling velocities are above 50 cm/s. LAA flow velocities in AF are characterized by irregular to and fro velocity waveforms (Fig. 42.3) of variable amplitudes. LAA velocities <20 cm/s are associated with increased presence of SEC and thrombus formation and a history of thromboembolic events.[23,50] Higher LAA emptying velocities suggest a favorable prognosis following cardioversion with a velocity of >40 cm/s associated with successful maintenance of normal sinus rhythm one year post cardioversion.[27]

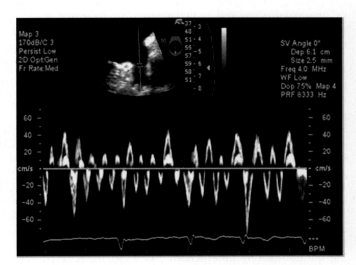

Figure 42.3 Reduced atrial emptying velocities in atrial fibrillation.

TEE plays an important role in clinical decision making for patients with AF requiring direct current (DC) cardioversion. The assessment of cardioversion using transesophageal echocardiography (ACUTE) study was a multicenter study of 1,222 patients with AF or atrial flutter of greater than 2 days duration, that compared a TEE guided strategy with a conventional anticoagulation management strategy.[26] Patients randomized to the TEE arm could proceed directly to cardioversion if no thrombus was detected and once therapeutic anticoagulation was achieved (typically within 24 h). Those found to have evidence of thrombus were not cardioverted and underwent 3 weeks of anticoagulation with warfarin before repeat TEE. If the thrombus had resolved, the patient received short-term heparin followed by DC cardioversion, and a continued 4 weeks of anticoagulation with warfarin. The conventional therapy group did not undergo TEE, and was anticoagulated with warfarin for 3 weeks prior to an attempted cardioversion followed by an additional 4 weeks of anticoagulation. There were no significant differences between the two groups in the composite endpoint of stroke, transient ischemic attack (TIA), or peripheral embolism with an overall very low rate noted (0.8% for the TEE group vs. 0.5% for the standard therapy group). However, the TEE guided therapy group had a significantly lower risk of bleeding and a shorter time to achieve NSR by study design.

Current guidelines recognize the use of TEE guided cardioversion as a class IIa recommendation for patients with AF for >48 h.[16] It should be emphasized that the absence of thrombi using the TEE approach does not obviate the use of anticoagulation prior to or following cardioversion. In earlier literature, it was felt that the presence of thrombus alone was the only source of potential embolus following successful cardioversion.[51] It is now understood that the period immediately following cardioversion is characterized by "stunned" atrial and LAA function. This is characterized by diminished LAA emptying velocities and increased SEC.[24] Atrial mechanical function returns several weeks following cardioversion. The risk of developing a thrombotic event rises to as high as 5.6% within the first week.[52–54] The risk appears similar and independent of the mode of cardioversion, and may occur with spontaneous, pharmacologic, or electrical cardioversion.[55–57] Hence, current guidelines advocate the use of anticoagulation with heparin prior to cardioversion and 4 weeks of warfarin following the procedure.[16]

In patients undergoing RFA, TEE allows direct visualization of all four PVs. Following the procedure, increased PV flow velocities may be indicative of PV stenosis, an infrequent but serious complication. High grade PV stenosis may be recognized on TEE by flow parameters, and is characterized by increased PV flow velocities (>1 m/s), turbulent aliasing blood flow (Fig. 42.4), and reduction in vessel diameter.[58]

4.1.3. Intracardiac echocardiography

Intracardiac Echocardiography (ICE) has evolved into an important imaging modality that facilitates several aspects of the RFA procedure. ICE allows direct and on-line anatomic evaluation. Standard fluoroscopy alone is prone to distortion of anatomical landmarks particularly if there is LA dilation. The intra-atrial septum may be directly visualized with ICE, providing safe transseptal access for catheter placement. The PV ostia are easily visualized, and PV anatomy well defined with ICE. This allows easier selection of appropriate catheter size, and accurate assessment of catheter position. PV anatomic variations can be identified and addressed in "real time." ICE improves safety in several ways. Catheter movement can be assessed using ICE, significantly reducing the fluoroscopy time needed. The exact interface between

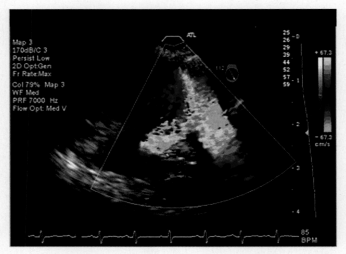

Figure 42.4 TEE evidence of pulmonary vein stenosis by color flow Doppler.

tissue and catheter may be assessed while radiofrequency energy is applied, helping to facilitate the appropriate titration of the energy dose (Fig. 42.5). The visualization of microbubbles is felt to be helpful in identifying suboptimal contact between the RFA catheter tip and the tissue (Fig. 42.6). Additionally, ICE is shown to be useful in identifying immediate procedural complications. Finally, Doppler interrogation of PV flow and LAA flow before and following RFA with ICE may be useful in quantifying atrial function and predicting outcomes.[59]

PV stenosis may be identified by PV narrowing with reduced diameter.[60] This has been poorly studied in the literature, with one study showing that changes in PV flow immediately post ablation were not predictive of the development of chronic PV stenosis.[61] Given that the esophagus is contiguous with the posterior wall of the left atrium, it has been suggested that use of ICE may aid in reducing the formation of an atrioesophageal fistula by ensuring the optimal amount of power and duration of ablation in this particular region.[62] Ingestion of a carbonated beverage may enhance esophageal visualization if such a complication is suspected. Finally, ICE offers monitoring for thrombi or pericardial effusions during the procedure, two other well-described complications of RFA.

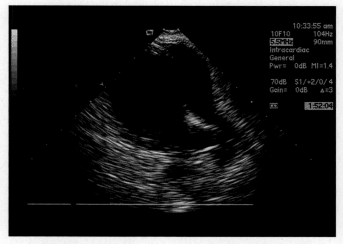

Figure 42.5 ICE demonstrating ablation catheter deployed in contact with pulmonary vein.

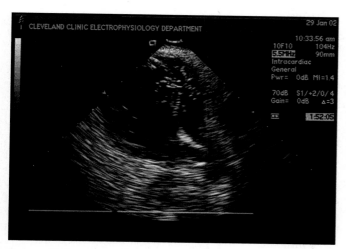

Figure 42.6 ICE images demonstrating microbubbles during ablation catheter positioning. The presence of microbubbles during RFA is suggestive of poor contact between the tip of the ablation catheter and PV tissue. This results in repositioning of the catheter to ensure better contact.

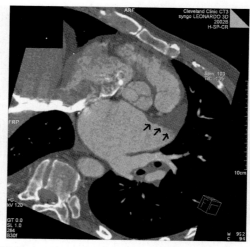

Figure 42.7 CT scan of patient with AF suggesting LAA thrombus.

4.2. Scintigraphic studies

Nuclear scintigraphy has a limited role in the management of patients with AF. Stress myocardial perfusion imaging may be indicated in patients requiring noninvasive detection of coronary artery disease or for an assessment of ejection fraction in patients with heart failure. The irregularity of AF can directly adversely affect the interpretability of such studies, particularly in the assessment of ventricular function. Multigated acquisition or MUGA uses ECG gating to correlate images of the cardiac blood pool with phases of the cardiac cycle based on R-R intervals. In perfusion imaging such as gated single photon emission computed tomography (SPECT), arrhythmias with variable R-R intervals can result in flickering of summed tomograms. When interpreted by computer algorithms, this may result in perfusion artifacts and errors in the assessment of myocardial thickening.[63,64] The concept of gating also applies to CT and MRI, and continues to pose diagnostic difficulties in patients with AF.

4.3. Multislice computed tomography

Multislice computed tomography (MDCT) provides detailed information regarding PV anatomy. It provides an offline assessment of PV and LA anatomy prior to RFA. It also serves similar potential utilities to ICE, in assessing the anatomical relationship between LA and esophagus, and in the detection of postablation complications. Prior CT-based studies have described the relationship of the posterior LA, coronary sinus, esophagus, and PVs.[65] Preablation CTs can provide information that may be crucial in avoiding esophageal injury. CT images have shown a close relationship between the LAA and proximal left circumflex artery. Circumflex artery occlusion during an attempted ablation within the coronary sinus has been reported.[66]

Studies evaluating the role of MDCT in patients undergoing RFA, have shown that thrombus may be identified.[67–69] These often appear as a filling defect in the LA or LAA on contrast-enhanced images. Several studies have looked at the ratio of Hounsfield units (HU) within the LAA relative to the measurement taken from a standard reference point, the ascending aorta (AA). This LAA/AA HU ratio has generally been found to inversely correlate with increasing grades of severe SEC and thrombus found on TEE.[68,70] The differentiation of severe SEC from thrombus has

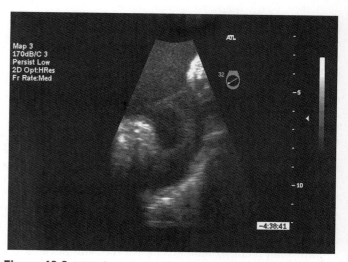

Figure 42.8 TEE of previous patient demonstrating LAA sludge.

not been reliably established with MDCT. Due to limitations, the detection of a filling defect on CT may falsely suggest thrombus rather than the severe degree of SEC or thrombus demonstrated by TEE. The absence of such a filling defect in addition to an increased LAA/AA HU ratio (>0.75) may be useful in excluding thrombus, although TEE remains the superior imaging modality for this indication. This is illustrated in Figures 42.7 and 42.8. Figure 42.7 demonstrates a CT scan with a clear filling defect in the LAA suggestive of thrombus. However, on closer inspection of the LAA by TEE (Fig. 42.8), it is clear that the defect is actually severe SEC or sludge and not thrombus.

MDCT has an important utility in detecting PV stenosis after RFA (Fig. 42.9). High grade stenoses particularly in multiple veins may be associated with symptoms and abnormal lung perfusion scans.[60] MDCT can delineate the lesions, with complete visualization of all four PVs achieved in all patients.

4.4. Magnetic resonance imaging

Cardiac MRI techniques, including magnetic resonance angiography (MRA), are becoming of increased utility in assessing cardiac function and imaging of the great vessels. MRI provides excellent resolution and allows a safe and noninvasive means of assessing soft tissue. It offers superior imaging for the assessment of

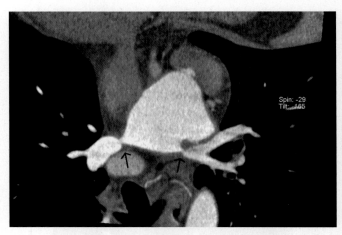

Figure 42.9 Evidence of bilateral pulmonary vein stenoses on CT. The arrows demonstrate stenoses of the right upper PV (*left arrow*) and the left inferior PV (*right arrow*). This patient went onto have angioplasties performed on both PVs.

cardiomyopathies, congenial heart disease, pericardial disease, and cardiac tumors and in assessing myocardial viability. It is more sensitive and specific compared to CT in the diagnosis of aortic dissection.[71]

The disadvantages of MRI include increased scan times and cost. Artifacts secondary to respiratory motion can be problematic. Cardiac MRI is incompatible, as a general rule, with pacemakers, defibrillators, and aneurysm clips. Like SPECT imaging, MRI relies on gating and is prone to variability in image quality and measurements in patients with AF. MRI is felt to have a very high sensitivity for LV thrombus over TTE and TEE.[72,73] There is limited data assessing the diagnostic potential of MRI with regard to thrombus formation in the LAA secondary to AF.[74,75] Thrombi residing in the LA or LAA may be visible on contrast and noncontrast MRI studies, however, the overall diagnostic accuracy of MRI compared to TEE may be limited (Fig. 42.10).

MRI is not routinely indicated for patients with AF, yet it has been studied in the population of patients undergoing RFA. MRI is of similar diagnostic utility to CT in such patients, providing important anatomic information on the preprocedural planning

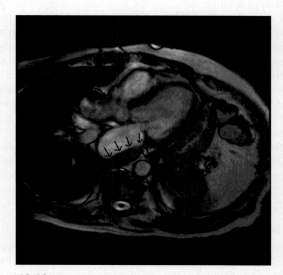

Figure 42.10 Left atrial thrombus evident on MRI. Layered thrombus is seen in the LA cavity as an area of low to intermediate signal intensity on this steady-state free precession cine image.

stage of the evaluation regarding PV and LA anatomical relations and variations.[76-78] Postprocedurally, MRI can be used to delineate PV anatomy, and similar to CT may aid in diagnosing PV stenosis.

5. IMAGING AND CLINICAL DECISION MAKING

5.1. Patients with newly diagnosed atrial fibrillation

Patients presenting with AF should have a thorough history and physical examination performed. AF should be confirmed by ECG, and may require additional Holter monitoring. The history should be focused on determining the onset and tolerability of symptoms, as well as identifying underlying factors, which may be cardiac (hypertension) or extracardiac (hyperthyroidism), that may contribute.

All patients should undergo TTE to assess for valvular heart disease, LVH, pericardial disease, pulmonary hypertension, and overt cardiomyopathy. Mitral stenosis and LV dysfunction found on TTE generally require anticoagulation and are TTE predictors of LAA thrombus (Table 42.3).[79] Clinical parameters such as a CHADS2 score may determine the need for anticoagulation.[20] Further imaging studies may be directed by patient symptoms and TTE findings, particularly if there is suggestion of underlying ischemia or cardiomyopathy in which case nuclear imaging, CT, or MRI may be helpful. Assessment of adequate rate control may require physiological testing including a 6-min walk test, exercise stress testing, or Holter monitoring. The general workup suggested by ACC guidelines is shown in Table 42.4.

TEE is generally not required in the immediate workup of newly diagnosed AF unless cardioversion is planned and facilitation of early cardioversion is desirable, rather than allowing for the 3 to 4 weeks of therapeutic anticoagulation in case of which TEE is not necessary.

5.2. Patients with atrial fibrillation requiring cardioversion

Patients who are hemodynamically unstable with evidence of angina, ischemia, or pre-excitation require prompt cardioversion. Electrical or chemical cardioversion may also be performed if the AF is of new onset and <48 h in duration. Special consideration to anticoagulation and/or TEE for further risk stratification should be given to patients with valvular heart disease, LV dysfunction or prior thromboembolic events, and AF of <48 h duration. For those with AF for >48 h, the advantages and disadvantages of conventional anticoagulation for 4 weeks must be considered. Advantages include a theoretical reduction in stroke rate from 5.6% to <2% and avoidance of performing TEE, which is invasive and may not be feasible in smaller community hospitals.[80-82] TEE offers the advantage of a reduced bleeding risk and earlier attainment of normal sinus rhythm with no difference in embolic complications.[26] The approach is summarized in Figure 42.11.

5.3. Patient with atrial fibrillation and stroke

The occurrence of stroke in patients with AF is usually on the basis of a cardioembolic event. ECG monitoring is crucial to confirming a diagnosis of AF if not evident on standard 12-lead ECG. The presence of AF alone is not sufficient to implicate a thrombus originating from the LA or LAA. Since AF is common in the elderly, there should always be consideration for other potential causes of stroke and all patients require a thorough workup.

TABLE 42.4

RECOMMENDED INITIAL EVALUATION OF PATIENT WITH AF BASED ON 2006 ACC GUIDELINES

Minimum evaluation

1. History and physical examination, to define

   Presence and nature of symptoms associated with AF

   Clinical type of AF (first episode, paroxysmal, persistent, or permanent)

   Onset of the first symptomatic attack or date of discovery of AF

   Frequency, duration, precipitating factors, and modes of termination of AF

   Response to any pharmacological agents that have been administered

   Presence of any underlying heart disease or other reversible conditions (e.g., hyperthyroidism or alcohol consumption)

2. Electrocardiogram, to identify

   Rhythm (verify AF)

   LV hypertrophy

   P-wave duration and morphology or fibrillatory waves

   Pre-excitation

   Bundle-branch block

   Prior myocardial infarction (MI)

   Other atrial arrhythmias

   To measure and follow the RR, QRS, and QT intervals in conjunction with antiarrhythmic drug therapy

3. Transthoracic ECG, to identify

   Valvular heart disease

   LA and RA size

   LV size and function

   Peak RV pressure (pulmonary hypertension)

   LV hypertrophy

   LA thrombus (low sensitivity)

   Pericardial disease

4. Blood tests of thyroid, renal, and hepatic function

   For a first episode of AF, when the ventricular rate is difficult to control

Additional testing

One or several tests may be necessary.

1. 6-min walk test

   If the adequacy of rate control is in question

2. Exercise testing

   If the adequacy of rate control is in question (permanent AF)

   To reproduce exercise-induced AF

   To exclude ischemia before treatment of selected patients with a type Ic antiarrhythmic drug

3. Holter monitoring or event recording

   If diagnosis of the type of arrhythmia is in question

   As a means of evaluating rate control

4. TEE

   To identify LA thrombus (in the LA appendage)

   To guide cardioversion

5. Electrophysiological study

   To clarify the mechanism of wide-QRS-complex tachycardia

   To identify a predisposing arrhythmia such as atrial flutter or paroxysmal supraventricular tachycardia

   To seek sites for curative ablation or AV conduction block/modification

6. Chest radiograph, to evaluate

   Lung parenchyma, when clinical findings suggest an abnormality

   Pulmonary vasculature, when clinical findings suggest an abnormality

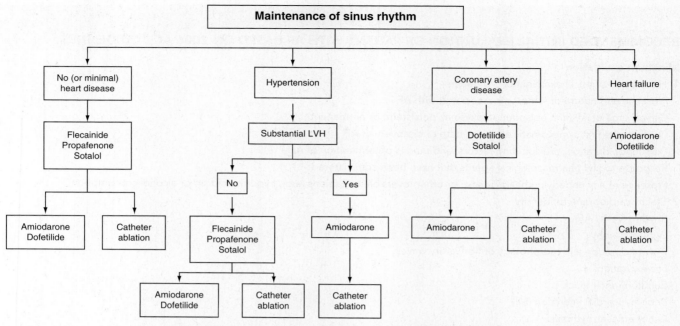

Figure 42.11 Approach to patient with AF needing cardioversion.

Most patients with AF suffering a stroke require anticoagulation with warfarin, and thus echocardiography often does not dramatically alter therapy. It is often useful in suggesting a mechanism of stroke. TTE is a reasonable starting point in all patients, and is superior to TEE at identifying LV thrombus. TEE is superior for detecting abnormalities of the intra-atrial septum including atrial septal aneurysm, patent foramen ovale, and atrial septal defect, which are considered risk factors for stroke. Such shunts may imply a paradoxical embolus. TEE provides direct visualization of the LAA, and may exclude thrombus in patients requiring cardioversion. Other LAA features on TEE associated with increased risk of stroke in patients with nonvalvular AF include dense spontaneous echo contrast, reduced LA peak flow velocities (≤20 cm/s), and complex aortic plaque.[83]

Aortic atheroma is related to increased stroke risk and frequently diagnosed on TEE. The risk of stroke is increased in patients with aortic atheroma and AF. In SPAF III, 35% of patients with AF had evidence of complex atheroma, that is, thick, mobile plaques. Risk of embolization increases based on plaque thickness (≥4 mm), mobility, presence of ulceration, and location, with risk increased if located in the AA.[50] SPAF III classified patients as having LA "abnormality" if there was LAA thrombus, dense SEC, or reduced LAA emptying velocities. Patients with LA abnormality had a 7.8% per year risk of stroke, while patients with complex aortic plaque had a risk of 12% per year. If patients had both features, their risk went up to 20.5% per year, suggesting that pathogenesis for stroke in these patients is multifactorial. The exact therapy for aortic atheroma is not entirely clear, and performing TEE solely to look for it is not an accepted indication.

6. FUTURE DIRECTIONS

Cardiac imaging is playing an important role in the diagnosis, management, and facilitation of therapeutic interventions for AF. Echocardiography remains the cornerstone of screening for significant structural heart disease and in facilitating cardioversion

through the exclusion of thrombus. As our electrical understanding of the arrhythmia improves, newer imaging modalities will play a central role in delineating important structures crucial for successful ablation and monitoring for complications.

REFERENCES

1. Go AS, Hylek EM, Phillips KA, et al. Prevalence of diagnosed atrial fibrillation in adults: national implications for rhythm management and stroke prevention: the AnTicoagulation and Risk Factors in Atrial Fibrillation (ATRIA) study. *JAMA.* 2001;285(18):2370–2375.
2. Feinberg WM, Cornell ES, Nightingale SD, et al. Relationship between prothrombin activation fragment F1.2 and international normalized ratio in patients with atrial fibrillation. Stroke Prevention in Atrial Fibrillation Investigators. *Stroke.* 1997;28(6):1101–1106.
3. Feinberg WM, Blackshear JL, Laupacis A, et al. Prevalence, age distribution, and gender of patients with atrial fibrillation. Analysis and implications. *Arch Intern Med.* 1995;155(5):469–473.
4. Kannel WB, Benjamin EJ Status of the epidemiology of atrial fibrillation. *Med Clin North Am.* 2008;92(1):17–40, ix.
5. Kannel WB, Abbott RD, Savage DD, et al. Epidemiologic features of chronic atrial fibrillation: the Framingham study. *N Engl J Med.* 1982;306(17):1018–1022.
6. Kannel WB, Abbott RD, Savage DD, et al. Coronary heart disease and atrial fibrillation: the Framingham study. *Am Heart J.* 1983;106(2):389–396.
7. Wolf PA, Abbott RD, Kannel WB. Atrial fibrillation: A major contributor to stroke in the elderly. The Framingham study. *Arch Intern Med.* 1987;147(9):1561–1564.
8. Wolf PA, Mitchell JB, Baker CS, et al. Impact of atrial fibrillation on mortality, stroke, and medical costs. *Arch Intern Med.* 1998;158(3):229–234.
9. Wolf PA, Abbott RD, Kannel WB. Atrial fibrillation as an independent risk factor for stroke: The Framingham study. *Stroke.* 1991;22(8):983–988.
10. Risk factors for stroke and efficacy of antithrombotic therapy in atrial fibrillation. Analysis of pooled data from five randomized controlled trials. *Arch Intern Med.* 1994;154(13):1449–1457.
11. Sanfilippo AJ, Abascal VM, Sheehan M, et al. Atrial enlargement as a consequence of atrial fibrillation. A prospective echocardiographic study. *Circulation.* 1990;82(3):792–797.
12. Welikovitch L, Lafreniere G, Burggraf GW, et al. Change in atrial volume following restoration of sinus rhythm in patients with atrial fibrillation: A prospective echocardiographic study. *Can J Cardiol.* 1994;10(10):993–996.
13. Simek CL, Feldman MD, Haber HL, et al. Relationship between left ventricular wall thickness and left atrial size: Comparison with other measures of diastolic function. *J Am Soc Echocardiogr.* 1995;8(1):37–47.
14. Appleton CP, Galloway JM, Gonzalez MS, et al. Estimation of left ventricular filling pressures using two-dimensional and Doppler echocardiography in adult patients with cardiac disease. Additional value of analyzing left atrial size, left atrial ejection fraction and the difference in duration of pulmonary venous and mitral flow velocity at atrial contraction. *J Am Coll Cardiol.* 1993;22(7):1972–1982.

15. Tsang TS, Barnes ME, Bailey KR, et al. Left atrial volume: Important risk marker of incident atrial fibrillation in 1655 older men and women. *Mayo Clin Proc.* 2001;76(5):467–475.

16. Fuster V, Ryden LE, Cannom DS, et al. ACC/AHA/ESC 2006 guidelines for the management of patients with atrial fibrillation—executive summary:a report of the American College of Cardiology/American Heart Association Task Force on Practice Guidelines and the European Society of Cardiology Committee for Practice Guidelines (Writing Committee to Revise the 2001 Guidelines for the Management of Patients With Atrial Fibrillation). *J Am Coll Cardiol.* 2006;48(4):854–906.

17. Tabata T, Grimm RA, Greenberg NL, et al. Assessment of LV systolic function in atrial fibrillation using an index of preceding cardiac cycles. *Am J Physiol Heart Circ Physiol.* 2001;281(2):H573–H580.

18. Grogan M, Smith HC, Gersh BJ, et al. Left ventricular dysfunction due to atrial fibrillation in patients initially believed to have idiopathic dilated cardiomyopathy. *Am J Cardiol.* 1992;69(19):1570–1573.

19. Gage BF, Waterman AD, Shannon W, et al. Validation of clinical classification schemes for predicting stroke: Results from the National Registry of Atrial Fibrillation. *JAMA.* 2001;285(22):2864–2870.

20. Go AS, Hylek EM, Chang Y, et al. Anticoagulation therapy for stroke prevention in atrial fibrillation: How well do randomized trials translate into clinical practice? *JAMA.* 2003;290(20):2685–2692.

21. Echocardiographic predictors of stroke in patients with atrial fibrillation: A prospective study of 1066 patients from 3 clinical trials. *Arch Intern Med.* 1998;158(12):1316–1320.

22. Tabata T, Grimm RA, Asada J, et al. Determinants of LV diastolic function during atrial fibrillation: beat-to-beat analysis in acute dog experiments. *Am J Physiol Heart Circ Physiol.* 2004;286(1):H145–152.

23. Al-Saady NM, Obel OA, Camm AJ. Left atrial appendage: structure, function, and role in thromboembolism. *Heart.* 1999;82(5):547–554.

24. Grimm RA, Stewart WJ, Maloney JD, et al. Impact of electrical cardioversion for atrial fibrillation on left atrial appendage function and spontaneous echo contrast: characterization by simultaneous transesophageal echocardiography. *J Am Coll Cardiol.* 1993;22(5):1359–1366.

25. Weigner MJ, Thomas LR, Patel U, et al. Early cardioversion of atrial fibrillation facilitated by transesophageal echocardiography: short-term safety and impact on maintenance of sinus rhythm at 1 year. *Am J Med.* 2001;110(9):694–702.

26. Klein AL, Grimm RA, Murray RD, et al. Use of transesophageal echocardiography to guide cardioversion in patients with atrial fibrillation. *N Engl J Med.* 2001;344(19):1411–1420.

27. Leung DY, Davidson PM, Cranney GB, et al. Thromboembolic risks of left atrial thrombus detected by transesophageal echocardiogram. *Am J Cardiol.* 1997;79(5):626–629.

28. Nagueh SF, Kopelen HA, Quinones MA. Assessment of left ventricular filling pressures by Doppler in the presence of atrial fibrillation. *Circulation.* 1996;94(9):2138–2145.

29. Klein AL, Murray RD, Grimm RA. Role of transesophageal echocardiography-guided cardioversion of patients with atrial fibrillation. *J Am Coll Cardiol.* 2001;37(3):691–704.

30. Pollick C, Taylor D. Assessment of left atrial appendage function by transesophageal echocardiography. Implications for the development of thrombus. *Circulation.* 1991;84(1):223–231.

31. Fatkin D, Herbert E, Feneley MP. Hematologic correlates of spontaneous echo contrast in patients with atrial fibrillation and implications for thromboembolic risk. *Am J Cardiol.* 1994;73(9):672–676.

32. Mugge A, Kuhn H, Nikutta P, et al. Assessment of left atrial appendage function by biplane transesophageal echocardiography in patients with nonrheumatic atrial fibrillation: Identification of a subgroup of patients at increased embolic risk. *J Am Coll Cardiol.* 1994;23(3):599–607.

33. Siostrzonek P, Koppensteiner R, Gossinger H, et al. Hemodynamic and hemorheologic determinants of left atrial spontaneous echo contrast and thrombus formation in patients with idiopathic dilated cardiomyopathy. *Am Heart J.* 1993;125(2 Pt 1):430–434.

34. Van Gelder IC, Crijns HJ, Blanksma PK, et al. Time course of hemodynamic changes and improvement of exercise tolerance after cardioversion of chronic atrial fibrillation unassociated with cardiac valve disease. *Am J Cardiol.* 1993;72(7):560–566.

35. Cappato R, Calkins H, Chen SA, et al. Worldwide survey on the methods, efficacy, and safety of catheter ablation for human atrial fibrillation. *Circulation.* 2005;11(9):1100–1105.

36. Vasan RS, Larson MG, Levy D, et al. Distribution and categorization of echocardiographic measurements in relation to reference limits: The Framingham Heart Study: formulation of a height- and sex-specific classification and its prospective validation. *Circulation.* 1997;96(6):1863–1873.

37. Pritchett AM, Jacobsen SJ, Mahoney DW, et al. Left atrial volume as an index of left atrial size: A population-based study. *J Am Coll Cardiol.* 2003;41(6):1036–1043.

38. Lang RM, Bierig M, Devereux RB, et al. Recommendations for chamber quantification: A report from the American Society of Echocardiography's Guidelines and Standards Committee and the Chamber Quantification Writing Group, developed in conjunction with the European Association of Echocardiography, a branch of the European Society of Cardiology. *J Am Soc Echocardiogr.* 2005;18(12):1440–1463.

39. Manning WJ, Weintraub RM, Waksmonski CA, et al. Accuracy of transesophageal echocardiography for identifying left atrial thrombi. A prospective, intraoperative study. *Ann Intern Med.* 1995;123(11):817–822.

40. Hwang JJ, Chen JJ, Lin SC, et al. Diagnostic accuracy of transesophageal echocardiography for detecting left atrial thrombi in patients with rheumatic heart disease having undergone mitral valve operations. *Am J Cardiol.* 1993;72(9):677–681.

41. Keren G, Bier A, Sherez J, et al. Atrial contraction is an important determinant of pulmonary venous flow. *J Am Coll Cardiol.* 1986;7(3):693–695.

42. Sohn DW, Song JM, Zo JH, et al. Mitral annulus velocity in the evaluation of left ventricular diastolic function in atrial fibrillation. *J Am Soc Echocardiogr.* 1999;12(11):927–931.

43. Hurrell DG, Oh JK, Mahoney DW, et al. Short deceleration time of mitral inflow E velocity: Prognostic implication with atrial fibrillation versus sinus rhythm. *J Am Soc Echocardiogr.* 1998;11(5):450–457.

44. Manning WJ, Leeman DE, Gotch PJ, et al. Pulsed Doppler evaluation of atrial mechanical function after electrical cardioversion of atrial fibrillation. *J Am Coll Cardiol.* 1989;13(3):617–623.

45. Yamada H, Donal E, Kim YJ, et al. The pseudorestrictive pattern of transmitral Doppler flow pattern after conversion of atrial fibrillation to sinus rhythm: Is atrial or ventricular dysfunction to blame? *J Am Soc Echocardiogr.* 2004;17(8):813–818.

46. Thomas L, Thomas SP, Hoy M, et al. Comparison of left atrial volume and function after linear ablation and after cardioversion for chronic atrial fibrillation. *Am J Cardiol.* 2004;93(2):165–170.

47. Seward JB, Khandheria BK, Freeman WK, et al. Multiplane transesophageal echocardiography: Image orientation, examination technique, anatomic correlations, and clinical applications. *Mayo Clin Proc.* 1993;68(6):523–551.

48. Agmon Y, Khandheria BK, Gentile F, et al. Echocardiographic assessment of the left atrial appendage. *J Am Coll Cardiol.* 1999;34(7):1867–1877.

49. Jue J, Winslow T, Fazio G, et al. Pulsed Doppler characterization of left atrial appendage flow. *J Am Soc Echocardiogr.* 1993;6(3 Pt 1):237–244.

50. Transesophageal echocardiographic correlates of thromboembolism in high-risk patients with nonvalvular atrial fibrillation. The Stroke Prevention in Atrial Fibrillation Investigators Committee on Echocardiography. *Ann Intern Med.* 1998;128(8):639–647.

51. Goldman M. The management of chronic atrial fibrillation. *Prog Cardiovasc Dis.* 1960;2:465–479.

52. Lown B, Perlroth MG, Kaidbey S, et al. "Cardioversion" of atrial fibrillation. A report on the treatment of 65 episodes in 50 patients. *N Engl J Med.* 1963;269:325–331.

53. Oram S, Davies JP. Further experience of electrical conversion of atrial fibrillation to sinus rhythm: Analysis of 100 patients. *Lancet.* 1964;1(7346):1294–1298.

54. Arnold AZ, Mick MJ, Mazurek RP, et al. Role of prophylactic anticoagulation for direct current cardioversion in patients with atrial fibrillation or atrial flutter. *J Am Coll Cardiol.* 1992;19(4):851–855.

55. Grimm RA, Leung DY, Black IW, et al. Left atrial appendage "stunning" after spontaneous conversion of atrial fibrillation demonstrated by transesophageal Doppler echocardiography. *Am Heart J.* 1995;130(1):174–176.

56. Falcone RA, Morady F, Armstrong WF. Transesophageal echocardiographic evaluation of left atrial appendage function and spontaneous contrast formation after chemical or electrical cardioversion of atrial fibrillation. *Am J Cardiol.* 1996;78(4):435–439.

57. Omran H, Jung W, Rabahieh R, et al. Left atrial chamber and appendage function after internal atrial defibrillation: A prospective and serial transesophageal echocardiographic study. *J Am Coll Cardiol.* 1997;29(1):131–138.

58. Schneider C, Ernst S, Bahlmann E, et al. Transesophageal echocardiography: A screening method for pulmonary vein stensis after catheter ablation of atrial fibrillation. *Eur J Echocardiogr.* 2006;7(6):447–456.

59. Donal E, Grimm RA, Yamada H, et al. Usefulness of Doppler assessment of pulmonary vein and left atrial appendage flow following pulmonary vein isolation of chronic atrial fibrillation in predicting recovery of left atrial function. *Am J Cardiol.* 2005;95(8):941–947.

60. Saad EB, Rossillo A, Saad CP, et al. Pulmonary vein stenosis after radiofrequency ablation of atrial fibrillation: functional characterization, evolution, and influence of the ablation strategy. *Circulation.* 2003;108(25):3102–3107.

61. Saad EB, Cole CR, Marrouche NF, et al. Use of intracardiac echocardiography for prediction of chronic pulmonary vein stenosis after ablation of atrial fibrillation. *J Cardiovasc Electrophysiol.* 2002;13(10):986–989.

62. Ren JF, Lin D, Marchlinski FE, et al. Esophageal imaging and strategies for avoiding injury during left atrial ablation for atrial fibrillation. *Heart Rhythm.* 2006;3(10):1156–1161.

63. Nichols K, Dorbala S, DePuey EG, et al. Influence of arrhythmias on gated SPECT myocardial perfusion and function quantification. *J Nucl Med.* 1999;40(6):924–934.

64. Nichols K, Yao SS, Kamran M, et al. Clinical impact of arrhythmias on gated SPECT cardiac myocardial perfusion and function assessment. *J Nucl Cardiol.* 2001;8(1):19–30.

65. Tsao HM, Wu MH, Chern MS, et al. Anatomic proximity of the esophagus to the coronary sinus: Implication for catheter ablation within the coronary sinus. *J Cardiovasc Electrophysiol.* 2006;17(3):266–269.

66. Takahashi Y, Jais P, Hocini M, et al. Acute occlusion of the left circumflex coronary artery during mitral isthmus linear ablation. *J Cardiovasc Electrophysiol.* 2005;16(10):1104–1107.

67. Gottlieb I, Pinheiro A, Brinker JA, et al. Diagnostic accuracy of arterial phase 64-slice multidetector CT angiography for left atrial appendage thrombus in patients undergoing atrial fibrillation ablation. *J Cardiovasc Electrophysiol.* 2008;19(3):247–251.

68. Patel A, Au E, Donegan K, et al. Multidetector row computed tomography for identification of left atrial appendage filling defects in patients undergoing pulmonary vein isolation for treatment of atrial fibrillation: Comparison with transesophageal echocardiography. *Heart Rhythm*. 2008;5(2):253–260.

69. Shapiro MD, Neilan TG, Jassal DS, et al. Multidetector computed tomography for the detection of left atrial appendage thrombus: A comparative study with transesophageal echocardiography. *J Comput Assist Tomogr*. 2007;31(6):905–909.

70. Kim YY, Klein AL, Halliburton SS, et al. Left atrial appendage filling defects identified by multidetector computed tomography in patients undergoing radiofrequency pulmonary vein antral isolation: A comparison with transesophageal echocardiography. *Am Heart J*. 2007;154(6):1199–1205.

71. Pohost GM, Hung L, Doyle M. Clinical use of cardiovascular magnetic resonance. *Circulation*. 2003;108(6):647–653.

72. Mollet NR, Dymarkowski S, Volders W, et al. Visualization of ventricular thrombi with contrast-enhanced magnetic resonance imaging in patients with ischemic heart disease. *Circulation*. 2002;106(23):2873–2876.

73. Srichai MB, Junor C, Rodriguez LL, et al. Clinical, imaging, and pathological characteristics of left ventricular thrombus: A comparison of contrast-enhanced magnetic resonance imaging, transthoracic echocardiography, and transesophageal echocardiography with surgical or pathological validation. *Am Heart J*. 2006;152(1):75–84.

74. Ohyama H, Hosomi N, Takahashi T, et al. Comparison of magnetic resonance imaging and transesophageal echocardiography in detection of thrombus in the left atrial appendage. *Stroke*. 2003;34(10):2436–2439.

75. Mohrs OK, Nowak B, Petersen SE, et al. Thrombus detection in the left atrial appendage using contrast-enhanced MRI: A pilot study. *AJR Am J Roentgenol*. 2006;186(1):198–205.

76. Jander N, Minners J, Arentz T, et al. Transesophageal echocardiography in comparison with magnetic resonance imaging in the diagnosis of pulmonary vein stenosis after radiofrequency ablation therapy. *J Am Soc Echocardiogr*. 2005;18(6):654–659.

77. Kato R, Lickfett L, Meininger G, et al. Pulmonary vein anatomy in patients undergoing catheter ablation of atrial fibrillation: Lessons learned by use of magnetic resonance imaging. *Circulation*. 2003;107(15):2004–2010.

78. Anselme F, Gahide G, Savoure A, et al. MR evaluation of pulmonary vein diameter reduction after radiofrequency catheter ablation of atrial fibrillation. *Eur Radiol*. 2006;16(11):2505–2511.

79. Ellis K, Ziada KM, Vivekananthan D, et al. Transthoracic echocardiographic predictors of left atrial appendage thrombus. *Am J Cardiol*. 2006;97(3):421–425.

80. Bjerkelund CJ, Orning OM. The efficacy of anticoagulant therapy in preventing embolism related to D.C. electrical conversion of atrial fibrillation. *Am J Cardiol*. 1969;23(2):208–216.

81. Roy D, Marchand E, Gagne P, et al. Usefulness of anticoagulant therapy in the prevention of embolic complications of atrial fibrillation. *Am Heart J*. 1986;112(5):1039–1043.

82. Moreyra E, Finkelhor RS, Cebul RD. Limitations of transesophageal echocardiography in the risk assessment of patients before nonanticoagulated cardioversion from atrial fibrillation and flutter: an analysis of pooled trials. *Am Heart J*. 1995;129(1):71–75.

83. Zabalgoitia M, Halperin JL, Pearce LA, et al. Transesophageal echocardiographic correlates of clinical risk of thromboembolism in nonvalvular atrial fibrillation. Stroke prevention in atrial fibrillation III investigators. *J Am Coll Cardiol*. 1998;31(7):1622–1626.

Ventricular Arrhythmias and Sudden Death

43

Luis J. Jimenez-Borreguero
Jose L. Merino

1. INTRODUCTION

1.1. Definition and epidemiology

Ventricular tachyarrhythmias (VTAs) are defined as rhythm disorders which originate from the ventricles, that is, by mechanisms with no participation of cardiac structures above the His bundle bifurcation. Several disorders are included in this term which range from ventricular ectopy to ventricular fibrillation. Single ventricular ectopy or premature ventricular contractions (PVCs) can be recognized as premature wide QRS complexes, which are not consistently preceded by P waves on the echocardiogram (ECG) or by his bundle activations at electrophysiological evaluation. PVCs can be the first manifestation of heart disease, but they are also often seen in a high proportion of the general population, especially those displaying left bundle branch block morphology and inferior axis. They have no or little influence in the long-term prognosis in this latter setting. Several definitions have been used for ventricular tachycardia (VT), but the most accepted is the demonstration of three or more consecutive PVCs at a rate >100 bpm.[1] VT is considered sustained when it last >30s or has to be terminated earlier due to homodynamic compromise. The second relevant consideration about VT characterization comes from the stable or changing morphology of the QRS complex. Monomorphic VT is that one showing no significant beat-to-beat change of the QRS complex morphology, typically is regular and commonly is the manifestation of a stable mechanism (Section 2). Polymorphic VT is defined as that one showing unstable QRS complexes with continuous change of morphology, duration, amplitude, and cycle length. Two types should be differentiated, multiform VT, in which no specific pattern is found, and torsade de pointes, in which the QRS complex polarity seems to gradually twist around the baseline and, most importantly, it is associated with prolonged QT interval during sinus rhythm. Ventricular flutter is characterized by regular QRS complex morphology at a rate of about 300 bpm with no isoelectric line between QRS complexes. Finally, ventricular fibrillation is a VTA with irregular QRS complexes at a rate of >300 bpm. Differentiation between ventricular fibrillation (VF) and polymorphic VT is made just by differences in ventricular rate, and, since both arrhythmias are irregular, the differences are often semantic and polymorphic. VT is the preferred term for nonsustained episodes and VF for the sustained ones. It is important to emphasize that recognition of the different types of VT has more than academic interest, since it gives important clues about their pathophysiology and treatment.

Sudden death (SD) is defined as that one which occurs suddenly, unexpectedly, not related to trauma and within 1 h from the symptoms onset or a change in clinical status. A 24-h time frame has been also used for SD definition which results in an increase of the proportion of SD among all causes of death and in a decrease in the percentage of cardiac causes among all SD mechanisms. The 1-h time frame has been applied for witnessed deaths and the 24-h for unwitnessed deaths in other studies. The incidence and relative frequency of SD among other mechanisms of death vary according to the definition used but it is between 10% and 20%, which makes it a major clinical and public health problem.[2] SD incidence also depends on the population studied. Patients with VT and left ventricular (LV) dysfunction due to ischemic heart disease have over 30% yearly incidence of SD, but this incidence is around 0.1% to 0.2% in the general population. However, these populations show an opposite relation when absolute numbers are considered due to the larger size of the general population.[3] This has important implications when designing strategies to reduce the impact of SD.

SD can be the result of different mechanisms, which include arrhythmias, nonarrhythmic cardiac disorders, and noncardiac disorders. However, VTA is considered to play the preponderant role. Probably the most frequent mechanism involved in sudden cardiac death (SCD) is polymorphic VT/ventricular fibrillation, since this is the most frequent VTA mechanism during myocardial ischemia. VTA can be also the result of other cardiac diseases, which will be discussed in the pathophysiology section. Finally, is important not to neglect the importance of nonarrhythmic mechanisms of SCD. This has been recently shown in implantable cardioverter/defibrillator (ICD) recipient populations, which show 28% of SCD, mostly due to electromechanical dissociation.[4]

1.2. Clinical presentation

1.2.1. Symptoms

The clinical presentation of VT is highly variable. VT presents in some patients with heart failure, hemodynamic collapse, and SCD; however, others complain of no or little symptoms. The determinants for poor VT tolerance are not well established and several factors have been implicated, including high heart rate, severe ventricular dysfunction, and large QRS complex width. Asymptomatic sustained VT may develop or aggravate ventricular dysfunction if it is fast enough. This phenomenon, which is denominated, tachycardia-induced cardiomyopathy develops in just few weeks if the heart rate is fast enough.

SCD presents by definition with no or few symptoms before death. However, some patients complained of chest pain shortly before death because an ischemic heart event is the most common trigger.

1.2.2. Outcome

Several studies have shown that long-term prognosis of patients with nontolerated VT is poor.[5] On the other hand, some investigators suggest that tolerated VT had a good prognosis. However, this impression was challenged by the data drawn from some registries, such as the Antiarrhythmics versus implantable defibrillators (AVID) registry, in which patients with tolerated VT and LV dysfunction showed even worse prognosis than those with nontolerated VT.[6] By contrast, the long-term outcome in patients with tolerated VT and structural heart disease (SHD) with no or little ventricular dysfunction is not well established. There are almost no data of patients with VT who were free of antiarrhythmic treatment, and now it is well known that many of these drugs have negative prognostic effect. Finally, the outcome of VT in patients without SHD is supposed to be similar to the general population. However, some investigators have reported isolated cases of SCD in this subpopulation. Whether these patients had incipient forms of SHD, such as arrhythmogenic right ventricular dysplasia (ARVD) or idiopathic dilated cardiomyopathy (IDCM), is a matter of discussion and warrants further research with novel imaging methods.

In general, the recurrence of SCD is high enough to ensure device preventive therapy.[7] The only exception is when SCD is associated with acute myocardial ischemia. Several studies have shown a favorable outcome with just coronary revascularization in patients with preserved LV function. Finally, the outcome of patients with SCD and no apparent SHD is unclear. In general, it is accepted that these patients merit ICD implantation. However, two different populations should be differentiated, those with identifiable primary electrical heart disease or channelopathy and those without an identifiable cause for SCD. SCD recurrence of the former is high enough to warrant ICD implantation and this therapy is even considered for asymptomatic patients with family history of SCD or other risks factors.[1] However, for the latter patients there are increasing evidences that SCD could be an isolated event, which most often is linked to a transient myocardial ischemic event.

2. PATHOPHYSIOLOGY

Monomorphic VTA should be differentiated from polymorphic VTA from the pathophysiology point of view. Monomorphic VT represents regular organized ventricular depolarization from the same site as a result of ectopic activity or stable macroreentry. However, polymorphic VT is considered the consequence of ventricular activation from multiple ventricular sites due to coexistent ectopy or multiple and unstable reentry phenomena. These differentiations are relevant, since monomorphic VT is seen in patients with focally driven arrhythmias without heart structural abnormalities or, in the case of macroreentry in patients with SHD and ventricular scars, which are responsible of the macroreentrant circuit. On the contrary, polymorphic VT is not necessarily associated with myocardial scars and is more often seen in acute "irritative" scenarios, such as myocardial ischemia, myocarditis, or ionic disturbance. Polymorphic VT is also typically seen in patients with myocardial channelopathies, such as the Brugada syndrome and the congenital long QT syndrome.

Necropsy studies have revealed that >80% of the patients dying suddenly had coronary artery disease (CAD), but only 40% of them showed signs of acute myocardial infarction (MI). This again suggests that myocardial ischemia and polymorphic VT/ventricular fibrillation play preponderant roles in SCD in Western countries. This scenario changes in patients dying suddenly under

35 years of age in whom hypertrophic cardiomyopathy (HCM) and ARVD are the most prevalent SCD causes and SCD is often the first manifestation of the diseases.[8]

2.1. Ischemic heart disease

Ischemic heart disease may present both polymorphic and monomorphic VTA. The first one is typically seen during myocardial ischemia, especially during the acute phase of MI. Monomorphic VT is also occasionally seen during acute MI but is almost restricted to patients with severe LV dysfunction or with concurrent old MI. Once the acute phase of MI has overcome, scar tissue replaces the necrotic myocardium and monomorphic VT due to macroreentry becoming the typical sustained VTA in this scenario. Scar tissue protects small strands of viable myocardium from the surrounding depolarization. These strands conduct slowly the activation front outside the scar so, when the impulse reaches normal myocardium, it is ready to be activated again and to recirculate the activation front to the entry of this slow conducting pathway (Fig. 43.1). Several initiatives have tried to identify these surviving strands of myocardium within the scar by noninvasive image techniques. This would probably be a promising area of research, which might provide both prognostic information and data to guide the ablation procedure.

Finally, is important to underline that the first 6 to 12 months are those with the greatest risk for VTA and SCD following MI, particularly in high-risk subgroups such as those with impaired ventricular function or ventricular aneurysms.

2.2. Cardiomyopathies

Most types of cardiomyopathies are associated with areas of scar and fibrosis which predispose patients to reentry and VTA, usually in the form of monomorphic VT. Contrary to ischemic heart disease, the distribution of these areas is not preponderant in the subendocardium and may be patchy and also affect the epicardium, especially in IDCM and Chagas disease. Recognition of the location of these areas by imaging techniques may have relevant implications since epicardial ablation through a pericardial access is now a well established technique in clinical practice. The pathological features of HCM are diverse and include hypertrophy and disarray of cardiac myocytes, increased interstitial collagen content, and thickening of the media of intramural coronary arteries. These changes are responsible for a high incidence of VTA, which presents both in the form of VT and direct ventricular fibrillation. ARVD typically shows areas of fibrosis and fat infiltration, mostly confined to the right

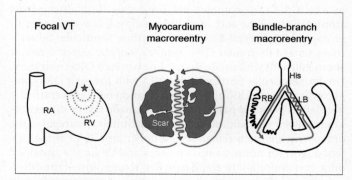

Figure 43.1 Monomorphic VT mechanisms. The site of origin of focal activation is depicted by a *red star*, activation front conduction by *discontinuous lines* and *red arrows* and slow conduction by *sinuous arrows*. See text for more details. RA, right atrium; RV, right ventricle; RB, right bundle branch; LB, left bundle branch.

ventricle but also affecting the left ventricle. These areas are responsible of slow conduction and reentry, leading to the high risk of monomorphic VT and SCD, especially during exercise. Finally, cardioskeletal muscular disorders, also known as neuromuscular disorders, are inherited cardiomyopathies in which both cardiac and skeletal muscles are affected. Cardiac involvement may lead to a form of nonischemic dilated cardiomyopathy with ventricular systolic dysfunction and risk of ventricular macroreentry phenomena. At the same time, some of these disorders, such as myotonic dystrophy which is the most common of them and has a prevalence of 1:8,000, affect predominantly the His-Purkinje system of the heart. This is probably the reason for the high incidence of bundle-branch reentry in this setting[9], a specific type of ventricular macroreentry (Fig. 43.1), which is often associated with SCD.[10]

2.3. Nonapparent structural heart disease

VTA can take place in patients without apparent SHD. As stated at the beginning of this section, inherited disorders of the cardiomyocite ion channels typically present with polymorphic VTA. These arrhythmias may be multiform, like in the Brugada syndrome, the catecholaminergic polymorphic VT, and the short QT syndrome, and show no specific pattern of initiation. On the other hand, *torsade de pointes* variant of polymorphic VT is typically seen in the long QT syndrome and typically is initiated by a short–long–short ventricular activation sequence.

Most monomorphic VTA in patients without apparent SHD can be placed in two groups: right ventricular (RV) outflow tract VT and fascicular VT. Outflow tract VT is the most common of them. This tachycardia typically presents in nonsustained repetitive runs and displays QRS complex left bundle-branch block configuration and inferior axis (Fig. 43.2). It has a focal mechanism that, in general, is due to trigger activity, although automatism and microreentry have also been reported in some patients (Fig. 43.2). It typically originates from the RV outflow tract, but more recently the site of the origin has been also found in the left ventricle. No significant structural heart abnormalities have been found in these patients although isolated reports have found subtle anatomical changes in the outflow tract demonstrated by cardiac magnetic resonance (CMR).[11]

Fascicular VT is less common and typically presents with long-lasting sustained episodes and displays QRS complex right bundle branch block configuration and superior axis. The most likely responsible mechanism is reentry, and it has been speculated about the potential participation of the left posterior fascicle of the left bundle branch of the His bundle and of anatomical structures, such a false tendon extending from the postero-inferior left ventricle to the septum.

3. DIAGNOSTIC EVALUATION

Physical examination could be normal in patients with suspicion to have episodes of VTA. Majority of patients with SCD have some form of SHD.[12] VTA and SCD are frequently associated to histologic disorders of the myocardium associated to several diseases such as MI, hypertrophic and dilated cardiomyopathies, RV dysplasia, myocarditis, or infiltrative diseases. Other scenarios for ventricular arrhythmias are functional disorders, such as those produced by myocardial ischemia without any evidence of permanent myocardial damage, or channelopathies such as Brugada syndrome, long or short QT, catecholamine-induced VT and others.

The chest X-ray provides a first evaluation of patients with SD and suspected tachyarrythmias. The assessment of the size and contours of the heart and great vessels in combination with the information from the personal and family history, anamnesis, physical examination, and ECG can give initial information about the probability to have SHD. Nevertheless, this information could not be enough to rule out ischemic heart disease or other SHDs with mild or hidden signs. Additional information provided by imaging techniques, stress testing, and coronary angiography is usually needed.

Noninvasive imaging allows to establish the diagnoses of several diseases associated to VTA and SCD (Table 43.1). Additionally, these techniques can provide in some cases important prognostic based on anatomical measurements such as LV ejection fraction (LVEF), wall thickness, and presence of aneurysms. Contrast enhancement CMR and its capability for detecting fibrosis in the myocardium provide a diagnostic tool to detect ischemic-induced scars as well as many infiltrative and inflammatory cardiomyopathies.

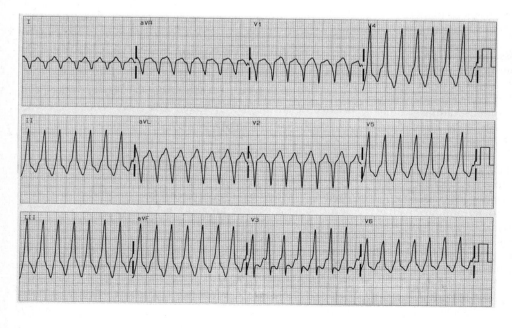

Figure 43.2 Twelve-lead ECG of idiopathic outflow tract VT, which originated from the left ventricle in this patient. Note the QRS complex left bundle branch configuration and inferior axis.

TABLE 43.1

EFFICACY OF IMAGING TECHNIQUES TO ASSESS STRUCTURAL HEART DISEASE RELATED WITH SUDDEN CARDIAC DEATH AND VENTRICULAR TACHYARRYTHMIAS

SHD		Echo	CMR	Nuclear	MDCT
LV function		++	+++	++	++
CAD	MI	+++	+++	+++	+
	Non-MI	+++	+++	+++	+++
Valvular		+++	+++		++
Cardiomyopahies	Dilated	+++	+++	+	+
	Infiltrative	++	+++		
	HCM	+++	+++	+	+
	ARVD	++	+++		+
Myocarditis		++	+++	++	
LV Aneurysms		+++	+++		+++
Isolated noncompaction ventricular myocardium		+++	+++		+
Coronary anomalous origin		++	++		+++

ARVD, arrythmogenic righ ventricular dysplasia; CMR, cardiac magnetic resonance; HCM, hypertrophic cardiomyopathy; MDCT, multidetector computed tomography.

3.1. Echocardiography

Transthoracic echocardiography is an inexpensive and widely available technique that is indicated in patients with VT when SHD is suspected (AHA, ACC, and ESC guidelines class I recommendation and evidence level B).[1] Echocardiography frequently finds normal structural heart, although other findings are LV or RV dysfunction or ventricular wall hypertrophy or valves diseases associated to VT or SCD.

When LV dilatation or systolic dysfunction is the only finding of the ECG in patients with VT or SCD, the differential diagnosis includes dilated cardiomyopathy and ischemic cardiomyopathy. An echocardiographic LV restrictive pattern detected by mitral and pulmonary vein diastolic flows and tissue Doppler in mitral annulus can serve for suspicion of restrictive cardiomyopathy. On the other hand, RV regional or global dysfunction or dilatation is considered to rely on as Task Force criteria for diagnosis of ARVD.

3.1.1. Coronary artery disease

CAD with or without MI could be associated to VT or SCD. Regional ventricular wall dysfunction demonstrated by 2D echocardiography may support the ECG suspicion of MI. Nevertheless, regional wall motion dysfunction alone may not distinguish subacute MI from chronic scar or from myocarditis or other myopathic processes. Inflammatory diseases of the myocardium may produce LV regional dysfunction indistinguishable from MI. The clinical history of chest pain and cardiovascular risk factors and complementary tests such as the ECG can sometimes help to make the appropriate interpretation of the echocardiographic findings. Invasive or CT coronary angiography may also contribute to make the differential diagnosis. Some cardiomyopathies produce myocite loss that can lead to segmental reduction of wall thickness that may mimic the presence of a scar.

Myocardial ischemia can be confirmed or ruled out by exercise echocardiography or myocardial perfusion imaging (MPI) in patients with VT or SCD and intermediate probability of having silent CAD when exercise ECG is less reliable because of left bundle branch block (LBBB), left ventricular hypertrophy (LVH),

ST-segment depression at rest, Wolff-Parkinson-White (WPW) syndrome, or digoxin use.[1] When patients are physically unable to perform a symptom limited exercise test, pharmacological stress testing with an imaging modality such as echocardiography, MPI, or CMR may be considered.[13] Exercise testing is recommended[13] for CAD detection in patients with non-sustained ventricular tachycardia (NSVT), without chest pain syndrome or angina equivalent in patients and with moderate to high Framingham coronary heart disease (CHD) risk.

VTA can be associated to a ventricular aneurysm in selected patients with MI: Resection of the aneurism may be chosen for VTA control.[1] A noninvasive evaluation to detect ventricular aneurysm in patients with history of MI and VTA or SCD may be done by echocardiography or CMR.

Variant angina is another ischemic entity that can be associated to SD, VT, or ventricular fibrillation. Coronary spasm is usually manifested as angina with transitory ST elevation. Moreover, cardiac arrest or syncope without angina is another way of presentation.[14,15] The mechanism of SD is transient myocardial ischemia that can cause ventricular tachyarrythmias, AV block, or asystole. Several investigators have proposed ergotamine stress echocardiography for the detection of coronary vasospasm in selected patients with selected variant angina.[16] However, there is not enough experience for the use of this test in patients with VT or SD.

3.1.2. Valvular disease

Severe aortic stenosis has a cumulative SCD risk of 15% to 20% in symptomatic patients[17] and 1% per year in asymptomatic patients.[18] Some hypothetic mechanisms may lead to SCD in aortic stenosis such as an abnormal Bezold–Jarisch reflex that produces arterial hypotension and bradycardia VTA, and atrioventricular conduction disturbances.[19]

Severe aortic stenosis associated to syncope or SCD is usually suspected by physical exam. Echocardiography may confirm the presence and severity of the stenosis, the repercussion in LV and aorta, and may differentiate it from subvalvular or supravalvular stenosis. In patients with good acoustic windows, 2D echocardiography usually provides information about the aortic leaflets number, thickness, calcification, commissural fusion, and valve stiffness. LV wall hypertrophy is another usual finding that is associated to severe aortic stenosis. Doppler echocardiography provides measurement of the peak and mean systolic velocities across the stenotic valve, and they serve for grading the severity of the stenosis. When LV function is impaired, the physical exam and Doppler velocity assessment may underestimate aortic stenosis severity (Chapter 27). In this case a calculation of the aortic valve area by the continuity method and/or dobutamine stress testing may clarify the severity of the aortic stenosis.

LV dysfunction and valve regurgitation. Severe valvular regurgitation may lead to SD in advance stages, usually associated to LV dysfunction. Significant aortic regurgitation can be assessed by physical examination and confirmed by echocardiography as the cause of LV dilatation and dysfunction. When significant mitral regurgitation coincides with LV dysfunction, echocardiography can provide additional information. Echocardiographic findings of rheumatic or myxomatous disease suggest intrinsic structural mitral valve disease as the primary cause of LV dysfunction. Secondary mitral regurgitation without structural valve abnormalities may be the result of ischemic papillary muscle dysfunction. In this case two mechanisms can contribute to the LV dilation and dysfunction: the regurgitant volume overload into the LV and the ischemic-myocardial injury. Echocardiography can detect papillary muscle dysfunction associated to an akinetic or dyskinetic wall segment as a cause of mitral regurgitation. Stress echocardiography can demonstrate a reduction in mitral regurgitation severity with low doses of dobutamine as a sign of myocardial viability in the wall segment where papillary muscle is implanted.

3.1.3. Dilated cardiomyopathies and myocardial inflammation

Acute myocardis is uncommonly associated with VT and conduction abnormalities as initial manifestation or during long-term follow-up.[20,21] Echocardiographic findings in the acute or chronic stages range from normal or mild LV regional wall motion abnormalities to global ventricular dysfunction in severe cases. Echocardiography alone performed at rest can distinguish neither the acute from the chronic stage nor the myocardis from other pathologies such as ischemic heart disease or other causes of dilated cardiomyopathy.

3.1.4. LV dysfunction and infiltrative diseases

Echocardiographic findings of LV diastolic dysfunction with preserved systolic function could be the first finding of infiltrative cardiomyopathies such as amyloidosis and hemochromatosis. Restrictive Doppler LV filling patterns are usually present in the advance stages of the disease. Echocardiographic LV restrictive patterns with preserved or mildly decrease ejection fraction, increased wall thickness, and increased myocardial echogenicity with a "granular sparkling" appearance (Fig. 43.3) are suggestive of amyloidosis when clinical and electrocardiographic findings are considered (Chapter 34).[22] Other types of restrictive cardiomyopathies include sarcoidosis, storage diseases, and endomyocardial fibrosis.

3.1.5. Nonischemic LV aneurysms

Idiopathic ventricular aneurysms may increase the risk of VTA and SCD.[23,24] The wall of LV aneurysms has a variable composition of collagen fibers and hypertrophied or normal myocytes. This

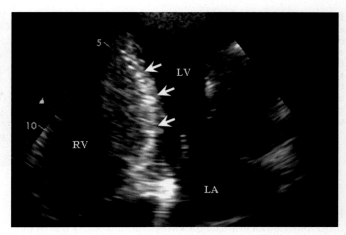

Figure 43.3 2D echocardiography in a four-chamber view where the interventricular septum shows hypertrophy and increased myocardial echogenicity with sparkling appearance *(arrows)*. LV restrictive pattern and preserved systolic ejection fraction suggest the diagnosis of amyloidosis. LA, left atrium; LV, left ventricle; RV, right ventricle.

histology could produce local conduction delay and dispersion of excitability and refractoriness as an arrhythmogenic substrate. Management of patients with idiopathic LV aneurysm and VTA or SCD has several options including aneurymectomy, implantation of ICD, VT ablation, or drug treatment.[24] Echocardiographic assessment of the aneurysm size and its possible association with mitral insufficiency and global LV dysfunction can contribute to the appropriate therapeutic decision.[24]

3.1.6. Isolated noncompacted ventricular myocardium

Althought investigators have reported no cases of VTA or SCD in children with *isolated noncompacted ventricular myocardium* (INVM),[25] other reports have demonstrated that INVM can be manifested as VTA (38%[26] to 47%[27]) or SCD (13% to 18%[28,29]). Fibrosis, trabeculation, and subendocardial ischemia could contribute to produce VTA.

Echocardiographic criteria for diagnosing INVM have been proposed by Jenni et al.[30] as absence of coexisting cardiac abnormalities; end-systolic ratio of the thickness of noncompacted layer to that of compacted layer of the LV wall >2 (in the short-axis view); predominant distribution in the apical and midventricular areas; and blood flow communication between the deep intertrabecular recesses and LV cavity as shown by Color Doppler[31] (Fig. 43.4A). Noncompaction of the right ventricle is more difficult to assess by echocardiography. The use of contrast echocardiography can contribute to a better demonstration of the deep intertrabecular recesses in communication with the ventricular cavity (Fig. 43.4B).[32]

3.1.7. Congenital diseases

VT, SD, or myocardial ischemia in adult life can be the first manifestation of patients with anomalous origin of the left coronary artery[33] from the pulmonary artery. This is a congenital anomaly that may course with heart failure during the first months of life. Children with enough collateral blood from the right coronary artery can reach the adult life without symptoms for many years.

Anomalous origin of coronary arteries can be detected by echocardiography or other imaging techniques. 2D and Doppler echocardiographies can show abnormal coronary artery origin into and from the pulmonary artery and intercoronary collateral signals within the ventricular septum.[34] Transesophageal echocardiography[35] may detect coronary anomalies and can be

Figure 43.4 A: Color Doppler echocardiography in a four-chamber view shows deep trabeculations with blood flow demonstrated in the recesses *(arrows)*. **B:** Contrast echocardiography in the same plane confirms the deep trabeculations *(arrows)* that are consistent with the diagnosis of isolated noncompacted cardiomyopathy. LV, left ventricle; RV, right ventricle.

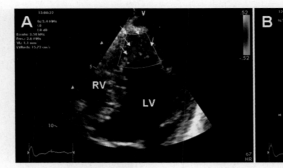

indicated when there is clinical suspicion. Nevertheless, echocardiography cannot evaluate the entire coronary artery tree as multidetector computed tomography (MDCT) or CMR (Fig. 43.5).

3.2. Magnetic resonance imaging

3.2.1. Coronary artery disease

Demonstration of myocardial ischemia by CMR can be possible using a vasodilator or dobutamine stress, and its high diagnostic accuracy for the detection of significant coronary disease has been demonstrated.[36] Indication of stress CMR is appropriate for evaluation of chest pain in patients with intermediate pretest probability of CAD, when ECG is uninterpretable or patient is enable to do exercise, or when prior tests are uninterpretable or equivocal (exercise, nuclear MPI, or stress echo).[37]

CMR imaging of gadolinium delayed enhancement (DE) provides an efficient tool to detect and quantify myocardial scar. DE may detect unrecognized myocardial scar consistent with MI, without other evidence of ischemic heart disease (Fig. 43.6) in older patients.[38] This imaging finding has demonstrated a strong association with major adverse cardiac events (MACE) including ventricular arrhythmias.[39] Some anatomic tissue heterogeneity observed in the periphery of myocardial scars is associated to an increase of the susceptibility to induction of ventricular arrhythmias in patients with prior MI and LV dysfunction.[40] When echocardiographic findings are in doubt, CMR can be chosen to rule out ventricular aneurysm in patients with history of MI and VTA or SCD.

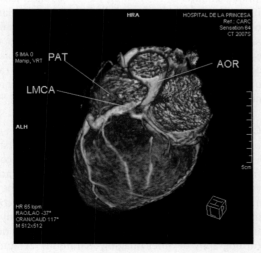

Figure 43.5 3D MDCT study of the heart where an anomalous origin of the left coronary artery from the pulmonary artery is demonstrated. AOR, aortic root; LMCA, left main coronary artery; PAT, pulmonary artery trunk.

3.2.2. Dilated cardiomyopathies and myocardial inflammation

LV and RV volumes, mass, structure, and function are well assessed by CMR as it provides high spatial resolution. CMR[41] is indicated when echocardiography does not offer accurate assessment of LV and RV functions and/or evaluation of structural changes.[1]

DE adds additional value in these patients. DE may help in distinguishing ischemic disease (Fig. 43.7) from nonischemic cardiomyopathies (Fig. 43.8).[42] The DE pattern for MI consists in hyperenhancement that always involves the subendocardium in selected segments of the ventricular wall, whereas segmental subendocardial involvement is rare in other myocardial diseases.[42,43] If delayed hyperenhancement respects the subendocardium, a nonischemic myocardial disease should be considered as the cause of the LV dysfunction.

VT could be the first manifestation of sarcoidosis without detectable systemic findings as reported by Usima et al.[44] A case report has showed a correlation between the focus of VT detected by electrophysiology induction and both the kinetic defects and DE in RV or LV walls.[45] In granulomatous diseases, both DE CMR and 18-FDG positron emission tomography (PET) can demonstrate inflammation of the ventricular wall.[46] Diagnosis of cardiac sarcoidosis in patients with ventricular arrhythmias has some therapeutic implications, since arrhythmia control includes treatment with high-dose steroids, antiarrhythmic drugs, ICD, or catheter ablation. Other cardiomyopathies secondary to inflammatory diseases such as Chagas disease may be associated to VT. DE CMR can detect focal abnormalities (Fig. 43.9). Diagnosis of acute myocarditis can often be confirmed by DE CMR (Fig. 43.10), which has a close correlation with myocardial biopsy.[47]

ARVD is characterized by fatty and fibrosis replacement of the myocardium with myocyte loss and ventricular arrythmias. It involves usually the RV, although the LV can also be affected. The diagnosis of ARVD is currently based on electrocardiographic and morphologic features as proposed by an international Task Force.[48] Anatomical criteria for diagnosis of ARVD include RV global or regional dysfunction and structural modifications that can be detected by echocardiography, angiography, or CMR.[48,49] The Task Force defines major and minor criteria. Major criteria are severe dilatation and RV dysfunction without or with mild LV involvement; localized RV aneurysms (akinetic or dyskinetic areas with diastolic bulging) and severe segmental dilatation of the RV. Minor criteria includes mild global dilatation or ejection fraction reduction of RV with normal LV; mild segmental dilatation of RV and regional RV hypokinesis. The reference method for the diagnosis of ARVD is the demonstration of fibrofatty replacement of the myocardium at either biopsy or autopsy. Original Task Force considers endomyocardial biopsy the method for demonstration of

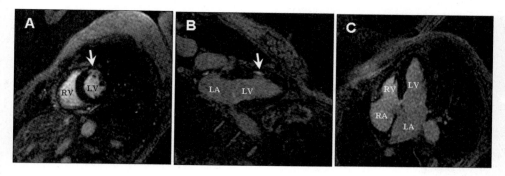

Figure 43.6 Late gadolinium enhancement CMR study in short axis (**A**), two-chamber (**B**) and four-chamber (**C**) views of the heart. A small area of subendocardial DE *(arrows)* is consistent with an unrecognized MI. LA, left atrium; LV, left ventricle; RA, right atrium; RV, right ventricle.

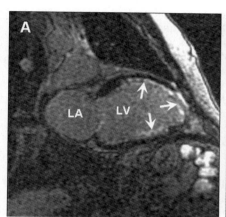
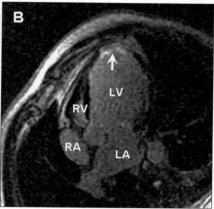

Figure 43.7 Patient with LV dysfunction. Delayed gadolinium enhancement CMR images in two- (**A**) and four- (**B**) chamber views of the heart that show subendocardial DE *(arrows)* consistent with ischemic cardiomyopathy. LA, left atrium; LV, left ventricle; RA, right atrium; RV, right ventricle.

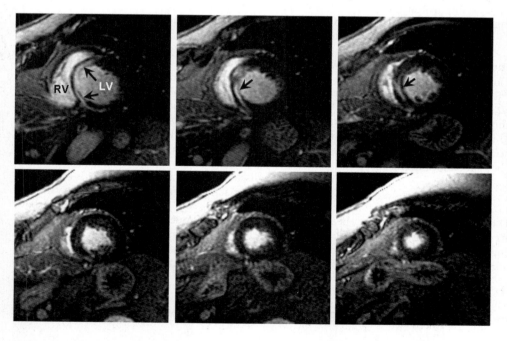

Figure 43.8 Patient with SCD and documented sustained VT. Echocardiography showed hypokinesis in the basal segment of the ventricular septum as the only finding. These images show delayed gadolinium enhancement in short-axis view of the heart from the ventricular base to the apex (from upper left to lower right figures). Spin echo images were normal for characterization of fat infiltration and acute inflammation. In this clinical context DE *(arrows)* that respects subendocardium in several areas represents nonischemic fibrotic tissue. Coronary angiography showed no significant coronary stenoses. These CMR findings suggest a previous inflammatory process such as myocarditis to be the primary disease. RV, right ventricle; LV, left ventricle.

fibrofatty replacement of the myocardium as a major criterion of ARVD. CMR can demonstrate fatty replacement of the myocardium (Fig. 43.11), although reproducibility, sensibility, and specificity for diagnosis of ARVD are limited.[50] Recent published series using CMR with DE has demonstrated fibrous infiltration of the myocardium in patients with ARVD.[51] CMR often avoids the misdiagnosis of ARVD often caused by echocardiographic imaging artefacts.[52]

3.2.3. LV dysfunction and infiltrative diseases
Diagnosis of cardiac amyloidosis by CMR is based on a DE pattern that demonstrates distribution over the entire subendocardial circumference and extend by varying degree into the neighboring myocardium (Fig. 43.12).[53] Vogelsberg et al.[54] have demonstrated that compared with myocardial biopsy this pattern has sensitivity and specificity of 80% and 94%, respectively, for diagnosing cardiac amyloidosis. They also have reported that 80% of patients

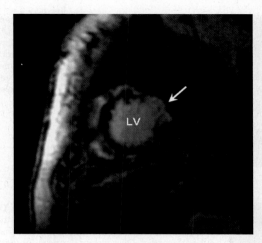

Figure 43.9 Late delayed gadolinium enhancement CMR study of a patient with LV dysfunction, nonsustained VT, positive serologic test for Trypanosoma Cruzi, and no evidence of CAD by catheterization. In the short-axis view of the heart a delayed hyperenhancement focus in the myocardium (arrow) is consistent with fibrosis in Chagas disease. LV, left ventricle.

with cardiac amyloidosis demonstrate DE in the papillary muscles. This is significantly more frequent compared with 11% in other cardiomyopathies.

The accumulation of iron in the myocardium in hemochromatosis could serve as an arrhythmogenic substrate that increases the risk for VT or SD.[55] Myocardial iron deposition can be reproducibly quantified using CMR T2* weight of the myocardium. This is a significant variable for predicting the need for treatment of ventricular dysfunction.[56]

3.2.4. Isolated noncompacted ventricular myocardium
CMR can contribute to the diagnosis of INVM[57] (Fig. 43.13) when echocardiography is unclear. A CMR ratio of noncompacted to compacted myocardium of >2.3 in diastole in any of the long-axis views may establish pathologic noncompaction, with sensitivity, specificity, positive and negative predictive values of 86%, 99%, 75%, and 99%, respectively.[58] A few reported cases of patients with INVM have described subendocardial scars using DE CMR.[59]

3.2.5. Valvular diseases
Valvular heart diseases associated to SD or VTA are usually well assessed by echocardiography. In patients with poor acoustic windows, CMR may be an alternative imaging test.[37] CMR may assess the severity of aortic stenosis by the calculation of valve area using

gradient echo sequences or by the calculation of flow velocity through the stenotic valve. Valvular regurgitation can be graded by the calculation of the regurgitant volume using phase contrast flow and steady state free precession (SSFP) LV cine sequences.

3.2.6. Congenital disorders
Patients with anomalous origin of the coronary arteries may be asymptomatic or may have an increase risk of SD. Although, CMR is indicated in patients with suspected anomalous origin of the coronary arteries[37], only few cases have reported the identification of an anomalous origin from the pulmonary artery.[60,61]

3.3. Nuclear scintigraphy
Silent ischemia detection is an objective in patients with ventricular arrhythmias who have an intermediate probability of having CHD by age, symptoms, and gender. Stress testing with nuclear MPI single-photon emission CT (SPECT) or 82-Rb or 13-N ammonia PET may be indicated when ECG is less reliable because of digoxin use, LVH, ST-segment depression at rest, WPW syndrome, or LBBB.[13] Myocardial perfusion SPECT or 18-FDG with 82-Rb PET can also be used to assess myocardial viability in patients with LV dysfunction and previous MI (Chapter 26).

Autopsy studies have demonstrated ischemic subendocardial lesions without CAD in patents with isolated noncompacted ventricular myocardium.[62] Perfusion with 13N ammonia PET and scintigraphy with thallium-201 have demonstrated transmural patchy perfusion defects and diminished coronary flow reserve in segments with noncompacted myocardium.[63]

3.4. Computed tomography
Indication of coronary angiography by CT is appropriate for evaluation of chest pain in patients with intermediate pretest probability of CAD when ECG is uninterpretable or patient is unable to exercise.[37] Nevertheless there is no incremental clinical benefit derived from imaging the coronary arteries by cardiac CT in patients with ventricular arrhythmias.[1]

VT, SD, or myocardial ischemia in adult life can be the first manifestation of patients with anomalous origin of the left coronary artery[33] from the pulmonary artery (Fig. 43.5). CT coronary angiography can demonstrate the abnormal origin of the coronary in the pulmonary artery.[64]

As previously discussed, the diagnosis of ARVD is established by the Task Force criteria. Although MDCT has not been validated for the diagnosis of ARVD, some cases of known ARVD have been reported using MDCT for detection of RV intramyocardial fat infiltration as low attenuation, increased RV trabeculation, and scalloping or enlargement of global, inlet or outflow tract RV dimensions.[65,66] Imaging artifacts can be produced by arrhythmias

Figure 43.10 DE CMR study of a patient with clinical suspicion of acute myocardis. Two-chamber (**A**) and short-axis (**B**) views show patched and subepicardial hyperenhancement in the LV inferior wall (arrows) that is typical of myocarditis. LV, left ventricle; LA, left atrium; RV, right ventricle.

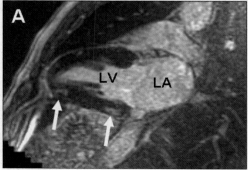
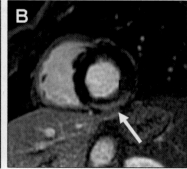

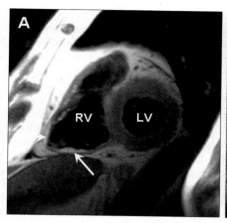
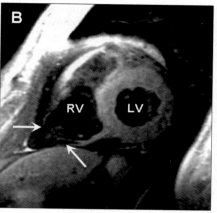

Figure 43.11 Spin echo CMR images without (**A**) and with fat suppression pulse (**B**) that show fat infiltration *(arrows)* in the RV wall in a patient with suspected arrythmogenic RV dysplasia. LV, left ventricle; RV, right ventricle.

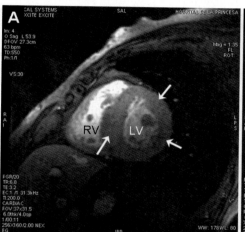
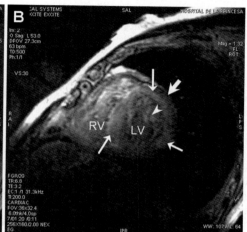

Figure 43.12 CMR short-axis views of the heart. **A:** Early enhancement of gadolinium shows homogeneous perfusion of the LV walls *(arrows)*. **B:** DE of gadolinium shows diffuse hyperhenhancement *(thin arrows)* that respects the lateral subepicardial layer *(thick arrowheads)*. The anterior papillary muscle is also hyperenhanced *(arrowhead)*. LV wall hypertrophy, preserved LV systolic function, and delayed hyperenhancement findings are consistent with cardiac amyloidosis. LV, left ventricle; RV, right ventricle.

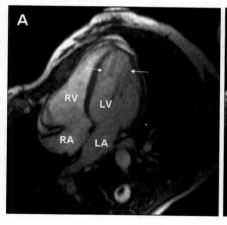
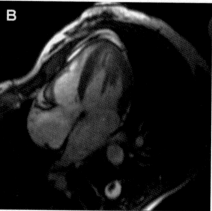

Figure 43.13 Four-chamber view of cine gradient echo CMR images in diastole (**A**) and systole (**B**) that show noncompaction in the apical segments of the left ventricle *(arrows)*. LA, left atrium; LV, left ventricle; RA, right atrium; RV, right ventricle.

or breathing motion during the CT exploration. Other causes of artifacts in the RV wall are produced by the leads and cables of pacemakers or implantable cardioverter-defibrillators.

4. SELECTING AND GUIDING THERAPY

Most of the information available about therapeutical management of VTA and SD prevention comes from patients with ischemic cardiomyopathy and, to a lesser extend, from IDCM patients. This is especially true with multicenter randomized trials. The evidence available from other less prevalent forms of SHD, such as HCM, noncompaction, or cardiac sarcoidosis, are scarce and the

therapeutical recommendations are extrapolated from the former mentioned clinical settings.

4.1. Antiarrhythmic drugs

Antiarrhythmic drugs were the only therapy for sustained VTA and for SD prevention in the past. However, the current type I antiarrhythmic drugs, such as flecainide and propafenone, are not recommended for VTA prevention in patients with SHD due to their potent myocardial depressor effects and because the Cardiac Arrhythmia Suppression Trial (CAST)[67] showed increased mortality in patients with ischemic ventricular dysfunction when treated with these drugs. Other type I antiarrhytmic drugs, such as quinidine, should when possible be avoided in patients with SHD due to the risk of facilitating polymorphic VT, especially in patients with heart failure or diuretic therapy, and because it has been associated with increased mortality. In general, type I antiarrhythmic drugs should be avoided in patients with SHD, when possible, due to their myocardial contractility depressor effect and to avoid AV block or bundle/branch block induction because His-Purkinje conduction disturbances are highly prevalent in patients with ventricular dysfunction. At the same time, type II and IV antiarrhythmic drugs—β-blockers and calcium antagonists—have been shown to be ineffective in suppressing induction and spontaneous recurrence of myocardial macroreentry VT, although, the beneficial hemodynamic effects of β-blockers in patients with SHD represent an indication for these drugs in patients with LV dysfunction. However, β-blockers and calcium antagonists should be considered first line therapy, at the same level than ablation, for idiopathic outflow tract VT and fascicular VT, respectively. In addition, β-blockers are the drugs of choice for VTA prevention in the long QT syndrome and in patient with catecholamine-induced polymorphic VT, and some type I drugs, such as quinidine or mexilitine, are often indicated to treat or prevent recurrent VTA in patients with Brugada syndrome or certain types of long QT syndrome (LQT3), respectively.

The effectiveness of type III drugs for secondary prevention of VTA in patients with SHD has been tested in several trials. The Electrophysiologic Study versus Electrocardiographic Monitoring (ESVEM) trial[68] compared the arrhythmic recurrence and outcome when antiarrhythmic therapy was selected by electrophysiological testing or Holter monitoring guidance in 486 patients with VT or VF, resuscitated from cardiac arrest or with unmonitored syncope. Antiarrhythmic drug therapy was consecutively and randomly chosen from seven compounds (imipramine, pirmenol, quinidine, procainamide, mexiletine, propafenone, and sotalol). There was a high recurrence of VTA in up to 51% of the patients at a 6-year follow-up with a mortality of 17%. Sotalol was the most effective drug with 35% VTA suppression (16% suppression for the other drugs, $p < 0.001$) at electrophysiological testing among the 234 patients evaluated. Patients on this drug showed the lowest VTA recurrence (risk ratio 0.43; $p < 0.001$) and mortality (risk ratio 0.50; $p = 0.004$) risks. However, the low suppression of inducibility and the high recurrence and mortality rates put the use of serial electrophysiological testing and Holter monitoring to select drug therapy into question, especially in patients with nonischemic cardiomyopathy in whom the reproducibility of electrophysiological and noninvasive testing is very low. The study also added further evidence against the use of type I antiarrhythmic drugs in patients with VTA and SHD.

The "Cardiac Arrest in Seattle: Conventional versus Amiodarone Drug Evaluation" (CASCADE) study[7] enrolled 228 patients with spontaneous ventricular fibrillation which was unrelated to acute MI or complex VTA. Patients were randomized to empiric amiodarone (100 to 400 mg) or to a variety of type I antiarrhythmic drugs selected by electrophysiologic testing. The study was stopped prematurely due to an unacceptable rate of VTA recurrence or death (35% at 2 years) in both groups, suggesting that VTA prevention in these patients should be by ICD implantation. Type I antiarrhythmic drug therapy was found to be an independent predictor of VTA recurrence.

According to the results of these trials, secondary prevention of VTA in SHD patients with type I antiarrhythmic drugs should be discouraged at the present time. Empiric amiodarone or electrophysiological/Holter guided sotalol is the most appropriate antiarrhythmic drug approach in such a patient. However, the low reproducibility of VT induction by electrophysiological testing in nonischemic SHD patients suggests the use of alternative therapies, such as ICD. In addition, pharmacological therapy is insufficient to reduce the mortality risk in those patients presenting with cardiac arrest.

4.2. Catheter ablation

Catheter ablation is highly effective in well defined substrates of macroreentry such as common atrial flutter or atrioventricular reentry due to accessory pathways. Ablation is less successful in other substrates, such as ventricular myocardial macroreentry, in which the circuit is less well defined and can be very complex in a 3D structure. Nevertheless, ablation feasibility has been demonstrated in selected patients with postinfarction VT because the arrhythmogenic area can be confined to a particular cardiac region. However, the frequent observation of persistent induction of other VT morphologies and the positive prognostic results of ICD for primary SD prevention in this population has limited the use of catheter ablation in ischemic cardiomyopathy. The situation is even more complex in nonischemic cardiomyopathy in which the substrate is poorly defined and not confined to a particular cardiac region. This would probably explain the paucity of publications on ablation in nonischemic cardiomyopathy. More recently, more aggressive approaches, consisting of the creation of lines of conduction block between the re-entrant circuit and an anatomical obstacle or normal myocardium by radiofrequency application, has been proposed as an alternative to focal radiofrequency application in patients with recurrent VT and frequent ICD discharges. At follow-up, most patients had a significant reduction of VT episodes. Therefore, at the present time, catheter ablation should be considered an adjunctive therapy to drugs, ICD, or both, in selected patients with SHD and incessant or frequent episodes of refractory VT.[1]

On the contrary, idiopathic VT has a fairly well defined arrhythmogenic substrate, which can be ablated with reasonable success rate around 90% and both with low recurrence and complication rates. Therefore, this therapeutic option should be offered to the patient from the first line. In addition, bundle-branch reentry VT is commonly seen in cardioskeletal muscular diseases, specially in myotonic dystrophy, and this VTA mechanism can be easily cured by ablation of the right bundle branch of the His bundle.

Finally, it is important to mention that small reports have shown the feasibility to ablate ventricular fibrillation, both in patients without and with SHD. The approach used is to target those PVCs which trigger ventricular fibrillation, rather than the arrhythmia maintaining substrate. Nevertheless, the risk of arrhythmia recurrence is not negligible and has restricted this indication to those patients with frequent ICD discharges despite antiarrhythmic drugs.

4.3. Surgical ablation

Surgical experience in ablation of VT is limited and most of the times based on isolated case reports for most VTA substrates. This therapy appears less successful for VT in patients with IDCM than in patients with ischemic heart disease, similar to that seen in catheter ablation. Nevertheless, coronary revascularization and heart transplantation are good alternatives for specific patients, like with the latter for those with end-stage SHD and recurrent VT.

4.4. Implantable cardioverter/defibrillator

ICD has been established as an accepted therapy for SD recurrence prevention and for certain types of sustained VT independent of the cause. Multicenter trials studying the role of ICD for secondary prevention of sustained VT have included patients with both ischemic and nonischemic cardiomyopathies. The first of these trials was the AVID trial,[5] which studied 1,016 patients resuscitated from near fatal ventricular fibrillation or tachycardia, with syncopal VT, or with severe LV dysfunction (ejection fraction of 40% or less) plus poorly tolerated VT. Patients were randomized to ICD implantation or to class III antiarrhythmic drugs (amiodarone in 96% of the patients). Survival was significantly ($p < 0.02$) better in the ICD group (75% vs. 64% at a 3-year follow-up). According to this trial, ICD should be implanted in SHD patients presenting with poorly tolerated VTA. Subsequently, two other trials published (The Canadian Implantable Defibrillator Study (CIDS) and the Cardiac Arrest Hamburg Study)[69,70] found a trend but no significant differences in overall survival between ICD and antiarrhythmic drugs in a similar population. Several reasons have been discussed to explain the differences in outcomes between the AVID trial and the other two, but the most plausible is the difference in sample sizes. Subanalysis of the CIDS and AVID trials found that the benefit of ICD was concentrated on patients with severe LV dysfunction. No benefit was detected in those with mild degrees of LV dysfunction. To date, no trial has studied the effect on survival of ICD, drugs, or no antiarrhythmic therapy in patients with well-tolerated sustained VT. However, the practice of ICD implantation is well established for patients with SHD, especially if they have ventricular dysfunction.

SCD primary prevention by ICD implantation has become an accepted practice in recent years. This has been extensively proved for ischemic cardiomyopathy patients (MADIT I and II trials, MUSTT trial).[71–73] However, the evidences is less compelling for nonischemic VT with trials showing either significant benefits (COMPANION, SCD-HeFT)[74,75] or no statistically significant differences of ICD compared with medical treatment (AMIOVIRT, CAT, DEFINITE).[76–78] Nevertheless ICD is recommended in patients with severe LV dysfunction and NYHA II-III functional class despite optimal medical treatment.[1] Evidence for SD primary prevention by ICD in arrythmogenic right ventricular cardiomyopathy (ARVC) and HCM patients are less solid and mostly based in expert consensus, which considers severe RV dilatation and dysfunction and LV involvement for the former and severe LV hypertrophy for the latter as risks factor supporting ICD implantation in addition to other risk factors.[1]

5. IMAGING AND PROGNOSIS

The assessment of LVEF by echocardiography or other imaging techniques provides information for the management and the prognosis of some group of patients with VTA or SCD.

Low LVEF is used to identify high-risk patients for selecting therapy to prevent sudden arrhythmic death, although most SCDs occur in patients with normal LVEF.[12] Prognosis of patients with nonsustained VT and LV dysfunction is worst compared with those with normal structural heart. The accuracy of LVEF noninvasive assessment is better for CMR[79] and radionuclide angiography (RNA) than for echocardiography,[12] although the latter is more widely utilized. RNA or CMR could be considered for LVEF assessment when echocardiography has poor acoustic windows. Although hemodynamically well-tolerated VT is associated with good prognosis in patients without SHD, it can also occur in patients with severe LV dysfunction. In asymptomatic patients with previous history of MI and current LVEF of ≤40%, there is a reasonable evidence for the indication of electrophysiology testing[1] as the frequency for induction of sustained VT is

high.[80] MADIT has demonstrated a relationship between EF and the inducibility of sustained VT in this group of patients.[81] The risk of SCD is more related to the underlying SHD and its severity than to the frequency or type of ventricular arrhythmias.[82] There is higher risk of SCD related to LV dysfunction in patients with previous MI and NSVT.[80] The assessment of size and morphology of myocardial scars or fibrosis as detected by DE CMR provides information on susceptibility to VTA in nonischemic dilated cardiomyopathy[83] as well as in patients with CAD.[84] Conversely, electrophysiologic testing for inducting VT has a low yield in dilated cardiomyopathies.[85] The prognostic value of stress CMR has been tested in 513 patients with known or suspected CAD.[86] An abnormal perfusion or a dobutamine stress CMR is an independent predictor that helps to identify patients at high risk for cardiac death or MI at 3 years of follow-up.

The identification of large ventricular aneurysms secondary to MI by echocardiography or CMR has prognostic consideration as they are associated to VTA. Resection of arrhythmogenic ventricular aneurisms may reduce or eliminate the associated ventricular arrhythmias and it can improve LV function in selected patients.[87]

Echocardiography and CMR may contribute to the risk evaluation in patients with HCM as LV hypertrophy with wall thickness ≥30 mm is considered as a major risk factor for VT or SCD. Other risk factors are prior cardiac arrest or spontaneously sustained VT; family history of premature or multiple HCM-related deaths; unexplained syncope; repetitive NSVT; and hypotensive blood pressure response during exercise test.[12] It is suggested that LV outflow dynamic gradient ≥30 mm Hg at rest assessed by Doppler echocardiography can be considered a minor risk factor for SCD in HCM.[88] Evidence of LV hypertrophy in patients with hypertension and without HCM is also associated with a higher rate of SCD.[89] Assessment of myocardial ischemia with ECG exercise testing, SPECT MPI, echocardiography, and CMR has proved to be difficult in patients with HCM.[12] The results of these tests as well as positron electron tomography have not showed a relationship with SCD risk. DE CMR can detect LV intramyocardial fibrosis in patients with HCM. Although the extent of hyperenhancement has been associated with progressive ventricular dilation and other markers of SCD[90], there are no significant differences in DE between patients with and without NSVT.[91]

Patients with asymptomatic severe aortic stenosis have 1% per year risk of SD.[92] Asymptomatic patients with severe aortic stenosis could have diverse ages, aortic valve velocities, and aortic valve areas. Abnormal exercise test results have shown to predict higher risk for SD in a series of 66 asymptomatic patients.[93] Exercise Doppler echocardiography in asymptomatic aortic stenosis has also been tested for its prognostic value.[94] An increase in mean pressure gradient by ≥18 mm Hg is associated with higher risk of cardiovascular events, including two cases of SD.[94] These findings are independent of the resting data of stenosis severity and independent of ECG changes induced by exercise.

6. FUTURE DIRECTIONS

Imaging technologies are continuously progressing. The 3D capability of tomography techniques such as CT and magnetic resonance imaging (MRI) allows for image guided electrophysiological testing and ablation procedures. Further studies need to evaluate the potential role of 3D echocardiography in this setting. The echocardiography assessment of LV diastolic or occult systolic dysfunction by 3D has to be validated in patients with SCD or VTA in order to detect early SHD.

MDCT technology is achieving lower radiation and better temporal resolution. These two advances will allow risk reduction and a better probability to obtain accurate images of the coronary arteries. The MDCT capability to detect myocardial scar and perfusion defects could play a future role in the assessment of MI or cardiomyopathies.

CMR has extended its indications, since DE and stress procedures have been applied to clinical practice. Myocardium characterization using DE CMR and T2 edema-weighted images would be a promising area for research which might provide both prognostic information for VTA or SCD and data to guide the ablation procedures in patients with MI and cardiomyopathies. CMR angiography for coronary evaluation is possible but its indications are under research. More advances are needed for a routine clinical use of CMR coronary angiography. Molecular MRI uses targeted contrast agents that usually are based in gadolinium or ultrasmall particles of iron oxide (USPIO). This technique has been demonstrated to be useful as a research tool for animal models of cardiovascular diseases. Its use in clinical practice may need long time until contrast agents could be tested enough in order to avoid human side effects.

Nuclear cardiology could play a role for molecular imaging in human. 18-FDG is a well known radiotracer used in clinical routine for molecular imaging of glucose. Future possible use of radiotracers based in ^{11}C could open new possibilities for molecular imaging of targeted aminoacids or peptides that could predict VTA. A large multicenter study is currently evaluating the use of metaiodobenzylguanidine (MIBG) as a maker of β-receptor density in heart failure density. Preliminary reports suggest that demonstration of reduced β-receptor density by this technique is associated with higher risk of VTA and SCD.

Multimodality imaging could take advantage of complementary techniques such as PET/CMR or PET/CT. CMR and CT offer better spatial and temporal resolution, whereas PET offers higher sensitivity for assessing metabolism and perfusion. The combination of both data in integrated and compressive images could take advantages to improve the accuracy of PET to detect small metabolic defects.

REFERENCES

1. Zipes DP, Camm AJ, Borggrefe M, et al. ACC/AHA/ESC 2006 guidelines for management of patients with ventricular arrhythmias and the prevention of sudden cardiac death: A report of the American College of Cardiology/American Heart Association Task Force and the European Society of Cardiology Committee for Practice Guidelines. *J Am Coll Cardiol*. 2006;48:e247–e346.
2. de Vreede-Swagemakers JJ, Gorgels AP, Dubois-Arbouw WI, et al. Out-of-hospital cardiac arrest in the 1990's: A population-based study in the Maastricht area on incidence, characteristics and survival. *J Am Coll Cardiol*. 1997;30:1500–1505.
3. Myerburg RJ, Kessler KM, Castellanos A. Sudden cardiac death: Epidemiology, transient risk, and intervention assessment. *Ann Intern Med*. 1993;119:1187–1197.
4. Mitchell LB, Pineda EA, Titus JL, et al. Sudden death in patients with implantable cardioverter defibrillators: The importance of post-shock electromechanical dissociation. *J Am Coll Cardiol*. 2002;39:1323–1328.
5. The Antiarrhythmics versus Implantable Defibrillators (AVID) Investigators. A comparison of antiarrhythmic-drug therapy with implantable defibrillators in patients resuscitated from near-fatal ventricular arrhythmias. *N Engl J Med*. 1997;337:1576–1583.
6. Anderson JL, Hallstrom AP, Epstein AE, et al. Design and results of the antiarrhythmics vs implantable defibrillators (AVID) registry. The AVID Investigators. *Circulation*. 1999;99:1692–1699.
7. Greene HL. The CASCADE Study: Randomized antiarrhythmic drug therapy in survivors of cardiac arrest in Seattle. CASCADE Investigators. *Am J Cardiol*. 1993;72:70F–74F.
8. Aguilera B, Suarez Mier MP, Morentin B. Arrhythmogenic cardiomyopathy as cause of sudden death in Spain. Report of 21 cases. *Rev Esp Cardiol*. 1999;52:656–662.
9. Merino JL, Carmona JR, Fernandez-Lozano I, et al. Mechanisms of sustained ventricular tachycardia in myotonic dystrophy: Implications for catheter ablation. *Circulation*. 1998;98:541–546.
10. Merino JL, Peinado R, Sobrino JA. Sudden death in myotonic dystrophy: The potential role of bundle-branch reentry. *Circulation*. 2000;101:E73.
11. Merino JL, Jimenez-Borreguero J, Peinado R, et al. Unipolar mapping and magnetic resonance imaging of "idiopathic" right ventricular outflow tract ectopy. *J Cardiovasc Electrophysiol*. 1998;9:84–87.
12. Goldberger JJ, Cain ME, Hohnloser SH, et al. American Heart Association; American College of Cardiology Foundation; Heart Rhythm Society. American Heart Association/American College of Cardiology Foundation/Heart Rhythm Society scientific statement on noninvasive risk stratification techniques for identifying patients at risk for sudden cardiac death: a scientific statement from the American Heart Association Council on Clinical Cardiology Committee on Electrocardiography and Arrhythmias and Council on Epidemiology and Prevention. *Circulation*. 2008;118:1497–1518.
13. Douglas PS, Khandheria B, Stainback RF, et al. ACCF/ASE/ACEP/AHA/ASNC/SCAI/SCCT/SCMR 2008 appropriateness criteria for stress echocardiography. *Circulation*. 2008;117:1478–1497.
14. Meisel SR, Mazur A, Chetboun I, et al. Usefulness of implantable cardioverter-defibrillators in refractory variant angina pectoris complicated by ventricular fibrillation in patients with angiographically normal coronary arteries. *Am J Cardiol*. 2002;89:1114–1116.
15. Seniuk W, Mularek-Kubadela T, Grygier M, et al. Cardiac arrest related to coronary spasm in patients with variant angina: A three-case study. *J Intern Med*. 2002;252:368–376.
16. Pálinkás A, Picano E, Rodriguez O, et al. Safety of ergot stress echocardiography for non-invasive detection of coronary vasospasm. *Coron Artery Dis*. 2001;12:649–654.
17. Sorgato A, Faggiano P, Aurigemma GP, et al. Ventricular arrhythmias in adult aortic stenosis: Prevalence, mechanisms, and clinical relevance. *Chest*. 1998;113:482–491.
18. Pellikka PA, Sarano ME, Nishimura RA, et al. Outcome of 622 adults with asymptomatic, hemodynamically significant aortic stenosis during prolonged follow-up. *Circulation*. 2005;111:3290.
19. Priori SG, Aliot E, Blomstrom-Lundqvist C, et al. Task force on sudden cardiac death of the European Society of Cardiology. *Eur Heart J*. 2001;22:1374–1450.
20. Cooper LT, Berry GJ, Shabetai R. For the Multicenter Giant Cell Myocarditis Study Group Investigators. Idiopathic giant-cell myocarditis: Natural history and treatment. *N Engl J Med*. 1997;336:1860–1866.
21. Kawai C. From myocarditis to cardiomyopathy: Mechanisms of inflammation and cell death: Learning from the past for the future. *Circulation*. 1999;99:1091–1100.
22. Picano E, Pinamonti B, Ferdeghini EM, et al. Two-dimensional echocardiography in myocardial amyloidosis. *Echocardiography*. 1991;8:253–259.
23. Paul M, Schäfers M, Grude M, et al. Idiopathic left ventricular aneurysm and sudden cardiac death in young adults. *Europace*. 2006;8:607–612.
24. Rajasinghe HA, Lorenz HP, Longaker MT, et al. Arrhythmogenic ventricular aneurysms unrelated to coronary artery disease. *Ann Thorac Surg*. 1995;59:1079–1084.
25. Ichida F, Hamanichi Y, Miyawaki T, et al. Clinical features of isolated noncompaction of the ventricular myocardium: Long-term clinical course, hemodynamic properties, and genetic background. *J Am Coll Cardiol*. 1999;34:233–240.
26. Chin TK, Perloff JK, Williams RG, et al. Isolated noncompaction of left ventricular myocardium: A study of eight cases. *Circulation*. 1990;82:507–513.
27. Ritter M, Oechslin E, Sütsch G, et al. Isolated noncompaction of the myocardium in adults. *Mayo Clin Proc*. 1997;72:26–31.
28. Chin TK, Perloff JK, Williams RG, et al. Isolated noncompaction of left ventricular myocardium: A study of eight cases. *Circulation*. 1990;82:507–513.
29. Oechslin E, Attenhofer Jost CH, Rojas JR, et al. Longterm follow-up of 34 adults with isolated left ventricular noncompaction. A distinct cardiomyopathy with poor prognosis. *J Am Coll Cardiol*. 2000;36(2):493–500.
30. Jenni R, Oechslin E, Schneider J, et al. Echocardiographic and pathoanatomical characteristics of isolated left ventricular noncompaction: A step towards classification as a distinct cardiomyopathy. *Heart*. 2001;86:666–671.
31. Chrissoheris MP, Ali R, Vivas Y, et al. Isolated noncompaction of the ventricular myocardium: Contemporary diagnosis and management. *Clin Cardiol*. 2007;30:156–160.
32. Agmon Y, Connolly HM, Olson LJ, et al. Noncompaction of the ventricular myocardium. *J Am Soc Echocardiogr*. 1999;12:859–863.
33. Angelini P, Velasco JA, Flamm S. Coronary anomalies: Incidence, pathophysiology, and clinical relevance. *Circulation*. 2002;105:2449–2454.
34. Yang YL, Nanda NC, Wang XF, et al. Echocardiographic diagnosis of anomalous origin of the left coronary artery from the pulmonary artery. *Echocardiography*. 2007;24:405–411.
35. Fernandes F, Alam M, Smith S, et al. The role of transesophageal echocardiography in identifying anomalous coronary arteries. *Circulation*. 1993;88:2532–2540.
36. Paetsch I, Jahnke C, Wahl A, et al. Comparison of dobutamine stress magnetic resonance, adenosine stress magnetic resonance, and adenosine stress magnetic resonance perfusion. *Circulation*. 2004;110:835–842.
37. Hendel RC, Patel MR, Kramer CM, et al. ACCF/ACR/SCCT/SCMR/ASNC/NASCI/SCAI/SIR 2006 appropriateness criteria for cardiac computed tomography and cardiac magnetic resonance imaging. *J Am Coll Cardiol*. 2006;48:1475–1497.
38. Barbier CE, Bjerner T, Johansson L, et al. Myocardial scars more frequent than expected: Magnetic resonance imaging detects potential risk group. *J Am Coll Cardiol*. 2006;48:765–771.
39. Kwong RY, Sattar H, Wu H, et al. Incidence and prognostic implication of unrecognized myocardial scar characterized by cardiac magnetic resonance in

diabetic patients without clinical evidence of myocardial infarction. *Circulation.* 2008;118:1011–1020.

40. Schmidt A, Azevedo CF, Cheng A, et al. Infarct tissue heterogeneity by magnetic resonance imaging identifies enhanced cardiac arrhythmia susceptibility in patients with left ventricular dysfunction. *Circulation.* 2007;115:2006–2014.

41. Grothues F, Smith GC, Moon JC, et al. Comparison of interstudy reproducibility of cardiovascular magnetic resonance with two-dimensional echocardiography in normal subjects and in patients with heart failure or left ventricular hypertrophy. *Am J Cardiol.* 2002;90:29–34.

42. McCrohon JA, Moon JC, Prasad SK, et al. Differentiation of heart failure related to dilated cardiomyopathy and coronary artery disease using gadolinium-enhanced cardiovascular magnetic resonance. *Circulation.* 2003;108:54–59.

43. Bello D, Shah DJ, Farah GM, et al. Gadolinium cardiovascular magnetic resonance predicts reversible myocardial dysfunction and remodeling in patients with heart failure undergoing beta-blocker therapy. *Circulation.* 2003;108:1945–1953.

44. Uusimaa P, Ylitalo K, Anttonen O, et al. Ventricular tachyarrhythmia as a primary presentation of sarcoidosis. *Europace.* 2008;10:760–766.

45. Redheuil AB, Paziaud O, Mousseaux E. Ventricular tachycardia and cardiac sarcoidosis: Correspondence between MRI and electrophysiology. *Eur Heart J.* 2006;27:1430.

46. Pandya C, Brunken RC, Tchou P, et al. Detecting cardiac involvement in sarcoidosis: A call for prospective studies of newer imaging techniques. *Eur Respir J.* 2007;29:418–422.

47. Mahrholdt H, Goedecke C, Wagner A, et al. Cardiovascular magnetic resonance assessment of human myocarditis: A comparison to histology and molecular pathology. *Circulation.* 2004;109:1250–1258.

48. McKenna WJ, Thiene G, Nava A, et al. Diagnosis of arrhythmogenic right ventricular dysplasia/cardiomyopathy. *Br Heart J.* 1994;71:215–218.

49. Corrado D, Fontaine G, Marcus FI, et al. Arrhythmogenic right ventricular dysplasia/cardiomyopathy: Need for an international registry. *Circulation.* 2000;101:e101–e106.

50. Tandri H, Castillo E, Ferrari VA, et al. Magnetic resonance imaging of arrhythmogenic right ventricular dysplasia: Sensitivity, specificity, and observer variability of fat detection versus functional analysis of the right ventricle. *J Am Coll Cardiol.* 2006;48:2277–2284.

51. Tandri H, Saranathan M, Rodriguez ER, et al. Noninvasive detection of myocardial fibrosis in arrhythmogenic right ventricular cardiomyopathy using delayed-enhancement magnetic resonance imaging. *J Am Coll Cardiol.* 2005;45:98–103.

52. Bomma C, Rutberg J, Tandri H, et al. Misdiagnosis of arrhythmogenic right ventricular dysplasia/cardiomyopathy. *J Cardiovasc Electrophysiol.* 2004;15:300–306.

53. Maceira AM, Joshi J, Prasad SK, et al. Cardiovascular magnetic resonance in cardiac amyloidosis. *Circulation.* 2005;111:186–193.

54. Vogelsberg H, Mahrholdt H, Deluigi CC, et al. Cardiovascular magnetic resonance in clinically suspected cardiac amyloidosis: Noninvasive imaging compared to endomyocardial biopsy. *J Am Coll Cardiol.* 2008;51:1022–1030.

55. Roest M, van der Schouw YT, de Valk B, et al. Heterozygosity for a hereditary hemochromatosis gene is associated with cardiovascular death in women. *Circulation.* 1999;100:1268–1273.

56. Anderson LJ, Holden S, Davis B, et al. Cardiovascular T2-star (T2*) magnetic resonance for the early diagnosis of myocardial iron overload. *Eur Heart J.* 2001;22:2171–2179.

57. Borreguero LJ, Corti R, de Soria RF, et al. Images in cardiovascular medicine. Diagnosis of isolated noncompaction of the myocardium by magnetic resonance imaging. *Circulation.* 2002;105:e177–e178.

58. Petersen SE, Selvanayagam JB, Wiesmann F, et al. Left ventricular non-compaction: Insights from cardiovascular magnetic resonance imaging. *J Am Coll Cardiol.* 2005;46:101–105.

59. Korcyk D, Edwards CC, Armstrong G, et al. Contrast-enhanced cardiac magnetic resonance in a patient with familial isolated ventricular non-compaction. *J Cardiovasc Magn Reson.* 2004;6:569–576.

60. Mesurolle B, Qanadli SD, Merad M, et al. Anomalous origin of the left coronary artery arising from the pulmonary trunk: Report of an adult case with long-term follow-up after surgery. *Eur Radiol.* 1999;9:1570–1573.

61. Su JT, Krishnamurthy R, Chung T, et al. Anomalous right coronary artery from the pulmonary artery: Noninvasive diagnosis and serial evaluation. *J Cardiovasc Magn Reson.* 2007;9:57–61.

62. Jenni R, Wyss CA, Oechslin EN, et al. Isolated ventricular noncompaction is associated with coronary microcirculatory dysfunction. *J Am Coll Cardiol.* 2002;39:450–454.

63. Weiford BC, Subbarao VD, Mulhern KM. Noncompaction of the ventricular myocardium. *Circulation.* 2004;109:2965–2971.

64. Waite S, Ng T, Afari A, et al. CT diagnosis of isolated anomalous origin of the RCA arising from the main pulmonary artery. *J Thorac Imaging.* 2008;23: 145–147.

65. Kantarci M, Bayraktutan U, Sevimli S, et al. Multidetector computed tomography findings of arrhythmogenic right ventricular dysplasia: A case report. *Heart Surg Forum.* 2008;11(1):E56–E58.

66. Bomma C, Dalal D, Tandri H, et al. Evolving role of multidetector computed tomography in evaluation of arrhythmogenic right ventricular dysplasia cardiomyopathy. *Am J Cardiol.* 2007;100:99–105.

67. Ruskin JN. The cardiac arrhythmia suppression trial (CAST). *N Engl J Med.* 1989;321:386–388.

68. Klein RC. Comparative efficacy of sotalol and class I antiarrhythmic agents in patients with ventricular tachycardia or fibrillation: Results of the Electrophysiology Study Versus Electrocardiographic Monitoring (ESVEM) Trial. *Eur Heart J.* 1993;14(suppl H):78–84.

69. Connolly SJ, Gent M, Roberts RS, et al. Canadian implantable defibrillator study (CIDS): A randomized trial of the implantable cardioverter defibrillator against amiodarone. *Circulation.* 2000;101:1297–1302.

70. Kuck KH, Cappato R, Siebels J, et al. Randomized comparison of antiarrhythmic drug therapy with implantable defibrillators in patients resuscitated from cardiac arrest: The Cardiac Arrest Study Hamburg (CASH). *Circulation.* 2000;102:748–754.

71. Moss AJ, Hall WJ, Cannom DS, et al. Improved survival with an implanted defibrillator in patients with coronary disease at high risk for ventricular arrhythmia. Multicenter Automatic Defibrillator Implantation Trial Investigators. *N Engl J Med.* 1996;335:1933–1940.

72. Moss AJ, Zareba W, Hall WJ, et al. Prophylactic implantation of a defibrillator in patients with myocardial infarction and reduced ejection fraction. *N Engl J Med.* 2002;346:877–883.

73. Buxton AE, Lee KL, Fisher JD, et al. A randomized study of the prevention of sudden death in patients with coronary artery disease. Multicenter Unsustained Tachycardia Trial Investigators. *N Engl J Med.* 1999;341:1882–1890.

74. Lindenfeld J, Feldman AM, Saxon L, et al. Effects of cardiac resynchronization therapy with or without a defibrillator on survival and hospitalizations in patients with New York Heart Association class IV heart failure. *Circulation.* 2007;115:204–212.

75. Bardy GH, Lee KL, Mark DB, et al. Amiodarone or an implantable cardioverter-defibrillator for congestive heart failure. *N Engl J Med.* 2005;352:225–237.

76. Strickberger SA, Hummel JD, Bartlett TG, et al. Amiodarone versus implantable cardioverter-defibrillator: Randomized trial in patients with nonischemic dilated cardiomyopathy and asymptomatic nonsustained ventricular tachycardia—AMIOVIRT. *J Am Coll Cardiol.* 2003;41:1707–1712.

77. Bansch D, Antz M, Boczor S, et al. Primary prevention of sudden cardiac death in idiopathic dilated cardiomyopathy: The Cardiomyopathy Trial (CAT). *Circulation.* 2002;105:1453–1458.

78. Kadish A, Dyer A, Daubert JP, et al. Prophylactic defibrillator implantation in patients with nonischemic dilated cardiomyopathy. *N Engl J Med.* 2004;350:2151–2158.

79. Bellenger NG, Davies LC, Francis JM, et al. Reduction in sample size for studies of remodeling in heart failure by the use of cardiovascular magnetic resonance. *J Cardiovasc Magn Reson.* 2000;2:271–278.

80. Schmitt C, Barthel P, Ndrepepa G, et al. Value of programmed ventricular stimulation for prophylactic internal cardioverterdefibrillator implantation in postinfarction patients preselected by noninvasive risk stratifiers. *J Am Coll Cardiol.* 2001;37:1901–1907.

81. Huikuri HV, Castellanos A, Myerburg RJ. Sudden death due to cardiac arrhythmias. *N Engl J Med.* 2001;345:1473–1482.

82. Nazarian S, Bluemke DA, Lardo AC, et al. Magnetic resonance assessment of the substrate for inducible ventricular tachycardia in nonischemic cardiomyopathy. *Circulation.* 2005;112:2821–2825.

83. Turitto G, Ahuja RK, Caref EB, et al. Risk stratification for arrhythmic events in patients with nonischemic dilated cardiomyopathy and nonsustained ventricular tachycardia: Role of programmed ventricular stimulation and the signal-averaged electrocardiogram. *J Am Coll Cardiol.* 1994;24:1523–1528.

84. Kannel WB, Thomas HE Jr. Sudden coronary death: The Framingham Study. *Ann N Y Acad Sci.* 1982;382:3–21.

85. Cannom DS, Prystowsky EN. Management of ventricular arrhythmias: Detection, drugs, and devices. *JAMA.* 1999;281:172–179.

86. Moon JC, McKenna WJ, McCrohon JA, et al. Toward clinical risk assessment in hypertrophic cardiomyopathy with gadolinium cardiovascular magnetic resonance. *J Am Coll Cardiol.* 2003;41:1561–1567.

87. Buxton AE, Lee KL, DiCarlo L, et al. Electrophysiologic testing to identify patients with coronary artery disease who are at risk for sudden death. Multicenter Unsustained Tachycardia Trial Investigators. *N Engl J Med.* 2000;342:1937–1945.

88. Bello D, Fieno DS, Kim RJ, et al. Infarct morphology identifies patients with substrate for sustained ventricular tachycardia. *J Am Coll Cardiol.* 2005;45:1104–1108.

89. Dimitrow PP, Klimeczek P, Vliegenthart R, et al. Late hyperenhancement in gadolinium-enhanced magnetic resonance imaging: Comparison of hypertrophic cardiomyopathy patients with and without nonsustained ventricular tachycardia. *Int J Cardiovasc Imaging.* 2008;24:77–83.

90. Milner PG, Dimarco JP, Lerman BB. Electrophysiological evaluation of sustained ventricular tachyarrhythmias in idiopathic dilated cardiomyopathy. *Pacing Clin Electrophysiol.* 1988;11:562–568.

91. Jahnke C, Nagel E, Gebker R, et al. Prognostic value of cardiac magnetic resonance stress tests: Adenosine stress perfusion and dobutamine stress wall motion imaging. *Circulation.* 2007;115:1769–1776.

92. Pellikka PA, Sarano ME, Nishimura RA, et al. Outcome of 622 adults with asymptomatic, hemodynamically significant aortic stenosis during prolonged follow-up. *Circulation.* 2005;111:3290–3295.

93. Amato MC, Moffa PJ, Werner KE, et al. Treatment decision in asymptomatic aortic valve stenosis: Role of exercise testing. *Heart.* 2001;86:381–386.

94. Lancellotti P, Lebois F, Simon M, et al. Prognostic importance of quantitative exercise Doppler echocardiography in asymptomatic valvular aortic stenosis. *Circulation.* 2005;112:I377–1382.

Atrioventricular, Intraventricular, and Interventricular Dyssynchrony

44

Avi Fischer
W. Lane Duvall

1. INTRODUCTION

Since the 1990s, studies have consistently demonstrated that cardiac resynchronization therapy (CRT) improves cardiac outcomes in patients with advanced congestive heart failure (HF), reduced left ventricular ejection fraction (LVEF), and an intrinsic conduction delay.[1,2] The underlying mechanisms of the beneficial effects of CRT have not been fully elucidated, but appear to be related to restored coordination of left and right ventricular (RV) contraction and relaxation.[2,3] The widespread acceptance of CRT has renewed interests in the evaluation and understanding of the mechanical effects associated with changes in atrioventricular (AV), interventricular, and intraventricular conduction.

2. PATHOPHYSIOLOGY

2.1. Normal conductive properties of the heart

Truly "physiologic" pacing maintains the normal sequence of atrial and ventricular activation by a complex and carefully choreographed affair. The coupling of excitation and contraction results in atrial activation followed by atrial contraction and ventricular activation that is followed by ventricular contraction. AV nodal tissue conducts impulses at a rate of approximately 1.3 to 1.7 m/s.[4] It takes approximately 80 ms for impulses to travel from the atrial side of the AV node to the ventricular side. This delay allows for optimal ventricular filling. Endocardial activation of the right ventricle starts near the insertion of the anterior papillary muscle approximately 10 ms after the onset of left ventricular (LV) activation. Activation occurs from apex to base in the septum and ventricular free walls. Depolarization occurs from endocardium to epicardium in a tangential and centrifugal fashion. Overall, the posterobasal segment of the left ventricle is the last portion of the heart to depolarize.

After isovolumic ventricular contraction, the aortic valve opens and the ejection phase occurs. As the pressure gradient across the aortic valve is greatest in the early portion of the ejection phase, emptying velocity is highest during this period. As the LV–aortic pressure gradient becomes increasingly negative, the aortic valve closes and isovolumic relaxation begins. Due to filling of the atrium during ventricular systole (when the mitral valve is open), atrial pressure is high. Coupled with a rapid decline in LV pressure, a positive AV pressure gradient is present during the early filling phase reflected by a large E-wave. As the pressure gradients reverse, as a result of atrial relaxation and ventricular contraction, the mitral valve closes. The importance of proper timing of atrial and ventricular contraction is a crucial determinant of pump function and cardiac output.

2.2. Dyssynchrony

HF may be caused by myocardial dysfunction or valvular dysfunction individually or in combination. Ventricular dyssynchrony has been proposed as a functional manifestation of HF.[5] Dyssynchrony has three major components: (a) electrical dyssynchrony consisting of interventricular or intraventricular conduction delays typically manifested as left bundle branch block (LBBB), (b) structural dyssynchrony consisting of disruption of myocardial collagen matrix impairing electrical conduction and mechanical efficiency, and (c) mechanical dyssynchrony consisting of regional wall motion abnormalities resulting in increased workload and stress, thereby compromising ventricular mechanics. Ventricular dyssynchrony has deleterious effects on cardiac function by reducing diastolic filling time,[6] diminishing the force of contraction,[7] increasing mitral regurgitation,[7] and causing postsystolic regional contraction.[8] The effects of ventricular dyssynchrony and CRT on the tissue level and molecular level are unknown.[9]

2.2.1. AV dyssynchrony

The importance of an appropriately timed atrial contraction in maintaining optimal cardiac output is well established, and because this interval influences both ventricular filling and closure of the AV valve, it is a determinant of ventricular performance. Atrial contraction precedes ventricular contraction allowing for the "atrial kick" contributing up as much as 20% of the filling volume of the ventricles. Optimally, atrial contraction must coincide with late diastole to produce maximal filling of the ventricle prior to the onset of ventricular systole. As a result of alterations in the timing of atrial conduction, primarily affecting the left atrium, LV filling may be reduced. A long PR interval will lead to fusion of early and late filling and a short PR interval, to suppression of atrial filling by the start of ventricular contraction.

2.2.2. V-V dyssynchrony

Mechanical activation of the ventricles depends on the rapid spread of electric signals via the His-Purkinje system that course through both ventricles. Normal activation occurs from the endocardium to the epicardium as well as from the apex to the base, and is nearly coincident in all regions of the left ventricle. In patients with LBBB, the total activation of the LV is prolonged with delayed activation and contraction of the lateral wall. In patients with HF, LV activation and contraction become dyssynchronous with regions of early and late contraction due to slowed or blocked conduction.[9] This is most commonly identified clinically by a prolonged QRS duration on the surface of electrocardiogram, but cardiac imaging provides an ideal method for measuring and quantifying the

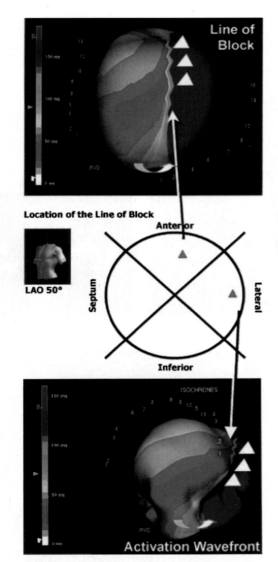

Figure 44.1 Reduction of conduction velocity and a line of block seen in four quadrants of the LV. (*Source*: Auricchio A, Fantoni C, Regoli F, et al. Characterization of left ventricular activation in patients with heart failure and left bundle-branch block. *Circulation.* 2004;109:1133–1139.

degree of LV dyssynchrony. The typical pattern seen with LBBB is early activation of the interventricular septum and late activation of the posterior and lateral walls.[6] Three-dimensional (3D) mapping studies have revealed long lines of block or slow conduction in hearts with LBBB (Fig. 44.1). The location and length of the lines of conduction block are variable, with delayed activation in different segments of the lateral wall of the LV.[10,11] Interestingly, the location of these lines of block is not fixed and may change, suggesting that they may in part be functionally determined rather than related to the areas of scar tissue.

3. IMAGING TECHNIQUES AND IDENTIFICATION OF DYSSYNCHRONY

3.1. Echocardiography

A number of echocardiographic parameters proposed as markers of mechanical dyssynchrony have been evaluated in small, mostly single center studies. These echocardiographic techniques range from simple M-mode echocardiography to more complex tissue Doppler imaging (TDI) and strain imaging. However, due to the large number of echocardiographic techniques that have been published, the difficulty in technical acquisition, the poor reproducibility of many of the parameters, and the lack of direct comparison studies, there is little consensus as to which technique or combination of techniques is optimal.

Perhaps the simplest approach to quantify LV dyssynchrony by echocardiography is the use of M-mode at the midventricular level to quantify the time delay from peak inward septal motion to peak inward posterior motion. The addition of color tissue Doppler to M-mode is a useful adjunct as changes in direction are color-coded which may aid in identifying the transition from inward to outward motion (Fig. 44.2). The M-mode delay between peak contraction of the septum and the inferior wall was studied, and a value of ≥ 130 ms was found to have a sensitivity of 100% and specificity of 63% for predicting LV reverse remodeling.[12,13] However, other groups have disputed the predictive value of this parameter.[14]

The use of conventional Doppler to measure the aortic pre-ejection interval as well as for calculating an interventricular mechanical delay based on the difference between the aortic and pulmonic pre-ejection intervals has also been shown to be predictive of response to CRT. Pre-ejection intervals are calculated by determining the delay from the beginning of the QRS to the onset of aortic ejection as visualized by pulse or continuous wave

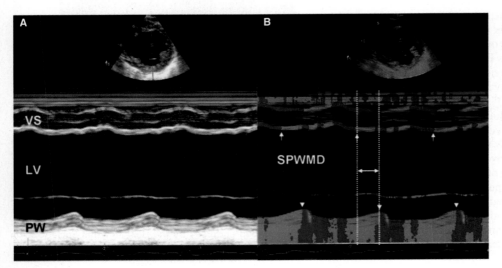

Figure 44.2 M-mode at the midventricular level with (**A**) and without (**B**) the addition of color tissue Doppler to M-mode demonstrating septal to posterior wall delay. (*Source*: Anderson LJ, Miyazaki C, Sutherland GR, et al. Patient selection and echocardiographic assessment of dyssynchrony in cardiac resynchronization therapy. *Circulation.* 2008;117:2009–2023.)

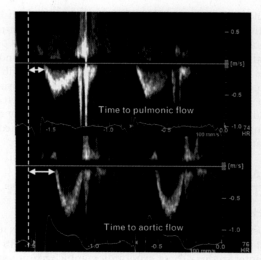

Figure 44.3 Conventional Doppler to measure the aortic and pulmonic pre-ejection interval. Pre-ejection intervals are calculated by determining the delay from the beginning of the QRS to the onset of ejection, while the interventricular mechanical delay is based on the difference between the aortic and pulmonic pre-ejection intervals. (*Source*: Gorcsan J, III. Role of echocardiography to determine candidacy for cardiac resynchronization therapy. *Curr Opin Cardiol*. 2008;23:16–22.)

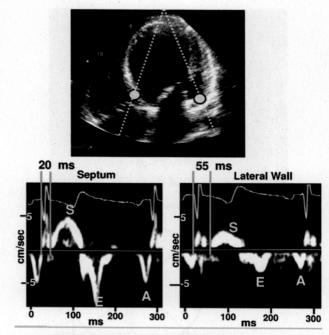

Doppler in the LVOT (Fig. 44.3). An interventricular mechanical delay of ≥ 40 ms[15] or > 49 ms[1] was found to predict greater improvement in echocardiographic parameters or clinical measures. An aortic pre-ejection time of > 160 ms was found to correlate with greater improvements in clinical outcomes such as quality of life and exercise capacity in patients with CRT devices.[16]

TDI to quantify longitudinal LV shortening velocities from the apical windows has the largest body of literature, is the principal method in clinical use, and uses two basic approaches: color-coded or pulsed TDI (Fig. 44.4A & B). Myocardial velocity curves, that measure the time from the onset of the QRS to the peak of systolic velocity, can be constructed online using pulsed TDI typically using two or four basal segments, or reconstructed offline from the color-coded TDI images using two to twelve segments. Early studies using TDI velocities of the basal segments imaged from the apical acoustic window found that LV dyssynchrony of >65 ms predicted improved clinical and echocardiographic response to CRT with high sensitivity and specificity of 80% to 92%.[17,18] Another basal segment approach involved used a composite index of interventricular and intraventricular dyssynchrony. A delay > 102 ms yielded a 88% accuracy in predicting improvement in LV function.[19] Perhaps, an approach that is more robust and more inclusive of the entire LV uses TDI to compile a 12-segment LV dyssynchrony index. This approach has been shown to identify patients who responded with reverse remodeling.[20–22] However, controversy remains as to the predictive value of this index.[23]

Tissue synchronization imaging (TSI) is a technique that automatically calculates the peak systolic velocities from TDI and displays the timing of peak systolic velocities as a red–green color map (Fig. 44.5). This allows for quick visualization of the earliest and latest activated segments while quantitative assessment is still possible. A single study evaluated the ability of TSI to predict response to CRT with a sensitivity of 82% and a specificity of 87%.[24]

Strain and strain rate imaging derived from color-coded TDI have the potential advantage of differentiating active myocardial contraction or deformation from passive translational movement. Using strain and strain rate imaging, the extent of LV dyssynchrony

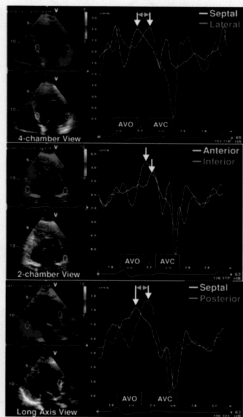

Figure 44.4 Myocardial velocity curves that measure the time from the onset of the QRS to the peak of systolic velocity can be constructed online using pulsed TDI (**top panels**) typically using two or four basal segments, or reconstructed offline from the color-coded TDI images (**bottom panels**) using 2 to 12 segments. (*Source*: Gorcsan J, III, Abraham T, Agler DA, et al. Echocardiography for cardiac resynchronization therapy: Recommendations for performance and reporting—a report from the American Society of Echocardiography Dyssynchrony Writing Group endorsed by the Heart Rhythm Society. *J Am Soc Echocardiogr*. 2008;21:191–213.)

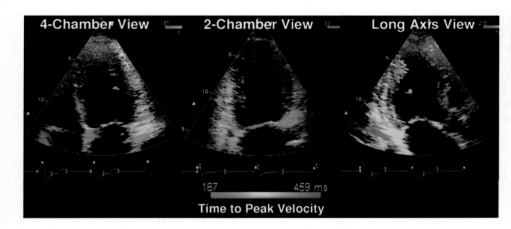

Figure 44.5 Tissue synchronization imaging from three apical views automatically calculates the peak systolic velocities from TDI and displays the timing of peak systolic velocities as a red–green color map. (*Source*: Bleeker GB, Yu CM, Nihoyannopoulos P, et al. Optimal use of echocardiography in cardiac resynchronisation therapy. *Heart*. 2007;93:1339–1350.)

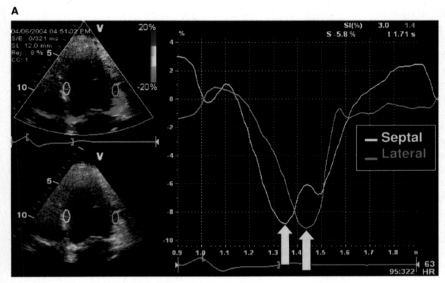

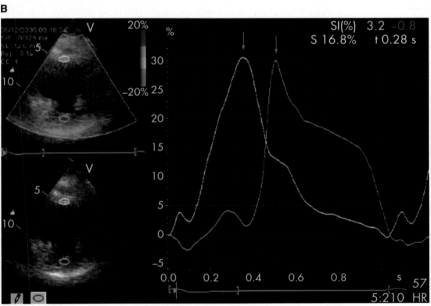

Figure 44.6 Strain imaging derived from color-coded TDI demonstrating longitudinal strain **(A)** and radial strain **(B)** in patients with dyssynchrony based on differences in peak strain in opposing walls. (*Source*: Gorcsan J, III, Abraham T, Agler DA, et al. Echocardiography for cardiac resynchronization therapy: Recommendations for performance and reporting–a report from the American Society of Echocardiography Dyssynchrony Writing Group endorsed by the Heart Rhythm Society. *J Am Soc Echocardiogr*. 2008;21:191–213. Bleeker GB, Yu CM, Nihoyannopoulos P, et al. Optimal use of echocardiography in cardiac resynchronisation therapy. *Heart*. 2007;93:1339–1350.)

can be quantified by measuring the time to peak systolic strain or strain rate similar to TDI (Fig. 44.6A & B). However, the acquisition is technically challenging because strain is also Doppler angle dependent and is difficult in patients with the spherical LV geometry often encountered in HF. Data as to the predictive value of this technique have been mixed, with Sogaard et al.[8,25] reporting that the extent of delayed longitudinal contraction at the base predicted improvement in LV function after CRT, while Yu et al.[22,26] demonstrated that parameters of strain rate were not useful to predict reverse remodeling in response to CRT. A small pilot study examining radial strain found that a delay of ≥ 130 ms was predictive in an improvement in stroke volume with CRT.[27]

Speckle tracking that is applied to routine grayscale echocardiographic images is a novel technique that can calculate myocardial strain, velocity, or displacement from 2D images, and unlike TDI it is not angle dependent. (Fig. 44.7A&B) Responders to CRT with an increase in LVEF had a greater disparity in opposing wall peak longitudinal systolic velocity[28] and in another study had a greater time difference in radial dyssynchrony based on peak septal to posterior wall strain.[29]

3D echocardiographic imaging in which the full volume of the left ventricle is captured over four cardiac cycles provides regional time–volume curves and a dyssynchrony index as well as ejection fraction (EF) (Fig. 44.8). Intuitively, a strategy of assessing 16 regional volumes rather than points or linear segments, may be more accurate in assessing LV regional and global dysfunction and dyssynchrony. In one study a 3D dyssynchrony index, defined as the standard deviation of the time taken to reach minimal regional volume for each of the LV segments, was found to accurately quantify global LV dyssynchrony and correlate with clinical improvement following CRT.[30] However, 3D imaging may be limited in many patients with suboptimal image quality. Furthermore, the low temporal resolution of 3D imaging makes difficult the detection of small regional differences in the timing of peak contraction and relaxation.

3.2. Magnetic resonance imaging

While most mechanical dyssynchrony analysis is based on echo-Doppler methods, these techniques may not provide the most comprehensive assessment of global dyssynchrony due to the limited nature of 2D views. Magnetic resonance imaging can provide high-resolution 3D circumferential and longitudinal myocardial activation data.[31] Tagged MRI was first utilized to demonstrate regional dyssynchrony[32,33] and later strain derived dyssynchrony indexes were employed (Fig. 44.9).[34] Velocity-encoded MRI has been compared to the standard tissue Doppler echocardiographic parameters, yields comparable information on LV dyssynchrony,[35] and magnetic resonance TSI has been shown to provide prognostic information as a predictor of mortality and morbidity after CRT.[36]

3.3. Scintigraphic methods
3.3.1. Gated myocardial perfusion single-photon emission computed tomography

LV dyssynchrony has been measured by phase analysis of gated single-photon emission computed tomography myocardial perfusion images using Fourier harmonic functions to approximate regional wall thickness changes over the cardiac cycle and to calculate the regional onset of mechanical contraction.[37] Five indices describing the phase dispersion of the onset of mechanical contraction have been studied and found to discriminate between patients with LV dysfunction, LBBB, RBBB, ventricular pacing, and normal controls (Fig. 44.10).[38] Subsequent work has shown good correlation with TDI[39] and reasonable accuracy in the ability to predict responders to CRT.[40] One disadvantage of this method, nevertheless, is its low

temporal resolution, making it difficult to recognize small differences in the timing of regional contractile events.

3.3.2. Gated blood pool scan

Phase analysis of gated blood pool radionuclide ventriculography has been used to quantify the timing of LV mechanical activation and synchronization even prior to the advent of biventricular pacing.[41,42] With the introduction of CRT, gated blood pool ventriculography has been used to quantify LV synchrony,[43,44] predict cardiac events based on the degree of interventricular and intraventricular dyssynchrony,[45] and measure the improvement in interventricular synchrony after biventricular pacing (Fig. 44.11A&B).[46] Like other scintigraphic methods, limited temporal resolution is a disadvantage of this method. Moreover, since radionuclide ventriculography is based on endocardial displacement, it is more prone to false positive findings in situations such as abnormal postoperative septal motion.

3.4. Dynamic nature of dyssynchrony

All of the aforementioned techniques evaluate dyssynchrony at rest, but exercise may change the presence and extent of ventricular dyssynchrony and may therefore affect the prognosis and response to CRT in a subset of HF patients.

In an initial study of exercise stress echocardiography in patients with HF using a 12segment TDI model, one third of patients had an increase in measured dyssynchrony, one third had a decrease, and one third had no change.[47] In a group of HF patients with a narrow QRS duration who were studied after exercise, one third of patients developed dyssynchrony that was not present at rest.[48] Exercise has been shown to unmask dyssynchrony in about 25% of patients, and correlates with changes in mitral regurgitation, stroke volume, and peak VO_2.[49] In other studies, the degree of dyssynchrony measured at peak exercise has been associated with LV reverse remodeling, and dobutamine stress echo has been also shown to unmask dyssynchrony in HF patients with both wide and narrow QRS durations.[50]

3.5. Imaging techniques in patient selection for CRT

Approximately, 20% of a generalized HF population has a prolonged QRS duration within the first year of diagnosis.[51] An important role of imaging techniques in identifying the presence of ventricular dyssynchrony is to predict the response and outcome after resynchronization therapy. Identifying patients with a wide QRS but no dyssynchrony is important as patients with no dyssynchrony appear to have a lower probability of response to CRT and a worse prognosis after CRT.[17] Other populations that may benefit from identification of dyssynchrony using the various available imaging techniques would be those patients who are not currently indicated for CRT but who might potentially benefit if they were found to have dyssynchrony. Included in this group of patients are those with a narrow QRS on the surface electrocardiogram[52] or those with a wide QRS but who have NYHA class II HF.[53] It is important to note however, that dyssynchrony imaging techniques were not used as entry criteria in the trials that established CRT as an effective therapy in patients with advanced congestive HF.

3.6. LV lead placement

LV lead placement is usually performed by a transvenous approach with pacing leads placed into branches of the coronary sinus. Cannulation of the coronary sinus with a guiding catheter is performed to facilitate lead implantation by providing support for the pacing leads. Coronary venography in the left anterior oblique and right anterior oblique projections assists in defining the branches as well as the angulation of side branches. The feasibility of transvenous

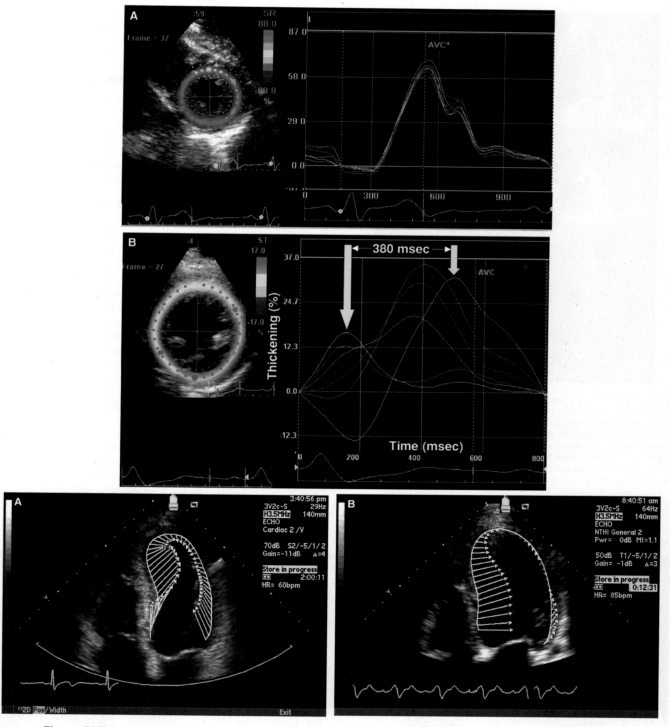

Figure 44.7 Two examples of speckle tracking applied to routine grayscale echocardiographic images that can calculate myocardial strain, velocity, or displacement from two-dimensional images. **Top panels:** Radial strain in a healthy individual and in a patient with heart failure and a left bundle branch block demonstrating dyssynchrony of peak segmental radial strain. **Bottom panels:** Velocity vector imaging (**A**) in a healthy individual and (**B**) in a patient with heart failure and a left bundle branch block demonstrating differences in velocity convergence. (*Source*: Gorcsan J, III, Abraham T, Agler DA, et al. Echocardiography for cardiac resynchronization therapy: Recommendations for performance and reporting–a report from the American Society of Echocardiography Dyssynchrony Writing Group endorsed by the Heart Rhythm Society. *J Am Soc Echocardiogr.* 2008;21:191–213.)

lead positioning is determined by anatomical and technical factors including venous anatomy, accessibility of the vein, pacing threshold, lead stability, and the absence of extracardiac stimulation. With current lead delivery systems, the ability to access specific coronary veins is not usually problematic.

Using current echocardiographic techniques, it is possible before device implantation to identify the site of latest activation of the LV, often the posterolateral region. Several studies have suggested the role and benefit for echocardiographic methods to direct LV lead placement through identification of the anatomic site of

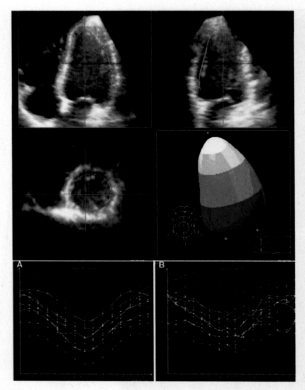

Figure 44.8 Three-dimensional echocardiographic assessment of 17-segment time–volume curves in a healthy patient with normal synchrony and in one with significant dyssynchrony. (*Source*: Gorcsan J, III, Abraham T, Agler DA, et al. Echocardiography for cardiac resynchronization therapy: Recommendations for performance and reporting–a report from the American Society of Echocardiography Dyssynchrony Writing Group endorsed by the Heart Rhythm Society. *J Am Soc Echocardiogr*. 2008;21:191–213.)

latest mechanical activation. Placing the LV lead at the site of latest velocity activation as identified by TDI was shown by two groups to be associated with a more favorable response to CRT.[54,55] Other echocardiographic techniques such as speckle tracking analyzing radial strain[29] and 3D echocardiography[56] have also been used to identify the presence of an optimal lead position that resulted in greater benefit of CRT. Finally, a strategy of combining preimplantation CT venography to visualize the cardiac venous system with tri-plane TSI to determine the area of latest mechanical activation demonstrated acute improvement in LV dyssynchrony and systolic function when the LV lead was able to be placed in the cardiac vein overlying the area of latest activation, while there was no acute improvement in patients with a mismatch.[57]

3.7. Imaging techniques in post-CRT assessment

The response to CRT may vary among individuals and efforts to reduce the number of nonresponders to this therapy are being explored. Factors contributing to nonresponse include inappropriate lead positioning (either due to displacement or unsuitable coronary veins), inadequate delivery of LV pacing, suboptimal device programming, or inappropriate patient selection. Noninvasive imaging techniques play an important role in patient management after implantation. As the AV and ventriculoventricular device settings closely interact with each other and may result in immediate hemodynamic changes, echocardiography has emerged over recent years as the technique of choice for postimplant optimization. Due to factors such as its time resolution, broad availability, low cost, and ability to evaluate changes in real time, echocardiography is now widely used clinically for this purpose.

3.7.1. AV optimization

The optimal programmed AV delay allows completion of the atrial contribution to diastolic filling resulting in the most favorable ventricular preload, and at the same time ensures that the ventricles are paced. Too short an AV delay will result in truncation of the contribution of atrial systole to ventricular filling by prematurely closing the mitral valve with ventricular contraction.

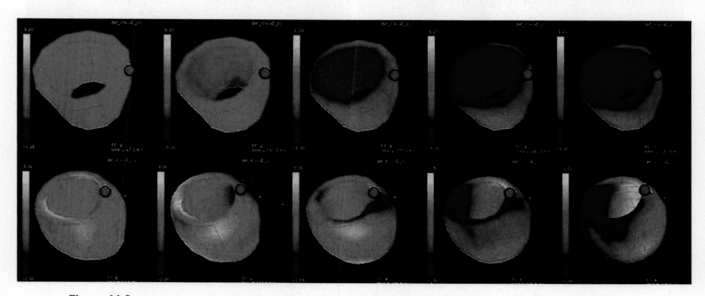

Figure 44.9 Magnetic resonance imaging can provide high-resolution 3D circumferential and longitudinal myocardial activation data. In data from Kass et al.[31] individual phases from the cardiac cycle showing the spatial and temporal evolution of 3D circumferential strain for a normal healthy human heart (**upper panels**) and a patient with severe cardiomyopathy and left bundle branch type conduction delay (**lower panels**). Time moves from left (end-diastole) to right (end-systole). During systolic contraction, the spatial and temporal distribution of circumferential strain are visualized by the color changes, where red corresponds to the neutral (end-diastolic) strain, blue is shortening, and yellow is lengthening or stretch.

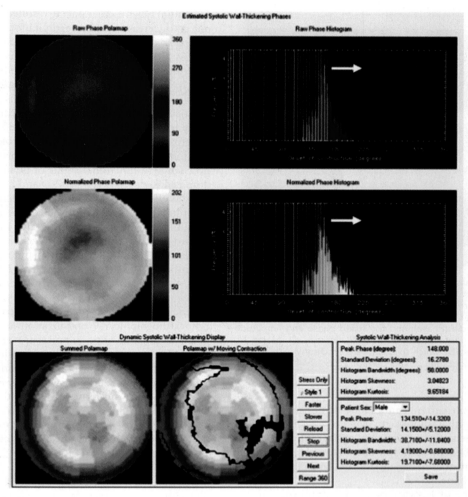

Figure 44.10 User interface of the phase analysis of gated single-photon emission computed tomography myocardial perfusion images using Fourier harmonic functions to approximate regional wall thickness changes over the cardiac cycle and to calculate the regional onset of mechanical contraction. (*Source:* Chen J, Henneman MM, Trimble MA, et al. Assessment of left ventricular mechanical dyssynchrony by phase analysis of ECG-gated SPECT myocardial perfusion imaging. *J Nucl Cardiol.* 2008;15:127–136.)

An AV delay that is too long may allow native conduction to occur and result in diastolic mitral regurgitation. (Fig. 44.12)

While AV synchrony is important (even in dual-chamber pacemakers[58]), routine echocardiographic optimization is not always performed due to lack of uniformity of optimization methods as well as time constraints in performing the optimization. While studies have demonstrated the benefits of AV optimization, Auricchio et al.[59] concluded that while AV optimization positively impacts hemodynamics, LV synchrony is much more important. When comparing patients with Doppler optimized AV intervals to a fixed AV interval, improvement in NYHA class and quality of life was seen, but no change in 6 min walking distance or EF.[60] Another larger study demonstrated that AV optimization enhanced LV hemodynamics in only a minority of patients and found only small differences in initial and postoptimization AV delays.[61]

Nonimaging guided settings such as empiric "out-of-the-box" AV delays or AV delay optimization algorithms based on ECG data[62] are commonly employed. Echocardiographic AV optimization utilizes pulsed Doppler of mitral inflow, and either pulsed or continuous wave Doppler of LV outflow tract is used in the Ritter[63] and iterative[64] AV optimization protocols. The Ritter method

attempts to optimally synchronize the termination of atrial contraction with the onset of ventricular systole by programming a short and then long AV delay and testing their impact on end-diastolic filling. The AV delay is then determined by correcting the long AV delay by the time shift from short and long Doppler tracings. The iterative method begins by programming a long AV delay and sequentially decreasing the delay to a minimum. The minimal AV delay that allows for adequate E and A wave separation and termination of the A wave 40 to 60 ms before the onset of the QRS is considered optimal. Alternatively, transaortic Doppler velocities as a surrogate for stroke volume can be measured at each AV delay with the maximal aortic time-velocity integral representing the optimal delay.

3.7.2. V-V optimization

The optimal programmed V-V delay allows for simultaneous mechanical activation of the right and left ventricles by adjusting the timing of the activation of the ventricular leads resulting in reduction in ventricular dyssynchrony. Utilizing the "out-of-the-box" V-V delay (simultaneous RV–LV excitation) may result in LV or lateral wall activation at a time that is inappropriate relative

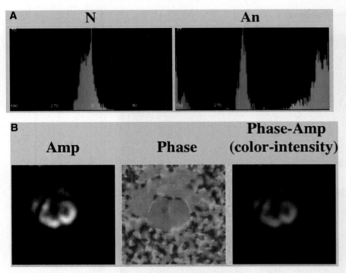

Figure 44.11 A: Phase histograms with examples of a normal, bell-shaped distribution in the Normal (N), with the typical biphasic distribution in the Abnormal (An). **B:** Images generated include the gray scale coded for amplitude image (Amp), the phase image color coded for regional phase angle (Phase), and the fused phase and amplitude images (Phase-Amp). (*Source*: O'Connell JW, Schreck C, Moles M, et al. A unique method by which to quantitate synchrony with equilibrium radionuclide angiography. *J Nucl Cardiol*. 2005;12:441–450.)

to RV excitation. While current studies have demonstrated mixed results, many show that subsets of patients benefit from V-V optimization. A systematic review of V-V optimization found no consistent trend of benefit from optimization, with small, single center studies demonstrating benefit and the larger, randomized studies showing no benefit.[65]

The first evidence of benefit from V-V optimization came from a small study by Sogaard et al.,[66] who demonstrated further improvement in LV function after V-V optimization. Bordachar et al.[67] and Naqvi et al.[68] demonstrated that optimized

sequential biventricular pacing resulted in increased cardiac output and decreased mitral regurgitation compared to simultaneous pacing. Several other small, nonrandomized studies found that V-V optimization resulted in increases in aortic velocity time integral and LV function.[69–71] The benefits of V-V optimization have also been demonstrated by gated blood pool radionuclide ventriculography with an analysis of LVEF at various interventricular delays.[72] In the larger multicenter, nonrandomized study InSync III, sequential biventricular pacing provided most patients with a modest increase in stroke volume and improvement in exercise capacity compared to simultaneous pacing, but no change in functional status or quality of life.[73] The two randomized trials (RHYTHM II ICD and DECREASE-HF) investigating the effects of V-V optimization demonstrated no improvement in NYHA class, 6 min walk times, and quality of life,[74] and no difference in stroke volume and LV function with a trend toward greater reduction in LV size with simultaneous pacing.[75] While small studies have demonstrated the beneficial effects of optimizing V-V settings, there is little consensus as to the utility of V-V optimization with regards to long-term clinical benefit.

3.7.3. Imaging techniques for optimizing V-V timing
Echocardiographic V-V optimization is the most commonly utilized imaging modality, and measures either surrogates for global cardiac function such as the aortic velocity time integral or indices of dyssynchrony. Optimization is performed by changing the V-V timing in a stepwise fashion, while measurements of aortic velocity time integral are recorded using pulsed or continuous wave Doppler. Gated blood pool radionuclide ventriculography has also been employed to optimize V-V timing by measuring LV function at various settings but this technique is not routinely used.[72]

4. FUTURE DIRECTIONS

The complex interplay between atrial and ventricular excitation and contraction is critical in determining cardiac output and function. Changes in the timing of AV as well as V-V conduction can have dramatic effects and understanding the role of

Figure 44.12 AV optimization with sensed AV delays (SAV) from 50 to 200 ms. Atrioventricular optimization using mitral inflow velocities. Sample volume is placed within mitral valve to see closure click. AV optimization may not be necessary if E and A waves are separated, and termination of A wave is before QRS onset or mitral closure click aligned with end of A and QRS complex. AV optimization is indicated if A wave is truncated or absent (AV delay too short), or E and A waves are merged (AV delay too long).

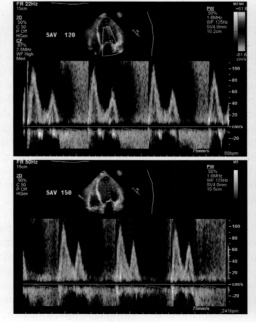

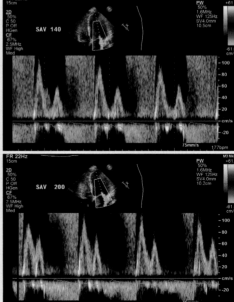

each of these components is critical. With advances in the imaging modalities available, we now are accumulating data useful in patient selection, lead placement, and optimization of CRT devices. At present, there is no consensus or gold standard for the evaluation and management of patients with dyssynchrony and CRT devices, as well as CRT device optimization has not been universally accepted. With the expanding understanding of the mechanisms important to "resynchronize" the ventricles with CRT and the interplay between atrial and ventricular conduction, we may ultimately favorably affect the outcome in patients who do not initially respond to CRT. Ongoing clinical trials testing the many existing techniques of optimizing CRT devices may shed additional light on techniques which are most useful to delay the progression of disease in those patients who have been implanted with CRT devices.

REFERENCES

1. Cleland JG, Daubert JC, Erdmann E, et al. The effect of cardiac resynchronization on morbidity and mortality in heart failure. *N Engl J Med.* 2005;352:1539–1549.
2. Linde C, Leclercq C, Rex S, et al. Long-term benefits of biventricular pacing in congestive heart failure: Results from the MUltisite STimulation in cardiomyopathy (MUSTIC) study. *J Am Coll Cardiol.* 2002;40:111–118.
3. Leclercq C, Kass DA. Retiming the failing heart: Principles and current clinical status of cardiac resynchronization. *J Am Coll Cardiol.* 2002;39:194–201.
4. Kupersmith J, Krongrad E, Waldo AL. Conduction intervals and conduction velocity in the human cardiac conduction system. Studies during open-heart surgery. *Circulation.* 1973;47:776–785.
5. Tavazzi L. Ventricular pacing: A promising new therapeutic strategy in heart failure. For whom? *Eur Heart J.* 2000;21:1211–1214.
6. Grines CL, Bashore TM, Boudoulas H, et al. Functional abnormalities in isolated left bundle branch block. The effect of interventricular asynchrony. *Circulation.* 1989;79:845–853.
7. Xiao HB, Lee CH, Gibson DG. Effect of left bundle branch block on diastolic function in dilated cardiomyopathy. *Br Heart J.* 1991;66:443–447.
8. Sogaard P, Egeblad H, Kim WY, et al. Tissue Doppler imaging predicts improved systolic performance and reversed left ventricular remodeling during long-term cardiac resynchronization therapy. *J Am Coll Cardiol.* 2002;40:723–730.
9. Spragg DD, Kass DA. Pathobiology of left ventricular dyssynchrony and resynchronization. *Prog Cardiovasc Dis.* 2006;49:26–41.
10. Fung JW, Yu CM, Yip G, et al. Variable left ventricular activation pattern in patients with heart failure and left bundle branch block. *Heart.* 2004;90:17–19.
11. Auricchio A, Fantoni C, Regoli F, et al. Characterization of left ventricular activation in patients with heart failure and left bundle-branch block. *Circulation.* 2004;109:1133–1139.
12. Pitzalis MV, Iacoviello M, Romito R, et al. Cardiac resynchronization therapy tailored by echocardiographic evaluation of ventricular asynchrony. *J Am Coll Cardiol.* 2002;40:1615–1622.
13. Pitzalis MV, Iacoviello M, Romito R, et al. Ventricular asynchrony predicts a better outcome in patients with chronic heart failure receiving cardiac resynchronization therapy. *J Am Coll Cardiol.* 2005;45:65–69.
14. Marcus GM, Rose E, Viloria EM, et al. Septal to posterior wall motion delay fails to predict reverse remodeling or clinical improvement in patients undergoing cardiac resynchronization therapy. *J Am Coll Cardiol.* 2005;46:2208–2214.
15. Yu CM, Bax JJ, Monaghan M, et al. Echocardiographic evaluation of cardiac dyssynchrony for predicting a favourable response to cardiac resynchronisation therapy. *Heart.* 2004;90(Suppl. 6):vi17–vi22.
16. Cazeau S, Bordachar P, Jauvert G, et al. Echocardiographic modeling of cardiac dyssynchrony before and during multisite stimulation: A prospective study. *Pacing Clin Electrophysiol.* 2003;26:137–143.
17. Bax JJ, Bleeker GB, Marwick TH, et al. Left ventricular dyssynchrony predicts response and prognosis after cardiac resynchronization therapy. *J Am Coll Cardiol.* 2004;44:1834–1840.
18. Yu CM, Chau E, Sanderson JE, et al. Tissue Doppler echocardiographic evidence of reverse remodeling and improved synchronicity by simultaneously delaying regional contraction after biventricular pacing therapy in heart failure. *Circulation.* 2002;105:438–445.
19. Penicka M, Bartunek J, De Bruyne B, et al. Improvement of left ventricular function after cardiac resynchronization therapy is predicted by tissue Doppler imaging echocardiography. *Circulation.* 2004;109:978–983.
20. Ansalone G, Giannantoni P, Ricci R, et al. Doppler myocardial imaging in patients with heart failure receiving biventricular pacing treatment. *Am Heart J.* 2001;142:881–896.
21. Yu CM, Fung WH, Lin H, et al. Predictors of left ventricular reverse remodeling after cardiac resynchronization therapy for heart failure secondary to idiopathic dilated or ischemic cardiomyopathy. *Am J Cardiol.* 2003;91:684–688.
22. Yu CM, Fung JW, Zhang Q, et al. Tissue Doppler imaging is superior to strain rate imaging and postsystolic shortening on the prediction of reverse remodeling in both ischemic and nonischemic heart failure after cardiac resynchronization therapy. *Circulation.* 2004;110:66–73.
23. El-Chami MF, Notabartolo D, Leon A, et al. Assessment of dyssynchrony index as a predictor of response to resynchronization therapy (abstr). *Circulation.* 2004;110:III-724–III-725.
24. Yu CM, Zhang Q, Fung JW, et al. A novel tool to assess systolic asynchrony and identify responders of cardiac resynchronization therapy by tissue synchronization imaging. *J Am Coll Cardiol.* 2005;45:677–684.
25. Sogaard P, Hassager C. Tissue Doppler imaging as a guide to resynchronization therapy in patients with congestive heart failure. *Curr Opin Cardiol.* 2004;19:447–451.
26. Yu CM, Gorcsan J III, Bleeker GB, et al. Usefulness of tissue Doppler velocity and strain dyssynchrony for predicting left ventricular reverse remodeling response after cardiac resynchronization therapy. *Am J Cardiol.* 2007;100:1263–1270.
27. Dohi K, Suffoletto MS, Schwartzman D, et al. Utility of echocardiographic radial strain imaging to quantify left ventricular dyssynchrony and predict acute response to cardiac resynchronization therapy. *Am J Cardiol.* 2005;96:112–116.
28. Cannesson M, Tanabe M, Suffoletto MS, et al. Velocity vector imaging to quantify ventricular dyssynchrony and predict response to cardiac resynchronization therapy. *Am J Cardiol.* 2006;98:949–953.
29. Suffoletto MS, Dohi K, Cannesson M, et al. Novel speckle-tracking radial strain from routine black-and-white echocardiographic images to quantify dyssynchrony and predict response to cardiac resynchronization therapy. *Circulation.* 2006;113:960–968.
30. Kapetanakis S, Kearney MT, Siva A, et al. Real-time three-dimensional echocardiography: A novel technique to quantify global left ventricular mechanical dyssynchrony. *Circulation.* 2005;112:992–1000.
31. Lardo AC, Abraham TP, Kass DA. Magnetic resonance imaging assessment of ventricular dyssynchrony: Current and emerging concepts. *J Am Coll Cardiol.* 2005;46:2223–2228.
32. McVeigh ER, Prinzen FW, Wyman BT, et al. Imaging asynchronous mechanical activation of the paced heart with tagged MRI. *Magn Reson Med.* 1998;39:507–513.
33. Curry CW, Nelson GS, Wyman BT, et al. Mechanical dyssynchrony in dilated cardiomyopathy with intraventricular conduction delay as depicted by 3D tagged magnetic resonance imaging. *Circulation.* 2000;101:E2.
34. Helm RH, Leclercq C, Faris OP, et al. Cardiac dyssynchrony analysis using circumferential versus longitudinal strain: Implications for assessing cardiac resynchronization. *Circulation.* 2005;111:2760–2767.
35. Westenberg JJ, Lamb HJ, van der Geest RJ, et al. Assessment of left ventricular dyssynchrony in patients with conduction delay and idiopathic dilated cardiomyopathy: Head-to-head comparison between tissue doppler imaging and velocity-encoded magnetic resonance imaging. *J Am Coll Cardiol.* 2006;47:2042–2048.
36. Chalil S, Stegemann B, Muhyaldeen S, et al. Intraventricular dyssynchrony predicts mortality and morbidity after cardiac resynchronization therapy: A study using cardiovascular magnetic resonance tissue synchronization imaging. *J Am Coll Cardiol.* 2007;50:243–252.
37. Chen J, Henneman MM, Trimble MA, et al. Assessment of left ventricular mechanical dyssynchrony by phase analysis of ECG-gated SPECT myocardial perfusion imaging. *J Nucl Cardiol.* 2008;15:127–136.
38. Trimble MA, Borges-Neto S, Smallheiser S, et al. Evaluation of left ventricular mechanical dyssynchrony as determined by phase analysis of ECG-gated SPECT myocardial perfusion imaging in patients with left ventricular dysfunction and conduction disturbances. *J Nucl Cardiol.* 2007;14:298–307.
39. Henneman MM, Chen J, Ypenburg C, et al. Phase analysis of gated myocardial perfusion single-photon emission computed tomography compared with tissue Doppler imaging for the assessment of left ventricular dyssynchrony. *J Am Coll Cardiol.* 2007;49:1708–1714.
40. Henneman MM, Chen J, Dibbets-Schneider P, et al. Can LV dyssynchrony as assessed with phase analysis on gated myocardial perfusion SPECT predict response to CRT? *J Nucl Med.* 2007;48:1104–1111.
41. Frais MA, Botvinick EH, Shosa DW, et al. Phase image characterization of ventricular contraction in left and right bundle branch block. *Am J Cardiol.* 1982;50:95–105.
42. Frais M, Botvinick E, Shosa D, et al. Phase image characterization of localized and generalized left ventricular contraction abnormalities. *J Am Coll Cardiol.* 1984;4:987–998.
43. Dinu C, Klein G, Morestin-Cadet S, et al. Gated blood pool tomoscintigraphy with 4-dimensional optical flow motion analysis quantifies left ventricular mechanical activation and synchronization. *J Nucl Cardiol.* 2006;13:811–820.
44. O'Connell JW, Schreck C, Moles M, et al. A unique method by which to quantitate synchrony with equilibrium radionuclide angiography. *J Nucl Cardiol.* 2005;12:441–450.
45. Fauchier L, Marie O, Casset-Senon D, et al. Interventricular and intraventricular dyssynchrony in idiopathic dilated cardiomyopathy: A prognostic study with fourier phase analysis of radionuclide angioscintigraphy. *J Am Coll Cardiol.* 2002;40:2022–2030.
46. Kerwin WF, Botvinick EH, O'Connell JW, et al. Ventricular contraction abnormalities in dilated cardiomyopathy: Effect of biventricular pacing to correct interventricular dyssynchrony. *J Am Coll Cardiol.* 2000;35:1221–1227.
47. Lafitte S, Bordachar P, Lafitte M, et al. Dynamic ventricular dyssynchrony: An exercise-echocardiography study. *J Am Coll Cardiol.* 2006;47:2253–2259.
48. Wang YC, Hwang JJ, Yu CC, et al. Provocation of masked left ventricular mechanical dyssynchrony by treadmill exercise in patients with systolic heart failure and narrow QRS complex. *Am J Cardiol.* 2008;101:658–661.

49. D'Andrea A, Caso P, Cuomo S, et al. Effect of dynamic myocardial dyssynchrony on mitral regurgitation during supine bicycle exercise stress echocardiography in patients with idiopathic dilated cardiomyopathy and 'narrow' QRS. *Eur Heart J.* 2007;28:1004–1011.

50. Chattopadhyay S, Alamgir MF, Nikitin NP, et al. The effect of pharmacological stress on intraventricular dyssynchrony in left ventricular systolic dysfunction. *Eur J Heart Fail.* 2008;10:412–420.

51. Shenkman HJ, Pampati V, Khandelwal AK, et al. Congestive heart failure and QRS duration: Establishing prognosis study. *Chest.* 2002;122:528–534.

52. Beshai JF, Grimm RA, Nagueh SF, et al. Cardiac-resynchronization therapy in heart failure with narrow QRS complexes. *N Engl J Med.* 2007;357:2461–2471.

53. Linde C. 12-Month results of the REVERSE study. In: American College of Cardiology. 2008 Scientific Sessions; 2008 April 01, 2008; Chicago; 2008.

54. Ansalone G, Giannantoni P, Ricci R, et al. Doppler myocardial imaging to evaluate the effectiveness of pacing sites in patients receiving biventricular pacing. *J Am Coll Cardiol.* 2002;39:489–499.

55. Murphy RT, Sigurdsson G, Mulamalla S, et al. Tissue synchronization imaging and optimal left ventricular pacing site in cardiac resynchronization therapy. *Am J Cardiol.* 2006;97:1615–1621.

56. Becker M, Hoffmann R, Schmitz F, et al. Relation of optimal lead positioning as defined by three-dimensional echocardiography to long-term benefit of cardiac resynchronization. *Am J Cardiol.* 2007;100:1671–1676.

57. Van de Veire NR, Marsan NA, Schuijf JD, et al. Noninvasive imaging of cardiac venous anatomy with 64-slice multi-slice computed tomography and noninvasive assessment of left ventricular dyssynchrony by 3-dimensional tissue synchronization imaging in patients with heart failure scheduled for cardiac resynchronization therapy. *Am J Cardiol.* 2008;101:1023–1029.

58. Mehta D, Gilmour S, Ward DE, et al. Optimal atrioventricular delay at rest and during exercise in patients with dual chamber pacemakers: A non-invasive assessment by continuous wave Doppler. *Br Heart J.* 1989;61:161–166.

59. Auricchio A, Stellbrink C, Block M, et al. Effect of pacing chamber and atrioventricular delay on acute systolic function of paced patients with congestive heart failure. The Pacing Therapies for Congestive Heart Failure Study Group. The Guidant Congestive Heart Failure Research Group. *Circulation.* 1999;99:2993–3001.

60. Sawhney NS, Waggoner AD, Garhwal S, et al. Randomized prospective trial of atrioventricular delay programming for cardiac resynchronization therapy. *Heart Rhythm.* 2004;1:562–567.

61. Kedia N, Ng K, Apperson-Hansen C, et al. Usefulness of atrioventricular delay optimization using Doppler assessment of mitral inflow in patients undergoing cardiac resynchronization therapy. *Am J Cardiol.* 2006;98:780–785.

62. Stellbrink C, Breithardt OA, Franke A, et al. Impact of cardiac resynchronization therapy using hemodynamically optimized pacing on left ventricular remodeling in patients with congestive heart failure and ventricular conduction disturbances. *J Am Coll Cardiol.* 2001;38:1957–1965.

63. Ritter P, Dib JC, Lelievre T. Quick determination of the optimal AV delay at rest in patients paced in DDD mode for complete AV block (abstr). *Eur J CPE.* 1994;4:A163.

64. Waggoner AD, Faddis MN, Osborn J. AV delay programming and cardiac resynchronization thereapy: Left ventricular diastolic filling indices and relation to stroke volume. *J Am Coll Cardiol.* 2005;45:99A.

65. Lim SH, Lip GY, Sanderson JE. Ventricular optimization of biventricular pacing: A systematic review. *Europace.* 2008;10:901–906.

66. Sogaard P, Egeblad H, Pedersen AK, et al. Sequential versus simultaneous biventricular resynchronization for severe heart failure: Evaluation by tissue Doppler imaging. *Circulation.* 2002;106:2078–2084.

67. Bordachar P, Lafitte S, Reuter S, et al. Echocardiographic parameters of ventricular dyssynchrony validation in patients with heart failure using sequential biventricular pacing. *J Am Coll Cardiol.* 2004;44:2157–2165.

68. Naqvi TZ, Rafique AM, Peter CT. Echo-driven V-V optimization determines clinical improvement in non responders to cardiac resynchronization treatment. *Cardiovasc Ultrasound.* 2006;4:39.

69. Fischer A, Hansalia R, Duvall W. Lack of predictors of optimal RV-LV delay as established by three dimensional echocardiography and aortic time velocity integrals. *J Cardiovasc Electrophys.* 2007;18:S2.

70. Parreira L, Santos JF, Madeira J, et al. Cardiac resynchronization therapy with sequential biventricular pacing: Impact of echocardiography guided V-V delay optimization on acute results. *Rev Port Cardiol.* 2005;24:1355–1365.

71. Valzania C, Biffi M, Martignani C, et al. Cardiac resynchronization therapy: Variations in echo-guided optimized atrioventricular and interventricular delays during follow-up. *Echocardiography.* 2007;24:933–939.

72. Burri H, Sunthorn H, Somsen A, et al. Optimizing sequential biventricular pacing using radionuclide ventriculography. *Heart Rhythm.* 2005;2:960–965.

73. Leon AR, Abraham WT, Brozena S, et al. Cardiac resynchronization with sequential biventricular pacing for the treatment of moderate-to-severe heart failure. *J Am Coll Cardiol.* 2005;46:2298–2304.

74. Boriani G, Muller CP, Seidl KH, et al. Randomized comparison of simultaneous biventricular stimulation versus optimized interventricular delay in cardiac resynchronization therapy. The Resynchronization for the HemodYnamic Treatment for Heart Failure Management II implantable cardioverter defibrillator (RHYTHM II ICD) study. *Am Heart J.* 2006;151:1050–1058.

75. Rao RK, Kumar UN, Schafer J, et al. Reduced ventricular volumes and improved systolic function with cardiac resynchronization therapy: A randomized trial comparing simultaneous biventricular pacing, sequential biventricular pacing, and left ventricular pacing. *Circulation.* 2007;115:2136–2144.

Aortic Atherosclerosis, Aneurysm and Dissection

45

Arturo Evangelista
Victor Pineda
Hug Cuellar

1. INTRODUCTION

1.1. Normal aorta

The aorta is the largest and strongest artery in the body; its wall comprises three layers: the thin inner layer or intima, a thick middle layer or media, and a rather thin outer layer, the adventitia. The endothelium-lined aortic intima is a thin, delicate layer and is easily traumatized. The media is composed of smooth muscle cells and multiple layers of elastic laminae that provide not only tensile strength but also distensibility, and elasticity, which play a vital circulatory role. The adventitia contains mainly collagen and carries the important vasa vasorum, which nourish the outer half of the aortic wall, including a major part of the media.

The elastic properties of the aorta contribute crucially to its normal function. However, elasticity and distensibility of the aorta decline with age. The loss of elasticity and aortic compliance probably account for the increase in pulse pressure commonly seen in the elderly and is accompanied by progressive dilatation of the aorta. This loss of elasticity is caused by structural changes, including an increase in collagen content and formation of intimal atherosclerosis.

1.1.1. Normal aortic dimensions

In the adult human, normal diameter is considered to be below 40 mm in the aortic root, 37 mm in ascending aorta, and 28 mm in the descending aorta. Although normal aortic dimensions should be normalized to body size, few studies refer to normal values indexed by body surface. In one study by transesophageal echocardiography (TEE), normal values of ascending aorta diameter ranged from 14 to 21 mm/m² and descending thoracic aorta diameter from 10 to 16 mm/m².[1] In a more recent study,[2] including 4,039 adult patients undergoing coronary artery calcium scanning, noncontrast gated cardiac computed tomography (CT) showed age, body surface area, gender, and hypertension to be directly associated with thoracic aorta dimensions. Mean diameters were 33 ± 4 mm for ascending aorta and 24 ± 3 mm for descending aorta. The corresponding upper limits of normal ascending and descending aortic diameters at the lower level of the pulmonary bifurcation were 41 and 30 mm, respectively. Male gender was a significant predictor only when interacting with age. In addition to hypertension, smoking was found to be an independent predictor associated only with an increase in descending aortic diameters.

1.2. Aortic diseases: epidemiology, pathogenesis and clinical presentation

1.2.1. Aortic atherosclerosis

Atherosclerosis is characterised by the development of multiple atheromatous plaques in the aorta wall and in the other arteries of great or medium caliber. Aortic atherosclerosis is well known to increase with advancing age and is related to traditional cardiovascular risk factors such as hypertension, hypercholesterolemia, diabetes mellitus, and smoking. The evidence accumulated in experimental studies during the past few decades indicates that atherogenesis initially involves the intima and is initiated by endocardial dysfunction with progression in the subendothelial space. The prevalence of aortic atheromas on TEE varies depending on the population studied. In a community study, aortic atheromas were present in 51% of randomly selected residents aged 45 years or older, with a greater prevalence in the descending aorta,[3] and complex atheromas were present in 7.6%. In patients with known significant carotid artery disease, the prevalence of aortic atheromas was 38%, and 92% in those with significant coronary artery disease.[4,5] Several studies have shown the association between aortic atheromas and embolic disease and stroke and peripheral embolism.[6–9] Complicated aortic atherosclerosis has been considered independent of other risk factors for stroke such as carotid disease or atrial fibrillation. In the Stroke Prevention in Atrial Fibrillation study, investigators reported that 35% of patients with "high risk" nonvalvular atrial fibrillation had complex aortic plaque (mobile, ulcerated size >4 mm).[10] However, although some studies suggested that aortic atherosclerosis is a high-risk factor for development of vascular events,[11] other studies showed that after adjustment for age and other risk factors, aortic atherosclerosis was not an independent predictor.[12]

Clots floating in the aorta frequently appear to originate from atherosclerotic plaque and have a high embolic risk. Another complication of aortic atherosclerosis is cholesterol embolization syndrome,[13] spontaneous or secondary to an invasive vascular procedure such as cardiac catheterization or placement of an intra-aortic balloon pump.[14,15] Similarly, ascending aorta and arch atheromas proved to be highly significant risk factors for intraoperative stroke.[16]

1.2.2. Aortic aneurysm

Aortic aneurysm is a pathologic dilatation of the aorta involving one or several segments. Aortic diameter exceeding 1.5 times the normal value is commonly considered to be an aneurysm. From a practical point of view, an aortic aneurysm is diagnosed when these diameters extend over 50 mm in ascending and over 40 mm in the descending aorta. Aneurysm of the ascending aorta most often results from cystic medial degeneration. The histologic changes lead to weakening of the aortic wall, which results in the formation of a fusiform aneurysm. Such aneurysms often involve the aortic root (annuloaortic ectasia) and may consequently result in aortic regurgitation. Major inherited connective tissue disorders such as Marfan syndrome, Ehler–Danlos, and others are known to cause aortic diseases. Annuloaortic ectasia is common in patients with Marfan syndrome, but this entity may also be present in patients with no apparent predisposing conditions.

Some cases of ascending aortic aneurysm are associated with an underlying bicuspid aortic valve. Nistri et al.[17] found that 52% of young people with normally functioning bicuspid aortic valves have echocardiographic evidence of aortic dilatation. Dilatation occurred most frequently at the level of the tubular portion of ascending aorta (44%), but 20% had dilatation at the sinus level.[18] Atherosclerosis is an unusual cause of ascending aortic aneurysms; when it is the etiology, there is usually evidence of atherosclerosis elsewhere. Proximal atherosclerotic aneurysms are typically fusiform and extend into the arch.

The predominant cause of aneurysm of the descending aorta is atherosclerosis. Cardiovascular risk factors are significantly associated with the presence of atherosclerotic aortic aneurysms. Hypertension is present in 60% of patients with atherosclerotic aortic aneurysm. Abdominal aortic aneurysms are much more common than thoracic aortic aneurysms. Men aged 65 and older screened by ultrasonography have a 4% to 9% prevalence of abdominal aortic aneurysm. The true incidence of thoracic aortic aneurysms is difficult to determine since many go undiagnosed. However, in a Mayo Clinic survey, the incidence in Olmstead County, Minnesota was 10.4 per 100,000 persons per year.[19]

The majority of aortic aneurysms are asymptomatic at the time of diagnosis and are discovered incidentally on imaging tests or, less frequently, on routine physical examination.

When patients with thoracic aortic aneurysms eventually experience symptoms, they tend to reflect direct compression of other intrathoracic structures; tracheal compression may generate wheezing, cough, or dyspnea; esophageal compression may result in dysphagia; and compression of the recurrent laryngeal nerve may cause hoarseness.

1.2.3. Acute aortic syndromes

Acute aortic syndromes include aortic dissection, intramural hematoma and penetrating ulcer. Aortic dissection is defined as the separation of the aortic media with presence of extraluminal blood within the layers of the aortic wall. The estimated incidence is 20 to 30 cases per million people per year. Different processes may produce rupture of the intima: (a) weakness of the aorta wall due to connective tissue diseases such as Marfan Syndrome, Edler–Danlos disease, bicuspid aortic valve, etc.; (b) mechanical stress induced from an aortic lesion secondary to jet impact as in aortic valve disease or aortic valve prosthesis; (c) atherosclerotic disease of the aortic wall; (d) iatrogenic lesions caused by catheters or surgery; (e) trauma; and (f) aortic inflammatory diseases.[20,21] Untreated systemic hypertension is encountered in almost 80% of cases of aortic dissection. Hypertension may not only directly weaken the aortic media, but may also initiate atherosclerosis of the vasa vasorum and thus intramural hemorrhage due to rupture of nutrient intramural vessels. Acute intramural hematoma is initiated by a vasa vasorum hemorrhage in medial wall layers. Intramural bleeding induces circular and longitudinal cleavage of the aortic wall. This entity involves the descending aorta in 65% of cases. It occurs typically in elderly patients (mean 65 to 70 years) with hypertension.[22] One important complication of aortic atherosclerosis is when the plaque evolves to a penetrating ulcer. This localized ulceration, a gaping communication between the lumen and the medial layer of the aorta, may result in intramural hematoma or aortic rupture.

Acute aortic syndromes have high mortality rates and require early medical and surgical treatment. Therefore, rapid and accurate diagnostic techniques, which can be applied in critically ill patients, are essential. It is important to identify the signs and symptoms of the disease to establish an early diagnosis. One of the most serious diagnostic errors is to confuse aortic dissection with myocardial infarction, especially if thrombolytic treatment is prescribed. This error can occur if it is not taken into account that the electrocardiogram may show myocardial infarction patterns in 10% of patients and signs of ischemia in 15%. On the other hand, although the chest X-ray has traditionally been considered to be always abnormal, recent series show that it can be normal in up to 20% of patients.[21]

1.2.4. Aortitis

Inflammatory diseases can destroy the medial layers of the aortic wall and lead to weakening of the aortic wall. Autoimmune diseases of the aorta can severely affect the vasa vasorum and decrease the blood supply of the media. Takayasu arteritis is a chronic inflammatory disease of unknown origin, which involves the aorta and its branches. This arteritis typically causes obliterative lesions of the aorta,[23] producing signs and symptoms of vascular insufficiency, but less often can produce aortic aneurysms. Takayasu arteritis typically affects young females. It occurs most often in the Asian population. The initial stages of the disease involve signs and symptoms of systemic inflammation. The second phase is vascular involvement. Once arterial obstruction develops, upper extremity claudication, stroke, dizziness, or syncope usually indicate aortic branch involvement. Hypertension is sometimes malignant and suggests narrowing of the aorta or renal arteries.

Giant cell arteritis tends to affect an older population but again females are affected far more often than males. When the aorta is affected, it may result in thoracic aortic aneurysm. Aside from these diseases, other aortitis such as in Behcet disease, Berger disease, Kawasaki disease, Reiter syndrome and some infectious processes have been described. Syphilis and other infections due to staphylococcus, salmonella, and mycobacteria, though less common, have been found to cause aortitis and mycotic aortic aneurysms.

2. PATHOPHYSIOLOGY

2.1. Aortic atherosclerosis

Aortic atheromas are characterized by irregular intimal thickening of at least 2 mm. The intima shows massive fibrosis and calcification and increased amounts of extracellular fatty acids. They often have superimposed mobile components, which are thrombi that have been shown to disappear with anticoagulation. The morphology of aortic atheromatous plaques is dynamic, with frequent formation and resolution of mobile components.[24] Based on their morphology, aortic atheromas are classified as either simple or complex plaques. These are atheromatous plaques that ulcerate and disrupt the elastic interna lamina, burrowing deeply into the aortic media and beyond.

2.2. Aortic aneurysms

Whatever the underlying cause, the development of an aneurysm is related to weakening of the media of the artery. Once dilatation begins, the enlargement tends to be progressive because lateral stress increases with widening of the lumen and slowing of the flow. According to Laplace law, wall stress correlates with pressure and radius and inversely with wall thickness, which signifies that hypertension is an important factor related to the development of aortic disease.[25] Additional degenerative changes are characterized by reduced cellularity and collagen fiber hyalinization. Furthermore, wall tension at constant arterial pressure increases with increasing diameter. Larger aneurysms expand more rapidly than small ones. Currently available evidence favors the view that cystic media necrosis is a marker of medial degeneration. In some instances, it reflects an intrinsic defect, as in Marfan syndrome, and in others may be indicative of the effect of long-standing hemodynamic stress, such as in hypertension. Aortic aneurysm results not from passive dilatation, but from a complex remodeling process involving both synthesis and breakdown of matrix proteins.

2.3. Acute aortic syndromes

In most aortic dissections, one tear or one or more entries are present in the aortic intima, resulting in an abnormal communication between the true aortic lumen and the split aortic media. With primary intimal dissection, the media is exposed to pulsatile aortic flow, probably creating a false aortic lumen and propagating a dissection, which is typically antegrade but sometimes retrograde from the site of the intimal tear.[26,27] The vast majority of aortic dissections originate in one of the two sites where the greatest hydraulic stress is located in ascending aorta, within several centimeters above the sinuses of Valsalva, and in descending aorta, just distal to the origin of the left subclavian artery at the site of the ligamentum arteriosum. Sixty-five percentage of intimal tears occur in the ascending aorta, 20% in the descending aorta, 10% in the aortic arch, and 5% in the abdominal aorta. Most dissections have a re-entry site and some communication sites throughout the descending aorta.

All mechanisms weakening the aorta's media layers via micro apoplexy of the vessel wall lead to higher wall stress, which can induce aortic dilatation, eventually resulting in intramural hemorrhage, aortic dissection, or rupture. In over 60% of hematomas, the location is in descending aorta and is frequently accompanied by other signs of aortic dissection. On occasions, localized zones of the hematoma, which break the intima, can be identified giving rise to saccular images that may be confused with penetrating ulcers. Hematomas and penetrating aortic ulcers may break through into the adventitia to form a pseudoaneurysm or may rupture freely into the mediastinum.

3. DIAGNOSTIC EVALUATION

3.1. Transthoracic echocardiography

Although transthoracic echocardiography (TTE) is not the technique of choice for overall assessment of the aorta, it is useful for the diagnosis and follow-up of some segments of the aorta. The use of all possible views is fundamental for correct assessment of the aorta by TTE. Using the parasternal view, it is possible to see the aortic root, the lower third of the ascending aorta, and also part of the descending thoracic aorta behind the left atrium. The right parasternal view permits visualization of the major part of the ascending aorta when the study is of good quality. The aortic arch, origin of the arch vessels, and proximal third of the descending aorta can be assessed from the suprasternal window. Finally, the distal portion of the thoracic aorta can be viewed using the modified apical view and the abdominal aorta from subcostal and abdominal approaches.

TTE may assess several parameters which evaluate the physical properties of the aorta wall.[27] Simultaneous diameter and blood pressure registration is essential for exact calculation of elastic parameters. Pressure registration at the aortic site cannot be determined noninvasively. However, close correlation of invasive and noninvasive determination of ascending aorta distensibility has been demonstrated.[28] Pulse wave velocity is considered a good surrogate for arterial distensibility, being correlated with direct measurements of arterial stiffness.[29] Pulse wave velocity is determined from serial determinations of pulsed Doppler recordings at the ascending, descending aorta, and femoral arteries (See Chapter 22).

3.1.1. Aortic atherosclerosis

TTE is limited for assessing aortic atherosclerosis but may play a role in the diagnosis of aortic arch atheromas using suprasternal harmonic imaging. Schwammenthal et al.[30] showed that adequate image quality could be achieved in 84% of cases. TTE represents not only an excellent screening test but provides complementary views of regions that may be blind spots for TEE. Both anatomical orientation and the location of detected atheromas with respect to the origin of the major aortic branches are more readily seen with TTE than TEE.

3.1.2. Aortic aneurysm

TTE is an excellent modality for imaging the aortic root,[31] which is important for patients with annuloaortic ectasia or Marfan syndrome. Since the predominant area of dilatation is in the proximal aorta, TTE often suffices for screening. This technique has seen tremendous success in the serial measurement of maximum aortic root diameters, evaluation of aortic regurgitation, and the timing of elective surgery. In addition, an aneurysm can arise in the sinus of Valsalva and is correctly seen both in long- and short-axis views. Several studies have shown the clinical usefulness of TTE in the measurement of aortic root in patients with aortic valvular disease, mainly in bicuspid aortic valve.[18,19]

Aortic root dimensions are assessed at end diastole in the parasternal long-axis view at four levels: annulus, sinuses of Valsalva, supra-aortic ridge, and proximal ascending aorta. Measurements ought to be made perpendicular to the long axis of the aorta with the use of the leading edge method. In these diseases, the right parasternal window obtained with the patient in the right lateral decubitus position allows us to visualize the ascending aorta and quantify the severity of aortic valve disease. Some experts[32] favor inner edge-to-inner edge diameter measurements to match those obtained by other methods of imaging the aorta, such as magnetic resonance imaging (MRI) and CT scanning. However, the normative data published in the literature were obtained using the leading edge technique. Two-dimensional (2D) aortic diameter measurements are preferable to M-mode (Fig. 45.1).

3.1.3. Acute aortic syndromes

TTE is a useful tool in the initial evaluation of patients with suspected acute cardiovascular disease and also aortic dissection.

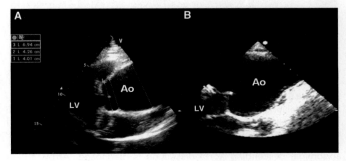

Figure 45.1 TE in parasternal long-axis view showing **(A)** ascending aorta aneurysm upper sinotubular junction; **(B)** annuloaortic ectasia with pyriform morphology. LV, left ventricle; Ao, aorta.

Demonstration of the presence of an intimal flap that divides the aorta into two lumina, the true and the false, forms the basis of the echocardiographic diagnosis of dissection. TTE has 78% to 100% sensitivity in ascending aorta dissection, but only 31% to 55% in the descending aorta. Specificity for type A aortic dissection was reported to range from 87% to 96% and for type B dissection 60% to 83%.[33-35] Thus, it constitutes an acceptable technique for type A dissection, but not for type B. However, these data are derived from old studies when the current imaging technology was not available. Recently, technological advances, in particular the introduction of harmonic imaging, have yielded improvements in TTE image quality (Fig. 45.2). However, the low negative predictive value of TTE does not permit the diagnosis of dissection to be ruled out, and further tests will be required. The value of TTE is also limited in patients with abnormal chest wall configuration, obesity, pulmonary emphysema, and in those on mechanical ventilation. These limitations prevent adequate decision-making, but have been overcome by TEE.

3.2. Transesophageal echocardiography

TEE is performed with 2.5 to 7.5 MHz transducers mounted on the distal end of a conventional gastroscope probe. Because of the close anatomical relationship between the esophagus and thoracic aorta, TEE allows visualization of the entire thoracic aorta except a blind area in the upper part of the ascending aorta near the right mainstem bronchus. The aortic valve, sinuses of Valsalva, and ascending aorta are well visualized by rotating the image plane to approximately 120 degrees in the long-axis view. The aortic arch is best imaged from a high esophageal position, starting with a short-axis view of the descending thoracic aorta. The descending thoracic aorta and proximal abdominal aorta are well seen by TEE. Any areas of abnormality are then examined in both long- and short-axis views.

3.2.1. Aortic atherosclerosis

TEE is a great method for evaluating aortic atheromas. It provides higher resolution images than TTE and has good interobserver reproducibility. TEE characterizes the plaque by measuring plaque thickness, ulceration, calcification, and superimposed mobile thrombi, thereby determining the embolic potential of each plaque. The advantages of TEE over other noninvasive modalities (CT and MRI) include its ability to assess the mobility of plaque in real time. The French Aortic Plaque in Stroke group showed that plaque thickness of ≥4 mm was significantly associated with increased stroke risk.[7,8] The presence of mobile lesions superimposed on aortic atheromas has been recognized to impart a high embolic risk. Other characteristics of the lesions seen on TEE, such as ulceration ≥2 mm in aortic plaques and noncalcified plaques, were also associated with higher risk of stroke. Grading systems used to classify aortic atherosclerosis are grade I = normal intimal thickening <3 mm; grade II = diffuse intimal thickening >3 mm; grade III = atheroma <5 mm; grade IV = atheromas >5 mm; and grade V = any mobile atheroma (Fig. 45.3A).[24]

Large mobile thrombi of the aorta are infrequent causes of systemic emboli and appear to be a complication of atherosclerosis. TEE is the best technique in the diagnosis and evolution of these large thrombi.[36] Optimal management of these complications remains to be defined, and anticoagulation therapy appears to be a logical approach, although surgical removal has been performed in cases with recurrent embolic events (Fig. 45.3B)

3.2.2. Aortic aneurysm

TEE is not the best technique for the measurement of aortic diameters. If the aorta is tortuous, TEE images may be difficult to interpret correctly. Cross-sectional images will appear ellipsoid in shape since the imaging plane passes through obliquely and not perpendicularly. TEE permits easy detection of thrombi and frequently demonstrates a slowly swirling spontaneous echo contrast due to reduced flow velocity in the dilated portion of the aorta. Whether fusiform or saccular, the lumen of an aneurysm frequently contains a laminated thrombus. CT and MRI are more useful than TEE in the assessment of aortic aneurysm.

3.2.3. Acute aortic syndrome

TEE has constituted a decisive advance in the diagnosis of aortic dissection. It can image the entire thoracic aorta except for a small portion of the distal ascending aorta near the proximal arch. Compared with other highly accurate diagnostic techniques (CT, MRI, etc.), echocardiography has the advantage of being applicable in any hospital department (emergency, intensive care, operating room, etc.), without the need to transfer the patient who is often in an unstable hemodynamic situation, monitored and with an intravenous line in place. The proximity

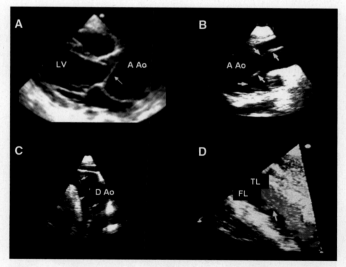

Figure 45.2 Aortic dissection by transthoracic echocardiography. **A:** Parasternal long-axis view showing intimal flap (*arrow*) in aortic root; **B:** Right parasternal view reveals intimal flap (*arrows*) in the upper part of ascending aorta; **C:** By suprasternal view intimal flap (*arrows*) in proximal descending thoracic aorta is visualized; and **D:** By subcostal view abdominal descending aorta dissection is diagnosed. *Arrow* shows a secondary communication between true (TL) and false lumen (FL); AAo, ascending aorta; DAo, descending aorta; LV, left ventricle; FL, false lumen; TL, true lumen.

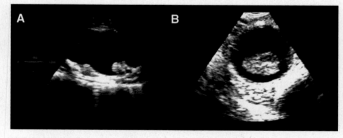

Figure 45.3 Transesophageal echocardiography showing the presence of **(A)** severe atherosclerosis (grade IV) in descending aorta; **(B)** large mobile thrombus in a patient with peripheral embolism.

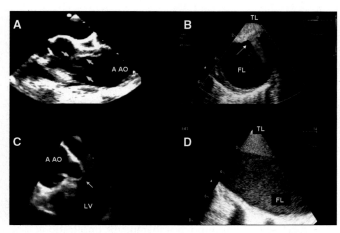

Figure 45.4 Aortic dissection by TEE. **A:** Longitudinal view of ascending aorta. *Arrows* show the mobile intimal flap in ascending aorta; **B:** Descending aorta dissection by transversal view. Color Doppler shows true lumen (TL) and a secondary communication (*arrow*) **C:** The intimal flap prolapse in the left ventricular outflow tract (*arrow*) is the mechanism of aortic regurgitation; and **D:** By contrast echocardiography true lumen is easily identified in difficult cases and gives information on false lumen flow volume.

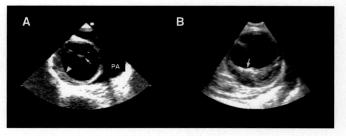

Figure 45.5 A: Intramural hematoma in ascending aorta (*head-arrows*). A reverberation into aorta lumen (*arrow*) could misdiagnose type A aortic dissection; **B:** Intramural hematoma in descending aorta. Arrow shows the presence of intimal calcification. PA, pulmonary artery.

of the esophagus to the aorta, without interference from the chest wall or lung, permits high-quality images to be obtained (Fig. 45.4).

Aortic Dissection. Since the first work published by Erbel et al.,[37] several studies have demonstrated the accuracy of TEE in the diagnosis of aortic dissection with sensitivity of 86% to 100%, specificity 90% to 100%, and negative predictive value 86% to 100%.[37-42] Our group published[43] one of the largest series (132 patients), with sensitivity and specificity of 96.8% and 100%, respectively. The low specificity of the technique described in some series such as that of Nienaber et al.[39] is explained by the fact that the majority of intraluminal images in the ascending aorta were considered diagnostic of dissected intima. Analysis of 8 large studies[37,39] showed that 14 of 435 patients (3.5%) with clinically suspected dissection were erroneously diagnosed as having ascending aorta dissection. Altogether, the experience accumulated in recent years demonstrates that the presence of an intraluminal linear echodensity in the ascending aorta alone should not be accepted as a dissection criterion. In the ascending aorta, particularly when dilated, linear reverberation artifacts are very common, being observed in 44% to 55% of studies.[43] Artifacts in the aortic root are caused by reverberation from the anterior wall of the left atrium or in the middle third of the ascending aorta by reverberations from the posterior wall of the right pulmonary artery (Fig. 45.5A). M-mode echocardiography is the most useful tool in the differential diagnosis between intimal flap and imaging reverberations.[43]

Intramural hematoma. TEE findings are circular or crescentic thickening (more than 5 mm) of the aortic wall (Fig. 45.5A) and there should be no flow within.[44] Diagnosis is straightforward in typical cases, but the hematoma may sometimes be mistaken for the presence of an intraluminal thrombus or a dissection with thrombosed false lumen. Displacement of intimal calcification caused by accumulation of blood within the aortic media is useful for differential diagnosis (Fig. 45.5B). Localized intimal ruptures are present in more than 30% of cases and most evolved to localized dissection (ulcerlike projections; ULP).

Penetrating aortic ulcer. The diagnosis of penetrating ulcers by TEE is based on the image of craterlike outpouching in the aortic wall, with jagged edges generally associated with extensive aortic atheroma.[45] Aortic wall thickening with inward displacement of intimal calcification is an indication of associated intramural hematoma.

The ideal diagnostic technique in acute aortic dissection should not only have high sensitivity and specificity but also permit assessment of the main anatomical and functional aspects of interest for its management.

(a) Intimal tear location: The intimal tear appears as a discontinuity of the intimal flap. TEE provides a direct image of the tear and permits its measurement. Erbel et al.[40] demonstrated a different evolutive pattern depending on the presence and location of the tear. TEE permits identification of the tear in 78% to 100% of cases.[37,40,42] Color Doppler can reveal the presence of multiple small communications between the two lumina, especially in descending aorta (Fig. 45.4B).[46] Anatomical controls showed that these images might correspond to the origin of intercostal or visceral arteries. Pulsed Doppler imaging flow velocities obtained through the intimal tear reflect the pressure gradient between the two lumina. It is important to differentiate these secondary communications from the main intimal tear. The latter is usually identified by 2D echocardiography, tends to measure more than 5 mm, and may be located in the proximal part of the ascending aorta in type A dissections and immediately after the origin of the left subclavian artery in type B dissections. On occasions, 2D echocardiography does not permit visualization of the intimal tear in the proximal part of the arch. In these cases, contrast echocardiography may help by showing a contrast flow in the false lumen directed toward the distal part of the arch.

(b) True lumen identification: In certain circumstances, identification of the true lumen is of special clinical interest. When the aortic arch is involved, the surgeon needs to know whether the supra-aortic vessels originate from the false lumen. Similarly, when the descending aorta dissection affects visceral arteries and ischemic complications arise, it may be important to identify the false lumen prior to surgery or endovascular treatment such as intimal fenestration or endoprosthesis implantation. Percutaneous intimal fenestration may be a therapeutic alternative when main artery branches originate from the false lumen.

On most occasions, distinction between true and false lumina is easy. The false lumen is usually larger and has less flow than the true lumen. M-mode shows how the intima moves toward the false lumen at the start of systole by expansion of the true lumen and thrombus is frequently observed in the false lumen. Use of ultrasound contrast may aid in the correct identification of the true lumen as long as there is differential flow between true and false lumina. Furthermore, contrast echocardiography is the best way to analyze false lumen flow (Fig. 45.4D).

(c) Diagnosis of complications: Appropriate diagnosis of dissection complications during the initial study may affect therapeutic decisions in the acute phase:

– Pericardial effusion and periaortic bleeding. Pericardial effusion is not always due to extravasation of blood from the aorta and may be secondary to irritation of the adventitia produced by the aortic hematoma or small effusion from the wall. In any event, the presence of pericardial effusion in an ascending aorta dissection is a sign of poor prognosis and suggests leakages from the false lumen into the pericardium. Echocardiography is the best diagnostic technique for estimating the presence and severity of tamponade. When acute or subacute bleeding involves a mediastinal hematoma, it is characterized by an increased distance between the esophagus and the aorta (>10 mm) or the left posterior atrial wall.[47] Periaortic hematoma and pleural effusions are best diagnosed by CT. The presence of periaortic hematoma has been related to an increase in mortality.[48]

– Aortic regurgitation is a frequent complication occurring in approximately 40% to 76% of patients. The diagnosis and quantification of aortic insufficiency severity can be correctly made with Doppler echocardiography, both TTE and TEE. Furthermore, TEE provides information on possible mechanisms that influence aortic insufficiency, which may greatly aid the surgeon in deciding to replace the aortic valve.[49] Several mechanisms may determine the onset of significant aortic insufficiency: (i) dilatation of the aortic annulus secondary to dilatation of the ascending aorta; (ii) rupture of the annular support and tear in the implantation of one of the valvular leaflets; (iii) in asymmetric dissections, the hematoma itself may displace a leaflet segment below coaptation level; (iv) prolapse of the intima in the outward tract of the left ventricle through the valvular orifice (Fig. 45.4C); and (v) previous aortic valvular disease. In a study conducted by Armstrong et al.,[50] aortic insufficiency was severe in 45% of ascending aorta dissections.

– Arterial vessel involvement. Diagnosis of involvement of the main arterial vessels of the aorta is important as it may explain some of the symptoms or visceral complications that accompany the dissection and aid election of an appropriate therapeutic strategy. TEE provides optimal imaging of the whole aorta and sometimes visualizes the upper part of the abdominal aorta. The origin of the left subclavian artery is easily observed. However, emergences of innominate and left carotid arteries remain inconsistently detected. In these cases, the TTE suprasternal view appears very useful. The right brachiocephalic trunk is one of the arterial branches most frequently affected. TEE is not a good technique for assessing supra-aortic branch involvement. In a recent work using multiplanar probes, sensitivity, specificity, and accuracy in the diagnosis of supra-aortic branch pathology were 60%, 85%, and 78%, respectively.[42] Involvement of coronary arteries in dissection has been considered to occur in 10% to 15% of cases, with the right coronary artery being most frequently affected. TEE shows the most proximal segment of the coronary arteries; thus,

it can be verified whether the coronary ostium originates in the false lumen or whether coronary dissection is present. In our experience, TEE permitted diagnosis of celiac trunk involvement, dissection or compression in 90% of cases, and superior mesenteric involvement in 64%. Visceral or peripheral malperfusion syndrome is a complication with high morbidity and mortality. Although echocardiography can be useful in diagnosing dissection of the supra-aortic trunks, celiac trunk and superior mesenteric artery, CT provides far more precise information. This technique is also irreplaceable for diagnosing renal and iliac artery disease. TEE, similarly to CT, can diagnose two types of circulation disorders of arterial branches: Dissection or dynamic obstruction of the intimal dissection at the ostium of the arterial branches leaving the aorta. Differentiating the two mechanisms has important therapeutic implications.

3.3. Computed tomography

CT is a well-established and widely used method for the diagnosis of aortic diseases. The end of the last century saw the advent of multidetector CT (MDCT) as a first-line diagnostic tool in aortic diseases.[51] The basic premise of MDCT is the simultaneous acquisition of data by at least two adjacent detector rows, in contrast to only one detector row in the first generation of helical CT. This results in a proportional increase in volume scanned per unit of time. The shorter scan time permits better vascular opacification with less contrast media. On the other hand, the detector arrays have gradually become thinner, with an increase in through-plane spatial resolution (virtual thickness of the MDCT image), in the range of 0.5 to 0.75 mm. The in-plane resolution (pixel size in the MDCT image) remains at about 0.4 mm, resulting in an isovolumetric voxel in submillimeter range. ECG-gating allows synchronization at a single point in the cardiac cycle of adjacent cardiac slabs scanned in consecutive heart beats, creating a motionless volumetric study of the heart.[52] This major breakthrough renders coronary MDCT angiography possible, and it is also useful for motionless imaging of the aorta root and may play a role in dynamic evaluation of aortic distensibility.

3.3.1. Non-contrast-enhanced aortic multidetector computed tomography

MDCT without contrast media is frequently used to detect hemorrhage and hematomas. Flowing blood and fresh hemorrhage have low attenuation values, around 10 to 20 HU. After a few minutes, the breakdown of erythrocytes allows layering of hemoglobin, which results in higher CT attenuation values due to its ferric content, around 40 to 70 HU.[53] A nonenhanced scan should be the first step in MDCT evaluation of acute aortic syndrome. Hyperdense mural thickening of the aortic wall in this context is diagnostic of acute mural hematoma. Semicircular hyperdense strands inside the lumen of an aortic aneurysm may correspond to fresh hemorrhage inside a mural thrombus, which heralds rupture of the aneurysm. Acute rupture of an aneurysm of the thoracic aorta may course with any combination of massive hemothorax, hemomediastinum and hematic pericardial effusion, as well as compression of vital structures.

3.3.2. Contrast-enhanced aortic multidetector computed tomography

The majority of injection protocols for aortic MDCT angiography involve an initial injection of iodinated contrast media at a fixed rate of 4 to 5 mL/s, followed by the injection of 30 to 50 mL of saline at a similar rate. The preferred injection route is via a superficial vein in the right forearm. Left-side routes should be avoided since nondiluted contrast flowing through the innominate venous trunk produces artifacts that may hinder evaluation of the supra-aortic arterial trunks.[54] The total contrast material volume may be fixed or adjusted to the characteristics of both the patient and the MDCT system used. As a general rule, 100 to 120 mL of contrast with a concentration of 320 to 400 mg/mL of iodine usually suffice to obtain an aortogram of diagnostic quality.

The arrival of the contrast bolus is dynamically tracked by a user defined region of interest placed at a single slice of the aorta. When acute aortic syndrome is clinically suspected, it is recommended to avoid tracking the descending aorta owing to the risk of monitoring the false lumen and losing the arterial phase of the true lumen. In cases of doubt, the test can be started by simple visual inspection of contrast arrival in the region of interest. A second optional examination of the aorta may be indicated a few seconds after the first aortogram. This optional phase is useful to assess slow flow within the false lumen of aortic dissections, study the hemodynamic repercussions of the flap in solid organs, and to detect low-flow contrast extravasation indicating aortic rupture.

3.3.3. ECG-gated contrast-enhanced aortic multidetector computed tomography

MDCT studies without cardiac synchronization present artifacts of cardiac motion (including the aortic root) and aortic pulsatility due to transmission of the systolic wave. Faster heart rates will show an increased frequency of artifacts along the ascending aorta. Pulsatility often hinders the reliable study of aortic root and coronary artery involvement in aortic dissection. ECG-gating is required to freeze the cardiac cycle with a limited temporal resolution, between 80 and 210 ms, but keeping an excellent spatial resolution. These characteristics are sufficient for morphological and dynamic studies of both aortic root and coronary arteries. However, ECG-gated MDCT is a technically complex examination, which requires a much slower table displacement than in standard non-gated MDCT. As a result, the examination time and, therefore, apnea increases up to a minimum of 15 s for a gated study of the thoracic aorta using 64-detector technology. An additional disadvantage of this technique is the increase in exposure to ionizing radiation, which may double up to values of 20 mSv when compared with a standard non-ECG-gated study.[55] These limitations recommend avoiding this technique in patients with acute disease, who are frequently dyspneic, and require a complete thoracoabdominal study. In this context, a conventional aortic MDCT provides equally solid results with much shorter examination times, no breathing artifacts and lower iodinated contrast load.

The "triple rule-out" examination is an ECG-gated thoracic MDCT, which has been proposed as an emergency room test in the diagnosis of patients with acute atypical chest pain and intermediate or low cardiovascular risk, with the aim of avoiding unnecessary admissions of patients without cardiovascular disease. In this context, a single MDCT test may be able to simultaneously rule out coronary disease, acute aortic disease and pulmonary embolism. There is currently insufficient evidence to support its usefulness, but recently developed MDCT models capable of significantly reducing exposure dose in gated studies will probably facilitate diffusion of the test.[56] A new application of ECG-gated aortic MDCT is the study of aortic wall distensibility, which can be obtained from aortic luminal area variations throughout the cardiac cycle.[57]

3.3.4. Aortic atherosclerosis

CT is useful for the detection of protruding aortic atheroma, especially in areas not visualized by TEE. In one small study, CT

yielded a sensitivity of 87%, specificity of 82%, and an overall accuracy of 84% in comparison to TEE.[58] Although CT can distinguish calcified plaque from fibrolipidic plaque, this method is less efficient than MRI for the characterization of atherosclerotic plaque composition,[59] and standard non-ECG-gated MDCT does not assess plaque mobility.

3.3.5. Aortic aneurysm

The multiplanar capacity of MDCT, together with its submillimetric spatial resolution, render it an excellent technique for the serial evaluation of both thoracic and abdominal aortic aneurysms. The study of aneurysms and their presurgical evaluation requires an MDCT angiography with iodinated contrast,[60] although it can be obviated in the control of aortic ectasia since the difference in radiological density between the aortic wall and adjacent tissue (adipose-connective mediastinal, retroperitoneal, and lung) is sufficient for correct border delimitation. Nevertheless, studies without endovenous contrast only permit measurement of the external adventitial diameter. In the clinical context of suspected rupture of a known aneurysm, it is recommended to begin the study with a nonenhanced examination, which allows easy detection of mediastinal hemorrhage or intrathrombus bleeding.

Measurements must adhere to a strict protocol that permits comparison between different imaging techniques as well as follow-up of the patient.[61] MDCT permits us to choose an imaging plane in any arbitrary space orientation; thus, it is possible to easily find the maximum aortic diameter plane, which must be doubly orthogonal to the longitudinal plane of the aortic segment (Fig. 45.6). The presence of intraluminal contrast permits us to delimit the intimal surface, and therefore it is necessary to distinguish between vascular lumen diameter and aortic diameter (including wall thickness). A further common presentation of data is a parasagittal, oblique maximum intensity projection (MIP) plane that passes through the aortic root, ascending aorta, aortic arch, and descending aorta. The MIP plane must have a thickness proportional to the aortic tortuosity to make sure that the maximum diameter is included in the image. This plane is easily reproducible and comparable in follow-up studies.

3.3.6. Acute aortic syndromes

The purpose of aortic MDCT is to provide a complete study that permits the differential diagnosis and characterization of the entities that course with acute aortic syndromes.[62] An initial non-enhanced thoracic examination is useful for the diagnosis of intramural hematoma and hemorrhagic complications of aortic dissection (hemopericardium and hemomediastinum). Attenuation values

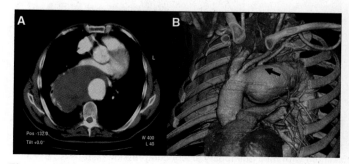

Figure 45.6 CT showing saccular aortic aneurysms. **A:** Axial image of a saccular aneurysm in distal thoracic aorta. Note large thrombus with adequate effective lumen; and **B:** Volume render of a MDCT aortography shows saccular aneurysms of aortic arch with left subclavian artery involvement (*arrow*).

of the fluid over 40 HU are considered diagnostic of hematic content.[54] Monitoring the bolus in the descending aorta should be avoided since partial or total placement of the region of interest in the false lumen will result in a low quality aortography. In this context, visual tracking of the arrival of contrast is preferable. The aortography must include the thoracic-abdominal region between the supra-aortic trunks and femoral arteries. We recommend having a third optional series in store, which can be started 20 seconds after the aortography if an aortic dissection is detected. This late phase study takes advantage of the still circulating contrast and is useful for distinguishing total false lumen thrombosis from total or partial filling of the false lumen through entry tears. The detector collimation (slice thickness) can be increased up to 2 to 3 mm to reduce the radiation dose.

– *Aortic dissection.* CT currently permits detection of the presence and extension of the intimomedial flap, measurement of flap thickness and its ratio to wall thickness, of the diameter ratio between the lumina and assessment of the degree of false lumen permeability (Fig. 45.7). A convex shape of the flap toward the true lumen indicates an ischemic configuration of the aortic dissection, with greater pressures and preferential flow in false lumen. MDCT delimitates the proximal extension of the dissection, the involvement of the aortic root, and the presence of hemopericardium (Fig. 45.7A).[54] An ECG-gated study permits us to assess the involvement of coronary arteries.[63,64] The dissection may extend distally to one iliac artery or both, ending in a cul-de-sac or rupturing into the true lumen. Detection and characterization of the intimal tear are essential for the treatment of aortic dissection, especially in Stanford type A aortic dissections. The entry tear in the ascending aorta can be large-sized and with a complex spiral morphology. The tachycardia and increased pulsatility of this zone in the acute patient can hinder visualization of the entry tear in conventional non-ECG-gated studies. In addition, MDCT permits detection of distal intimal ruptures (re-entry tears), which will be decisive in the evolution of the false lumen.

MDCT is irreplaceable in its capacity to study visceral artery involvement and for optimal therapy planning (Fig. 45.8). The relationship of the flap regarding the arterial branch can be summarized in the following configurations[63,64]: (a) branch origin in the false lumen with no flap involvement. The visceral perfusion depends on the flow dynamics of the false lumen; (b) origin in the true lumen, with no flap involvement. Adequate perfusion is not guaranteed, especially if there is proximal/upstream dynamic obstruction of the true lumen; (c) origin in the true lumen with dynamic obstruction and ischemic configuration, where the flap prolapses in the ostium of the branch and obstructs flow; (d) fixed obstruction in which the intimal dissection may stop in the bifurcation, wrest the intima from the ostium or extend through the vessel; and (e) mixed obstruction with ischemic configuration and simultaneous extension of the flap.

A further strong point of MDCT is the study of involved visceral organs. The inclusion of a late series adds dynamic information about organ perfusion and visceral ischemia, which is necessary for treatment and predicts patient outcome.[65] A cerebral vascular accident is associated with increased early mortality in dissected patients. A CT scan of the head may be performed additionally if neurologic involvement is suspected. The most frequently involved supra-aortic branches are the innominate artery and the left common carotid artery. The left subclavian artery is less frequently affected than the right subclavian artery. The characteristic pattern of dissection propagation consists in involvement of the left-sided branches of the descending thoracic and abdominal aorta. The left kidney is the organ at greater risk of ischemia. Kidney failure and mesenteric infarct have been identified by different groups as risk factors for early death in patients with dissection. If the dissection only affects the intercostal arteries on one side (generally the left), the contralateral arteries perfuse the spinal cord. Bilateral involvement will result in a medullary infarct. The absence of a re-entry tear in the distal aorta or its branches may collapse the true lumen from the pressure or thrombosis of the false canal and jeopardize perfusion through the true lumen (Fig. 45.7B). Lower limb ischemia has been described in up to 26% of patients with dissection.

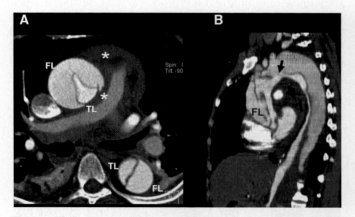

Figure 45.7 A: Axial MDCT image shows an almost circular flap involving the ascending aorta and extending to the descending aorta. Notice the hyperdense hematic pericardial effusion and hemomediastinum with mild pulmonary artery compression (*asterisks*); **B:** Parasagittal MPR (multiplanar reformation) of type A aortic dissection with involvement of descending and abdominal aorta. The *black arrow* marks the location of entry tear in the upper part of ascending aorta and total thrombosis of the distal part of descending aorta with partial true lumen compression. TL, true lumen; FL, False lumen.

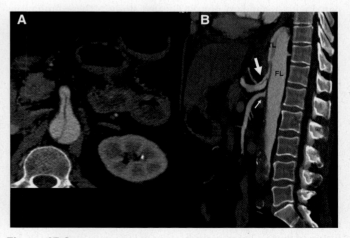

Figure 45.8 A: Axial MDCT shows dissection flap in abdominal aorta extending into the superior mesenteric artery; **B:** Sagittal MPR image shows involvement of the abdominal aorta. In this case, fixed obstruction of the celiac trunk (*arrow*), with flap extending into the proximal vessel and dynamic obstruction of the superior mesenteric artery, with curtainlike false lumen compressing true lumen at the arterial branch ostium. Note absence of enhanced blood at the distal aortic true lumen (*small arrow*). TL, true lumen; FL, False lumen.

– *Intramural hematoma.* In the acute setting, intramural hematoma is distinguished from dissection by its concentric and vertical involvement versus the descending spiral morphology of dissection, as well as by its high attenuation in a non-enhanced MDCT. On imaging follow-up of intramural hematoma, the appearance of ULP is frequently observed, as ulcers that rupture the intima and communicate the aortic lumen with the thrombosed medial wall hematoma (Fig. 45.9).[66]

– *Penetrating atherosclerotic* ulcer. The lesion disrupts the interna elastic media burrowing deeply into the aortic media and generating in some cases subintimal hematoma. The involvement is focal, preferentially located in the mid and distal thoracic aorta, despite the existence of ulcers in abdominal aorta (Fig. 45.10). This lesion is less frequently seen in the aortic root and ascending aorta, probably because they are relatively preserved from atherosclerosis.[67] Outside the context of acute aortic syndrome, the diagnosis of penetrating ulcers should be made with caution, since the degree of penetration of the intima in an atheromatous plaque cannot always be distinguished by MDCT.

3.4. Magnetic resonance imaging

MRI is a noninvasive imaging technique that permits the most complete study of aortic disease. It offers morphologic, functional, and biochemical information. Technological advances that have implied the implementation of faster gradients, newer sequences, and ultrafast MR angiography have led to MRI being the modality of choice for imaging aortic diseases. Conventional ECG-gated spin echo imaging and cine gradient echo have earned MRI the reputation of being the ideal tool for evaluating the aorta. Contrast-enhanced 3D MR angiography permits rapid acquisition and multiplanar imaging with minimal dephasing artifacts. Phase contrast imaging is another technique that enables flow in the great vessels to be evaluated with accurate quantification of peak velocity, and forward and regurgitant flow.

3.4.1. Black-blood sequences

Blood circulating through the aorta is black on conventional spin echo and turbo spin echo sequences owing to the signal emptying produced by the transit time effect of moving blood in the short phase. These sequences provide great morphologic information on the aortic wall and adjacent structures. T1- or T2-weighted images are useful for characterization of wall tissue, permitting assessment of the hematic content of the intramural hematoma or the lipid content of the atherosclerosed plaque. Postcontrast T1 imaging with fat suppression is useful in the diagnosis of some entities such as aortitis or mycotic aneurysms. ECG-triggered, breath-hold TSE has been the cornerstone of black-blood MRI for aortic disease. A double inversion-recovery technique is used to abolish the blood signal. The black-blood appearance is the result of nulling of the blood flowing into the slice by the first 180° inversion pulse at a specific inversion time (IT). Imaging occurs during mid to late diastole and the entire image is acquired over several heartbeats. Spin echo single-shot (HASTE or SS-FSE) sequences permit correct morphologic assessment of the aorta with very rapid acquisition times.[68]

3.4.2. Cine-MRI sequences

Cine-MR images are acquired using gradient echo sequences that provide excellent contrast between blood and surrounding tissue without the use of contrast agents. Contrast-to-noise depends on T2/T1 differences, which with short repetition times (TR) are high for blood and low for tissues. Given their high temporal resolution, it is possible to obtain images of multiple phases of the heart cycle and visualize blood flow both in systole and diastole. Gradient echo sequences generate images of brilliant blood. The emptying signal determines turbulent flow in hemodynamically significant stenosis or valvular regurgitation that may be useful in the detection of aortic coarctation or valvular disease. Steady-state free precession sequences (True fast imaging with steady state precession (FISP) Fiesta or Balanced fast field echo (FFE)) are those more commonly used. They, are normally used for the functional study of cardiac chambers, although their use is widely extended to the study of the aorta. Their main characteristic is that they permit high-contrast images with very short acquisition times since they have very low TR.[69] Velocity-encoded cine-MRI sequences (phase-contrast cine-MRI) provide great functional information owing to their capacity to quantify flow. Quantification of both

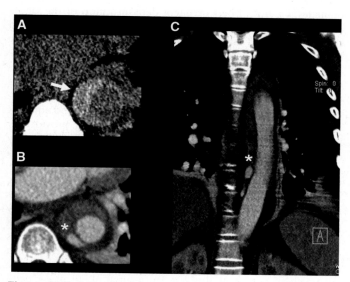

Figure 45.9 A: Axial source image from a nonenhanced MDCT scan in a patient with acute aortic syndrome. Arrow shows a hyperdense wedge in the descending aorta wall, which is the hallmark of intramural hematoma. Note its circular morphology. **B:** By enhanced MDCT angiography, the hematoma appears less dense than the aortic lumen. Asterisk marks the point of a small intimal tear causing a localized leak from the aortic lumen into the aortic media. **C:** Coronal MPR reformatted image shows type B intramural hematoma and the medial leak (*asterisk*).

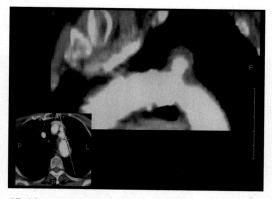

Figure 45.10 Parasagittal oblique MPR image of a MDCT aortography showing a penetrating aortic ulcer in the distal part of the aortic arch. Note its neck and protruding hypodense margins. The small inset shows the parasagittal imaging plane projected from the axial source image.

flow velocity and volume permits physiopathologic assessment of blood flow alterations in different aortic diseases. With this technique, the information is processed using signal magnitude images and phase images. Signal magnitude images are in brilliant blood and offer better anatomic assessment, while phase images show a map of flow velocities and direction. Using postprocessing techniques, it is possible to obtain curves of flow versus time, velocity versus time, and peak velocity versus time. In this manner, the hemodynamic repercussion can be quantified in different situations such as aortic coarctation or valvular disease, and also in the analysis of flow patterns in true and false lumina of aortic dissection. A more detailed explanation of MRI sequences and image acquisition protocols is available in Chapter 10)

3.4.3. Contrast-enhanced MR angiography

Contrast-enhanced MR angiography (CE-MRA) images are obtained by T1-weighted 3D gradient echo sequences following endovenous contrast administration, utilizing the shortening effect of T1 of contrast with gadolinium. These sequences offer important anatomic information on both the aorta and main vessels originating from it. This technique is suitable for the depiction of abnormalities such as penetrating atherosclerotic ulcers, dissection, coarctation, and aneurysm. The acquired images must be re-evaluated by postprocess MIP and MPR. By the application of ultrarapid spoiled gradient echo sequences in steady-state precession and the implantation of acquisition techniques in parallel, we can obtain multiphasic time-resolved 3D MRA images with high temporal and spatial resolution.[70] These sequences are very useful in aortic dissection or shunts. In multiphasic time-resolved 3D MRA sequences, contrast injection is started at the same time as the image acquisition, utilizing the first set of images as a mask for the posterior subtraction using postprocessing techniques and MIP and MPR reconstructions.

3.4.4. Atherosclerosis

MRA sequences are highly useful for the detection of aortic atheromatosis, although they offer only information on the repercussion of the plaque in the aorta lumen in the form of stenosis, which occurs in advanced stages of the disease. For only detection of atheromatous plaques, alterations occurring in the aortic wall must be observed. TSE sequences in black blood are very useful in the identification and characterization of the plaque and for distinguishing its constituent components in vivo. Being composed of cholesterol esters, the lipid nucleus has a short T2 and will be hypointense in T2-weighted images, while the fibrous capsule is hyperintense in T2-weighted images compared to the lipid nucleus.[71] Fayad et al.[72]

showed that MRI evaluation of the aorta compared well with TEE imaging for the assessment of aortic atherosclerotic plaque thickness, extent, and composition. Furthermore, high resolution noninvasive MRI demonstrates regression of aortic atherosclerotic lesions due to lipid lowering by simvastatin (Chapter 23).[72,73]

One promising aspect to be considered is the capability of MRI to detect inflammatory activity of atheromatous plaque with the administration of contrast media. Inflammatory phenomena that determine the accumulation of macrophages can be demonstrated as hyperenhancement of gadolinium chelates in the plaque. This enhancement is also produced with the use of other contrasts such as ultrasmall superparamagnetic particles of iron oxides by macrophages of the atheromatous plaque.[74,75]

3.4.5. Aortic aneurysms

The basic information to be obtained is aortic diameter and aneurysm extension and their relationships with the main arterial branches. CE-MRA offers excellent demonstration of the whole aortic anatomy and is very efficacious for the identification and characterization of aneurysms. It is recommendable to combine MRA images with spin echo in black-blood images, which are very useful for detecting alterations in the wall and adjacent structures that could go unnoticed if only MRA images are acquired. In mycotic aneurysm, postcontrast T1-weighted images permit identification of inflammatory changes in the aortic wall and adjacent fat, secondary to bacterial infection. The information provided by MRA in aortic aneurysm assessment is similar to that offered by current CT equipment with multidetections. Both methods permit us to accurately determine aortic diameters in sagittal plane. Furthermore, preprocessing techniques (MIP, MPR, and rendering volume) facilitate visualization of the aorta in its entirety together with the relationship of its principal branches and are highly useful when planning treatment (Fig. 45.11). The advantage of MRI over CT is that it is a nonionizing technique that permits serial follow-up studies to be conducted innocuously. For correct monitoring, it is necessary to measure aortic diameter in the same location and same spatial plane. The sagittal plane allows us to obtain more reproducible measurements. The combination of information obtained on aneurysm morphology and functional data provided by cine-MRI sequences aids understanding of the physiopathology of aneurysmal dilatation. When the aneurysm affects the ascending aorta, it is recommended to conduct a functional study through the aortic valve using cine-MRI sequences to rule out associated valvular disease that may be related to aortic dilatation. Recently, MRI has been established as an accurate noninvasive tool for the assessment of aortic distensibility and pulse

Figure 45.11 Saccular atherosclerotic aneurysm. Volume-rendering images by contrast-enhanced MR angiography show a saccular aneurysm of the aortic arch and its relationship with supra-aortic branches.

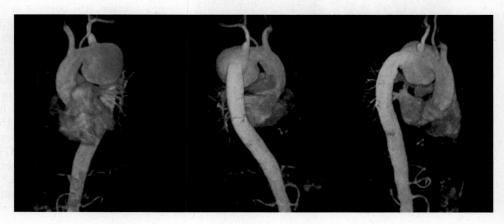

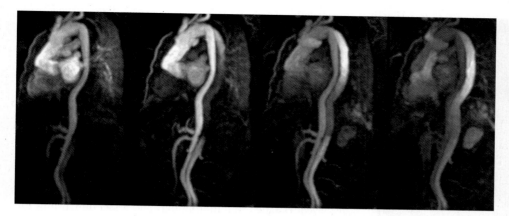

Figure 45.12 Surgically-treated type A aortic dissection with patent false lumen in descending aorta. Time-resolved sagittal maximum-intensity-projection angiograms show time course of enhancement of both lumina. Note the proximal and distal simultaneous inflow of the false lumen.

wave velocity. These methods have been used to assess aortic elasticity in patients with Marfan syndrome, bicuspid aortic valve, or aortic aneurysms.[76]

3.4.6. Acute aortic syndrome

Aortic dissection. The diagnosis of aortic dissection is based on the demonstration of the intimal flap that separates the true from the false lumen. Both black-blood images and CE-MRA images show the presence of the intimal flap. Contrast CE-MRA has proved to be superior to black-blood sequences in the assessment of dissection extension and supra-aortic trunk involvement. Owing to the limitation of this technique to visualize the aorta wall and adjacent structures, the study protocol of aortic dissection should include black-blood sequences to rule out wall structure alterations.

For planning surgery or endovascular repair, it is very useful to demonstrate the course of the flap, entry tear location, false lumen thrombosis, aortic diameter, and main arterial trunk involvement by postprocessed techniques with MPR, MIP, volume rendering, etc. It is mandatory to always visualize the image source of the CE-MRA since the flap may not be seen on volumetric reconstruction.[77] Above all, in type B dissections (Stanford type B), it is important to acquire images with wide field of view that include the whole aorta from the arch to the aortic bifurcation. Time-resolved MRA provides additional functional information compared to conventional MRA. The dynamic assessment of blood flow in entry tears is the main advantage of time-resolved MRA. The longer resolution times of conventional MRA, around 20 s, do not permit correct demonstration of dynamic changes in blood flow through the different entry tears. On the other hand, the different timing in contrast enhancement in both lumina implies that one of the lumina remains partially contrasted with the use of long resolution time sequences. By applying rapid MRA sequences, we obtain multiple continuous acquisitions, succeeding in visualizing both lumina with maximum contrast concentration in different phases, which facilitates their morphologic assessment (Fig. 45.12).[78] In ascending aorta dissections (Stanford type A), it is recommendable to include cine-MRI sequences on the left ventricular outflow tract in the study protocol to rule out valvular regurgitation.

Intramural hematoma. Although greater availability and rapidity favor the use of CT in acute disease, MRI plays a major role in the diagnosis of intramural hematoma. The greater contrast among tissues offered by MRI permits small intramural hematomas, which may go unnoticed by CT, to be detected.[79] The

typical finding that permits diagnosis by MRI is the presence of wall thickening of the hyperintense aorta on T1-weighted black-blood sequences. In hyperacute phase, the hematoma shows an isointense signal in T1-weighted images and a hyperintense signal in T2-weighted images (Fig. 45.13). From the first 12 to 24 h, the change from oxyhemoglobin to metahemoglobin determines a hyperintense signal in T1- and T2-weighted images, which, with fat suppression, are useful to differentiate periaortic fat from intramural hematoma. On occasions, mural thrombi may present a semilunar morphology that mimicks the morphology of the intramural hematoma, rendering the differential diagnosis by CT or TEE difficult. This differentiation is easier by MR since mural thrombosis shows a hypointense or isointense signal in both T1-and T2-weighted sequences (Fig. 45.14).

Penetrating ulcer. The diagnosis of penetrating ulcer by MRI is based on the identification of adherence to the aortic wall, with a craterlike appearance, in MRI sequences. Black-blood sequences may show disruption of the intima with extension of the ulcer to the media, which is thickened, and may be associated with the formation of an intramural hematoma. It may be difficult to differentiate penetrating ulcer from the typical forms of dissection. The differential diagnosis should be established between arteriosclerotic ulcers that penetrate

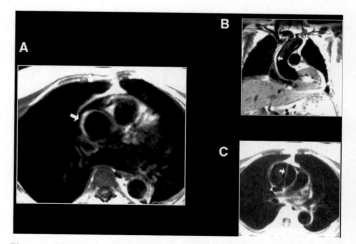

Figure 45.13 Type A aortic intramural hematoma. **A:** Axial and **B:** Coronal T1-weighted black-blood image shows a thin intramural hematoma (*arrow*) formation in ascending aorta. **C:** Follow-up axial T1-weighted black-blood image obtained 6 months later shows a new aortic dissection (*arrow*) in ascending aorta.

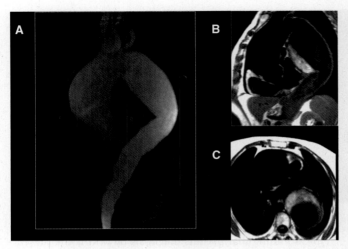

Figure 45.14 Intramural hematoma diagnosed by MRI. Sagittal oblique MIP reformation of contrast-enhanced MRA shows an aneurysm in ascending and proximal descending thoracic aorta **(A)**; T1-weighted black-blood image shows eccentric thickening of the anterior wall of the descending aorta with increased signal intensity, indicating intramural hematoma in sagittal **(B)** and axial **(C)** views.

the middle layer and ulcerlike images that develop from a localized dissection of an intramural hematoma that appears as a pseudoaneurysm located in the area of the former intramural hematoma. Prognosis of these ulcerlike images is clearly more benign than that of symptomatic arteriosclerotic ulcers.

3.4.7. Aortitis

Spin echo in black-blood sequences is useful to identify the wall thickening produced in aortitis of diverse causes. In the initial stages of Takayasu arteritis, short inversion-time, inversion-recovery (STIR), and postcontrast T1-weighted sequences are particularly useful. Inflammatory changes in initial phases are reflected with contrast hyperuptake and hyperintensity secondary to the wall edema in STIR sequences (Fig. 45.15). In advanced stages of the disease, CE-MRA details the presence of stenosis in the aorta and its main branches secondary to the fibrous changes that appear in chronic phase.

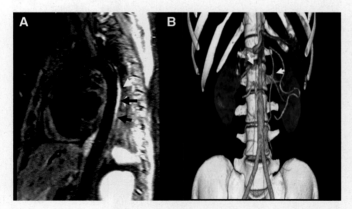

Figure 45.15 Takayasu arteritis. **A:** Initial stage. Sagittal STIR image by MRI shows thickening of the aorta wall with increased signal (*arrow*), suggesting wall edema; **B:** Advanced stage. Anterior view of a volume render from a MDCT angiography. Notice the small thoracoabdominal aortic luminal diameter with normal size at the infrarenal segment. Arrows show proximal renal artery stenosis.

3.5. Intravascular ultrasound

Intravascular ultrasound employs the same principles as conventional ultrasound in a catheter-based technology. It is an invasive technique using a percutaneous sheath delivery system over a guide wire. Current phased-array intravascular catheters for aortic dissection utilize frequencies of around 10 MHz. The best images are obtained on withdrawal rather than insertion and when the catheter is parallel to the vessel. The ultrasound beam is then directed at 90 degrees to the luminal surface. One limitation of intravascular ultrasound (IVUS) is the blind spot in the immediate vicinity of the catheter. Longitudinal reconstruction of the IVUS images provides further understanding. The images are stacked and a longitudinal view similar to an angiogram is displayed. Detailed wall morphology and vessel dimensions can then be viewed in the cross-sectional images.

There is valuable information that can be obtained by IVUS such as identification of the proximal entry point and the distal extent of dissection, the relationship of the false lumen with the major aortic vessels, and the measurement of aortic dimensions during endovascular treatment. When using IVUS in a suspected thoracic dissection it is conventional to insert the catheter using a retrograde femoral approach. IVUS is useful in the endovascular management of dissection and some experts consider this technique the method of choice. The use of intravascular ultrasound has been advocated to complement angiographic information in endovascular therapy. In patients with classic forms of aortic dissection, this catheter-based imaging tool provides crisp visualization of the intimal-medial flap. This technique appears particularly well suited to delineate the most distal extent of abdominal aortic dissection.[80] Sensitivities and specificities of close to 100% have been reported.[81] IVUS may also help to distinguish the true from false lumen when it is difficult to make this distinction. Branch involvement appears to be better defined with IVUS than with TEE or with CT.[80,81] In addition, the precise mechanism of vessel compromise (dissection intersecting and narrowing of the vessel origin versus ostium spared by the dissection but covered by a prolapsing flap) may be clarified by IVUS.

3.6. Nuclear metabolic imaging

Findings of preliminary animal experimental studies showed that FDG PET may depict and quantify the macrophage content within aortic plaques. Using fused PET/CT images, Tatsumi et al.[82] showed that FDG uptake frequently occurs in the aortic wall in humans. The tracer uptake site was mostly distinct from the location of the site of calcification. The frequency of FDG uptake was significantly higher in patients 55 or older and tended to be higher in women with a history of cardiovascular disease. PET/CT may be depicting the metabolic activity of atherosclerosis changes.[83] More detailed description of the role of PET-FDG for the evaluation of aortic atherosclerosis is available in Chapter 23.

3.7. Diagnostic strategies
3.7.1. Aortic atherosclerosis

TEE and MRI are powerful noninvasive tools for visualizing aortic atheromas. In patients with stroke or peripheral embolism, TEE is the technique of choice since it affords excellent assessment of the size and mobility of complicated plaques. MR imaging can noninvasively distinguish various components of the plaque such as fibrous cap, lipid core, and thrombus, thereby assessing plaque stability. In T2-weighted images, fibrous cap and thrombus are seen as a high-intensity signal, and lipid core is seen as a low-intensity signal. Unlike TEE, MRI can visualize the entire thoracic aorta including the small section of ascending aorta, which is obscured by the tracheal air column. Also, serial MRI can be used to monitor progression and regression of atheromatous plaques after lipid-lowering therapy. The limitations of MRI imaging include its cost, reduced ability to assess plaque mobility, and its contraindication in patients with pacemaker or defibrillator.

3.7.2. Aortic aneurysm

Aneurysms affecting the aortic root can be correctly assessed by TEE if the echocardiographic window is adequate. The excellent reproducibility of measurements at this level and information from other parameters such as aortic regurgitation severity, ventricular function, etc., facilitate appropriate follow-up. TEE will only be warranted when the acoustic window is poor or when the type of surgical treatment (repair or valve replacement) is considered. Both TTE and TEE have limitations for adequate measurement of distal ascending aorta diameters, aortic arch, and descending aorta. However, contrast-enhanced CT scanning and MRI very accurately detect the size of thoracic aortic aneurysms. Axial images often cut through the ascending aorta off-axis, resulting in a falsely large aortic diameter. Nevertheless, when the axial data are reconstructed into 3D images (CT angiography), one can measure the tortuous aorta in true cross section and obtain an accurate diameter. Such 3D imaging should then always be used to follow such patients over time. MRI may be preferred, however, for the follow-up of younger patients, since it avoids the need for ionising radiation.

3.7.3. Acute aortic syndromes

The role of imaging techniques has changed substantially in recent years. Until 15 years ago, it was usual to perform diagnostic aortography. This technique was later shown to lead to a 20% rate of false-negative diagnoses, especially in thrombosed type A dissections and intramural hematoma.[3] A recently published meta-analysis[51] showed diagnostic accuracy to be practically the same (95% to 100%) for CT, TEE, and MRI. Most shortcomings are due to user interpretation errors rather than the technique itself. The analysis of the International Registry of Aortic Dissection (IRAD)[21] showed that CT is the most frequently used imaging technique (61%), followed by echocardiography (33%), angiography (4%) and MRI (2%). The main advantage of CT is its wide availability, accuracy, and rapidity (Table 45.1). However, echocardiography also plays an important role in diagnosis, mainly of type A dissection. TTE with harmonic imaging might be of particular value since it is a rapid and easily available imaging modality. TTE is a noninvasive test that is perfectly tolerated, easily performed at the patients' bedside, and rapid. Although harmonic imaging has improved the sensitivity of TEE in visualizing intimal flap dissection, it does not make it possible to definitively rule out acute aortic syndrome.

TABLE 45.1
COMPARING THE DIAGNOSTIC VALUE OF IMAGING TECHNIQUES IN AORTIC DISSECTION

	TTE/TEE	MDCT	MRI	Angiography	IVUS
Sensitivity	+++	+++	+++	++	+++
Specificity	+++	+++	+++	++	+++
Classification	+++	+++	+++	+	++
Tear localization	+++	+++	++	+	+
Aortic regurgitation	+++	–	++	++	–
Pericardial effusion	+++	+++	+++	–	–
Mediastinal hematoma	++	+++	+++	–	+
Side branch involvement	++	+++	++	+++	+++
Coronary artery involvement	++	+++	++	+++	++
X-ray exposure	–	++	–	+++	–
Patient comfort	+	+++	+	+	+
Follow-up studies	++	+++	+++	–	–
Intraoperative availability	+++	–	–	(+)	(+)

TTE/TEE, transthoracic/transoesophageal echocardiography; MDCT, multidetector computed tomography; MRI, magnetic resonance imaging; IVUS, intravascualr ultrasound.

In our experience, the best combination for correctly diagnosing acute aortic dissection and its complications is CT and TTE. Ascending aortic dissections should be examined by TEE when serious diagnostic questions arise following CT or when hemodynamic instability makes it inadvisable to transfer the patient. The role of TEE, once the syndrome has been diagnosed by CT, depends on the quality of study and whether it is a disease of the ascending or descending aorta. In cases of ascending aorta involvement, it is fundamental to locate the entry tear before considering surgical treatment. In our opinion, if the diagnosis appears to be definitive by CT, a transthoracic study should always be performed to assess the presence and etiology of the aortic insufficiency, pericardial effusion, and ventricular function (Fig. 45.16). Similarly, it is easy to obtain information on the dissection of supra-aortic vessels using the suprasternal approach. In hospitals with cardiac surgery and sufficient experience in TEE, it may be performed as a first-choice diagnostic technique, since its information suffices in the majority of cases to indicate the

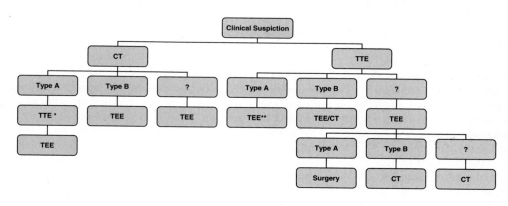

Figure 45.16 Diagnostic test algorithm in clinical suspicion of acute aortic syndrome. T = E*T if TTE information is definitive, TEE may be performed in the operating room before surgery.

most appropriate medical or surgical treatment. Patients should be strongly sedated and hemodynamic monitoring constant during the procedure. Ideally, in type A aortic syndrome, TEE should be performed immediately prior to surgery in the operating room under general anesthesia to avoid an increase in blood pressure that may favor an aortic rupture, and the results assessed intraoperatively. When the disease affects only the descending aorta, TEE is recommended when the patient is hemodynamically stable and pain-free. Hemokinetic information, location of entry and re-entry sites, partial thrombosis, and maximum diameter of the false lumen may aid the decision to implant an endoprosthesis with the aim of closing the intimal tear.

CT is certainly an efficient diagnostic imaging modality for intramural hematoma. Detection is based on the high-attenuation signal of acute bleeding. If only images after contrast enhancement are acquired, the aortic wall thickening may simulate atheromatous involvement of the aorta. Therefore, every aortic examination for an acute aortic syndrome requires images before and after intravenous contrast enhancement. The management strategy of thoracic pain suggestive of acute aortic syndrome frequently includes at least two imaging techniques. This strategy could be mandatory for detecting intramural hematoma and may explain why the incidence rate varies from 5% to 30% in the series reported in the literature.[22,84] In stable patients with doubtful intramural hematoma diagnosis by CT, MRI is the technique of choice as the hyperintense signal in the aortic wall can facilitate a correct diagnosis. CT is better than TEE for detection of aortic ulcers, particularly if they are small. It is efficient for the evaluation of their penetration and bleeding inside or outside the aortic wall. MRI is accurate for the investigation of aortic ulcers, especially for intramural hemorrhage-complicating ulcers and is indicated if renal failure is present.

TEE, CT, and MRI are also very useful in the diagnosis of traumatic aortic lesions such as intimal dissection medial laceration, pseudoaneurysm, or periaortic hemorrhage.[85,86] The selection of the imaging test depends on the hemodynamic unstability of the patient and the availability and experience of the centre. TEE offers excellent information on the aortic wall lesions, but both, CT and MR, have an advantage because of their wider field of vision.

4. SELECTING AND GUIDING THERAPY

Aortic root pathology is now accepted as the most common cause of aortic valve incompetence. The diameter of the sinotubular junction is 10% to 15% smaller than the diameter of the annulus. The upper part of the valve commissures is attached just below the sinotubular junction and the diameter of the aorta at this level approximates to that of the annulus. The noncoronary sinus is the largest of the three sinuses. The length of the base of the leaflets is approximately 1.5 times longer than the length of its free margin.

4.1. Ascending aorta aneurysm surgery

Valve insufficiency appears because dilatation of the root and/or sinotubular junction will displace the valve commissures outwards so that the leaflet edges cannot coapt in diastole. Conventional treatment of aortic regurgitation caused by a dilated, aneurysmal aortic root is replacement of the ascending aorta using a synthetic graft, replacement of the aortic valve with a mechanical prosthesis (the graft and prosthesis are usually combined as a "composite graft"), and reimplantation of the coronary arteries. In selected cases without sinuses dilatation, the valve and ascending aorta may be replaced separately. The geometric relationships

of the aortic root have been shown to be consistent over a wide range of sizes, an important point when surgical reconstruction is considered. Patients who have aortic root pathology and normal aortic valve leaflets are suitable for a remodeling procedure. It is imperative that perioperative TEE be used in these patients. This will provide the surgeon with important information regarding the morphology of the aortic root and also the dimensions of the aortic annulus and severity of any aortic regurgitation. If the aortic annulus is also dilated (>28 mm) on echocardiography during perioperative measurement, the remodeling procedure can be combined with a surgical annuloplasty. TEE must also be used following the procedure to ensure that there is no residual aortic regurgitation.

The functional classification of aortic root abnormalities responsible for aortic regurgitation attempts to provide a simple guide to aid the diagnosis of major abnormalities so that corrective surgical techniques can then be applied.[87] The classification applied by TEE information is based on the assessment of leaflet function and root anatomy. In type I abnormalities, the leaflet motion seems normal and the leaflets themselves appear structurally normal. Aortic regurgitation is due to the enlargement of one or both of the areas supporting the leaflets. The outward displacement of the commissures is responsible for a decreased coaptation of the aortic cusps causing central aortic regurgitation. Abnormalities in the type I group are further subdivided into type Ia, aneurysm of the ascending aorta as in atherosclerotic aneurysm; type Ib, aneurysm of the aortic root, as in Marfan syndrome; type Ic, isolated dilatation of the annulus although it is often associated with type Ib; and type Id, perforation of the leaflets due to traumatic or infective processes. In type II lesions, one or more of the cusps prolapse below the level of normal coaptation, the prolapse may sometimes form part of a degenerative process related to aging and hypertension, late state of Ib lesions, or regurgitant bicuspid lesions. In this type of lesion, the direction of the aortic regurgitation jet is toward the mitral valve or the septum. In type III lesions, one or more cusps do not reach the opposing cusps because their motion is restricted by fibrosis or calcification; they are present in rheumatic or degenerative disease of the elderly. In type Ia, aortic regurgitation reduction is usually achieved by replacing the ascending aorta with an appropriately sized Dacron graft. Type Ib lesions are treated by an aortic-sparing operation, the reimplantation technique (David operation). In this procedure, the native aortic cusps and their commissures are reimplanted inside a tubular Dacron graft. In type Ic lesions, the most appropriate surgical procedure may be a partial subcommissural annuloplasty, associated with a sinotubular junction plasty. Type Id are treated by patch closure. In type II lesions, cusp prolapse is treated by plication of the free margin if the cusp is priable, and in bicuspid aorta valve resection of the diseased area of the valve may be necessary. Type III lesions often need aortic valve replacement. Furthermore, some studies have shown that functional anatomy defined by TEE is strongly and independently predictive of valve repairability and postoperative outcome.[87]

4.2. Surgery in type A aortic syndrome

Two key questions need to be answered by TEE prior to deciding on the most appropriate technique for repairing an acute type A (types I and II) dissection: What is the size of the aortic root and what is the condition of the aortic valve? If the ascending aorta and aortic root diameters are normal without downstream displacement of the coronary ostia and with no commissural detachment of the aortic valve leaflets or other acute or chronic pathological changes of the leaflets, a tubular graft is usually anastomosed to the sinotubular ridge. Whenever one or more commissures are detached, the valve needs to be resuspended prior to graft insertion. If valve reconstruction appears unsafe, or if obvious congenital or acquired abnormalities are present, it is generally better to replace the valve before a supracommissural graft is inserted.

An acute type A dissection in a previously ectatic proximal aorta requires a different approach. In such circumstances, including most patients with Marfan syndrome, implantation of a composite graft (aortic valve prosthesis plus ascending aortic tube graft) is recommended. Valve-sparing operations are more complicated and time-consuming than composite grafting and should be performed by surgeons who have wide experience in such procedures in elective cases.

4.3. Endovascular therapy in descending aorta

The submillimetric multiplane capacity of MDCT permits topographic planning of endovascular prosthesis implantation, both in descending thoracic aorta and abdominal aorta. MDCT also has a role in the planning of endovascular fenestration of the flap in cases of organic ischemia due to the flap obstruction.[88] The minimum requirements for endoprosthesis implantation are (a) the endoprosthesis must cover the damaged zone and a minimum of 15 mm of healthy aorta. If sufficient proximal neck is not available, the origin of the left subclavian artery is covered providing there is good contralateral vertebral circulation, or a protective carotid-subclavian bypass is performed; (b) maximum landing zone diameter of 40 mm; and (c) absence of thrombus or circumferential atheroma in landing zone.

The rationale for endovascular treatment of aortic dissection was originally based on evidence in the literature of the protective effect of false lumen thrombosis against false lumen expansion. Closure of the entry tear of a type B dissection may promote both depressurization and shrinkage of the false lumen, with subsequent thrombosis, remodeling and stabilization of the aorta.[89,90] In aortic dissection, successful fenestration provides a re-entry tear for the dead-end false lumen back into the true lumen which allows expansion of the true lumen and improvement in the flow of arterial branches connected to the true lumen.

Visceral and supra-aortic vessel involvement can be detected by MDCT documenting true or false lumen supply. Axial and MPR images provide an overall view of the aortic dissection and demonstrate the anatomic relationships between the flap and adjacent great vessels. Measurements for sizing stent graft should be assessed in MIP reconstruction and SSD (shaded surface display) since being the most accurate and reliable in multiplanar measurements, MIP and SSD preserve the variable enhancement patterns of the lumina and are more sensitive for visualization of the flap and entry sites. MDCT is better to investigate the extension of aortic dissection toward visceral arteries and the mechanisms of visceral ischemia. MDCT and TEE both will help identify the best route and therapeutic strategy for endovascular or surgical treatment of organ malperfusion. The search for entry sites may be instrumental in decision making.

TEE can be highly useful in the operating room to guide correct stent positioning in type B aortic dissection and visualizing safe advancement of the stent graft device in the true lumen and its position in front of the entry site.[91,92] Stent deployment can be monitored by fluoroscopy using TEE probe as a marker facing the selected area, thereby avoiding the need for repeated contrast medium injections. After stent deployment, TEE with color-Doppler is more sensitive than angiography in identifying endoleak (usually velocity >100 cm/s). TEE guidance of balloon inflation

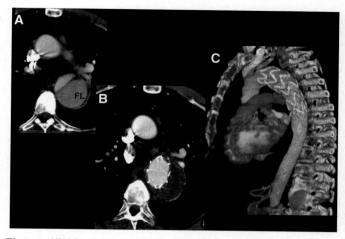

Figure 45.17 Descending aorta dissection treated by stent-graft implantation. **A:** Axial CT shows a type B aortic dissection with large false lumen (FL); **B:** After endografting total thrombosis of the false lumen was visualized; and **C:** Volume render showing the proximal struts of the stents correctly placed distal to the origin of subclavian artery. No flow outside the stent is seen with patent branch vessels of the aorta.

can detect complete balloon expansion. Monitoring of thrombus formation is a direct sign of the success of the procedure.

IVUS is useful in guiding endovascular surgery. In particular, in identifying the origin of the dissection and the extent; the relationship of the false lumen to the major vessels; confirming correct deployment of the stent; and ensuring none of the great vessels have been compromised by the stent. One limitation of IVUS is the blind spot in the immediate vicinity of the catheter. However this is not generally a problem as the probe can be rotated within the vessel lumen so the vessel wall can be clearly seen. Another limitation is reflections of air bubbles trapped in the prosthetic material, and its inability to obtain good images beyond the metallic material. Intraluminal phased-array imaging is increasingly accepted for cardiac applications. Bartel et al.[93] showed that intraluminal phased-array imaging may be superior to IVUS and TEE in detecting communications between the true and false lumens, and it is also highly useful as a guiding tool for emergency intimal flap fenestration.

CT and MR are standard in the follow-up phase and are satisfactory in identifying false lumen thrombosis and detecting the presence of endoleaks (Fig. 45.17).

5. IMAGING AND PROGNOSIS

5.1. Aortic aneurysm

The size of the aorta is the principal predictor of aortic rupture or dissection.[94] In a large retrospective study gathering thoracic aortic aneurysms from different etiologies, the risk of rupture or dissection was 6.9% per year and, including death, was 15.6% per year for a size >60 mm. The odds ratio for rupture increased 27-fold compared with lower values.[94] The mean rate of growth for all thoracic aneurysms was 1 mm/year. The rate of growth was significantly greater for aneurysms of the descending aorta, 1.9 mm/year, than those of the ascending aorta, 0.7 mm/year. In addition, dissected thoracic aneurysms grew significantly more rapidly (1.4 mm/year) than nondissected aneurysms (0.9 mm/year). The mean rupture rate was only 2% per year for aneurysms less than 50 mm in diameter, rising slightly to 3% for aneurysms with diameter of 50 to 59 mm, but increasing sharply to 7%

per year for aneurysms 60 mm or larger. In a more recent study, Davies et al.[95] showed, from a series of 410 patients, that aortic size index is a significant predictor of aortic rupture. The authors recommended elective operative repair before the patient enters the zone of moderate risk with an aortic size index >2.75 cm/m^2.

The clinical importance of maximum aortic diameter in the indication for prophylactic surgical treatment implies taking measurements as accurately as possible. In studies comparing the reproducibility of the three techniques, echocardiography, CT, and MRI, interobserver variability varies and increases with aortic diameter. It is essential for the same observer to compare measurements side by side using the same anatomic references. Tomographic scans in a situation where the aorta does not lie perpendicular to the plane of the scan produce an elliptical image with a major (maximum) and minor (minimum) diameter. In most natural history studies of aneurysm expansion, the minimum diameter has been reported to avoid the effect of convolution. However, MDCT permits us to define a plane in any arbitrary space orientation and easily find the orthogonal plane to the vessel walls. Measurements should be taken on MPR images. The systematic use of this approach showed interobserver variability of 2.8 ± 4.4 mm, significantly lower than that obtained with axial images (4.0 ± 5.1 mm).

5.2. Acute aortic syndrome

Along with age, signs, and/or symptoms of organ malperfusion and clinical instability, fluid extravasation into the pericardium and periaortic hematoma have poor prognosis in acute phase.[96] After discharge, variables related to greater aortic dilatation were entry tear size, maximum descending aorta diameter in subacute phase, and the high pressure pattern in false lumen. Maximum aortic diameter in subacute phase[97] was a significant predictor of progressive dilatation since, according to Laplace law, maximum aortic diameter is the factor influencing increased wall stress.

MRI appears to be the technique of choice for following patients treated medically or surgically in acute aortic syndrome. MRI avoids exposure to ionizing radiation or nephrotoxic contrast agents used for CT and is less invasive than TEE. The large field of view of MRI permits visualization of anatomical landmarks in order to take measurements at an identical level of the aorta. Furthermore, the integrated study of anatomy and physiology of blood flow can provide very interesting data to clarify the mechanisms responsible for aortic dilatation. Time-resolved MRA can provide additional dynamic information of blood flow in entry tears. Velocity-encoded cine-MR sequences have a promising role in the functional assessment of aortic dissection through the quantification of flow in both lumina and the possibility of establishing hemodynamic patterns of progressive dilatation risk. This technique together with time-resolved MRA should provide new and highly useful physiopathologic understanding to determine the best therapeutic management in each case.

CT is the technique most frequently performed to follow-up aortic dissection. CT has excellent reproducibility in aortic diameter measurements and accuracy in detecting signs of leakages at anatomoses/stent sites and permits vessel malperfusion assessment (Fig. 45.18). Regular controls of the aorta should be made at 3, 6, and 12 months after the acute event, followed by yearly examination.

TEE provides prognostic information in acute type A dissection beyond that provided by clinical risk variables. A flap confined to ascending aorta or a completely thrombosed false lumen showed a protective role.[97] Finally, increased false lumen pressure was another important factor implying false lumen enlargement.

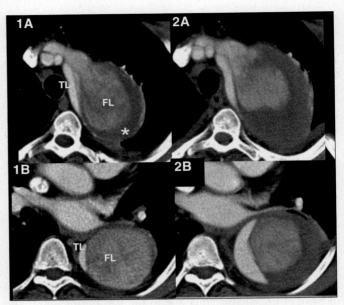

Figure 45.18 Follow-up of type B aortic dissection by MDCT. **1A:** Axial source image shows predominant enhancement of the true lumen (TL) and a large false lumen (FL) with mural thrombus (*asterisk*); **1B:** Axial image at a lower level; **2A:** Five months later, MDCT shows severe increase of the aortic size due to false lumen expansion, with an increase of the peripheral thrombus; and **2B:** Axial MDCT image at the **1B** level shows dramatic increase of both false lumen and true lumen and caudal extension of the thrombus.

The high false lumen pressure was due, in the majority of cases, to a large entry tear without distal emptying flow or re-entry site of similar size. It is often difficult to identify the distal discharge communication; thus, indirect signs of high false lumen pressure such as true lumen compression,[98] partial thrombosis of the false lumen[99] or the velocity pattern of the echocardiographic contrast in false lumen should be considered.[100]

The evolution of intramural hematoma to reabsorption, aneurysm formation, or dissection (Fig. 45.19).[84] Intramural hematoma regressed completely in 34% of patients, progressed to aortic dissection in 12% and to aneurysm in 20%, and evolved to pseudoaneurysm in 24% (Fig. 45.20). Given their wider field of view, MRI and CT are better than TEE in defining this

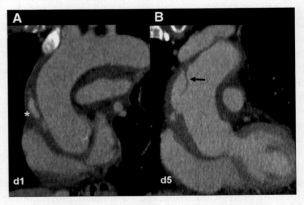

Figure 45.19 Evolution of acute type A intramural hematoma. **A:** Oblique coronal MPR image shows acute type A intramural hematoma with a small leak in the media (*asterisk*). **B:** Five days later, CT shows enlargement of the tear and progression of the leak, expanding the aortic diameter and separating an intimomedial flap (*arrow*) evolving to a localized dissection.

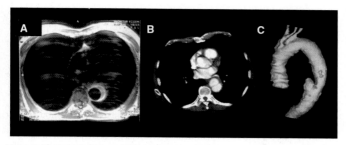

Figure 45.20 Intramural hematoma in descending aorta by MRI **(A)**, which evolves at 6 months to localized dissection shown by MDCT **(B)**, and progressive pseudoaneurysm formation by volume render MDCT **(C)**.

dynamic evolution. MRI is able to diagnose the intramural bleeding evolution and new asymptomatic intramural rebleeding episodes.

The natural history of penetrating aortic ulcer is unknown. Like intramural hematoma, several evolutive possibilities have been described. Many patients with penetrating ulcer do not need immediate aortic repair but do require close follow-up with serial imaging studies, by CT or MRI, to document any disease progression. Although many authors have documented the propensity for aortic ulcers to develop progressive aneurysmal dilatation, the progression is usually slow. Spontaneous, complete aortic rupture may occur. Some aortic ulcers are an incidental finding, similar to saccular aneurysms. In these cases, size and enlargement are the only predictors of complications.

6. FUTURE DIRECTIONS

The considerable advances in imaging techniques have greatly increased our understanding of aortic diseases. The clinical usefulness of each imaging modality for the diagnosis of the different aortic diseases is well established. The availability, cost/benefit ratio, and additive value of each technique determine its indications. MRI offers the greatest morphologic and dynamic information on the aorta. Nevertheless, CT has the advantage of availability and excellent spatial resolution. TTE continues to be the technique most used in clinical practice for aortic root assessment and TEE is highly useful in unstable patients and in the preoperative control of acute aortic syndromes. New advances such as time-resolved 3D phase contrast velocity (4D-flow) in MRI, ECG-gated MDCT, or the use of contrast in echocardiography studies will permit further improvement in the diagnosis and better definition of the biomechanical properties of the aortic wall, which without doubt will further understanding of the prognosis and management of aortic diseases.

REFERENCES

1. Drexler M, Erbel R, Müller U, et al. Measurement of intracardiac dimension and structures in normal young adult subjects by transesophageal echocardiography. *Am J Cardiol*. 1990;65:1491–1496.
2. Wolak A, Gransar H, Thomson LEJ, et al. Aortic size assessment by noncontrast cardiac computed tomography: Normal limits by age, gender, and body surface area. *J Am Coll Cardiol: Cardiovasc Imag*. 2008;1:200–208.
3. Agmon Y, Khanderia BK, Meissner I, et al. Relation of coronary artery disease and cerebrovascular disease with atherosclerosis of the thoracic aorta in the general population. *Am J Cardiol*. 2002;89:262–267.
4. Demopoulos LA, Tunick PA, Bernstein NE, et al. Protruding atheromas of the aortic arch in symptomatic patients with carotid artery disease. *Am Heart J*. 1995;129:40–44.
5. Tunich PA, Kronzon I. Atheromas of the thoracic aorta: Clinical and therapeutic update. *J Am Coll Cardiol*. 2000;35:545–554.
6. Nishino M, Masugata H, Yamada Y, et al. Evaluation of thoracic aortic atherosclerosis by transesophageal echocardiography. *Am Heart J*. 1994;127:336–344.
7. Vaduganathan P, Ewton A, Nagueh SF, et al. Pathologic correlates of aortic plaques, thrombi and mobile "aortic debris" imaged in vivo with transesophageal echocardiography. *J Am Coll Cardiol*. 1997;30:357–363.
8. Laperche T, Laurian C, Roudaut R, et al. Mobile thromboses of the aortic arch without aortic debris. *Circulation*. 1997;96:288–294.
9. Dressler FA, Craig WR, Castello R, et al. Mobile aortic atheroma and systemic emboli: Efficacy of anticoagulation and influence of plaque morphology on recurrent stroke. *J Am Coll Cardiol*. 1998;31:134–138.
10. Blackshear JL, Pearce LA, Hart RG, et al. Aortic plaque in atrial fibrillation. Prevalence, predictors, and thromboembolic implications. *Stroke*. 1999;30:834–840.
11. Dàvila-Román VG, Murphy SF, Nickerson NJ, et al. Atherosclerosis of the ascending aorta is an independent predictor of long-term neurologic events and mortality. *J Am Coll Cardiol*. 1999;33:1308–1316.
12. Meissner I, Khandheria BK, Sheps SG, et al. Atherosclerosis of the aorta: Risk factor, risk marker, or innocent bystander? *J Am Coll Cardiol*. 2004;44:1018–1024.
13. Hyman BT, Landas SK, Ashman RF, et al. Warfarin-related purple toes syndrome and cholesterol microembolization. *Am J Med*. 1987;82:1233–1237.
14. Karalis DG, Quinn V, Victor MF, et al. Risk of catheter-related emboli in patients with atherosclerotic debris in the thoracic aorta. *Am Heart J*. 1996;131:1149–1155.
15. Fukumoto Y, Tsutsui H, Tsuchihashi M, et al. The incidence and risk factors of cholesterol embolization syndrome, a complication of cardiac catheterization: A prospective study. *J Am Coll Cardiol*. 2003;42:211–216.
16. Van der Linden J, Hadjinikolaou L, Bergman P, et al. Postoperative stroke in cardiac surgery is related to the location and extent of atherosclerotic disease in the ascending aorta. *J Am Coll Cardiol*. 2001;38:131–135.
17. Nistri S, Sorbo MD, Marin M, et al. Aortic root dilatation in young men with normally functioning bicuspid aortic valves. *Heart*. 1999;82:19–22.
18. Nkomo VT, Enriquez-Sarano M, Ammash NM, et al. Bicuspid aortic valve associated with aortic dilatation. A community-based study. *Arterioscler Thromb Vasc Biol*. 2003;23:351–356.
19. Bickerstaff LK, Pairolero PC, Hollier LH, et al. Thoracic aortic aneurysms: A population-based study. *Surgery*. 1982;92:1103–1108.
20. Erbel R, Alfonso F, Boileau C, et al. Diagnosis and management of aortic dissection. Recommendations of the Task Force on aortic dissection, European Society of Cardiology. *Eur Heart J*. 2001;22:1642–1681.
21. Hagan PG, Nienaber CA, Isselbacher EM, et al. The international registry of acute aortic dissection (IRAD). *JAMA*. 2000;283:897–903.
22. Evangelista A, Mukherjee D, Mehta R, et al. Acute intramural hematoma of the aorta. A mistery in evolution. *Circulation*. 2005;111:1063–1070.
23. Ishikawa K. Diagnostic approach and proposed criteria for the clinical diagnosis of Takayasu's arteriopathy. *J Am Coll Cardiol*. 1988;12:964–972.
24. Montgomery DH, Ververis JJ, Mcgorisk G, et al. Natural history of severe atheromatous disease of the throracic aorta: A transesophageal echocardiographic study. *J Am Coll Cardiol*. 1996;27:95–101.
25. Davies RR, Gallo A, Coady MA, et al. Novel measurement of relative aortic size predicts rupture of thoracic aortic aneurysms. *Ann Thorac Surg*. 2006;81:169–177.
26. Evangelista A, González-Alujas MT. Pathophisiology of aortic dissection. In: Rousseau H, Verhoye J-P, Heautot J-F, eds. *Thoracic Aortic Diseases*. Berlin: Springer; 2006.
27. Baumgartner D, Baungartner C, Matyas G, et al. Diagnostic power of aortic elastic properties in young patients with Marfan syndrome. *J Thorac Cardiovasc Surg*. 2005;129:730–739.
28. Stefanadis C, Stratos C, Boudoulas H, et al. Distensibility of the ascending aorta: Comparison of invasive and non-invasive techniques in healthy men and in men with coronary artery disease. *Eur Heart J*. 1990;11:990–996.
29. Farrar DJ, Bond MG, Riley WA, et al. Anatomic correlates of aortic pulse wave velocity and carotid artery elasticity during atherosclerosis progression and regression in monkeys. *Circulation*. 1991;83:1754–1763.
30. Schwammenthal E, Schwammenthal Y, Tanne D, et al. Transcutaneous detection of aortic arch atheromas by suprasternal harmonic imaging. *J Am Coll Cardiol*. 2002;39:1127–1132.
31. Roman MJ, Devereux RB, Kramer-Fox R, et al. Two-dimensional echocardiographic aortic root dimensions in normal children and adults. *Am J Cardiol*. 1989;64:507–512.
32. Brooke BS, Habashi JP, Judge DP, et al. Angiotens II blockade and aortic-root dilatation in Marfan's Syndrome. *N Engl J Med*. 2008;358:2787–2795.
33. Victor MF, Mintz GS, Kotler MN, et al. Two dimensional echocardiographic diagnosis of aortic dissection. *Am J Cardiol*. 1981;48:1155–1159.
34. Granato JE, Dee P, Gibson RS. Utility of echocardiography in suspected ascending aortic dissection. *Am J Cardiol*. 1985;56:123–129.
35. Iliceto S, Antonelli G, Biasdco G, et al. Two-dimensional echocardiographic evaluation of aneurysms of the descending thoracic aorta. *Circulation*. 1982;66:1045–1049.
36. Avegliano G, Evangelista A, Elorz C, et al. Acute peripheral arterial ischemia and suspected aortic dissection. Usefulness of transesophageal echocardiography in differential diagnosis with aortic thrombosis. *Am J Cardiol*. 2002;90:674–677.
37. Erbel R, Engberding R, Daniel W, et al. Echocardiography in diagnosis of aortic dissection. *Lancet*. 1989;1:457–461.
38. Chirrillo F, Cavallini C, Longhini C, et al. Comparative diagnostic value of transesophageal echocardiography and retrograde aortography in the evaluation of thoracic aortic dissection. *Am J Cardiol*. 1994;74:590–595.
39. Nienaber CA, von Kodolitsch Y, Nicolas V, et al. The diagnosis of thoracic aortic dissection by noninvasive imaging procedures. *N Engl J Med*. 1993;328:1–9.
40. Erbel R, Oelert H, Meyer J, et al. Effect of medical and surgical therapy on aortic dissection evaluated by transesophageal echocardiography. Implications for prognosis and therapy. *Circulation*. 1993;87:1604–1615.

41. Sommer T, Fehske W, Holzknecht N, et al. Aortic dissection: A comparative study of diagnosis with spiral CT, multiplanar transesophageal echocardiography, and MR imaging. *Radiology.* 1996;199:347–352.

42. Keren A, Kim CB, Hu BS, et al. Accuracy of biplane and multiplane transesophageal echocardiography in diagnosis of typical acute aortic dissection and intramural hematoma. *J Am Coll Cardiol.* 1996;28:627–636.

43. Evangelista A, García del Castillo H, González-Alujas T, et al. Diagnosis of ascending aortic dissection by transesophageal echocardiography: Utility of M-mode in recognizing artifacts. *J Am Coll Cardiol.* 1996;27:102–107.

44. Song JK, Kim HS, Kang DH, et al. Different clinical features of aortic intramural hematoma versus dissection involving the ascending aorta. *J Am Coll Cardiol.* 2001;37:1604–1610.

45. Vilacosta I, San Roman JA, Aragoncillo P, et al. Penetrating atherosclerotic aortic ulcer: Documentation by transesophageal echocardiography. *J Am Coll Cardiol.* 1998;32:83–89.

46. Mohr-Kahaly S, Erbel R, Rennollet H, et al Ambulatory follow-up of aortic dissection by transesophageal two-dimensional and color-coded Doppler echocardiography. *Circulation.* 1989;80:24–33.

47. Le Bret F, Ruel P, Rosier H, et al. Diagnosis of traumatic mediastinal hematoma with transesophageal echocardiography. *Chest.* 1994;105:373–376.

48. Mukherjee D, Evangelista A, Nienaber CH, et al. Implications of periaortic hematoma in patients with acute aortic dissection. *Am J Cardiol.* 2005;96:1734–1738.

49. Movsowitz HD, Levine RA, Hilgenberg AD, et al. Transesophageal echocardiographyc description of the mechanisms of aortic regurgitation in acute type A aortic dissection: Implications for aortic valve repair. *J Am Coll Cardiol.* 2000;36:884–890.

50. Armstrong WF, Bach DS, Carey L, et al. Spectrum of acute dissection of the ascending aorta: A transesophageal echocardiography study. *J Am Soc Echocardiogr.* 1996;9:646–656.

51. Shiga T, Wajima Z, Apfel CC, et al. Diagnostic accuracy of transesophageal echocardiography, helical computed tomography, and magnetic resonance imaging for suspected thoracic aortic dissection. systematic review and meta-analysis. *Arch Intern Med.* 2006;166:1350–1356.

52. Cody DD, Mahesh M. Technologic advances in multidetector CT with a focus on cardiac imaging. *Radiographics.* 2007;27:1829–1837.

53. Shanmuganathan K, Mirvis SE, Sover ER. Value of contrast-enhanced CT in detecting active hemorrhage in patients with blunt abdominal or pelvic trauma. *Am J Roentgenol.* 1993;161:65–69.

54. Sebastià C, Pallisa E, Quiroga S, et al. Aortic dissection: Diagnosis and follow-up with helical CT. *Radiographics.* 1999;19:45–60.

55. Einstein AJ, Henzlova MJ, Rajagopalan S. Estimating risk of cancer associated with radiation exposure from 64-slice computed tomography coronary angiography. *JAMA.* 2007;298:317–323.

56. Stillman AE, Oudkerk M, Ackerman M, et al. Use of multidetector computed tomography for the assessment of acute chest pain: A consensus statement of the North American Society of Cardiac Imaging and the European Society of Cardiac Radiology. *Eur Radiol.* 2007;17:2196–2207.

57. Zhang J, Fletcher JG, Vrtiska TJ, et al. Large-vessel distensibility measurement with electrocardiographically gated multidetector CT: Phantom study and initial experience. *Radiology.* 2007;245:258–266.

58. Tenenbaum A, Garniek A, Shemesh J, et al. Dual-helical CT for detecting aortic atheromas as a source of stroke: Comparison with transesophageal echocardiography. *Radiology.* 1998;208:153–158.

59. Fuster V, Fayad ZA, Moreno PR, et al. Atherothrombosis and high-risk plaque: Part II: Approaches by noninvasive computed tomographic/magnetic resonance imaging. *J Am Coll Cardiol.* 2005;46:1209–1218.

60. Posniak HV, Olson MC, Demos TC, et al. CT of thoracic aortic aneurysms. *Radiographics.* 1990;10:839–855.

61. Cayne NS, Veith FJ, Lipsitz EC, et al. Variability of maximal aortic aneurysm diameter measurements on CT scan: Significance and methods to minimize. *J Vasc Surg.* 2004;39:811–815.

62. Yoshida S, Akiba H, Tamakawa M, et al. Thoracic involvement of type A aortic dissection and intramural hematoma: Diagnostic accuracy comparison of emergency helical CT and surgical findings. *Radiology.* 2003;228:430–435.

63. Johnson TR, Nikolaou K, Becker A, et al. Dual-source CT for chest pain assessment. *Eur Radiol.* 2008;18:773–780.

64. Williams DM, Lee DY, Hamilton BH, et al. The dissected aorta: Part III. Anatomy and radiologic diagnosis of branch-vessel compromise. *Radiology.* 1997;203:37–44.

65. Vernhet H, Serfaty JM, Serhal M, et al. Abdominal CT angiography before surgery as a predictor of postoperative death in acute aortic dissection. *Am J Roentgenol.* 2004;182:875–879.

66. Lee YK, Seo JB, Jang YM, et al. Acute and chronic complications of aortic intramural hematoma on follow-up computed tomography: Incidence and predictor analysis. *J Comput Assist Tomogr.* 2007;31:435–440.

67. Hayashi H, Matsuoka Y, Sakamoto I, et al. Penetrating atherosclerotic ulcer of the aorta: Imaging features and disease concept. *Radiographics.* 2000;20:995–1005.

68. Vignaux OB, Augui J, Coste J, et al. Comparison of single-shot fast spin-echo and conventional spin-echo sequences for MR imaging of the heart: Initial experience. *Radiology.* 2001;219:545–550.

69. François CJ, Carr JC. MRI of the thoracic aorta. *Magn Reson Imaging Clin N Am.* 2007;15:639–651.

70. Finn JP, Baskaran V, Carr JC, et al. Thorax: Low-dose contrast-enhanced three-dimensional MR angiography with subsecond temporal resolution—initial results. *Radiology.* 2002;224:896–904.

71. Bitar R, Moody AR, Leung G, et al. In vivo identification of complicated upper thoracic aorta and arch vessel plaque by MR direct thrombus imaging in patients investigated for cerebrovascular disease. *Am J Roentgenol.* 2006;187:228–234.

72. Fayad ZA, Nahar T, Fallon JT, et al. In vivo magnetic resonance evaluation of atherosclerotic plaques in the human thoracic aorta. *Circulation.* 2000;101:2503–2509.

73. Corti R, Fayad ZA, Fuster V, et al. Effects of lipid-lowering by simvastatin on human atherosclerotic lesions. A longitudinal study by high-resolution, noninvasive magnetic resonance imaging. *Circulation.* 2001;104:249–252.

74. Briley-Saebo KC, Shaw PX, Mulder WJ, et al. Targeted molecular probes for imaging atherosclerotic lesions with magnetic resonance using antibodies that recognize oxidation-specific epitopes. *Circulation.* 2008;117:3206–3215.

75. Briley-Saebo KC, Mulder WJ, Mani V, et al. Magnetic resonance imaging of vulnerable atherosclerotic plaques: Current imaging strategies and molecular imaging probes. *J Magn Reson Imaging.* 2007;26:460–479.

76. Nollen GJ, Groenink M, Tijssen JGP, et al. Aortic stiffness and diameter predict progressive aortic dilatation in patients with Marfan syndrome. *Eur Heart J.* 2004;25:1146–1152.

77. Kunz RP, Oberholzer K, Kuroczynski W, et al. Assessment of chronic aortic dissection: Contribution of different ECG-gated breath-hold MRI techniques. *Am J Roentgenol.* 2004;182:1319–1326.

78. Fattori R, Bacchi-Reggiani L, Bertaccini P, et al. Evolution of aortic dissection after surgical repair. *Am J Cardiol.* 2000;86:868–872.

79. Nienaber CA, von Kodolitsch Y, Petersen B, et al. Intramural hemorrhage of the thoracic aorta: Diagnostic and therapeutic implications. *Circulation.* 1995;92:1465–1472.

80. Weintraub AR, Erbel R, Gorge G, et al. Intravascular ultrasound imaging in acute aortic dissection. *J Am Coll Cardiol.* 1994;24:495–503.

81. Yamada E, Matsumura M, Kyo S, et al. Usefulness of a prototype intravascular ultrasound imaging in evaluation of aortic dissection and comparison with angiographic study, transesophageal echocardiography, computed tomography and magnetic resonance imaging. *Am J Cardiol.* 1995;75:161–165.

82. Tatsumi M, Cohade C, Nakamoto Y, et al. Fluodeoxyglucose uptake in the aortic wall at PET/CT: Possible findings for active atherosclerosis. *Radiology.* 2003;229:831–837.

83. Okane K, Ibaraki M, Toyoshima H, et al. 18FDG accumulation in atherosclerosis: Use of CT and MR co-registration of thoracic and carotid arteries. *Eur J Nucl Med Mol Imaging.* 2006;33:589–594.

84. Evangelista A, Domínguez R, Sebastià C, et al. Long-term follow-up of aortic intramural hematoma. Predictors of outcome. *Circulation.* 2003;108:583–589.

85. Fattori R, Celletti F, Descovich B, et al. Evolution of post-traumatic aneurysm in the subacute phase: Magnetic resonance imaging follow-up as a support of the surgical timing. *Eur J Cardiothorac Surg.* 1998;13:582–587.

86. Smith MD, Cassidy JM, Souther S, et al. Transesophageal echocardiography in the diagnosis of traumatic rupture of the aorta. *N Engl J Med.* 1995;332:356–362.

87. de Waroux JB, Pouleur AC, Goffinet C, et al. Functional anatomy of aortic regurgitation. Accuracy, prediction of surgical repairability, and outcome implications of transesophageal echocardiography. *Circulation.* 2007;116 (Suppl. I):I-264–I-269.

88. Muhs BE, Vincken KL, van Prehn J, et al. Dynamic cine-CT angiography for the evaluation of the thoracic aorta; insight in dynamic changes with implications for thoracic endograft treatment. *Eur J Vasc Endovasc Surg.* 2006 Nov;32(5):532–536.

89. Nienaber Ch, Fattori R, Lund G, et al. Nonsurgical reconstruction of thoracic aortic dissection by stent-graft placement. *N Engl J Med.* 1999;340:1539–1545.

90. Dake MD, Kato N, Mitchell RS, et al. Endovascular stent-graft placement for the treatment of acute aortic dissection. *N Engl J Med.* 1999;340:1546–1552.

91. Koschyk DH, Nienaber CA, Knap M, et al. How to guide Stent-graft implantation in type B aortic dissection? Comparison of angiography, transesophageal echocardiography and intravascular ultrasound. *Circulation.* 2005;112 (Suppl. I):I-260–I-264.

92. Rocchi G, Lofiego C, Biagini E, et al. Transesophageal echocardiography-guided algorithm for stent-graft implantation in aortic dissection. *J Vasc Surg.* 2004;40:880–885.

93. Bartel T, Eggebrecht H, Müller S, et al. Comparison of diagnostic and therapeutic value of transesophageal echocardiography, intravascular ultrasonic imaging, and intraluminal phased-array imaging in aortic dissection with tear in the descending thoracic aorta. *Am J Cardiol.* 2007;99:270–274.

94. Davies RR, Goldstein LJ, Coady et al. Yearly ruptured or dissection rates for thoracic aortic aneurysms; simple prediction based on size. *Ann Thorac Surg.* 2002;73:17–27.

95. Davies RR, Gallo A, Coady MA, et al. Novel measurement of relative aortic size predicts rupture of thoracic aortic aneurysms. *Ann Thorac Surg.* 2006;81:169–177.

96. Tsai TT, Nienaber CA, Eagle KA. Acute aortic syndromes. *Circulation.* 2005;112:3802–3813.

97. Bossone E, Evangelista A, Isselbacher E, et al. Prognostic role of transesophageal echocardiography in acute type A aortic dissection. *Am Heart J.* 2007;153:1013–1020.

98. Immer FF, Krahenbuhl E, Hagen U, et al. Large area of the false lumen favors secondary dilatation of the aorta after acute type A aortic dissection. *Circulation.* 2005;112:(Suppl. I) I-49–52.

99. Tsai TT, Evangelista A, Nienaber CA, et al. Partial thrombosis of the false lumen in patients with acute type B aortic dissection. *N Engl J Med.* 2007;357:349–359.

100. Kronzon I, Tunick PA. Atheromatous disease of the thoracic aorta: Pathologic and clinical implications. *Ann Intern Med.* 1997;126:629–637.

Pulmonary Hypertension

Samer J. Khouri
Utpal Pandya

46

1. INTRODUCTION

Pulmonary hypertension (PH) is a complex disease characterized by constant elevation of mean pulmonary arterial pressure (mPAP). A commonly used definition of PH is an mPAP >25 mm Hg at rest or >30 mm Hg with exercise, in the setting of normal or reduced cardiac output and normal pulmonary wedge pressure <15 mm Hg.[1,2] Through the past decade, tremendous advances have been made in the understanding, diagnosis, and treatment of PH. Despite these advances, PH remains a debilitating and progressive disease. The pathophysiology of PH is complex. The need to organize these heterogeneous groups of diseases under one umbrella, to standardize the diagnostic evaluation, and to facilitate communication of patient care has lead the effort to classify PH in different categories. Dresdale et al.[3] initially proposed the term primary PH in 1951. In 1973, the first World Health Organization (WHO) Conference attempted the first classification of PH. The main classification was divided into primary or secondary PH based on identifiable cause of PH.[4] This was followed by reclassification in the second WHO Conference in Evian, France. This meeting proposed to aggregate patients into more homogenous groups.[5] The third WHO Conference was held in Venice in 2003, where the terms primary and secondary PH were replaced by idiopathic pulmonary arterial hypertension (IPAH), familial PAH (FPAH), and associated PAH (APAH) to reflect the advances in the understanding of disease pathology, histopathology features, natural history, and response to therapy (Table 46.1).[6]

1.1. Clinical presentation

PH patients present with nonspecific symptoms and are frequently misdiagnosed and treated for other conditions that are more common.[7] In 1981, the National Institute of Health (NIH) initiated a national registry to characterize the PH natural history, pathogenesis, and treatments.[8] This registry showed that the mean interval from the onset of symptoms to diagnosis was 2 years. However, the increase in awareness of PH and the availability of noninvasive echocardiography to more easily assess systolic right ventricular (RV) pressure (and consequently, systolic pulmonary pressure) have served to facilitate diagnosis. Table 46.2 summarizes the prevalence of symptoms and physical findings in PH. Shortness of breath was found in 60% of patients at the initial presentation, with 98% prevalence at the time of diagnosis. Other symptoms include fatigue, chest pain, near syncope, syncope, and leg edema (Table 46.2). PH is more prevalent among women, with a female-to-male ratio of 1.7:1 and mean age of 36 ± 15 years.[8] Thus, active and young patients who have dyspnea and fatigue might dismiss their symptoms and thereby delay the diagnosis of the disease.

On physical examination, accentuation of the pulmonary component (P2) of the second heart sound is the most prevalent sign and was found in 93% of patients. An S4 gallop is noted in 38% of patients. An S3 gallop is reported in 23% of patients associated with elevated right atrial pressure (RAP) (13 mm Hg compared to 9 mm Hg, $p < 0.001$) and reduced cardiac index. Tricuspid regurgitation can be encountered in 40% of patients as well as an early diastolic high-pitched (Graham Steel) murmur of pulmonary insufficiency in 13%.

Also, an early systolic ejection click can be heard, along with a midsystolic ejection murmur caused by the turbulence of trans-valvular flow and a palpable left parasternal lift produced by RV hypertrophy.[9] In addition to cardiac findings many other physical examination findings can be seen, such as a prominent "A" wave of the jugular vein, hepatojugular reflex, lower extremity edema, and cyanosis.[7,8,10] Since PH can be associated with many diseases, such as connective tissue disease (CTD), portal hypertension, and HIV or associated with left heart disease, lung diseases and/or hypoxemia,[11] the symptoms and physical findings of these diseases can be prominent and should lead to the screening for PH.[1] The prognosis of patients with PAH depends on the functional class (FC) (Table 46.3), exercise endurance, and hemodynamics, where most of these variables depend on the RV function and the development of RV failure.[12]

2. PATHOGENESIS OF PULMONARY HYPERTENSION

The pulmonary vasculature is a low pressure system with a normal systolic pulmonary arterial pressure (sPAP) of 18 to 25 mm Hg, end diastolic PAP of 6 to 10 mm Hg, and an mPAP of 12 to 16 mm Hg.[10] The hallmark of PH is persistent elevation of mPAP >25 mm Hg.[1] The pathogenesis of PH is not completely understood, but many histological, biological, and genetic factors of PH have been defined. Plexiform lesions are the histologic sine qua non of patients with IPAH and FPAH. They result from proliferation of monoclonal endothelial cells, smooth muscle cells, and an accumulation of circulating cells (e.g., macrophages and progenitor cells).[10,13,14] These observations suggest that the vascular bed in patients with PH is different from normal people and is affected by gene mutations that control proliferation, apoptosis, and differentiation of these cells.[14]

Several genotypes were found to be associated with PH. Bone morphogenic protein receptor II (BMPR-2),[15] Activin-like kinase type-1,[16] and 5-hydroxytryptamine transporter[17] genes are implicated in the development of IPAH and FPAH. The complex pathophysiology of PH is mediated by endogenous factors, which

655

TABLE 46.1

CLINICAL CLASSIFICATION OF PH (VENICE 2003)

Group 1. Pulmonary arterial hypertension (PAH)

Idiopathic (IPAH)

Familial (FPAH)

Associated with (APAH)

    Connective tissue disease (CTD)
    Congenital systemic-to-pulmonary shunts
    Portal hypertension
    HIV infection
    Drugs and toxin

Other (thyroid disorders, glycogen storage disease, Gaucher disease, hereditary hemorrhagic telangiectasia, hemoglobinopathies, myeloproliferative disorders, and splenectomy)

Associated with significant venous or capillary involvement
    Pulmonary veno-occlusive disease (PVOD)
    Pulmonary capillary hemangiomatosis (PCH)

Persistent PH of the newborn

Group 2. PH with left heart disease

    Left-sided atrial or ventricular heart disease

    Left-sided valvular heart disease

Group 3. PH associated with lung diseases and/or hypoxemia

    Chronic obstructive pulmonary disease

    Interstitial lung disease

    Sleep-disordered breathing

    Alveolar hypoventilation disorders

    Chronic exposure to high altitude

    Developmental abnormalities

Group 4. PH due to chronic thrombotic and/or embolic disease

    Thromboembolic obstruction of proximal pulmonary arteries

    Thromboembolic obstruction of distal pulmonary arteries

    Nonthrombotic pulmonary embolism (tumor, parasites, foreign material)

Group 5. Miscellaneous

    Sarcoidosis, histiocytosis X, lymphangiomatosis, compression of pulmonary vessels (adenopathy, tumor, fibrosing mediastinitis)

Source: Adapted from Simonneau G, Galie N, Rubin LJ, et al. Clinical classification of pulmonary hypertension. *J Am Coll Cardiol*. 2004;43(12 Suppl S):5S–12S.

TABLE 46.2

SYMPTOMS AND PHYSICAL FINDINGS OF PATIENTS WITH PULMONARY ARTERIAL HYPERTENSION

Symptoms	Initial symptom (%)	At diagnosis (%)	Findings	Percentage of patients
Dyspnea	60	98	Accentuation of P2	93
Fatigue	19	73	Tricuspid regurgitation	40
Chest pain	7	47	Right-sided S4	38
Near syncope	5	41	Peripheral edema	32
Syncope	8	36	Right-sided S3	23
Leg edema	3	37	Cyanosis	20
Palpitations	5	33	Pulmonic insufficiency	13

Source: Adapted from Rich S, Dantzker D, Ayers S. Primary pulmonary hypertension. A national prospective study. *Ann Intern Med*. 1987;07:216–223.

TABLE 46.3

RISK FACTORS AND ASSOCIATED CONDITIONS FOR PAH AND CLASSIFIED ACCORDING TO THE STRENGTH OF EVIDENCE

A. *Drugs and Toxins*
1. Definite
   Aminorex
   Fenfluramine
   Dexfenfluramine
   Toxic rapeseed oil
2. Very likely
   Amphetamines
   L-tryptophan
3. Possible
   Meta-amphetamines
   Cocaine
   Chemotherapeutic agents
4. Unlikely
   Antidepressants
   Oral contraceptives
   Estrogen therapy
   Cigarette smoking

B. *Demographic and medical conditions*
1. Definite
   Gender
2. Possible
   Pregnancy
   Systemic hypertension
3. Unlikely
   Obesity

C. Diseases
1. Definite
   HIV infection
2. Very likely
   Portal hypertension/liver disease
   Collagen vascular diseases
   Congenital systemic-pulmonary-cardiac shunts
3. Possible thyroid disorders

Source: Adapted from the Simonneau G, Galie N, Rubin LJ, et al. Clinical classification of pulmonary hypertension. *J Am Coll Cardiol.* 2004;43 (12 Suppl S):5S–12S.

lead to abnormal cell proliferation and pulmonary vascular constriction. These pathways include: (a) the prostacyclin pathway, where prostacyclin is a potent pulmonary vasodilator and inhibits pulmonary vascular remodeling. The deficiency of prostacyclin in the lung leads to the development of prostacyclin analogs as a target of treatment for patients with PH[18]; (b) the endothelin-1 pathway, where endothelin-1 is a very potent pulmonary vasoconstrictor. Its level is found to be elevated in patients with PH; (c) the nitric oxide (NO) pathway, where NO stimulates cyclic guanosine monophosphate (cGMP) in the vascular smooth muscle and induces vascular relaxation. The phosphodiesterase family of enzymes causes rapid degradation of cGMP. Inhibiting these enzymes can possibly sustain the NO effect and maintain vasodilatation. Targeting these pathways showed significant clinical benefit. In addition, other mediators may play a role in the development of future therapies like serotonin and angiotensin II. Furthermore, Alpha-1 adrenergic blockade lowers the pulmonary vascular resistance (PVR), whereas beta-receptor blockade does not change the PVR.[10]

3. CLASSIFICATION OF PULMONARY HYPERTENSION

In the Evian classification, there were five categories in which PH was grouped based on specific therapeutic intervention.[5] A few changes were proposed at the third WHO Conference in Venice (Table 46.1), which include (a) discontinuing the term "Primary Pulmonary Hypertension," (b) reclassification of PVOD and PCH, and (c) reassessment of the classification of congenital systemic to pulmonary shunts.[11]

3.1. Idiopathic pulmonary arterial hypertension

By definition, IPAH has no known etiology. It is a rare disorder with an incidence of 2 to 5 per million per year,[2] affecting the young (mean age 37) with a female (1.7:1) preponderance.[8] Despite the histologic characterization of plexiform lesions, it is a diagnosis of exclusion. The proposed mechanism and pathway that lead to phenotype transformation of the pulmonary arteries include exposure to a number of identified risk factors (Table 46.3). Once initiated, the cascade of events leads to angioproliferative response in endothelial cells with medial thickening due to vascular smooth muscle hypertrophy and proliferation. Simultaneously, increased pulmonary vascular reactivity with vascular constriction and in situ thrombosis occurs.[13,19]

3.2. Familial pulmonary arterial hypertension

FPAH composes 6% of patients with PAH according to the NIH registry, with the same female-to-male ratio. The pattern of inheritance is autosomal dominant with variable penetration.[20] BMPR-2 mutation was identified as a cause of FPAH in 50% to 90% of patients,[21] but fewer than 20% of individuals with BMPR-2 mutation develop FPAH.[22] Other genetic mutations have been identified. Nonetheless, the loss of function or dysfunction of a single mutation like BMPR-2 and the loss of downstream signaling are not sufficient by themselves to lead to PAH. A combination of multiple genetic defects and multiple signal transduction abnormalities is required for the pathogenesis of PAH.[14,23] The clinical course, natural history, and outcome of FPAH are identical to IPAH.

3.3. Associated pulmonary arterial hypertension

Multitude of diseases may manifest elevations in PAP, wherein assessing and following the pulmonary pressures are integral to clinical care. CTD, especially scleroderma and CREST syndrome, are associated with PAH. CREST is an acronym for the five main features: Calcinosis, Raynaud phenomena, Esophageal dysmotility, Sclerodactyly, and Telangiectasia. CREST syndrome is a limited form of scleroderma associated with antibodies against centromeres and usually spares the lungs and kidneys. Annual screening with echocardiography is recommended due to 30% incidence of APAH with scleroderma and 50% with CREST syndrome. Mixed CTD might be associated with APAH in as many as 66% of patients. APAH was reported with other connective diseases, but with a much lower incidence. The histopathology of APAH with CTD is similar to the IPAH. Medical therapy is similar to IPAH, but prognosis is worse. APAH is also associated with many congenital heart diseases (Table 46.4).

The histopathology is similar with better prognosis compared to other forms of pulmonary arterial hypertension. In the Swiss HIV study, 0.6% of patients had APAH. Other factors, which can cause PAH, include drugs and toxins such as aminorex, fenfluramine, and dexfenfluramine. Other diseases that are associated with PAH include thyroid disorders, glycogen storage disease, Gaucher disease, hereditary hemorrhagic telangiectasia, hemoglobinopathies, myeloproliferative disorders, and splenectomy.

3.4. Pulmonary venous hypertension associated with left heart disease

A variety of cardiac diseases can cause elevated pulmonary venous pressure and consequently, PVH. These diseases include cardiomyopathies, mitral and aortic valve disease, and pericardial disease. The elevation of pulmonary pressure is associated with a poor cardiac prognosis.[24] PAH is increased proportionally with the increase of wedge pressure and when the transpulmonary gradient (mPAP—pulmonary wedge pressure) continues to be low, <12 mm Hg. When the wedge pressure exceeds 25 mm Hg, the PAH increases disproportionally and the transpulmonary gradient increases due to vasoconstriction and possibly other hormonal factors. The histopathology of these patients is similar to IPAH and this group might benefit from PAH specific treatment.[10] Management of PVH should focus on the primary cardiac etiology. Multiple small studies were done in patients with left heart disease. Prostacyclin analogs and endothelin-1 receptor antagonists (ETRA) were associated with worse outcome or increased mortality. Trials with phosphodiestrase-5 (PDE5) inhibitors, sildenafil, are limited, and short-term studies are promising but concern about long-term adverse events continues to limit their use.[25]

3.5. Pulmonary hypertension associated with lung diseases and/or hypoxemia

Chronic obstructive pulmonary disease (COPD) is associated with mild PH (mPAP, 25 to 34 mm Hg) in 50.2%, moderate (mPAP, 35 to 45 mm Hg) and severe (mPAP >45 mm Hg) in 9.8% and 3.7% of patients, respectively.[26] Advanced interstitial lung disease is associated with PH in 32% of patients, where there is a linear correlation between mPAP and outcomes with higher PH associated with a greater risk of mortality.[27] The prevalence of PH in patients with obstructive sleep apnea (OSA) (mPAP >20 mm Hg) is around 20%. Most cases are mild with mPAP generally 25 to 30 mm Hg. PH is most strongly associated with other risk factors, such as left-sided heart disease, parenchymal lung disease, nocturnal desaturation, and obesity.[27]

3.6. Pulmonary hypertension due to chronic thrombotic and/or embolic disease

The diagnosis of chronic thromboembolic disease is on the rise due to increased ability to diagnose this disease and the availability of effective therapy, including medical and surgical approaches like endarterectomy. For a more detailed discussion, please refer to Chapter 47.

4. DIAGNOSTIC EVALUATION

The initial phase of evaluation for patients with PH is detection of PH which is done by physical examination, chest X-ray (CXR), electrocardiography (ECG), and echocardiography before proceeding to more specific tests to characterize the type and the etiology of PH[1] (Fig. 46.1). The ECG may show occasional right heart hypertrophy, right atrial enlargement, and right-axis deviation, but the sensitivity and specificity of ECG are low.[8,28] The CXR may give an indication for RV, right atrial, and pulmonary artery enlargement or associated causes of PH such as hyperinflation in patients with COPD, or kyphosis and fibrosis for patients with restrictive lung disease. Further testing should be done to establish the diagnosis and etiology of PH. These tests should be applied in a systematic way and be based on clinical suspicion.

4.1. Echocardiography

Transthoracic echocardiography is the cornerstone in the evaluation of patients with PH. When PH is the indication for the test or is the major finding, the basic elements that should be documented in every echocardiographic report are estimation of sPAP or its surrogate, the RV systolic pressure (RVSP) (in the absence of pulmonary stenosis), the right atrial size, RV size and function, and the presence or absence of pericardial effusion. These results establish and guide the diagnosis of PH and help in the assessment of the degree of PH severity and long-term prognosis. Consequently, a comprehensive echocardiographic study is essential, especially at the initial evaluation where identification of left ventricular systolic and diastolic function, left ventricle (LV) size and wall thickness, mitral and aortic valve abnormalities, and pericardial disease are important to rule out pulmonary venous hypertension (PVH) as a cause of PH. In addition, it is paramount to evaluate for the presence of any congenital heart disease, in particular for the presence of an intracardiac shunt.

With the advancement of echocardiography instrumentation, real-time 3D echocardiography becomes feasible, and estimation of RV volume, function, and ejection fraction is becoming more accurate and reliable. Recently, more attention has been focused on studying the RV function and hemodynamic parameters, especially with the development of reliable treatment options for PH. Noninvasive assessment of PVR and mean pulmonary

TABLE 46.4
CLASSIFICATION OF CONGENITAL SYSTEMIC-TO-PULMONARY SHUNTS

1. Type
    Simple
    Atrial septal defect (ASD)
    Ventricular septal defect (VSD)
    Patent ductus arteriosus (PDA)
    Total or partial unobstructed anomalous pulmonary venous return
    Complex
        Truncus arteriosus
        Single ventricle with unobstructed pulmonary blood flow
        Atrioventricular septal defects

2. Dimensions
    Small (ASD ≤2.0 cm and VSD ≤1.0 cm)
    Large (ASD >2.0 cm and VSD >1.0 cm)

3. Associated extracardiac abnormalities

4. Correction status
    Noncorrected
    Partially corrected (age)
    Corrected: spontaneously or surgically (age)

Source: Adapted from the Simonneau G, Galie N, Rubin LJ, et al. Clinical classification of pulmonary hypertension. *J Am Coll Cardiol.* 2004;43 (12 Suppl. S):5S–12S.

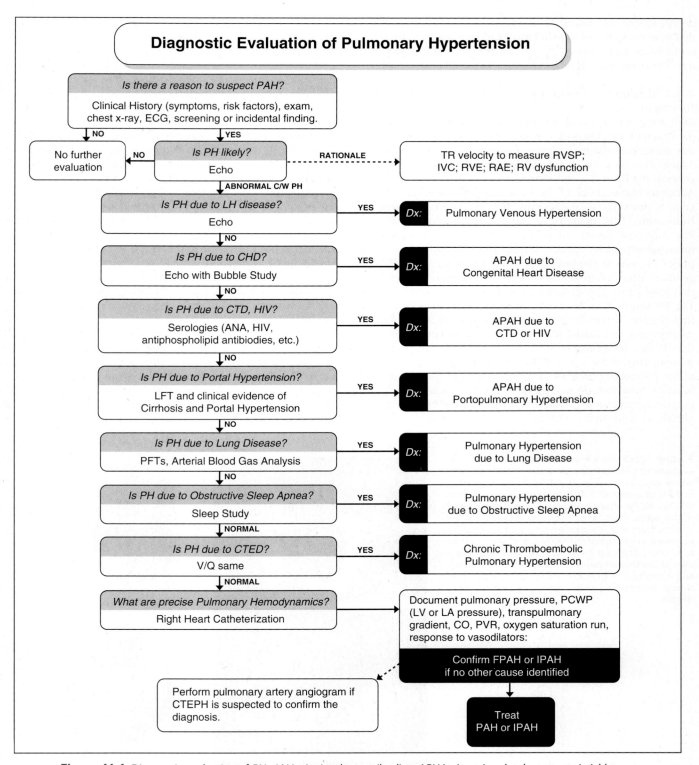

Figure 46.1 Diagnostic evaluation of PH. ANA, Antinuclear antibodies; APHA, Associated pulmonary articrial hypertension; CHD, Congenital heart disease; CO, Cardiac output; CTD, Connective tissue disease; CTED, Chronic thromboembolic disease, CTEPH, Chronic thromboembolic pulmonary hypertension; Dx, Diagnosis; ECG, Electrocardiography; FPAH, Famillial pulmonary arterial hypertension; HIV, Human immunodeficiency virus; IPAH, Idiopathic pulmonary arterial hypertension; IVC, Inferior vena cava; LA, Left atrial; LH, Left heart; LV, Left ventricular; LFT, Liver function test; RVE, Right ventricular enlargement; RVSP, Right ventricular systolic pressure; RV, Right ventriuclar; TR Velocity, Peak velocity of TR jet; V/Q, Perfusion/ventilation scan.

artery pressure are a few of the new echocardiographic parameters that have evolved and hopefully will soon be integrated into the echocardiographic report, as the data is being studied and validated by many investigators.

4.1.1. Evaluation of right ventricle morphology and function

Evaluating RV size and function is extremely important for patients with PH. Quantitative and qualitative assessment of RV size remains challenging due to the complex geometric shape, which does not match any simple mathematical model. In general, the RV is crescent shaped and wrapped around the LV. Adequate visualization of the RV requires multiple echocardiographic views. The RV wall is thin <0.5 cm. The RV thickness can be measured from many views and from 2D or M-mode images. The American Society of Echocardiography recommends the measurement of RV thickness from the subcostal view at the peak of R-wave at the level of chordae tendineae.[29] The RV can generate pressure of 45 to 50 mm Hg. Pressure higher than that level cannot be generated except with a hypertrophic RV. The RV response to long-term pressure overload is concentric hypertrophy. This mechanism will ultimately fail and lead to RV enlargement and finally RV failure. It is important to consider that RV failure can also occur in the case of infarction, ischemia, or myopathy of the right ventricle without significant elevation of the pulmonary pressure and PVR.[10] Most of the RV size and function assessment is qualitative in the day-to-day echocardiographic laboratories. The right ventricle and RV outflow can be visualized from many standard views. These views include the right inflow view, the short-axis view at the level of aortic valve, the short-axis view at the level of papillary muscles, the apical four-chamber view, and the subcostal four-chamber view.

A qualitative assessment of RV size can be obtained easily from a true apical four-chamber view (Fig. 46.2A). RV diameter at mid ventricle (RVD2) or the area of the RV should be smaller than the LV. Moderate enlargement occurs when the diameter or the RV area is equal to the LV and severe enlargement exists when these parameters exceed the size and dimension of LV.[29] Furthermore, widening of the RV apical angle is a marker of structural abnormality and RV dysfunction. From the apical four-chamber view, the RV apical angle is defined by two diverging lines. The first line is aligned parallel to the most linear portion of the endocardium contiguous with the distal RV free wall, while the second line is aligned with the endocardium of the interventricular septum close to the RV apex. The RV apical angles, both in systole and diastole, were found to have very strong linear correlation with RV end-systolic area ($R = 0.89$, $p < 0.0001$) and end-diastolic area ($R = 0.81$, $p < 0.0001$).[30] The RV outflow tract (RVOT) and pulmonary artery are best viewed and measured from short axis at the level of the aortic valve (Fig. 46.2B).

With RV pressure overload due to elevated PH, the RV wall thickness increases and hypertrophy occurs. The septal motion becomes paradoxical due to the shift of the center of mass from LV to RV. The septal curvature in the short axis at the level of papillary muscle becomes flattened during systole (D-shape) and resumes its normal curvature during diastole. In volume overload, the septal flattening occurs at diastole (Fig. 46.3).[31]

Figure 46.2 Transthoracic echocardiogram to evaluate the RV function. **A:** Apical four-chambers, where you can measure basal RV diameter (RVD1), mid RV diameter (RVD2), and base to apex length (RVD3). **B:** Parasternal short-axis view at the level of the aortic valve, where you can measure the RV outflow tract at the subpulmonary region (RVOT1), pulmonic valve annulus (RVOT2), and main pulmonary artery diameter (PA1). **C:** Parasternal short-axis view at the level of papillary muscles, septal motion, and evaluation of pressure and/or volume overload is best appreciated in this view. See text for more details.

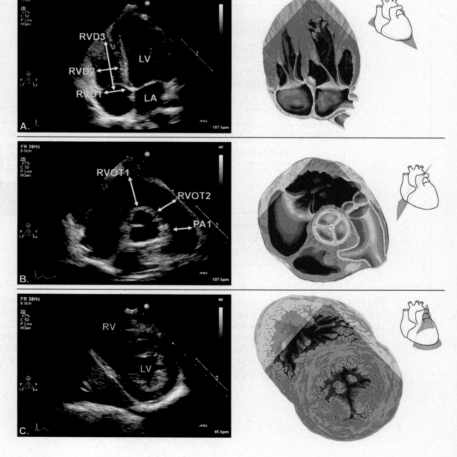

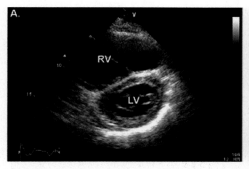

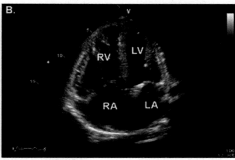

Figure 46.3 Echocardiograms from patients with severe PH. **A:** Short-axis view at the level of papillary muscles showed flattening of the ventricular septum (D-shape). **B:** RV is severely dilated and larger than LV.

The assessment of RV function is usually visual and qualitative. The lack of a simple geometric shape restricts adequate assessment of RV function. Several surrogates were developed to assess the RV function which include: (a) excursion of the tricuspid annulus, which moves toward the apex during systole by 1.5 to 2.0 cm in normal individuals, and any excursion less than 1.5 cm is associated with poor outcome.[32] (b) peak RV strain and time-to-peak RV strain are univariate predictors of mild PH.[33] (c) RV peak annulus systolic velocity by tissue Doppler imaging (TDI) is limited and it has a poor correlation with RV systolic function.[34] (d) RV fractional area change, which is measured from the apical four-chamber view, provides a reasonable estimation of RV function and correlates well with RV ejection fraction measured by cardiac magnetic resonance (CMR).[29] (e) The RV tei-index correlates well with severe RV dysfunction and abnormal hemodynamic parameters.[35]

With the development of echocardiographic equipment, especially the 3D echocardiogram and the increased recognition of RV role in multiple cardiopulmonary diseases, re-emphasis on RV quantitative assessment has captured more attention and interest of the investigators. Because 3D echocardiography is able to visualize and detect the RV shape and volume without geometric assumption, it overcomes the inherent limitation of 2D echocardiography.[36] Gopal et al.[37] were among the first to assess RV size and function with RT3D echo and compare it to CMR. They found a good correlation using two methods to assess the RV parameters, with superiority of the disk summation method over apical rotation.

There is a very little data published regarding the right atrium (RA) size, area, and volume. The data that is available is consistent with area and volume similar that of the left atrium (area ≤20 cm² and volume ≤21 mL/m²).[29] Pericardial effusion, right atrial enlargement, and septal displacement are the parameters that reflect the severity of RV failure and predict adverse outcome in patients with PAH.[38]

4.1.2. Evaluation of right ventricular hemodynamic parameters

One of the most important values of Doppler echocardiography is its ability to noninvasively quantify the velocity of blood flow

and consequently, the hemodynamic parameters. In patients with arterial PH, its value comes from: (a) establishing the diagnosis, the severity, and the prognosis of patients with PH; (b) the ease of remeasuring the hemodynamic parameters for longitudinal follow-up; (c) to observe the hemodynamic response to medical therapy. The following section will review the evaluation of RAP, sPAP, mPAP, and PVR.

Evaluation of right atrial pressure. The right atrium is an essential part of the right heart. Estimating the RAP is an important task because it is a core component in calculating the pulmonary pressure and RVSP. There are several parameters that can be reflective of elevated pressure in the right atrium like enlargement of the coronary sinus,[39] hepatic vein, and leftward bowing of interatrial septum. Assessment of inferior vena cava (IVC) diameter and its dynamic response to respiration, however, are the best tools that are currently available to assess RAP (Fig. 46.4). The American Society of Echocardiography recommends viewing the IVC from the subcostal window and measuring it 1 to 2 cm from its junction with the right atrium in the left decubitus position.[29] The normal IVC diameter is <1.7 cm. The diameter of the IVC is dynamic and responsive to the change in respiration. There are several parameters that are recommended to assess the RAP and they are summarized in Table 46.5.

In some special populations, we should be careful in assessing RAP. Highly trained athletes can have an enlarged IVC at about 2.3 ± 0.46 cm compared to age control matched subjects. These athletes have normal response to respiration with >50% collapse of their IVC.[41] An IVC <12 mm diameter and spontaneous collapse suggest intravascular depletion.[42] In mechanically-ventilated patients, there is a poor correlation between IVC assessment and RAP, but IVC <12 mm still predicts 10 mm Hg or less.[43]

Several other techniques were developed to assess RAP from hepatic vein flow, TDI, velocity of the tricuspid valve lateral annulus (*E/E* ratio), and isovolumic relaxation time calculated from TDI tricuspid annulus velocity. These parameters can distinguish a mean RAP in a dichotomous way, but with relatively low sensitivity and low specificity.[43]

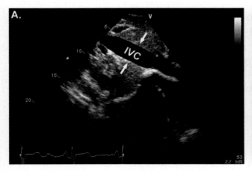

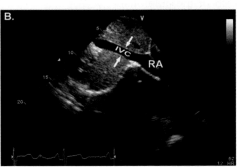

Figure 46.4 Evaluation of RAP from subcostal view using IVC diameter and a brief sniff. **A:** Patient with severe PH and IVC diameter of 2.2 cm, with brief sniff (**B**), IVC collapses <50% consistent with 15 mm Hg RAP.

TABLE 46.5
IVC PARAMETERS TO ASSESS RAP

RAP from IVC diameter with normal respiration[40]

RAP (mm Hg)	IVC Diameter (mm)	IVC collapse (%)
5	<20	>50
10	<20	<50
15	≥20	>50
20	≥20	>50

RAP from IVC diameter and a brief sniff[29]

0–5	<17	>50
6–10	>17	>50
10–15	>17	<50
>15	>17	Plethoric

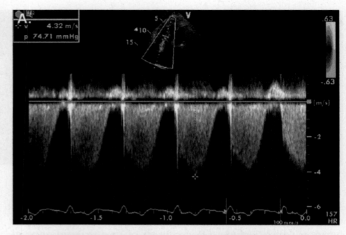

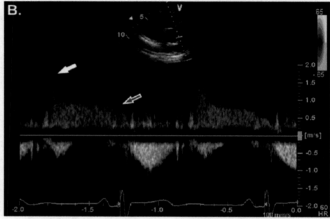

Evaluation of systolic pulmonary arterial pressure. Peak sPAP is the main and first hemodynamic parameter for the right ventricle that was evaluated and integrated in clinical practice. The modified Bernoulli equation $(4V^2)$ is the most validated equation to assess sPAP.[44,45] This equation calculates the value of the peak systolic pressure gradient of the tricuspid regurgitant jet, $4(TRV_{max})^2$, where TRV_{max} is the maximal tricuspid regurgitation velocity (Fig. 46.5). It is recommended to use multiple views to find the maximal velocity.[46] By adding the RAP to the tricuspid gradient, we derive the RVSP. The sPAP is equal to RVSP with the assumption of no gradient across the pulmonic valve.

$$RVSP = 4 \times (TRV_{max})^2 + RAP \qquad \text{(Eq. 46.1)}$$

There are several factors limiting the detection of the tricuspid regurgitant jet. Some of these factors are due to the patient's underlying disease, such as COPD, where the position of heart is displaced behind the sternum and the ability for detection is decreased.[47] Other factors depend on the prevalence of PH in a certain segment of the population. Agitated air–saline mixture (10% air and 90% normal saline) improves the detection of PAH. Also, it improves the correlation of the assessment of sPAP from $(r = 0.64)$ to $(r = 0.86)$. The use of 10% air, 10% blood, and 80% normal saline increases further the correlation $(r = 0.92)$.[48]

Evaluation of mean pulmonary arterial pressure. The third WHO Conference established the definition of PAH as an elevated mPAP greater than 25 mm Hg, so the ability to noninvasively calculate the mPAP is of great clinical importance. RV catheterization is the gold standard for assessment of PH and mPAP. The occurrence of the dicrotic notch of the pulmonary pressure waveform approximates the early maximal pulmonary valve insufficiency (PVI_{max}) (Fig. 46.5).[49] Since we can derive intracardiac pressures applying the modified Bernoulli equation, we can calculate the pulmonary valve gradient at that point by adding RAP. The correlation that we can achieve is statistically significant $(r = 0.93)$.

$$mPAP = 4 \times (PVI_{max})^2 + RAP \qquad \text{(Eq. 46.2)}$$

Chemla et al. studied the relationship between sPAP and mPAP. They demonstrated that the sPAP and mPAP are strongly related over an mPAP range of 10 to 78 mm Hg with excellent correlation

Figure 46.5 Assessment of RV hemodynamic parameters. **A:** Patient with severe PH who has an increased tricuspid valve regurgitant jet velocity $(TRV_{max} = 4.32 \, m/s)$ and maximum gradient of 75 mm Hg. To calculate sPAP using modified Bernoulli equation, you add RAP of 15 mm Hg (Fig. 46.3) and obtain a sPAP of 90 mm Hg. **B:** Doppler at the RVOT from the parasternal short-axis view at the level of the aortic valve. Early or maximal velocity of pulmonary valve insufficiency (PVI_{max}) (*solid arrow*) to calculate mPAP, and late pulmonary valve insufficiency (*empty arrow*) that is useful to calculate the diastolic pulmonary pressure using modified Bernoulli equation. See text for more details.

$(r^2 = 0.98)$, using high fidelity catheter. Using a regression analysis, a new formula was proposed and was confirmed with prospective measurement on 15 patients.[50]

$$mPAP = 0.61 \, sPAP + 2 \, mm \, Hg \qquad \text{(Eq. 46.3)}$$

Using this equation, an mPAP of more than 25 mm Hg corresponds with a sPAP of 38 mm Hg, This value more accurately defines PH, compared to the standard 30 mm Hg that is used in many catheterization laboratories.

Evaluation of pulmonary vascular resistance. PVR is an essential factor in the assessment of patients with PH. It helps in evaluating the severity of disease, prognosis, outcome, and response to therapy. Usually, PVR is assessed in the catheterization laboratory, but with the advance of Doppler echocardiography, many formulas have been proposed. The PVR is calculated invasively by the ratio of transpulmonary pressure (mPAP—wedge pressure) to transpulmonary flow (cardiac output). Abbas et al.[51] proposed a new formula based on extrapolation of invasive data, where TRV correlates with transpulmonary pressure and TVI of RVOT correlates with transpulmonary flow. The RVOT is interrogated using 1 to 2 mm pulsed wave Doppler sample at the pulmonary valve. Continuous wave Doppler can be used to obtain TVR. The ratio TRV: TVI of RVOT has been shown to correlate with PVR with a correlation factor of (r = 0.93). A simplified equation derived from linear regression is:

$$PVR \text{ (wood unit)} = 10 \times TRV/TVI_{RVOT} \qquad \text{(Eq. 46.4)}$$

Bland–Altman analysis has showed satisfactory agreement between the PVRs that were calculated by catheterization and Doppler echocardiography.

4.2. Nuclear imaging

Nuclear imaging can be an important part of evaluating patients with PH. The ventilation/perfusion (V/Q) scan plays an essential role in evaluating patients with chronic thromboembolic PH and it is going to be reviewed in detail in Chapter 10. Radionuclide angiography (RNA) or radionuclide ventriculography is a noninvasive and highly reproducible method to assess the RV volumes and global and regional systolic function. Two techniques are used to perform RNA, the equilibrium method or multigated acquisition and the first pass technique. Evaluation of the RV ejection fraction is best obtained with first pass due to better temporal resolution and RV count to background ratio. One advantage of RNA is its dependency on radioisotope count rather than on any geometric shape to assess the RV volumes and EF. However, spatial resolution is limited with both first pass and equilibrium methods. The need for ionizing radiation and iodine contrast and the absence of hemodynamic information limit the routine application of this test for the routine evaluation of PH patients.

4.3. Computed tomography

Computed tomography imaging is an X-ray based procedure where tomographic images are produced based on a rotational radiation source around the patients. The density of the soft tissue and blood is similar, so coronary arteries and cardiac cavities cannot be delineated without using contrast agent. Chest CT angiogram (CTA) findings in patients with PH include RV and RA enlargement (Fig. 46.6), RV hypertrophy, enlarged proximal pulmonary vessels and pruning of distal ones, calcification, and possible pulmonary artery aneurysm.[52] Assessment of RV volumes and function requires ECG gating, which increases radiation dosage.

The 64-multi-detector computed tomography (MDCT) scanners have higher temporal and spatial resolution. Plumhans et al.[53] recently compared the RV functional and volume parameters by using 64-MDCT to 1.5T CMR. They found an excellent correlation with CMR, end diastolic volume (r = 0.99), end systolic volume (r = 0.98), stroke volume (r = 0.98), and EF (r = 0.97). Bland–Altman plots showed no systemic variation between MDCT and CMR. The need for ionizing radiation and iodine contrast and the absence of hemodynamic information also limit the routine application of this test for the routine evaluation of PH patients.

4.4. Magnetic resonance imaging

CMR is a well-established technique with numerous cardiovascular applications. As discussed in Chapter 7, CMR requires specialized receiver coils, pulse sequencing, and gating methods. No side effect is reported for CMR, but there are few limitations. These limitations include claustrophobia in 2% of patients and interference from ferromagnetic objects. The pump that is used for prostanoid infusion in patients with PH is incompatible with CMR and should not be in the scanning room. Furthermore, the need for sustained breath-holding and steady heart rhythms makes imaging difficult in sicker PH patients. CMR finding in patients with PH include RV and RA enlargement, RV hypertrophy (Fig. 46.7, Movies 46.1, 46.2), enlarged proximal pulmonary vessels (Fig. 46.8) and pruning (Fig. 46.9, movie 46.3) of distal ones, reduced stroke volume, cardiac output, and pulmonary arteries distensibility. The steady-state free precession pulse (SSFP) is the preferred pulse sequence for acquisition of volumetric, morphologic, mass, and functional data to assess the RV and LV. The high accuracy of this technique made it the gold standard to evaluate the RV morphology. Phase contrast velocity mapping sequences are used to measure velocity to calculate hemodynamic parameters including CO, SV, and QP/QS in patients with known or suspected congenital heart disease.[54,55] In this regard, CMR is superior to echocardiography, since it allows to detect shunt lesions outside of the conventional limited echocardiographic acoustic windows, including anomalous pulmonary venous return and intrapulmonary shunts.

4.5. Right heart catheterization

Despite all the hemodynamic data that can be obtained by noninvasive testing, right heart catheterization should be done to confirm the diagnosis and to rule out PVH, especially that using

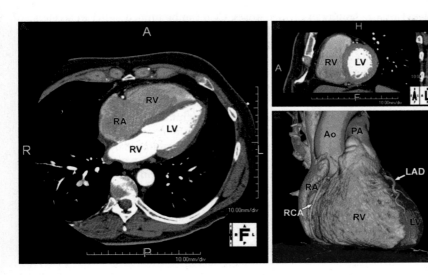

Figure 46.6 Cardiac CTA obtained by 64-MDCT. **A:** Axial view shows right atrial and ventricular enlargement in patients with PAH. **B:** Short axis of the heart showed RV bigger than LV. **C:** 3D volume-rendering image of the RV. Ao, Aorta; LA, Left atrium, LAD, left arterior descending artery; LV, left verticle; RA, right atrium; RCA, right coronery artery; RV, right ventricle.

END-DIASTOLE   **END-SYSTOLE**

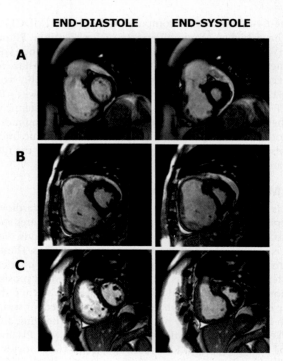

Figure 46.7 SSFP CMR images obtained at end-diastole and end-systole in a patient with moderate (**A, Movie 46.1**), moderately-severe (**B**) and severe (**C, Movie 46.2**) PH. Notice the different degrees of RV enlargement, RV hypertrophy, and end-systolic septal shift.

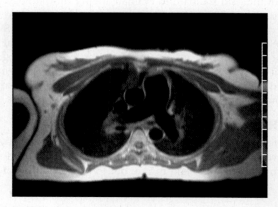

Figure 46.8 Axial HASTE CMR image showing severely dilated main and right pulmonary arteries in a patient with severe PH.

prostanoids or ETRA are associated with increased mortality in patients with left heart disease. To diagnose PAH from the hemodynamic standpoint, all three criteria should be present (mPAP ≥ 25 mm Hg, pulmonary wedge pressure ≤15 mm Hg, PVR >3 Wood units).

After the venous saturation and cardiac output, an acute vasoreactivity test can be performed. To acutely induce decrease in PVR, a fast acting, short-duration pulmonary vascular dilator is used. IV epoprostenol, IV adenosine, or inhaled NO is commonly used.[2] The contraindications for performing the vasoreactivity test include low cardiac output or left heart failure. A positive responder to vasodilators, based on retrospective data of patients on CCB, are defined as a reduction of mPAP by at least 10 mm Hg to a value of 40 mm Hg or less, with an increased or unchanged cardiac output.[56]

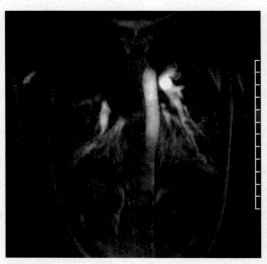

Figure 46.9 Pulmonary angiogram coronal image showing dilated proximal pulmonary arteries with distal pruning (**Movie 46.3**).

5. SELECTING AND GUIDING THERAPY

Over the last decade, remarkable advances have occurred in the understanding, diagnosis, and treatment of PH (Fig. 46.10). In addition to conventional therapy, three groups of specific medications have been developed and approved by the food and drug administration (FDA) for treatment of PH, including prostanoids, ETRA, and phosphodiesterase-5 inhibitors. Several other potential therapeutic targets are under investigation.

5.1. Conventional medical therapy

The conventional medical therapy consists of calcium channel blockers (CCB), oxygen supplementation, anticoagulation, digoxin, and diuretics. CCB should be used only if the acute vasoreactivity test during right heart catheterization is positive, and it is contraindicated in patients with acute decompensated right heart failure, low cardiac output, and low systemic blood pressure. Rich et al.[57] were the first who showed the benefit of high dose CCB in patients with IPAH. Only 12.8% of patients with PAH have a positive vasoreactivity test and 6.8% have a long-term response to CCB.[56] Nifedipine or diltiazem can be used based on patients' heart rate (HR). For HR <100, nifedipine is used up to 240 mg/day, and for HR >100 diltiazem is used up to 720 mg orally in divided doses. CCB can be titrated either in accelerated fashion while the patient is in the hospital with a right heart catheter in, or slowly as an outpatient. CCB should not be used empirically to treat PAH in the absence of demonstrated positive vasoreactivity test.[11]

Oxygen supplemental therapy is proven to be beneficial in patients with COPD, right heart failure, and chronic hypoxia where long-term survival is significantly improved.[58] Based on improved mortality and morbidity rates in patients with COPD and because hypoxia is a very potent pulmonary vasoconstrictor,[59] the oxygen therapy is used widely in patients with PH and hypoxia to maintain oxygen saturation >90%.[11,60] The oxygen therapy in patients with Eisenmenger syndrome is still controversial. Patients with OSA and PH need continuous positive airway pressure rather than oxygen therapy.

There is no randomized control trial for patients with PAH and anticoagulation therapy, but many prothrombotic abnormalities are found in these patients in addition to in situ thrombosis.[13] One small prospective study and three retrospective studies

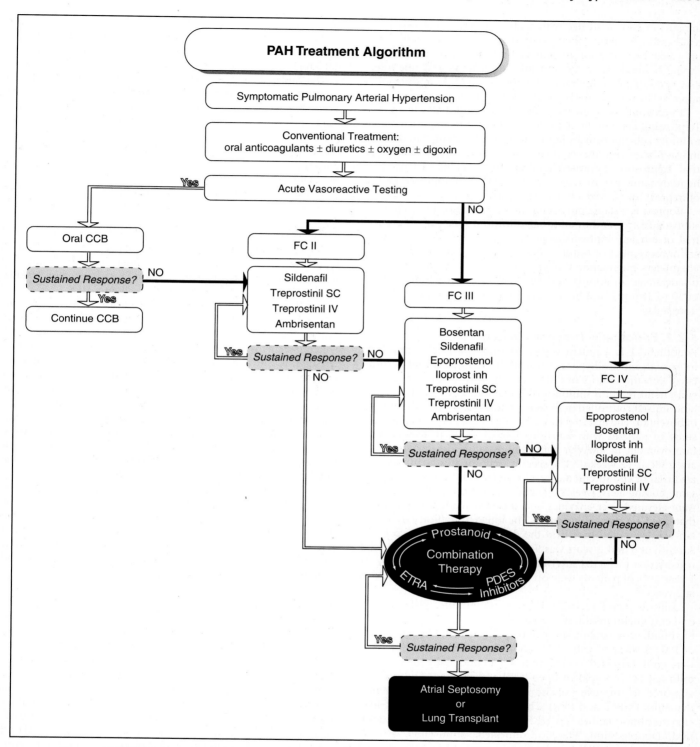

Figure 46.10 PAH treatment algorithm. CCB, Calcium-channel blocker, FC, Functional class; IV, Intravenous; SC, Subcutaneoul PDES, Phosphodiestrase-5 inhibitors; ETRA, Endothelim-1 receptor antagonists.

showed improved survival of patients with PAH receiving warfarin.[61] Based on these reports, many experts use anticoagulation for these patients. Diuretics and digoxin are used mainly for the management of volume overload and right heart failure.

5.2. Specific medical therapy

The specific medical therapy is aimed at reversing some aspects of the pathology of PH. It includes the three groups of cellular targets that were approved by the US FDA.

5.2.1. Prostanoids

Prostacyclin is synthesized in the vascular endothelium from the arachidonic acid. It promotes vascular relaxation, inhibition of smooth muscle growth, and decreased platelet aggregation. Prostacyclin analogs are also called prostanoids. Epoprostenol is the first prostanoid that was used in patients with PAH and in a prospective, open label, and randomized clinical trial in patients with IPAH and APAH due to CTD.[18] This trial showed improved exercise capacity, quality of life, hemodynamic parameters, and mortality in patients who are treated with continuous intravenous epoprostenol and conventional therapy compared to conventional therapy only. Because of its short half-life of 3 to 6 min, an infusion pump should be used for continuous infusion (intravenous line infection is the main complication for this therapy). Epoprostenol is approved by the FDA for FC III and IV PAH patients.

Treprostinil is a prostacyclin analog with half-life of 3 h. Treprostinil is more stable in room temperature and it is feasible to infuse subcutaneously, but up to 85% of patients can develop infusion site pain and erythema. In a multicenter randomized trial, treprostinil improved modestly the walking distance and hemodynamic parameters.[62] Recently, the FDA approved IV use of treprostinil, in addition to its subcutaneous use.

Iloprost is a stable prostanoid that can be used intravenously, subcutaneously, and in an inhaled form. A randomized clinical trial of inhaled iloprost was performed with significant statistical improvement of 6-min walking distance and hemodynamic parameters, but no mortality improvement.[63] The most important disadvantage for iloprost is the short duration of action (half-life of 20 to 25 min), and the frequent requirement of 6 to 9 inhalations a day.

5.2.2. Endothelin-1 receptor antagonists

Endothelin-1 is a potent vasoconstrictor and might contribute to smooth muscle hypertrophy with a blood level that is correlated with the severity of PAH.[64] Bosentan is the first unselective endothelin receptor inhibitor of both isoform ET_A and ET_B. Two randomized controlled trials were performed to assess the efficacy of bosentan. The first trial was a double-blind, placebo-controlled study of patients with function class III or IV. It demonstrates improvement in 6MWD, and hemodynamic parameters mPAP and PVR at 12 weeks.[65] The second trial, the Bosentan randomized trial of endothelin antagonist therapy (BREATH-1), had the same finding at 16 weeks. The main side effect, in the two trials, were elevated liver enzymes and the FDA made a requirement that these are checked monthly. The long-term efficacy of bosentan was examined based on the data from previous two trials. Survival at 1 and 2 years was 96% and 88.5% compared to NIH registry that predicted survival at 69% and 57%, respectively. At 1 year 78% of patients were on bosentan monotherapy and 55% at 2 years.[66]

Ambrisentan is a selective ET_A receptor inhibitor and is the second endothelin inhibitor to receive approval by the FDA. A double-blind, dose-ranging study of 64 patients with idiopathic PAH or PAH associated with CTD, anorexigen use, or HIV infection were randomized to receive ambrisentan once daily for 12 weeks followed by 12 weeks of open-label ambrisentan. Ambrisentan appeared to improve exercise capacity, symptoms, and hemodynamics (mPAP and PVR). The incidence and severity of liver enzyme abnormalities is 3.1%.[67] Ambrisentan in PAH, Randomized, Double-Blind, Placebo-Controlled, Multicenter, Efficacy Study 1 and 2 (ARIES-1 and ARIES-2) randomized 202 and 192 patients, respectively, to placebo or ambrisentan (ARIES-1, 5 or 10 mg; ARIES-2, 2.5 or 5 mg) orally once daily for 12 weeks. The primary end point for each study was change in 6-min walk distance from baseline to week 12. The 6-min walk distance increased in all ambrisentan groups. In 280 patients completing 48 weeks of treatment with ambrisentan monotherapy, the improvement from baseline in 6-min walk at 48 weeks was 39 m.[68]

5.2.3. Phosphodiestrase-5 inhibitors

NO stimulates cyclic guanosine 3'-5' monophosphate (cGMP) in the vascular smooth muscle and induces vascular relaxation.

Phosphodiesterase type 5 (PDE5) is highly expressed in the pulmonary vasculature and causes rapid degradation of cGMP. Inhibiting PDE5 can possibly sustain the NO effect and help to improve vascular dilatation in patients with PAH.

The Sildenafil use in PAH (SUPER) study randomized 278 patients with symptomatic PAH to placebo or sildenafil for 12 weeks.[69] Patients were IPAH, APAH (due to CTD or repair congenital heart disease) in WHO FC II and III. Sildenafil reduced the mean pulmonary artery pressure, improved the WHO FC, and were associated with side effects such as flushing, dyspepsia, and diarrhea. Among the 222 patients completing 1 year of treatment with sildenafil monotherapy, the improvement at 1 year in 6MWD was 51 m.[69] Based on this study and a follow-up open label study, the FDA approved Sildenafil for treatment of patients with PAH.

5.3. Surgical therapy

Two surgical procedures are performed for patients with PH, atrial septostomy, and lung transplant. Pulmonary thromboendarterectomy provides a potential surgical cure for patients with CTEPH and will be discussed in more detail in Chapter 10.

Atrial septostomy is a palliative procedure for patients with severe PH to decompress the right heart congestion and improve cardiac output. This procedure was based on a report of patients with IPAH, where patients who had patent foramen ovale (PFO) had a better survival outcome than patients without PFO.[70] The criteria to perform this procedure are patients with most advanced PAH and include those with severe FC III or IV, a history of recurrent syncope, or refractory right heart failure. Patients with most advanced PAH, defined by elevated PVR, atrial oxygen saturation <80% at rest, and severe right heart failure (low CO and elevated RAP), appear to die or worsen with atrial septostomy.[71] Atrial septostomy tends to result in improved hemodynamic and 6MWD for short period of time, but this procedure is associated with high mortality (>10%).

Lung transplant is the ultimate therapy for patients with PAH. The development of effective therapy for PAH such as the prostanoids changes the natural history of this disease and has altered the criteria for lung transplant. The treatment with epoprostenol is viewed as a bridge or an alternative to transplant for many patients with PAH,[72] where transplant should not be considered until the failure of medical therapy.[71]

6. IMAGING AND PROGNOSIS

Survival in patients with PH depends on the etiology of the disease, where patients with PAH due to scleroderma have worse prognosis than IPAH and APAH due to congenital heart disease.[12] The estimated median survival from the time of diagnosis is 2.8 years, and 1- and 5- year survival rate are only 68% and 34%, respectively.[8,10,12] More than 70% of patients with PAH will die of right heart failure, and most of the remainder die due to arrhythmia. Most of the main predictors of poor prognosis in PAH are related to the development of RV failure.[12,38] From the imaging standpoint, echocardiography and CMR play a key role in the evaluation of right heart function and long-term prognosis. One of most relevant findings in patients with IPAH is the detection of pericardial effusion, where it had negative prognostic implications. Right atrial volume index and RV tei-index have also been correlated with bad outcomes.[12]

7. FUTURE DIRECTIONS

Significant work lies ahead to further improve the survival and outcome of patients with PAH. Many genetic mutations have been identified. With a greater understanding of its role in the pathogenesis of PAH, the better outcome we can achieve. Three cellular targets were identified and medical therapy was found to be effective by targeting these pathways. More targets were identified including potassium channel, serotonin regulation, and tyrosine kinase. Many clinical studies are underway to assess the effectiveness of these new therapies. The interaction between these pathways and the combination therapy are also under very active investigation. Measuring the effectiveness of these therapies and monitoring the outcome, especially with accurate noninvasive diagnostic imaging modalities such as CMR and real-time 3D echo, should improve individual patient's outcome and future drug development.

ACKNOWLEDGMENTS

The authors wish to thank Blair Grubb, MD and Diane McCarthy for their careful review and comments, and Tonya Floyd-Bradstock, our medical illustrator, for her hard work on our diagrams and figures.

REFERENCES

1. Barst RJ, McGoon MD, Torbicki A, et al. Diagnosis and differential assessment of pulmonary arterial hypertension. *J Am Coll Cardiol.* 2004;43(12):40–47.
2. McLaughlin M, Vallerie V, McGoon M, et al. Pulmonary arterial hypertension. *Circulation.* 2006;114:1417–1431.
3. Dresdale D, Schultz M, Michtom R. Primary pulmonary hypertension. I. Clinical and hemodynamic study. *Am J Med.* 1951;11:686–705.
4. Hatano S, Strasser T. *Primary Pulmonary Hypertension: Report on a WHO Meeting.* Geneva: World Health Organization; 1975:7–45.
5. Fishman A. Clinical classification of pulmonary hypertension. *Clin Chest Med.* 2001;22:385–391.
6. Simonneau G, Galie N, Rubin LJ, et al. Clinical classification of pulmonary hypertension. *J Am Coll Cardiol.* 2004;43(12 Suppl S):5S–12S.
7. Hegewald M, Markewitz B, Elliott C. Pulmonary hypertension: Clinical manifestations, classification, and diagnosis. *Int J Clin Pract.* 2007;61 (Suppl 156):5–14.
8. Rich S, Dantzker D, Ayers S. Primary pulmonary hypertension. A national prospective study. *Ann Intern Med.* 1987;107:216–223.
9. McGoon MD, Gutterman D, Steen V, et al. Screening, early detection, and diagnosis of pulmonary arterial hypertension: ACCP evidence-based clinical practice guidelines. *Chest.* 2004;126:14–34.
10. Rich S, McLaughlin VV. *Pulmonary Hypertension.* 8th Ed. Philadelphia, PA: WB Saunders; 2008.
11. Badesch DB, Abman SH, Ahearn GS, et al. Medical therapy for pulmonary arterial hypertension: ACCP evidence-based clinical practice guidelines. *Chest.* 2004;126:35–62.
12. McLaughlin VV, Presberg KW, Doyle R, et al. Prognosis of pulmonary arterial hypertension (ACCP Evidence-Based Clinical Practice Guidelines). *Chest.* 2004;126:78S–92S.
13. Tuder M, Rubin M, Marecki P, et al. Pathology of pulmonary hypertension. *Clin Chest Med.* 2007;28:23–43.
14. Yuan J, Rubin LJ. Pathogenesis of pulmonary arterial hypertension: The need for multiple hits. *Circulation.* 2005;111:534–538.
15. Aldred M, Brannon CA, Conneally PM, et al. Heterozygous germline mutations in BMPR2, encoding a TGF-β receptor, cause familial primary pulmonary hypertension. *Nat Genet.* 2000;26:81–84.
16. Loscalzo J. Genetic clues to the cause of primary pulmonary hypertension. *N Engl J Med.* 2001;345(5):367–371.
17. Eddahibi S, Humbert M, Fadel E, et al. Serotonin transporter overexpression is responsible for pulmonary artery smooth muscle hyperplasia in primary pulmonary hypertension. *J Clin Invest.* 2001;108(8):1141–1150.
18. Barst RJ, Rubin LJ, Long W, et al. A comparison of continuous intravenous epoprostenol (prostacyclin) with conventional therapy for primary pulmonary hypertension. *N Engl J Med.* 1996;334:296–301.
19. Lee S-D, Shroyer KR, Markham NE, et al. Monoclonal endothelial cell proliferation is present in primary but not secondary pulmonary hypertension. *J Clin Invest.* 1998;101(5):927–934.
20. Newman JH, Wheeler L, Lane K, et al. Mutation in the gene for bone morphogenetic protein receptor II as a cause of primary pulmonary hypertension in a large kindred. *N Engl J Med.* 2001;345(5):319–324.
21. Newman JH, Trembath RC, Morse JA, et al. Genetic basis of pulmonary arterial hypertension. *J Am Coll Cardiol.* 2004;43(12, Suppl S):33S–39S.
22. Thomson J, Machado R, Pauciulo M, et al. Sporadic primary pulmonary hypertension is associated with germline mutations of the gene coding BMPR-II, a receptor member of the TFG-beta family. *J Med Genet.* 2000;37(10):741–745.
23. Machado RD, James V, Southwood M, et al. Investigation of second genetic hits at the BMPR2 Locus as a modulator of disease progression in familial pulmonary arterial hypertension. *Circulation.* 2005;111:607–613.
24. Ghio S, Gavazzi A, Campana C, et al. Independent and additive prognostic value of right ventricular systolic function and pulmonary artery pressure in patients with chronic heart failure. *J Am Coll Cardiol.* 2001;37:183–188.
25. Oudiz R. Pulmonary hypertension associated with left-sided heart disease. *Clin Chest Med.* 2007;28:233–241.
26. Thabu G, Dauriat G, Stern JB, et al. Pulmonary hemodynamics in advanced COPD candidates for lung volume reduction surgery or lung transplantation. *Chest.* 2005;127(5):1531–1536.
27. Lettieri CJ, Nathan SD, Barnett SD, et al. Prevalence and outcomes of pulmonary arterial hypertension in advanced idiopathic pulmonary fibrosis. *Chest.* 2006;129(3):746–752.
28. McGoon MD, Gutterman D, Steen V, et al. Screening, early detection, and diagnosis of pulmonary arterial hypertension. *Chest.* 2008;126:14S–23S.
29. Lang RM, Bierig M, Devereux RB, et al. Recommendations for chamber quantification: A report from the American Society of Echocardiography's Guidelines and Standards Committee and the Chamber Quantification Writing Group, developed in conjunction with the European Association of Echocardiography, a branch of the European Society of Cardiology. *J Am Soc Echocardiogr.* 2005;18:1440–1463.
30. Lopez-Candales A, Dohi K, Iliescu A, et al. An abnormal right ventricular apical angle is indicative of global right ventricular impairment. *Echocardiography.* 2006;23(5):361–368.
31. Otto CM. *Textbook of Clinical Echocardiography.* 2nd Ed. Philadelphia, PA: WB Saunders; 2000.
32. Severino S, Caso P, Cicala S, et al. Involvement of right ventricle in left ventricular hypertrophic cardiomyopathy: Analysis by pulsed doppler tissue imaging. *Eur J Echocardiogr.* 2000;2:281–288.
33. Lopez-Candales A, Rajagopalan N, Dohi K, et al. Abnormal right ventricular myocardial strain generation in mild pulmonary hypertension. *Echocardiography.* 2007;24:615–622.
34. JKjaergaard J, Sogaard P, Hassager C. Right ventricular strain in pulmonary embolism by doppler tissue echocardiography. *J Am Soc Echocardiogr.* 2004;17(11):1210–1212.
35. Vonk M, Sander M, van den Hoogen F, et al. Right ventricle Tei-index: A tool to increase the accuracy of non-invasive detection of pulmonary arterial hypertension in connective tissue diseases. *Eur J Echocardiogr.* 2007;8:317–321.
36. Hung J, Lang R, Flachskampf F, et al. 3D echocardiography: A review of the current status and future directions. *J Am Soc Echocardiogr.* 2007;20:213–233.
37. Gopal AS, Chukwu EO, Iwuchukwu CJ, et al. Normal values of right ventricular size and function by real-time 3-dimensional echocardiography: Comparison with cardiac magnetic resonance imaging. *J Am Soc Echocardiogr.* 2007;20:445–455.
38. Raymond RJ, Hinderliter AL, Willis PW, et al. Echocardiographic predictors of adverse outcomes in primary pulmonary hypertension. *J Am Coll Cardiol.* 2002;39(7):1214–1219.
39. Mahmud E, Raisinghani A, Keramati S, et al. Dilation of the coronary sinus on echocardiogram: Prevalence and significance in patients with chronic pulmonary hypertension. *J Am Soc Echocardiogr.* 2001;14:44–49.
40. Sciomer S, Magri D, Badagliacca R. Non-invasive assessment of pulmonary hypertension: Doppler-echocardiography. *Pulm Pharmacol Ther.* 2007;20:135–140.
41. Goldhammer E, Mesnick N, Abinader EG, et al. Dilated inferior vena cava: A common echocardiographic finding in highly trained elite athletes. *J Am Soc Echocardiogr.* 1999;12:988–993.
42. Kircher BJ, Himelman RB, Schiller NB. Noninvasive estimation of right atrial pressure from the inspiratory collapse of the inferior vena cava. *Am J Cardiol.* 1990;66:493–496.
43. Lee KS, Abbas AE, Khandheria BK, et al. Echocardiographic assessment of right heart hemodynamic parameters. *J Am Soc Echocardiogr.* 2007;20:773–782.
44. Currie P, Seward J, Chan K, et al. Continuous waver Doppler determination of right ventricular pressure: A simultaneous Dopper-catheterization study in 127 patients. *J Am Coll Cardiol.* 1985;6:750–756.
45. Skjaerpe T, Hatle L. Noninvasive estimation of systolic pressure in the right ventricle in patients with tricuspid regurgitation. *Eur Heart J.* 1986;7(8):704–170.
46. Abramson SV, Burke JB, Pauletto FJ, et al. Use of multiple views in the echocardiographic assessment of pulmonary artery systolic pressure. *J Am Soc Echocardiogr.* 1995;8(1):55–60.
47. Arcasoy SM, Christie JD, Ferrari VA, et al. Echocardiographic assessment of pulmonary hypertension in patients with advanced lung disease. *Am J Respir Crit Care Med.* 2003;167:735–740.
48. Jeon D-S, Luo H, Iwami T, et al. The usefulness of a 10% air-10% blood-80% saline mixture for contrast echocardiography: Doppler measurement of pulmonary artery systolic pressure. *J Am Coll Cardiol.* 2002;39:124–129.
49. Abbas AE, Fortuin FD, Schiller NB, et al. Echocardiographic determination of mean pulmonary artery disease. *Am J Cardiol.* 2003;92:1373–1376.
50. Chemla D, Castelain V, Humbert M, et al. New formula for predicting mean pulmonary artery pressure using systolic pulmonary artery pressure. *Chest.* 2004;126:1313–1317.
51. Abbas AE, Fortuin FD, Schiller NB, et al. A simple method for noninvasive estimation of pulmonary vascular resistance. *J Am Coll Cardiol.* 2003;41(6):1021–1027.
52. AboulHosn J, Oudiz R. Congenital heart disease and computed tomography. In: Budoff MJ, Shinbane JS, eds. *Cardiac CT Imaging: Diagnosis of Cardiovascular Disease.* London: Springer-Verlag; 2006:221–238.
53. Plumhans C, Muhlenbruch G, Rapaee A, et al. Assessment of global right ventricular function on 64-MDCT compared with MRI. *Am J Roentgenol.* 2008;190(5):1358–1361.

54. Lorenz CH. Right ventricular anatomy and function in health and disease. In: Manning WJ, Pennell DJ, eds. *Cardiovascular Magnetic Resonance*. New York, NY: Churchill Livingstone; 2002.

55. Mcclure L, Peacock A. Imaging of the heart in pulmonary hypertension. *Int J Clin Pract*. 2007;61(Suppl 156):15–26.

56. Sitbon O, Humbert M, Jais X, et al. Long-term response to calcium channel blockers in idiopathic pulmonary arterial hypertension. *Circulation*. 2005;111:3105–3111.

57. Rich S, Brundage BH. High-dose calcium channel-blocking therapy for primary pulmonary hypertension: Evidence for long-term reduction in pulmonary arterial pressure and regression of right ventricular hypertrophy. *Circulation*. 1987;76(1):135–141.

58. Long term domiciliary oxygen therapy in chronic hypoxic cor pulmonale complicating chronic bronchitis and emphysema. Report of the Medical Research Council Working Party. *Lancet*. 1981;1(8222):681–686.

59. Weissmann N, Tadic A, Hanze J, et al. Hypoxic vasoconstriction in intact lungs: A role for NADPH oxidase-derived H_2O_2? *Am J Physiol Lung Cell Mol Physiol*. 2000;279:L683–L690.

60. Badesch DB, Abman SH, Simonneau G, et al. Medical therapy for pulmonary arterial hypertension. *Chest*. 2007;131:1917–1928.

61. Alam S, Palevsky H. Standard therapies for pulmonary arterial hypertension. *Clin Chest Med*. 2007;28:91–115.

62. Simonneau G, Barst RJ, Galie N, et al. Continuous subcutaneous infusion of treprostinil, a prostacyclin analogue, in patients with pulmonary arterial hypertension. *Am J Respir Crit Care Med*. 2002;165:800–804.

63. Olschewski H, Simonneau G, Galie N, et al. Inhaled iloprost for severe pulmonary hypertension. *N Engl J Med*. 2002;347(5):322–329.

64. Rubens C, Ewert R, Halank M, et al. Big endothelin-1 and endothelin-1 plasma levels are correlated with the severity of primary pulmonary hypertension. *Chest*. 2001;120:1562–1569.

65. Channick RN, Simonneau G, Sitbon O, et al. Effects of the dual endothelin-receptor antagonist bosentan in patients with pulmonary hypertension: A randomised placebo-controlled study. *Lancet*. 2001;358:1119–1123.

66. McLaughlin VV, Sitbon O, Badesch DB, et al. Survival with first-line bosentan in patients with primary pulmonary hypertension. *Eur Respir J*. 2005;25:244–249.

67. Galie N, Badesch DB, Oudiz R, et al. Ambrisentan therapy for pulmonary arterial hypertension. *J Am Coll Cardiol*. 2005;46(3):529–535.

68. Galie N, Olschewski H, Oudiz R, et al. Ambrisentan for the treatment of pulmonary arterial hypertension. *Circulation*. 2008;117:3010–3019.

69. Galie N, Ghofrani H, Torbicki A, et al. Sildenafil citrate therapy for pulmonary arterial hypertension. *N Engl J Med*. 2005;353:2148–2157.

70. Glanville A, Burke C, Theodore J, et al. Primary pulmonary hypertension. Length of survival in patients referred for heart-lung transplantation. *Chest*. 1987;91:675–681.

71. Doyle R, McCrory DC, Channick R, et al. Surgical treatments/interventions for pulmonary arterial hypertension. *Chest*. 2004;126:63S–71S.

72. Conte J, Gaine S, Orens J, et al. The influence of continuous intravenous prostacyclin therapy for primary pulmonary hypertension on the timing and outcome of transplantation. *J Heart Lung Transplant*. 1998;17(7):679–685.

Pulmonary Embolism

47

Samer J. Khouri
Dawn-Alita Hernandez

1. INTRODUCTION

Pulmonary embolism (PE) is part of a larger syndrome that includes the formation of thrombus and its distal consequences of embolization. Venous thromboembolism (VTE) refers to a spectrum of disorders that include deep venous thrombosis (DVT) of extremities and pelvic veins, the embolic events arising from them such as PE and chronic thromboembolic disease (CTED), and chronic thromboembolic pulmonary hypertension (CTEPH).

From the clinical standpoint, PE is divided into three main groups: massive, submassive, and nonmassive or small PE. Massive PE is associated with shock and/or hypotension (defined as systolic blood pressure <90 mm Hg). Submassive PE is a subgroup defined as PE with right ventricle (RV) dysfunction (as identified by echocardiography) and no systemic hypotension. Otherwise, a nonmassive or small PE would be diagnosed.[1]

Studying and preventing PE cannot be done without focusing on its root cause, the deep venous thrombosis. VTE and its complication, the PE, remain an important cause of mortality and morbidity in hospitalized patients despite rigorous screening tools and refined imaging techniques aimed at primary prevention of these disorders. Thus, 25% to 50% of patients with first-time VTE have an idiopathic condition, without a readily identifiable risk factor. Early mortality after VTE is strongly associated with the presentation as PE, advanced age, cancer, or underlying cardiovascular disease.[2]

1.1. Epidemiology

1.1.1. Epidemiology of the acute pulmonary embolism

While many studies have been dedicated to racial, socioeconomic, and environmental disparities in both incidence and outcome of VTE and PE, the most common contributing factors are listed in Table 47.1. Much effort has been dedicated to determining relative risks for thrombogenesis for each category listed. In each of these risk factors, Virchow triad, which includes hypercoagulability, venous stasis, and vascular endothelial damage, remains the driving force for clot formation.

Depending on a patient's risk factors, escalating VTE prophylaxis therapy should be employed. While all patients should be screened for DVT risk, not all patients will be candidates for pharmacologic DVT prophylaxis due to contraindications to anticoagulant therapy. PE remains the most common cause of acute cor pulmonale and accounts for an estimated 650,000 deaths per year or 10% of patients who die in hospitals in the United States, making it the third overall cause of cardiovascular

death (behind acute coronary syndrome and cerebrovascular accidents).[2,3] Recent studies have detected PE in 15% of routine biopsies with only 30% of these cases diagnosed correctly antemortem.[4]

The overall cost of VTE in health care in dollars is about $17,500, $18,900, and $25,600 annually per patient with DVT, PE, and combination of DVT and PE, respectively. This cost is further increased with recurrent DVT or PE. Considering that 10% to 40% of hospitalized patients die from their initial PE, early detection and appropriate treatment of this high-risk population renders the potential for both clinical and economic benefits.[5]

1.1.2. Epidemiology of the chronic thromboembolic pulmonary hypertension

Although all patients with acute PE may have elevation of their mean pulmonary arterial pressure (mPAP) in the acute setting, not all patients will have persistent pulmonary hypertension (PH). In fact, patients with a single PE may recover over the space of months and ultimately have minimal evidence of their previous PE.[6,7] Patients developing CTEPH can be grouped into two groups; those with known PE and recurrence versus those who present with primary diagnosis of PH without documented history of VTE/PE. In particular, patients sent for evaluation of pulmonary arterial hypertension (PAH) should be evaluated for chronic thrombosis.

While the exact number of patients with CTEPH is not known, it is estimated that up to 2,500 patients per year with dyspnea have chronic thrombus formation and resultant PH.[6] Interestingly, patients with prothrombotic factors such as protein C and protein S deficiency and antithrombin II defects do not comprise the majority of CTEPH.[8] The only prothrombotic risk factor for development of CTEPH is lupus anticoagulant, which accounts for approximately one quarter of patients.[9]

1.1.3. Epidemiology venous thromboembolism

DVT occurs for the first time in 100 persons per 100,000 each year in the United States and rises exponentially from five cases per 100,000 in patients <15 years old to >500 cases per 100,000 persons at 80 years of age. One third of patients with symptomatic DVT manifest PE, whereas two thirds of them manifest DVT alone.[2] DVT of extremities is divided into deep and superficial venous thrombus formation (Fig. 47.1). DVT of the lower extremities is the cause of PE in >80% of patients. DVT of the lower extremities is defined as thrombus formation proximal to the popliteal veins. Because popliteal veins have a high rate of propagation to proximal veins, they are typically included in the DVT subset despite their superficial anatomy. However, superficial venous thrombus formation has been studied and is treated as equivalent to DVT

TABLE 47.1

RISK FACTORS FOR PULMONARY EMBOLISM

Factors increasing risk for pulmonary embolism		
Lower risk	*Moderate risk*	*Higher risk*

▪ Between ages of 41 and 60 years
▪ Planned minor surgery
▪ Obesity
▪ Hypertension
▪ Inflammatory bowel disease
▪ Lower extremity edema
▪ Varicose veins
▪ Smoking
▪ Oral contraceptives
	▪ Between ages of 61 and 74 years
	▪ Major surgery
	▪ Critical illness
	▪ Malignancy
	  (*Present or previous; excluding skin.*)
	▪ Immobility *(for 72 h)*
	▪ Factors present within last 30 days:
	  – Central venous acess
	  – Immobilizing cast
		▪ Age 75 years or older
		▪ Surgery plus morbid obesity
		▪ Elective knee or hip replacement
		▪ Factors present within last 30 days
		  – Multiple traumas
		  – Stroke
		  – Hip, pelvis, or femur fracture
		▪ History of DVT/PE
		▪ Family history of thrombosis
		▪ Additional risk factors
		  – CHF MI
		  – Chronic lung disease
		  – History of stroke

Source: Adapted from Kucher N, Goldhaber S. Management of massive pulmonary embolism. *Circulation.* 2005;112(2):e28–e32; Kucher N, Sophia K, Rene Q, et al. Electronic alerts to prevent venous thromboembolism among hospitalized patients. *N Engl J Med.* 2005;352(10):969–977.

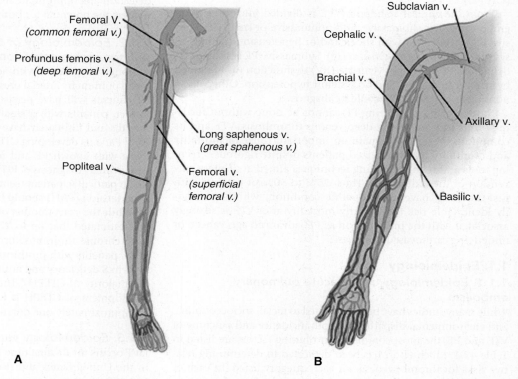

Figure 47.1 The diagram illustrates the upper (**B**) and lower (**A**) extremity deep (light blue) and superficial (dark blue) venous systems (see text for details). (Adapted from Lang RM, Bierig M, Devereux RB, et al. Recommendations for chamber quantification; A report from the American Society of Echocardigraphy's Guidelines and Stantdards Committee and the Chamber Quantification Writing Group, developed in conjunction with the European Association of Echocardiography, a branch of the European Society of Cardiology. *J Am Soc Echocardiogr.* 2005;18:1440–1463.)

in special cases where (i) the patient is symptomatic (pain, swelling) or (ii) the patient is at high risk for developing DVT, as the superficial venous thrombus may herald previous or future clot formation.

In the upper extremities, deep venous system is considered in all vessels proximal to the basilic and cephalic veins, including internal jugular veins. Upper extremity DVT formation is "effort induced" in about one quarter of cases, also known as Paget-von Schrötter syndrome.[10] This syndrome, characterized by an intrinsic anatomical defect, leads to chronic venous insufficiency and ultimately DVT formation of the upper extremities at the thoracic

inlet and costoclavicular space. The majority of the remaining cases of upper extremity DVT are considered secondary and are related to indwelling catheters or devices, decreased protein C and S levels or activity, or obstruction from secondary anatomical abnormalities (e.g., malignancy, irradiation, trauma). Initially, upper extremity DVT was felt to be innocuous, but recent investigations suggest that 20% of upper extremity DVT results in PE.[10] In addition, up to 30% of diagnosed PE patients have no evidence of lower extremity DVT. Some investigations recommend examination of the upper extremities in these patients, which may lead to diagnosis of upper extremity DVT.

1.2. Clinical presentation

Presentation of VTE is variable and can be divided into symptomatic and asymptomatic patients. It is unknown exactly how many asymptomatic VTE events occur annually, but it has been proposed that as many as 1 million patients have undiagnosed DVT. Classic symptoms of DVT include pain and/or swelling of the extremity involved. Up to 10% of patients will go on to develop postthrombotic syndrome (PTS).[11,12] PTS is characterized by chronic pain, swelling, discoloration of the skin, and even ulcer development. Patients with PTS develop chronic venous insufficiency and associated ulcers, which do not heal well and may become chronically infected. Compression stockings of the affected limb, in conjunction with anticoagulation, may assist in prevention of PTS; however, PTS can develop in up to 2 years after acute DVT formation.

While in some cases, in situ thrombus formation may occur in the pulmonary arteries, PE classically develops as a complication of DVT formation. At the time of an acute occlusion of segmental or subsegmental pulmonary arteries, patients may be asymptomatic. However, symptoms typically described by patients with PE include pleuritic chest pain, generalized anxiety with dyspnea, palpitations, and/or tachycardia. In addition to classic pleuritic chest pain, patients present with a variety of other symptoms including syncope, presyncope, convulsion, shock, and cardiopulmonary arrest (Table 47.2). These presenting symptoms are usually sudden in onset and may dissipate within 30 min to several hours. Ultimately, if the injury progresses to pulmonary infarct, the patient may develop fever and exquisite chest pain (both pleuritic and intensified with palpation/pressure) within hours to days after the initial PE.

Wheezing, a less classical presentation, which does not respond to β-agonist inhalers or which abates too quickly to attribute to the onset of action of inhalers, may be a clinical sign of CTEPH. CTEPH patients with no history of VTE usually present with symptoms similar to patients with pulmonary arterial hypertension (Chapter 46 for details). Patients may present with a variety of physical examination findings including split second heart sound (S2) with increased intensity of P2, RV S4 gallop, tricuspid regurgitation (TR) (holosystolic) murmur, and lower extremity edema and ascites. Patients who have progressed to decompensated cor pulmonale will present with elevated jugular venous pressure (JVP) with increased v wave.

2. PATHOPHYSIOLOGY

While the pathophysiology of both acute and chronic VTE will be discussed here, special underlying pathologies such as vasculitis, iatrogenic thrombosis, and inherited and acquired thrombophilic states inherently increase the risk of thrombus formation. This necessitates consideration for specific medical therapy in those patients who are target to these pathologies. The coagulation cascade and development of resultant PH remain unchanged.

2.1. Acute pulmonary embolism

In the case of acute PE, PH develops via two main mechanisms; mechanical obstruction and hypoxia-induced vasospasm. In the lung, unlike the rest of the systemic arterial vascular bed, hypoxia induces vasospasm.[13–15] This is thought to be an autoregulation designed to decrease perfusion to relatively hypoventilated alveolar units or lobules. In the case of PE, as tissue hypoxia develops, resultant venous return is increasingly deoxygenated and acidotic. These two factors, mechanical obstruction and hypoxia-induced vasospasm, drive PA pressures higher in a vicious cycle. If the thromboembolic burden is high enough or if the thrombus propagates, the RV may ultimately fail to deliver adequate volumes to the left ventricle, a situation known as acute cor pulmonale with resultant depressed cardiac output. Depending on how acutely cor pulmonale develops and whether the right heart can adapt, the patient may present with symptoms from syncope to refractory hypotension to acute cardiopulmonary arrest (sudden death).

2.2. Chronic thromboembolic pulmonary hypertension

PH arising from CTED has been less well investigated than acute pulmonary embolus. In contrast to acute PE, CTEPH is more difficult to identify as symptoms are more insidious. Dyspnea on exertion is the main presenting symptom. With the progressive embolization, the pulmonary pressures rise, and the RV compensates with hypertrophy. Ultimately, the intraventricular pressure exceeds perfusion capabilities of the right coronary artery and angina develops. With further progression, the RV output diminishes and patients may present with presyncope or syncope with exertion.

Two primary natural histories have been described leading to CTEPH. In patients with acute PE, it is estimated that up to 0.5% to 4.0% will progress to CTEPH.[16,17] In the case of patients without recurrent PE, PH likely develops due to flow-limiting stenoses, which do not resolve with incorporation of the thrombus into the vessel wall. Because CTEPH develops when >30% of pulmonary vasculature is flow-limited, it stands to reason that patients at greatest risk for developing PH are those in whom larger arteries (segmental and greater) are involved. CTEPH may also develop in the setting of recurrent PE. When evaluating a patient for CTEPH, ventilation/perfusion scan (V/Q scan) is still recommended as a screening tool. In the case of patients with acute PE, Wartski demonstrated that as many as 66% of patients still had persistent defects at 90 days post acute event and only 8% had obstruction of >50% pulmonary vascular bed.[7] Therefore, it stands to reason that factors influencing development of CTEPH include a combination of recurrent thromboembolic events and the ability to form collateral blood vessels.

TABLE 47.2

PRESENTING SYMPTOMS SUGGESTIVE OF PULMONARY EMBOLISM (PE) AND/OR CHRONIC THROMBOEMBOLIC PULMONARY HYPERTENSION (CTEPH)

Signs and symptoms of PE and CTEPH	
Acute VTE/PE	CTEPH
Dyspnea (acute)	Acrocyanosis
CP (pleuritic or atypical)	Progressive dyspnea
Tachycardia/palpitations	Pulmonary bruits – up to 10% (may be confused with wheeze)
Syncope	Cor pulmonale
Cardiopulmonary arrest/death	– Ascites
Hemodynamic collapse	– JVD
Hemoptysis	– Lower extremity edema
Lower extremity edema	Fatigue
	Syncope and Presyncope

2.3. Deep venous thrombosis

DVT involves deposition of fibrin clot, platelets, RBC, and leukocytes in the intravascular bed via coagulation cascade. As described above, DVT usually forms in the setting of interrupted or languid blood flow in larger vessels of the upper or lower extremity. In the absence of perturbed blood flow, inflammation and/or underlying coagulopathy may be involved. In particular, protein C and S depleted states may lead to thrombosis. These may be heritable (as in protein C and S deficiency) or acquired (as in liver failure, disseminated intravascular coagulopathy (DIC), or antiphospholipid antibody syndrome).[18]

As with acute PE, DVT antithrombotic agents are utilized to accelerate intrinsic antithrombin activity in attempts to alleviate obstruction of the vessel and decrease propagation of thrombus formation. In the case of DVT, the target of therapy is early resolution and stability of thrombus to decrease incidence of PE and PTS, by decreasing venous valvular dysfunction and stabilizing the thrombus within the vessel.[12,19]

3. DIAGNOSTIC EVALUATION

At instances where a patient arrives with an acute thromboembolic event, it is essential to quickly establish accurate diagnosis of PE. In screening a patient to determine if further imaging is required, a normal serum D-dimer effectively rules out acute PE.[20,21] (In cases of CTEPH, D-dimer is only helpful if there is ongoing or acute thromboembolic disease and may be normal in patients within the periods of quiescence between thrombotic events.) For those patients with elevated serum D-dimer or those suspected of CTEPH, imaging studies are the main method of diagnosis (Fig. 47.2). Currently, imagery modalities include extremity Doppler and B-mode ultrasound (Duplex), pulmonary angiography, extremity venograms, pulmonary computed tomography angiogram (CTA), echocardiogram, and V/Q scans. More recently, magnetic resonance imaging (MRI) has also been employed though it is not yet considered a mainstay of diagnosis. Though many advances have been made in diagnosis of VTE/PE, none of the tests replaces sound clinical judgment and the choice of test often requires careful consideration.

3.1. Transthoracic echocardiography

Visualization of pulmonary arteries and pulmonary thromboembolism is very limited with transthoracic echocardiography (TTE). However, PE causes an acute increase in RV afterload that can lead to right ventricular dilatation, dysfunction, and occasionally hemodynamic compromise and failure if it is associated with massive PE. The prognostic relevance of RV function was established through a number of registries.[22,23] The patients with significant embolization and >30% lung involvement are associated with RV dysfunction.[24] Overall, 40% to 60% of patients with acute PE have normal RV function depending on their presentation and associated risk and the size of the emboli. Because of the high prevalence of normal RV function in patients with small PE, TTE is not a good tool to establish the PE diagnosis.[25] The main benefit of TTE comes from risk stratification of PE patients and establishing the high risk patients who might benefit from more aggressive management.[26,27] Many studies and registries have demonstrated that patients with acute pulmonary embolus and RV dysfunction have a poorer prognosis.[22,23]

3.1.1. Conventional transthoracic echocardiography and Acute pulmonary embolism

The mortality rate associated with massive PE can be as high as 30%, submassive PE is between 5% and 10%, and small PE mortality is <5%. The submassive PE is defined as PE with RV dysfunction and no systemic hypotension.[1] The value of TTE is

Figure 47.2 Diagnostic algorithm for pulmonary embolism.

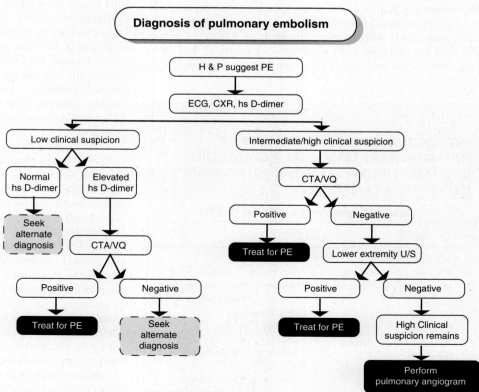

realized by identifying those patients with RV dysfunction who have higher mortality. McConnell et al.[28] were among the first who analyzed regional right ventricular function abnormalities in acute PE. They identified a distinctive pattern of segmental wall motion abnormalities in the apical-four chambers, with akinesis of the middle segment of the RV free wall and normal motion for the apical and basal apex. The sensitivity, specificity, positive and negative predictive values were 77%, 94%, 71%, and 96% respectively. Casazza et al.[29] analyzed 201 consecutive patients with either submassive PE or RV infarction. The value of McConnell sign in this study was less impressive with no value to differentiate PE from RV infarction where it was associated with both diseases.

Kjaergaard et al.[30] attempt to quantify the RV dysfunction measures (Table 47.3), where they analyze the RV diameter, RV to left ventricle (RV:LV) ratio, TR max velocity, PA acceleration time, and tricuspid annulus motion (TAM). Univariate logistic regression analysis was done using the presence or absence of PE as an outcome. All of the RV parameters were related to PE outcome. However, the sensitivity, specificity, and predictive values of TTE parameters were too low to be an alternative diagnostic method to establish the PE diagnosis alone.[30] Fremont et al.[31] analyzed a registry of 1,416 patients and found that RV:LV end-diastolic diameter ratio of ≥0.9 has a sensitivity and specificity of 72% and 58%, respectively, to predict hospital mortality. Chung et al.[32] found that TAM correlates best with PE extent ($r = -0.65$). TAM with <2.0 cm had sensitivity, specificity, and positive and negative predictive values of 75%, 84%, 75%, and 79%, respectively. The follow-up of these patients revealed that RV:LV end-diastolic diameter ratio and RV ejection area returned to normal within 6 weeks and TAM normalized within 3 to 6 months.[32]

As the echocardiographic parameters for RV dysfunction are valuable but have limited diagnostic and prognostic values,

biomarker elevations in patients with PE have the same limitation. Elevation of cardiac troponins I and T are associated with severe PE.[27] This elevation is most likely due to RV dysfunction and hemodynamic instability. More recently, brain natriuretic peptide and N-terminal probrain natriuretic peptide were found to be elevated in patients with PE, due to the same mechanism and have the same prognostic values.[26] A new algorithm was proposed to identify patients at low risk, medium risk, and high risk based on combined troponin T and RV function (Table 47.3), where group I are low risk with negative biomarkers and normal RV function, group II are intermediate risk with either positive biomarkers or RV dysfunction, and group III are high-risk patients with positive biomarkers and RV dysfunction. The third group is associated with significantly higher in-hospital morbidity and mortality.[26]

Long-standing PH due to CTE tends to increase RV afterload and can lead to significant RV hypertrophy (RV wall thickness) and chronic PH. The process of RV remodeling and the cardiac parameters that can be derived are similar to other causes of PH, which were discussed in detail in Chapter 46. Whenever underlying chronic PH is suspected, care should be taken to rule out either recurrent PE or CTEPH. Successful pulmonary endarterectomy (PEA) leads to a significant reduction of RV size and function.[33]

3.1.2. Tissue doppler indices and acute pulmonary embolism

Conventional Doppler echocardiography is applied to fast-flowing blood. The velocity and direction of blood flow are calculated by measuring the frequency shift of returning echoes and comparing them to the frequency of emitted ultrasound. The signal that is coming from blood has high velocity and low amplitude. To eliminate noise from adjacent structures, filters exclude low

---

TABLE 47.3

THE UPPER TABLE SHOWS THE RESULT OF UNIVARIATE LOGISTIC REGRESSION OF TRANSTHORACIC ECHOCARDIOGRAPHIC VARIABLES COMPARING PATIENTS WITH PULMONARY EMBOLISM TO PATIENTS WITHOUT PULMONARY EMBOLISM ON THE VENTILATION/PERFUSION SCAN

Prognostic value of echocardiography Variable (cut-off)	OR	95% CI	P Value
RV anatomy			
RV diameter, (3.1 cm)	2.99	1.83–4.90	< .0001
RV/LV ratio (0.78)	82.9	15.1–4.52	< .0001
RV pressure			
TR max velocity, (2.8 m/s)	4.19	2.17–8.08	< .0001
PA ac time, (89 ms)	0.96	0.95–0.97	< .0001
RV function			
TAM (1.9 cm)	0.50	0.30–0.85	< .01

Prognostic value of echocardiography and troponin Variable			
Cardiac troponin T combined with echocardiography			
Group 1: TnT negative, echo negative	–	–	–
Group 2: TnT positive, echo negative	3.70	0.76–18.18	0.107
Group 3: TnT negative, echo positive	5.56	0.97–31.99	0.055
Group 4: TnT positive, echo positive	10.00	2.14–46.80	0.004

Note: The lower table shows the odds ratio of the biomarkers combined with echocardiography compared to group 1. CI, confidence intervals; OR, odds ratio; RV, right ventricle; TR, tricuspid regurgitation; PAT, pulmonary artery acceleration time; TAM, tricuspid annulus motion. TnT troponin T.
Source: Adapted from Binder L, Burkert P, Manfred O, et al. N-terminal pro-brain natriuretic peptide or troponin testing followed by echocardiography for risk stratification of acute pulmonary embolism. *Circulation.* 2005;112:1573–1579; Kjaergaard J, Bente KS, Jens OL, et al. Quantitative measures of right ventricular dysfunction by echocardiography in the diagnosis of acute nonmassive pulmonary embolism. *J Am Soc Echocardiogr.* 2006;19(10):1264–1271.

velocity, high-amplitude signals. Tissue Doppler imaging (TDI) application removes the high-pass filter. The signals returning from blood are thus excluded, and the low velocity, high-amplitude echoes returning from cardiac tissue can be analyzed. Color TDI measures mean velocities derived from each pixel location, whereas pulsed-wave TDI measures peak velocities in the sample volume.[34]

The information acquired from color TDI can be used to derive TDI indices. In addition to tissue velocity, strain and strain rate are two important indices. Strain is a measure of myocardial deformation, and strain rate is a measure of the rate of myocardial deformation over time. Because these indices are quantifiable, they have the potential of overcoming reproducibility in assessing RV wall motion and overcome the effects of both translation and tethering.[35,36] Most of the RV evaluations with TDI were done using apical four-chambers and longitudinal tissue velocity, strain, and strain rate.[37]

Early case reports of right ventricular strain analysis in massive PE showed good reproducibility with TDI quantification of RV motion.[38] The midsegment of the RV free wall initially had low or even positive strain in three patients which gradually normalized during the period of observation after thrombolysis. These changes were not seen in the apical and basal segments of the RV free wall where the strain values were normal. The findings were in concordance with the McConnell sign in PE.[38] Other investigators were not able to reproduce these findings.[32] Table 47.4 shows the values of longitudinal TDI indices in normal healthy patients and in patients with submassive PE, where there were no significant different between these two groups.

Non-Doppler two-dimensional strain imaging is a new echocardiographic method to measure strain and strain rate. It analyzes the motion of the myocardium by tracking speckles or the natural acoustic markers. Because this technique is not dependent on TDI, it is angle independent.[39] Teske et al.[40] compared the TDI versus the non-Doppler derived strain in patients with normal and abnormal RV function, and they found that they correlate moderately well for strain ($r = 0.73$) and strain rate correlates better ($r = 0.90$). No data is yet available for this technique in patients with acute PE.

3.2. Transesophageal echocardiography

Most patients with VTE, PE, and CTEPH do not specifically require the more invasive form of echocardiography or transesophageal echocardiography (TEE), for diagnosis and management of their PH. However, TEE may be required to adequately assess the RV for technical reasons (e.g., patient's body habitus or mechanical ventilation) and may be used to directly visualize the thromboembolus in the main PA. In some cases, TEE may help determine surgical and/or catheter directed approach of embolectomy.

3.3. Vascular ultrasound

DVT is the main cause of PE. Lower extremities DVT are the cause of PE in >80% of cases. The annual incidence of DVT in the United States is 2.5 million cases. Around 25% of untreated DVT will lead to PE. In a study by Maki et al.,[41] 2,026 consecutive vascular ultrasounds were reviewed retrospectively. Acute DVT was found in 269 (9.9%) cases. Of these 269 cases, DVT was isolated to the superficial femoral vein in 60 (22.3%) cases. The remaining 209 cases (77.7%) showed thrombus that extended into the common femoral, the popliteal veins, or both. Vascular ultrasound with Doppler imaging or Duplex scan is almost always sufficient to establish the diagnosis of DVT, and venogram

TABLE 47.4

PEAK REGIONAL MYOCARDIAL VELOCITY AND PEAK SYSTOLIC STRAIN IN HEALTHY INDIVIDUALS AND PATIENTS ON DAY ONE POST ACUTE PE, NO SIGNIFICANT DIFFERENCE WAS NOTED BETWEEN HEALTHY INDIVIDUALS AND PATIENT WITH ACUTE PE (DATA DERIVED FROM IMAGES ACQUIRED IN THE APICAL FOUR-CHAMBER VIEW)

Segment	RV lateral wall healthy individuals	RV lateral wall acute PE – Day 1
Peak TDI S-wave velocity, cm/s		
Basal	9.1 ± 2.5	9.3 ± 2.5
Mid	7.3 ± 3.2	7.2 ± 2.4
Apical	4.4 ± 2.7	5.1 ± 2.0
Peak TDI E-wave velocity, cm/s		
Basal	9.3 ± 3.7	7.0 ± 2.8
Mid	7.4 ± 3.2	5.4 ± 2.6
Apical	5.0 ± 2.1	3.7 ± 1.7
Peak TDI A-wave velocity, cm/s		
Basal	11.4 ± 4.2	10.0 ± 2.4
Mid	8.9 ± 4.3	7.6 ± 3.0
Apical	4.7 ± 2.3	4.7 ± 2.7
Peak systolic strain, %		
Basal	3.1 ± 13	27 ± 9
Mid	2.3 ± 11	28 ± 12
Apical	34 ± 10	24 ± 10

TDI, tissue Doppler imaging; PE, pulmonary embolism; S-wave, the systolic wave of wall motion; E'-wave, the early diastolic wave of wall motion; A'-wave, the atrial contraction wave and its effect on wall motion.
Source: Adapted from Chung T, Louise E, Robert M, et al. Natural history of right ventricular dysfunction after acute pulmonary embolism. *J Am Soc Echocardiogr.* 2007;20(7):885–894; Perk G, Tunick PA, and Kronzon I. Non-Doppler two-dimensional strain imaging by echocardiography—from technical considerations to clinical applications. *J Am Soc Echocardiogr.* 2007;20:234–243.

is primarily employed when the patient needs an intervention, such as deploying an inferior vena cava (IVC) or superior vena cava (SVC) filter. In other cases, such as suspected SVC syndrome or in the diagnosis of pelvic vein thrombosis, venogram may be necessary to establish the diagnosis and for the planning stages of intervention, such as endovascular stent placement or localized thrombolytic infusion. In a prospective study, 126 legs in 117 patients suspected of having DVT or PE were examined with duplex scanning and conventional contrast venography as a gold standard.[42] The sensitivity and specificity of duplex scanning were 90.6% and 94.6%, respectively.

The B-mode, color flow, and pulse Doppler are essential elements of the Duplex scan for the assessment of the ultrasound venous examination. The venous blood flow characteristic in a normal vein is continuous, unidirectional, and phasic flow (Fig. 47.3A). The flow stops with Valsalva maneuver and augments with distal compression (Figs. 47.3B & C).

The normal B-mode of the vein includes thin, smooth, and invisible wall and has an anechoic lumen that is compressible (Figs. 47.4A & B). Less than 14 days is defined as the timing for acute thrombosis. It is distinguished by low echogenicity or anechogenicity (Figs. 47.3C & D). Veins with recent thrombosis are generally distended and larger than the arteries. Lack of compressibility is the most characteristic finding of the acute DVT. Doppler flow is absent if the vein occlusion is complete. If there is subtotal occlusion or recanalization of the thrombus, the pulse Doppler would be continuous but not phasic, with minimal or no response for Valsalva maneuver or distal compression.

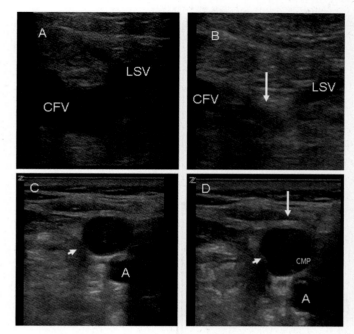

Figure 47.4 **A**: A normal common femoral vein (CFV) at the site where long saphenous vein (LSV) drainage. **B**: The arrow refers to the compression applied by the sonographer that led to complete obliteration of the CFV as normal response. **C**: The jugular vein is dilated and had low echogenic material consistent with acute thrombosis. **D**: The arrow refers to the pressure applied by the sonographer and the lack of compressibility of the vein with acute DVT. Figure A shows the Doppler of the same patients with no flow in the jugular vein.

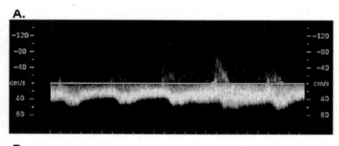

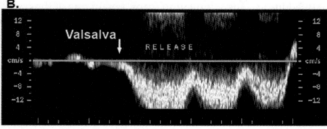

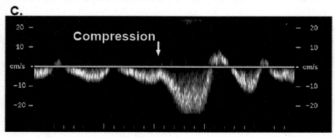

Figure 47.3 The upper panel (**A**) shows normal, continuous, unidirectional venous flow, and the lower panel (**B**) shows no flow in patients during Valsalva maneuver (Before the arrow) and then, release and continuing normal venous flow. (**C**) Normal venous flow, then distal compression starting at the arrow site with augmentation of venous flow.

During subacute and chronic phase, the thrombus becomes more echogenic and then starts to canalize and dissolve. The size of the vein will then return to normal size or even smaller than the artery. The vein wall becomes thickened and the residual thrombus fuses to the wall, and the risk of embolization decreases. The rate of resolution of DVT was evaluated by Caprini et al.[11] The rate of normalization at 6 months after diagnosis was 78% in the common femoral vein, 70% in the superficial femoral vein, and 75% in the popliteal vein. The average number of days necessary for these thrombi to become stable was 10.7 days, and damage to the vessel wall or venous valves was documented in 44% of the patients.

3.4. Nuclear ventilation/perfusion imaging

Nuclear ventilation/perfusion imaging or lung scintigraphy, is one of the first imaging techniques available for diagnosis of PE. Imaging results depend highly on the proper administration of the test and interpretation of the results. Lung scintigraphy involves injection of 1.0 to 5.0 millicurie of technetium (^{99m}Tc) labeled macroaggregated human serum albumin with particle diameter not exceeding $150\,\mu$ (ideally 10 to $90\,\mu$). Patients with significant PH or right-to-left shunt should have reduced doses (100,000 particle dose instead of traditional adult 150,000 to 500,000 particle dose).

Ideally, the patient should lie supine for 10 min prior to injection and during the infusion. Slow infusion minimizes turbulence and the patient is encouraged to take deep breaths and/or cough prior to and during administration. This allows for recruitment of all areas of atelectasis. Imaging should begin immediately post injection and in the upright position. Six views are usually obtained from the scintillation camera: Anterior, posterior, right

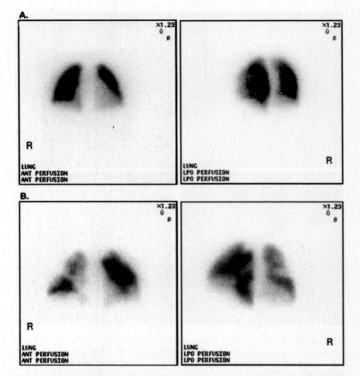

Figure 47.5 The upper two images are anterior and left posterior oblique perfusion lung images showing normal perfusion. The lower two images are also anterior and left posterior oblique perfusion lung images in patient with shortness of breath. The upper left lobe has perfusion defect (*back arrow*) that is consistent with pulmonary embolism. ANT, anterior; LPO, left posterior oblique; R, right.

and left posterior oblique, and either lateral or anterior oblique views. Ventilation imaging may be made with xenon (^{133}Xe), 10 to 30 millicuries. Alternatively, ^{99m}Tc labeled diethylenetriamine pentaacetic acid may be nebulized with oxygen.

While perfusion scintillation may be performed without ventilation scan (Fig. 47.5), traditional studies rely on diagnosis of V/Q mismatches to diagnose PE in the acute phase. Difficulties in determining the accuracy of diagnosis arise because interpretation and utilization of V/Q scans require an in-depth knowledge of anatomy of the lung and its variations, strict criteria for diagnosing V/Q mismatches, and an understanding of pretest and post-test probabilities.

The most thorough prospective investigation into the accuracy of interpretation criteria of V/Q scans, known as the Prospective Investigation of Pulmonary Embolism Diagnosis (PIOPED),[43]

coupled pretest estimation of risk with experienced interpreting radiologists to investigate some of the technical issues involved in interpretation of V/Q. Criteria for determining test stratification into normal/low, intermediate, and high probability for PE were defined by PIOPED as follows:

Low risk is defined as, (a) matched defects with normal chest X-ray, (b) perfusion defect with much larger chest X-ray abnormality, (c) small perfusion defects with normal chest X-ray, (d) nonsegmental perfusion defects (hilum, aorta, heart borders), and (e) multiple matched V/Q abnormalities with normal CXR. Intermediate probability is defined as, (a) one moderate or two large mismatched perfusion defects, (b) one matched defect with normal chest X-ray, or (c) unable to clearly place in low or high probability groups. High probability is defined as two or more large mismatched segmental defects.

Difficulty arises because >72% of studies are found to be intermediate probability of PE with 20% to 80% likelihood of PE. Table 47.5 shows probability of PE based on pretest and posttest probabilities from the PIOPED study. Unfortunately, there was no standardization of how clinicians determined pretest probability of PE, adding to the question of accuracy in real-life scenarios. Despite this, current recommendations are that V/Q scan be used in those patients unable to undergo pulmonary CTA due to renal impairment or other contraindication and possibly as a baseline for determining future events. Several other trials assessed the feasibility of V/Q scan to assess PE. The European guidelines to diagnose PE provide a review of the value of lung scintigraphy scan to diagnose PE as follows: 25% of patients with suspected PE will have normal perfusion scan and no anticoagulation therapy needed; 25% of patients will have high probability perfusion lung scan and therapy should be instituted; the reminder of patients will need further diagnostic evaluation.[1] This approach was supported by subanalysis of PIOPED II, where Sostman et al.[44] analyzed the sensitivity and specificity of V/Q scan and found after exclusion of patients with intermediate or low probability that the sensitivity of a high probability (PE present) scan finding was 77.4%, while the specificity of very low probability or normal (PE absent) scan finding was 97.7%.

In addition, lung scintillation scans remain one of the tests of choice in establishing CTEPH. While echocardiography is a first step in establishing PH, V/Q scan has a major and pivotal role in distinguishing large occlusive disease like CTEPH from small-vessel pulmonary vascular disease such as idiopathic pulmonary arterial hypertension, and normal V/Q scan excludes CTEPH.[45] The presence of multiple, small, subsegmental defects make small-vessel PH more likely. However, lobar and segmental perfusion defect or mismatched V/Q scan is not specific to CTEPH.

TABLE 47.5

PROBABILITY OF PE BEFORE AND AFTER TEST RESULTS FROM THE PIOPED STUDY

Pretest clinical suspicion	Likelihood of pulmonary embolism			
	Interpretation of V/Q scan			
	Normal (%)	Low (%)	Intermediate (%)	High (%)
Low	2	4	16	56
Intermediate	6	16	28	88
High	0	40	66	96

External vascular compression, pulmonary venoocclusive disease, pulmonary capillary hemangiomatosis, fibrosing mediastinitis, and pulmonary vasculitis can present in a similar pattern and are indistinguishable from CTEP.[46]

3.5. Computed tomography angiogram

Original data from PIOPED were collected to attempt to accurately establish diagnosis and prognosis for patients with acute PE.[43] At that time, V/Q scans and pulmonary angiogram were the primary modalities for detection of PE. Subsequently, spiral computed tomography (CT) and lower extremity venogram were developed using iodinated contrast and volumetric data collection of pulmonary vasculature.

The interpretation requires knowledge of pulmonary vasculature anatomic variations. Current protocols involve injecting 80 to 125 mL of iodinated contrast at a flow rate of 3 to 5 mL/s in a single breath hold. The pulmonary vascular tree can be scanned at peak pulmonary opacification after an average 15 s delay. The curser of the CT software should be placed in the PA for detection of radiodensity. A Hounsfield unit of 180 should be detected before acquisition is started. Imaging is usually performed with 120 kV, 210 to 250 mA, a slice thickness of 3 mm, a table speed of 5 mm s^{-1} (pitch 1.7).[1] Accuracy of diagnosis relies on proper reconstruction of images collected from each detector, which is protocol dependent (i.e., collimation width, scan delay, reconstruction width, and pitch of scanner unique for PE protocol). Current CTA employs postprocessing techniques such as surface and volume three-dimensional rendering of vessels, multiplanar reformatting, and maximum intensity projections to assist with diagnosis. A pulmonary CTA scan is interpreted as positive for PE when a vessel is completely or partially occluded, has mural defects at vessel wall or central thrombus and surrounded by contrast (Fig. 47.6). The accuracy of multidetector CTA for the diagnosis of acute PE has been reported recently by PIOPED II investigators. Stein et al. analyzed 824 patients with a reference diagnosis of PE (stein 06). The sensitivity and specificity of pulmonary CTA were 83% and 96%, respectively. Performing a CT venogram with pulmonary CTA increased the sensitivity of diagnosed PE to 90% and specificity was 95%.[47]

CTEPH findings on pulmonary CTA include mosaic perfusion of the lung parenchyma, central PA enlargement, right atrial and ventricle enlargement, the presence of collateral vessels arising from systemic pulmonary circulation, eccentric and calcified thrombus, abrupt cutoff of segmental or lobar arteries, and irregularities of PA diameter (Fig. 47.7).

Studies utilizing spiral CT alone to diagnose PE are reported to have a sensitivity ranging from 53% to 100% and specificity from 78% to 100%.[48,49] The broad range in sensitivity in these studies demonstrates the difficulties with pulmonary CTA interpretation and techniques, and CTA sensitivity diminishes beyond the level of first-order segmental PA branches. In addition, techniques can contribute to decreased sensitivity and specificity. Spiral CT is excellent for the diagnosis of central or lobar PE, however, the value of spiral CT to diagnose subsegmental PE is limited.[1] Multidetector CT improved the resolution and the visualization of segmental and subsegmental arteries.[46]

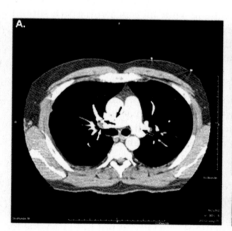
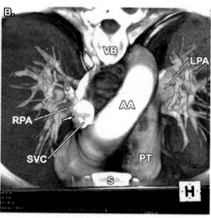

Figure 47.6 A: Axial chest CTA shows multiple small clots in the right and left pulmonary arteries (*black arrows*) in patient with acute submassive PE. **B**: Three-dimensional rendering of the chest that is cropped from above showed a thrombus in the SVC (*white arrow*) that is the source of the PE. RPA, Right pulmonary artery; SVC, Superior vena cava; VB, vertebral body; AA, Aortic arch; S, Sternum; PT, Pulmonary trunk; LPA, Left pulmonary artery.

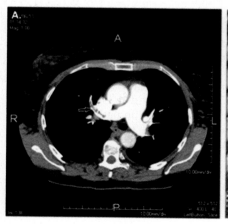
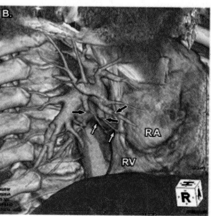

Figure 47.7 A: An axial chest CTA shows a calcified thrombus (*Black arrow*) in the right pulmonary artery in patient with chronic thromboembolic pulmonary hypertension (CTEPH). **B**: Three-dimensional rendering of the right pulmonary arteries shows complete occlusion of the pulmonary artery branches (*white arrows*) with the development of smaller collateral arteries (*black arrows*) in the same patients. RA, right atrium; RV, right ventricle.

3.6. Magnetic resonance imaging

Though not one of the more traditional modalities utilized to diagnose PE, MRI protocols can be utilized with reasonable accuracy. In one study, three protocols were utilized to maximize sensitivity and specificity and compared a triple technique MRI protocol (real-time MRI, MR perfusion imaging, and MR angiography) with 16-MDCT. In this study, sensitivities were examined for lobar, segmental, and subsegmental PE when compared to 16-MDCT utilizing all techniques in under 10 min.[50,51]

The main drawbacks of MRI studies include length of time needed to complete the examination and inaccessibility to patient. In addition, MRI protocols designed to study vascular images may miss alternative diagnoses, such as emphysema, which may not be missed on MDCT techniques as suggested by this same study. For patients with end-stage renal disease requiring hemodialysis, substituting MRI is not a viable option as a condition known as nephrogenic systemic fibrosis is associated with gadolinium contrast agents.

3.7. Pulmonary angiogram

Pulmonary angiogram remains the gold standard for diagnosis of PE. Despite this, pulmonary angiogram is a less commonly employed strategy for diagnosis of PE. Landmark studies of PIOPED and PIOPED II compared accuracy of V/Q scan, CTA and the gold standard, and pulmonary angiogram, after asking clinicians to rank pretest likelihood that the patient had PE (low 0% to 19%, medium 19% to 28%, and high >29%). In the PIOPED II study,[52,53] patients assigned pretest low to moderate risk underwent rapid ELISA D-dimer screening. This study did not further test patients with negative D-dimer, as false negative is between 0.7% and 2%. Currently, serum laboratory data (D-dimer with >90% sensitivity) coupled with radiographic (CTA) or nuclear (V/Q scan) studies have largely replaced pulmonary angiography for diagnosis of patients with acute PE.[44,47,53] Concerns with complications from contrast are greater in pulmonary angiography than in CTA due to the load necessary for diagnosis. In addition, perforation of the RV or PA in pulmonary angiography is not present in the CTA techniques utilized for diagnosis of PE. Pulmonary angiography also requires additional expertise, equipment, and time, as well as radiation exposure to the evaluating team. Pulmonary angiogram has historically been utilized in patients with intermediate probability on V/Q scan, but with high risk of complication from anticoagulation or in determining when to administer thrombolytics. Subsequent to the advent of multidetector spiral CTA scanners and further studies supporting the diagnostic criteria for PE of less invasive echocardiogram, pulmonary angiogram has been largely utilized to assist in direct visualization of thrombosis and catheter directed thrombolytic infusion or in preoperative evaluation prior to surgical embolectomy or PEA. In particular, pulmonary angiogram is advantageous in that it allows the operator to visualize segmental and subsegmental lesions, which may be missed on CTA or V/Q scan or conversely, to identify lesions which may have nonflow limiting stenosis that may be overestimated due to signal averaging in CTA.

4. SELECTING AND GUIDING THERAPY

4.1. Medical therapy

4.1.1. Prophylaxis of venous thromboembolism

The mainstay of initial management of VTE remains primary prevention. Currently, most facilities continue to utilize primarily unfractionated heparin (UFH) or low molecular weight heparins (LMWH) for prophylaxis of VTE. Current recommendations are that all patients be considered for LMWH over UFH where possible, due to the lower incidence of heparin-induced thrombocytopenic (HIT) associated with LMWHs.[54] While up to 15% of patients may develop thrombocytopenia initially with heparin administration, typically platelet counts do not drop below 100,000 and the patient is at no increased risk of thrombus formation.[55,56]

While attempts should be made to use LMWH in prophylaxis for VTE, not all patients are candidates for LMWH. In addition, there are several contraindications to pharmacologic DVT prophylaxis. In these cases, compression stockings, pneumatic compression devices, early ambulation, and possible IVC filter placement should be considered.

4.1.2. Medical therapy of pulmonary embolism

After the patients have been diagnosed with a thromboembolic event, they should be divided first into two groups: physiologically stable and unstable patients. All patients should be considered for full anticoagulation dosing of LMWH or UFH. While LMWH has a lower incidence of HIT, it is longer acting and may only partially be reversed with protamine, should bleeding complications develop. For this reason, the form of acute anticoagulation for each patient should be carefully considered. Warfarin therapy should not be employed in the acute phases of VTE. In addition, care should be taken to provide adequate supplemental oxygen therapy (resting, ambulatory, and nocturnal) in the acute PE patients as hypoxia will exacerbate their PH and/or acute cor pulmonale.

In the case of the physiologically unstable patient (i.e., severe hypoxia, respiratory failure, or hemodynamic instability), care should be administered and ideal therapy initiated within an hour of presentation. Patients with life-threatening VTE should be considered for thrombolytic therapy with tissue plasminogen activator (tPA). Thrombolytics may be delivered systemically or through catheter directed therapy.[57–59]

Other indications for tPA administration include severe right ventricular strain or failure on echocardiogram, refractory hypoxia. Administration of tPA has no benefit in the patient with CTEPH, except in the setting of an acute thromboembolic event as most clots have been endothelialized and thrombolytics are not effective in reversing the resultant PH or cor pulmonale (Table 47.6).

4.1.3. Medical therapy of chronic thromboembolic pulmonary hypertension

PEA is the main therapy for CTEPH, but medical therapy is indicated in a number of situations.[60] (a) PEA is not indicated due to distal small-vessel thromboembolic disease, (b) as a bridge for PEA, (c) patients with residual PH post-PEA, and (d) when surgery is contraindicated due to significant comorbidities.

CTEPH conventional therapy (chapter 46) focuses on symptomatic relive of RV failure symptoms with no significant outcome improvement, this therapy includes diuretics, digoxin, anticoagulation, and calcium channel blockers. However, lifelong anticoagulation therapy is indicated to prevent recurrent PE recurrence.[61] There is a significant data emerging about the benefit of the selective therapy for PH in patients with CTEPH, which include prostacyclin analogs (prostanoids), endothelin receptor antagonist (ETRA), and phosodiestrase-5 (PDE-5) inhibitors.

Epoprostenol is an intravenous form of prostacyclin analogs studied in 11 patients with CTEPH, and median follow-up of 12.4 month showed that epoprostenol may improve exercise tolerance, functional class and clinical status,[62] Presurgery infusion

TABLE 47.6

THROMBOLYTICS IN ACUTE PULMONARY EMBOLISM

Indications for considering tPA	Relative contraindications	Absolute contraindications

▪ Hemodynamic collapse
▪ Uncontrolled hypertension
▪ If low bleeding risk:
  – Marked dyspnea
  – Hypoxia.
  – Elevated troponin.
  – RV dysfunction on echo and RV enlargement to >90% on CTA
	▪ Uncontrolled hypertension
	▪ Recent ischemic CVA (*<3 months*)
	▪ H/O peptic ulcer disease
	▪ Anticoagulation therapy
	▪ Recent surgery (*<2 weeks*)
		▪ Intracranial disease (*mass. hemorrhage, AVMi*)
		▪ Active internal bleeding
		▪ Hemorrhagic CVA
		▪ Dissecting aortic aneurysm
		▪ Recent head trauma
		▪ Pregnancy

of epoprostenol was studied with various protocols from 6 weeks to 24 months and these reports showed hemodynamic improvements and good surgical outcomes.[63,64]

Endothelin-1 plasma level is elevated in patients with CTEPH, which is one of the most vasoconstrictor substances.[65] Hoeper et al.[66] performed an open-label multicenter study to evaluate the safety and efficacy of the dual ETRA bosentan in 19 patients with inoperable CTEPH for 3 months. Pulmonary vascular resistance, 6-min walking distance (6MWD), mPAP, and cardiac index all were improved. Forty-seven patients with inoperable CTEPH underwent evaluation after 1 year of bosentan therapy by Hughes et al.,[67] where significant improvements were noted with 6MWD, hemodynamics and functional classification. One-year survival was 96%. Pepke-Zaba et al.[68] performed a bosentan study in a multicenter, prospective, double-blind, placebo-controlled study of 157 patients with inoperable CTEPH or PH after PEA. At 16 weeks of therapy, bosentan showed a significant improvement in 6MWD and functional class. Sildenafil is a PDE-5 inhibitor that also showed a significant improvement of hemodynamic and 6MWD in patients with inoperable CTEPH.[69,70]

4.2. Invasive and surgical therapy

4.2.1. Embolectomy

Currently, there are two main methods of embolectomy in use for thromboembolic disease: percutaneous and open. In the case of acute DVT or PE, percutaneous catheter directed embolectomy may be as effective as traditional surgical embolectomy and has much less associated risk. This involves directly cannulating the PA or other vessel involved and attempting to aspirate the thrombus with an angiographic catheter. Several types of catheter have been investigated and the use of catheter-based embolectomy is still primary, and most PE and DVT are treated noninvasively.

Current percutaneous catheters use rheolytic, aspiration, or fragmentation techniques to lyse the thromboembolus. Preliminary studies show percutaneous catheter embolectomy has success similar to that of surgical embolectomy and is associated with significantly less morbidity.[6,54,71] Standard fragmentation catheters with directed thrombolytic agents have a success rate of 95%, while the Greenfield catheter, rheolytic AngioJet and the Hydrolyser catheters and the Amplatz catheters have success rates as high as 100% in small studies. In these studies, primary complications were major bleeding at the insertion site (2%), perforation of the RV, and minor bleeding (8%). Thrombolytic infusion (in situ) did not appear to increase overall bleeding risk. This suggests that in most cases a combination of tPA and direct aspiration of the thrombus should be performed.[71]

4.2.2. Pulmonary Endarterectomy

PEA is the treatment of choice and often curative for patients with CTEPH.[72] The selection criteria for PEA according to the guideline of American College of Chest Physicians are the following: (a) NYHA functional class II or IV, (b) a preoperative pulmonary vascular resistance of >300 dyn s cm^{-5}, (c) surgical accessible thrombus in the lobar or segmental arteries, and (d) no severe comorbidities.[73] Initial, postoperative mortality was high, but with the improvement of the technique the mortality went down to 4.4% in the most recent report.[72] However, 10% to 15% of patients with CTEPH continue to have significant PH post endarterectomy.[46]

5. IMAGING AND PROGNOSIS

Although V/Q scans and MDCT are the modalities most commonly utilized to diagnose PE, neither correlates well with outcomes. The modality of choice for prognosis and for treatment decision tree, as previously discussed, is echocardiogram with Doppler images. Echocardiogram findings with prognostic value include RV:LV ratio, RV function, and TAM.

6. FUTURE DIRECTIONS

While pulmonary angiogram still remains the gold standard for diagnosis of acute PE, important advances are being made in CTA in hopes of replacing the more invasive techniques. Current techniques in the development for advancing the accuracy of diagnosis of PE include increased number of detectors and change in contrast injection. The 64 detector helical CT attempts to increase both sensitivity and specificity of detecting PE by decreasing artifact created by signal averaging in reconstruction of both volumetric reconstructions and conventional imaging. Other attempts at changing protocols of collimation width, pitch, scan delay, and reconstruction have improved the quality of imaging, but largely not changed the overall accuracy of CTA significantly. On the horizon, a triple-rule-out multidetector row CT technique is in development to attempt to combine simultaneous evaluation of the coronary arteries, pulmonary arteries, and aorta.

ACKNOWLEDGMENT

The authors wish to thank Dr. Utpal Pandya and Diane McCarthy for their careful review and comments, and Tonya Floyd-Bradstock, our medical illustrator, for her hard work on our diagrams and figures.

REFERENCES

1. Task Force on Pulmonary Embolism, E.S.o.C., et al., Guidelines on diagnosis and management of acute pulmonary embolism. *Eur Heart J.* 2000;21:1301–1336.
2. White RH. The epidemiology of venous thromboembolism. *Circulation.* 2003;2003(107):I-4–I-8.
3. Silverstein M, et al. Trends in the incidence of deep vein thrombosis and pulmonary embolism: A 25-year population-based study. *Arch Intern Med.* 1998;6:585–593.
4. Kakkar A, Vasishta R. Pulmonary embolism in medical patients: An autopsy-based study. *Clin Appl Thromb Hemost.* 2008;14(2):159–167.
5. MacDougall DA, Feliu AL, Boccuzzi SJ, et al. Economic burden of deep-vein thrombosis, pulmonary embolism, and post-thrombotic syndrome. *Am J Health-Syst Pharm.* 2006;20:S5–S15.
6. Manecke GR, Wilson WC, Auger WR, et al. Chronic thromboembolic pulmonary hypertension and pulmonary thromboendarterectomy. *Semin Cardiothorac Vasc Anesth.* 2005;9(September):189–204.
7. Wartski M, Collignon M. Incomplete recovery of lung perfusion after 3 months in patients with acute pulmonary embolism treated with antithrombotic agents. THESEE Study Group. Tinzaparin ou Heparin Standard: Evaluation dans l'Embolie Pulmonaire Study. *J Nucl Med.* 2000;41(6):1043–1048.
8. Fedullo P, Auger W, Channick R, et al. Chronic thromboembolic pulmonary hypertension. *Clin Chest Med.* 1995;16(2):353–374.
9. Wolf M, Boyer-Neumann C, Parent F, et al. Thrombotic risk factors in pulmonary hypertension. *Eur Respir J.* 2000;15(2):395–399.
10. Bernardi E, Pesavento R, Prandoni P. Upper extremity deep venous thrombosis. *Semin Thromb Hemost.* 2006;32(7):729–736.
11. Caprini J, Botteman M, Stephens J. Economic burden of long-term complications of deep vein thrombosis after total hip replacement surgery in the United States. *Value Health.* 2003;6:59–74.
12. Vonk-Noordegraaf A, Lankhaar J-W, Gotte M, et al. Magentic resonance and nuclear imaging of the right ventricle in pulmonary arterial hypertension. *Eur Heart J.* 2007;9(Suppl. H):H29–H34.
13. Waypa GB, Schumacker PT. Oxygen sensing in hypoxic pulmonary vasoconstriction: Using new tools to answer an age-old question. *Exp Physiol.* 2008;93(1):133–138.
14. Weir EK, Lopez-Barneo J, Buckler KJ, et al. Acute oxygen-sensing mechanisms. *N Engl J Med.* 2005;353(19):2042–2055.
15. Weissmann N, Sommer N, Schermuly RT, et al. Oxygen sensors in hypoxic pulmonary vasoconstriction. *Cardiovasc Res.* 2006;71(4):620–629.
16. Fedullo P, Auger W, Kerr K, et al. Chronic thromboembolic pulmonary hypertension. *N Engl J Med.* 2001;345(20):1465–1472.
17. Pengo V, Lensing A, Prins M, et al. Incidence of chronic thromboembolic pulmonary hypertension after pulmonary embolism. *N Engl J Med.* 2004;350:2257–2264.
18. Hooper WC, Evatt BL. The role of activated protein C resistance in the pathogenesis of venous thrombosis. *Am J Med Sci.* 1998;316(2):120–128.
19. Bullano M, Willey V, Hauch O, et al. Longitudinal evaluation of health plan cost per venous thromboembolism or bleed events in patients with a prior venous thromboembolism event during hospitalization. *J Manage Care Pharm.* 2005;11(8):663–673.
20. Ginsberg J, Wells P, Kearon C, et al. Sensitivity and specificity of a rapid whole-blood assay for D-dimer in the diagnosis of pulmonary embolism. *Ann Intern Med.* 1998;129(12):1006–1011.
21. Wells PS, Owen C, Doucette S, et al. Does this patient having deep vein thrombosis? *JAMA.* 2006;295:199–207.
22. Goldhaber SZ, Visani L, De Rosa M. Acute pulmonary embolism: Clinical outcomes in the International Cooperative Pulmonary Embolism Registry (ICOPER). *Lancet.* 1999;353:1386–1389.
23. Kasper W, Konstantinides S, Geibel A, et al. Management strategies and determinants of outcome in acute major pulmonary embolism: Results of a multicenter registry. *J Am Coll Cardiol.* 1997;30:1165–1171.
24. Chung T, Emmett L, Khoury V, et al. Atrial and ventricular echocardiographic correlates of the extent of pulmonary embolism in the elderly. *J Am Soc Echocardiogr.* 2006;19:347–353.
25. Wolde MT, Sohne M, Quak E, et al. Prognostic value of echocardiographically assessed right ventricular dysfunction in patients with pulmonary embolism. *Arch Intern Med.* 2004;164:1685–1689.
26. Binder L, Pieske B, Olschewski M. N-terminal pro-brain natriuretic peptide or troponin testing followed by echocardiography for risk stratification of acute pulmonary embolism. *Circulation.* 2005;112:1573–1579.
27. Konstantinides S, Geibel A, Olschewski M, et al. Importance of cardiac troponins I and T in risk stratification of patients with acute pulmonary embolism. *Circulation.* 2002;106:1263–1268.
28. Mcconnell MV, Solomon S, Rayan ME, et al. Regional right ventricular dysfunction detected by echocardiography in acute pulmonary embolism. *Am J Cardiol.* 1996;78:469–473.
29. Casazza F, Bongarzoni A, Capozi A, et al. Regional right ventricular dysfunction in acute pulmonary embolism and right ventricular infarction. *Eur J Echocardiogr.* 2005;6:11–14.
30. Kjaergaard J, Schaadt BK, Lund JO, et al. Quantitative measures of right ventricular dysfunction by echocardiography in the diagnosis of acute nonmassive pulmonary embolism. *J Am Soc Echocardiogr.* 2006;19(10):1264–1271.
31. Fremont B, Pacouret G, Jacobi D, et al. Prognostic value of echocardiographic right/left ventricular end-diastolic diameter ratio in patients with acute pulmonary embolism. *Chest.* 2008;133:358–362.
32. Chung T, Emmett L, Mansberg R, et al. Natural history of right ventricular dysfunction after acute pulmonary embolism. *J Am Soc Echocardiogr.* 2007;20(7):885–894.
33. Menzel T, Krann T, Bruckner A, et al. Quantitative assessment of right ventricular volumes in severe chronic thromboembolic pulmonary hypertension using transthoracic three-dimensional echocardiography: Changes due to pulmonary thromboendarterectomy. *Eur J Echocardiogr.* 2002;3:67–72.
34. Otto CM. *Textbook of Clinical Echocardiography.* 2nd Ed. Philadelphia, PA: WB Saunders Company; 2000.
35. Di Salvo G, Pacileo G, Caso P, et al. Strain rate imaging is a superior method for the assessment of regional myocardial function compared with Doppler tissue imaging: A study on patients with transcatheter device closure of atrial septal defect. *J Am Soc Echocardiogr.* 2005;18(5):398–400.
36. Voigt J, Exner B, Schmiedehausen K, et al. Strain-rate imaging during dobutamine stress echocardiography provides objective evidence of inducible ischemia. *Circulation.* 2003;107(16):2120–2126.
37. Pellerin D, Sharma R, Elliott P, et al. Tissue Doppler, strain, and strain rate echocardiography for the assessment of left and right systolic ventricular function. *Heart.* 2003;89:iii9–iii17.
38. Kjaergaard J, Sogaard P, Hassager C. Right ventricular strain in pulmonary embolism by Doppler tissue echocardiography. *J Am Soc Echocardiogr.* 2004;17(11):1210–1212.
39. Kjaergaad J, Sogaard P, Hassager C. Quantitative echocardiographic analysis of the right ventricle in healthy individuals. *J Am Soc Echocardiogr.* 2006;9:1365–1372.
40. Teske A, De Boeck BW, Olimulder M, et al. Echocardiographic assessment of regional right ventricular function: A head-to-head comparison between 2-dimensional and tissue doppler-derived strain analysis. *J Am Soc Echocardiogr.* 2008;21(3):275–283.
41. Maki D, Kumar N, Nguyen B, et al. Distribution of thrombi in acute lower extremity deep venous thrombosis: Implications for sonography and CT and MR venography. *Am J Roentgenol.* 2000;175(5):1299–1301.
42. van Ramshorst B, Legemate D, Verzijlbergen J, et al. Duplex scanning in the diagnosis of acute deep vein thrombosis of the lower extremity. *Eur J Vasc Surg.* 1991;5(3):255–260.
43. The pioped investigators. Value of the ventilation/perfusion scan in acute pulmonary embolism. Results of the prospective investigation of pulmonary embolism diagnosis (PIOPED). *JAMA.* 1990;263(20):2753–2759.
44. Sostman HD, Stein PD, Gottschalk A, et al. Acute pulmonary embolism: Sensitivity and specificity of ventilation-perfusion scintigraphy in PIOPED II study. *Radiology.* 2008;246(3):941–946.
45. Fishman AJ, Moser KM, Fedullo PF. Perfusion lung scans vs pulmonary angiography in evaluation of suspected primary pulmonary hypertension. *Chest.* 1983;84(6):679–683.
46. Auger WR, Kim NH, Kerr KM, et al. Chronic thromboembolic pulmonary hypertension. *Clin Chest Med.* 2007;28(1):255–269, x.
47. Stein PD, Fowler SE, Goodman LR, et al. Multidetector computed tomography for acute pulmonary embolism. *New Engl J Med.* 2006;354(22):2317–2327.
48. Carman TL, Deitcher SR. Advances in diagnosing and excluding pulmonary embolism: Spiral CT and D-dimer measurement. *Cleve Clin J Med.* 2002;69(9):721–729.
49. Eng J, Krishnan JA, Segal JB, et al. Accuracy of CT in the diagnosis of pulmonary embolism: A systematic literature review. *AJR.* 2000;183:1819–1827.
50. Kluge A, Mueller C, Strunk J, et al. Experience in 207 combined MRI examinations for acute pulmonary embolism and deep vein thrombosis. *AJR.* 2006;186(6):1686–1696.
51. Kluge A, Luboldt W, and Bachmann G. Acute pulmonary embolism to the subsegmental level: Diagnostic accuracy of three MRI techniques compared with 16-MDCT. *Am J Roentgenol.* 2006;187(1):W7–W14.
52. Gottschalk A, Stein PD, Goodman LR, et al. Overview of prospective investigation of pulmonary embolism diagnosis II. *Semin Nucl Med.* 2002;32(3):173–182.
53. Stein PD, Woodard PK, Weg JG, et al. Diagnostic pathways in acute pulmonary embolism: Recommendations of the PIOPED II investigators. *Am J Med.* 2006;119(12):1048–1055.
54. Martel N, Lee J, Wells PS. Risk for heparin-induced thrombocytopenia with unfractionated and low-molecular-weight heparin thromboprophylaxis: A meta-analysis. *Blood.* 2005;106(8):2710–2715.
55. Greinacher A. Antigen generation in heparin-associated thrombocytopenia: The nonimmunologic type and the immunologic type are closely linked in their pathogenesis. *Semin Thromb Hemost.* 1995;21(1):106–116.
56. Chong BH, Castaldi PA. Platelet proaggregating effect of heparin: Possible mechanism for non-immune heparin-associated thrombocytopenia. *Aust N Z J Med.* 1986;16(5):715–716.
57. Kucher N. Catheter embolectomy for acute pulmonary embolism. *Chest.* 2007;132(2):657–663.
58. Digonnet A, Moya-Plana A, Aubert S, et al. Acute pulmonary embolism: A current surgical approach. *Interact Cardiovasc Thorac Surg.* 2007;6(1):27–29.
59. Irwin RS. ed. Antithrombotic and thrombolytic therapy: American College of Chest Physicians Evidenced-Based Clinical Practice Guidelines. 8th Ed. *Chest.* (Suppl.) 2008;133:367S–968S.
60. Bresser P, Pepke-Zaba J, Jais X, et al. Medical therapies for chronic thromboembolic pulmonary hypertension. *Proc Am Thorac Soc.* 2006;3:594–600.
61. Hoeper MM, Mayer E, Simonneau G, et al. Chronic thromboembolic pulmonary hypertension. *Circulation.* 2006;113(16):2011–2020.
62. Scelsi L, Ghio S, Campana C, et al. Epoprostenol in chronic thromboembolic pulmonary hypertension with distal lesions. *Ital Heart J:* (Official Journal of the Italian Federation of Cardiology). 2004;5(8):618–623.

63. Bresser P, Fedullo PF, Auger WR, et al. Continuous intravenous epoprostenol for chronic thromboembolic pulmonary hypertension. *Eur Respir J*: (*Official Journal of the European Society for Clinical Respiratory Physiology*). 2004;23(4):595–600.

64. Ono F, Nagaya N, Okumura H, et al. Effect of orally active prostacyclin analogue on survival in patients with chronic thromboembolic pulmonary hypertension without major vessel obstruction. *Chest*. 2003;123(5):1583–1588.

65. Reesink H, Lutter R, Kloek J, et al. Hemodynamic correlates of endothelin-1 in chronic thromboembolic pulmonary hypertension. *Eur Respir J*. 2004;24:111s.

66. Hoeper MM, Kramm T, Wilkens H, et al. Bosentan therapy for inoperable chronic thromboembolic pulmonary hypertension. *Chest*. 2005;128(4):2363–2367.

67. Hughes R, George P, Parameshwar J, et al. Bosentan in inoperable chronic thromboembolic pulmonary hypertension. *Thorax*. 2005;60(8):707.

68. Pepke-Zaba J, Mayer E, Simmoneau G, et al. Bosentan for inoperable chronic thromboembolic pulmonary hypertension: A randomised, placebo-controlled trial—BENEFIT. *Thorax*. 2007;62(Suppl 3):S30.

69. Ghofrani HA, Schermuly RT, Rose F, et al. Sildenafil for long-term treatment of nonoperable chronic thromboembolic pulmonary hypertension. *Am J Respir Crit Care Med*. 2003;167(8):1139–1141.

70. Sheth A, Park JES, Ong YE, et al. Early haemodynamic benefit of sildenafil in patients with coexisting chronic thromboembolic pulmonary hypertension and left ventricular dysfunction. *Vascul Pharmacol*. 2005;42(2):41–45.

71. Skaf E, Beemath A, Siddiqui T, et al. Catheter-tip embolectomy in the management of acute massive pulmonary embolism. *Am J Cardiol*. 2007;99(3): 415–420.

72. Jamieson SW, Kapelanski DP, Sakakibara N, et al. Pulmonary endarterectomy: Experience and lessons learned in 1,500 cases. *Ann Thorac Surg*. 2003;76(5):1457–1462; discussion 1462–1464.

73. Doyle R, McCrory DC, Channick R, et al. Surgical treatments/interventions for pulmonary arterial hypertension: ACCP evidence-based clinical practice guidelines. *Chest*. 2004;126:63–71.

Cerebrovascular Disease

48

Anthony A. Bavry
Samir R. Kapadia

1. INTRODUCTION

Stroke is the most feared and serious manifestation of cerebrovascular disease. Only heart disease and cancer are responsible for more deaths. It is estimated that nearly six million Americans are living after a stroke which makes this disease the leading cause of disability in this country.[1] Approximately, three quarters of a million Americans have a new or recurrent stroke each year with estimated direct health care costs of at least $40 billion. Interestingly, women are responsible for roughly two thirds of stroke deaths. Given the scope and severity of stroke, the understanding and management of carotid and cerebrovascular disease is unquestionably a significant public health priority.

The clinical presentation of a neurological disorder depends on the underlying disease process. Symptoms are protean and can highly overlap various neurological diseases. For this reason, it is necessary for the practitioner to have a high index of suspicion for a given neurological disease and perform a thorough history and physical examination. Noninvasive imaging serves an invaluable role in promptly and safely establishing a diagnosis, determining prognosis, and guiding therapy.

In addition to stroke, there are numerous neurological conditions that are responsible for considerable morbidity and mortality, many of which are only rarely encountered in clinical practice. A detailed description on these conditions is beyond the scope of this chapter. Rather, the intent of this chapter is to provide an overview of the commonly used neurological imaging tools, namely computed tomography (CT), magnetic resonance imaging (MRI), carotid ultrasound, and brain perfusion imaging. This chapter will also highlight several clinical disorders for which neurological imaging plays a valuable role: carotid artery atherosclerotic disease, intracranial aneurysm, arteriovenous malformation (AVM), carotid artery dissection, and thrombosis of the cerebral veins and sinuses. Some invasive carotid/cerebral angiograms will be displayed in order to illustrate large and small vessel anatomy (Figs. 48.1–48.3).

2. ETIOLOGY AND PATHOPHYSIOLOGY

Extracranial atherosclerosis. Roughly one fifth of the stroke burden is caused by atherosclerotic extracranial disease.[1] It is important to keep in mind that even in the presence of carotid artery disease, lacunar and cardioembolic strokes (i.e. an etiology other than large vessel atherosclerosis) are responsible for 38% to 45% of ipsilateral strokes.[2] There is a strong predilection for atherosclerosis to develop in the proximal internal carotid artery, although the common carotid artery is occasionally involved (Fig. 48.4).

The distal common carotid artery can become diseased at the site of prior carotid endarterectomy. This section will focus on the association between carotid artery stenosis and stroke.

Two of the strongest patient and anatomic predictors of stroke after the diagnosis of carotid artery disease are symptom status (e.g., recent stroke or transient ischemic attack) and the severity of the lesion (e.g., severely stenotic lesions carry a greater risk of stroke than less severe stenoses).[2] Lastly, the rate of adverse events associated with a given surgeon and hospital for percutaneous or surgical revascularization needs to be considered. Among asymptomatic patients with <60% internal carotid stenosis, the 5-year risk of ipsilateral stroke is 8% compared with 16% for stenoses >60%.[3]

Intracranial aneurysms. The prevalence of intracranial aneurysms has increased with the widespread application of neurological imaging. Brain imaging is usually performed due to a variety of symptoms such as heachache or seizure; however, asymptomatic aneurysms are also increasingly being discovered.

Since aneurysms are relatively uncommon, affecting approximately 2% of the worldwide population, knowledge on their natural history is slowly accumulating.[4] Ruptured or symptomatic aneurysms are often treated expeditiously through surgical or endovascular techniques. Asymptomatic aneurysms are often smaller, and therefore, surveillance imaging is especially important in this group to guide the need and timing of aneurysm repair. A prospective study in over 4,000 patients documented a higher rupture rate according to size and location of the aneurysm.[5] For example, aneurysms in the posterior circulation are more likely to rupture for unclear reasons than those in the anterior circulation. The 5-year rupture rate for a 7 to 12 mm aneurysm in the posterior circulation is 15%, compared with 2.6% for a similarly sized aneurysm in the anterior circulation. Within the anterior circulation, an aneurysm <7 mm has a rupture rate of 0% compared with 40% for those >25 mm. Within the posterior circulation, rupture rates are 2.5% versus 50%.

Arteriovenous malformation. AVMs are a relatively uncommon congenital cerebral malformation that is due to an abnormal communication between the arterial and venous circulations. More precisely, AVMs are comprised of a tangle of abnormal veins and arteries of varying sizes, without interconnecting capillaries. AVMs are the second most common cause of intracerebral hemorrhage (approximately 10% of cases), after intracranial aneurysm. In approximately half of the cases, AVMs present as a bleeding episode, although they can also present with seizure, focal neurological deficit, headache, or they are incidentally discovered.[6,7] AVMs are more likely to bleed during the second and third decades of life. Our knowledge of the natural history and optimal

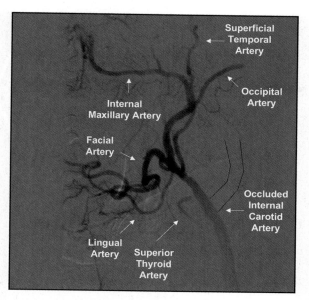

Figure 48.1 Common carotid artery angiogram that reveals the major branches of the external carotid artery. Note the occluded internal carotid artery.

treatment of AVMs remains relatively incomplete. For example, a recent cohort study on the management of AVMs in Scotland, documented a greater risk of a poor outcome among patients who underwent interventional treatment versus conservative management.[8] In this study, patients who underwent interventional treatment were younger (40 years versus 55 years), more often presented with seizure (60% vs. 39%), had fewer comorbidities (3 vs. 4), and had smaller AVM (52% vs. 35%). All treatment modalities were represented; embolization, gamma-knife radiosurgery, surgical excision, and aneurysm coiling. The results of the United States National Institutes of Health ARUBA (A Randomized trial of Unruptured Brain AVM) study are forthcoming.[9]

Carotid artery dissection. Carotid and vertebral artery dissection is an uncommon cause of stroke overall, although it is a frequent cause of stroke in young and middle-aged patients (Fig. 48.5).[10] This disease process has become increasingly recognized with the advent of noninvasive imaging. Dissection is thought to be initiated by a subintimal tear which results in intramural hematoma, or alternatively primary intramural hematoma may occur. This can produce stenosis and/or aneurysm.

Dissection is distinctly not an atherosclerosis process. Arteriopathy is often considered, although it is found in only a minority of patients. Ehlers–Danlos syndrome type IV is the most common

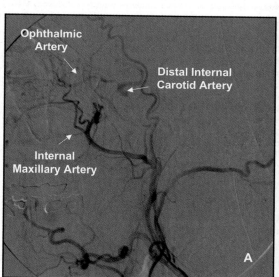

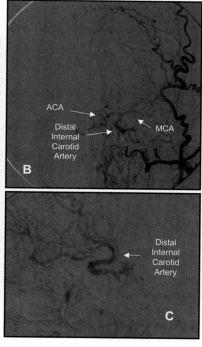

Figure 48.2 Collaterals from the external carotid artery to the distal internal carotid artery through the ophthalmic artery (**Panel A**). **Panel B** (frontal view) with reconstitution of the distal internal carotid artery and filling of the left anterior cerebral artery (ACA) and left middle cerebral artery (MCA). **Panel C** (oblique view) with slightly delayed view.

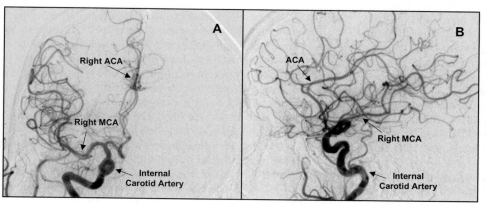

Figure 48.3 Intracranial angiography of the anterior circulation. **Panel A** shows the distal right internal carotid artery in anteroposterior projection. The distal right internal carotid artery bifurcates into the right middle cerebral artery (MCA) and right anterior cerebral artery (ACA). There is no significant intracranial atherosclerosis. Note the "pseudoaneurysm" in the distal internal carotid artery at the tip of the *lower arrow*. This reflects tortuosity in the vessel, which is unfolded in the lateral projection (**Panel B**) and reinforces the importance of multiple projections.

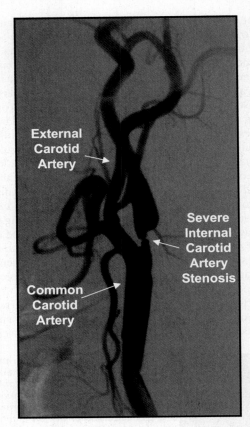

Figure 48.4 Common carotid artery angiography. High magnification view shows the distal bifurcation of the common carotid artery into the external and internal carotid arteries. A severe stenosis is noted in the proximal internal carotid artery.

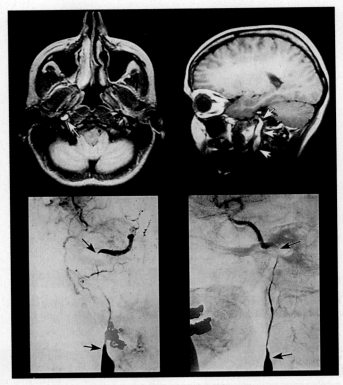

Figure 48.5 Findings on magnetic resonance imaging and angiography in a 37-year-old woman with a dissection of the internal carotid artery. On T1-weighted magnetic resonance imaging, an axial view (**upper left-hand panel**) and a sagittal view (**upper right-hand panel**) show a subacute intramural hematoma in the wall of the right internal carotid artery (*white arrows*). On magnetic resonance angiography, a frontal view (**lower left-hand panel**) and a lateral view (**lower right-hand panel**) show a corresponding long segment of high-grade stenosis extending from about 2 cm distal to the carotid bulb to the base of the skull (*black arrows*). (Reprinted from Schievink WI. Spontaneous dissection of the carotid and vertebral arteries. *N Engl J Med.* 2001;344:898–906, with permission.)

connective tissue disorder, followed by Marfan syndrome, polycystic kidney disease, and osteogenesis imperfecta type I. A minority of patients have at least one family member with a carotid or vertebral artery dissection. Changes resembling fibromuscular dysplasia can be seen on angiography, and cystic medial necrosis is often observed at autopsy; however, both of these are nonspecific. Ultrastructural abnormalities in dermal connective tissue have been documented in the majority of patients with carotid and vertebral dissection. It is unknown why the carotid and vertebral arteries can be at risk of dissection, although it is thought that the highly mobile extracranial portion of these arteries may produce shearing forces.

A precipitating event to carotid and vertebral dissection is often documented. Examples include hiking, painting a ceiling, sneezing, and chiropractic manipulation. For chiropractic manipulation, dissection has been estimated to occur in 1 of every 20,000 spinal manipulations. Symptoms can be vague, although half of the patients will have unilateral orbital or facial pain and the majority of patients will have a unilateral headache. This may progress to cerebral or retinal ischemic symptoms which have been documented in 50% to 90% of patients.

Invasive carotid angiography has been considered the gold standard for the diagnosis of this condition. This can reveal spiral dissection extending from the proximal internal carotid to the petrous region, where the carotid artery enters the skull. MR angiography is quickly replacing this modality as the gold standard due to its high resolution. MR angiography can show intramural hematoma, stenosis, and aneurysm, although the dissection is not directly visualized. MRI can also show cerebral

edema. CT angiography is also being used to diagnose dissection, although experience with this modality is relatively limited. Carotid duplex can be performed which will give indirect data by showing an abnormal flow pattern.

The treatment of dissection consists of anticoagulation, although no randomized trials have been conducted to support this approach. Initially, this would consist of intravenous heparin, followed by coumadin and aspirin long term. Rarely, if there are persistent or stuttering neurological symptoms, patients can be referred for carotid stenting or surgical bypass of the carotid artery. Overall, most patients with dissection do well with full recovery, although the mortality rate is approximately 5%.

Thrombosis of the cerebral veins and sinuses. Thrombosis of the cerebral veins and sinuses is a rare neurological condition, affecting an estimated 3 to 4 individuals per million.[11] Similar to carotid dissection, thrombosis of the sinuses is typically observed in young women, while it is characteristically not seen in children and the elderly. Since the most common symptom of this condition, headache, is very nonspecific, a high index of suspicion must exist to correctly make its diagnosis. With the advent of high-resolution neuroimaging techniques (Fig. 48.6), the incidence of the disease has increased in the last decade.

Thrombosis of the cerebral veins will produce symptoms related to localized cerebral edema; however, it is rare to only have thrombosis of the cerebral veins. Pathologically, there is

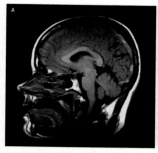
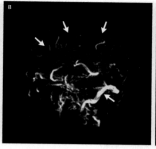
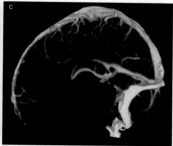

Figure 48.6 In **Panel A**, a T1-weighted MRI scan provides a sagittal view of a hyperintense signal in the thrombosed superior sagittal sinus (*black arrows*). In **Panel B**, a magnetic resonance venogram reveals the absence of a signal in the superior sagittal sinus (*upper white arrows*) and a normal flow signal in the transverse and sigmoid sinuses (*lower white arrow*) as well as in a number of veins. In **Panel C**, an image obtained by CT venography shows reconstruction of a normal cerebral venous system. This view provides the normal appearance of the major sinuses, including the straight sinus and the cortical and deep cerebral veins. (Reprinted from Stam J. Thrombosis of the cerebral veins and sinuses. *N Engl J Med.* 2005;352:1791–1798, with permission.)

often an overlap between thrombosis of the veins and sinuses, where the latter results in intracranial hypertension. Such patients may experience headache and/or neurological signs.

A cause or predisposing condition is discovered in the majority of cases. Many patients will have a genetic or acquired prothrombotic disorder. An example of the former includes the prothrombin gene mutation, while examples of the latter include pregnancy and the puerperium. Other associations include infections (otitis, mastoiditis, and sinusitis), oral contraceptives, and mechanical causes (includes head trauma, internal jugular vein catheterization, and lumbar puncture).

3. DIAGNOSTIC EVALUATION

3.1. Computed tomography

With modern technology, CT scanners are now capable of obtaining sections as thin as 0.5 to 1 mm at a speed of 0.5 to 1 s per rotation allowing complete studies of the brain in as little as 2 to 10 s. Radiation exposure depends on the dose used, but is normally between 3 and 5 cGy for a routine brain CT study. Use of iodinated contrast allows accurate delineation of the blood vessels (CT angiogram) and identifies breach of blood brain barriers.

CT scan is the preferred mode of imaging in patients with suspected acute stroke to assess for bleeding and to provide triage to the next level of care. In many ways this serves a similar role as the electrocardiogram in patients presenting with acute chest pain. Iodinated contrast injection is not indicated while assessing for intracranial bleeding.

In more chronic situations, the CT scan can help to define the size, location, and to some extent chronicity of an infarct. The location and shape of infarction along with clinical presentation can help to identify the potential mechanism of a stroke. A wedge-shaped infarct may suggest an embolic event, whereas a lacunar infarct may suggest spontaneous thrombosis of small vessels in hypertensive patients.

CT can be useful for establishing the differential diagnosis of cerebrovascular disease. CT is a frontline imaging test, especially in a patient with a suspected acute or chronic neurological disorder due to the speed, noninvasive nature, and accuracy of this test in establishing a diagnosis. CT of the head is useful to evaluate for neoplastic, vascular, or degenerative diseases. A patient who presents with the triad of urinary incontinence, gait instability, and cognitive impairment, might be expected clinically to have the condition of normal pressure hydrocephalus. It is important to consider and make this diagnosis, since it is readily treatable

by shunting. CT reveals enlarged ventricles out of proportion to cerebral atrophy (Fig. 48.7). Lumbar puncture confirms normal opening pressure. This is in contrast to enlarged ventricles with generalized cerebral atrophy that would be expected with Alzheimer dementia. While neurological imaging of patients with Alzheimer dementia is relatively nonspecific, this disorder has a predilection for degeneration of the mesial temporal lobe structures. The absence of temporal lobe atrophy in a patient with dementia suggests a diagnosis other than Alzheimer dementia.[12] Causes of neck pain that could be assisted diagnostically with CT include cervical disc disease, spinal stenosis, cord compression, and tumor infiltration of the brachial plexus.

CT scanning has several advantages over MRI. It is readily available and imaging can be accomplished very rapidly. Diagnosis of acute bleeding is better with CT scanning. It is particularly helpful when hyperperfusion syndrome is suspected in patients undergoing carotid revascularization (Fig. 48.8). Patients with metal implants or on life support equipment are not suitable for MRI.

Although CT scanning provides excellent resolution for most of the brain structures, posterior fossa imaging can be compromised by bone artifacts. In many situations, contrast enhancement is also

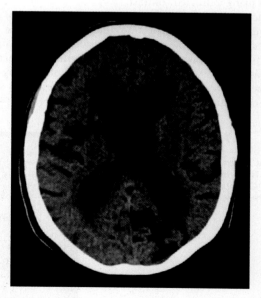

Figure 48.7 Computed tomography of the brain reveals bilateral ventricular enlargement. Lumbar puncture revealed normal opening pressure, consistent with normal pressure hydrocephalus.

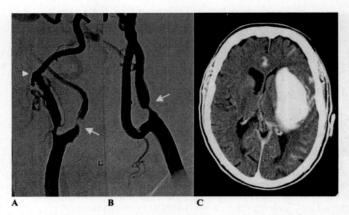

Figure 48.8 Panel A shows a 90% stenosis in the left internal carotid artery. Slow filling of the distal internal carotid artery is evident. **Panel B** shows an 80% stenosis in the right internal carotid artery. **Panel C** is a CT scan of the brain 1 h after carotid artery stenting which shows a large intracranial hemorrhage. (Reprinted from Abou-Chebl A. Intracranial hemorrhage and hyperperfusion syndrome following carotid artery stenting. *J Am Coll Cardiol.* 2004;43:1596–1601, with permission.)

necessary which may pose an issue in patients with renal insufficiency. Further, an acute infarct is not seen on CT scan for several hours.

3.2. Computed tomography angiography

CT angiography provides excellent definition of neck and intracranial vessels in a noninvasive way. It is extremely helpful to diagnose obstructive disease of carotid arteries at the bifurcation and to precisely define the anatomy of the vessel before and after the stenosis. This is sometimes important in the planning of percutaneous or surgical revascularization. Carotid artery atherosclerosis is typically associated with significant calcification. Although this causes blooming artifact and some overestimation of the lesion severity, in most cases accurate diagnosis can be reached. However, routine use of CT scanning in the assessment of carotid stenosis is not recommended because vascular ultrasound provides a noninvasive and very reliable functional estimation of stenosis severity without using iodinated contrast.

Intracranial anatomy of obstructive and aneurysmal disease can be defined by CT angiography including the Circle of Willis. Selective cerebral angiography is indicated when intervention is planned or when flow related information is needed in some cases of collateral circulation. Timing of imaging can be optimized for venous filling if the clinical presentation suggests venous circulation pathology.

3.3. Vascular ultrasound

Vascular ultrasound is an excellent imaging modality to evaluate the carotid anatomy and flow dynamics. Vascular ultrasound is noninvasive, has no known risk, and it is readily available. Ultrasound is commonly used for imaging the common carotid, internal, and external carotid arteries. "B-mode" or gray scale is used to define arterial wall anatomy such as the presence of plaque (Fig. 48.9). Ulcerated plaque has been suggested as a risk factor for future neurologic events.[13] Gray scale is not able to estimate lesion severity, therefore Doppler is used instead (Fig. 48.10). Doppler waveforms are interrogated along the length of the artery to document flow velocity patterns. Various criteria have been proposed for estimating lesion severity based on peak systolic and diastolic velocities (Table 48.1).

There several conditions where limitation of the Doppler criteria are well recognized. In cardiovascular diseases leading to reduced cardiac output due to valvular heart disease, coronary artery disease,

TABLE 48.1
VARIOUS ULTRASOUND CRITERIA FOR DETERMINING SEVERITY OF CAROTID ARTERY STENOSIS

Stenosis Severity	Strandness Criteria	Stenosis Severity	Cleveland Clinic Criteria
Normal	PSV < 125 Flow reversal in bulb	0% to 19%	PSV < 105 No plaque
1% to 15%	PSV ≤ 125 No flow reversal in bulb	20% to 39%	PSV < 105 Visible plaque
16% to 49%	PSV < 125 Marked spectral broadening	40% to 59%	PSV 105 to 159 Visible plaque
50% to 79%	PSV > 125 EDV < 140	60% to 79%	PSV > 160 EDV < 135
80% to 99%	PSV > 125 EDV > 140	80% to 99%	PSV > 240 EDV ≥ 135

PSV = peak systolic velocity, EDV = end diastolic velocity.
Adapted from Ziada KM, Olin JW. Noninvasive evaluation of arterial disease. In Casserly IP, Sachar R, Yadav JS, eds. *Manual of Peripheral Vascular Intervention.* Philadelphia, PA: Lippincott Williams & Wilkins; 2005:8–35.

Figure 48.9 Grayscale imaging (**left panel**) reveals an ulcerated plaque within the right internal carotid artery (ICA). The plaque is bordered by *white and green arrows*. Color imaging (**right panel**) confirms the presence of flow within the plaque.

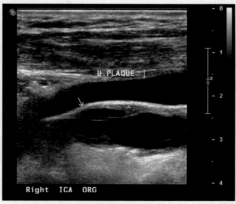
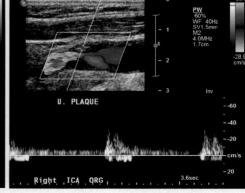

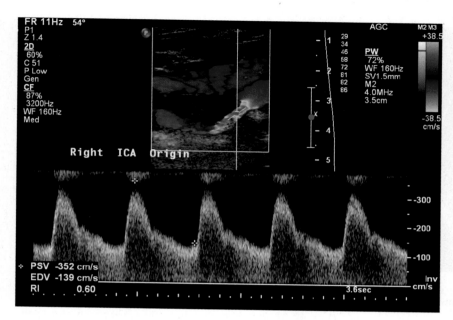

Figure 48.10 Doppler imaging of the right internal carotid artery (ICA). The waveform indicates flow throughout diastole characteristic of the low-resistance vascular bed of the brain. The peak systolic velocity (PSV) is 352 cm/s and the end diastolic velocity (EDV) is 139 cm/s. Together, these velocities suggest an internal carotid stenosis of 80% to 99%. Also note the presence of turbulent flow within the stenosis.

or other causes of cardiomyopathy, there is decreased velocity of blood flow in the common carotid artery. In these situations, how much flow acceleration should be considered significant is not well defined. Aortic stenosis adds another variable due to flow acceleration in the ascending aorta. Ostial lesions of the carotid origins from the arch or tandem lesions also make the distal lesions difficult to assess. There are no criteria currently available for in-stent restenosis.

Doppler flow assessment can also be performed to evaluate proximal intracranial vessels. It provides additional functional flow information in patients with stroke. It is also a good tool to monitor flow or look for constant embolization.

3.4. Magnetic resonance imaging

MRI is the result of an interaction between hydrogen protons in biologic tissues, the magnet (typically 1.5 T with availability of 3 to 8 T for specific protocols), and energy in the form of radiofrequency waves of a specific frequency introduced by coils placed next to the area of interest. The main magnet imparts slight changes in the magnetic field throughout the imaging volume. The coils deliver specific radiofrequency to transiently excite hydrogen protons. As the protons return to equilibrium energy state (relaxation), they release radiofrequency energy (the echo), which is detected by the coils to generate an MR image. This image consists of a map of the distribution of hydrogen protons, with signal intensity determined by both the density of hydrogen protons as well as differences in the relaxation times to equilibrium (relaxation rate) of hydrogen protons on different molecules (see Chapter 6).

Two relaxation rates, T1 and T2, influence the signal intensity of the image. The T1 relaxation time is the time measured in milliseconds for 63% of the hydrogen protons to return to their normal equilibrium state, while the T2 relaxation is the time for 63% of the protons to become dephased owing to interactions among nearby protons. Fat and subacute hemorrhage has higher signal intensity than brain on T1 weighted images. Structures containing more water, such as cerebrospinal fluid and edema, have lower signal intensity on T1 weighted images and higher signal intensity on T2 weighted images. T2 weighted images are more sensitive than T1 weighted images to edema, demyelination, infarction, and chronic hemorrhage, while T1 weighted imaging is more sensitive to subacute hemorrhage and fat-containing structures.

Contrast MRI is performed with a paramagnetic Gadolinium contrast which reduces the T1 and T2 relaxation times of nearby water protons, resulting in a high signal on T1-weighted images and a low signal on T2-weighted images. A rare complication, nephrogenic systemic fibrosis, has recently been reported in patients with renal insufficiency who have been exposed to Gadolinium contrast agents.[14] Diffusion-weighted imaging assesses microscopic motion of water molecules in the brain tissue. Restriction of motion appears as relatively high signal intensity on diffusion-weighted images. Diffusion-weighted imaging is the most sensitive technique for detection of acute cerebral infarction of <7 days duration. It also helps to define encephalitis and abscess formation.

Perfusion MRI is performed after a rapid intravenous bolus of gadolinium contrast material. In patients with stroke, perfusion imaging can help to identify the territory at risk. In the setting of reduced blood flow, a prolonged mean transit time of contrast but normal or elevated cerebral blood volume in the tissue may indicate tissue supplied by slow collateral flow that is at risk of infarction.

MRI provides enhanced contrast resolution compared with CT. MRI is useful for diagnosing most disorders; however, it is relatively limited due to its cost and availability as well as the expense and time of performing a study. Abnormal CT scans have been reported in only 30% to 40% of patients with multiple sclerosis,[15] therefore MRI has largely replaced CT in the assessment of this disorder. This disease most commonly affects young women from the age of 20 to 35 years. It is an inflammatory demyelinating disease of the central nervous system that is characterized by relapses and remissions of neurological signs. On T1 imaging, multiple sclerosis brain lesions appear dark and on T2 imaging they appear bright (Fig. 48.11). Lesions can appear discrete or confluent. The differential diagnosis for brain lesions that appear to be due to multiple sclerosis include normal variant, vasculitides such as systemic lupus erythematosous, migraine associated lesions, Lyme disease, acute disseminated encephalomyelitis, emboli, and brain metastases. This differential illustrates that the diagnosis of multiple sclerosis is clinical first and requires a careful history and physical examination.

3.5. Magnetic resonance angiography

MR angiography provides a flow map of the arteries rather than anatomical definition of the wall of the arteries like in the CTA (Fig. 48.5). One of the most frequently used techniques is the

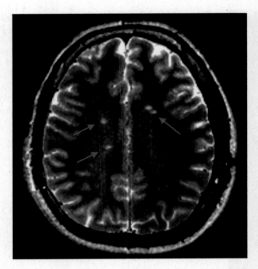

Figure 48.11 MR of the brain with T2 weighting showing bright plaques (*red arrows*) within the periventricular weight matter characteristic of multiple sclerosis.

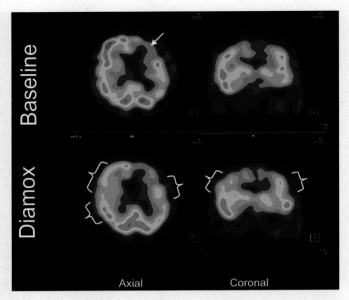

Figure 48.12 Brain perfusion study. The upper panels reveal perfusion at rest, while the **lower panels** reveal perfusion after the administration of the cerebral vasodilator acetazolamide. The *arrow* represents an area of decreased perfusion at rest consistent with a previous left frontal lobe infarction. The *brackets* represent areas of decreased perfusion at stress (cerebral vasodilatation) and are consistent with decreased reserve in the territories the bilateral middle cerebral arteries. Invasive coronary angiography revealed an occluded right common carotid artery and left internal carotid artery. His anterior circulation was supplied by the vertebral arteries (i.e., posterior circulation) by pial collaterals. The distal left internal carotid artery was also collateralized by the left external carotid artery (internal maxillary artery) to ophthalmic artery.

time-of-flight imaging. In this technique, the suppression of non-moving tissue is achieved to provide a low-intensity background for the high signal intensity of flowing blood in each section. This highlights arterial or venous structures without using specific contrast. Another technique, phase-contrast MR angiography, is based on velocity and direction of flow; however, this requires increased acquisition time. MR angiography can also be acquired during infusion of contrast material. Advantages include faster imaging times (1 to 2 min vs. 10 min), fewer flow-related artifacts, and higher resolution images. Contrast-enhanced MR angiography has become the standard for extracranial vascular MR angiography.

MR angiography has lower spatial resolution compared with digital substraction angiography. This limits its usefulness in small-vessel abnormalities, such as vasculitis and distal vasospasm. Another limitation is the inability to see within a stented segment. MR angiography is not reliable in differentiating complete from near-complete occlusions. Due to the longer acquisition time, motion of the patient or of the anatomic structures creates artifacts. Despite this, MR angiography has proved useful in the evaluation of the extracranial carotid and vertebral arteries as well as of larger-caliber intracranial arteries and dural sinuses. It has also proved useful in the noninvasive detection of intracranial aneurysms and vascular malformations.

3.6. Brain perfusion imaging

Single photon emission computed tomography or brain perfusion imaging is used to obtain functional information of the brain (Fig. 48.12).[16] Brain perfusion imaging complements the structural/anatomical information obtained from CT and MRI. The most widely used radiopharmaceutical is [99m]Technetium and the cerebral vasodilator is acetazolamide. A common indication of brain perfusion studies is to assess the functional reserve of the brain, determine prognosis, and help guide decisions regarding revascularization.[17,18] Brain perfusion is also used to determine epileptogenic foci prior to epileptic surgery, allow for early detection of dementia, and obtain prognosis after traumatic brain injury.

4. SELECTING AND GUIDING THERAPY

4.1. Endarterectomy

Carotid endarterectomy was introduced in 1954, therefore it is the therapy against which carotid stent revascularization is compared. The NASCET (North American Symptomatic Carotid Endarterectomy Trial) randomized patients with an internal carotid artery stenosis within 4 months of a stroke or transient ischemic attack to carotid endarterectomy versus medical management.[19] The investigators reported that for lesions >70%, the risk of any ipsilateral stroke within 5 years of enrollment was 9% in the surgical group and 26% in the medical group for an absolute risk reduction of 17% ($p < 0.001$). Benefit was still present, although diminished among patients with a stenosis 50% to 69%. Among these patients, the 5-year risk of stroke was 16% with surgery and 22% with medical therapy ($p = 0.045$).[20] Carotid endarterectomy has also been studied in asymptomatic patients with carotid artery stenosis.[3] These patients were generally in good health and so they were suitable for randomization to surgery or optimal medical management. The risk of perioperative morbidity and mortality was <3%, which serves as a good benchmark for evaluating a hospital for carotid endarterectomy. At a median follow-up of 2.7 years, the risk of ipsilateral stroke or any stroke or death within the perioperative period was 5.1% for surgery versus 11% for medical management.

4.2. Percutaneous stenting

Despite the proven superiority of carotid endarterectomy over medical management for severe carotid artery stenosis, many patients are poor candidates for surgery due to extensive comorbidities. The SAPPHIRE (Stenting and Angioplasty with Protection in Patients at High Risk for Endarterectomy) trial was designed to test the noninferiority of carotid artery stenting with embolic protection versus carotid endarterectomy in high-risk patients.[21,22] High-risk criteria included significant cardiac disease (congestive heart failure, abnormal stress test, or need for open heart surgery), severe pulmonary artery disease, contralateral carotid artery occlusion, contralateral laryngeal nerve palsy, previous radiation therapy to the neck, restenosis after endarterectomy, or age >80 years. Symptomatic patients had to have a stenosis of at least 50%, while asymptomatic patients had to have a stenosis of at least 80%. At 1 year of follow-up, the incidence of the primary endpoint (death, stroke, or myocardial infarction within 30 days or death or ipsilateral stroke between 31 days and 1 year) was 12% in the carotid stent group versus 20% in the surgical group ($p = 0.004$ for noninferiority and $p = 0.053$ for superiority).[21] At 3 years of follow-up, major or minor ipsilateral stroke occurred in 7.4% of the carotid stent arm and 6.3% of the carotid endarterectomy group. Considering any stroke in any location, the stroke incidence was 10.1% in the stenting group and 10.7% in the surgical group ($p = 0.99$).[22]

Two recent trials have raised questions about carotid stenting in symptomatic patients. In the SPACE trial, a planned noninferiority randomized trial of carotid stenting and CEA, the stroke risk of carotid stenting was similar to CEA despite only 27% use of EPD in the trial.[23] However, the authors surprisingly concluded that carotid stenting should not be used in widespread terms. The results of this outdated trial do not support this conclusion. EVA-3S had very inexperienced endovascular operators and many different devices.[24] Carotid stenting had worse outcomes compared to CEA in this study, but this is expected if very inexperienced operators perform carotid stenting. On the other hand, CEA had better than expected results in this study. A significant number of strokes happened in the patients not treated with embolic protection or with unsuccessful stenting. This study highlights that proper training is essential for good outcomes with carotid stenting.

4.3. Medical therapy

Medical therapy and risk factory modification should be given to all patients with carotid artery atherosclerotic disease. Patients with mild carotid artery stenosis (e.g., <50%), will be principally managed medically. For every 10 mm Hg reduction in systolic blood pressure, the risk of stroke is reduced by one third.[25] Angiotensin-converting enzyme inhibitors (e.g., ramipril) appear to be especially important in reducing stroke risk.[26] Statin medications have been associated with a nearly 20% reduction in the risk of all strokes.[27] Medical therapy should be used in conjunction with revascularization strategies in all patients.

5. FUTURE DIRECTIONS

Up to the present time, carotid and cerebrovascular imaging has mainly focused on the precise delineation of anatomy. For example, with internal carotid artery disease, noninvasive imaging modalities have attempted to determine the degree of stenosis, which is often accurate and reliable when compared with invasive angiography. In the future, it is likely that imaging will have a complementary role in the determination of the functional and prognostic significance of a lesion by incorporating other characteristics such as plaque volume and composition.[28] By identifying 'vulnerable plaques,' it may be possible to more accurately determine which patients would derive the most benefit from revascularization and stroke prevention measures. It is possible that some patients with minimal degree of carotid stenosis, although with a "vulnerable plaque" would derive benefit from revascularization, while other patients with more severe stenosis and a stable lesion may not benefit as much. MRI can be enhanced with intravenous injection of ultrasmall iron oxide particles. These particles are accumulated by monocytes/macrophages. Since these cells accumulate within atheromatous plaques, this might be an additional mechanism to identify 'vulnerable plaques.' Another imaging modality involves the use of annexin A5 which binds to apoptotic cells. Studies have revealed that patients who have a transient ischemic attack display more annexin A5 uptake in the culprit vessel. In summary, there are numerous, noninvasive imaging modalities that are being developed to study the functional and prognostic significant of a given vessel which may help to more precisely direct therapy to those most likely to benefit.

REFERENCES

1. Stroke Statistics – American Heart Association. Available at http://www.strokeassociation.org/presenter.jhtml?identifier=4725 Accessed September, 2008.
2. Inzitari D, Eliasziw M, Gates P, et al. The causes and risk of stroke in patients with asymptomatic internal-carotid-artery stenosis. North American Symptomatic Carotid Endarterectomy Trial Collaborators. *N Engl J Med.* 2000;342: 1693–700.
3. Executive Committee for the Asymptomatic Carotid Atherosclerosis Study. Endarterectomy for asymptomatic carotid artery stenosis. *JAMA.* 1995;273: 1421–1428.
4. Qureshi AI, Janardhan V, Hanel RA, et al. Comparison of endovascular and surgical treatments for intracranial aneurysms: An evidence-based review. *Lancet Neurol.* 2007;6:816–825.
5. Wiebers DO, Whisnant JP, Huston J III, et al. Unruptured intracranial aneurysms: Natural history, clinical outcome, and risks of surgical and endovascular treatment. *Lancet.* 2003;362:103–110.
6. Brown RD, Jr, Wiebers DO, Torner JC, et al. Frequency of intracranial hemorrhage as a presenting symptom and subtype analysis: A population-based study of intracranial vascular malformations in Olmsted Country, Minnesota. *J Neurosurg.* 1996;85:29–32.
7. Stapf C, Mast H, Sciacca RR, et al. The New York Islands AVM Study: Design, study progress, and initial results. *Stroke.* 2003;34:e29–e33.
8. Wedderburn CJ, van Beijnum J, Bhattacharya JJ, et al. Outcome after interventional or conservative management of unruptured brain arteriovenous malformations: A prospective, population-based cohort study. *Lancet Neurol.* 2008;7:223–230.
9. Brown RD Jr. Unruptured brain AVMs: To treat or not to treat. *Lancet Neurol.* 2008;7:195–196.
10. Schievink WI. Spontaneous dissection of the carotid and vertebral arteries. *N Engl J Med.* 2001;344:898–906.
11. Stam J. Thrombosis of the cerebral veins and sinuses. *N Engl J Med.* 2005; 352:1791–1798.
12. George AE, de Leon MJ, Stylopoulos LA, et al. CT diagnostic features of Alzheimer disease: Importance of the choroidal/hippocampal fissure complex. *Am J Neuroradiol.* 1990;11:101–107.
13. O'Donnell TF Jr, Erdoes L, Mackey WC, et al. Correlation of B-mode ultrasound imaging and arteriography with pathologic findings at carotid endarterectomy. *Arch Surg.* 1985;120:443–449.
14. Todd DJ, Kay J. Nephrogenic systemic fibrosis: An epidemic of gadolinium toxicity. *Curr Rheumatol Rep.* 2008;10:195–204.
15. Jacobs L, Kinkel WR. Computerized axial transverse tomography in multiple sclerosis. *Neurology.* 1976;26:390–391.
16. European Association of Nuclear Medicine Procedure Guidelines for Brain Perfusin SPET using 99mTc-labelled Radiopharmaceuticals. Available at http://www.eanm.org/scientific_info/guidelines/gl_neuro_spet_radio.pdf Accessed September, 2008.
17. Kuroda S, Kamiyama H, Abe H, et al. Acetazolamide test in detected reduced cerebral perfusion reserve and predicting long-term prognosis in patients with internal scarotid artery occlusion. *Neurosurgery.* 1993;32:912–918.
18. Cikrit DF, Dalsing MC, Lalka SG, et al. The value of acetazolamide single photon emission computd tomography scans in the preoperative evaluation of asymptomatic critical carotid stenosis. *J Vasc Surg.* 1999;30:599–605.
19. North American Symptomatic Carotid Endarterectomy Trial Collaborators. Beneficial effect of carotid endarterectomy in symptomatic patients with high-grade carotid stenosis. *N Engl J Med.* 1991;325:445–453.
20. Barnett HJ, Taylor DW, Eliasziw M, et al. Benefit of carotid endarterectomy in patients with symptomatic moderate or severe stenosis. North American Symptomatic Carotid Endarterectomy Trial Collaborators. *N Engl J Med.* 1998;339:1415–1425.
21. Yadav JS, Wholey MH, Kuntz RE, et al. Protected carotid-artery stenting versus endarterectomy in high-risk patients. *N Engl J Med.* 2004;351:1493–1501.
22. Gurm HS, Yadav JS, Fayad P, et al. Long-term results of carotid stenting versus endarterectomy in high-risk patients. *N Engl J Med.* 2008;358:1572–1579.
23. Ringleb PA, Allenberg JR, Berger J, et al. 30 day results from the SPACE trial of stent-protected angioplasty versus carotid endarterectomy in symptomatic patients: A randomised non-inferiority trial. *Lancet.* 2006;368:1239–1247.
24. Mas JL, Chatellier G, Beyssen B, et al. Endarterectomy versus stenting in patients with symptomatic severe carotid stenosis. *N Engl J Med.* 2006;355: 1660–1671.
25. Lawes CM, Bennett DA, Feigin VL, et al. Blood pressure and stroke: An overview of published reviews. *Stroke.* 2004;35:776–785.
26. Bosch J, Yusuf S, Pogue J, et al. Use of ramipril in preventing stroke: Double blind randomized trial. *BMJ.* 2002;324:1–5.
27. O'Regan C, Wu P, Arora P, et al. Statin therapy in stroke prevention: A meta-analysis involving 121,000 patients. *Am J Med.* 2008;121:24–33.
28. Kwee RM, van Oostenbrugge RJ, Hofstra L, et al. Identifying vulnerable carotid plaques by non-invasive imaging. *Neurology.* 2008;70:2401–2409.

Renal Artery Disease

49

Manisha Das
Debabrata Mukherjee

1. INTRODUCTION

Renal artery disease is a common entity in a certain category of patients and may be associated with significant mortality and morbidity.[1] Atherosclerotic renal artery stenosis (RAS) is also an independent predictor of death.[1,2] Early diagnosis and appropriate treatment of renal artery disease may improve renal function, morbidity, and mortality. Developments in the field of imaging over the last few decades have facilitated the diagnosis and therapy for patients with renal artery disease. However, the guidelines are not clear regarding which imaging modalities are optimal for RAS diagnosis and in guiding therapy for this patient population. This chapter will provide an overview of RAS, the different imaging modalities currently available, and insight on selecting appropriate diagnostic tests, therapy, and follow-up.

1.1. Epidemiology

RAS is the most common cause for secondary hypertension and may be due to atherosclerosis, fibromuscular dysplasia (FMD), or systemic diseases involving the renal arteries. FMD is typically seen in young and middle-aged females, and accounts for about 10% of cases. Approximately 90% of RAS cases are atherosclerotic in nature.[3,4] The prevalence of atherosclerotic RAS increases with age and is commonly associated with other comorbid conditions including diabetes, peripheral arterial disease, coronary artery disease, hypertension, and dyslipidemia. Atherosclerotic RAS is a progressive disease that may occur alone or in combination with hypertension and ischemic kidney disease.[4] Keith et al. suggested that renovascular disease is more common in white than black populations in all age groups, but this fact has not been confirmed in other series.[5]

RAS is a common and progressive disease in patients with atherosclerosis. The incidence of RAS in the general population is 0.1% considering all age groups. A population-based study using duplex ultrasound in elderly patients (>65 years) showed that the prevalence of significant RAS was 6.8%, with 9.1% in men, 5.5% in women, 6.9% in whites, and 6.7% in blacks.[6]

The prevalence of any atherosclerotic RAS in patients undergoing cardiac catheterization may vary up to 30% by screening renal angiography.[7] The incidence of hemodynamically significant RAS (>50% lumen occlusion) among elderly people or those with diffuse atherosclerotic vascular diseases may vary from 11% to 18%.[8] In the United States, 12% to 14% of patients in whom dialysis is initiated have been found to have significant RAS.[9] RAS is also common in patients diagnosed with peripheral vascular disease; the prevalence varies from 22% to 59%.[10-13] The prevalence of RAS was found to be 53% in 295 patients undergoing necropsy

and up to 74% in age groups >70 years.[14] Atherosclerotic RAS is a rapidly progressive disease. During a follow-up period of 12 to 60 months, RAS progressed from 36% to 71% of patients, with 16% having total occlusion of the renal arteries. Patients with long segments of disease and multiple diseased segments had worse disease progression.[15-18]

1.2. Clinical presentation

The clinical features of RAS fall into two categories depending on renal or extrarenal involvement. The renal involvement could lead to renovascular hypertension (RVH), which along with pre-existing essential hypertension, can result in significant renal damage and loss of renal mass. Mailloux et al.[19] reviewed the causes of end-stage renal disease (ESRD) in 683 patients who entered into their dialysis program over a 20-year period. Eighty-three patients (12%) had documented RAS as a cause of ESRD. The extrarenal features that are associated with RAS are recurrent angina, myocardial infarction, and uncontrolled hypertension leading to flash pulmonary edema, stroke, or aortic dissection.

Renovascular disease should be clinically suspected if one or more of the following are present (Table 49.1):

A. Hypertension

1. New onset hypertension before age 30 or after 55 years of age: Essential hypertension usually presents between ages 30 and 55. FMD should be suspected in patients presenting with severe hypertension before 30 years of age, especially in young and middle-aged women with no family history of hypertension. After 55 years of age, one of the most common causes of secondary hypertension is due to atherosclerotic process involving the renal arteries.

2. Previously well controlled, hypertension becomes difficult to control: In patients with well-controlled hypertension on a certain antihypertensive regimen, if blood pressure (BP) suddenly becomes uncontrolled, suspect secondary causes including renovascular disease, which can superimpose on previously diagnosed essential hypertension.

3. Hypertension resistant to medical therapy: Resistant hypertension is defined as failure to control BP below 140/90, with at least three antihypertensive medications (including a diuretic), which have different mechanism of action, despite patient compliance. In this patient population, RVH should strongly be suspected. Dustan et al. have shown that 72% of patients with atherosclerotic renovascular disease and 65% of patients with FMD present with resistant

TABLE 49.1
CLINICAL FEATURES SUGGESTIVE OF RAS

1. Hypertension diagnosed before the age of 30 or after age 55, without any family history of hypertension
2. Accelerated hypertension: in a compliant patient with more than three antihypertensive medications
3. Resistant hypertension: poorly controlled hypertension, with three or more medications of different class of action including a diuretic
4. Acute renal failure or worsening renal function in a patient treated with ACEI or ARB
5. Recurrent acute pulmonary edema without any explainable cause
6. Hypertension with hypokalemia
7. Hypertension with end organ damage
8. Bruit over abdominal aorta or over renal arteries
9. Difference in kidney size of >1.5 cm or any kidney size <9 cm
10. Hypertension in a patient with extensive atherosclerotic involvement like peripheral vascular disease

Source: Adapted from Mukherjee D, *ACC Current Journal Review*, 2003.

TABLE 49.2
COMPARISON OF ATHEROSCLEROTIC RAS AND FMD

	Atherosclerotic RAS	FMD
Etiology	Atherosclerotic involvement of renal arteries	Multiple proposed etiology—genetic, hormonal factors. Smoking and hypertension are associated with FMD
Incidence	90% of all RAS	10% of RAS
Imaging	Usually smooth or shelflike narrowing	Beaded or "string of pearl" appearance, rarely smooth narrowing
Angio-graphic appearance	Usually involves proximal 2 cm of renal artery	Usually involves distal two-thirds and branch points of renal arteries
Treatment	PTCA and stent placement	PTCA and/ or stent placement
Outcome	Progressive disease; high incidence of reocclusion after balloon angioplasty.	Good angiographic outcome after PTCA and/ or stent

hypertension.[20] However, renovascular disease can present with mild, moderate, severe, or no hypertension.[21]

4. Malignant or accelerated hypertension: RVH is common in patients with hypertension and end-organ damage such as hypertensive retinopathy, nephropathy, etc.
5. Hypertension and concomitant peripheral arterial disease: Patients with generalized atherosclerosis have significantly higher prevalence of RAS.

B. Signs

1. Hypertension with end-organ damage, for example, papilledema, heart failure, acute renal failure
2. Systolic or diastolic bruit in the epigastrium, bruit over the abdominal aorta (lateralizing bruit over the renal arteries is more specific, but is not a common finding)
3. Recurrent acute (flash) pulmonary edema

C. Abnormal laboratory findings

1. Acute renal failure or creatinine elevation with angiotensin-converting enzyme inhibitors (ACEI) or angiotensin receptor blockers (ARB)
2. Chronic renal insufficiency with mild proteinuria and bland urinary sediment
3. Azotemia in a patient with uncontrolled hypertension
4. Azotemia in an elderly patient with atherosclerosis
5. Hypertension with hypokalemia (secondary hyperaldosteronism due to elevated renin)

2. PATHOPHYSIOLOGY

Renal artery disease includes four different disease categories (RAS, renal artery aneurysm, arteriovenous (AV) fistula, and thromboembolic disease). Several systemic diseases can also involve renal arteries.

2.1. Renal artery stenosis

The two more common causes of RAS are atherosclerotic involvement of renal arteries and FMD (Table 49.2).

2.1.1. Atherosclerotic involvement

Approximately 90% of RAS cases are secondary to atherosclerosis and involve the ostium and the proximal portion of the main renal artery, with plaque extending into the perirenal aorta.[3,4] Atherosclerosis could be localized to renal arteries or may be part of a generalized process that frequently involves the proximal 2 cm of the renal arteries. These lesions often involve the intima of the vessel and present as eccentric plaques. Rarely, it can present as circumferential lesions and destroy the intima. Sometimes, complicated plaques will present as dissecting hematoma and subsequent thrombosis of the entire vessel.

RAS may cause either ostial or nonostial lesions. Ostial lesions are classified as those lying within 5 mm of the vessel origin, and nonostial lesions are classified as those lying >5 mm from the vessel origin.[73] The degree of stenosis is based on the ratio of the diseased segment to the reference segment (which could be proximal to the diseased segment or the distal segment excluding the poststenotic dilatation).[74]

2.1.2. Fibromuscular dysplasia

FMD describes a noninflammatory, nonatherosclerotic condition where stenotic lesions intervene with aneurysmal outpouching of vessel. Leadbetter and Burkland originally described this condition in 1938.[22] FMD comprises <10% of all cases of renovascular disease. Although the exact pathophysiology is not known, congenital dysplasia and maldevelopment of the fibrous, muscular, and elastic tissues of the renal artery are presumed to be responsible for its development. FMD is a multisystem disease involving renal and extrarenal arteries. Other possible etiologies may include genetic predisposition, mechanical, and hormonal factors. Cigarette smoking and history of hypertension are associated with an increased risk for this condition. Presentation could be asymptomatic to multisystem involvement, as patients with FMD clinically resemble patients suffering from necrotizing

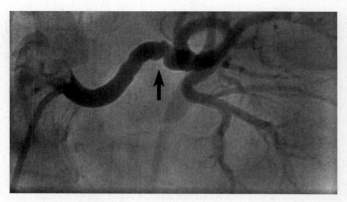

Figure 49.1 Renal angiogram showing "string of pearl" appearance of the left renal artery suggestive of FMD in a woman with resistant hypertension.

vasculitis.[23] McCormack et al.[24] described the histological entity of FMD in 1958. If there is strong suspicion clinically, angiography is the best modality to evaluate FMD (Fig. 49.1). Depending on the histological and angiographic features, FMD has been classified into the following subtypes:

Primary Intimal Fibroplasia occurs most often in children and young adults. Histopathologically, it shows accumulation of collagen inside the internal elastic lamina. Aneurysmal dilatation and dissecting hematoma to the outer media is sometimes seen as a complication. Angiographically, these lesions appear to have smooth contour with focal stenosis. Progressive renal artery obstruction and ischemic renal atrophy may be seen as a complication. This disease process can involve the contralateral kidney or the other vessels as a part of disease process.

Medial Fibroplasia is the most common type of FMD, and occurs most often in women 25 to 50 years of age. Histopathologically, the internal elastic lamina is lost and thickened areas of muscle are replaced by collagen. Alternate areas of thinned media and micro aneurysm formation angiographically resemble a "string of beads" mostly involving the distal two-thirds of renal arteries and their branches. The course of the disease process is usually slow, so decline in size of the kidneys or loss of renal function occurs slowly.

Perimedial Fibroplasia, also known as "Girlie disease," is less common than the previous types and is mostly seen in men and women 15 to 30 years old. Angiographically, there will be an appearance of "beading" and the bead size never exceeds the normal caliber of the vessel. Collateral circulation is frequent with this condition as opposed to medial fibroplasias. This disease condition progresses rapidly and ultimately leads to ischemic renal atrophy if treated by medical therapy alone.

Fibromuscular Hyperplasia is the rarest form of FMD and is frequently seen in children and young adults. The renal artery will show concentric thickening of smooth muscles and fibrous tissue. Angiographically, there is smooth narrowing of the renal artery and branch points, looking similar to intimal fibroplasias. Long-term follow-up of these patients shows progressive renal artery occlusion and loss of renal function.

2.2. Renal artery aneurysm

Renal artery aneurysm is a less common entity contributing to RVH. As described by Poutasse, there are four different types of renal artery aneurysm: saccular, fusiform, intrarenal, and dissecting.[24,25] Renal artery aneurysms can lead to resistant hypertension; they have a potential for rupture, especially in pregnant women, if the aneurysm size is >2 cm and if they are noncalcified.

2.3. Arteriovenous fistula

The renal AV fistula is a relatively uncommon lesion and most cases are discovered as an incidental finding during angiographic evaluation of renovascular disease. The clinical finding varies from hematuria, predominantly diastolic hypertension, or high-output cardiac failure. The etiology could be congenital or cirsoid fistula (about one-fourth of cases), and angiographically presents as multiple small interconnecting AV channels, early filling of renal veins, and/or delayed filling of distal vasculature. Idiopathic fistulas are relatively less common and could be secondary to venous erosion of a pre-existing renal artery aneurysm. The most common cause of AV fistula is iatrogenic kidney trauma sustained during needle biopsy, blunt or penetrating trauma, or secondary to erosion caused by tumor, inflammation, or postrenal surgery complications.[26]

2.4. Thromboembolic disease

The embolism of renal arteries could result as a complication of rheumatic heart disease, infective endocarditis, postcardiac surgery, repair of aortic aneurysm, or during cardiac catheterization. Thrombosis of renal arteries is less common and is often associated with polycythemia Vera, intimal fibroplasias, tumor, trauma, localized arteritis, and rarely, after umbilical arterial catheterization in a newborn. Occasionally, blunt trauma to the kidney can result in intimal dissection and subsequent thrombotic occlusion of the renal artery.

2.5. Systemic diseases

Systemic diseases including middle aortic syndrome, Takayasu arteritis, and neurofibromatosis are associated with RAS. Sometimes neural tissue, diaphragmatic crura, or muscle bundles will compress the renal arteries externally.

2.6. Renal artery stenosis of transplanted kidney

Finally, RAS is not uncommon in transplanted kidneys (Fig. 49.2). The incidence is about 6.6%.[27] A study by

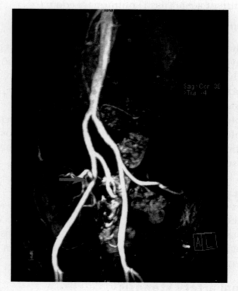

Figure 49.2 MR angiogram with gadolinium using T2 HASTE coronal view of transplanted kidney. There is an area of narrowing >50% at the site of anastomosis of the transplanted kidney and the external iliac artery.

Sutherland et al. showed that atherosclerotic risk factors, risk of allograft rejection, and type of anastomotic surgical procedure were not different between groups with and without RAS.[27] Diagnosis and management follow the same algorithm as native RAS.

3. IMAGING OF RENAL ARTERIES FOR DIAGNOSTIC EVALUATION

Careful selection of appropriate imaging modalities is crucial for diagnosing the particular grade of renovascular disease. The grade determines which patients will benefit from intervention and also helps in monitoring postintervention follow-up and disease progression. Ultrasound, nuclear scintigraphy, computed tomography (CT), magnetic resonance (MR), and catheter angiography, have been used to evaluate renal artery disease (Table 49.3). The objectives of various imaging modalities are:

1. To establish the anatomic diagnosis of RAS (identification of main renal artery and accessory renal arteries)
2. To assess physiologic changes distal to the diseased segment and in the renal parenchyma
3. To evaluate hemodynamic significance of RAS and to differentiate reversible from irreversible kidney damage as a consequence of RAS; this will essentially provide guidance for revascularization
4. To identify additional pathology such as abdominal aortic aneurysm, dissection, renal masses, etc., that will impact management of renal artery disease.

The advantages and disadvantages of each imaging modality are shown in Table 49.4.

3.1. Duplex ultrasonography

Comprehensive renal ultrasonography (USG) with B-mode spectral sampling and color-flow imaging with Doppler is the initial screening technology of choice. It is safe, inexpensive, and widely available. USG can provide a significant amount of useful information in the form of renal size assessment and images of the renal arteries; it can also measure blood flow velocities and pressure waveforms. This imaging modality will not only diagnose RAS but may also give the functional significance. Color-Doppler flow imaging will show turbulence in the area of stenosis in the renal artery. Spectral sampling proximal to the narrowed area will show spectral widening and increased velocity. Figures 49.3 and 49.4 are examples of RAS diagnosed by ultrasound.

The following ultrasound criteria are used to diagnose significant the proximal RAS with a high degree of accuracy:

1. The ratio of peak systolic velocity between the main proximal renal artery and the aorta is indicative of luminal narrowing. A ratio >3.5, for example, corresponds to 60% luminal narrowing.[28,29]
2. The magnitude of the peak systolic velocity (PSV) at the narrowed segment correlates with the degree of luminal narrowing; for example, peak velocities of 150 and 180 cm/s correspond to luminal narrowing of 50% and 60%, respectively (Figs. 49.3 and 49.4).[30,31]
3. Turbulent flow in the poststenotic area is a marker of significant obstruction in the renal arteries.
4. If the renal arteries are visualized but no Doppler signal is detected "total occlusion" should be suspected.

Other Doppler ultrasound criteria have been described in the literature and are presumed to corroborate with degree of narrowing. One is intrarenal spectral Doppler change distal to the stenosis, known as "tardus-parvus phenomenon", these abnormalities include slow systolic acceleration and decreased resistive index (RI).[32-35]

Other criteria used (although they do not necessarily correspond with angiographic severity) are loss of early systolic peak (ESP), acceleration rate <3 m/s[2], acceleration index >4, acceleration time to systolic peak >0.07 s, a >5% difference in the RI between the two

TABLE 49.3
RATIONALE OF CURRENTLY AVAILABLE TESTS FOR RENAL ARTERY DISEASE

Physiologic studies involving renin-angiotensin system	Rationale
Blood tests	
Peripheral PRA	Measures the level of renin-angiotensin system activity
Captopril stimulated PRA	Stimulated release of renin from stenotic kidney
Renal vein renin activity (invasive)	Lateralization of the involved kidney
Imaging studies to evaluate differential renal perfusion	
Pre- and post-captopril nuclear imaging with technetium-99m labeled mertiatide (^{99m}Tc MAG3) or pentetic acid (DTPA) (Renography, and estimation of fractional flow to each kidney)	Captopril-mediated fall in filtration pressure of the stenotic kidney only leading to amplified difference in renal perfusion and allows estimation of fall in fractional flow/GFR in each kidney
Imaging to evaluate the renal artery anatomy	
Doppler USG	Visualization of kidneys and renal arteries, estimates size/anatomy of kidneys, measures flow velocity, and calculates RI to assess the severity of the stenosis
CTA	Visualization of kidneys, renal arteries, and perirenal aorta, estimates size/anatomy of kidneys
MRA	Visualization of kidneys, renal arteries, and perirenal aorta, estimates size/anatomy of kidneys

Source: Adapted from Safian RD, Textor SC, Renal Artery Stenosis. *N Engl J Med.* 2001;344(6):431–442.

TABLE 49.4

RELATIVE ADVANTAGES AND DISADVANTAGES OF DIFFERENT MODALITIES OF RENAL ARTERY IMAGING

	Duplex ultrasound	CT angiogram	MRI/MR angiogram	Nuclear (captopril renogram)	Renal angiogram
Advantages	Safe, inexpensive, and widely available, no need for nephrotoxic contrast use	Anatomy of the kidney—size, degree of RAS, contralateral kidney—can be evaluated	1. Precisely defines the renal anatomy, size of the kidney, renal and accessory renal arteries, and their origin, angulation, and course 2. No exposure to iodinated contrast or radiation 3. Estimation of GFR	1. Can measure GFR and blood flow of an individual kidney 2. Safe, noninvasive, no use of contrast agents	The gold standard imaging modality: accurate and can proceed to intervention if RAS is hemodynamically significant
Disadvantages	1. Dependent on operator experience 2. Resolution depends on patient body habitus (obese) or presence of bowel gas	1. Exposure to iodinated contrast 2. Exposure to ionizing radiation 3. Sometimes, difficult to image the distal vessels or branch points or heavily calcified vessels	1. Metallic implants create artifacts 2. Nephrogenic systemic fibrosis in patients with reduced GFR (Cr CL <30)	1. Less accurate and high false negative results if there is significant renal failure, bilateral RAS, or chronic ACEI use	1. Invasive procedure—complications may include hematoma, pseudoaneurysm, or atheromatous embolization 2. Contrast-induced nephropathy
Sensitivity	60%–97%	90%–98%	88%–100%	90%	100%
Specificity	85%–99%	85%–94%	71%–99%	79%	100%
Contrast use	Usually none	Iodinated (70–150 mL)	Gadolinium	No	Iodinated
Stent and artifact	No	No	Yes	No	No
Invasive tests	No	No	No	No	Yes

Figure 49.3 Bilateral RAS diagnosed by Duplex ultrasound in a patient with uncontrolled hypertension despite multiple antihypertensive medications.

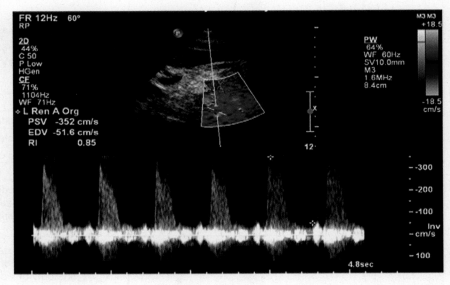

kidneys and a pulsatility index >0.12.[32–40] The change in waveform distal to the area of stenosis depends on multiple factors, including compliance of the vessel rather than only degree of pressure drop. These criteria are mainly applicable for proximal RAS, not a branch lesion or narrowing of the accessory renal artery.

Duplex ultrasound can be used to calculate the An RI, which is a prognostic marker for patients who will benefit after revascularization.[41] The RI is defined as the ratio of PSV (V_{max}, in centimeters per second) and the end-diastolic velocity (V_{min}, in centimeters per second), such that:

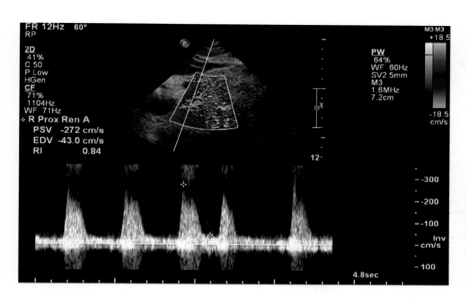

Figure 49.4 Bilateral RAS diagnosed by Duplex ultrasound, in a patient with uncontrolled hypertension despite multiple antihypertensive medications.

$$RI = [1 - (V_{min} \div V_{max})] \times 100 \qquad (Eq.\ 49.1)$$

The RI values are taken as the average of two to three measurements in segmental arteries from the upper, middle, and lower third of each kidney (Figs. 49.3 and 49.4). An RI value >80 in patients with RAS is associated with poor outcome after revascularization (percutaneous coronary intervention with or without stents as well as surgical revascularization); those patients may not show any improvement of BP or renal function after revascularization.[42] Higher RI is corroborated with parenchyma damage or small vessel disease associated with long-standing hypertension leading to nephrosclerosis or glomerulosclerosis.

Ultrasound is also useful tool to monitor renal artery patency after percutaneous or surgical revascularization. The presence of metal in stents does not create any artifact by ultrasound, but is a potential problem with magnetic resonance imaging (MRI) or magnetic resonance angiography (MRA).

The major drawback of ultrasound is a 15% to 20% failure rate to adequately visualize the renal arteries, due to either operator inexperience or technical issues such as obesity or the presence of bowel gas. The results are highly dependent on operator expertise. While interpretation is consistently accurate in nonatheromatous involvement of renal arteries. Sometimes, the accessory renal arteries may be missed and mild stenosis is difficult to detect.

A size difference of >1.5 cm between the two kidneys on ultrasound is potentially indicative of significant RAS. The reported sensitivity ranges from 60% to 97%, and specificity from 85% to 99%. Because of technical difficulties and the time-consuming nature of the procedure, Doppler studies may be replaced by other noninvasive methods of imaging the renal arteries, however Doppler ultrasound is still widely used as the first-line screening test to evaluate RAS. The new development of tissue harmonic imaging and the use of echo contrast agents have been shown to improve visualization of the renal arteries and to significantly reduce the number of equivocal examinations.[43,44]

3.2. Nuclear imaging of renal arteries/captopril renogram

Renal functional assessment by radionuclide scintigraphy indirectly evaluates renal function (glomerular filtration rate [GFR] of individual kidneys). It involves the use of radiotracers such as [99m]technetium-mercaptoacetyltriglycine (^{99m}Tc-MAG3) or Tc Diethylenetriamine pentaacic acid (^{99m}Tc-DTPA). Conventional

^{99m}Tc-MAG3 renography allows evaluation of the split function of the kidneys (contribution of each kidney to overall function). A difference in split function is an indirect evidence of RAS. Radionuclide imaging is performed before and 1 h after administration of 50 mg of captopril. In unilateral RAS, the renal function deteriorates acutely after captopril administration in the affected kidney, whereas in the unaffected (nonstenotic) kidney the function remains unchanged.

Nuclear imaging is a safe, noninvasive method to assess renal size, blood flow, and excretory function. The use of an ACEI in conjunction with renography (captopril challenge scintigraphy) removes angiotensin II-mediated vasoconstriction, which increases the difference in GFRs of the stenotic kidney and the contralateral kidney.

A positive scan indicates the presence of RVH with hemodynamically significant RAS. Abnormalities suggestive of a positive scan are shown in Figures 49.5 and 49.6, and include:

1. A delayed time to maximal activity of >11 min after captopril administration
2. Significant asymmetry between peak activities of both kidneys
3. Cortical retention of radioactivity after captopril administration
4. After ACEI administration, marked reduction in GFR is suggestive of RAS.

Use of this imaging modality is limited as false negative results arise in the presence of bilateral stenosis or with chronic use of ACEI. Impaired renal function also reduces the specificity of the examination. Due to these limitations, this method is not widely used as a first-line test for noninvasive diagnosis of RAS.

Captopril renography has been reported to be of value in identifying patients in whom BP is likely to decrease after successful correction of RAS, with a sensitivity of 92% (range 84% to 100%) and a specificity of 78% (range 62% to 100%).[45-51] However, this approach is less accurate in patients with renal impairment, bilateral RAS, or with RAS in a solitary kidney.[45] Figures 49.5 and 49.6 show precaptopril and postcaptopril renograms from a patient with documented RAS and MR angiogram confirming the diagnosis (Fig. 49.7).

3.3. Positron emission tomography (PET) imaging

PET imaging can measure renal blood flow with use of ^{15}O-labeled water, ^{13}N-labeled ammonia, rubidium-82, and copper-labeled

Figure 49.5 Baseline captopril renogram (before captopril administration) in a patient with suspected RAS, showing bilateral symmetrical renal uptake.

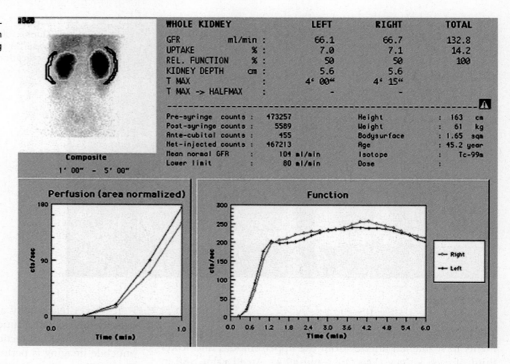

Figure 49.6 Postcaptopril administration after 48 h, bilateral reduction in GFR is consistent with bilateral renovascular disease; left kidney is affected worse than the right kidney.

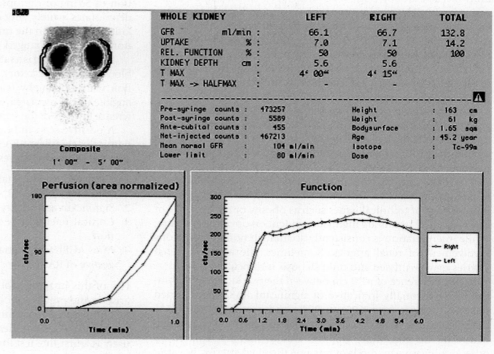

pyruvaldehyde-bisN4-methylthiosemicarbazone (PTSM) tracers. Renal blood flow can also be quantified using a modified microsphere kinetic model.[48] PET is not widely available, however, and the majority of these tracers require generation by an on-site cyclotron, further limiting their routine use for evaluating renal artery disease.

3.4. Computed tomographic angiography (CTA)

The introduction of multislice CT with three-dimensional (3D) reconstructions has made this method an important noninvasive means of identifying RAS and for evaluation after revascularization (Fig. 49.8). This modality can image the aorta at the same time.

The advantages of CTA are the following:

1. The size and shape of the kidneys and the presence of accessory renal arteries are easily diagnosed with contrast-enhanced CTA.
2. The degree of stenosis is usually classified as significant (>50% lesion) or nonsignificant (<50%) lumen narrowing; CTA accurately identifies the location of the lesion (ostial, truncal, and pseudotruncal)[52]; and degree of calcification is well visualized.
3. The related abnormalities associated with renovascular disease (e.g., poststenotic dilation, decreased size of the ipsilateral kidney, and delayed enhancement) corroborate the diagnosis of renovascular disease.[53]

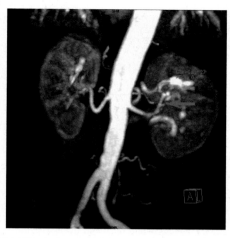

Figure 49.7 MR angiogram of the previous patient with gadolinium showing "beaded appearance" of the mid-distal segment of the left renal artery suggestive of FMD. Notice the smoothly narrowing, <50% luminal obstruction 4 mm from the origin of the right renal artery. Gadolinium uptake was delayed in the left kidney compared to the right kidney.

contrast medium. Because CTA of the renal arteries requires the use of 70 to 150 mL of iodinated contrast, the procedure is contraindicated in patients with severe contrast allergy. Furthermore, the use of contrast in patients with impaired renal function can result in contrast-induced nephropathy. The most effective means of preventing this is by prior hydration. With regard to image analysis, Rubin et al. showed that maximum intensity projection offers greater sensitivity (92%) than volume-rendering display (59%).[54] However, Johnson et al. showed that volume-rendering provides greater specificity (99%) than maximum intensity projection (87%).[55] Axial and spatial resolutions are improved with the use of a 64-slice CT scanner with <1 mm slice thickness. The use of 256-slice systems (currently used only for research) should further reduce the amount of iodinated contrast required to generate diagnostic-quality images.

3.5. Magnetic resonance angiography/magnetic resonance imaging

The evolution of MRA from flow-enhanced (time-of-flight or the phase-contrast) sequence to T1-weighted contrast-enhanced acquisitions (Figs. 49.9 and 49.10; Table 49.5) has increased

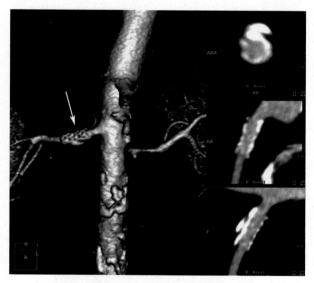

Figure 49.8 One year after right renal stent placement, a patient had a decline in BP control. An abdominal CTA was performed using automated trigger bolus at 125 Hounsfield units with the region of interest in the suprarenal abdominal aorta. 80 mL of Omnipaque 350 contrast followed by 50 mL of saline both at a rate of 4 mL per s were used for arterial opacification. The volume rendered image **(left)** confirms the presence of a right renal stent *(arrow)* in a calcific renal artery, and is also suggestive of mildleft RAS. Orthogonal curved planar reconstructions **(right)** examine the right renal artery relative to a reconstructed path in lateral, superior, and AP projections (1-mm thickness), and demonstrate a patent stent. (Adapted from Goldman C, Sanz J. CT angiography of the abdominal aorta and its branches with protocols. In: Mukherjee D, Rajagopalan S. *CT and MR Angiography of the Peripheral Circulation.*)

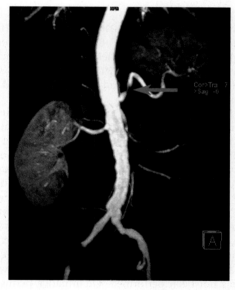

Figure 49.9 MR angiogram showing left RAS in a patient with accelerated hypertension.

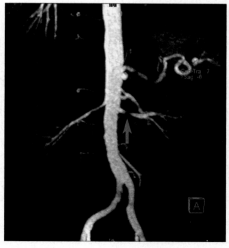

Figure 49.10 MR angiogram showing severe stenosis of the left renal artery *(arrow)* and positive "string sign."

4. Metal stents and in-stent restenosis are better imaged and show fewer artifacts with CTA compared to MRI/MRA.
5. CTA may help to accurately delineate distal lesions like FMD of the renal arteries.

One limitation to this imaging modality is that image interpretation may be difficult in heavily calcified arteries. Another major limitation of CTA is that it involves use of ionizing radiation and iodinated

TABLE 49.5

GRADING OF RAS BASED ON 3D CE-MRA AND 3D PHASE-CONTRAST MRA

Grade	3D CE MRA	3D PC MRA
Normal (0%–24%)	Normal	Normal
Mild (25%–49%)	Mild stenosis	Normal
Moderate (50%–75%)	Moderate stenosis	Stenosis ± dephasing
Severe (75%–99%)	Stenosis >75%	Severe dephasing
Occlusion	Optimum image quality but cannot find renal artery	Optimum image quality but cannot find renal artery

3D, three-dimensional; CE, contrast enhanced; PC, phase contrast; MRA, magnetic resonance angiography.
Source: Adapted from Dong Q, Chabra S, Prince MR, et al. MRA of abdominal aorta and renal and mesenteric arteries. In: Higgins CB, De Roos A, eds. *MRI and CT of the Cardiovascular System*. 1st Ed. Philadelphia, PA: Lippincott Williams & Wilkins; 2003:393–414.

the sensitivity (from 88% to 100%) and specificity (from 71% to 99%) for diagnosing RAS.[56-64] Both sensitivity and specificity are higher in patients with atherosclerotic RAS and lower in patients with FMD (Figs. 49.11A&B). Current MRA sequences offer shorter acquisition times and higher spatial and temporal resolutions.[65,66]

Renal Perfusion: MRA can quantify renal perfusion. The degree of renal perfusion depends on both the arterial flow rate and local factors, such as regional blood volume and vasoreactivity. Perfusion determination will vary according to the type of contrast agent used. Absolute quantification of parenchymal perfusion can be assessed with diffusible (i.e., Gadolinium or Gd-chelates)[67] or purely intravascular contrast agents (i.e., iron oxide particles).[68] Renal perfusion can alternatively be measured using pulsed arterial spin labeling (or spin tagging) using endogenous water as a diffusible tracer.[69] This technique can generate a perfusion-weighted image by the subtraction of an image in which inflowing spins have been labeled from an image in which spin labeling has not been performed. Quantitative perfusion maps can then be calculated when T1 of the tissue and efficiency of labeling are known. A 50% decrease of cortical perfusion has been described in severe (80%) RAS.[68]

Captopril-Enhanced Filtration Studies with Gd–MRA: Gd as a contrast agent behaves as a glomerular tracer. After the intravenous infusion of a bolus of Gd, it is possible to follow its intrarenal transit during breath holding. This transit begins with a vasculointerstitial phase producing a cortical, then a medullary enhancement of signal intensity also known as T1-shortening effect. The tubular phase is characterized by a drop of signal intensity (T2-shortening effect) within the external medulla that extends centripetally toward the papilla, and finally a ductal phase characterized by late low-signal intensity within the internal medulla and the renal collecting system. In RVH as with scintigraphy, the normal contrast kinetics are altered by captopril on the side of the stenosis, thus inducing a delay or disappearance of the tubular and ductal phases or a late T2 effect extending across the whole kidney.[70]

Blood Oxygen Level Dependent (BOLD) Imaging: This relatively new technology may be useful to evaluate renal

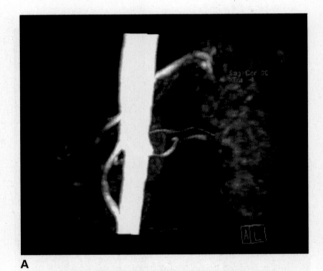

A

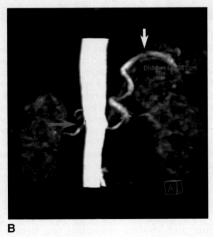

B

Figure 49.11 A, B: MR angiogram showing atherosclerotic narrowing of the origin of bilateral renal arteries (50% luminal narrowing of the right renal artery and 60% of the left renal artery). The renal arteries of both sides, starting from mid-distal segments also show changes suggestive of FMD.

physiology and pathophysiology, especially renal parenchymal disease. This modality uses the paramagnetic effect of deoxyhemoglobin also known as the BOLD effect, and has the benefits of producing angiograms without using iodinated contrast or radiation (compared to CTA or catheter angiography). Enhancement with Gd-based contrast has generally been replaced by noncontrast enhanced techniques due to contrast-associated nephrogenic systemic fibrosis in patients with moderate to end-stage renal failure.[71] A Food and Drug Administration alert limits the use of Gd in patients with reduced creatinine clearance (<30 mL/min).

MRI and gadolinium-based MRA are useful tools to monitor RAS patients both anatomically and hemodynamically after renal revascularization.[72]There are two important limitations of MRA/MRI. First, patients with metallic implants such as pacemakers, defibrillators, cochlear implants, metallic prostheses, and spinal cord stimulators are not candidates for MRI/MRA. Secondly, claustrophobic patients cannot be imaged in the regular MRI, and open MRI has limited availability.

3.6. Renal arteriography and digital subtraction angiography

These imaging modalities are the "gold standard" for diagnosing renal artery disease.[75] They should not be used as a screening tool for evaluation of RAS, but if other noninvasive tests are inconclusive, and in the setting of high clinical suspicion, catheter angiography is recommended. These tests may be ideal to evaluate FMD and lesions involving distal segments or branch points of renal artery. During angiography, pressure gradients can be measured across areas of stenosis to determine hemodynamic significance where there is doubt, and therapeutic procedures such as percutaneous transluminal angioplasty (PTA) or stenting can be carried out at the same time (Figs. 49.12 and 49.13).

As an invasive technique, there is a small amount of risk involved from the arterial puncture and from manipulation of the catheter and wire. Angiography uses iodinated contrast and therefore entails radiation-related risk. In patients at high risk of contrast-related nephropathy, including patients with renal impairment or contrast allergy, carbon dioxide (Fig. 49.14) or Gd may be used as nonnephrotoxic contrast agents.

3.7. Laboratory tests and other evaluation techniques

The presence of a positive laboratory test is helpful in diagnosing RAS when clinical suspicion is high (Table 49.5). The value of elevated plasma renin activity (PRA) to diagnose RVH is limited secondary to low sensitivity (57%) and specificity (66%) as well as high false negative (43%) and false positive (34%) rates. Elevated PRA could be present in 15% of all patients with essential hypertension.[75] Sensitivity and specificity are much increased when PRA is measured both before and 60 min after [captopril 50 mg Per Oral (PO)]. The false positive rate in patients with essential hypertension is 1.8%.[76-78] Another laboratory test, renal vein renin ratio, is the ratio of renin production from the renal vein of the stenotic kidney to that from the normal kidney. Renin production could be altered by some antihypertensive medications. If a patient is not taking an ACEI, it could be added prior to renin estimation to increase the sensitivity and specificity of the test. In unilateral RAS, a renal vein renin level >1.5:1 indicates a positive test. This test has limited sensitivity and specificity in

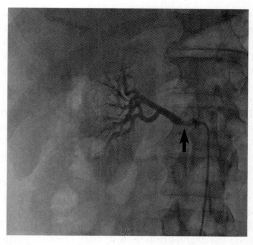
Figure 49.12 Renal angiogram of a patient showing hemodynamically significant right ostial RAS.

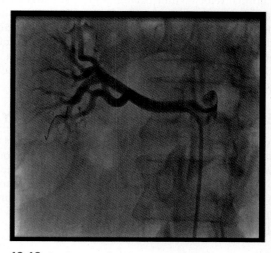
Figure 49.13 Angiogram showing successful stent placement in the previous patient.

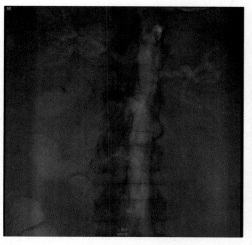
Figure 49.14 CO_2 renal angiogram of a patient with impaired renal function. The angiogram shows stenosis at the origin of the right renal artery.

identifying which patients with hypertension will show benefit after revascularization and how much benefit may be expected.

Anatomic Evaluation: The best anatomic evaluation is done by CTA and MRA. These can accurately diagnose the degree of RAS, the perirenal structures, and the abdominal aorta. Poststenotic dilatations (>20%) are considered a marker for severe RAS, although this has not been confirmed in any large clinical series.

Renal Parenchymal Changes: The renal parenchymal damage corresponds with severity and duration of RAS. Renal length difference between two kidneys >1 cm is a measure of significant renal parenchymal damage.[79] Revascularization is not indicated if any individual kidney length is <7 cm. Mounier-Vehier et al. showed that cortical atrophy measured by cortical thickness <8 mm or cortical volume <800 mm^2 are earlier to show changes before permanent damage.[80]

Renal Hemodynamics by MRI: 3D phase contrast MRI can discriminate the degrees of RAS. MRI signal intensity corresponds with flow velocity. Any obstruction in flow will result in severe dephasing in MR signals with these sequences. The degree of dephasing also correlates with the gradient across the obstruction. A normal velocity–time curve shows an ESP followed by an incisura, followed by a lower midsystolic peak (MSP). Mild RAS is defined by diminished height of ESP. Moderate RAS (>50%) is defined by complete loss of ESP and diminished height of MSP. High-grade stenosis corresponds with complete flattening of ESP and MSP and no or minimum systolic velocity. These results correspond to the angiographic findings.[81,82]

4. SELECTING AND GUIDING THERAPY

The goals of treating renovascular disease are to control BP in patients with RVH, to preserve or salvage kidney function, and to prevent flash pulmonary edema, recurrent angina, and heart failure. The modalities of therapy currently available are medical therapy and revascularization (either percutaneous or surgical). No large prospective randomized control trial has shown one modality to be better than another.

4.1. Revascularization

Revascularization is indicated for unilateral or bilateral RAS with at least 70% luminal narrowing and if at least one of following is present (Table 49.6):

TABLE 49.6

CURRENT INDICATIONS FOR RENAL ARTERY REVASCULARIZATION

1. Resistant or accelerated hypertension with more than three antihypertensive medications including a diuretic and presence of unilateral or bilateral RAS
2. RAS and recurrent acute pulmonary edema without any explainable cause
3. Dialysis-dependent renal failure and presence of hemodynamically significant bilateral RAS or unilateral RAS with a solitary functional kidney
4. Chronic renal insufficiency (creatinine >2 mg/dL) and hemodynamically significant bilateral RAS or unilateral RAS with a solitary functioning kidney.

Source: Adapted from Mukherjee D. Renal Artery Stenosis: Who to Screen and How to Treat? *ACC Curr J Rev.* 2003;12(3):70–75.

---

1. Inability to control BP with adequate antihypertensive regimen
2. Chronic renal insufficiency not from any reason other than bilateral RAS or unilateral RAS in a solitary kidney; in order to restore renal function by maintaining renal blood flow when medical therapy fails
3. Dialysis-dependent renal failure not from any reason other than bilateral RAS or unilateral RAS in a solitary kidney
4. Severe angina, recurrent flash pulmonary edema secondary to uncontrolled hypertension from RAS and not from active ischemia, and heart failure.

The current standard for revascularization in most patients is PTA with stent placement across the stenosis. Angioplasty without stent placement is commonly used for nonatheromatous involvement of renal arteries such as FMD. Revascularization by surgical reconstruction is generally done only in patients with complicated renal artery anatomy or in patients who require pararenal aortic reconstructions for aortic aneurysms or severe aortoiliac occlusive disease.

4.2. Medical therapy

The principle of medical therapy in renovascular disease is to control hypertension and treat secondary cardiac risk factors. Therapy may include lipid management with statins, use of antiplatelet agents such as aspirin or clopidogrel, cessation of smoking, and control of diabetes. Because the incidence of coronary artery disease is very high in these patient populations, they should undergo screening for coronary artery disease. Medical therapy is indicated for patients whether or not they are candidates for revascularization. After starting with one antihypertensive medication with optimum dose, if BP is not at goal, another medication from a different pharmacological class may be added. Combination therapy with multiple antihypertensive agents is required for most patients, with ACEI or ARBs, calcium-channel blockers, and β-blockers. Patients treated solely with medical therapy should have periodic (every 3 months) assessment of renal function, along with duplex ultrasound evaluation.

Patients with unilateral RAS should be started on an ACEI or diuretic and their dose should be titrated to keep BP at goal. For patients with bilateral RAS, ACEI should be avoided, as they can predispose irreversible renal failure. Studies done in patients with renovascular disease showed that captopril is effective in RVH in >90% cases.[83]

4.3. Percutaneous interventions

In 1978, Gruntzig first used percutaneous transluminal coronary angioplasty (PTCA) successfully in a patient with RAS to control hypertension.[84] Revascularization is indicated in patients with hemodynamically significant (>70%) bilateral RAS or hemodynamically significant RAS in a single functioning kidney, or if they have significant gradient (peak gradient >20 mm Hg and mean gradient >10 mm Hg). Percutaneous interventions in such patients may restore renal function or treat RVH unless irreversible damage has already occurred.

Patients who show significant improvement after revascularization are those who have bilateral RAS, with creatinine level >1.5 but <2.5 mg/dL, proteinuria <1 g/day, preserved renal length (at least >7 cm) and difference in renal length >1.5 cm, worsening of renal function with ACEI, and renal RI <80 (Fig. 49.15).

The benefit of revascularization in unilateral RAS with a normally functioning contralateral kidney is not well established. If the opposite kidney is functioning but still has parenchyma damage, there could be some benefit from intervention. Complete bilateral occlusion of renal arteries most often leads to irreversible kidney

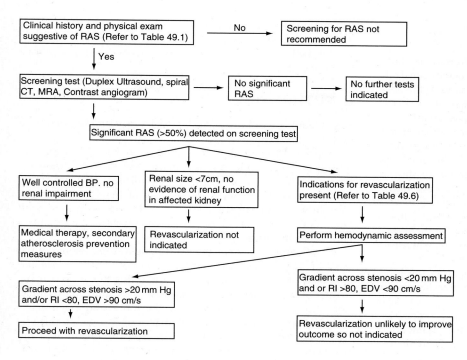

Figure 49.15 Flow diagram for imaging of renal artery disease. Algorithm for the detection and treatment of renal artery stenosis. RAS, renal artery stenosis; CT, computed tomography; MRA, magnetic resonance angiography; BP, blood presssure; RI, renal artery resistive index ([1-end-diastolic-velocity divided by maximal systolic velocity] x 100); EDV, end-diastolic velocity. (Reproduced with permission from Mukherjee D, *ACC Curr J Rev.* 2003).

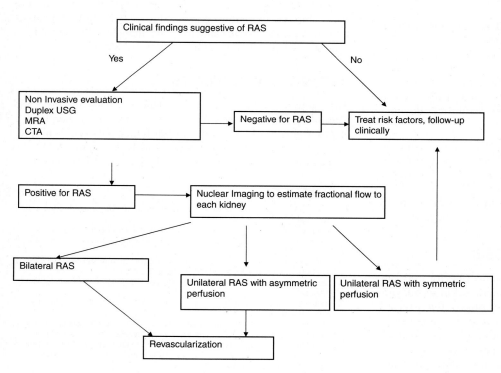

Figure 49.16 The sequential imaging modalities in a patient with suspected RAS.

damage, but some of the glomeruli could still be functioning based on perfusion maintained by collateral circulation (Fig. 49.16).

4.4. Medical therapy versus balloon angioplasty

A few small randomized controlled trials compared medical therapy with balloon angioplasty (BA) in hemodynamically significant RAS. The DRASTIC (Dutch Renal Artery Stenosis Intervention Cooperative) trial randomized 106 patients diagnosed with RAS involving at least 50% of the lumen, serum creatinine ≤2.3 mg per dL, and hypertension, to either medical management or BA.[85] BP reduction was statistically significant (systolic BP 179±25 to 169±28 mm Hg, $p < 0.001$; and diastolic BP 104±10 to 99±12 mm Hg, $p < 0.001$) in the angioplasty group compared to the medical therapy group. There was significant ($n = 22$, 44% of patients) crossover at the end of 3 months, from the medical therapy group to the BA group (14 patients with uncontrolled hypertension taking more than three antihypertensive medications and eight patients with worsening renal function). In this study, 16% of patients in the medical therapy group had significantly progressive RAS and occlusion. However, there was no significant difference in BP between the two groups at the end of 12 months.

4.5. Balloon angioplasty versus renal artery stenting

BA for atherosclerotic RAS results in high procedure success but a significant restenosis rate of up to 50%.[86,87] Bulky and calcified atherosclerotic plaques in the renal arteries often extend to the adjacent aorta. Angioplasty of these lesions without stents results in significant recoiling, which presents clinically as restenotic lesions.

On the other hand, few randomized trials comparing the results of renal artery stents have shown superior results compared to BA alone.[88,89] A study by Dorros et al. involving 85 patients with atherosclerotic RAS and hypertension showed higher procedure success rate, more cost effectiveness, and a lower restenosis rate (14% in the stent group compared to 48% in the BA group; $p < 0.01$). The BA group showed 90% patency at 6 months, 62% of BA patients required a stent placement, and 57% of patients required a second or third procedure, whereas in the stent group 12% patients needed a second procedure.

A meta-analysis by Leertouwer et al.[90] comparing the long-term effect of BA versus renal artery stent placement has shown superior results in the stent group (procedure success rate 98% compared to 77% in BA group, $p < 0.001$; restenosis rate 17% compared to 26% in BA group, $p < 0.001$). Overall, renal artery angioplasty is associated with major complications in about 10% to 15% of patients and a mortality rate of about 1%[91-94] and high rate of restenosis.[93]

BA is the treatment of choice for FMD as it provides high procedure success and relatively lower restenosis rate.[95]

4.6. Surgical revascularization

Renal artery surgery has complication rates of 8% to 11% and a death rate of 2% to 8%[91,96,97]; therefore, surgical revascularization is not commonly performed unless one of the following is present:

1. Recurrent restenosis or failed revascularization or complications during/after percutaneous revascularization procedure
2. Branch vessel disease or distal disease (such as FMD) not amenable to percutaneous revascularization
3. Simultaneous aortic surgery (aneurysm repair or severe aortoiliac disease) if not possible to repair percutaneously.

5. IMAGING AND PROGNOSIS

Doppler: Calculation of the end-diastolic velocity and renal artery RI from the flow velocities may predict clinical outcomes after renal artery revascularization. A value of RI >80 is associated with poor outcome after revascularization as it is suggestive of parenchymal disease, whereas a value of <80 is associated with satisfactory clinical outcome after revascularization.[41]

MRA: The 3D phase-contrast MRI method allows the measurement of renal blood flow distal to the stenosis. Binkert et al.[98] reported that a renal flow index (renal flow in mL per min divided by renal volume in cm³) of <1.5 mL/min/cm³ is a predictor of successful outcome of revascularization, the improvement of hypertension, renal function, or kidney survival after revascularization.

The following criteria, in general, can help determine whether a kidney is salvageable or not:

1. Sudden occlusion of a renal artery often results in irreversible kidney damage, whereas gradual occlusion will result in development of collateral circulation. Angiographic demonstration of collateral circulation on the side of renal artery occlusion is an indicator of viable kidney.

2. Renal biopsy showing well-preserved glomeruli.
3. Kidney size >9 cm.
4. Normal kidney function on intravenous pyelogram or isotope renography.

6. FUTURE DIRECTIONS

Several advances in imaging technologies may improve detection of RAS in the future.

Doppler Ultrasonography (USG): Doppler study with contrast agents (echo bubbles) is a method to increase diagnostic accuracy. The use of contrast agents will also give functional assessment of the kidneys by analysis of renal time-intensity wash-in/wash-out curves.[43] The use of ACEI such as captopril with Doppler USG as an agent for "stress test" increases the sensitivity and specificity of RAS.[99]

PET Imaging of Kidneys: Future applications of molecular renal imaging are likely to involve studies of tissue hypoxia and apoptosis in renovascular disease, monitoring the molecular signatures of atherosclerotic plaques, measuring endothelial dysfunction, and response to balloon revascularization and restenosis.

MRI/MRA to Evaluate Renal Arteries: The newer imaging technologies of noncontrast MRI with the use of breath-hold and navigator-gated noncontrast Steady State Free Precession (Nav SSFP) MRA protocols are equally effective for the evaluation of RAS compared to contrast-enhanced MRA (CE-MRA). Sensitivity and negative predictive value for detecting RAS with Nav SSFP is satisfactory with an acceptable specificity of 85%.[100]

ACKNOWLEDGMENTS

The authors would like to acknowledge Suman Jana, MD and Donna Gilbreath, MA, for their assistance in editing, Lisa Pauley, RT(R), James Buck, MD, and Carina Butler, MD for their assistance in retrieving the MRI images, and Partha Sinha, MD, who helped obtain nuclear images at the University of Kentucky.

REFERENCES

1. Conlon PJ, Athirakul K, Kovalik E, et al. Survival in renal vascular disease. *J Am Soc Nephrol.* 1998;9(2):252–256.
2. Kennedy DJ, Colyer WR, Brewster PS, et al. Renal insufficiency as a predictor of adverse events and mortality after renal artery stent placement. *Am J Kidney Dis.* 2003;42(5):926–935.
3. McLaughlin K, Jardine AG, Moss JG. ABC of arterial and venous disease. Renal artery stenosis. *BMJ.* 2000;320(7242):1124–1127.
4. Safian RD, Textor SC. Renal-artery stenosis. *N Engl J Med.* 2001;344(6): 431–442.
5. Keith TA III. Renovascular hypertension in black patients. *Hypertension.* 1982;4(3):438–443.
6. Hansen KJ, Edwards MS, Craven TE, et al. Prevalence of renovascular disease in the elderly: A population-based study. *J Vasc Surg.* 2002;36(3):443–451.
7. Harding MB, Smith LR, Himmelstein SI, et al. Renal artery stenosis: Prevalence and associated risk factors in patients undergoing routine cardiac catheterization. *J Am Soc Nephrol.* 1992;2(11):1608–1616.
8. Weber-Mzell D, Kotanko P, Schumacher M, et al. Coronary anatomy predicts presence or absence of renal artery stenosis. A prospective study in patients undergoing cardiac catheterization for suspected coronary artery disease. *Eur Heart J.* 2002;23(21):1684–1691.
9. United States Renal Data System (USRDS). *1997 Annual Data Report.* Bethesda, MD: U.S. Department of Health and Human Services, National Institutes of Health, National Institute of Diabetes and Digestive Diseases; 1997.
10. Choudhri AH, Cleland JG, Rowlands PC, et al. Unsuspected renal artery stenosis in peripheral vascular disease. *BMJ.* 1990;301(6762):1197–1198.
11. Missouris CG, Papavassiliou MB, Khaw K, et al. High prevalence of carotid artery disease in patients with atheromatous renal artery stenosis. *Nephrol Dial Transplant.* 1998;13(4):945–948.
12. Swartbol P, Thorvinger BO, Parsson H, et al. Renal artery stenosis in patients with peripheral vascular disease and its correlation to hypertension. A retrospective study. *Int Angiol.* 1992;11(3):195–199.
13. Wilms G, Marchal G, Peene P, et al. The angiographic incidence of renal artery stenosis in the arteriosclerotic population. *Eur J Radiol.* 1990;10(3):195–197.

14. Hunt JC, Sheps SG, Harrison EG Jr et al. Renal and renovascular hypertension. A reasoned approach to diagnosis and management. *Arch Intern Med.* 1974;133(6):988–999.
15. Meaney TF, Dustan HP, McCormack LJ. Natural history of renal arterial disease. *Radiology.* 1968;91(5):881–887.
16. Schreiber MJ, Pohl MA, Novick AC. The natural history of atherosclerotic and fibrous renal artery disease. *Urol Clin North Am.* 1984;11(3):383–392.
17. Tollefson DF, Ernst CB. Natural history of atherosclerotic renal artery stenosis associated with aortic disease. *J Vasc Surg.* 1991;14(3):327–331.
18. Wollenweber J, Sheps SG, Davis GD. Clinical course of atherosclerotic renovascular disease. *Am J Cardiol.* 1968;21(1):60–71.
19. Mailloux LU, Napolitano B, Bellucci AG, et al. Renal vascular disease causing end-stage renal disease, incidence, clinical correlates, and outcomes: A 20-year clinical experience. *Am J Kidney Dis.* 1994;24(4):622–629.
20. Dustan HP, Humphries AW, Dewolfe VG, et al. Normal arterial pressure in patients with renal arterial stenosis. *JAMA.* 1964;187:1028–1029.
21. Olin JW, Piedmonte MR, Young JR, et al. The utility of duplex ultrasound scanning of the renal arteries for diagnosing significant renal artery stenosis. *Ann Intern Med.* 1995;122(11):833–838.
22. Leadbetter W, Burkland C. Hypertension in unilateral renal disease. *J Urol.* 1938;39(5):611–626.
23. Olin JW. Syndromes that mimic vasculitis. *Curr Opin Cardiol.* 1991;6:768–774.
24. McCormack L, Hazard J, Poutasse E. Obstructive lesions of the renal artery associated with remediable hypertension. *Am J Pathol.* 1958;34:582.
25. Poutasse EF. Renal artery aneurysms. *J Urol.* 1975;113(4):443–449.
26. Novick AC. Renal artery aneurysm and arteriovenous malformation. In: Novick AC, Straffon RA, ed. *Vascular Problems in Urologic Surgery.* Philadelphia, PA: WB Saunders; 1982.
27. Sutherland RS, Spees EK, Jones JW, et al. Renal artery stenosis after renal transplantation: The impact of the hypogastric artery anastomosis. *J Urol.* 1993;149(5):980–985.
28. Kohler TR, Zierler RE, Martin RL, et al. Noninvasive diagnosis of renal artery stenosis by ultrasonic duplex scanning. *J Vasc Surg.* 1986;4(5):450–456.
29. Taylor DC, Kettler MD, Moneta GL, et al. Duplex ultrasound scanning in the diagnosis of renal artery stenosis: A prospective evaluation. *J Vasc Surg.* 1988;7(2):363–369.
30. Helenon O, el Rody F, Correas JM, et al. Color Doppler US of renovascular disease in native kidneys. *Radiographics.* 1995;15(4):833–854; discussion 854–865.
31. Strandness DE, Jr. Duplex imaging for the detection of renal artery stenosis. *Am J Kidney Dis.* 1994;24(4):674–678.
32. Conkbayir I, Yucesoy C, Edguer T, et al. Doppler sonography in renal artery stenosis. An evaluation of intrarenal and extrarenal imaging parameters. *Clin Imaging.* 2003;27(4):256–260.
33. Nchimi A, Biquet JF, Brisbois D, et al. Duplex ultrasound as first-line screening test for patients suspected of renal artery stenosis: Prospective evaluation in high-risk group. *Eur Radiol.* 2003;13(6):1413–1419.
34. Schwerk WB, Restrepo IK, Stellwaag M, et al. Renal artery stenosis: Grading with image-directed Doppler US evaluation of renal resistive index. *Radiology.* 1994;190(3):785–790.
35. Stavros AT, Parker SH, Yakes WF, et al. Segmental stenosis of the renal artery: Pattern recognition of tardus and parvus abnormalities with duplex sonography. *Radiology.* 1992;184(2):487–492.
36. Baxter GM, Aitchison F, Sheppard D, et al. Colour Doppler ultrasound in renal artery stenosis: Intrarenal waveform analysis. *Br J Radiol.* 1996;69(825):810–815.
37. Kliewer MA, Tupler RH, Carroll BA, et al. Renal artery stenosis: Analysis of Doppler waveform parameters and tardus-parvus pattern. *Radiology.* 1993;189(3):779–787.
38. Kliewer MA, Tupler RH, Hertzberg BS, et al. Doppler evaluation of renal artery stenosis: Interobserver agreement in the interpretation of waveform morphology. *Am J Roentgenol.* 1994;162(6):1371–1376.
39. Lafortune M, Patriquin H, Demeule E, et al. Renal arterial stenosis: Slowed systole in the downstream circulation—experimental study in dogs. *Radiology.* 1992;184(2):475–478.
40. Oliva VL, Soulez G, Lesage D, et al. Detection of renal artery stenosis with Doppler sonography before and after administration of captopril: Value of early systolic rise. *AJR Am J Roentgenol.* 1998;170(1):169–175.
41. Mukherjee D, Bhatt DL, Robbins M, et al. Renal artery end-diastolic velocity and renal artery resistance index as predictors of outcome after renal stenting. *Am J Cardiol.* 2001;88(9):1064–1066.
42. Radermacher J, Chavan A, Bleck J, et al. Use of Doppler ultrasonography to predict the outcome of therapy for renal-artery stenosis. *N Engl J Med.* 2001;344(6):410–417.
43. Lencioni R, Pinto S, Napoli V, et al. Noninvasive assessment of renal artery stenosis: Current imaging protocols and future directions in ultrasonography. *J Comput Assist Tomogr.* 1999;23(Suppl. 1):S95–100.
44. Williams GJ, Macaskill P, Chan SF, et al. Comparative accuracy of renal duplex sonographic parameters in the diagnosis of renal artery stenosis: Paired and unpaired analysis. *Am J Roentgenol.* 2007;188(3):798–811.
45. Fommei E, Ghione S, Hilson AJ, et al. Captopril radionuclide test in renovascular hypertension: A European multicentre study. European Multicentre Study Group. *Eur J Nucl Med.* 1993;20(7):617–623.
46. Geyskes GG, de Bruyn AJ. Captopril renography and the effect of percutaneous transluminal angioplasty on blood pressure in 94 patients with renal artery stenosis. *Am J Hypertens.* 1991;4(12 Pt 2):685S–689S.
47. Harward TR, Poindexter B, Huber TS, et al. Selection of patients for renal artery repair using captopril testing. *Am J Surg.* 1995;170(2):183–187.
48. Mann SJ, Pickering TG, Sos TA, et al. Captopril renography in the diagnosis of renal artery stenosis: Accuracy and limitations. *Am J Med.* 1991;90(1):30–40.
49. Prigent A. The diagnosis of renovascular hypertension: The role of captopril renal scintigraphy and related issues. *Eur J Nucl Med.* 1993;20(7):625–644.
50. Setaro JF, Chen CC, Hoffer PB, et al. Captopril renography in the diagnosis of renal artery stenosis and the prediction of improvement with revascularization. The Yale Vascular Center experience. *Am J Hypertens.* 1991;4(12 Pt 2):698S–705S.
51. Datseris IE, Bomanji JB, Brown EA, et al. Captopril renal scintigraphy in patients with hypertension and chronic renal failure. *J Nucl Med.* 1994;35(2):251–254.
52. Kaatee R, Beek FJ, Verschuyl EJ, et al. Atherosclerotic renal artery stenosis: Ostial or truncal? *Radiology.* 1996;199(3):637–640.
53. Fleischmann D. Multiple detector-row CT angiography of the renal and mesenteric vessels. *Eur J Radiol.* 2003;45(Suppl. 1):S79–87.
54. Rubin GD, Dake MD, Napel S, et al. Spiral CT of renal artery stenosis: Comparison of three-dimensional rendering techniques. *Radiology.* 1994;190(1):181–189.
55. Johnson PT, Halpern EJ, Kuszyk BS, et al. Renal artery stenosis: CT angiography—comparison of real-time volume-rendering and maximum intensity projection algorithms. *Radiology.* 1999;211(2):337–343.
56. Bakker J, Beek FJ, Beutler JJ, et al. Renal artery stenosis and accessory renal arteries: Accuracy of detection and visualization with gadolinium-enhanced breath-hold MR angiography. *Radiology.* 1998;207(2):497–504.
57. De Cobelli F, Vanzulli A, Sironi S, et al. Renal artery stenosis: Evaluation with breath-hold, three-dimensional, dynamic, gadolinium-enhanced versus three-dimensional, phase-contrast MR angiography. *Radiology.* 1997;205(3):689–695.
58. Fain SB, King BF, Breen JF, et al. High-spatial-resolution contrast-enhanced MR angiography of the renal arteries: A prospective comparison with digital subtraction angiography. *Radiology.* 2001;218(2):481–490.
59. Hany TF, Debatin JF, Leung DA, et al. Evaluation of the aortoiliac and renal arteries: Comparison of breath-hold, contrast-enhanced, three-dimensional MR angiography with conventional catheter angiography. *Radiology.* 1997;204(2):357–362.
60. Rieumont MJ, Kaufman JA, Geller SC, et al. Evaluation of renal artery stenosis with dynamic gadolinium-enhanced MR angiography. *Am J Roentgenol.* 1997;169(1):39–44.
61. Tello R, Thomson KR, Witte D, et al. Standard dose Gd-DTPA dynamic MR of renal arteries. *J Magn Reson Imaging.* 1998;8(2):421–426.
62. Thornton J, O'Callaghan J, Walshe J, et al. Comparison of digital subtraction angiography with gadolinium-enhanced magnetic resonance angiography in the diagnosis of renal artery stenosis. *Eur Radiol.* 1999;9(5):930–934.
63. Volk M, Strotzer M, Lenhart M, et al. Time-resolved contrast-enhanced MR angiography of renal artery stenosis: Diagnostic accuracy and interobserver variability. *Am J Roentgenol.* 2000;174(6):1583–1588.
64. Wilman AH, Riederer SJ, King BF, et al. Fluoroscopically triggered contrast-enhanced three-dimensional MR angiography with elliptical centric view order: Application to the renal arteries. *Radiology.* 1997;205(1):137–146.
65. Masunaga H, Takehara Y, Isoda H, et al. Assessment of gadolinium-enhanced time-resolved three-dimensional MR angiography for evaluating renal artery stenosis. *Am J Roentgenol.* 2001;176(5):1213–1219.
66. Van Hoe L, De Jaegere T, Bosmans H, et al. Breath-hold contrast-enhanced three-dimensional MR angiography of the abdomen: Time-resolved imaging versus single-phase imaging. *Radiology.* 2000;214(1):149–156.
67. Vallee JP, Lazeyras F, Khan HG, et al. Absolute renal blood flow quantification by dynamic MRI and Gd-DTPA. *Eur Radiol.* 2000;10(8):1245–1252.
68. Schoenberg SO, Aumann S, Just A, et al. Quantification of renal perfusion abnormalities using an intravascular contrast agent (part 2): Results in animals and humans with renal artery stenosis. *Magn Reson Med.* 2003;49(2):288–298.
69. Calamante F, Thomas DL, Pell GS, et al. Measuring cerebral blood flow using magnetic resonance imaging techniques. *J Cereb Blood Flow Metab.* 1999;19(7):701–735.
70. Grenier N, Trillaud H, Combe C, et al. Diagnosis of renovascular hypertension: Feasibility of captopril-sensitized dynamic MR imaging and comparison with captopril scintigraphy. *AJR Am J Roentgenol.* 1996;166(4):835–843.
71. Wiginton CD, Kelly B, Oto A, et al. Gadolinium-based contrast exposure, nephrogenic systemic fibrosis, and gadolinium detection in tissue. *Am J Roentgenol.* 2008;190(4):1060–1068.
72. Carlos RC, Prince MR, Ward JS, et al. Renal anatomic changes on magnetic resonance imaging and gadolinium-enhanced magnetic resonance angiography after renal revascularization. Original investigation. *Invest Radiol.* 1998;33(9):660–669.
73. Baumgartner I, von Aesch K, Do DD, et al. Stent placement in ostial and nonostial atherosclerotic renal arterial stenoses: A prospective follow-up study. *Radiology.* 2000;216(2):498–505.
74. Dong Q, Chabra S, Prince MR, et al. MRA of abdominal aorta and renal and mesenteric arteries. In: Higgins CB, De Roos A, eds. *MRI and CT of the Cardiovascular System.* 1st Ed. Philadelphia, PA: Lippincott Williams & Wilkins; 2003:393–414.
75. Bloch MJ, Basile J. Clinical insights into the diagnosis and management of renovascular disease. An evidence-based review. *Minerva Med.* 2004;95(5):357–373.
76. Canzanello VJ, Textor SC. Noninvasive diagnosis of renovascular disease. *Mayo Clin Proc.* 1994;69(12):1172–1181.

77. Mann SJ, Pickering TG. Detection of renovascular hypertension. State of the art: 1992. *Ann Intern Med.* 1992;117(10):845–853.
78. Wilcox CS. Use of angiotensin-converting-enzyme inhibitors for diagnosing renovascular hypertension. *Kidney Int.* 1993;44(6):1379–1390.
79. Zhang HL, Schoenberg SO, Resnick LM, et al. Diagnosis of renal artery stenosis: Combining gadolinimum-enhanced three-dimensional magnetic resonance angiography with functional magnetic resonance pulse sequences. *Am J Hypertens.* 2003;16(12):1079–1082.
80. Mounier-Vehier C, Lions C, Devos P, et al. Cortical thickness: An early morphological marker of atherosclerotic renal disease. *Kidney Int.* 2002;61(2):591–598.
81. Schoenberg SO, Bock M, Kallinowski F, et al. Correlation of hemodynamic impact and morphologic degree of renal artery stenosis in a canine model. *J Am Soc Nephrol.* 2000;11(12):2190–2198.
82. Schoenberg SO, Knopp MV, Bock M, et al. Combined morphologic and functional assessment of renal artery stenosis using gadolinium enhanced magnetic resonance imaging. *Nephrol Dial Transplant.* 1998;13(11):2738–2742.
83. Case DB, Atlas SA, Marion RM, et al. Long-term efficacy of captopril in renovascular and essential hypertension. *Am J Cardiol.* 1982;49(6):1440–1446.
84. Gruntzig A, Kuhlmann U, Vetter W, et al. Treatment of renovascular hypertension with percutaneous transluminal dilatation of a renal-artery stenosis. *Lancet.* 1978;1(8068):801–802.
85. van Jaarsveld BC, Krijnen P, Pieterman H, et al. The effect of balloon angioplasty on hypertension in atherosclerotic renal-artery stenosis. Dutch Renal Artery Stenosis Intervention Cooperative Study Group. *N Engl J Med.* 2000;342(14):1007–1014.
86. Plouin PF, Darne B, Chatellier G, et al. Restenosis after a first percutaneous transluminal renal angioplasty. *Hypertension.* 1993;21(1):89–96.
87. Sos TA, Pickering TG, Sniderman K, et al. Percutaneous transluminal renal angioplasty in renovascular hypertension due to atheroma or fibromuscular dysplasia. *N Engl J Med.* 1983;309(5):274–279.
88. Dorros G, Prince C, Mathiak L. Stenting of a renal artery stenosis achieves better relief of the obstructive lesion than balloon angioplasty. *Cathet Cardiovasc Diagn.* 1993;29(3):191–198.
89. van de Ven PJ, Kaatee R, Beutler JJ, et al. Arterial stenting and balloon angioplasty in ostial atherosclerotic renovascular disease: A randomised trial. *Lancet.* 1999;353(9149):282–286.
90. Leertouwer TC, Gussenhoven EJ, Bosch JL, et al. Stent placement for renal arterial stenosis: Where do we stand? A meta-analysis. *Radiology.* 2000;216(1):78–85.
91. Erdoes LS, Berman SS, Hunter GC, et al. Comparative analysis of percutaneous transluminal angioplasty and operation for renal revascularization. *Am J Kidney Dis.* 1996;27(4):496–503.
92. Pattison JM, Reidy JF, Rafferty MJ, et al. Percutaneous transluminal renal angioplasty in patients with renal failure. *Q J Med.* 1992;85(307–308):883–888.
93. Ramsay LE, Waller PC. Blood pressure response to percutaneous transluminal angioplasty for renovascular hypertension: An overview of published series. *BMJ.* 1990;300(6724):569–572.
94. Sos TA. Angioplasty for the treatment of azotemia and renovascular hypertension in atherosclerotic renal artery disease. *Circulation.* 1991;83(Suppl. 2):I162–166.
95. Slovut DP, Olin JW. Fibromuscular dysplasia. *N Engl J Med.* 2004;350(18):1862–1871.
96. Libertino JA, Bosco PJ, Ying CY, et al. Renal revascularization to preserve and restore renal function. *J Urol.* 1992;147(6):1485–1487.
97. Van Damme H, Lombet P, Creemers E, et al. Surgery for occlusive renal artery disease: Immediate and long-term results. *Acta Chir Belg.* 1995;95(1):1–10.
98. Binkert CA, Debatin JF, Schneider E, et al. Can MR measurement of renal artery flow and renal volume predict the outcome of percutaneous transluminal renal angioplasty? *Cardiovasc Intervent Radiol.* 2001;24(4):233–239.
99. Rene PC, Oliva VL, Bui BT, et al. Renal artery stenosis: Evaluation of Doppler US after inhibition of angiotensin-converting enzyme with captopril. *Radiology.* 1995;196(3):675–679.
100. Maki JH, Wilson GJ, Eubank WB, et al. Steady-state free precession MRA of the renal arteries: Breath-hold and navigator-gated techniques vs. CE-MRA. *J Magn Reson Imaging.* 2007;26(4):966–973.

Peripheral Arterial Disease

John P. Reilly

50

1. INTRODUCTION

Peripheral vascular disease can refer to all noncoronary vascular diseases in aggregate, but typically refers to vascular diseases of the lower extremities. Renovascular and cerebrovascular, including carotid disease, are typically each considered separately. Although public awareness of peripheral vascular disease remains disproportionately low compared to coronary and cerebrovascular diseases, it is equally associated with increased morbidity and mortality. The risk factors and therefore patient populations at risk for peripheral arterial disease (PAD) are similar for those with cardiovascular disease. Thus, the cardiovascular specialist must be familiar with the presentation, evaluation, and therapeutic options for patients with peripheral vascular diseases.

2. EPIDEMIOLOGY

The incidence and prevalence of PAD has been well studied in several populations at varying degrees of risk. An important determinant of the measured incidence and prevalence of disease is the definition used for the presence of disease. In fact, most people with PAD are ignorant of their disease and remain asymptomatic, thus those studies that rely on patient reported symptoms would underestimate the true prevalence of the disease. Some of these studies relied on patient reported symptoms, while other studies relied on noninvasive imaging as a more sensitive indicator of disease. The World Health Organization (WHO) Rose questionnaire is a standardized questionnaire developed to elicit and characterize claudication symptoms. The Framingham Heart Study employed the Rose questionnaire to identify those among its cohort of 5,209 men and women aged 28 to 62 years who had intermittent claudication.[1] The questionnaire was administered every 2 years, beginning in 1948. Among those 30 to 44 year old, the annual incidence of PAD, as defined by claudication by the Rose questionnaire, was 0.06% of men and 0.03% of women. This increased to 0.6% and 0.5% among men and women, respectively, between the ages of 65 and 74 years. The Edinburgh Artery Study examined 1,592 men and women aged 55 to 74 years of age. Symptoms of claudication were assessed using the WHO questionnaire, but the presence of disease was assessed using Ankle–brachial index (ABI) and change in ankle pressure after hyperemia. The 5-year cumulative incidence of PAD was 15.5 per 1,000 patient years.[2] A study of over 8,000 Israeli men followed over 21 years revealed an incidence of 4.3%.[3]

Criqui et al. examined the prevalence of PAD in an unselected population in southern California.[4] The University of California at San Diego had completed a population study on hyperlipidemia and recruited 613 patients from this cohort, about half of whom had hyperlipidemia. This study employed the Rose questionnaire, physical examination of bilateral pulses, and medical history in conjunction with noninvasive testing. ABI, Doppler flow velocities, as well as responses to hyperemia were measured in all subjects. Patients were defined as having large vessel PAD if their ABIs were ≤ 0.8, or flow velocity was abnormal. Using these noninvasive imaging criteria, the prevalence of large vessel PAD for the overall population was 11.7%. The National Health and Nutrition Examination Survey (NHANES) was a cross-sectional survey of over 9,000 subjects, and ABIs were obtained in 2,174 of them. This study defined an ABI ≤ 0.9 to be abnormal and diagnostic of PAD. Using this definition, the prevalence of PAD was 4.3% among subjects ≥40 years of age.

One of the largest cohorts studied to examine the prevalence of PAD was the PAD Awareness, Risk and Treatment: New Resources for Survival (PARTNERS) study.[5] Recruiting from 350 primary care practices across the United States, 6,979 patients underwent ABI to determine the prevalence of PAD. To be eligible for the study, potential subjects had to be 70 years of age or older, or between the ages of 50 and 69 years with a history of cigarette smoking or diabetes. A prior history of PAD was accepted as establishing the diagnosis or an ABI ≤ 0.9 during screening. In this population, the prevalence of PAD was determined to be 29% (Figs. 50.1 and 50.2).

The most common cause of PAD is atherosclerosis, thus, the risk factors for coronary artery disease (CAD) are shared with PAD. Hypertension, hypercholesterolemia, diabetes mellitus, and tobacco use, all increase the risk of developing PAD, as do unconventional risk factors like hyperhomocystinemia or elevated levels of C-reactive protein. However, the dominant risk factor for PAD is a history of tobacco use. In fact, smoking is two to three times more likely to cause PAD as compared to CAD.[6] Approximately 80% of patients with PAD are current or former smokers.[7,8] Smoking increases the risk of PAD and claudication from two to ten times as compared to those who have never smoked.[8–10]

Diabetes mellitus increases the risk of PAD to nearly the same degree as a history of tobacco use. Nearly one in five people with PAD has diabetes.[11] Diabetes is known to be a risk for CAD, including the smaller distal vessels. Similarly, among patients with diabetes and PAD, the smaller infrapopliteal vessels are more likely to be significantly involved. These smaller caliber, infrapopliteal vessels become diffusely diseased, which is why patients with diabetes are at increased risk of developing critical limb ischemia and of requiring limb amputation.[12–14] Some reports estimate that diabetics are at a 15-fold increased risk for lower extremity amputation.[15]

Each of the lipid abnormalities that are associated with an increase in atherosclerotic heart disease has been shown to increase the risk of PAD. Increasing levels of cholesterol are

Prevalence of PAD

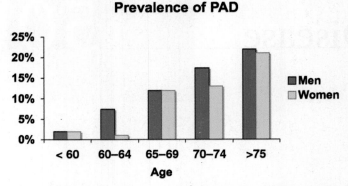

Figure 50.1 Prevalence of peripheral arterial disease (PAD). (Adapted from Criqui MH. The prevalence of peripheral arterial disease in a defined population. *Circulation.* 1985;71(3):510–515.)

Prevalence of PAD

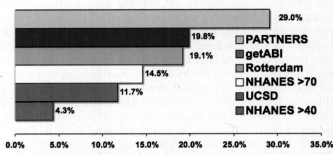

Figure 50.2 Prevalence of peripheral arterial disease across a series of population studies.

correlated with increasing incidence of PAD.[16,17] Lower levels of high-density lipoprotein (HDL) and higher levels of low-density lipoprotein are found in patients with PAD as compared to matched controls without PAD.[7,17,18] Although a causal relationship between hyperhomocystinemia and elevated C-reactive protein to atherosclerosis is less well established, both are associated with increased risk of PAD. Hyperhomocystinemia carries a two- to three-fold risk for PAD as compared to normal levels

of homocysteine.[19,20] The Physicians Health Study revealed that those with the highest levels of C-reactive protein were at twice the risk of developing PAD.[21]

3. CLINICAL PRESENTATION

The majority of patients with PAD are asymptomatic. This absence of symptoms is the underlying fact that determined the methods of prevalence studies that employed objective noninvasive studies, such as the ABI, to define the presence of disease. While Criqui et al. found a 11.7% rate of PAD by performing ABI, intermittent claudication was present in only 2.1% of men and 1.7% of women.[4] In the San Luis Valley Diabetes Study which included mostly Hispanic and white diabetic patients, PAD was defined by an ABI < 0.94. In this study a history of claudication was rare despite a 13.7% prevalence of PAD.[22] In the Edinburgh Artery Study, symptoms of claudication were present only 4.5% of the time.[23]

The classic symptoms of lower extremity PAD is claudication (see Chapter 19). Generally, there is sufficient blood flow at rest and the individual does not experience any discomfort. With the increased demand of movement or exercise, the individual with claudication experiences discomfort, pain, weakness, or fatigue in specific muscle groups. Most commonly, the calf muscles are the first to become involved, although these symptoms may then extend proximally. The muscle groups involved are determined by the level of occlusive disease. Stenosis of the common or superficial femoral artery produces claudication of the calf. If the stenosis is more proximal, such as terminal aorta or iliac disease, the individual will experience symptoms at the hips, buttocks, and thighs as well as the calf muscles. Those with infrapopliteal disease may experience pain or numbness of the feet, although, as there are three vessels below the knee, this disease must be extensive to produce claudication on the basis of isolate infrapopliteal disease. The examiner should carefully evaluate if the symptoms are asymmetric, that is, if one leg experiences discomfort to a greater degree or with a lesser effort, as PAD will often be asymmetric. Importantly, the symptoms are reproducible with similar levels of exertion and are promptly relieved with rest. Two classification systems qualify the severity of ischemia, Fontaine and Rutherford, and create a standardized language in which clinicians can communicate to one another (Table 50.1). Changes of body position

TABLE 50.1

TWO COMMONLY USED CLASSIFICATION SYSTEMS TO QUALIFY THE SEVERITY OF ISCHEMIA IN PATIENTS WITH PERIPHERAL ARTERIAL DISEASE

	Fontaine		Rutherford	
Stage	*Characteristics*	*Grade*	*Category*	*Characteristics*
I	Asymptomatic	0	0	Asymptomatic
IIa	Mild claudication	I	1	Mild claudication
IIb	Mod-severe claudication	I	2	Moderate claudication
		I	3	Severe claudication
III	Ischemic rest pain	II	4	Ischemic rest pain
		III	5	Minor tissue loss
IV	Ulceration or gangrene	IV	6	Ulceration or gangrene

will have no effect on vascular causes of claudication, and if the individual must sit down, or bend over to relieve symptoms, claudication is not the cause of the discomfort.

There are many causes of lower extremity pain or weakness that may be confused with claudication or "pseudoclaudication." Nerve root compression, spinal stenosis, arthritis, chronic compartment syndrome, venous claudication, and symptomatic Baker cyst may each present with symptoms that mimic true claudication. The astute clinician must be wary of elements of the history that suggest that the discomfort does not arise from insufficient circulation. Symptoms that are not promptly relieved by rest suggest arthritis, spinal stenosis, or radicular pain. Pain at rest may occur with arthritis as well as with symptomatic Baker cysts. Spinal stenosis typically requires a change in position, such as sitting down, leaning over at the waist, or bending over a shopping cart, to relieve discomfort. Intermittent claudication occurs at the same level of exertion consistently; radicular pain often occurs nearly immediately after onset of exertion, the pain of spinal stenosis may begin after prolonged standing, the onset of arthritic pain is variably related to exertion.

As opposed to the patient with claudication, the patient with critical limb ischemia (CLI) has insufficient perfusion to sustain the limb at rest; left untreated, such ischemia would require limb amputation within 6 months. Patients with CLI experience pain at rest, ulcers, and ischemic gangrene. Rest pain in CLI is often exacerbated when the patient is supine and may improve by dangling the foot over the edge of the bed, for example. Narcotics are often required for relief of pain. Patients with neuropathy, such as that which is secondary to diabetes or ischemia, may not experience severe pain despite presenting with CLI. Patients may present with CLI as their first manifestations of PAD, although patients who are followed for claudication may subsequently present with CLI. Atherosclerotic arterial disease is the most common cause of CLI, and this disease is frequently diffuse and affects more than one anatomic level. The infrapopliteal vessels are almost uniformly involved. Thromboangiitis obliterans (Berger disease), vasculitis, thromboembolic or atheroembolic events, and trauma, popliteal entrapment may also critically impair circulation and produce CLI. Vasospastic disease, severely low cardiac output states, and diabetes may all impair microvascular blood flow, thereby exacerbating CLI.

Careful examination of pulses is imperative during examination of limbs with critical ischemia in order to determine the likely level of stenosis or occlusion. When dependent, the extremity develops rubor that quickly blanches upon elevation, sluggish capillary filling is present. Livido reticularis suggests atheroembolic disease as a cause of CLI. Ulcers should be carefully examined; arterial ulcers are painful and tender to the touch unless neuropathy clouds the scenario. The surrounding tissue often has concomitant cellulitis. Venous ulcers are typically located over the malleoli as opposed to ulcers of arterial origin.

The presentation of CLI may be of acute or chronic onset and CLI typically refers to the latter; those patients with acute critical limb ischemia are managed significantly differently from those who present chronically, so they are distinguished as having acute limb ischemia. When obtaining the history from the patient with CLI, the duration and onset of symptoms are the most important elements of the history. There is an extensive potential for collateral development to the lower leg through the internal iliac and profunda femoral arteries. This collateral bed allows obstructive disease to develop on multiple levels before the balance is finally tipped in the patient with CLI and enough ischemia is present to threaten the limb's viability. Patients with acute limb ischemia, by contrast, have not had sufficient time to develop this collateral circulation when a sudden, new obstruction creates limb threatening ischemia. The distinction between acute limb ischemia and CLI is important because

the acutely ischemic limb must be recognized and urgently revascularized. Pain, paralysis, parasthesia, pulselessness, and pallor are the classic five "P's" that aid in identifying patients with acutely ischemic limbs. The ischemic limb is also subjectively and objectively cool (poikliothermia) to the patient and clinician, respectively.

Atheroembolic or thromboembolic disease is often a cause of the acutely ischemic limb as these phenomena produce a sudden obstruction to flow that may cause acute limb ischemia. At bifurcation or trifurcation points in the arterial system, there is a sudden reduction in the caliber of the vessel, as opposed to more gradual tapering in nonbranching segments. Emboli are commonly found in these bifurcations or trifurcations due to this sudden change in vessel caliber. The source of these emboli may be from the heart or aneurysms more proximal in the arterial tree. In situ thrombotic occlusion superimposed on pre-existing plaque is another mechanism for the sudden development of an ischemia producing lesion.

4. OUTCOMES

The natural history of limb ischemia has not been extensively studied. The limbs of patients who present with claudication generally have a good prognosis. Claudication in isolation does not increase the risk of limb loss through 10 years of follow-up.[24] Abnormal ABI and a history of diabetes mellitus were each a predictor of the development of ischemic ulcers or rest pain in these patients with claudication. By definition, patients with CLI are at greatly increased risk of limb loss. The number and extent of stenotic lesions, as well as the potential for successful revascularization, determine the likelihood of loss of limb. Patients with acute limb ischemia must be promptly evaluated for evidence of a threatened limb, such as paralysis or anesthesia, and referred for rapid revascularization as appropriate. Among patients who present with CLI, 25% will undergo major limb amputation within the following year.[25]

There is considerable overlap among populations with CAD, cerebrovascular disease and PAD. Atherosclerosis is a systemic disease that affects the entire vascular system. Approximately, one out of four people with CAD have vascular disease in multiple vascular territories.[26,27] Sixty percent of people with PAD also have evident atherosclerosis in coronary or cerebrovascular arteries. Patients with PAD are at increased risk for myocardial infarction (MI) and cerebrovascular accident (CVA).[25] The severity of PAD has been shown to directly correlate with severity of carotid artery disease, so the 40% increased incidence of ischemic neurologic events among those with PAD is not surprising.[28] The Edinburgh Artery Study confirmed this relationship between increasing severity of PAD and increased incidence of transient ischemic attacks (TIA) and stroke, a four to five fold increase compared to those without PAD.[29] The risk for MI is increased 20% to 60%, and there is a two to six fold increase in coronary death.[28-33] Those patients who present with CLI are arguably among the sickest patients across all specialties and subgroups. During the first year after presentation with CLI, the mortality rate is 25% and increases to as high as 45% in those patients with CLI who undergo limb amputation (Fig. 50.3).[33-36]

5. PATHOPHYSIOLOGY

Atherosclerosis is the most common cause of obstructive PAD worldwide. As was mentioned above, the usual risk factors for atherosclerotic CAD also increase the risk for PAD. Atherosclerosis is a systemic disease that effects the coronary and cerebrovascular circulations as detailed above.[25-27] As a systemic disease, it affects large and small vessels of the peripheral arterial

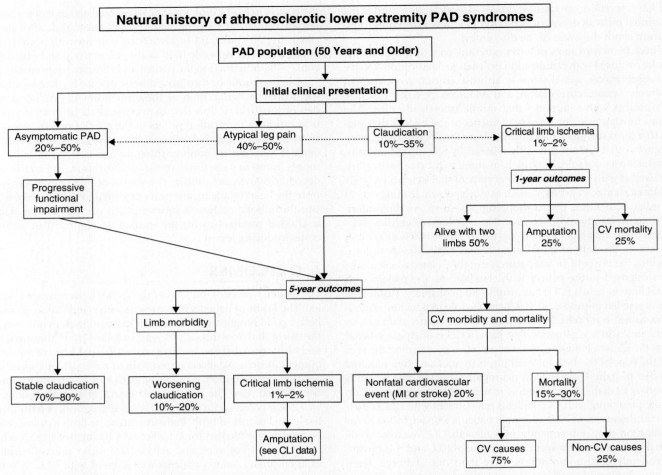

Figure 50.3 This algorithm demonstrates the natural history of PAD, the upper half describes the initial presentation with PAD. The lower half demonstrates outcomes 5 years after initial presentation. (Adapted from Hirsch AT, Haskal ZJ, Hertzer NR, et al. ACC/AHA 2005 Practice Guidelines for the management of patients with peripheral arterial disease (lower extremity, renal, mesenteric, and abdominal aortic): A collaborative report from the American Association for Vascular Surgery/Society for Vascular Surgery, Society for Cardiovascular Angiography and Interventions, Society for Vascular Medicine and Biology, Society of Interventional Radiology, and the ACC/AHA Task Force on Practice Guidelines (Writing Committee to Develop Guidelines for the Management of Patients With Peripheral Arterial Disease): Endorsed by the American Association of Cardiovascular and Pulmonary Rehabilitation; National Heart, Lung, and Blood Institute; Society for Vascular Nursing; TransAtlantic Inter-Society Consensus; and Vascular Disease Foundation. *Circulation*. 2006;113(11):e463–e654.

circulation. Other systemic diseases may also affect the circulation: degenerative, dysplastic, inflammatory, in situ thrombosis, and thromboembolism.

Several vasculidities can effect the peripheral arterial system at each level. The inflammatory response thickens the arterial wall with resulting obstruction. The aorta, and first- and second-order branches of the aorta may be affected by giant cell arteritis (Takayasu's), Behçet syndrome, and arthropathy associated vasculitis. Muscular arteries and their branches may be affected by Kawasaki disease, Wegener granulomatosis, Churg–Strauss syndrome, polyarteritis nodosa, or giant cell arteritis. Vasculitis of the smallest vessels occurs with systemic inflammatory diseases such as rheumatoid arthritis, systemic lupus erythematosus, serum sickness, and other autoimmune diseases. Obstructive disease in large- and medium-sized vessels affected by vasculitis may need to be treated by surgical or endovascular revascularization, however, the underlying inflammatory process must be treated with immune modulation. In small vessel vasculits, anti-inflammatory pharmaceutical therapy may be the only treatment.

Young smokers are the population at risk for thromboangiitis obliterans, also known as Buerger disease. The pathologic process results in obliteration of the smaller arteries and arterioles, typically the infropopliteal vessels. In some cases, superficial veins may be involved as well. Fibromuscular dysplasia is most commonly associated with renovascular disease, however, this dysplastic disease may also effect the carotid, vertebral, and iliac arteries.[37]

Thrombus plays an important role in the atherosclerotic process, both in situ thrombosis and embolic thrombus. Conditions that increase the propensity to form in situ clot include malignancies, inflammatory bowel disease, nephrotic syndrome, serum lupus anticoagulant, serum anticardiolipan antibody, protein C deficiency, antithrombin III deficiency, and mutations of factor V Leiden or of prothrombin.[38] Thromboembolic disease can cause symptoms due to arterial obstruction in patients with atherosclerotic arteries and in those with normal arteries of the lower extremities. The source of large emboli may be the left atrial appendage in those with atrial fibrillation, the left ventricle in cardiomyopathy or post-MI, or the aorta in patients with abdominal aortic aneurysm. Small emboli may originate from cardiac sources described above, from aneurysms of smaller arteries or from ruptured arterial plaque.[39–41] Embolic clot will typically become lodged at branching points in the arterial tree as these points result in rapid reduction in vessel caliber, often precluding the passage of the embolus. Thromboembolism is a discrete event as opposed to the development of atherosclerotic plaque. The sudden nature of the obstruction precludes the development of collateral circulation in patients who did not have sufficient obstruction to drive the development of collaterals prior to the embolic event.[40] Thus, many patients with acute limb ischemia have a thromboembolism as the underlying inciting event.

6. DIAGNOSTIC EVALUATION

A diagnostic algorithm for the evaluation of patients with suspected PAD is shown in Figure 50.4. The relative benefits and limitations of noninvasive diagnostic tests are summarized in Figure 50.5.

6.1. Ankle–brachial index

The ABI is the single most valuable diagnostic tool for the evaluation of PAD. It is simple to perform, noninvasive and risk free. The results of the ABI are both diagnostic of and prognostic for PAD. The cardiovascular specialist must understand the ABI and how it is performed (Fig. 50.6).

An ABI ≤ 0.9 is abnormal and diagnostic of obstructive peripheral arterial disease, therefore, an abnormal ABI has been used in epidemiologic studies as the definition for the presence of PAD. As discussed above, the UCSD study of hyperlipidemia, the NHANES and PARTNERS studies all employed the ABI as a screening tool to uncover the prevalence of PAD in their respective populations.[42] The ABI is inversely proportional to the degree of stenosis, or total "burden" of stenosis, and indirectly correlates with the severity of symptoms. An ABI that is ≤0.9 is consistent with symptoms of intermittent claudication, ABI measurements between 0.71 and 0.9 suggest mild obstruction, and those with measurements between

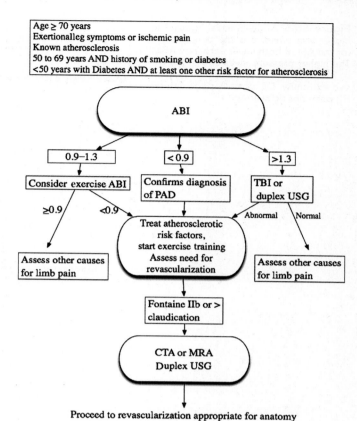

Figure 50.4 Diagnostic algorithm for the evaluation of symptomatic and asymptomatic patients at high risk for peripheral arterial disease (PAD). CTA, computer tomography angiogram; MRA, magnetic resonance angiography; ABI, ankle–brachial index; TBI, toe–brachial index.

	Benefits	Limitations
ABI	Can be office based Diagnoses presence of PAD when <0.9	Medial Calcinosis may produce non-compressible vessels (Diabetics, Renal failure, elderly)
ABI with Exercise	Increase sensitivity for Iliac disease Correlate symptoms with ABI	Requires treadmill
Duplex USG	Diagnose and image PAD Useful for revascularization patients Surgical graft surveillance	Pelvic vessels may be difficult to image due to bowel gas Dense Calcium may cause shadowing
CTA	Assess lesion anatomic characteristics Assess eligibility for revascularization Quick and Reproducible Imaging of stents and clips	Ionizing Radiation Iodinated contrast may
MRA	Assess lesion anatomic characteristics Assess eligibility for revascularization Stents produce artifact Implants preclude MRA (PPM, ICD, etc.)	May overestimate stenosis Stents produce artifact Implants preclude MRA (PPM, ICD, etc.)

Figure 50.5 Benefits and limitations of noninvasive tests used for the evaluation of peripheral arterial disease.

Figure 50.6 Ankle–brachial index. The higher arm pressure is the denominator for the ABI of both lower extremity ABIs. The higher pressure measured in the DP or PT is the denominator for their respective extremity. DP, dorsalis pedis artery; PT, posterior tibial artery.

$$Right\ ABI = \frac{Higher\ right\ ankle\ pressure}{Higher\ arm\ pressure}$$

$$Right\ ABI = \frac{Higher\ left\ ankle\ pressure}{Higher\ arm\ pressure}$$

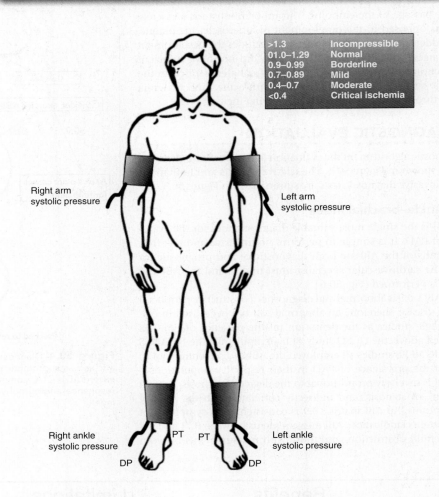

>1.3	Incompressible
01.0–1.29	Normal
0.9–0.99	Borderline
0.7–0.89	Mild
0.4–0.7	Moderate
<0.4	Critical ischemia

Right arm systolic pressure

Left arm systolic pressure

Right ankle systolic pressure

Left ankle systolic pressure

PT   PT

DP   DP

0.41 and 0.7 have moderate obstruction. Those patients with ABIs ≤ 0.4 have severe obstructive disease consistent with CLI. Although the ABI is proportional to the degree of obstruction, by itself it is not sufficient to make the diagnosis of claudication. The presence of symptoms in patients with obstructive disease is dependent on the strength of collateral circulation and the time course over which these obstructions develop.

The ABI can be readily performed in a physician office with a manual blood pressure cuff and handheld Doppler probe. The systolic blood pressure is measured manually in each arm, the higher value is then used as the denominator. Patients who have PAD may have obstructive disease of the subclavian artery, reducing the measured pressure, which is why the single highest pressure is used to calculate the ABI for both lower extremities. The cuff is then placed above the ankle, and the systolic pressures at the dorsalis pedis and posterior tibialis arteries are measured using the Doppler probe. The higher value measured at the ankle is then used as the numerator to calculate the ABI for the respective lower extremities. Performing the ABI can be done even more simply, using an automated blood pressure cuff.

Although the ABI is an excellent tool for the diagnosis of PAD, it is also an excellent predictor of all-cause mortality. In a study among the population of a university affiliated community hospital, McKenna et al. found that those with an ABI < 0.85 had a

relative risk for total mortality of 2.36 (95% confidence interval [CI] 1.60 to 3.48), after adjusting for other variables. As the ABI decreased, the mortality increased with a p value < 0.0001 for this trend. With respect to specific cause of death, the ABI was inversely proportional to cardiac death, not with noncardiac causes. Those with normal ABI had no increased risk of mortality and had a relative risk 1.14 (CI 0.78 to 1.61). Those with an ABI < 0.4 had a markedly increased risk of death, with a relative risk of mortality of 4.49 (CI 3.52 to 5.64).[43] These results were corroborated by Vogt et al. in a study of 1537 patients in the Systolic Hypertension in the Elderly Program, and about one quarter of the population had an ABI < 0.9 and these patients had an age- and gender-adjusted relative risk for total mortality of 3.8 (95% CI 2.1 to 6.9). The relative risk for mortality from CHD was 3.24 (95% CI 1.4 to 7.5), and for mortality from cardiovascular disease was 3.7 (95% CI 1.8 to 7.7). Results were similar when those who were known to have cardiovascular disease at the baseline exam were excluded from the analysis.[32]

If sufficient collaterals have developed to compensate for a stenosis, the resting ABI may be normal. Those patients with symptoms suggestive of PAD whose ABI is normal should undergo ABI measurement after exercise. The arteriolar dilatory response to exercise reduces vascular resistance, reducing the systolic pressure in the lower extremity, thereby lowering the ABI. In other patients, particularly those with diabetes or renal failure, the infrapopliteal vessels may become calcified and incompressible, artificially increasing the ABI. Thus, an ABI ≥ 1.3 does not exclude PAD. In these cases, a toe–brachial index (TBI) should be employed. Small cuffs are used to compress the digital arteries, which are spared the calcification of the infrapopliteal vessels, and the TBI is calculated in the same manner as the ABI.

As an extension of the ABI, the vascular laboratory may be asked to perform segmental pressure measurements. Plethysmographic cuffs are placed on the upper and lower thighs, and upper and lower portions of the lower legs. Analogous to the ABI, these lower extremity pressures may be indexed against the brachial artery. Segmental pressure measurements provide the additional information of localizing the stenosis; a pressure gradient between the brachial artery pressure and the upper thigh suggests aortic or iliac stenosis, when the gradient is between the upper and lower thighs, the lesion will be found in the superficial femoral artery (SFA). A 20 mm difference in pressures is generally accepted as significant.

6.2. Vascular ultrasound

The cardiovascular specialist is well acquainted with the merits and potential for ultrasound evaluation through their familiarity with echocardiography. Ultrasonography displays anatomic vascular details in grayscale images. In addition to displaying vessel lumen narrowing, plaque can be visualized, allowing the assessment of the degree of calcification (Fig. 50.7). Ultrasound also displays aneurysm, arterial dissection, lymphatic disease, soft tissue impingement, and popliteal entrapment. Although the imaging capability of ultrasound entices, combining this anatomic imaging with physiologic information derived by Doppler measurements of blood velocity, is what strengthens the role of duplex ultrasonography (see Chapter 3). Duplex ultrasound is widely available, relatively inexpensive, noninvasive, and risk free. When needed, it can be performed at the bedside for hospitalized patients. Imaging quality and interpretability is dependent upon the skill and effort of the ultrasonographer performing the exam, therefore may be variable.

Peak systolic velocities are measured at identified stenoses and in the segment immediately proximal to the stenosis (Figs. 50.8–50.10). If the velocity within the stenosis is twice that of the proximal segment, the lesion is interpreted to be at least 50% stenotic.[44,45] Some investigators have attempted to use velocity measurements to distinguish lesions between 50% and 75% and those between 75%

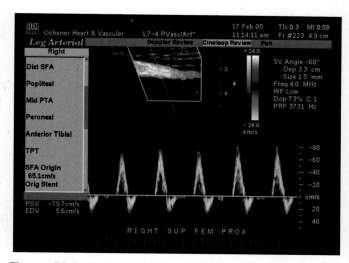

Figure 50.8 Pulse Doppler recording in the normal superficial femoral artery (SFA) demonstrates a velocity pattern that is similar to an invasive arterial tracing. With obstruction this pattern becomes blunted distal to the stenosis.

and 99%.[46,47] Totally occluded vessels have no flow, thus the Doppler measured velocity for 100% lesions is zero. The sensitivity and specificity for the detection of a ≥50% stenosis from the iliac to the popliteal artery is 90% to 95%. The diagnostic accuracy of Duplex imaging is impaired when the vessel is difficult to image, such as excessive bowel gas for pelvic vessels or dense calcification causing shadowing of acoustic waves. If significant tortuosity of the vessel causes the sonographer to obtain an inadequate Doppler signal, for example, if the Doppler probe is perpendicular to blood flow, the accuracy of the study will be negatively effected.

In most cases, the diagnosis of obstructive PAD can be made without duplex ultrasound, as history, physical exam, and an abnormal ABI should establish the diagnosis. Duplex ultrasound should be employed in those patients who may benefit from revascularization. From the ultrasound exam the location and degree of stenosis can be determined and can predict suitability for endovascular repair in 84% to 92% of cases.[48,49] Duplex ultrasonography has also been used to select the appropriate infrapopliteal vessel for distal anastamosis of surgical bypass grafts.[50,51] In patients who

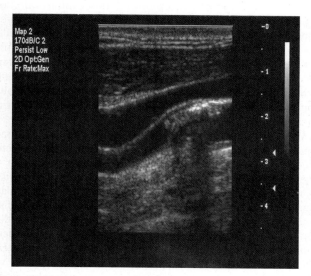

Figure 50.7 Vascular ultrasound demonstrating grayscale image of vessel as well as plaque present within the wall, although lumen is preserved.

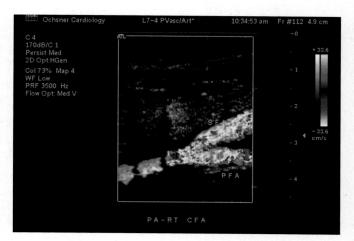

Figure 50.9 Duplex ultrasound of the bifurcation of the right common femoral artery (CFA) into the superficial femoral artery (SFA) and the profunda femoris (PFA). Color coding of Doppler derived flow velocities demonstrates turbulent flow at the bifurcation resulting in a mosaic of red and blue. This turbulent flow suggests stenosis at the bifurcation.

Figure 50.10 Color Duplex ultrasound on the left demonstrates a stent (*white arrow*) with focal in stent restenosis demonstrated by the turbulent flow (*thin arrow*). **Right panel** demonstrates increased velocity through the restenotic segment.

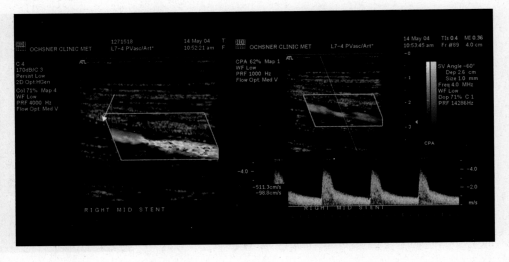

have had surgical revascularization with venous conduits, surveillance duplex ultrasonography is routinely employed in an effort to monitor graft patency. This surveillance is more sensitive for the development of graft threatening lesions than history, physical exam, or ABI.[52-56] In one report, grafts with abnormal duplex exams that were revised had a 90% patency rate at one year, that was similar to those patients with normal duplex exams at surveillance. By contrast, those with abnormal duplex exams that were not revised had a patency rate of 66%.[54] Although neither widely adapted nor studied, a similar policy of surveillance following endovascular intervention may improve long-term patency.

6.3. Computed tomographic angiography

With the development of multidetector computed tomography (MDCT) scanners noninvasive peripheral angiography has become possible. As the ability of the CT scanner to cover larger territories more quickly has improved, the scanner can keep up with a bolus of intravenous contrast dye as it flows through the aorta to the lower extremities (see Chapters 8 and 10). This test is minimally invasive requiring the insertion of an intravenous catheter in a superficial vein, typically in the antecubital fossa. As opposed to invasive angiography there is no requirement for observed recovery after the procedure and no risk of significant bleeding. Patients are still exposed to ionizing radiation and intravenous contrast dye and the attendant risks of these exposures. Patients with previous contrast dye allergies must be premedicated with antihistamine and steroids prior to undergoing CT angiography. A prior history of renal insufficiency, diabetes mellitus, contrast-induced nephropathy, heart failure, or dehydration increases the potential for contrast-induced nephropathy.[57-59] One report would suggest that intravenous contrast agent may be less deleterious to renal function than the intra-arterial injection required for traditional angiography.[60]

Unlike imaging with magnetic resonance (MR), the presence of implants, such as permanent pacemakers and implantable cardiac defibrillators, pose no contraindication for CT angiography. The presence of surgical clips or prosthetic joint implants may cause some artifact, however, this usually is limited to the immediate adjacent structures and does not prevent interpretation of the study.

CT angiography produces images that correlate well with conventional invasive angiography. Lawrence et al. performed single detector CTA in six patients suspected of PAD who were scheduled to undergo digital subtraction angiography (DSA).

Forty-eight arterial segments were compared from the inguinal ligament to the proximal calf. Twenty-six of twenty-eight occlusions or obstructions greater than 50% were correctly identified. This resulted in a sensitivity of 92.9%, a specificity of 96.2%, and diagnostic accuracy of 95.5%.[61] Riecker et al.[62] similarly examined single detector CT angiography with helical acquisition compared to DSA. Examining images between the groin and mid calf, CT angiography was 94% to 100% sensitive for the detection of occlusion and 98% to 100% specific. Sensitivity and specificity for the detection of stenoses ≥75% was 67% to 84% and 94% to 100%, respectively. Rubin et al.[63] compared CT angiography performed with a four detector CT scanner with DSA and found 100% concordance between the two modalities among the 24 patients studied. In addition, CT angiography successfully imaged 26 vessels that were not seen on DSA due to tight upstream stenoses producing slow flow. Similarly, Martin et al. examined 41 patients with both modalities and found an 87% sensitivity and 98% specificity for stenoses, while the sensitivity and specificity for occlusion was 92% and 97%, respectively. One hundred and ten additional segments were visualized on MDCT that were not seen by DSA.[64] Contrast injection for CT angiography occurs over 15 to 20 s, such that collateralized vessels and vessels that fill slowly due to stenoses have a greater opportunity to be visualized compared to short-duration contrast injections performed immediately before DSA acquisition. The interpretation of CT angiograms is bolstered by the ability to manipulate the acquired images to evaluate the angiogram in an infinite number of angles, even rotational digital subtraction angiograms have a finite number of angles that may be reviewed. In addition to the lumen of the angiogram, CT angiography allows evaluation of the vessel wall and the surrounding parenchymal structures (Figs. 50.11 and 50.12).

When performed properly, CT angiography can replace traditional invasive angiography; thus it is an excellent tool to define which patients are potential candidates for revascularization. CT angiography can identify the location and degree of stenosis. It provides excellent characterization of the lesion, length, diameter, side branches, plaque composition, and runoff vessels distal to the stenosis to be revascularized. In patients with an indication for revascularization, CT angiography should be considered prior to the procedure. CT angiography should also be considered when a vasculitis is being considered in order to evaluate the vessel wall, which cannot be performed by conventional angiography. Similarly, obstruction secondary to extrinsic compression,

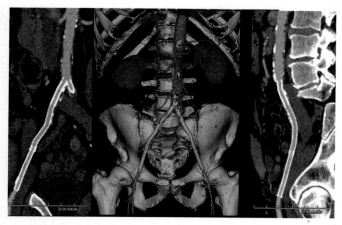

Figure 50.11 Middle panel: A three-dimensional reconstruction of the aorta through the abdomen and pelvis demonstrates bilateral iliac stenting from the origin or the common iliac to the distal external iliac. This image also demonstrates that the common femoral arteries are spared, and a benign angulation of the terminal aortic bifurcation which is amenable to revascularization. **Left and right panels:** Patent stents in left and right iliac arteries, respectively.

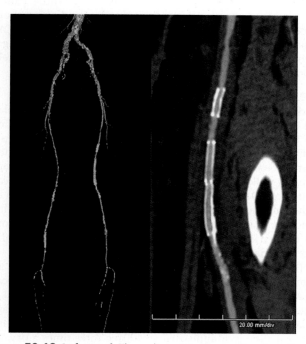

Figure 50.12 Left panel: Three-dimensional reconstruction of aorta with runoff angiography. The distal aorta through to the infrapopliteal arteries are displayed for evaluation, including left superficial femoral artery stents with mild in-stent restenosis, **right panel**.

such as popliteal obstruction secondary to a Baker cyst, can be readily evaluated by CT imaging, which is not restricted to looking at the lumen of the vessels.

6.4. Magnetic resonance angiography

Magnetic resonance angiography (MRA) can be used to evaluate for the location and degree of stenosis. Unlike CT angiography, MRA depicts the vessels, more similar to conventional angiography. Several techniques are employed to allow MRA, two-dimensional time of flight, three-dimensional imaging, bolus chase, and contrast-enhanced imaging with gadolinium. Recently, gadolinium

has been implicated as the cause of nephrogenic systemic fibrosis (NSF), which is a debilitating disease that affects the skin, muscle, and internal organs. While gadolinium had once been considered a less nephrotoxic option for digital subtraction angiography, patients with acute or chronic renal insufficiency with a glomerular filtration rate less than 30 mL/min should not receive gadolinium. Thus, a noncontrasted technique or another imaging modality should be employed.

Comparison of MRA and conventional angiography reveals a high degree of correlation. The sensitivity and specificity of MRA to detect lesions more than 50% obstructed have been reported between 90% and 100% using conventional angiography as the control.[65] As discussed above about CTA, some reports suggest that MRA may be a better test to demonstrate the patency of infrapopliteal vessels in patients with CLI. In twenty-four patients with diabetes and CLI, nearly 40% had pedal vessels, which had escaped detection by conventional angiography.[66] Other reports dispute this claim, and it is logical that the basis of this claim is dependent upon the quality of each study.[67–69]

MRA does not require exposure to the ionizing radiation that CT and conventional angiography require. Also, iodinated contrast must be used for all conventional and CT angiograms. While the safety of gadolinium for contrast enhancement is now in doubt, by employing newer imaging pulse sequences, MRA can be accomplished without the injection of an intravenous contrast agent. Patients with permanent pacemakers, implanted defibrillators, and some cerebral clips preclude performing an MR exam. Metal clips and stents may cause sufficient artifact to significantly reduce accuracy. Turbulent flow in a stenosis may cause overestimation of severity. Retrograde collateral flow may create significant artifact in time of flight studies.

MRA and CT angiography provide the same information, the location and degree of stenosis, with the caveats mentioned above. The degree of accuracy when compared to conventional angiography is similar. A comparison of MRA with gadolinium with CT angiography with a 16-slice scanner reveals greater interobserver agreement for MRA.[70,71] Calcification impaired interobserver agreement, particularly in infrapopliteal vessels in CTA studies. This as well as the ability to repeat image acquisition multiple times after contrast injections to evaluate collateral flow without the need for added radiation exposures, are advantages of MRA. Higher spatial resolution for visualization of small caliber vessels and ease of acquisition, on the other hand, are superior advantages of CTA.

7. TREATMENT

Atherosclerosis is the dominant cause of PAD and is a systemic disease. Patients with PAD have an increased risk of cardiovascular events, such as death, MI, and stroke.[25–32] Treatment of their underlying cardiovascular risk factors is of paramount importance in reducing the morbidity and mortality among patients with PAD. This treatment should include therapy for lipid abnormalities, hypertension, and diabetes. Lifestyle modification should include daily aerobic exercise and elimination of cigarette smoking. These treatments are beneficial for all patients with PAD regardless of clinical scenario: asymptomatic or claudication.

Patients with PAD are regarded as "high risk" for future cardiovascular event when considering the National Cholesterol Education Program Adult Treatment Panel III guidelines for lipid therapy. The goal of treatment is to achieve an LDL of 100 mg/dL, although if PAD is associated with other risk factors for atherosclerosis, that goal should be less than 70 mg/dL. Statin therapy reduces the likelihood of MI and death due to cardiovascular cause by approximately 30%.[72] Retrospective analysis of the Scandanavian Simvastatin Survival Study found that the development or worsening of claudication was reduced with simvastatin, a result that was supported in a prospective trial of atorvastatin which found that the walking distance to the onset of claudication was longer on statin therapy.[73,74] Antihypertensive therapy reduces the risk of stroke, heart failure, and death so should be used when treating patients with PAD. There is no evidence that beta-blockers adversely effect claudicants, as they have been shown to reduce the risk of MI and death they should be prescribed as indicated. Angiotensin-converting enzyme inhibitors were studied in the Heart Outcomes Prevention Evaluation study, including more than 4,000 patients with PAD. Ramipril reduced the risk of major adverse cardiovascular event by 25%, as it did in the overall population.[75] Caution is advised when treating patients with CLI, as distal perfusion may be dependent upon blood pressure. Those patients with PAD who quit smoking have a lower risk of death, MI, and amputation than those who continue to smoke, so smoking cessation must be encouraged.[76]

Antiplatelet therapy is a cornerstone treatment for atherosclerotic diseases. Antiplatelet therapy produces a 22% reduction in odds of MI, stroke, or vascular death among patients with PAD.[77] This benefit is equally shared among claudicants, those with endovascular or surgical revascularization. An analysis of a spectrum of aspirin doses revealed that although higher doses of aspirin resulted in greater reductions in vascular events, this was at the expense of increased intracranial or gastrointestinal bleeding.[77] Doses smaller than 75 mg did not afford significant protection against vascular events, and doses greater than 325 mg significantly increased bleeding risk, so 75 to 325 mg should be prescribed to patients with lower extremity PAD. One prospective trial compared aspirin to clopidogrel in patients with a history of vascular disease. The event rate for cardiovascular events was reduced by 8.7%; among PAD patients, clopidogrel reduced this risk by 24% more than aspirin.[78] This additional benefit was achieved without increased bleeding risk. Patients with PAD should receive antiplatelet therapy, aspirin, or clopidogrel, to reduce their risk of MI, stroke, and vascular death.

Antcoagulation therapy with warfarin or derivative thereof has not been shown to be beneficial on balance. There is a paucity of data specifically addressing anticoagulation therapy for PAD, although much may be inferred from data on CAD. Again, the risk reduction for vascular events is coupled with increased risk of bleeding. Treatment with goal International Normalized Ratio (INR) of 2.8 to 4.8 was associated with a 4.5-fold increase in major bleeding, although a significant reduction for death and for MI was achieved. With goal INR between 2 and 3, no significant reduction was achieved for stroke or death nor for MI, but bleeding increased nearly eightfold.[79] One trial specifically examining the benefit of aspirin versus warfarin for infrainguinal graft patency showed no significant difference.

7.1. Management of asymptomatic patients

Unlike the ischemia discovered by an abnormal stress test, an abnormal ABI or other noninvasive vascular study does not demand specific treatment. Aside from the lifestyle and risk factor modifications discussed in Section 7, there is no therapy indicated for the patient without symptoms or signs of lower extremity PAD. Some patients with PAD will have concomitant neuropathy which may be secondary to diabetes or their PAD. The feet of these patients should be carefully examined for signs of CLI, such as absent pulses, ulcer, or gangrene.

7.2. Management of symptomatic patients

7.2.1. Exercise training

For patients with discomfort in the legs when walking, claudication, the initial treatment is more walking. In the most recent ACC/AHA guidelines for the treatment of PAD, exercise training receives a Class I indication as the initial treatment modality for patients with claudication.[80,81] The mechanisms for the benefit derived from exercise training are not completely understood, are likely multifactorial, and include improvement in muscle metabolism, endothelial function, muscular strength, and alteration in gait. Exercise[82] training results in improvement in pain-free walking time and maximal walking time. In order to be of benefit, exercise must be performed for at least 30 min and occur at least three times a week. Benefit has been reported to occur as early as 1 month after initiating training and to continue to improve for 6 months. Treadmill exercise is the best form of exercise to relieve lower extremity claudication; treadmill speed and resistance should initially be set to provoke claudication at three to five minutes. When the patient develops moderate claudication, the patient is allowed to rest until symptoms resolve and then should exercise again. As the population with claudication frequently has concomitant CAD, an exercise stress test should be performed prior to initiating exercise training. Those patients who develop ischemia prior to limitation by claudication should undergo appropriate further evaluation for obstructive CAD. Supervised exercise is considered superior to patients walking on their own, and this can be accommodated in most cardiac rehabilitation programs.

7.2.2. Pharmacologic therapy

Cilostazol is a phosphodiesterase inhibitor, and it inhibits platelets and vasodilates. It has been shown to have beneficial effects on HDL and triglycerides. Cilostazol has also been shown to inhibit smooth muscle cell proliferation and reduce restenosis after coronary intervention.[82] Cilostazol has also been shown to improve walking distance by 40% to 60%.[83] Patients are typically started on 50 mg twice daily and increased to 100 mg twice a day if the individual is tolerant of the side effects, which may include headache, diarrhea, palpitations, and dizziness. Cilostazol should not be used in patients with heart failure as there is a potential for excess mortality (FDA black box warning).

Pentoxifylline is a derivative of methylxanthine that acts as a hemorheologic agent. It has been shown to have a statistically significant improvement in pain-free and maximal walking distances.[84,85] The magnitude of benefit is not as great as that of cilostazol, thus it is considered a second line agent to cilostazol. Pentoxifylline is administered as 400 mg three times a day, and has no black box warning. It is generally well tolerated although dyspepsia, nausea, diarrhea, and sore throat have been reported.

7.2.3. Revascularization

Patients with intermittent claudication that limits their vocation or activities important to their lifestyle (Fontaine IIb) may be considered for revascularization therapy. As discussed above, ACC/AHA guidelines recommend a trial of exercise training and pharmacologic therapy as initial therapy for claudication.

Individuals with Fontaine IIb claudication who are considered for revasclarization will undergo further diagnostic testing to determine if they are eligible for revascularization and for which type of revascularization they may be eligible. If surgical revascularization is being considered, then identification of the level of stenosis and the patency of the runoff vessels distal to the anticipated point of distal anastamosis is sufficient information.

A surgical bypass creates a proximal anastamosis in a segment that is relatively spared, and then creates a distal anastomosis that is also similarly spared. The exact length, degree, and morphology of the stenosis are less important considerations. Identification of healthy segments for anastomosis and good runoff of the infrapopliteal vessels are important determinants of short- and long-term successes. Duplex ultrasound and segmental pressures will localize the level and degree of stenosis, but to fully evaluate the patient for revascularization an angiogram is necessary. When considering endovascular revascularization, the exact location, length, degree, and morphology of the stenosis are important predictors of success. In addition, tortuosity of vessels proximal to the lesion and the angulation of the aortic bifurcation having an appropriate vessel to obtain vascular access determine the technical difficulty for endovascular revascularization. Angiography will provide these details to decipher the likelihood of success for endovascular therapy. A noninvasive angiogram with CTA or MRA provides this roadmap to identify which patients should not be offered endovascular therapy before performing an invasive angiogram. The relative merits and faults of these two techniques are discussed earlier in the chapter, but the experience with each technique at the practitioner's institution will be an important determinant of which modality to use.

Endovascular treatment of PAD employs expanding balloons and stents most commonly, although mechanical and laser atherectomy, cutting balloons, cryoangioplasty, and thrombectomy are used as adjunctive therapies. Technology for endovascular therapy continues to improve and evolve. The common iliac artery has the most durable results after endovascular therapy; the response and durability worsen, the more distal in the vascular tree the intervention is performed. Lesion specific characteristics such as longer lesions, serial stenoses, and poor runoff vessels distal to the point of balloon or stent predict poor long-term success. Smoking, renal failure, and diabetes are patient characteristics that are also associated with lower durability of results. The Trans-Atlantic Society Consensus (TASC) Working Group developed a scheme to classify lesions, categorizing them into which may be most appropriate for endovascular therapy and which may be most appropriate for surgical revascularization. These categories are meant to reflect the relative likelihood for success and of risk, thus this scheme provides a good framework, but the expertise of the operator may increase or decrease the likelihood of success, thus affecting the decision for surgical versus endovascular therapy.

Surgical revascularization is associated with greater morbidity and mortality than percutaneous endovascular procedures.[86,87] The threshold to operate on an individual for claudication, then, is higher as compared to PTA/stent. An appropriate preoperative evaluation should be performed, given the high prevalence of coronary and cerebrovascular diseases in this population.[26,27] As with endovascular therapy, surgical therapy for iliac disease has a higher likelihood of long-term success than bypass for femoral artery disease, particularly if the distal anastomosis is below the knee. The conduit material is also an important determinant of success for femoral artery bypass; autologous vein having better durability then polytetrafluoroethylene (PTFE) synthetic graft. The 5-year patency rate for venous bypass grafts is 80%, for PTFE with distal anastomosis above the knee 75%, and for PTFE with a distal anastomosis below the knee 65%.[88]

Patients who present with CLI frequently have critical stenoses at more than one level of the vascular tree, iliac, and femoral, or femoral and tibial. Due to the extensive nature of the disease, both methods of revascularization face a greater challenge to restore flow. CLI progresses to tissue necrosis, thus evaluation and treatment for CLI must be rapid. Patients who present with acute limb threatening ischemia must be evaluated and treated on an emergent basis, with efforts to achieve complete revascularization to the foot promptly. Patients who present with subacute or chronic CLI should be treated promptly, but may not require emergent revascularization. These patients may initially be treated for upstream or inflow stenosis, and subsequently undergo revascularization of outflow stenosis. For all patients with CLI, the arterial anatomy, clinical presentation, and comorbid conditions will determine whether surgical or endovascular therapy is initiated in efforts to salvage the limb.

8. FUTURE DIRECTIONS

Peripheral arterial disease is a significant cause of morbidity, and due to the prevalence of coexisting coronary and cerebrovascular diseases, patients with PAD are at increased risk for mortality. The cardiovascular specialist must be cognizant of PAD and its presentations, and remain vigilant for evidence of its presence. The physician who is well versed in PAD and the techniques for the evaluation thereof will gain insight into the patient's vascular health. Imaging methods have revolutionized the detection and management of PAD. The ABI is one of the most cost-effective methods, easy to apply to large-scale populations, and able to predict not only limb outcomes but also cardiac and neurovascular events. Efforts should continue to incorporate the ABI as a routine component of a routine health assessment in middle age and elderly men and women with cardiovascular risk factors. Once the disease is established, advanced three-dimensional anatomical imaging with CT and MR should be aimed to be performed using less contrast in the future. Further validation of dynamic imaging protocols may help very soon to evaluate limb perfusion and anatomy reliably within a single study.

REFERENCES

1. Kannel WB, Skinner JJJ, Schwartz MJ. Intermittent claudication: Incidence in the Framingham Study. *Circulation.* 1970;41:875–883.
2. Leng GC, Lee AJ, Fowkes FG, et al. Incidence, natural history and cardiovascular events in symptomatic and asymptomatic peripheral arterial disease in the general population. *Int J Epidemiol.* 1996;25(6):1172–1181.
3. Bowlin SJ, Medalie JH, Flocke SA, et al. Intermittent claudication in 8343 men and 21-year specific mortality follow-up. *Ann Epidemiol.* 1997;7(3):180–187.
4. Criqui MH. The prevalence of peripheral arterial disease in a defined population. *Circulation.* 1985;71(3):510–515.
5. Hirsch AT. Peripheral arterial disease detection, awareness and treatment in primary care. *JAMA.* 2001;286(11):1317–1324.
6. Price JF, Mowbray PI, Lee AJ, et al. Relationship between smoking and cardiovascular risk factors in the development of peripheral arterial disease and coronary artery disease: Edinburgh Artery Study. *Eur Heart J.* 1999;20:344–353.
7. Meijer WT, Hoes AW, Rutgers D, et al. Peripheral arterial disease in the elderly: The Rotterda Study. *Arterioscler Thromb Vasc Biol.* 1998;18:185–192.
8. Smith GD, Shipley MJ, Rose G. Intermittent claudication, heart disease risk factors, and mortality. The Whitehall Study. *Circulation.* 1990;82:1925–1931.
9. Bowlin SJ, Medalie JH, Flocke SA, et al. Epidemiology of intermittent claudication in middle-aged men. *Am J Epidemiol.* 1994;140:418–430.
10. Kannel WB, McGee DL. Update on some epidemiologic features of intermittent claudication: The Framingham Study. *J Am Geriatr Soc.* 1985;33(1):13–18.
11. Hiatt WR, Hoag S, Hamman RF. Effect of diagnostic criteria on the prevalence of peripheral arterial disease. The San Luis Valley Diabetes Study. *Circulation.* 1995;91:1472–1479.
12. Dormandy JA, Murray GD. The fate of the claudicant–a prospective study of 1969 claudicants. *Eur J Vasc Surg.* 1991;5(2):131–133.
13. McDaniel MD, Cronenwett JL. Basic data related to the natural history of intermittent claudication. *Ann Vasc Surg.* 1989;3(3):273–277.
14. Most RS, Sinnock P. The epidemiology of lower extremity amputations in diabetic individuals. *Diabetes Care.* 1983;6(1):87–91.
15. Bild DE, Selby JV, Sinnock P, et al. Lower-extremity amputation in people with diabetes. Epidemiology and prevention. *Diabetes Care.* 1989;12(1):24–31.
16. Ingolfsson IO, Sigurdsson G, Sigvaldason H, et al. A marked decline in the prevalence and incidence of intermittent claudication in Icelandic men 1968–1986: A strong relationship to smoking and serum cholesterol–the Reykjavik Study. *J Clin Epidemiol.* 1994;47(11):1237–1243.

17. Murabito JM, D'Agostino RB, Silbershatz H, et al. Intermittent claudication. A risk profile from The Framingham Heart Study. *Circulation.* 1997;96:44–49.
18. Horby J, Grande P, Vestergaard A, et al. High density lipoprotein cholesterol and arteriography in intermittent claudication. *Eur J Vasc Surg.* 1989;3:333–337.
19. Boushey CJ, Beresford SA, Omenn GS, et al. A quantitative assessment of plasma homocysteine as a risk factor for vascular disease. Probable benefits of increasing folic acid intakes. *JAMA.* 1995;274(13):1049–1057.
20. Graham IM, Daly LE, Refsum HM, et al. Plasma homocysteine as a risk factor for vascular disease. The European Concerted Action Project. *JAMA.* 1997;277(22):1775–1781.
21. Ridker P, Cushman M, Stampfer M, et al. Plasma concentration of C-reactive protein and risk of developing peripheral vascualr disease. *Circulation.* 1998;97:425–428.
22. Hiatt WR, Marshall JA, Baxter J, et al. Diagnostic methods for peripheral arterial disease in the San Luis Valley Diabetes Study. *J Clin Epidemiol.* 1990;43(6):597–606.
23. Fowkes FG, Housley E, Macintyre CC, et al. Reproducibility of reactive hyperaemia test in the measurement of peripheral arterial disease. *Br J Surg.* 1988;75(8):743–746.
24. Muluk SC, Muluk VS, Kelley ME, et al. Outcome events in patients with claudication: A 15-year study in 2777 patients. *J Vasc Surg.* 2001;33(2):251–257; discussion 257–258.
25. Weitz JI, Byrne J, Clagett GP, et al. Diagnosis and treatment of chronic arterial insufficiency of the lower extremities: A critical review. *Circulation.* 1996;94(11):3026–3049.
26. Bhatt DL, Steg PG, Ohman EM, et al. International prevalence, recognition, and treatment of cardiovascular risk factors in outpatients with atherothrombosis. *JAMA.* 2006;295(2):180–189.
27. Ohman EM, Bhatt DL, Steg PG, et al. The REduction of Atherothrombosis for Continued Health (REACH) Registry: An international, prospective, observational investigation in subjects at risk for atherothrombotic events-study design. *Am Heart J.* 2006;151(4):786 e781–e710.
28. Zheng ZJ, Sharrett AR, Chambless LE, et al. Associations of ankle-brachial index with clinical coronary heart disease, stroke and preclinical carotid and popliteal atherosclerosis: The Atherosclerosis Risk in Communities (ARIC) Study. *Atherosclerosis.* 1997;131:115–125.
29. Leng GC, Lee AJ, Fowkes FG, et al. Incidence, natural history and cardiovascular events in the general population. *Int J Epidemiol.* 1996;25:1172–1181.
30. Smith GD, Shipley MJ, Rose G. Intermittent claudication, heart disease risk factors, and mortality. The Whitehall Study. *Circulation.* 1990;82:1925–1931.
31. Kornitzer M, Dramaix M, Sobolski J, et al. Ankle/arm pressure index in asymptomatic middle-aged males: an independent predictor of ten-year coronary heart disease mortality. *Angiology.* 1995;46(3):211–219.
32. Vogt MT, Cauley JA, Newman AB, et al. Decreased ankle/arm blood pressure index and mortality in elderly women. *JAMA.* 1993;270(4):465–469.
33. Criqui MH, Langer RD, Fronek A, et al. Mortality over a period of 10 years in patients with peripheral arterial disease. *N Engl J Med.* 1992;326(6):381–386.
34. Luther M. The influence of arterial reconstructive surgery on the outcome of critical limb ischaemia. *Eur J Vasc Surg.* 1994;8:682–689.
35. Kazmers A, Perkins AJ, Jacobs LA. Major lower extremtiy amputation in Veteran Affairs medical centers. *Ann Vasc Surg.* 2000;14:216–222.
36. Dormandy JA, Heeck L, Vig S. The fate of patients with critical leg ischemia. *Semin Vasc Surg.* 1999;12:142–147.
37. Luscher TF, Lie JT, Stanson AW, et al. Arterial fibromuscular dysplasia. *Mayo Clin Proc.* 1987;62(10):931–952.
38. Lee R. Factor V Leiden: A clinical review. *Am J Med Sci.* 2001;322(2):88–102.
39. Kottke-Marchant K. Genetic polymorphisms associated with venous and arterial thrombosis: an overview. *Arch Pathol Lab Med.* 2002;126(3):295–304.
40. Dormandy J, Heeck L, Vig S. Acute limb ischemia. *Semin Vasc Surg.* 1999;12:148–153.
41. Lillicrap D. The genetics of venous and arterial thromboembolism. *Curr Atheroscler Rep.* 2001;3:209–215.
42. Hirsch AT, Criqui MH, Treat-Jacobson D, et al. Peripheral arterial disease detection, awareness, and treatment in primary care. *JAMA.* 2001;286(11):1317–1324.
43. McKenna M, Wolfson SK, Kuller LH. The ratio of ankle and arm arterial pressure as an independent predictor of mortality. *Atherosclerosis.* 1991;87(2–3):119–128.
44. Moneta GL, Yeager RA, Lee RW, et al. Noninvasive localization of arterial occlusive disease: A comparison of segmental Doppler pressures and arterial duplex mapping. *J Vasc Surg.* 1993;17(3):578–582.
45. Pinto F, Lencioni R, Napoli V. Peripheral ischemic occlusive arterial disease: Comparison of color Doppler pressure and arterial duplex mapping. *J Vasc Surg.* 1996;17:578–582.
46. Sacks D, Robinson ML, Marinelli DL, et al. Peripheral arterial Doppler ultrasonography: Diagnostic criteria. *J Ultrasound Med.* 1992;11(3):95–103.
47. Whelan JF, Barry MH, Moir JD. Color flow Doppler ultrasonography: Comparison with peripheral arteriography for the investigation of peripheral vascular disease. *J Clin Ultrasound.* 1992;20(6):369–374.
48. Edwards JM, Coldwell DM, Goldman ML, et al. The role of duplex scanning in the selection of patients for transluminal angioplasty. *J Vasc Surg.* 1991;13(1):69–74.
49. van der Heijden F, Legemate D, van Leeuwen M. Value of duplex scanning in the selection of patients for percutaneous transluminal angioplasty. *Eur J Vasc Surg.* 1993;7:71–76.
50. Ascher E, Mazzariol F, Hingorani A, et al. The use of duplex ultrasound arterial mapping as an alternative to conventional arteriography for primary and secondary infrapopliteal bypasses. *Am J Surg.* 1999;178(2):162–165.
51. Proia RR, Walsh DB, Nelson PR, et al. Early results of infragenicular revascularization based solely on duplex arteriography. *J Vasc Surg.* 2001;33(6):1165–1170.
52. Bandyk DF, Schmitt DD, Seabrook GR, et al. Monitoring functional patency of in situ saphenous vein bypasses: The impact of a surveillance protocol and elective revision. *J Vasc Surg.* 1989;9(2):286–296.
53. Laborde AL, Synn AY, Worsey MJ, et al. A prospective comparison of ankle/brachial indices and color duplex imaging in surveillance of the in situ saphenous vein bypass. *J Cardiovasc Surg (Torino).* 1992;33(4):420–425.
54. Mattos MA, van Bemmelen PS, Hodgson KJ, et al. Does correction of stenoses identified with color duplex scanning improve infrainguinal graft patency? *J Vasc Surg.* 1993;17(1):54–64.
55. Mills JL, Harris EJ, Taylor LM, Jr., et al. The importance of routine surveillance of distal bypass grafts with duplex scanning: A study of 379 reversed vein grafts. *J Vasc Surg.* 1990;12(4):379–386.
56. Taylor PR, Tyrrell MR, Crofton M, et al. Colour flow imaging in the detection of femoro-distal graft and native artery stenosis: Improved criteria. *Eur J Vasc Surg.* 1992;6(3):232–236.
57. Mehran R, Aymong ED, Nikolsky E, et al. A simple risk score for prediction of contrast-induced nephropathy after percutaneous coronary intervention: Development and initial validation. *J Am Coll Cardiol.* 2004;44(7):1393–1399.
58. Mehran R, Nikolsky E. Contrast-induced nephropathy: Definition, epidemiology, and patients at risk. *Kidney Int Suppl.* 2006;100:S11–15.
59. Nikolsky E, Aymong ED, Dangas G, et al. Radiocontrast nephropathy: Identifying the high-risk patient and the implications of exacerbating renal function. *Rev Cardiovasc Med.* 2003;4(Suppl 1):S7–S14.
60. Lufft V, Hoogestraat-Lufft L, Fels LM, et al. Contrast media nephropathy: Intravenous CT angiography versus intraarterial digital subtraction angiography in renal artery stenosis: A prospective randomized trial. *Am J Kidney Dis.* 2002;40(2):236–242.
61. Lawrence JA, Kim D, Kent KC, et al. Lower extremity spiral CT angiography versus catheter angiography. *Radiology.* 1995;194(3):903–908.
62. Riecker O, Duber C, Schmiedt W. Prospective comparison of CT angiography of the legs with intrarterialdigital subtraction angiography. *Am J Roentgenol.* 1996;182:269–276.
63. Rubin GD, Schmidt AJ, Logan LJ, et al. Multi-detector row CT angiography of lower extremity arterial inflow and runoff: Initial experience. *Radiology.* 2001;221(1):146–158.
64. Martin ML, Tay KH, Flak B, et al. Multidetector CT angiography of the aortoiliac system and lower extremities: A prospective comparison with digital subtraction angiography. *Am J Roentgenol.* 2003;180:1085–1091.
65. Nelemans PJ, Leiner T, de Vet HC, et al. Peripheral arterial disease: A meta-analysis of the diagnostic performance or MR angiography. *Radiology.* 2000;217:105–114.
66. Kreitner KF, Kalden P, Neufang A, et al. Diabetes and peripheral arterial occlusive disease: Prospective comparison of contrast enhanced three dimensional MR angiography with conventional digital subtraction angiography. *Am J Roentgenol.* 2000;174:171–179.
67. Leyendecker JR, Elsass KD, Johnson SP, et al. The role of infrapopliteal MR angiography in patients undergoing optimal contrast angiography for chronic limb-threatening ischemia. *J Vasc Interv Radiol.* 1998;9:545–551.
68. Oser RF, Picus D, Hicks ME, et al. Accuracy of DSA in the evaluation of patency of infrapopliteal vessels. *J Vasc Interv Radiol.* 1995;6:589–594.
69. Hartnell G. MR angiography compared with digital subtraction angiography. *Am J Roentgenol.* 2000;175:1188–1189.
70. Ouwendijk R, de Vries M, Pattynama PM, et al. Imaging peripheral arterial disease: A randomized controlled trial comparing contrast-enhanced MR angiography and multi-detector row CT angiography. *Radiology.* 2005;236(3):1094–1103.
71. Ouwendijk R, Kock MC, Visser K, et al. Interobserver agreement for the interpretation of contrast-enhanced 3D MR angiography and MDCT angiography in peripheral arterial disease. *AJR Am J Roentgenol.* 2005;185(5):1261–1267.
72. Sacks FM, Pfeffer MA, Moye LA, et al. The effect of pravastatin on coronary events after myocardial infarction in patients with average cholesterol levels. Cholesterol and Recurrent Events Trial investigators. *N Engl J Med.* 1996;335(14):1001–1009.
73. Mohler ER, III, Hiatt WR, Creager MA. Cholesterol reduction with atorvastatin improves walking distance in patients with peripheral arterial disease. *Circulation.* 2003;108(12):1481–1486.
74. Pedersen TR, Kjekshus J, Pyorala K, et al. Effect of simvastatin on ischemic signs and symptoms in the Scandinavian simvastatin survival study (4S). *Am J Cardiol.* 1998;81(3):333–335.
75. Yusuf S, Sleight P, Pogue J, et al. Effects of an angiotensin-converting-enzyme inhibitor, ramipril, on cardiovascular events in high-risk patients. The Heart Outcomes Prevention Evaluation Study Investigators. *N Engl J Med.* 2000;342(3):145–153.
76. Jonason T, Bergstrom R. Cessation of smoking in patients with intermittent claudication. Effects on the risk of peripheral vascular complications, myocardial infarction and mortality. *Acta Med Scand.* 1987;221(3):253–260.
77. Collaborative meta-analysis of randomised trials of antiplatelet therapy for prevention of death, myocardial infarction, and stroke in high risk patients. *BMJ.* 2002;324(7329):71–86.

78. A randomised, blinded, trial of clopidogrel versus aspirin in patients at risk of ischaemic events (CAPRIE). CAPRIE Steering Comittee. *Lancet.* 1996;348: 1329–1339.

79. Anand SS, Yusuf S. Oral anticoagulants in patients with coronary artery disease. *J Am Coll Cardiol.* 2003;41(4 Suppl. S):62S–69S.

80. Hirsch AT, Haskal ZJ, Hertzer NR, et al. ACC/AHA 2005 Practice Guidelines for the management of patients with peripheral arterial disease (lower extremity, renal, mesenteric, and abdominal aortic): A collaborative report from the American Association for Vascular Surgery/Society for Vascular Surgery, Society for Cardiovascular Angiography and Interventions, Society for Vascular Medicine and Biology, Society of Interventional Radiology, and the ACC/AHA Task Force on Practice Guidelines (Writing Committee to Develop Guidelines for the Management of Patients With Peripheral Arterial Disease): endorsed by the American Association of Cardiovascular and Pulmonary Rehabilitation; National Heart, Lung, and Blood Institute; Society for Vascular Nursing; TransAtlantic Inter-Society Consensus; and Vascular Disease Foundation. *Circulation.* 2006;113(11):e463–e654.

81. Hirsch AT, Haskal ZJ, Hertzer NR, et al. ACC/AHA 2005 guidelines for the management of patients with peripheral arterial disease (lower extremity, renal, mesenteric, and abdominal aortic): Executive summary a collaborative report from the American Association for Vascular Surgery/Society for Vascular Surgery, Society for Cardiovascular Angiography and Interventions, Society for Vascular Medicine and Biology, Society of Interventional Radiology, and the ACC/AHA Task Force on Practice Guidelines (Writing Committee to Develop Guidelines for the Management of Patients With Peripheral Arterial Disease) endorsed by the American Association of Cardiovascular and Pulmonary Rehabilitation; National Heart, Lung, and Blood Institute; Society for Vascular Nursing; TransAtlantic Inter-Society Consensus; and Vascular Disease Foundation. *J Am Coll Cardiol.* 2006;47(6):1239–1312.

82. Tsuchikane E, Fukuhara A, Kobayashi T, et al. Impact of cilostazol on restenosis after percutaneous coronary balloon angioplasty. *Circulation.* 1999;100(1): 21–26.

83. Money SR, Herd JA, Isaacsohn JL, et al. Effect of cilostazol on walking distances in patients with intermittent claudication caused by peripheral vascular disease. *J Vasc Surg.* 1998;27(2):267–274.

84. Lindgarde F, Jelnes R, Bjorkman H, et al. Conservative drug treatment in patients with moderately severe chronic occlusive peripheral arterial disease. Scandinavian Study Group. *Circulation.* 1989;80(6):1549–1556.

85. Porter JM, Cutler BS, Lee BY, et al. Pentoxifylline efficacy in the treatment of intermittent claudication: Multicenter controlled double-blind trial with objective assessment of chronic occlusive arterial disease patients. *Am Heart J.* 1982;104(1):66–72.

86. Franco CD, Goldsmith J, Veith FJ, et al. Management of arterial injuries produced by percutaneous femoral procedures. *Surgery.* 1993;113(4):419–425.

87. Lumsden AB, Miller JM, Kosinski AS, et al. A prospective evaluation of surgically treated groin complications following percutaneous cardiac procedures. *Am Surg.* 1994;60(2):132–137.

88. Hunink MG, Wong JB, Donaldson MC, et al. Patency results of percutaneous and surgical revascularization for femoropopliteal arterial disease. *Med Decis Making.* 1994;14(1):71–81.

Incidental Extracardiac Findings in Cardiovascular Imaging Tests

51

Patricia Carrascosa
Carlos Capuñay

1. INTRODUCTION

Cardiac imaging is one of the most rapidly growing fields in medicine. Several noninvasive imaging modalities such as ultrasound (US), nuclear medicine, and magnetic resonance imaging (MRI) are in constant improvement and expansion of their clinical applications. More recently, contrast-enhanced cardiac computed tomography (CT) has been widely adopted as an alternative to invasive angiography to define the coronary anatomy.[1-5]

Cross-sectional cardiac imaging modalities not only provide information on the cardiac structure, but also other organs that are included in the examination field, such as portions of lungs, mediastinum, great vessels, spine, and upper abdomen. Unexpected extracardiac findings with variable clinical significance can be observed in a considerable percentage of patients,[6-8] and for that reason, physicians who analyze cardiac studies should be trained to recognize pathological findings in other thoracic or abdominal organs. When feasible, a combined reading of the exams by a radiologist and a cardiologist undoubtedly assures the best diagnostic performance.

Noncardiac incidental findings can be divided in clinically nonsignificant and significant findings, depending on the requirement of additional follow-up or further investigation. For a practical approach, findings are classified by organs, focusing on the most common ones. In this chapter, we will review common extracardiac findings that may be encountered in a thoracic examination. Depending on the type of study been performed, the imaging physician should also become familiar with the anatomy and pathology of the neck, abdomen, and pelvis, which are beyond the scope of this chapter.

2. PATHOPHYSIOLOGY

2.1. Lung parenchyma

Lung parenchymal findings are easier to characterize by CT than by MR imaging due to the higher spatial resolution of the former. Lung nodules and masses that are "hot" or hyperactive in scintigraphic studies usually represent infection or malignancy. US has no value, since its penetration through air is limited. Based on their appearance, CT findings can be classified into four categories: increase in lung opacity, decrease in lung opacity, nodular patterns, and linear patterns.

2.1.1. Increase in lung opacity

Generally, the lung attenuation will increase due to tissue or blood increment or to a decrease in air volume. Depending on the degree of lung involvement, three types of augmented lung opacity can be recognized: consolidation, ground-glass opacity, and pulmonary nodules or masses. *Consolidation* is described as an increase in lung parenchyma attenuation that obscures the vessels and airways margins; it reflects the replacement of the alveoli air by other component such as exudates, transudates, blood, cells, etc.[9] When the lumen of the airways contains air, these airways become visible as an air bronchogram. The radiological significance of the term "consolidation" is widely broad and unspecific. Consolidations can be focal or multifocal; diffuse or segmental in distribution; nodular (Figs. 51.1–51.3). Margins are usually blurred except when they contact an adjacent anatomic structure or fissure.[10-12] Table 51.1 summarizes the differential diagnosis.

The term *ground-glass opacity* describes a hazy increase in lung opacity with preservation of the vascular and bronchial margins. Ground-glass opacity not always reflects a pathologic condition.[9] Physiologic ground-glass attenuation can be seen in the dependent lung areas or on expiratory CT scans. The presence of ground-glass opacity in subacute and chronic diseases often indicates active stage of the disease, especially in the absence of lung fibrosis.[13,14] Table 51.2 summarizes the differential diagnosis.

Pulmonary nodules are defined as spherical, well-defined edge opacities of up to 3 cm in diameter.[15-17] They can be solid or semisolid ("ground glass nodules"), solitary or multiple (Figs. 51.4 and 51.5). Although the last distinction is very helpful to reduce the potential differential diagnosis (Table 51.3), it requires exploration of the entire thorax including the apices. Table 51.4 summarizes the differential diagnosis.

In general, the smaller the size of a nodule, the more likely it is to be benign. A nodule with a diameter <1 cm is called a small nodule, whereas one larger in size is defined as a large nodule (Fig. 51.6). Micronodules are considered not >7 mm. The term mass is used for lesions >3 cm in size. A total of 80% of benign nodules are <2 cm in diameter; however, 15% of malignant nodules are <1 cm and 42% are <2 cm in diameter.[15]

Well-defined, smooth margins are characteristics of benign nodules; nevertheless, these features are not diagnostic. Almost 21% of malignant nodules have well-defined margins. Nodules with irregular, spiculated margins or lobulations are likely to be malignant (Fig. 51.7).[15,17]

Solid, soft tissue density or nonsolid, ground-glass density nodules are seen at CT in both benign (55%) and malignant (20%) etiologies. The presence of fat tissue attenuation (–40 to –20 HU) is a reliable sign of hamartoma, and can be seen at CT in almost 50% of the cases (Fig. 51.8). Pseudocavitation and air bronchogram within a nodule are usually found in malignant lesions

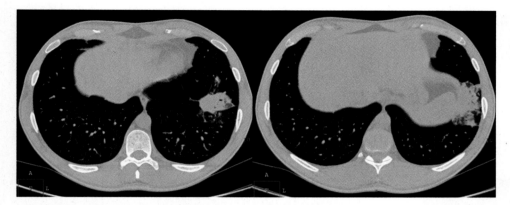

Figure 51.1 Focal, subpleural consolidation in the left lower lobe. There is also accentuation of interlobular septa.

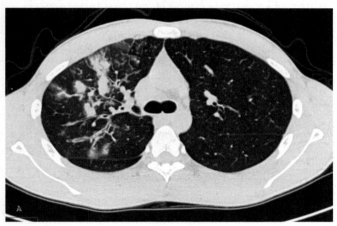

Figure 51.2 Centrilobular airspace nodules, centrilobular branching lines, and tree-in-bud patterns, are common findings of infectious disease. There is also bronchial wall and interlobular septa thickening.

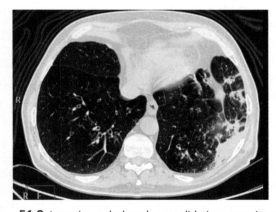

Figure 51.3 Irregular subpleural consolidation associated with pleural thickening.

TABLE 51.1
MAIN DIFFERENTIAL DIAGNOSIS OF LUNG CONSOLIDATION

Acute
Pulmonary infection
Pulmonary edema
Pulmonary hemorrhage
Acute respiratory distress syndrome
Acute interstitial pneumonia
Radiation pneumonitis
Subacute/chronic
Bronchioalveolar carcinoma
Lymphoma
Eosinophilic pneumonia
Vasculitis
Lipoid pneumonia
Interstitial lung disease
Hypersensitivity pneumonitis
Sarcoidosis

TABLE 51.2
MAIN DIFFERENTIAL DIAGNOSIS OF GROUND-GLASS OPACITY

Acute
Pulmonary infection
Pulmonary edema
Pulmonary hemorrhage
Acute respiratory distress syndrome
Acute interstitial pneumonia
Radiation pneumonitis
Subacute
Hypersensitivity pneumonitis
Interstitial lung disease
Vasculitis
Bronchoalveolar carcinoma
Lipoid pneumonia
Sarcoidosis

(bronchoalveolar cell carcinoma; lymphoma) (Fig. 51.9). The presence and pattern of calcification also help in the differentiation between benign and malignant nodules; nonetheless, 38% to 63% of benign nodules are not calcified. Central, laminated, and solid calcifications are typically present in benign, postinfection nodules (Fig. 51.10). Central, lobulated calcification is characteristic of chondroid calcification in a hamartoma. Pulmonary carcinoid tumors and lung cancers may also be calcified in a diffuse and amorphous pattern. When calcification is not apparent at visual assessment, the determination of CT attenuation values within the nodule is recommended. An attenuation value of 200 HU is often a good cutoff value between calcified (>200 HU) and noncalcified (<200 HU) nodules. Malignant nodules show greater contrast enhancement than benign ones.[15-18] Malignant nodules usually demonstrate increased perfusion and metabolic activity in single photon emission computed tomography (SPECT) and positron emission tomography (PET) studies (Fig. 51.11).

Figure 51.4 Axial CT, coronal MPR, and axial MIP images showing a round, calcified nodule in the posterior segment of the right upper lobe, adjacent to the major fissure (*arrows*).

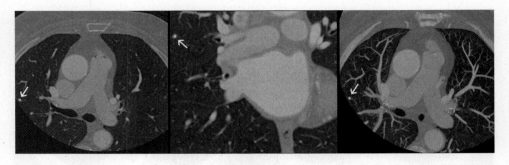

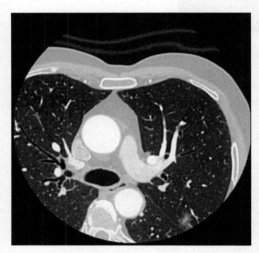

Figure 51.5 Poor-defined, ground-glass opacity in the left upper lobe, adjacent to the major fissure.

TABLE 51.3
DIFFERENTIAL DIAGNOSIS OF NODULES BASED ON THE DISTRIBUTION PATTERN

(Peri)lymphatic distribution
Sarcoidosis
Lymphangitic spread of tumor
Silicosis
Coal miners' pneumoconiosis
Amyloidosis
Lymphoproliferative diseases (lymphoma and lymphocytic interstitial pneumonia)

Centrilobular Distribution
Bronchiolitis[a]
Bronchopneumonia
Allergic bronchopulmonary aspergillosis[a]
Hypersensitivity pneumonitis
Organizing pneumonia[a]
Bronchoalveolar carcinoma[a]
Asbestosis
Vasculitis
Pulmonary hemorrhage

Random Distribution
Infections (TB, fungus)
Metastases

[a]Can show tree-in-bud pattern.

2.1.2. Decrease in lung opacity

Lung attenuation will decrease when the amount of air abnormally increases (air trapping), the vascular blood volume decreases (hypoperfusion) or lung tissue is destroyed and loss of lung tissue occurs.[19] Lung destruction is most frequently the

TABLE 51.4
DIFFERENTIAL DIAGNOSIS OF PULMONARY NODULES OR MASSES

Solitary	Multiple
Infective	
Granuloma	Granulomas
Lung Abscess	Lung Abscesses
Round pneumonia	Round pneumonias
	Septic infarcts
Inflammatory	
Rheumatoid arthritis	Rheumatoid arthritis
Sarcoidosis	Sarcoidosis
Wegener granulomatosis	Wegener granulomatosis
Lipoid pneumonia	
Congenital	
Arteriovenous malformation	Arteriovenous malformation
Sequestration	
Neoplastic	
Bronchial carcinoma	Metastasis
Solitary metastasis	Lymphoma
Carcinoid	Kaposis sarcoma
Hamartoma	Bronchoalveolar carcinoma
Lymphoma	
Miscellaneous	
Lung infarct	Lung infarcts
Intrapulmonary lymph node	Mucoid impactions
Mucoid impaction	
Round atelectasis	

result of pulmonary emphysema. Low-attenuation lung changes can appear as lung cysts or cystlike structures, be well-defined, circumscribed, and rounded with a thin wall (<3 mm thick). Cysts usually contain air but may also contain liquid or solid material. Table 51.5 summarizes the differential diagnosis.

The most frequent cause of cystic lung changes is endstage pulmonary fibrosis (*honeycombing*), characterized by air-filled cystic spaces, with a diameter ranging from several millimeters to centimeters and a thin, fibrous tissue wall (1 to 3 mm). They are distributed in a peripheral subpleural location, predominantly in the lower pulmonary lobes (Fig. 51.12).[19–22] *Pneumatoceles* are

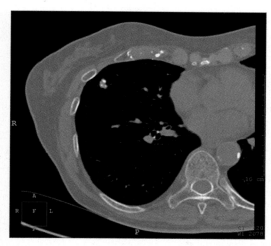

Figure 51.6 Small, partially-calcified nodule in the right upper lobe.

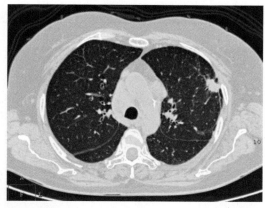

Figure 51.7 Axial CT image with lung window through the left upper lobe shows a subpleural, irregular, spiculated lesion. The appearance is highly suggestive of a primary lung carcinoma.

thin-walled air-filled spaces associated with pulmonary infections or posttraumatic laceration.[23]

Bronchiectasis, when perpendicular to the scan plane, can simulate lung cysts. Bronchiectasis is defined as localized, irreversible bronchial dilatation, with thickening of the bronchial wall.[24] Bronchial dilatation is considered when the diameter of the bronchus is greater than the diameter of the adjacent pulmonary artery branch (bronchus/artery ratio >1). Classically, bronchiectasis is classified into: (i) cylindrical bronchiectasis with a straight, regular outlines that end abruptly; (ii) cystic or bronchiectasis with bronchial ballooned appearance that may have air-fluid levels;

and (iii) varicose bronchiectasis with bronchus dilatation and interspersed sites of relative constriction (Fig. 51.13).[22,25]

Pulmonary *emphysema* is characterized by an irreversible, abnormal enlargement of the alveoli distal to the terminal bronchiole, accompanied by the destruction of their walls.[22] This increase in air content and loss of lung structure generate a decrease in lung attenuation. Four types of emphysema can be recognized, based on the anatomic distribution of these areas of lung destruction. In centrilobular emphysema, the CT shows areas of decreased attenuation within the central parts of the secondary lobules (Fig. 51.14). Emphysematous areas are interspersed within the normal parenchyma. In panlobular emphysema, the CT shows a homogeneous decrease in attenuation in the entire secondary lobule (Fig. 51.15). Paraseptal emphysema involved secondary lobules adjacent to the visceral pleura or fissures (Fig. 51.16). Bullous emphysema is characterized by large air-containing areas with thin walls, usually associated with any type of emphysema (Fig. 51.17).[26,27]

2.1.3. Nodular pattern

A nodular pattern is characterized by multiple nodular opacities <3 cm. The CT assessment of the nodular pattern is based on the nodule characteristics and its distribution. According to their borders (sharp or blurred) or density (solid or ground glass), lung nodules are classified into interstitial nodules and airspace nodules. The size, presence of calcification, and cavitations are also valuable. Location of the nodules allows the distinction between perilymphatic, centrilobular, and random distribution patterns.[22,28,29]

Airspace nodules can present not only as small centrilobular nodular opacities but also as a cluster of small nodules. Centrilobular nodules associated with intralobular branching lines are called the tree-in-bud pattern. Borders are usually ill defined, and the density varies between ground glass to soft tissue depending on the grade of involvement. When the entire pulmonary nodule is affected, large nodules as well as ground-glass opacity and consolidation can appear. In Table 51.6 the most common causes of airspace nodules are summarized.

Interstitial nodules are usually sharply defined with soft tissue attenuation. They are related to a nodular cellular proliferation and associated to diseases with vascular or lymphatic distribution. Conglomeration or growth of interstitial nodules can develop into larger nodules or masses. Table 51.7 shows the different diseases that can be associated with interstitial nodules.

Distribution of the nodules allows the distinction between perilymphatic, centrilobular, and random distributions. Airspace nodules are predominantly present among diseases that involve the airways and surrounding airspaces, while interstitial nodules are mainly related to diseases that are spread by or located near the lymphatics or the blood vessels.

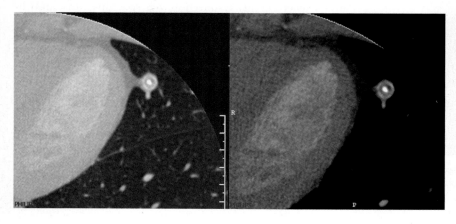

Figure 51.8 Magnified images through the lingula imaged with narrow and wide windows, respectively, show a well-defined nodule with a central large calcification surrounded by fat, consistent with the diagnosis of a pulmonary hamartoma.

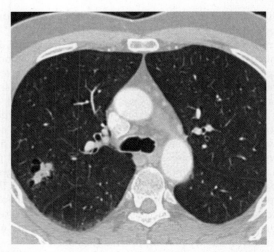

Figure 51.9 Axial CT image with lung window through the right upper lobe shows an irregular, pseudocavitated lesion. The appearance is suggestive of a malignant nodule.

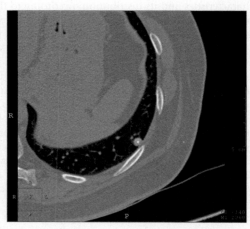

Figure 51.10 Small, round, well-defined margin nodule with subpleural location in the left lower lobe. It shows a round, central "benign" calcification.

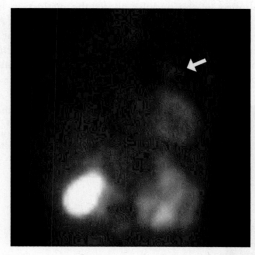

Figure 51.11 Left upper lobe mass (*arrow*) showing increased ^{99}Tc sestamibi uptake found incidentally during a myocardial perfusion SPECT study.

TABLE 51.5
CYSTIC AND CYSTLIKE LUNG DISEASES

Lung cysts
Pulmonary fibrosis, end-stage disease (honeycombing)
Lymphangiomyomatosis
Langerhans histiocytosis
Lymphocytic interstitial pneumonia
Bronchogenic cyst
Pulmonary cyst
Pneumatocoeles

Cystlike lesions (cavitary nodules)
Langerhans histiocytosis
Metastasis
Septic embolism
Wegener granulomatosis
Pulmonary aspergillosis
Rheumatoid arthritis
TB
Bronchiectasis

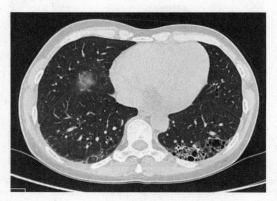

Figure 51.12 Predominately peripheral (and basal) septal thickening and honeycombing, with traction bronchiectasis in several areas of the left lower lobe.

A nodular pattern with perilymphatic distribution has peribronchovascular, subpleural, centrilobular nodules, and/or nodules in the interlobular septa. They are typically well-defined, soft tissue nodules with patchy distribution, easily recognized when subpleural in location or in relation to the fissures (Fig. 51.18).

Centrilobular nodular opacities can result from bronchiolar and peribronchiolar diseases, from vascular and perivascular diseases, and from perilymphatic diseases. These nodular opacities can be associated with intralobular branching lines, creating the tree-in-bud pattern, indicator of small airway disease and almost always reflecting airway infection, but sometimes may also be seen in its absence.

Random distribution occurs as the result of the random location of the nodules in relation to the structures of the secondary pulmonary lobule, also associated with a bilateral and symmetric distribution through the lungs. This distribution is the result of a vascular spread of the disease.

2.1.4. Linear pattern

Linear opacities can develop when the interstitium is thickened (peribronchovascular tissue; interlobular septa), when the lymphatics or perilymphatic tissue is affected, when blood vessels increase in diameter, or when airways walls are thickened. Irregular septal thickening may indicate the development of fibrosis (Fig. 51.19).[22,28]

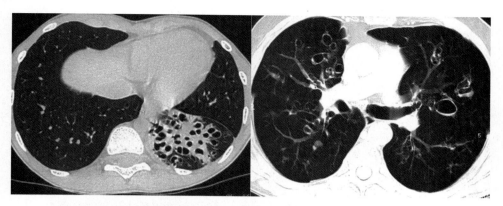

Figure 51.13 Axial CT images demonstrating multiple dilated, thick-walled bronchi in the left lower lobe (**left**) and multiple cystic bronchiectasis (**right**).

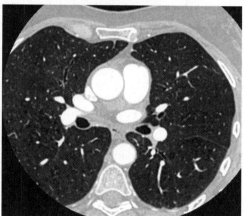

Figure 51.14 Centrilobular emphysema.

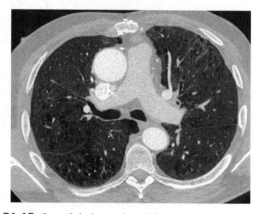

Figure 51.15 Centrilobular and panlobular emphysema.

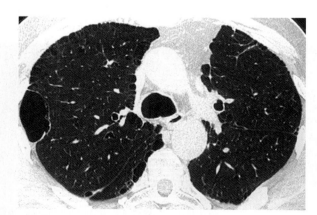

Figure 51.16 Paraseptal emphysema.

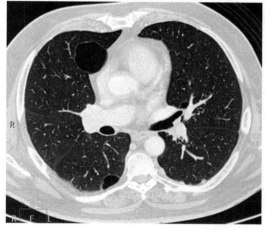

Figure 51.17 Large bullae with a diameter larger than 1 cm in the right upper lobe, adjacent to the mediastinum. There is also a small one in the upper segment of the right lower lobe in subpleural location.

TABLE 51.6
AIRSPACE NODULES: DIFFERENTIAL DIAGNOSIS

Infectious bronchiolitis and bronchopneumonia
Smoking related parenchymal lung disease
Hypersensitivity pneumonitis
Bronchioloalveolar carcinoma[a]
Organizing pneumonia[a]
Pulmonary edema
Pulmonary hemorrhage

[a]Nodules, masses, or consolidation can be associated.

TABLE 51.7
INTERSTITIAL NODULES: DIFFERENTIAL DIAGNOSIS

Sarcoidosis[a]
Lymphangitic carcinomatosis
Lymphoma[a]
Silicosis and coal workers' pneumoconiosis[a]
Amyloidosis
Langerhans cell histiocytosis
Bronchiolitis
Haematogenous metastases[a]
Vasculitis[a]
Miliary infection

[a]Nodules or masses can be associated.

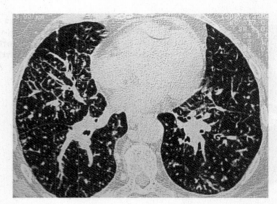

Figure 51.18 Nodular pattern with (peri) lymphatic distribution shows peribronchovascular, subpleural, centrilobular nodules, and nodules in the interlobular septa.

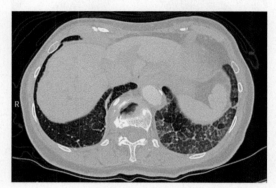

Figure 51.19 Intralobular linear opacities and interlobular septal thickening through the left lower lung, causing a fine reticular pattern.

2.2. Pleural findings

Pleural effusions are the most common pleural abnormality.[30,31] When the rate of fluid production is increased or when reabsorption is impaired, pleural effusions developed. CT is of limited value in distinguishing transudates from exudates. However, with transudates, pleural thickening and/or enhancement is not typically seen on CT, while thickening of the parietal pleura almost always indicates an exudate.[32] Most pleural effusions are of homogeneous, waterlike attenuation (Fig. 51.20); higher density effusions are almost always exudates and those with a density similar to soft tissue are suggestive of hemothorax. On MRI, transudates are hypointense on T1 weighting and hyperintense on T2 weighting (Fig. 51.21); subacute or chronic hemorrhage shows high signal with T1 and T2.[33] By US, pleural effusions are hypoechoic,

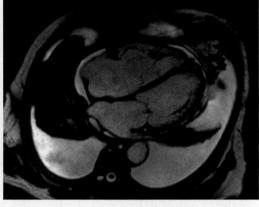

Figure 51.21 Large bilateral pleural effusions on T2-weighted MR image. Fluid shows high signal intensity. There is also pericardial effusion.

semilunar in appearance and may have septae, loculations, and/or floating echo dense material, usually atelectatic lung. On scintigraphic studies, pleural and pericardial effusions appear as areas void of radioactive signal (Fig. 51.22).

Pleural thickening may be focal or diffuse, and is usually the result of a preceding inflammatory or infectious process. Other benign causes include prior surgery, trauma, radiation therapy, and asbestos exposure. Malignant etiology should be suspected when nodularity, circumferential pleural thickening, or thickness over 1 cm is seen.[33-35]

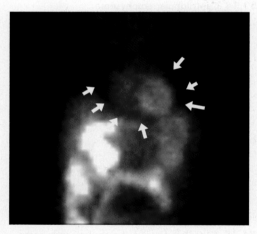

Figure 51.22 Pericardial effusion (*arrows*) noticed in a myocardial perfusion SPECT study.

Figure 51.20 Bilateral pleural effusion, larger on the left side. There are focal, irregular areas of consolidation and interstitial thickening in the upper segment of left lobber lobe.

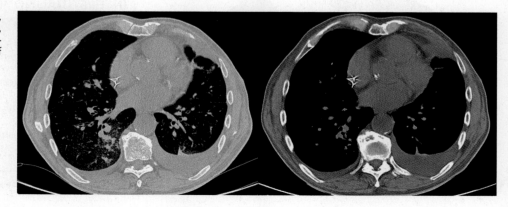

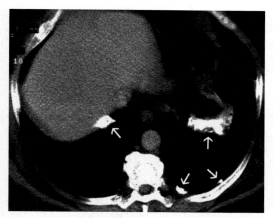

Figure 51.23 Large bilateral pleural calcifications (*arrows*).

Pleural calcification may be a result of prior infection, hemorrhage, or as the result of asbestos exposure. Symmetric, bilateral distribution of calcified plaques on the diaphragm is almost pathognomonic of asbestos-related pleural disease (Fig. 51.23).

The most common benign tumors of the pleura are lipomas and localized fibrous tumors, while metastases are the most common form of malignancy. CT is useful in defining the location and extent of pleural lesions and in evaluating the underlying lung parenchyma.[31,34,35] MRI may be also useful, especially for the evaluation of infiltration of the chest wall or diaphragm. High signal intensity (SI) relative to intercostal muscles on T2-weighted images and on contrast-enhanced T1-weighted images strongly favors malignancy.[36,37]

2.3. Mediastinal diseases

Mediastinal abnormalities can be vascular and nonvascular. Differential diagnosis of nonvascular mediastinal masses on CT is usually based on the location and identification of the structure from which it is arising. However, it is also important to remember that most lesions can be seen in any part of the mediastinum (Table 51.8). For that reason, determination of the attenuation of mediastinal masses is extremely important in their differential diagnosis.[38–40] Masses can be grouped into: fat density lesions; low-density lesions (greater than fat, but less than muscle); high-density lesions (greater than muscle); and contrast-enhancing lesions (increased attenuation following the injection of contrast) (Table 51.9).

Vascular abnormalities are basically related to the aorta and pulmonary arteries, although venous abnormalities (pulmonary veins; systemic veins) can be found.

2.3.1. Thymus

The thymus lies in the upper anterior mediastinum and extends inferiorly to the base of the heart. From the age of 15 to about 25 years old, the thymus is recognizable as a triangular or bilobed structure outlined by mediastinal fat. At this age the thymus begins to involute, and in the adults it is no longer recognizable as a soft tissue structure, because of progressive fatty involution. With complete thymic involution, the anterior mediastinum appears to be entirely filled with fat, slightly higher than that of subcutaneous fat. In adult subjects a thickness of 1.3 cm is considered the maximum allowable normal value. On MRI, the normal thymus appears homogeneous, of intermediate SI on T1-weighted images, and of high SI on T2 relaxation times.

TABLE 51.8

DIFFERENTIAL DIAGNOSIS OF MEDIASTINAL MASSES BASED ON THEIR LOCATION

Prevascular space
Thymic masses
Germ cell tumors
Thyroid abnormalities
Hodgkin lymphoma

Cardiophrenic Angle
Lymph node masses
Pericardial cyst
Morgagni hernia
Fatty masses

Pretracheal Space
Lymph node masses
Thyroid abnormalities
Vascular abnormalities

Aortopulmonary Window
Lymph node masses
Vascular abnormalities (aorta or pulmonary artery)

Subcarinal Space
Lung carcinoma
Esophageal masses

Paravertebral Region
Neurogenic tumor
Meningocele
Extramedullary hematopoiesis
Hernias
Esophageal masses
Lymph node masses
Thymic mass (Thymic carcinoma)

TABLE 51.9

DIFFERENTIAL DIAGNOSIS OF MEDIASTINAL MASSES BASED ON THEIR ATTENUATION

Fat attenuation masses
Lipomatosis
Thymolipoma
Teratoma
Lipoma
Liposarcoma
Fatty hernias
Lymph node enlargement (rarely; Whipple disease)

Low-attenuation masses
Congenital or acquired cysts (bronchogenic, esophageal duplication, pericardial)
Necrotic tumors (lymphoma, cystic thymoma, germ cell tumors)
Thoracic meningocele
Cystic goiter
Dilated, fluid-filled esophagus

High-attenuation masses
Calcified lymph nodes
Lymphoma (after treatment)
Calcified primary neoplasms
Calcified goiter
Calcified vascular lesions

Enhancing masses
Carcinoid tumors
Lymphangiomas
Hemangiomas
Paraganglioma
Inflammatory disease with enhancing lymph nodes
Metastatic tumor

Figure 51.24 Small, round, well-defined hypodense lesion in the anterior mediastinum corresponding to a thymoma (*arrows*).

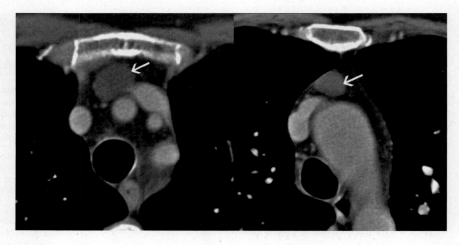

Thymic masses represent almost 20% of primary mediastinal tumors, including thymic hyperplasia, thymoma, thymic carcinoma, thymic cyst, thymolipoma, and lymphoma.

Thymoma is the most common primary thymic tumor, accounting for 15% of primary mediastinal masses, most common in patients aged 50 to 60 years. Typically on CT, thymomas appear as homogeneous sharply demarcated and oval, round, or lobulated soft tissue attenuation masses. Rarely, they appear cystic. Clear delineation of fat planes surrounding a thymoma is an indicator of the absence of extensive local invasion. Invasive thymomas accounts for 30% of all thymomas. They are significantly larger with irregular contours, and have a higher prevalence of focal low attenuation areas on CT scans (Fig. 51.24).

On MRI, thymomas demonstrate SI similar to that of muscle on T1-weighted images, and SI higher than that of muscle and similar to that of fat on T2-weighted images. Postcontrast homogeneous and moderate enhancement is often observed.

2.3.2. Thyroid

Intrathoracic extension of thyroid abnormalities occurs in nearly 10% of patients with thyroid disease, usually representing direct contiguous growth into the mediastinum of a goiter, but also can be secondary to thyroid enlargement associated with thyroiditis or thyroid carcinoma. In 80% of cases, an enlarged thyroid extends into the anterior mediastinum, although posterior mediastinal goiters constitute approximately 20% of cases (Fig. 51.25). Mediastinal thyroid masses usually appear inhomogeneous and cystic on CT regardless of their cause.

On MRI, most focal pathologic processes have prolonged T2 values and they are easily identified on T2-weighted images and on enhanced sequences.

2.3.3. Lymph nodes

The majority of mediastinal lymph nodes are located in relation to the trachea and main bronchi, and serve to drain the lungs. Mediastinal lymph node abnormalities most commonly involve the pretracheal space, subcarinal space, and aortopulmonary window, although they can be seen in any mediastinal compartment. By CT, lymph nodes are round or elliptical, soft tissue nodules surrounded by mediastinal fat. The size of normal nodes varies with their location. The least diameter of a lymph node should generally be used when measuring its size, considering 10 mm as the upper limit of normal for the majority of the mediastinal lymph nodes, with the exception of the subcarinal region (12 mm).

Enlargement of lymph nodes is a common CT finding in a broad spectrum of diseases; larger the node, the more likely it indicates a significant abnormality. Lymph nodes >20 mm more often reflect the presence of neoplasm, granulomatous disease, or infection, and should be considered potentially significant (Fig. 51.26). Calcification of lymph nodes is commonly seen in granulomatous diseases or fungal infections, but may be associated

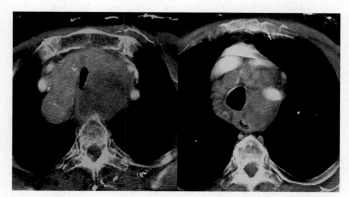

Figure 51.25 Intrathoracic extension of the thyroid, representing direct contiguous growth into the mediastinum of a goiter. There is compression and right displacement of the trachea.

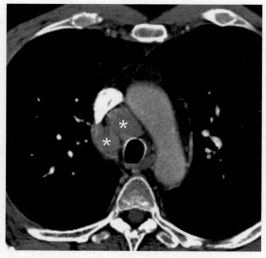

Figure 51.26 Enlarged mediastinal lymph nodes in the upper right paratracheal space (*asterisks*).

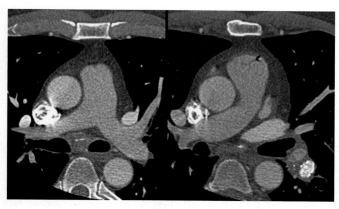

Figure 51.27 Enlarged subcarinal and left hilar lymph nodes, the last one being grossly calcified.

with other entities (Fig. 51.27). Low-attenuation lymph nodes classically reflect the presence of necrosis, and are commonly present in patients with tuberculosis (TB), fungal infections, and neoplasms.

MR is comparable to CT in visualization of mediastinal lymph nodes, especially when they are embedded in mediastinal fat or adjacent to blood vessels. Nevertheless, MRI is unable to detect calcification.

2.3.4. Aorta

The appearance of the aorta is characteristic, consisting of an ascending segment, a transverse segment or arch, and a descending segment. As measured in >100 normal subjects,[41] the mean diameter of the proximal ascending aorta is 3.6 cm (range 2.4 to 4.7 cm), the distal ascending aorta is 3.51 cm (range 2.2 to 4.6 cm), the proximal descending aorta is 2.63 cm (range 1.6 to 3.7 cm), and the distal descending aorta is 2.42 cm (range 1.4 to 3.3 cm). Usually, the innominate artery arises as the first branch of the arch. The second branch is the left common carotid artery, and the left subclavian artery is the last arch branch arising from the posterosuperior portion of the aortic arch.

A wide variety of congenital anomalies of the aorta can be present. The most common one, found in nearly 0.5% of the normal population, is the aberrant right subclavian artery originating from the posterior portion of a normal left-sided arch, crossing the mediastinum from left-to-right, lying posterior to the trachea and esophagus.[42] The origin of the anomalous artery is dilated in up to 60% of cases (Kommerell diverticulum). Other congenital anomalies include a right-sided aortic arch with or without aberrant left subclavian artery and a double aortic arch. Coarctation of the aorta consists of a focal narrowing in the proximal descending thoracic aorta, usually in the region of the ductus arteriosus.

Acquired aortic disease is commonly secondary to atherosclerotic disease. Aortic atherosclerotic plaques are common findings on cardiac imaging. Thoracic aneurysms secondary to atherosclerosis are fusiform dilatations of a segment of the aorta, usually containing mural thrombus and calcification of the aortic wall. Aortic aneurysm is defined as an irreversible dilatation of the aorta. In the thoracic aneurysms, one or more aortic segments can be involved. Measuring the size of a thoracic aortic aneurysm from multidetector computed tomography (MDCT) and MRI studies must be carried out on true short-axis images of the aneurysm obtained from multiplanar reformats at a workstation. Typical aortic dissections produce an intimomedial tear at the areas of greatest hydraulic stress, that is, the right lateral wall of the

ascending aorta[43] or the descending aorta distal to the left subclavian artery origin. Dailey et al.[44] refined the aortic dissection classification into a more clinically point of view as dissections involving the ascending aorta as Stanford A and, those distal to the left subclavian artery, as type B. Acute Stanford A proximal dissections account for 75% of all cases of aortic dissection. Atypical aortic dissections include aortic intramural hematoma (IMH) and penetrating atherosclerotic ulcer.[45]

Noncontrast CT findings on calcium scoring images may show displacement of intimal calcification from the aortic wall, usually a diagnostic sign of **aortic dissection**. Besides, noncontrast CT images provide important information that may be obscured with intravenous contrast such as the presence of blood in the mediastinum or pleural or pericardial spaces in cases of ruptured aortic dissection. On both contrast-enhanced CT and MR images, the identification of an intimomedial flap that separates two lumens or a strandlike structure that projects into the opacified lumen are classically seen (Fig. 51.28). In most cases, the true lumen is smaller in size and usually enhanced to a greater degree than the false lumen, has an oval configuration, and it rarely presents thrombus. The possibility of branch vessel involvement must be ruled out.[45,46,47]

Aortic IMH represents localized hemorrhage confined to the aortic media.[45,48] CT appearance of acute IMH in noncontrast images is pathognomonic, demonstrating a crescent-shaped area along the wall of the aorta that has higher attenuation than the vascular lumen. Intimal calcifications may be medially displaced, and pleural and pericardial effusions are common, associated findings. On contrast-enhanced CT images, the crescent-shaped area that represents the hematoma will not enhance, and it appears hypodense in comparison to the enhanced lumen. An intimal flap is absent. The MR characteristics of IMH depends both on the age of the hematoma and on the pulse sequence used. Classic signs are the identification of focal crescent wall thickening without evidence of intimal flap.[48] Acute IMH is usually isointense on T1-weighted spin echo (SE) or double inversion recovery (IR) images; subacute IMH is hyperintense from methemoglobin. A complete description of imaging findings of aortic pathologies is available in Chapter 45.

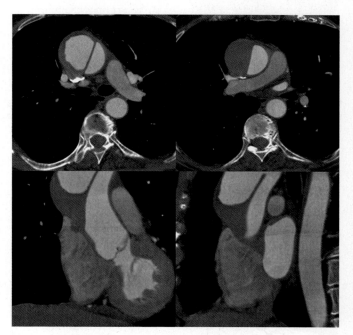

Figure 51.28 Stanford type A aortic dissection. The false lumen is partially thrombosed.

2.3.5. Pulmonary arteries

MDCT allows direct visualization of intra-arterial clot. CT findings in acute pulmonary embolism include vascular abnormalities and pleuroparenchymal findings. On contrast-enhanced images, pulmonary embolism appears: (a) as filling defects within the vessel lumen; the filling defects may be serpiginous; (b) the artery may show a cutoff or appears completely nonopacified. The most common pleuroparenchymal findings are segmental and/ or subsegmental atelectasis (Fig. 51.29). Pulmonary infarction is generally reported to occur in only 10% of cases.[49-53] A complete description of imaging findings in pulmonary embolism is available in chapter 47.

2.4. Diaphragm

Common pathways that allow communication between the abdomen and thorax are the aortic and esophageal hiatuses. Herniation of the stomach through the esophageal hiatus is a common finding in adults (Fig. 51.30). This acquired abnormality is secondary to laxity and stretching of the phrenoesophageal ligament and widening of the esophageal hiatus. Another potential pathway is the persistence of the embryonic pleuroperitoneal canal (Bochdalek hernia), 90% of cases on the left side (Fig. 51.31). Herniation may also occur in the anterior portions of the diaphragms, resulting in a paracardiac mass (Morgagni hernia). These defects are associated with protrusion of omental or even retroperitoneal fat.[54-57]

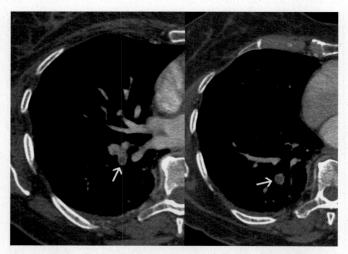

Figure 51.29 Pulmonary embolism. Presence of small filling defects within the vessel lumen at the segmental artery of the right lower lobe (*arrows*).

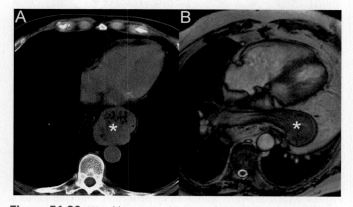

Figure 51.30 Hiatal hernia on CT (**A**) and MR (**B**) images (*asterisks*).

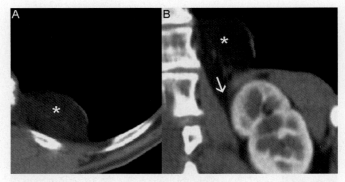

Figure 51.31 Bochdalek hernia. Axial (**A**) and coronal MPR (**B**) CT images showing posterior left diaphragmatic defect (*arrow*) with protrusion of omental fat (*asterisks*).

2.5. Breast

Although CT is not used in the daily practice for the evaluation of breast pathology, this anatomic area is always included in the cardiac CT field of view. Size and normal anatomy vary according to sex and age. In young women, the breast is mainly compound of glandular parenchyma of soft tissue attenuation, with fat tissue increasing with the age, replacing the parenchyma. In men, the amount of breast parenchyma and fat tissue are limited. Attention to the presence of calcification or breast nodules should be focused during the image interpretation. Calcifications may vary from subtle, punctate to large ones (Fig. 51.32). Benign breast lesions, such as fibroadenomas, are usually round or oval in shape, have regular, well-defined contours, and CT density is lower than the adjacent parenchyma, with an increase in density of <30 HU after the injection of intravascular contrast. Malignant lesions have irregular, spiculated borders and significant postcontrast enhancement with an increase in density of >60 HU. Lesions with an enhancement between 30 and 60 HU are difficult to differentiate between benign and malignant diseases, and other criteria should be analyzed, such as the size and delineation of the tumor. Malignant breast masses usually demonstrate increased perfusion and metabolic activity on SPECT and PET (Fig 51.33).

Differentiating masses as cystic or solid is the traditional role of US in the workup of breast masses, being an overlap in sonographic findings between benign and malignant solid breast

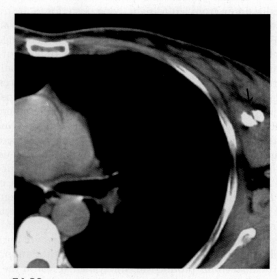

Figure 51.32 Large calcifications in the left breast parenchyma (*arrow*).

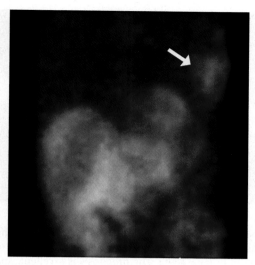

Figure 51.33 Large breast mass (*arrow*) demonstrating increased ^{99}Tc sestamibi uptake during a myocardial perfusion study.

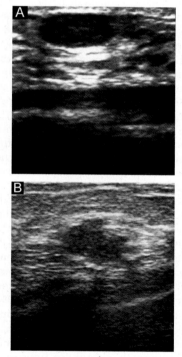

Figure 51.34 Breast ultrasound showing (**A**) a well-defined, benign nodule (fibroadenoma) and (**B**) an irregular shape, spiculated margins (intraductal carcinoma).

lesions. Malignant features include an irregular shape, ill-defined or spiculated margins, marked hypoechogenicity associated to attenuating distal echoes and punctate calcifications, and an anterior–posterior diameter greater than the transverse diameter (Fig. 51.34).

On MR images, incidentals findings on breast tissue are difficult to categorize, especially for the poor SI and small field of view of the region.

2.6. Liver lesions

2.6.1. Hepatic cysts

Simple hepatic or congenital cysts are benign developmental lesions that do not communicate with the biliary tree. They seem to originate from a hamartomatous tissue. Hepatic cysts are a common finding, being found in 1% to 3% of routine liver examinations. They may sometimes behave as space-occupying masses, displacing intrahepatic vessels and sometimes the biliary tree leading to jaundice, and causing swelling of the hepatic margin. Rarely do they cause pain, and symptoms disappear after percutaneous aspiration. Simple hepatic cysts can be solitary or multiple. Their size is very much variable, frequently <5 cm. They tend to increase in number and size with age. Usually, they have a serous content, rarely they may present as "complicated" cysts due to the presence of hemorrhage or inflammation. Solitary hepatic cysts occur more frequently in women in fourth to fifth decade. Their sizes range from few millimeters up to 20 cm; the content may be serous. Developmental anomalies and retention are the main etiologies.[58–63]

The typical appearance of a single cyst at sonography is of an anechoic, round, or ellipsoid structure, characterized by the absence of an own wall and an increased acoustic signal behind (Fig. 51.35). In some occasions, there can be lateral acoustic shadows. Rarely, it can present septa or calcifications. Color Doppler analysis may be helpful in excluding the presence of vessels. In plain CT, they usually have the appearance of cystic lesions, well-defined, with no evident wall. They have a homogeneous and hypoattenuating content with attenuation values similar to water (<20 HU) that do not modify their density with endovenous contrast (Fig. 51.36). Higher attenuation values (>20 HU) are present in cysts with hemorrhage or inflammation inside (complicated cysts).[58,61,64] At MRI, hepatic cysts have homogeneous, very low SI on T1-weighted images and homogeneous, very high SI on T2-weighted images, similar to the water SI (Figs. 51.37 and 51.38). This increase allows differentiation of these lesions from metastatic disease. The wall is never seen, and no enhancement is present after administration of gadolinium. In case of complication such as intracystic hemorrhage, there is high SI, sometimes with a fluid–fluid level, on both T1- and T2-weighted images when mixed blood products are present. Fat-saturation sequences may be helpful in confirming the blood content.[61,63]

Differential diagnosis of simple cysts includes choledochal cysts, necrotic metastasis and echinococcal cysts.

2.6.2. Hemangiomas

Hemangiomas are the most common benign tumors of the liver. Their size ranges from a few millimeters to several centimeters. When size increases, they can have cystic degeneration. The female-to-male ratio has been reported from 2:1 to 5:1. They occur at all

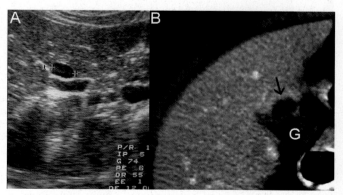

Figure 51.35 Hepatic cyst. **A**: On ultrasound, the lesion is characterized as an anechoic, round structure, with absence of an own wall and an increased acoustic signal behind in the left. **B**: On CT, the lesion is hypodense, with contrast enhancement (*arrow*). G, gallbladder.

Figure 51.36 Small, round, well-defined margins hypodense lesions in the liver. They do not show contrast enhancement, compatible to hepatic cyst (*arrows*).

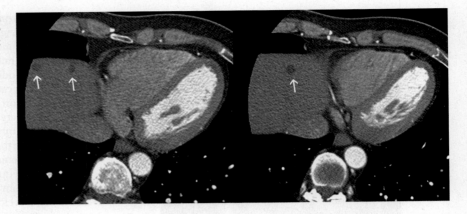

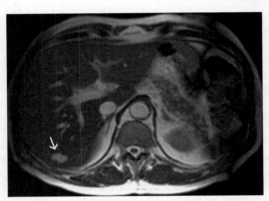

Figure 51.37 Small, lobulated, well-defined margins hyperintense lesion on T2-weighted MR images in the right liver lobe, compatible to hepatic cyst (*arrow*).

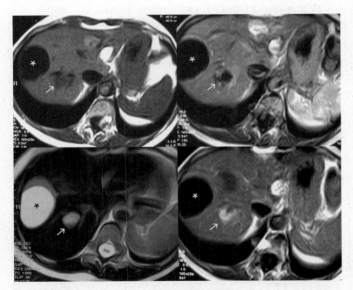

Figure 51.38 Round, well-defined margins hypointense lesion on T1-weighted images, hyperintense on T2-weighted images in the right liver lobe (VIII segment), and compatible to hepatic cyst (*asterisks*). There is also another focal, nodular lesion, hyperintense on T2-weighted images that shows globular, peripheral contrast enhancement compatible to hemangioma (*arrows*).

a single layer of flat endothelium. The septa between the spaces are often incomplete. Blood vessels and arteriovenous shunting may be seen in large septa. The prognosis is excellent, apart from exceptionally giant lesions. The most common type is the cavernous hemangiomas, which have the tendency to develop thrombosis, hyalinization, and occasional calcification.[65,66] By US, hemangiomas appear as echogenic masses of uniform density, less than 3 cm in diameter with acoustic enhancement and sharp margins (Fig. 51.39). A hypoechoic center may be present, but is not frequent a hypoechoic halo. They may have an atypical pattern if bigger than 3 cm, appearing as hypo- or iso-echoic. On color Doppler, no vascular pattern is observed as intralesional flow is too slow to be revealed. By CT, in general, they appear as a hypodense uniform image. Rarely, there are hyperdense areas similar to calcium, indicating regressive tissue changes. After contrast administration there is a peripheral nodular enhancement with concentric interflow that leads to isodense zone in 15 to 20 min after injection. The kinetic behavior pattern can be attributed to the accumulation of contrast in cavernous spaces and slow flow migration of contrast medium with pools of blood contained in those spaces. For that reason large hemangiomas require more time to become homogenous. On the other hand, small hemangiomas enhance quickly (Fig. 51.40).[67–69]

Most hemangiomas have a homogeneous appearance and smooth, well-defined margins by MRI. On long T2-weighted sequences, they have a significantly greater contrast-to-noise ratio than cancer. MR allows detection of almost all hemangiomas over 1 cm in diameter, with an overall accuracy of 90%. Today, gadolinium administration with dynamic serial imaging is done in all cases. Hemangiomas have the following features: (a) peripheral hyperintense nodules with a nonintact ring immediately after contrast administration; (b) progressive centripetal enhancement that is most intense at 90 s (persistent homogeneous enhancement

ages. The vast majority of hemangiomas remain clinically silent. Hemangiomas are commonly small (<4 cm) and single, but may also be multiple and may occasionally occupy a very large segment of the liver. Microscopically, hemangiomas are composed of blood-filled spaces of variable size and shape and are lined by

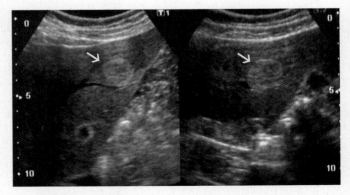

Figure 51.39 Echogenic mass of uniform density, less than 3 cm in diameter with sharp margins, compatible to hemangioma (*arrow*).

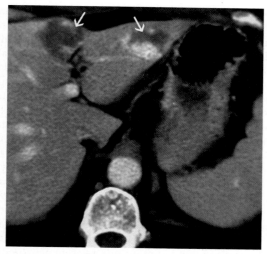

Figure 51.40 Round, well-defined lesions in the left hepatic lobe with peripheral nodular enhancement, typically of liver hemangiomas (*arrows*).

without heterogeneous or peripheral washout). Therefore, using a combination of T2-weighted images with serial dynamic post-gadolinium sequences, MR is a reliable imaging modality for the diagnosis of hemangiomas (Figs. 51.38 and 51.41).[66,70]

2.6.3. Steatosis

Hepatic steatosis (fatty metamorphosis) is the result of excessive accumulation of triglycerides within hepatocytes. It occurs frequently in obese patients. Other etiologies are Cushing syndrome, diabetes mellitus, alcoholic liver disease, chronic infection, chemotherapy, tetracycline treatment, and corticoid use. Fatty liver develops in a setting of heterozygous hypobetalipoproteinemia, and this entity should be considered a possible cause. In general, there is an increase in the organ size. Although it is most commonly a diffuse process, fatty metamorphosis frequently is nonuniform or focal.[71-73] Diffuse fatty infiltration reveals a hyperechoic pattern throughout the liver by US, to the point of masking the normally hyperechoic portal vein wall (Fig. 51.42).

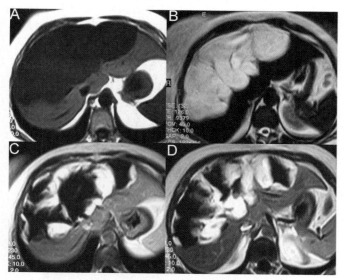

Figure 51.41 Large, lobulated lesion, hypointense lesion on T1-weighted (**A**) hyperintense on T2-weighted images (**B**) that shows globular, peripheral enhancement on postcontrast T1-weighted images (**C,D**) compatible to gigantic hemangioma.

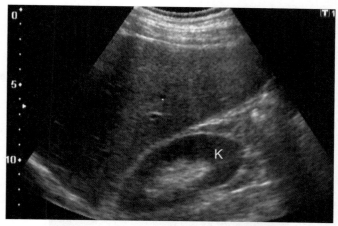

Figure 51.42 Diffuse fatty infiltration (steatosis) reveals a hyperechoic pattern throughout the liver. K, right kidney.

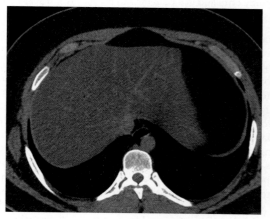

Figure 51.43 Steatosis. Liver CT attenuation value is lower than that of the blood vessels.

Increased hepatic fat content produces a diffuse reduction in mean hepatic CT attenuation value. On images obtained without intravenous contrast, the diagnosis can be done when the liver attenuation value is lower than the blood vessels and the spleen (Fig. 51.43).[74,75] By MRI, SE sequences are relatively insensitive in detecting fatty infiltration. Chemical shift imaging using in-phase and out-of-phase (opposed-phase) spoiled gradient-echo sequences distinguishes proton signals from water and fat. Imaging with fat and water protons in-phase results in their signals being additive, while opposed-phase imaging leads to their cancellation. Thus, on opposed-phase images normal liver parenchyma has an isointense signal and fat appears hypointense and these sequences are useful to detect liver fat. In-phase and opposed-phase gradient-echo sequences provide complementary diagnostic information. On postcontrast images, simple fat deposition enhances in a pattern similar to normal liver parenchyma.[76,77] Differential diagnosis includes amyloidosis, glycogen storage diseases, and inflammation granuloma. Chronic liver disease is commonly associated with splenomegaly (Fig 51.44).

2.7. Adrenal glands

The adrenal glands are paired suprarenal, retroperitoneal organs that are surrounded by a variable amount of retroperitoneal fat. A variety of pathologic processes can affect the adrenal glands. Adrenal masses are common, estimated to occur in 9% of the population. However, the adrenal gland is also a common site of

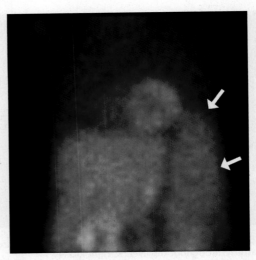

Figure 51.44 Splenomegaly noted in a ⁹⁹Tc sestamibi myocardial perfusion study obtained in a patient with chronic liver disease (*arrows*).

metastasis, particularly from lung carcinoma. Thus, differentiating an adrenal mass as benign or malignant is critical in the oncology patient, since it will greatly affect patient treatment and prognosis. A major problem in clinical practice is to differentiate an adrenal adenoma from other tumors, usually a metastasis. Although most adenomas are small, homogeneous and smooth in borders, while metastases are larger heterogeneous, have an irregular outline, there is overlap in some cases. Two specific imaging characteristics are useful in differentiating adrenal adenomas from nonadenomas. Adenomas have increased lipid content and a more rapid contrast washout compared to nonadenomatous lesions. CT and MR allow the differentiation between them. Most adrenocortical adenomas contain considerable lipid (lipid rich), but the amount of fat is still significantly less than in a myelolipoma. About 20% of adenomas contain little or no lipid. Also infrequently, a cortical carcinoma and metastasis can contain sufficient fat but these tend to be large and irregular in outline at initial presentation.[78–81] By US, the abnormal adrenals are obviously easier to be seen if enlarged. The measurements should be performed at the level of the widest portion of each pole. Multiple criteria are important in the assessment of their size. They may present as unilateral symmetrical enlargement, asymmetrical unilateral enlargement, bilateral symmetrical enlargement, or bilateral asymmetrical enlargement. Symmetry is relative to the cranial and caudal pole of one adrenal. Adenomas are solid, homogeneous lesions, with echogenicity similar to renal parenchyma. A size >4 cm is suspicious for malignancy. Most carcinomas or adrenal metastasis are similar in appearance to adenomas, especially if small. Adrenal hyperplasia presents as bilateral, diffuse enlargement or multiple small nodules. Infection involvement of the adrenals (TB, Histoplasmosis, cytomegalovirus (CMV)) looks similar to hyperplasia. Myelolipoma are usually highly echogenic lesions. The pheochromocytoma presents as a large, solid lesion with cystic areas of necrosis and hemorrhage. Nuclear scintigraphy with meta-iodo benzylguanidine (MIBG) is particularly useful to diagnose this tumor. At CT, certain imaging findings are helpful in differentiating benign from malignant lesions. Larger lesions have a greater likelihood of being malignant. In particular, lesions >4 cm in diameter tend to be either metastasis or a primary adrenal carcinoma. Change in lesion size is a useful indicator of malignancy because adenomas are slow growing and tend not to change the size. The shape of

the adrenal gland can also be helpful in predicting malignancy.[79,82] Currently, there are two main CT criteria (histologic and physiologic) used to differentiate benign adenomas from malignant adrenal masses. Intracellular lipid content of the adrenal mass represents the anatomic difference between adenomas and metastases, and differences in vascular enhancement patterns represent the physiologic difference. Adenomas have abundant intracytoplasmic fat in the adrenal cortex and thus have low attenuation at CT. Conversely, metastases have little intracytoplasmic fat and thus do not have low attenuation at nonenhanced CT. In nonenhanced CT, due to their fat content, most adenomas have lower attenuation values than malignant tumors. A threshold of 10 HU has 71% sensitivity and 98% specificity for characterizing adrenal masses (Fig. 51.45). The specificity approached 100% when other features such as adrenal size, shape, and change in lesion size were considered. When measuring the attenuation of the adrenal gland, it is important to use as large a region of interest as possible to fill the gland, but to not include adjacent periadrenal fat.[80] As a rough guide, adrenal tumors having a CT density of 0 HU or less can be assumed to be benign, and those having a density >20 HU can be assumed to be malignant. It is those with intermediate densities that present a diagnostic dilemma. For most tumors, both CT and MR yield similar results in differentiating adenomas from nonadenomas. Lesions measuring >10 HU on unenhanced CT can be characterized with chemical shift MR or with contrast washout enhancement. Washout is equal to initial enhanced attenuation minus delayed enhanced attenuation. More rapid washout is a characteristic finding in a majority of adenomas (compared to nonadenomas). Mean CT attenuation measured at specific time delays postcontrast (10 to 30 min), is lower for adenomas than for nonadenomas. Loss of 50% of the attenuation value of the adrenal mass at delayed CT is specific for an adenoma, <50% washout is indicative of either a metastasis or an atypical adenoma. Percentage of washout is typically calculated by the following formula: (1–delayed enhanced HU value/initial enhanced HU value) × 100. Lipid-poor adenomas (30%) cannot be differentiated from nonadenomas by their precontrast attenuation values; however, they have enhancement and washout characteristics similar to those of more typical lipid-rich adenomas.[83–85] By MRI signal intensities of both benign and malignant tumors vary, presumably due to their inhomogeneous histologic appearance. In general, metastases and carcinomas

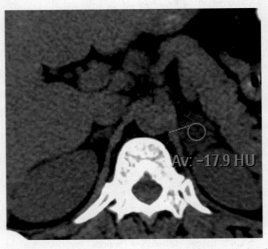

Figure 51.45 Nodular enlargement of the left adrenal gland due to a low density (−17.9 HU) lesion, compatible to an adrenal adenoma.

contain larger amounts of fluid than fat. However, there is a significant overlap in T1 and T2 SI between adenomas and metastases, and thus SI is not useful to reliably differentiate between them. Enhancement patterns have also been investigated as a mean of differentiating benign adrenal adenomas from metastases, and, similar to their appearance at CT, adenomas vigorously enhance and exhibit early washout of contrast material compared with metastases on MR images. Adenomas appear bright on T2-weighted images.[85] Chemical shift imaging is an MRI technique used to detect lipid within an organ, and is the most sensitive method for differentiating adenomas from metastases.[86–88] To obtain chemical shift images, two breath-hold T1-weighted acquisitions are performed. The first uses a short echo time (2.2 m/s at 1.5 T) when the fat and water protons are out of phase, and a second in-phase acquisition uses a longer echo time (4.4 m/s). On out-of-phase images, there is signal drop-off in adenomas due to the intravoxel signal cancellation of the lipid and water protons. Thus, on out-of-phase images, the adenoma appears darker than on in-phase images. In adrenal masses that do not contain lipid (e.g., metastases), there is no significant signal loss on out-of-phase images, and thus the SI of the adrenal gland is the same on in-phase and out-of-phase images. With the chemical shift technique, the sensitivity and specificity for differentiating adenomas from metastases range from 81% to 100% and 94% to 100%, respectively (Fig. 51.46). Nonfunctioning adenomas range from hypointense to mostly isointense to liver parenchyma on both T1- and T2-weighted sequences, and show mild-to-moderate postcontrast enhancement (Fig. 51.47). Most adenomas contain insufficient fat to produce a major change on fat-suppressed MR images, and a major decrease in intensity should suggest a myelolipoma. Nevertheless, chemical shift MR is useful in differentiating lipid-rich adenomas from nonadenomas. This technique is insensitive in characterizing lipid-poor adenomas.[81,85] The adrenal-to-spleen ratio is a useful measurement. Metastases have an adrenal-to-spleen ratio >0.8, while most adenomas have a lower ratio. An overlap exists, however, and the ratio is of limited value in establishing the benign or malignant nature of an adrenal lesion. Some investigators prefer muscle as their standard. Most adenomas are isointense to muscle or spleen on in-phase spoiled gradient echo images, and appear hypointense on opposed phase images. With a chemical shift technique, most adenomas have a loss of SI on opposed-phase images while most benign nonadenomas, pheochromocytomas, and metastases do not. Loss in SI in bone marrow in an adjacent vertebral body is a useful confirmation of this technique. With a tendency of adrenal adenomas to contain fat and the high

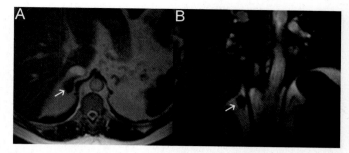

Figure 51.47 Nodular enlargement (*arrow*) of the right adrenal gland on axial (**A**) and coronal (**B**) T1-weighted MR images.

sensitivity of opposed-phase imaging for detecting fat, in a setting of a known malignancy, and an adrenal tumor, MR can be sufficient to differentiate these entities and save the patients from a biopsy. Another option is to use a SI index, defined as: (SI in-phase–SI opposed-phase)/SI in-phase. This index differentiates adenomas, metastases, and pheochromocytomas with a cutoff value of 11.2% to 16.5%.

For most tumors, both CT and MR yield similar results in differentiating adenomas from nonadenomas. Lesions measuring >10 H on unenhanced CT can be characterized with chemical shift MRI or with contrast washout. Lipid-poor adenomas cannot be differentiated from nonadenomas by their precontrast attenuation values; however, they have enhancement and washout characteristics similar to those of more typical lipid-rich adenomas. Contrast-enhanced MR of adrenal adenomas can be distinguished from malignancies by their characteristic initial homogeneous capillary blush followed by a rapid washout. Postcontrast MR reveals peak enhancement of most adrenal adenomas during the early phase, followed by a relatively rapid washout; most metastases exhibit a slower washout. Exceptions include pheochromocytomas, which show little washout and granulomas which reveal minimal enhancement.[86–88]

2.8. Spine
2.8.1. Degenerative disease
The spine has different articulations: the discovertebral and apophyseal joints in throughout the spine, the costotransverse and costocorporeal joints in the thoracic spine. Of these, the discovertebral joint is fibrocartilaginous in type and others are synovial. Based on the principal site of involvement, discovertebral degeneration can be divided into discovertebral osteoarthritis and spondylosis deformans. The former osteoarthritis affects the nucleus pulposus with diffuse condensation of peridiscal bones. On the other hand, the degenerative change of the apophyseal and costovertebral joints is considered to be a classical osteoarthritis, since these joints are synovial.[89–91] Discovertebral osteoarthritis manifests the narrowing of the intervertebral space, endplate sclerosis, and focal osteophytes by CT. Occasionally, compression fracture may be superimposed on an endplate. By contrast, spondylosis deformans is characterized by multiple osteophytes, often prominent, formed in the lateral and anterior edges of the endplates. The discovertebral changes are narrowing of the intervertebral spaces and endplate scleroses (Figs. 51.48 and 51.49).[90,91] Scintigraphic manifestations of discovertebral osteoarthrosis include tracer uptake in the vertebral endplates and marginal spurs with significant diminution of the intervertebral space. The endplates are affected in pairs. The osteophytes in spondylitis deformans are represented scintigraphically by beaklike uptake of various sizes and intensities at the lateral or

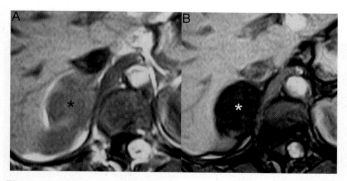

Figure 51.46 Right adrenal adenoma. Chemical shift MRI technique, in-phase (**A**) and out-of-phase (**B**) images. The lesion appears darker on out-of-phase images than on in-phase images, characteristic of adrenal adenomas (*asterisk*).

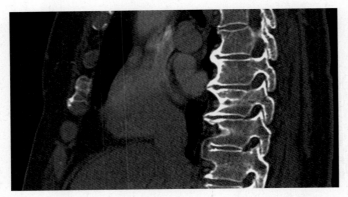

Figure 51.48 Degenerative changes in the dorsal spine. Anterior osteophytes.

anterior edges of the vertebral bodies.[90] By MRI, degenerative disease may lead to SI changes in the marrow immediately adjacent to the intervertebral discs, which are often referred to as discogenic vertebral or endplate changes. There are three types of endplate changes previously classified by Modic et al.[89] Type 1 change represents proliferation of fibrovascular tissues, which replace the normal marrow. This can be seen as hypointensity on T1-weighted images and hyperintensity on T2-weighted images. Type 2 change represents the proliferation of fatty marrow, and is seen as hyperintensity on both T1-weighted and T2-weighted fast SE sequences. Type 3 change represents the replacement of marrow by dense bone, and is therefore hypointense on both T1 and T2-weighted images. The disc itself is often hyperintense and enhances in discitis, but maintains low SI and lack of enhancement in degenerative disc disease. Osteophytes are frequently placed near endplates of the vertebral bodies, and may be situated anteriorly, laterally, or posteriorly. Osteophytes in the anterior and lateral aspects of the spine are common in the older population. These changes are often called spondylosis deformans. They are thought to be an attempt to increase the surface area to help reduce the stress of axial loading. Patients with these types of osteophytes are regularly asymptomatic. On the other hand, posterior osteophytes are often associated with disc disease. Habitually, disc disease and osteophyte coexist, and together are simply called disc-osteophyte complex resulting in narrowing of the spinal canal or neural foramina.[89-91]

2.8.2. Disc pathology

In normal young patients, the disc is hyperintense on T2-weighted images. With aging, the annulus fibrosis thickens. The core of the disc will contain increased fibrous material, leading to decreased SI on T2-weighted images. However, the disc height should be preserved. When disc degeneration occurs, loss of both disc height and the high SI on T2-weighted images appear. Although, this loss of high T2 SI is often described as disc desiccation. Degenerative discs may calcify and may lead to negative pressure within the disc, trapping of gas, often nitrogen. This is described as the vacuum phenomenon (hypointense on both T1- and T2-weighted images).[89-92]

Disc degeneration may lead to displacement of the disc material beyond the normal intervertebral disc space, usually through radial disruption of the annulus fibrosis. Normal disc space is defined craniocaudally by the vertebral body endplates and circumferentially by the ring apophysis of the vertebral bodies. Disc displacement may be described as a bulge or herniation, depending on the percentage of circumference involved. Disc bulging refers to diffuse displacement of disc material beyond the normal disc space, and covers >50% of the normal disc space circumference.[92] Disc displacement covering 50% or less of the circumference is called herniation, which may be further subcategorized into broad-based herniation (covering 25% to 50% of disc space circumference) and focal herniation (covering <25% of the circumference). Disc protrusion and extrusion are terms that describe the shapes of herniation; migration refers to displacement of disc material away from the site of extrusion, regardless of continuity. Very often, disc extrusion is seen associated with superior or inferior migration of disc material.[89,92]

3. FUTURE DIRECTIONS

Currently, most imaging equipment manufacturers are developing automated tools to aid in the detection and characterization of incidental findings. Automatic detection of lung nodules has been adopted by many radiology practices. Given the high prevalence of lung nodules and the importance of defining changes in size during serial studies, these tools may become essential part of CT and MR workstations.

Detecting and reporting incidental findings is a subject of controversy. Some argue that many incidental findings lead to repetitive unnecessary testing. However, malignancy is often detected incidentally and often while curable. Physicians must remember their ethical responsibility to provide the best possible care to their patients. This responsibility should include reporting potentially life-threatening incidental findings.

Figure 51.49 Degenerative disease with dorsal scoliosis.

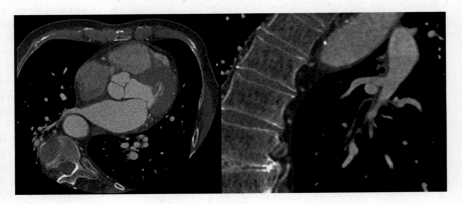

REFERENCES

1. Prat-Gonzalez S, Sanz J, Garcia MJ. Cardiac CT: Indications and limitations. *J Nucl Med Technol.* 2008;36(1):18–24.
2. Wilson GT, Gopalakrishnan P, Tak T. Noninvasive cardiac imaging with computed tomography. *Clin Med Res.* 2007;5(3):165–171.
3. Janne d'Othée B, Siebert U, Cury R, et al. A systematic review on diagnostic accuracy of CT-based detection of significant coronary artery disease. *Eur J Radiol.* 2008;65(3):449–461.
4. Dewey M, Rutsch W, Schnapauff D, et al. Coronary artery stenosis quantification using multislice computed tomography. *Invest Radiol.* 2007;42(2):78–84.
5. Raff GL, Gallagher MJ, O'Neill WW, et al. Diagnostic accuracy of noninvasive coronary angiography using 64-slice spiral computed tomography. *J Am Coll Cardiol.* 2005;46(3):552–557.
6. Haller S, Kaiser C, Buser P, et al. Coronary artery imaging with contrast-enhanced MDCT: Extracardiac findings. *Am J Roentgenol.* 2006;187(1):105–110.
7. Gedik GK, Ergün EL, Aslan M, et al. Unusual extracardiac findings detected on myocardial perfusion single photon emission computed tomography studies with Tc-99m sestamibi. *Clin Nucl Med.* 2007;32(12):920–926.
8. Onuma Y, Tanabe K, Nakazawa G, et al. Noncardiac findings in cardiac imaging with multidetector computed tomography. *J Am Coll Cardiol.* 2006;48(2):402–406.
9. Austin JH, Müller NL, Friedman PJ, et al. Glossary of terms for CT of the lungs: Recommendations of the Nomenclature Committee of the Fleischner Society. *Radiology.* 1996;200:327–331.
10. Itoh H, Murata K, Konishi J, et al. Diffuse lung disease: Pathologic basis for the high-resolution computed tomography findings. *J Thorac Imaging.* 1993;8:176–188.
11. Leung AN, Miller RR, Müller NL. Parenchymal opacification in chronic infiltrative lung diseases: CT-pathologic correlation. *Radiology.* 1993;188:209–214.
12. Naidich DP, Zerhouni EA, Hutchins GM, et al. Computed tomography of the pulmonary parenchyma: Part 1: Distal air-space disease. *J Thorac Imaging.* 1985;1:39–53.
13. Remy-Jardin M, Remy J, Giraud F, et al. Computed tomography assessment of ground-glass opacity: Semiology and significance. *J Thorac Imaging.* 1993;8:249–264.
14. Miller WT Jr, Shah RM. Isolated diffuse ground-glass opacity in thoracic CT: Causes and clinical presentations. *Am J Roentgenol.* 2005;184:613–622.
15. Erasmus JJ, Connolly JE, McAdams HP, et al. Solitary pulmonary nodules: Part I. Morphologic evaluation for differentiation of benign and malignant lesions. *Radiographics.* 2000;20(1):43–58.
16. Khouri NF, Meziane MA, Zerhouni EA, et al. The solitary pulmonary nodule. Assessment, diagnosis, and management. *Chest.* 1987;91(1):128–33.
17. Viggiano RW, Swensen SJ, Rosenow EC. III. Evaluation and management of solitary and multiple pulmonary nodules. *Clin Chest Med.* 1992;13(1):83–95.
18. Erasmus JJ, McAdams HP, Connolly JE. Solitary pulmonary nodules: Part II. Evaluation of the indeterminate nodule. *Radiographics.* 2000;20(1):59–66.
19. Webb WR, Stein MG, Finkbeiner WE, et al. Normal and diseased isolated lungs: High-resolution CT. *Radiology.* 1988;166:81–87.
20. Primack SL, Hartman TE, Hansell DM, et al. End-stage lung disease: CT findings in 61 patients. *Radiology.* 1993;189:681–686.
21. American Thoracic Society (ATS), the European Respiratory Society (ERS) and the World Association of Sarcoidosis and Other Granulomatous Disorders. Statement on sarcoidosis: Joint Statement of the American Thoracic Society (ATS), the European Respiratory Society (ERS) and the World Association of Sarcoidosis and Other Granulomatous Disorders (WASOG) adopted by the ATS Board of Directors and by the ERS Executive Committee, February 1999. *Am J Respir Crit Care Med.* 1999; 160:736–755.
22. Müller NL, Fraser RS, Lee KS, et al. *Diseases of the Lung: Radiologic and Pathologic Correlations.* Philadelphia, PA: Lippincott Williams & Wilkins, 2003.
23. Colling J, Allaouchiche B, Floccard B, et al. Pneumatocele formation in adult Escherichia coli pneumonia revealed by pneumothorax. *J Infect.* 2005;51(3):e109–e111.
24. Kumar NA, Nguyen B, Maki D. Bronchiectasis: Current clinical and imaging concepts. *Semin Roentgenol.* 2001;36:41–50.
25. Sibtain NA, Padley SPG. HRCT in small and large airways diseases. *Eur Radiol.* 2004;14:L31–L43.
26. Morgan MDL, Strickland B. Computed tomography in the assessment of bullous lung disease. *Br J Dis Chest.* 1984;78:10–25.
27. Kazerooni EA, Whyte RI, Flint A, et al. Imaging of emphysema and lung volume reduction surgery. *Radiographics.* 1997;17:1023–1036.
28. Bessis L, Callard P, Gotheil C, et al. High-resolution CT of parenchymal lung disease: Precise correlation with histologic findings. *Radiographics.* 1992;12:45–58.
29. Johkoh T, Müller NL, Ichikado K, et al. Perilobular pulmonary opacities: High-resolution CT findings and pathologic correlation. *J Thorac Imaging.* 1999;14:172–177.
30. Medford A, Maskell N. Pleural effusion. *Postgrad Med J.* 2005; 81:702–710.
31. Arenas JJ, et al. Evaluation of CT findings for diagnosis of pleural effusions. *Eur Radiol.* 2000;10:681–690.
32. Williford ME, et al. Computed tomography of pleural disease. *Am J Roentgenol.* 1983;140:909–914.
33. Falaschi F, et al. Usefulness of MR signal intensity in distinguishing benign from malignant pleural disease. *Am J Roentgenol.* 1996;166:963–968.
34. Rusch VW, Godwin JD, Shuman WP. The role of computed tomography scanning in the initial assessment and the follow-up of malignant pleural mesothelioma. *J Thorac Cardiovasc Surg.* 1988;96:171–177.
35. Kinoshita T, Ishii K, Miyasato S. Localized pleural mesothelioma: CT and MR findings. *Magn Reson Imaging.* 1997;15:377–379.
36. Patz EF, et al. Malignant pleural mesothelioma: Value of CT and MR imaging in predicting resectability. *Am J Roentgenol.* 1992;159:961–966.
37. Falaschi F, et al. Usefulness of MR signal intensity in distinguishing benign from malignant pleural disease. *Am J Roentgenol.* 1996;166:963–968.
38. Kim Y, Lee KS, Yoo JH, et al. Middle mediastinal lesions: Imaging findings and pathologic correlation. *Eur J Radiol.* 2000;35:30–38.
39. Glazer HS, Molina PL, Siege MJ, et al. Pictorial essay. High-attenuation mediastinal masses on unenhanced CT. *Am J Roentgenol.* 1991;156:45–50.
40. Glazer HS, Siege MJ, Sagel SS. Pictorial essay. Low-attenuation mediastinal masses on CT. *Am J Roentgenol.* 1989;152:1173–1177.
41. Aronson DJ, Glazer HS, Madsen K, et al. Normal thoracic aortic diameters by computed tomography. *J Comput Assist Tomogr.* 1984;8:247–250.
42. Edwards J. Anomalies of derivatives of the aortic arch system. *Med Clin North Am.* 1948;32:925–949.
43. Vilacosta I, Roman JA. Acute aortic syndrome. *Heart.* 2001; 85:365–368.
44. Dailey PO, Trueblood HW, Stinson EB, et al. Management of acute aortic dissections. *Ann Thorac Surg.* 1970;10:237–247.
45. Macura KJ, Corl FM, Fishman EK, et al. Pathogenesis in acute aortic syndromes: Aortic dissection, intramural hematoma, and penetrating atherosclerotic aortic ulcer. *Am J Roentgenol.* 2003;181:309–316.
46. Zhan MF, Zhou QZ, Xiao HM, et al. Acute aortic dissection with intimal intussusception: MRI appearances. *Am J Roentgenol.* 2006;186:841–843.
47. Le Page MA, Quint LE, Sonnad SS, et al. Aortic dissection: CT features that distinguish true lumen from false lumen. *Am J Roentgenol.* 2001;177:207–211.
48. Murray JG, Manisali M, Flamm SD, et al. Intramural hematoma of the thoracic aorta: MR image findings and their prognostic implications. *Radiology.* 1997;204:349–355.
49. van Strijen MJ, de MW, Schiereck J, et al. Single-detector helical computed tomography as the primary diagnostic test in suspected pulmonary embolism: A multicenter clinical management study of 510 patients. *Ann Intern Med.* 2003;138:307–314.
50. Tsai KL, Gupta E, Haramati LB. Pulmonary atelectasis: A frequent alternative diagnosis in patients undergoing CT-PA for suspected pulmonary embolism. *Emerg Radiol.* 2004;10:282–286.
51. Schoepf UJ, Costello P. Multidetector-row CT imaging of pulmonary embolism. *Semin Roentgenol.* 2003;38:106.
52. Remy-Jardin M, Bahepar J, Lafitte JJ, et al. Multi-detector row CT angiography of pulmonary circulation with Gadolinium-based contrast agents: Prospective evaluation in 60 patients. *Radiology.* 2006;238:1022–1035.
53. Remy-Jardin M, Mastora I, Remy J. Pulmonary embolus imaging with multislice CT. *Radiol Clin North Am.* 2003;41:507.
54. Panicek DM, Benson CB, Gottlieb RH, et al. The diaphragm: Anatomic, pathologic, and radiologic considerations. *Radiographics.* 1988;8:385–425.
55. Gale ME. Bochdalek hernia: Prevalence and CT characteristics. *Radiology.* 1985;156:449–452.
56. Weinshelbaum AM, Weinshelbaum EI. Incarcerated adult Bochdalek hernia with splenic infarction. *Gastrointest Radiol.* 1982;7:287–289.
57. LaRosa JRDV, Esham RH, Morgan SL. Diaphragmatic hernia of Morgagni. *South Med J.* 1999;92:409–411.
58. Murphy BJ, Casillas J, Ros PR, et al. The CT appearance of cystic masses of the liver. *Radiographics.* 1989;9:307–322.
59. Singh Y, Winick AB, Tabbara SO. Multiloculated cystic liver lesions: Radiologic-pathologic differential diagnosis. *Radiographics.* 1997;17:219–224.
60. Mergo PJ, Ros PR. Benign lesions of the liver. *Radiol Clin North Am.* 1998;36: 319–331.
61. Mortelé KJ, Ros PR. Cystic focal liver lesions in the adult: Differential CT and MR imaging features. *Radiographics.* 2001;21(4):895–910.
62. Precetti S, Gandon Y, Vilgrain V. Imaging of cystic liver diseases. *J Radiol.* 2007;88(7–8 Pt 2):1061–1072.
63. Horton KM, Bluemke DA, Hruban RH, et al. CT and MR imaging of benign hepatic and biliary tumors. *Radiographics.* 1999;19(2):431–451.
64. Federle MP, Filly RA, Moss AA. Cystic hepatic neoplasms: Complementary roles of CT and sonography. *AJR Am J Roentgenol.* 1981;136:345–348.
65. Leslie DF, Johnson CD, MacCarty RL, et al. Distinction between cavernous hemangiomas of the liver and hepatic metastases on CT: Value of contrast enhancement patterns. *AJR Am J Roentgenol.* 1995;164:625–629.
66. Whitney WS, Herfkens RJ, Jeffrey RB, et al. Dynamic breath-hold multiplanar spoiled gradient-recalled MR imaging with gadolinium enhancement for differentiating hepatic hemangiomas from malignancies at 1.5 T. *Radiology.* 1993;189:863–870.
67. Leslie DF, Johnson CD, MacCarty RL, et al. Single-pass CT of hepatic tumors: Value of globular enhancement in distinguishing hemangiomas from hypervascular metastases. *AJR Am J Roentgenol.* 1995;165:1403–1406.
68. Stephens DH, Johnson CD. Benign masses of the liver. In: Silverman PM, Zeman RK, eds. *CT and MRI of the Liver and Biliary System.* New York, NY: Churchill Livingstone, 1990:93–127.
69. Whitehouse RW. Computed tomography attenuation measurements for the characterization of hepatic haemangiomas. *Br J Radiol.* 1991;64:1019–1022.
70. Tung GA, Vaccaro JP, Cronan JJ, et al. Cavernous hemangioma of the liver: Pathologic correlation with high-field MR imaging. *AJR Am J Roentgenol.* 1994;162:1113–1117.
71. Alpers DH, Sabesin M. Fatty liver: Biochemical and clinical aspects. In: Shiff L SE, ed. *Diseases of the Liver.* Philadelphia, PA: JB Lippincott Co, 1982:813.
72. Friedman A, Johns T, Levy D, et al. Cirrhosis, other diffuse disease, portal hypertension, and vascular disease. In: Friedman AC, ed. *Radiology of the Liver, Biliary Tract, Pancreas and Spleen.* Baltimore, MD: Williams & Wilkins, 1987:69.
73. Brawer MK, Austin GE, Lewin KJ. Focal fatty change of the liver, a hitherto poorly recognized entity. *Gastroenterology.* 1980;78:247–252.

74. Bydder GM, Chapman RW, Harry D, et al. Computed tomography attenuation values in fatty liver. *J Comput Assist Tomogr.* 1981; 5:33–35.

75. Kawata R, Sakata K, Kunieda T, et al. Quantitative evaluation of fatty liver by computed tomography in rabbits. *AJR Am J Roentgenol.* 1984;142:741–746.

76. Rosen BR, Carter EA, Pykett IL, et al. Proton chemical shift imaging: An evaluation of its clinical potential using an in vivo fatty liver model. *Radiology.* 1985;154:469–472.

77. Stark DD, Bass NM, Moss AA, et al. Nuclear magnetic resonance imaging of experimentally induced liver disease. *Radiology.* 1983; 148:743–751.

78. Kenney PJ, Wagner BJ, Rao P, et al. Myelolipoma: CT and pathologic features. *Radiology.* 1998;208:87–95.

79. Korobkin M. Combined unenhanced and delayed enhanced CT for characterization of adrenal masses. *Radiology.* 2002;222:629–633.

80. Korobkin MCT. Characterization of adrenal masses: The time has come. *Radiology.* 2000;217:629–632.

81. Korobkin M, Giordano TJ, Brodeur FJ, et al. Adrenal adenomas: Relationship between histologic lipid and CT and MR findings. *Radiology.* 1996;200:743–747.

82. Krestin GP, Friedmann G, Fischbach R, et al. Evaluation of adrenal masses in oncologic patients: Dynamic contrast-enhanced MR vs CT. *J Comput Assist Tomogr.* 1991;15:104–110.

83. Peña CS, Boland GW, Hahn PF, et al. Characterization of indeterminate (lipid-poor) adrenal masses: Use of washout characteristics at contrast-enhanced CT. *Radiology.* 2000;217(3):798–802.

84. Boland GW, Hahn PF, Peña C, et al. Adrenal masses: Characterization with delayed contrast-enhanced CT. *Radiology.* 1997;202(3):693–696.

85. Mayo-Smith WW, Boland GW, Noto RB, et al. State-of-the-art adrenal imaging. *Radiographics.* 2001;21(4):995–1012.

86. Mayo-Smith WW, Lee MJ, McNicholas MM, et al. Characterization of adrenal masses (_5 cm) by use of chemical shift MR imaging: Observer performance versus quantitative measures. *AJR Am J Roentgenol.* 1995;165:91–95.

87. Bilbey JH, McLoughlin RF, Kurkjian PS, et al. MR imaging of adrenal masses: Volume of chemical-shift imaging for distinguishing adenomas from other tumors. *AJR Am J Roentgenol.* 1995;164:637–642.

88. Outwater EK, Siegelman ES, Radecki PD, et al. Distinction between benign and malignant adrenal masses: Value of T1-weighted chemical-shift MR imaging. *AJR Am J Roentgenol.* 1995;165:579–583.

89. Modic MT, Masaryk TJ, Ross JS, et al. Imaging of degenerative disc disease. *Radiology.* 1988;168:177–186.

90. Olsen WL, Chakeres DW, Berry I, et al. Spine and spinal cord trauma. In: Manelfe C, ed. *Imaging of the Spine and Spinal Cord.* New York, NY: Raven Press; 1992:413–416.

91. Resnick D, Niwayama G. Degenerative disease of the spine. In: Resnick D ed. *Diagnosis of Bone and Joint Disorders,* 3rd Ed. Philadelphia, PA: WB Saunders; 1995:1372–1462.

92. Fardon DF, Milette PC. Nomenclature and classification of lumbar disc pathology: Recommendations of the Combined Task Forces of the North American Spine Society, American Society of Spine Radiology, and American Society of Neuroradiology. *Spine.* 2001;26:E93–E113.

Page numbers followed by a "f" indicate figures; page numbers followed by a "t" denote tables.